A SYSTEM OF PRACTICAL MEDICINE

Volume I: Pathology and General Diseases

PREFACE.

The present work has been undertaken in the belief that by obtaining the co-operation of a considerable number of physicians of acknowledged authority, who should treat subjects selected by themselves, there could be secured an amount of practical information and teaching not otherwise accessible. It was determined to restrict the selection of authors to those of this country—including Canada—not from any want of recognition of the importance of the studies of certain special subjects by European investigators, but because it was felt that the proper time had arrived for the presentation of the whole field of medicine as it is actually taught and practised by its best representatives in America.

It is a matter of importance also that a comprehensive study shall be made of the various forms of disease as occurring among our highly composite population and under our varied and peculiar climatic influences. Of course, in the present work comparative studies of this kind must occupy a subordinate position; yet it cannot fail to enhance both its interest and its value to have the various forms of disease as they occur in this country discussed by those among us who are confessedly the most competent and experienced.

The force of these observations must have been felt by the distinguished men to whom I made application, for with scarcely an exception they joined cordially in the laborious undertaking. I take the greatest pleasure in testifying to the courtesy which has marked all our relations, and which has lessened materially the labor and strain inevitable in the production of such a work.

To ensure greater accuracy in the revision of the large amount of proof-sheets, as well as to relieve me of some of the details connected with the editorial work, I associated with myself Dr. THOMAS HOLMESCATHCART, and, after sudden illness had cut short his very promising career, I was fortunate in securing the assistance of Dr. LOUIS STARR for the same purpose.

In order to render the work as valuable as possible to the general practitioner, its scope has been made as comprehensive as could be done without exceeding the limits prescribed by the nature of the undertaking. This will be particularly noted in the section on Gynæcology, where is presented a series of articles by eminent specialists upon the subjects of chief importance to the general practitioner, written with special reference to their constitutional relations and their bearings on associated morbid conditions, while, among the general diseases, a full article on puerperal fever has properly been included. Important articles will also be found on Tracheotomy, the Diseases of the Rectum and the Anus, and those of the Bladder and the male sexual organs. Comprehensive sections have further been provided, from the pens of distinguished specialists, upon medical ophthalmology, medical otology, and on skin diseases, presenting these large and complicated subjects in a clear and practical light and with special reference to their relations to general medical practice. In the presentation of such subjects as hydrophobia, glanders, and anthrax care has been taken to ensure the full discussion of these affections, not only as occurring in man, but also in the lower animals, since it is highly important to provide the physician with authoritative information on at least such points of Veterinary Science as have a direct practical bearing on morbid processes in man.

In view of the intimate relations of all questions of hygiene to the causation and prevention of disease, in regard to which medical men are constantly consulted, and are, indeed, often obliged to assume weighty responsibilities, interesting articles on Drainage and Hygiene have been provided.

In order to avoid repetition and confusion, and at the same time to secure a comprehensive presentation of the subjects of General Pathology and of General Etiology, Symptomatology, and Diagnosis, considerable space has been devoted to their full discussion. The chapter on General Morbid Processes will be found to convey distinct and conservative teaching on all points included under that comprehensive title, and will thus supply a solid basis for the subsequent discussions of special morbid conditions. In any work on General Medicine at the present day frequent allusion must be made to the relations of various low organisms to morbid processes. This question—or rather the series of questions which arise in connection with this subject, and which at present form the most fruitful topic of discussion and of investigation—will be found treated by different authors in various places and from various standpoints. No attempt has been made to secure uniformity of views upon a matter which is still *sub judice*, and which demands much more skilful and critical investigation before its true scientific position has been finally determined. It has even been felt to be desirable to allow a certain amount of repetition, which has naturally resulted from the introduction of this discussion, not only in the chapter on General Etiology, but in connection with the causation of scarlatina, diphtheria, hydrophobia, pyæmia, puerperal fever, and phthisis.

Throughout the work the chief purpose of the editor and of his collaborators, to furnish a concise and thoroughly practical system of medicine, has compelled the omission of bibliographical lists, of numerous references, and of extended discussions of theoretical views or of controverted questions, in order that more space might be devoted to clear descriptions of disease and to a full presentation of the subjects of diagnosis and treatment. If it should seem, in consequence, that inadequate recognition has been made of the labors of others, it must be borne in mind that ample quotations and numerous references were inadmissible in such a work as the present.

The classification and nomenclature which have been adopted are those recommended by the Royal College of Physicians of England and by the American Medical Association. Charts and tables have been inserted wherever they were needed to elucidate the text, but after mature reflection it was felt necessary to omit all illustrations that were not imperatively required, although many original drawings and paintings of high value were offered with the articles.

THE EDITOR.

OCTOBER, 1884.

GENERAL MORBID PROCESSES.[1]
INFLAMMATION; THROMBOSIS AND EMBOLISM; EFFUSIONS; DEGENERATIONS; TUBERCULOSIS; MORBID GROWTHS.

BY REGINALD H. FITZ, M.D.

[1] In the preparation of this subject full and free use has been made of the following works: *Die Cellular Pathologie*, Virchow, 4te Auflage, Berlin, 1871; *Handbuch der Allgemeinen Pathologie*, Uhle und Wagner, 7te Auflage, Leipzig, 1876; *Handbuch der Allgemeinen Pathologie als Pathologische Physiologie*, Samuel, Stuttgart, 1879; *Vorlesungen über Allgemeine Pathologie*, Cohnheim, 2te Auflage, Berlin, 1882; *Lehrbuch der Pathologischen Anatomie*, Birch-Hirschfeld, 2te Auflage, 1er Band, Leipzig, 1882; *Lehrbuch der Allgemeinen und Speciellen Pathologischen Anatomie*, Ziegler, 1er und 2er Theil, Jena, 1882 and 1883.

GENERAL MORBID PROCESSES.

Disease is to be regarded as representing the result of a series of processes called morbid or pathological, from the fact that they are manifested by disturbances in the organism.

The processes concerned are the same in kind as those essential to health, but they are modified in time, place, or quantity.

Morbid processes, therefore, are to be considered as modified physiological processes tending to cause disease.

All physiological processes are subject to certain variations which tend to produce disturbances in the functions of the body. In the healthy organism this tendency is checked by the automatic regulators of the functional activity of the various organs, to the importance of which Virchow[2] long ago called attention. By their action the influence of external agents is controlled within certain limits. The lids close and prevent injury to the eye. Sneezing, coughing, and vomiting bring about the expulsion of noxious irritants. Sweating aids in neutralizing the injurious effects of exposure to high temperatures. Rapid respiration permits a sufficient cleansing of the blood in rarefied atmospheres. When the limits, within which the regulation of physiological processes is possible, are exceeded, such processes become pathological and disease begins. A morbid process, therefore, is usually incapable of recognition till disease is present. It may exist and disease be unsuspected and denied. A diminished blood-supply may be one link in the process which eventually leads to the production of disturbances. [p. 36]Another link is to be found in the fatty degeneration resulting from this lack of blood.

[2] *Handbuch der Speciellen Pathologie und Therapie,* Virchow, 1er Band, p. 15, Erlangen, 1854.

Such a degeneration may have long existed in the walls of a blood-vessel, and yet the individual appear in the best of health. The sudden rupture of the weakened wall results in death or disease. With the manifestation of the disturbances which render the condition of the vessel obvious the individual is said to be diseased.

In most instances, however, the morbid process makes itself early apparent. Disturbances of nutrition, formation, or function soon become sufficient in quantity to attract attention from the resulting discomfort, and the presence of disease is then recognized. The latter is thus essentially a conventional term, and begins when the morbid processes occasion a sufficient degree of inconvenience.

The process is never at a standstill. It either tends toward a return to the physiological conditions, or its course is in the direction of their destruction. As physiological processes are absolutely dependent upon the vitality of the elements of the tissues, so those which have become pathological cease to exist with the death of such elements. In the dead body there is no disease, although its results remain, and furnish the most efficient means of identifying the processes which occasioned them.

In the study of morbid processes, therefore, one must appreciate the normal conditions and manifestations of life in the individual. Physiological laws govern pathological phenomena, and the latter must always be submitted to the tests furnished by the former.

Just as little, however, as the study of anatomy familiarizes the student with the anatomical changes resulting from diseased processes, does the study of physiology accustom the student to the features of disease. Pathological processes must be studied by themselves and for themselves, although the means which are employed may be the same as those used in physiological research.

It is evident that the exactness of method which is the demand of the physiological investigator cannot be secured by the pathologist. The material of the latter lies farther, beyond his control. Nevertheless, much of the ground to be gone over is common, and the object sought for is essentially the same—the knowledge of the conditions necessary to maintain life.

In an introduction to the study of disease there are certain processes which deserve early recognition. They are both the cause and the result of disease, and may occur in various diseases, either limited to one organ or present in a series of organs. Their treatment at present obviates the necessity of repetition, and prepares the reader for the special consideration of their occurrence in the various structures and systems of the body.

These processes are named in virtue of some prominent characteristic, and each is made up of a complex series of conditions and disturbances. In part, they represent modifications in the circulation of blood and lymph; in part, they consist of nutritive derangements, whose consequences appear as the various degenerations, or as the additions to the body, the new formations.

The processes and groups of processes in question are those included under the following heads: inflammation; thrombosis and embolism; effusions; degenerations; tuberculosis; and morbid growths.

[p. 37]

Inflammation.

Inflammation is characterized now, as in the time of Galen, by the presence of redness, heat, swelling, and pain. The disturbance of function, added to modern definitions, is to be regarded either as a result or a cause, or both, of the variously modified physiological processes whose sum is the inflammation.

The redness of inflammation is obviously dependent upon the presence of an increased quantity of blood. This is readily apparent in the direct observation of the blood-vessels of an inflamed, transparent part of the body, as the mesentery of the frog or rabbit, or the tongue and webbed foot of the former animal. The redness of inflammation consequently demands the presence of blood-vessels in the affected region, and becomes all the greater the more vascular the part—*i.e.* the richer it is in such vessels.

Redness does not suffice for the existence of inflammation, for it may be found in the absence of other evidence of the latter. The diffused redness, often extensive, of birth-marks, that from venous obstruction or temporary congestions, from vaso-motor disturbances—the section of the sympathetic furnishing a well-known instance—are examples of non-inflammatory redness. Inflammation may even be present without redness, as may be constantly observed in the occurrence of parenchymatous inflammation and of the chronic interstitial varieties.

The heat of inflammation is one of the most important clinical features, yet not indispensable, as appears from its absence in chronic interstitial forms of inflammation. In the acute varieties of inflammation an elevated temperature is constant, and its observation and record furnish a most valuable means of determining the beginning and progress of an inflammation, which, for a time, may furnish but little additional evidence.

The heat of inflammation is the prominent characteristic of inflammatory fever, and it is the study of this variety of fever of late years which has resulted in an intelligible and relatively satisfactory theory concerning fevers in general. Information of much value is to be found in the recent work of Wood,[3] which contains abundant historical information, as well as extensive original observations and conclusions.

[3] *Fever: A Study in Morbid and Normal Physiology*, H. C. Wood, A.M., M.D., Philadelphia, 1880. (Reprint from the *Smithsonian Contributions to Knowledge*, No. 357.)

Inflammatory fevers are distinguished from idiopathic forms. The latter variety includes the occurrence of fever as an attribute of the disease concerned, the more characteristic symptoms of which follow the febrile outbreak. Local inflammatory processes may take place during the progress of the disease with its fever, but such processes are co-effects of the cause of the latter, rather than its cause. Most of those diseases in which fever occurs as one of the joint effects of the cause of the disease, are included among the infective or zymotic classes.

The inflammatory fevers are those attending an acute inflammatory process, and are secondary to, and occasioned by, the latter. The type of this variety is seen in the fever occurring during the progress of a wound, whether its course is toward healing or extension. Such [p. 38]traumatic fevers are characterized as septic or aseptic; the former including the conditions of septicæmia and pyæmia. The aseptic traumatic fevers, as described by Volkmann,[4] are those which pursue their course with an elevated temperature, but without most of the other febrile phenomena.

[4] *Beiträge zur Chirurgie*, Leipzig, 1875, p. 24; *Sammlung Klinischer Vorträge*, No. 121, Genzmer und Volkmann.

Fever in general is characterized by a combination of disturbances in the physiological processes of the body. Such processes are those concerned in the production and dissipation of heat, in respiration and circulation, digestion and secretion, and in mental, motor, and other sensorial action. Such disturbances are manifested by a persistent elevation of temperature, an increased destruction of tissue, a quickened and modified pulse, accelerated breathing, increased thirst, diminished appetite, and diminished quantity and altered quality of the secretions. The sensorial disturbances include wakefulness and stupor, headache, delirium, twitchings, cramps, and other symptoms indicative of functional impairment of the nervous system.

Of all these manifold evidences of fever, the elevation of temperature is the one whose cause, range, and results have been most carefully and critically investigated. No record of a case in which fever is present is regarded as complete without the chart of the daily variations in temperature, respiration, and circulation. The practical value of such records is thus admitted, and in the experiments relating to the origin of animal heat the observations of temperature are as essential as the chemical analyses, each of which supplements the other.

The more accurate determination of the heat produced in the body is obtained either by the use of the calorimeter (an apparatus for measuring the collected heat liberated from the body) or by estimating the quantity of heat produced in the destruction of the constituents of the body from quantitative analyses of the discharged carbonic acid and urea. The results of such investigations are regarded by Rosenthal[5] as possessing only a relative value, but justify the conclusion that most of the heat produced in the organism results from the oxidation of its constituents.

[5] *Hermann's Handbuch der Physiologie*, Leipzig, 1882, iv. 2, 375.

For the preservation of health it is essential that this heat should be removed from the body in such quantity that the temperature of the latter shall not vary to any considerable extent, for any considerable time, from 37.2° C. (98.4° F.). The removal of the heat is mainly accomplished by its radiation or conduction into a surrounding cooler medium, and by the evaporation of moisture from the surface of the body. Too great a removal of heat results in death from freezing, while too great an accumulation of heat terminates fatally from the effects of an unduly elevated temperature. To ensure the normal range of temperature, constantly changing relations must exist between the production of heat and its dissipation. The cooler the surroundings, the more must heat be produced, or the less must heat be evolved from the body.

An increased production of heat is obvious under conditions of climate demanding prolonged exposure to low temperature. An abundantly fatty diet promotes the formation of heat, while suitable clothing checks its dissipation. Although it is claimed by Liebermeister that sudden exposure to cold stimulates heat-production, Rosenthal[6] disputes this [p. 39]statement, and maintains that it is still to be regarded as doubtful whether the production of heat can be varied to suit the demands of sudden and temporary changes of temperature. With the admission of this doubt, the regulation of the temperature of the body, under the circumstances just referred to, is mainly accomplished through the influence of agencies favoring or checking the loss of heat. Since heat is largely brought to the surfaces of the body by the circulating blood, modifications in the fulness and rapidity of this superficial current produce corresponding differences in the amount of heat and moisture presented. Such variations are considered to be accomplished through the action of the vaso-motor nervous system, whose differing effects are apparent in the pale, cool skin and the flushed, warm surface.

[6] *Op. cit.*, 413.

The search for the regulation of such vaso-motor action has led to the view that the production of heat, as well as its dissipation, may be influenced from a nervous centre. Wood[7] claims that the result of experiments made by him proves the existence of such a heat-centre in or above the pons. Although admitting the possibility of its being a muscular vaso-motor centre, he regards it rather as an inhibitory heat-centre, which acts, as suggested by Tscheschichin, by repressing the chemical changes in the constituents of the body through which heat is produced.

[7] *Op. cit.*, 254.

This view is objected to by Rosenthal,[8] on the ground that the facts are not universally agreed upon, and their interpretation is somewhat vague. Even the increased production of heat as determined by Wood, if admitted, may be regarded as the result of a modified circulation.

[8] *Op. cit.*, 442.

The preservation of a normal range of temperature in general is to be recognized as the result of variations in the relation of heat-production to heat-dissipation. The causes which influence this relation may act from without or from within, and are regarded as producing their effect by means of the vaso-motor nervous system. The causes which act from within are those concerned in the febrile elevation of temperature. Whether the latter is associated with, or independent of, inflammatory processes, the question of first importance relates to the modification of physiological conditions. The causes of the physiological production of heat and its dissipation have already been referred to, and the same elements demand consideration in the pathological range of temperature so striking in fever.

Relatively accurate inductions with regard to the origin of febrile heat were first rendered possible by the experiments of Billroth and Weber. These observers found that the introduction of putrid material into the circulation of animals produced fever. It was afterward shown that various substances, not necessarily of a putrid character, might produce the same result.

From measurements with the calorimeter of the heat produced, it was concluded by Wood[9] that in the fever of pyæmic dogs more heat was produced than in healthy, fasting dogs, although less than in high-fed, healthy dogs. An increased production of heat in the fevered animal is thus obvious, as his capacity to receive and assimilate food is considerably less than that of a high-fed, healthy dog. The calculations of Sanderson, referred to by Wood,[10] based upon the analyses of eliminated carbonic [p. 40]acid and urea, show that the febrile human subject produces very much more heat than the fasting, though less than the fully-fed, healthy, man.

[9] *Op. cit.*, 236.
[10] *Op. cit.*, 239.

An increased production of heat in fever is generally admitted, although it alone is not to be regarded as the essential feature in the elevated range of the temperature. The fasting man or animal under ordinary circumstances is not febrile, and an increased production of heat from full feeding in health, equal to that observed in fever, not being associated with fever, it is apparent that the retention of the produced heat is of importance for the existence of fever. Although it has been shown by various observers that more heat is dissipated during fever than in health, this increased loss is not in proportion to the increased production of heat. A persistent elevation of temperature is the necessary result. This elevation is subject to daily and hourly differences, as is the temperature of the healthy individual. These variations in the range of the febrile temperature are apparently due to an agency like that which dominates the course of normal temperatures—viz. a varying action of the vaso-motor nervous apparatus, as well as of that controlling the secretion of sweat, now permitting, now checking, the dissipation of the produced heat.

For the existence of the elevated temperature of fever, therefore, there is demanded the presence of an agent within the body which, as stated by Wood,[11] shall act "upon the nervous system which regulates the production and dissipation of animal heat—a system composed of diverse parts so accustomed to act continually in unison in health that they become, as it were, one system and suffer in disease together." It may be that there exists, as claimed by Wood and Tscheschichin, a heat-centre independent of the vaso-motor and other centres, through which heat is dissipated, or it may be, as maintained by Rosenthal, that the vaso-motor system alone is concerned in the regulation of temperature. Such action may be inhibitory or excitant, according to the views of the one or the other author, without affecting the main question as above stated.

[11] *Op. cit.*, 255.

The elevation of temperature suffices to explain for the most part certain of the other phenomena of fever, as thirst, digestive disturbances, increased respiration, and emaciation. A coincident affection of various cerebro-spinal centres is demanded to explain the altered action of the heart and the numerous nervous symptoms which are to be found in fever. The agent producing such manifold effects is obviously no unit. It may be introduced from without or it may arise within the body, and its transfer to the nervous centres is undoubtedly accomplished through the circulation.

Among those agents which act from without are to be included the specific causes of infective diseases. It is probable that these produce the fever, as they occasion other symptoms of the disease, and their action may be regarded as direct, or indirect through the secondary products of their own vital changes. In the light of the existing facts the products of minute organisms developed outside the human body may give rise to fever when introduced, without the organism, into the body. The history of septicæmia contains numerous illustrations of the pyrogenetic properties of material produced in connection with wounded surfaces of the body exposed to the action of minute organisms. The introduction of blood of the same, or of a different animal, into the [p. 41]circulation of a given animal is followed by fever, as is the injection of considerable quantities of water into the blood-vessels. The same is true of various chemical substances.

It is further obvious that the agents producing fever may arise within the body. The fever resulting from the deprivation of water, and from the destruction of tissues, are instances of the probable origin of pyrogenetic substances from the rapid metamorphosis of tissues.

It is suggested by Samuel[12] that under given circumstances the fever may be sanatory. This view is based upon the probability that certain parasitic organisms are destroyed at such temperatures as may be produced within the body. The growth of the bacillus of malignant pustule takes place most vigorously at a temperature of 30.5° C. (95° F.), while its development is feeble at 40° C. (104° F.). The bacillus of tuberculosis, as shown by Koch, thrives at temperatures between 37° C. (98.6° F.) and 38° C. (100.4° F.), but its growth ceases at temperatures above 41° C. (105.8° F.). The spiral fibre of relapsing fever, which is present in the blood in great abundance at the beginning of the febrile onset, disappears at the close, the temperature being 42° C. (107.6° F.). It is not to be found in the intervals between the febrile paroxysms, but reappears a few hours before the recurrence of the fever. The history of intermittent fever suggests a similar relation between its cause and the febrile periods.

[12] *Op. cit.*, 155.

The value of pain as evidence of inflammation is merely relative. Its existence depends upon the presence of sensitive nerves, and those inflammations are the least painful which occur in parts where such nerves are fewest.

The pain of inflammation is attributable to the pressure upon the nerves of that product of the inflammation known as the exudation. This pressure becomes all the greater the more abundant the exudation, or the greater the obstruction offered to its diffusion throughout the inflamed part. The intense pain resulting from inflammation of the fascia or of the periosteum is thus explained, while an inflammation of the loose connective tissue may be diffused over a wide area with little or no pain. In the chronic varieties of inflammation, where the exudation is but scanty, and its accumulation extended over a long period of time, there may be no pain during the entire course of the inflammation.

Swelling remains for consideration as the most important of the four cardinal symptoms. Like the others, its presence is not absolutely essential. It may exist at one time in the course of the inflammation, and may be absent at another. Even a diminution in the size of an organ may suggest the existence of an inflammation, for the yellow and cirrhotic atrophies of the liver give evidence, respectively, of an acute and chronic inflammation of this organ.

The swelling of an inflamed part is due to the presence of an increased quantity of blood, and lymph, and to the exudation. These constituents of the swelling are not of equal importance. Although the quantity of blood in the part is increased, no considerable swelling is produced, provided the flow of blood and lymph from the part be unobstructed. The current of lymph through the larger lymphatics may be greatly increased, yet a decided swelling be absent, unless there is an obstruction to the passage of lymph from the inflamed region.

[p. 42]The exudation is the most essential element of the swelling, and our knowledge of its origin and fate includes the most important features of the general pathology of the processes concerned.

The inflammatory exudation is represented by the accumulation, outside the blood-vessels, of material previously within them. The prevailing views concerning the manner of origin of this exudation, and its relation to inflammatory processes, are essentially due to the rediscovery by Cohnheim of the forgotten observation of Addison, that white blood-corpuscles pass through the apparently intact walls of the blood-vessels.

In the observation of the mesentery or other transparent part of a suitable animal, the changes taking place in inflammation are, at the outset, limited to the blood-vessels and their immediate vicinity. The vessels become dilated and the rapidity of the flow within them is soon diminished. In the veins particularly the white blood-corpuscles separate in considerable numbers from the general current and line the wall in constantly-increasing numbers, while the red corpuscles are borne along the middle of the stream. The white corpuscles stagnate, stick to the wall for a longer or shorter time, and often change their place, while the red corpuscles are in constant and progressive motion. In the capillaries a considerable number of white corpuscles are found in contact with the wall, but numbers of red corpuscles are associated with them. The formation of the exudation now begins by the passage of white corpuscles through the apparently intact wall of the veins and capillaries, especially of the former. Limited numbers, under ordinary circumstances, of red corpuscles also make their way through the walls of the capillaries. This is the phenomenon of emigration, and is associated with the amoeboid movements of the white corpuscles.

With the passage outward of the white and red corpuscles there is also the effusion of liquid material. Both the liquid and solid constituents continually escape and spread in all directions beyond the wall, following the course of the least resistance. It is probable that this course is defined by the pre-existing spaces within the tissues of the part, the lymph-spaces. The exudation is more abundant in parts richly provided with blood-vessels and in those containing the larger spaces; it is diminished where the vessels are less numerous or the surrounding parts more resistant, with smaller and fewer lymph-spaces. The resulting swelling is the less when ready opportunities for the diffusion and removal of the exudation by lymphatics and veins are presented, and when the material appears upon surfaces over which it may flow away.

The liquid portion of the exudation represents something more than the transuded blood-serum, and a certain practical importance results from the distinction drawn between an exudation and a transudation. Such a distinction is especially called for when the inflammatory or non-inflammatory origin of considerable quantities of fluid in the larger cavities of the body is concerned. From a recent contribution to our knowledge of this subject by Reuss[13] the following information is derived: The percentage of albumen is always greater in exudations than in transudations, and is more constant in the former than in the latter. It increases with the severity of the inflammation, being highest in the ichorous forms, less in the purulent, and least in the serous exudations. When an [p. 43]inflammatory exudation is found to contain less albumen than usual, the existence of a transudation with secondary inflammation is suggested, or the exudation may have taken place in a hydræmic individual. A sufficient number of exceptions are met with, however, to interfere with the absolute nature of this test.

[13] *Deutsches Archiv für Klinische Medicin*, 1879, xxiv. 583.

The coagulation of an inflammatory exudation apparently depends upon the contained white blood-corpuscles; the more numerous (within certain limits) these are in a serous exudation, the more abundant is the formation of fibrin. The cellular element likewise is that which in abundant liquid exudations characterizes them as purulent. Although it is generally agreed that most of the corpuscles of pus are emigrated white blood-corpuscles, it is not necessary to admit that all are of this nature. The cells present in an inflamed part include those pre-existing, as well as those which escape from the vessels. The former are the wandering cells of the connective tissues, as well as the fixed variety, the epithelial cells of the surface of a mucous membrane in addition to the subjacent connective-tissue cells. Amoeboid cells outside the blood-vessels have been seen to divide, and it is possible that such duplication may serve as the method of formation of a certain number of pus-corpuscles. The statements concerning the proliferation of the fixed connective-tissue cells and of epithelium are derived from appearances, and are interpretations of these appearances, not observations of a process.

The changes taking place along the walls of the blood-vessels being the feature of prime importance in the observation of the progress of an inflammation, numerous investigators have directed their attention to the determination of the nature of the changes in the vessel wall by means of which the escape of the corpuscles is permitted. Arnold represents the most strenuous advocates of the stomata theory, according to which the leucocytes pass through canals normally existing in the wall. By means of the silver method of staining, and by injections of various insoluble pigments into the blood-current, certain results are met with, which give color to the view that pores and canals are present upon and in the walls of the vessels, analogous to those found in the diaphragm. As the latter have been shown to be in direct communication with the lymphatic system of tubes and spaces, so the walls of the blood-vessels have been assumed to present similar channels of communication.

The prevailing views at the present time are in favor of the artificial nature of the stomata and pores in the walls of the blood-vessels. An increased porosity of the vascular wall in inflammation is necessary for the occurrence of the exudation, but such porosity is regarded rather as a physical condition permitting an observable filtration, and a filtration of solids as well as liquids.

In this connection reference should be made to the observation of Winiwarter, who has demonstrated that colloid material, a solution of gelatin, passes through the vascular wall in inflammation more readily—*i.e.* under less pressure—than through the normal wall of the blood-vessel.

The causes of inflammation are to be regarded as those which produce an increased porosity of the vessel wall without causing its death, for no exudation escapes from a dead vessel, its contents becoming clotted.

These causes may act from without or from within, primarily affecting [p. 44]the tissues outside the vessels, or exerting their action, at the outset, upon the wall itself. The usual histological relation of vessels and surrounding tissues is such that both are simultaneously affected. The occurrence of an inflammation in non-vascular parts, however, as the cornea, from irritation of its centre, the part farthest removed from the surrounding blood-vessels, shows that the affection of the vessels may be indirect as well as direct. This indirect action is to be regarded as taking place through the agency of nerves or through that of the nutritive currents. That nervous influence alone does not suffice to transmit the effect of an applied cause is apparent from the absence of inflammation of the cornea which has become anæsthetized by section of the trigeminus nerve. With the protection of the cornea from external irritation there is an absence of inflammation.

The consideration of the final symptom of inflammation, the disturbance of function, which has been added in recent times, belongs to special rather than general pathology. It varies according to the seat of the inflammation, the disturbed function of the brain or heart differing from that of the liver or kidney. The clinical importance of this symptom of inflammation is greater than of all the rest, as it is the one whose presence is constant and indispensable.

An inflammation may exist, as already stated, without heat, redness, or pain. The swelling may escape observation from the limited quantity of the exudation and other causative agents, or from the inaccessibility of the inflamed part to physical examination. The disturbance of function, however, becomes early apparent, and is present throughout the course of the inflammation. A knowledge of its nature enables the seat of the latter to be recognized, and its variations furnish a desired test of the efficiency of therapeutic agents.

The causes of inflammation may be divided into the traumatic, toxic, parasitic, infectious, dyscrasic or constitutional, and trophic.

The traumatic causes are those which act mechanically, producing an injury to tissues by pressure, crushing, tearing, stretching, and the like. Others represent modifications in temperature, thermic agencies, and include extremes of cold as well as of heat. The chemicals whose action is direct, as caustic, include a third variety of the traumatic causes. Such chemicals are applied to surfaces, cutaneous or mucous, and comprise the active element producing the perforating ulcer of the stomach and duodenum, as well as such substances as potash or sulphuric acid which may have been swallowed intentionally or accidentally.

The toxic group of causes is closely allied to the chemical variety of the traumatic agencies. It includes chemicals whose action is indirect, through absorption in a diluted form rather than from direct application in a concentrated condition. Such chemicals are derived from without, as arsenic, phosphorus, and antimony; or may be formed within the body, and the latter include the chemical products of putrefactive changes—in the urine, for instance—and, with considerable probability, certain of the active agents of blood-poisoning in septic diseases. It is not unlikely that some of the inflammatory affections met with among the so-called constitutional diseases, as rheumatism and gout, may owe their origin to the production of chemical substances within the body, excessive in quantity if not changed in quality.

[p. 45]The parasitic causes of inflammation are both animal and vegetable, and act upon the surfaces of the body or within its deeply-seated parts. Some of the animal parasites act locally at their place of entrance, while others produce but slight disturbances in this region, their effects usually resulting from the transfer of their offspring to remote parts of the body. The vegetable parasites are for the most part the various fungi, which act locally upon the skin or on those transitional surfaces lying between skin and mucous membrane. The resulting parasitic inflammations are known as favus, sycosis, ringworm, thrush, etc. The border-line between such parasitic diseases and those included among the infective diseases is somewhat arbitrarily drawn. Parasites in the limited sense act chiefly as foreign bodies, while the effect of minute vegetable organisms is rather that of ferments, in virtue of their products. Such a distinction is of relative value merely, as the micrococci and bacteria are capable of acting in other ways than by the production of septic material.

The infectious causes of inflammation are for the most part parasitic in their nature, although the discovery and identification of the parasite are in most of these inflammations assumed rather than demonstrated. The relation of the anthrax bacillus to malignant pustule no longer admits of a doubt, mainly in consequence of the researches of Koch. This investigator has been enabled to establish a definite etiological relation between the septicæmia of certain animals and accompanying minute vegetable organisms. His recent discovery of the bacillus of tuberculosis definitely removes the tubercular process from the group of dyscrasic or constitutional affections to that of the infective diseases. The constant presence of minute organisms in relapsing fever, leprosy, malaria, typhoid fever, diphtheria, erysipelas, and numerous other affections associated with, if not characterized by, inflammatory conditions, renders extremely probable the closest pathological relation between such diseases and a microscopic organism. That an inflammatory process may be regarded of infectious origin, it is necessary, according to Koch,[14] that a characteristic organism should be found in all cases of the disease, and in such numbers and distribution as to account for all the phenomena of the disease in question.

[14] *Untersuchungen über die Aetiologie der Wundinfectionskrankheiten*, 1878, 27.

These organisms may act in virtue of their growth and the consequent demand for oxygen, as seems probable in certain cases of malignant pustule, where the affected individual dies with symptoms of asphyxia. Their operation may also be like that of ferments, which produce chemical material whose effect may be remote from the immediate presence of the minute organism. They may likewise, in connection with their colonization in various parts of the body, act more immediately upon the walls of the blood-vessels, and produce that increased porosity which is so essential a factor in inflammation.

The discovery of the immediate cause of the various infective diseases, as measles, scarlatina, variola, cholera, dysentery, mumps, whooping cough, cerebro-spinal meningitis, and numerous other epidemic and endemic affections, still remains a question for the future. The constant association of microbia with any or all of such diseases is but one fact in connection with them, and such a discovery is to be regarded merely as a step forward, to be followed by others, each of which represents not only an advance, but confirms the position attained.

[p. 46]The dyscrasic or constitutional causes of inflammation are those which, though long established, appear less demanded as our knowledge advances. Regarded as the result of an alteration in the composition of the blood, it is obvious that such changes may arise from the introduction, from without, of wholly foreign material. The dyscrasia may also represent modifications in the relative proportion of the normal constituents of the blood. In the former series are included what, for the most part, have already been referred to under the toxic and infectious causes of inflammation. The dyscrasiæ from lead, alcohol, and the like belong to this series. Still more important are the poisons, the virus of tuberculosis and scrofula, of leprosy and syphilis. The dyscrasiæ known as anæmia, leucæmia, uræmia, icterus, and diabetes are to be regarded less as inflammatory causes than as predisposing conditions which favor the action of other groups of causes.

The trophic causes of inflammation are those whose action is supposed to take place through the influence of nerves. Although, as has already been stated, a faulty innervation of tissues is an important element in favoring the action of various inflammatory causes, there remain certain forms of inflammation where the disturbance of nervous action seems to be the essential feature. The occurrence of an acute peripheral gangrene soon after certain traumatic or inflammatory lesions of the brain or spinal cord, of articular inflammation following chronic affections of the cerebro-spinal axis, are instances in point. The origin and distribution of herpes zoster, the occurrence of sympathetic ophthalmia and symmetrical gangrene, suggest a predominant disturbance of innervation as the exciting cause. At the same time, it is desirable to call attention to the recent observations of MacGillavray, Leber, and others,[15] which suggest that a sympathetic ophthalmia is due to the extension of a septic choroiditis along the lymph-spaces of the optic nerve. It is further apparent that in certain so-called trophic inflammations, as the pneumonia after section of the pneumogastric, and the inflammation of the eye following paralysis of the trigeminus, the paralysis of the nerve is a remote, rather than an immediate cause, of the inflammation. There still remain, however, a number of localized inflammations whose origin is so intimately connected with nervous disturbances as to demand, for the present at least, a corresponding classification.

[15] Wadsworth's "Report of Recent Progress in Ophthalmology," *Boston Medical and Surgical Journal*, 1882, cvi. 517.

The course of an inflammation is often indicated by the predominance of certain symptoms, which, for the most part, indicate a condition of the individual acted upon rather than a peculiarity of the cause. The sthenic inflammations take place in robust individuals with powerful hearts and an abundant supply of blood. In such persons a strong pulse, high fever, and an injection of the superficial blood-vessels suggested, in former times, the necessity of bloodletting as the essential therapeutic agent. The sthenic form of inflammation was most commonly associated with pneumonia, where the obstruction to the passage of blood through the lungs was an important cause of the superficial injection of the blood-vessels.

The asthenic inflammations, on the contrary, are those occurring in feeble individuals, debilitated in consequence of pre-existing disease, exposure, or habits. A weak heart, low febrile temperature, and [p. 47]superficial pallor, characterize the asthenic inflammations, which show a frequent tendency to become localized in the more dependent parts of the body, the force of the circulation being too feeble to overcome the effect of gravitation.

In the typhoidal inflammations are associated those symptoms which are so prominent in the severe varieties of typhoid fever. These are the predominant symptoms: hebetude or low, muttering delirium, picking at the bed-clothes, involuntary evacuations, stertor, and the like. The nervous disturbances are associated with a feeble pulse and a dusky hue of the skin.

The constituents of an inflammatory exudation are frequently used as a basis of classification, and characterize the inflammation from the anatomical point of view. As the exudation is complex in its composition, the predominant element is made use of to designate the variety, and in doubtful cases a combined adjective indicates the presence of the two most abundant constituents. As the exudation is directly derived from the blood and contains serum in addition to white and red corpuscles, the serous, purulent, and hemorrhagic varieties of exudation naturally arise. The fibrinous and diphtheritic inflammations relate to the presence of membranes or false membranes. Finally, there are the productive inflammations, resulting in the new formation of tissue, and the destructive inflammations, where losses of substance occur.

Serous inflammations are most frequent in those parts of the body where the structure contains the largest lymph-spaces. The so-called serous cavities of the body offer the most favorable opportunities for the accumulation, as well as for the exudation, of the inflammatory product; then follow the regions of the larger lymph-spaces, according to the size and number of the latter.

The serous inflammations may also arise from the epithelial coverings of the body, as the cutaneous, alimentary, and respiratory surfaces. The serous exudations of the skin are those present in vesicles, blisters, or bullæ, which owe their limitation to the resistance offered to the spreading of the liquid inflammatory product by the coherent epidermis. Serous inflammations of the alimentary canal may assume a vesicular character, although, from the structure of its mucous membrane and the macerating influence of its contents, the vesicles are apt to be of an extremely transitory character.

The more important serous inflammations of the intestines are those manifested by profuse watery evacuations, the extreme form of which is to be found in cholera.

Serous inflammation of the lungs accompanies the more severe forms, and usually represents but a limited and circumscribed affection, associated with more abundant cellular and fibrinous products.

Serous inflammations of the peritoneum, pleura, pericardium, tunica vaginalis, and central ventricles often give rise to the presence of enormous quantities of fluid, whose partial removal from many of the cavities concerned by operative measures frequently represents a most beneficial result of treatment.

The smaller lymph-spaces of the connective tissue in various parts of the body are the frequent seat of the inflammatory oedema, so called, whose presence is an important indication of the direction assumed by a[p. 48]spreading inflammation, as well as a suggestion of the frequent virulence of its cause.

In general, the serous inflammations are to be regarded as less severe than other varieties, or as representing an early stage of what later may be otherwise characterized by a change in the nature of the products.

The purulent variety of inflammation is present when the exudation is abundantly cellular. As has already been stated, such cells are, for the most part, white blood-corpuscles. The purulent exudation, like the serous variety, may appear either on surfaces, when the term secretion is applied, or within the lymph-spaces of the connective tissue over a considerable space, when the pus is said to be infiltrated. When the infiltration is more circumscribed and the walls of the affected lymph-spaces are destroyed, so that adjoining cavities are thrown into larger holes, an abscess is present, from whose wall pus is constantly derived, while the inflammation is progressive.

The attention of the surgeon, in particular, has been directed to the isolation of the immediate cause of suppurative inflammation, and the modern, antiseptic, treatment of wounds is essentially based upon the view of the infectious origin of pus. The frequent presence of microbia in purulent exudation where no precautions are taken to exclude their admission, and their frequent absence or presence in minute quantities where such precautions are taken, have suggested that through their influence an inflammatory exudation is likely, if not actually compelled, to become purulent.

Whether the microbia or their products are the cause of most suppurative inflammations may be regarded as an open question. It is generally admitted, however, that, as a rule, an inflammation becomes purulent in consequence of the presence of an infective agent; in other words, that most pus is of an infectious origin and possesses infectious attributes. The labors of Lister in insisting upon the exclusion of all possible putrefactive agencies in the treatment of wounds have met with universal approval, and the basis of his treatment remains fixed, although different methods have been devised for its enforcement.

His researches, and those stimulated by his work, have resulted in the establishment of principles which affect the whole field of theoretical as well as practical medicine.

Although most pus may be considered as due to the action of a virus introduced from without, and capable of indefinite progressive increase within the body, all pus is not to be regarded as of infectious origin. There are pyrogenetic agencies, like petroleum, turpentine, and croton oil, which, introduced into the body, produce suppurative inflammation without the association of microbia.

A bland pus is usually in a state of beginning putrescence, so that it is only relatively bland, and acquires extreme virulence when long exposed to putrefactive agencies. It is possible that those agencies producing an ichorous pus are the same or different from those present in bland pus. The ichorous exudation contains less corpuscles than bland pus, is more fluid, less opaque, strongly alkaline, of a greenish color, and of offensive odor.

In hemorrhagic inflammation the exudation contains large numbers of red blood-corpuscles. The occurrence of this form is sometimes associated[p. 49]with peculiarities of the cause, as is obvious from the epidemics of hemorrhagic small-pox, measles, scarlatina, and cerebro-spinal meningitis. It is also associated with peculiarities of the individual, as in such epidemics all cases are not equally hemorrhagic, and in scurvy the hemorrhages are attributable to the abnormal conditions to which the sufferers are exposed. Hemorrhagic exudations are also met with in those inflammations of serous surfaces accompanying the outcropping of tubercular and cancerous or sarcomatous growths. In all cases a hemorrhagic exudation represents a grave complication, and when found in serous cavities has a certain diagnostic, as well as prognostic, importance.

Fibrinous inflammations are characterized by the presence in the exudation of considerable quantities of fibrin. As the prevailing theory of the formation of fibrin demands fibrino-plastic as well as fibrinogenous material, both are to be sought for in the exudation. The latter is present in the liquid portion of the exudation; the existence of the former, as well as that of the ferment, is dependent upon the presence of the white blood-corpuscles. The more numerous these, within certain limits, the more abundant the formation of fibrin. As their death appears essential for the fibrinous coagulation, the latter is most constantly met with in those parts of the body where the white blood-corpuscles are quickest separated from influences favoring their life. The farther removed they are from the blood-vessels, the more likely is their early death. Fibrinous exudations are therefore frequent and abundant in cellular and serous (sero-cellular) inflammation of the great serous cavities of the body. The clotted fibrin appears as false membrane lying upon the serous surface, either smooth or rough, tripe-like, or as villosities projecting above the surface, and again as bands, fibrinous adhesions, stretching across the cavity and uniting opposed surfaces.

The frequent occurrence of fibrinous exudations on the mucous membranes of the larynx and trachea, accompanied by the suffocative symptoms known as croup, has led to the use of the term croupous inflammation as synonymous with fibrinous inflammation, and its application to various parts of the body where croupous—*i.e.* suffocative—symptoms are not in question. Croupous inflammation, when used, is to be considered as an anatomical term, indicating merely the production of fibrin, and, for the avoidance of confusion, it is preferable to substitute fibrinous for croupous when such inflammations are described.

The disease, croup, it is well known, may exist without a croupous—that is, fibrinous—inflammation, as is familiarly recognized in the constant use of the terms spasmodic, membranous, and diphtheritic croup.

Fibrinous inflammation of the mucous membrane of the larger air-passages is much more frequently met with than that of mucous membranes elsewhere, as of the intestines, uterus, and bladder. The pseudo-membranous inflammations of the latter tracts are more commonly the result of the catarrhal and diphtheritic varieties than of the fibrinous form. Fibrinous exudations on mucous surfaces, according to Weigert, can only take place when the epithelium is destroyed. Hence those causes which give rise to the destruction or detachment of the epithelium are alone capable of producing a fibrinous inflammation of mucous membranes, and a fibrinous laryngitis, trachitis, and bronchitis may result from [p. 50]the local application of such irritants as steam or ammonia, as well as occur in the diseases croup and diphtheria.

Fibrinous exudations may also be present within tissues, especially in those whose meshes are wide, provided the essential elements of coagulation are present. The coagulative necrosis of various organs, to be more fully mentioned hereafter, is closely allied to fibrinous clotting, the fibrino-plastic element being derived from the death of the parenchymatous cells of the part.

In the existence of a fibrinous pneumonia the conditions are somewhat analogous to those present in the fibrinous inflammation of serous surfaces and of the areolar connective tissue. There is present an abundantly cellular exudation, held in the place of its origin, the cells undergoing rapid death and surrounded by a wall whose superficial cells resemble in structure, if not in origin, the endothelial cells lining the smaller lymph-spaces of connective tissue, as well as the larger cavities within the same, known as serous cavities.

The diphtheritic inflammation is no more to be confounded with the disease diphtheria than is the fibrinous inflammation with the disease croup. Although diphtheria owes its name to the frequent presence of an apparent membrane, it may be said that the latter is not essential to the existence of the former. Diphtheria, like croup, is an affection in which various exudations may be present, and the anatomical product alone does not suffice in all instances for the recognition of the disease. In croup there may be a swollen mucous membrane, with a slight superficial mucous exudation, or a more abundant exudation of desquamated epithelium and mucus, as well as a fibrinous false membrane. In diphtheria the same varieties of exudation may occur, and in addition the diphtheritic exudation may also be present. The latter, however, is not limited to the disease diphtheria, for its presence is apparent in other mucous membranes than that of the air-passages, and in the pharyngeal mucous membrane in other diseases than diphtheria. A diphtheritic conjunctivitis, enteritis, cystitis, and endometritis are recognized. The cutaneous surfaces of the body may also furnish a diphtheritic exudation. The diphtheritic inflammations of wounds and of variolous eruptions are instances in point.

The characteristics of a diphtheritic inflammation are the presence within the tissues of a clotted exudation, which is associated with a defined swelling and death of the part. The exudation contains not only dead leucocytes and interlacing fibres, but is also provided with abundant granular material, much of which presents the well-known peculiarities of microscopic organisms. The apparent false membrane is thus dead, infiltrated tissue, which may be torn away from the continuous unaffected tissue, leaving a raw, rough surface, but not peeled from a comparatively smooth surface, as in other forms of pseudo-membranous inflammation.

The frequent association of a superficial false membrane, corresponding in area with that of the deeper-seated changes, in which cells and fibres may be present, is to be recognized. The diphtheritic process, however, is localized within, and not upon, the tissues affected. The diphtheritic exudation represents a local death, a necrosis, of the part concerned, and the result has frequently been compared with the death consequent upon the action of a caustic.

[p. 51]The immediate cause of a diphtheritic inflammation is now generally attributed to the action of microbia which enter the tissue from without, and in their growth beneath the surface produce not only the local, but also the remote, constitutional disturbances which are associated with a diphtheritic inflammation. The investigations of Wood and Formad[16] point to ordinary putrefactive organisms as a sufficient cause for the diphtheritic inflammation of diphtheria, while other observers demand a specific organism as the exciting cause. The occurrence of diphtheritic inflammations in various parts of the body, in regions, as the intestine, where putrefactive processes are constantly present, and in the bladder and uterus, where the phenomena of putrefaction are often associated with diphtheritic inflammation, suggest the efficacy of ordinary putrefactive agencies in producing the latter. As all microbia found in putrefaction are not alike, and as the properties of certain, differ from those of others, and as our knowledge of the effects of all is but fragmentary, the characteristics of specific germs for a diphtheritic inflammation of one part of the body, or of all parts of the same, must still be regarded as not proven.

[16] *Research on Diphtheria for the National Board of Health*, 1880, Supplement No. 7.

Productive inflammations are those which result in the new formation of tissues. One of the frequent products of inflammation is fibrous tissue, which, at first abundantly cellular, later becomes more vascular, and is finally transformed into a tissue whose fibres predominate over its cells. This formation of a cicatricial tissue demands further recognition when the termination of inflammation is considered.

In a more limited sense certain inflammations are called productive when multiple circumscribed new formations, as cancer, sarcoma, tubercle, and the like, arise in connection with the ordinary products of inflammation. Such new formations are of frequent occurrence in serous membranes, and a tuberculous pericarditis or a cancerous peritonitis, indicates that a growth of tubercles or cancerous nodules has taken place, in addition to a more or less abundant exudation with various proportions of serum fibrin and cells. This association of ordinary and transitory inflammatory products with the formation of more permanent tissues may be found within organs as well as upon surfaces. A tubercular arachnitis or lepto-meningitis presents the various products of an inflammation of the pia mater with an abundant formation of tubercles. In like manner, a tubercular pneumonia, or a tubercular nephritis suggests an association of neoplastic growth and inflammation, in the lung and kidney. Such a relation offers a basis for the theory in favor of the inflammatory origin of tumors, and is, in part at least, a cause for the frequent consideration of tubercles as mere inflammatory products, wholly cellular or cellular and fibrous, subject to the same modifications as take place during the course of ordinary inflammations.

Even if tuberculous and scrofulous inflammations are regarded as inflammatory processes, modified by a specific cause and by peculiarities of the individual, the cancerous and sarcomatous inflammations are still to be considered as representing an association of inflammatory disturbances and specific new formations, the cause of the latter not being the cause of the former. As ordinary inflammations of the regions concerned may take place in the absence of the neoplasms, so may the [p. 52]specific growth appear in the same regions without anatomical or clinical evidence of inflammation.

The classification of inflammation as to its products is supplemented by distinctions drawn with reference to the seat. The exudations may be superficial or deep-seated; they may lie within the cells, parenchyma, of an organ, or within the interstitial tissue of the same.

The product of superficial inflammations may lie on the surface, as in the case of inflamed mucous membranes, or immediately below the surface, as in numerous cutaneous inflammations, of which erysipelas may serve as the type. The term catarrhal, applied to superficial inflammations, carries with it the idea of displacement, flowing, of the exudation. The product of a catarrhal inflammation must be largely liquid, that such a displacement may readily take place, and the catarrhal exudation is chiefly composed of an excess of those elements which are present in the normal, physiological secretion from the membrane concerned. Mucus therefore represents a frequent constituent of the catarrhal exudation, and mucous as well as muco-purulent catarrhs of the gastro-intestinal, bronchial, genito-urinary, and other mucous membranes are recognized. The catarrhal inflammation of the respective membranes usually represents the mildest form, as it demands an intact epithelium, and a ready removal of the inflammatory product.

As the cause of a catarrhal inflammation may occasion a destruction of the epithelium or a necrosis of the mucous membrane, the frequent association of catarrhal with fibrinous or diphtheritic inflammations is obvious. In such cases the clinical importance of the latter varieties gives them the precedence in the designation of the inflammation. The retention of the catarrhal products is the frequent cause of permanent disturbances of a more or less serious nature. These result in part from the mechanical obstruction offered to the function of parts beyond the seat of obstruction, as pulmonary atelectasis; and in part from the changes taking place in the retained product. Purulent otitis media with its dangerous or fatal results, and gangrene of the lung terminating in septic pleurisy, are not infrequent instances of severe disturbances from putrefaction of the retained products of a primarily catarrhal inflammation. A cheesy degeneration of the catarrhal cells leads to a surrounding fibrous, or destructive, inflammation, with a corresponding diminution in the function of the organ affected.

Of the deep-seated varieties of inflammation, that requiring special mention is the phlegmonous form. This runs its course within the less dense fibrous tissue known as the areolar or cellular tissue. The term cellulitis is usually employed by English writers to indicate the seat and nature of the process, and although the use of the term cellular tissue is rapidly becoming obsolete, the convenience of cellulitis favors the retention of the latter name.

The exudation lies within the larger lymph-spaces, and is therefore sometimes designated as the result of a lymphangitis, the deep-seated, wider lymph-spaces being concerned rather than those more superficial. Certain forms of phlegmonous inflammation are of decidedly infectious origin, and, when seated subcutaneously, are known as phlegmonous erysipelas, being thus distinguished from the simple erysipelas, whose seat is defined by the small superficial lymph-spaces of the skin.

[p. 53]Infective forms of cellulitis are also frequently met with in the loose, sub-peritoneal tissue of the pelvis. The infectious element usually proceeds from the uterus, and excites the malignant oedema of the broad ligament, the septic parametritis, or the pelvic cellulitis, according as the lymph-spaces inflamed lie nearer the fundus or cervix, and as the direction of the current is upward toward the spine, or outward toward the sub-peritoneal lymphatics of the pelvic wall.

Parenchymatous inflammation is present when the exudation is taken into the cells of an organ, or when the changes dependent upon inflammation of an organ take place within its functionally important cells. Virchow originally used the term parenchymatous inflammation in contradistinction to secretory inflammation, the changes in the former occurring within the elements of the tissues, while in the latter the exudation made its appearance on the surface of the organ.

Parenchymatous inflammation is manifested by a degeneration of the cells affected. This may terminate in their destruction through the conversion of their protoplasm into fat-drops, fatty degeneration; although more frequently a simple accumulation of albuminoid granules (granular degeneration) occurs. The latter represents a transitory condition, from which a return to the normal state readily takes place. This form of inflammation is met with in those organs which present a sharply-defined contrast between the functionally important cells and the connective tissue which surrounds them. The liver, kidneys, heart, spleen, pancreas, and glands in general, are consequently the most frequent seat of parenchymatous inflammation.

Opposed to this variety is the interstitial inflammation. The exudation of the latter remains within the connective-tissue framework of the organ. It is essentially cellular in character, and the number of cells is comparatively small. With their presence and the possibility of their nutrition a permanent increase in the quantity of the fibrous tissue of the organ is permitted. This becomes relatively greater in the course of time, and the parenchymatous cells become degenerated and absorbed. Interstitial inflammations are likely to become chronic in character, and, from the outset, are usually associated with parenchymatous changes.

An important clinical distinction is drawn with reference to the duration of an inflammation. Acute inflammations are those whose course is rapid, whose progress is associated with graver disturbances of function, and with a greater prominence of the cardinal symptoms. The chronic forms occupy more time in their progress, the functional disturbances, though severe, are injurious more from their protracted persistence, than their temporary violence, while redness, swelling, heat, and pain are symptoms of trifling prominence.

The exudation in acute inflammation, if recovery takes place, is rapidly removed from the place of its origin, while in the chronic variety it tends to become a part of the region in which it lies, or, if removed, slowly disappears, and may be constantly replaced. Acute inflammations may become chronic, and the chronic variety is liable to acute exacerbations.

The distinction between acute and chronic inflammations is essentially one of convenience, and, when considered from the anatomical point of view, relates rather to the persistence of the results. These may be [p. 54]present as a variously modified exudation or as a degenerated condition of the parenchyma of the organ or tissue affected.

Inflammation terminates in resolution, production, or destruction.

For resolution to occur it is necessary that the causes of inflammation cease to act, either by their removal or their isolation, and that their results be removed. With the removal of the results there is often associated the removal of the cause. That such may take place it is necessary that the function of the vessel walls be so restored that the exudation ceases to escape. Inflammatory products already outside the vessels, if present on surfaces with external outlets, are carried along in the course of the excretions. If they lie within the cavities of the body not opening externally, their removal is accomplished through the medium of the circulating lymph and blood, by absorption. The liquid portion of the exudation becomes a part of the circulating fluids of the body. The fibrin is converted into a granular detritus, which eventually disappears from the place of its formation. The leucocytes may return to the blood-vessels or enter the lymphatics; the latter course probably being the one taken by the larger number of the corpuscles. Many undergo a fatty degeneration, and as they lie in lymph-spaces their conversion into an emulsion permits a removal of the mechanical obstruction to the flow of lymph through the spaces in which they were accumulated. The red blood-corpuscles are destroyed, their pigment being dissolved by the surrounding fluid and removed in the course of the circulation and excretions, or it becomes transformed into granules or crystals, which may remain in the place of their formation, or be transferred, within amoeboid cells, to remote parts of the body.

When the exudation is abundant, as in the great lymph-sacs of the body—the several serous cavities—and especially when the openings in the walls of these sacs are obstructed or the currents within them are feeble, absorption takes place with great difficulty, and demands a long interval of time. The fibrinous and cellular portion of such an exudation frequently becomes converted into a caseous mass, from a partial fatty degeneration and inspissation. This mass becomes isolated from the cavity in which it lies, usually at the most dependent portion, by the formation of a capsule of connective tissue. It may subsequently become infiltrated with lime salts, calcified, and thus remain comparatively inert throughout the life of the individual.

The productive termination of inflammation is manifested by the new formation of connective tissue. This tissue is variously designated, as the inflammatory process is limited to the surfaces of the body exposed to the air, or the surfaces of cavities and organs, or as it lies within organs or the deep-seated parts of the body. In numerous instances it becomes a permanent constituent of the body, and, as time is usually essential for its formation, its occurrence is indicative of a chronic, rather than an acute inflammation. Certain chronic inflammations are progressive in character, the production of connective tissue being continuous, with perhaps occasional intermissions, as in the chronic interstitial inflammations of organs and tissues. The new-formed tissue, which at the outset is rich in cells, becomes in time more fibrous, and associated with this change in structure is a physical modification, manifested by its shrinkage. This new formation may fill a gap resulting from the destruction of tissue in [p. 55]the progress of an inflammation, when it is present as cicatricial tissue—the scar which is usually met with upon the surfaces of the body or of certain of its organs. When opposed surfaces are united by the new-formed tissue, the term adhesion is applied; the adhesions being present as fibrous bands, cords, or membranes. The pericardial milk-spots and thickenings, the tendinous or semi-cartilaginous, indurated patches of serous membranes and of the intima of arteries, are all regarded as manifestations of a chronic inflammation of these tissues. With the localization of the inflammation in the outer walls of the bronchi and blood-vessels a thickening of the external sheath results, called a peri-bronchitis, arteritis, or phlebitis, as the case may be.

The new formation of blood-vessels is essential for the production and preservation of this connective tissue, and both arise from pre-existing tissues. Pus-corpuscles represent the simple cellular product of an inflammation, and their existence is but transitory. With the new formation of blood-vessels imbedded in abundant cells there exists a granulation-tissue, likewise transitory, but out of which arises the permanent fibrous tissue. The question is still mooted as to the part played by exuded white blood-corpuscles in the production of the permanent results of inflammation. It is generally conceded, especially since the observations of Ziegler, that they are capable of transformation into lasting constituents of tissue, into blood-vessels as well as into cells and fibres. Whether all the resulting permanent products of inflammation are dependent upon their activity, or whether the pre-existing fixed elements participate, is still to be considered undecided.

What, at present, appears most probable is, that from exuded leucocytes there arise, in the course of several days, larger cells—epithelioid or endothelioid—which are eventually associated with still larger cells, more irregular in shape, and provided with projecting filaments, giant-cells. Both varieties may result from the enlargement of leucocytes by fusion or by the assimilation of nutriment. The epithelioid cells eventually become fusiform or stellate, and their projections, as well as those of many of the giant-cells, become fibrillated. The fibrils of adjoining cells, becoming united, are thus transformed into a meshwork of fibrous bundles enclosing irregular spaces, while the nuclei of the cells, with the immediately surrounding protoplasm, remain upon these bundles as the permanent cells of the new-formed tissue. The blood-vessels arise from pre-existing vessels, chiefly capillaries, and probably are also formed from the cells present in the exudation. The former method is indicated by the projection of solid sprouts from the wall of a capillary, which may unite, forming arches, and communicate with sprouts from neighboring capillaries, thus forming bridges. Both arches and bridges then become hollowed and admit the circulating blood. Ziegler maintains that the projections of the larger epithelioid cells and giant-cells become elongated, and eventually fused with capillaries, or the projections from capillaries. When this fusion is accomplished the cells become hollowed, their cavities communicating with those of the blood-vessels. These epithelioid cells, whose formation and transformation are of such importance in the history of productive inflammation, are designated by Ziegler as formative cells, and are frequently derived from the exuded white blood-corpuscles, though not identical with them.

[p. 56]The inflammations not terminating in resolution or production, end in the destruction of the part. This result occurs when the nutrition of the inflamed territory is so diminished, by the changes in and around the vessels, as to become insufficient for its preservation. As the nutriment is derived through the blood-vessels, the more complete and the more permanent the stagnation in them the more likely is death to result. This event also depends upon the quantity and quality of the exudation. The more abundantly cellular the latter, the more likely is an abscess or ulcer to result.

As most abundantly cellular exudations are considered to be dependent upon the presence of putrefactive agencies, those inflammations of a predominant putrid character (gangrenous inflammations) are those terminating in destruction. The dead product is present as a slough or sequestrum, when dead soft or hard tissues are detached, entire or in part, from the living; or as a granular detritus contained in a more or less abundant liquid. The inflammatory process producing the slough and sequestrum is characterized as a gangrenous inflammation of soft parts or a caries of bone, while the process resulting in the formation of the granular detritus, and which has no necessary connection with putrefactive agencies, is called a softening, from the physical condition of its result.

Thrombosis and Embolism.

A blood-clot formed within a blood-vessel during life is called a thrombus. The entire process of which the thrombus is the essential element is designated thrombosis.

These terms were introduced by Virchow[17] to avoid the confusion which resulted from regarding the process and result as synonymous with inflammation of the vessel. All writers, even at present, do not adhere to this strictness of meaning. For a thrombus of the vulva indicates a clot of extravasated blood within the connective tissue of the labium; in like manner, a vaginal thrombus is the effused and clotted blood in the loose connective tissue surrounding the vagina. These exceptions are gradually disappearing, and the word hæmatoma, tumor composed of clotted blood, is being substituted in both instances. A cancerous thrombus represents a mass of cancerous tissue whose growth is extended along the course of a vessel, its wall having been penetrated. In general, however, the term thrombus, unless otherwise qualified, is used as first stated.

[17] *Handbuch der Speciellen Pathologie und Therapie*, Erlangen, 1854, i. 159.

Although thrombosis is commonly a morbid process, it is not uniformly so. Its physiological significance is illustrated by the part it takes in the closure of the umbilical and uterine vessels, after childbirth. The surgeon makes use of it in his efforts to overcome certain of the ill effects of amputation, and to accomplish a cure of such local diseases as aneurism, where it is deemed important to diminish the supply of blood.

The thrombus being a blood-clot, it is composed, like the latter, of fibrin and blood-corpuscles. It is presumable that the fibrinous part of a thrombus owes its origin to the same conditions which determine the presence of fibrin in blood removed from the vessels during life or in that within the vessels after death.

[p. 57]According to A. Schmidt,[18] the blood and other fluids, in which clotted fibrin makes its appearance, contain two generators, called fibrino-plastic and fibrinogenous. The former is considered to be paraglobulin, a substance contained mainly in the white blood-corpuscles, while the fibrinogenous generator is held in solution in the plasma of the blood. When these materials are acted upon by a third, the fibrin ferment, clotting takes place and fibrin is formed. It is thought that the ferment is intimately connected with the white blood-corpuscles, for with the microscope coagulation is seen to advance as these become destroyed, and where the leucocytes are most abundant, there coagulation advances most rapidly. The elements of clotted fibrin are always present in circulating blood, but Brücke has shown that blood remains fluid, under ordinary circumstances, because of its constant contact with the normal vascular wall.

[18] Rollett, *Hermann's Handbuch der Physiologie*, Leipzig, 1880, iv. 1, 114.

The general causes of thrombosis are those which produce an abnormal condition of the endothelium, a rapid destruction of the white blood-corpuscles, or a stagnation of the blood. With the presence of one of these causes there is often conjoined another, and the conditions under which they are present are conveniently used in the classification of thrombi.

Although stagnation of the blood is often an important immediate cause of its coagulation, it is apparent, from the investigations of Durante[19] and others, that stagnant blood clots in the living vessels only when their endothelium is in an abnormal condition. With the co-existence of abnormal endothelium and stagnant blood, thrombi form with greater frequency and become more voluminous in a given interval of time.

[19] *Wiener Medizinische Jahrbucher*, 1871, 321.

The importance of the death of white blood-corpuscles in the formation of thrombi is generally admitted, and is especially insisted upon by Weigert. According to the observations of Zahn, the nucleus of certain thrombi is the result of the death of these leucocytes and their accumulation upon an altered intima. The experiments of Naunyn, Köhler, and others show that a thrombus may be rapidly produced by the injection into the blood of fibrino-plastic substances, and of those through which free hæmoglobin is admitted into the circulation. The former may be expressed from a fresh blood-clot; the latter may be obtained by thawing frozen blood, or by injecting such material (bile-acids, for instance) into the circulating blood as rapidly destroys the red blood-corpuscles. Although Weigert lays special stress upon the destruction of white blood-corpuscles in the formation of the thrombus, it appears, from the experiments above referred to, that indirectly the destruction of the red corpuscles is also of importance.

Although largely made up of fibrin, a thrombus also contains blood-corpuscles, both red and white, and the appearance of the mass is modified according to the variations in the relative proportions of these constituents.

Zahn[20] divides thrombi, according to their color, into red, white or colorless, and mixed varieties. The red owes its color to a large number of red blood-corpuscles, while the white and mixed forms contain various proportions of white blood-corpuscles and fibrin and a diminished number[p. 58]of red corpuscles. The cause of this difference in the color of thrombi is to be sought for in their method of origin. When blood clots slowly in a dish, the heavier red corpuscles settle to the bottom, and the lighter white corpuscles form a superficial layer. Stagnant blood clotting rapidly furnishes a uniformly red mass. The red thrombus, like the red clot, is the result of the rapid coagulation of stagnant blood. The white thrombus, on the contrary, largely composed of white blood-corpuscles, represents a constantly increasing deposition of these from flowing blood. The mixed thrombi arise from a combination of both conditions, and are usually white at the outset. Thrombi formed in the heart and larger arteries are usually white, those in the auricular appendages and on venous valves are mixed, while red thrombi are more common in arteries and veins, since the conditions favoring their origin are more frequently met in such vessels.

[20] *Virchow's Archiv*, 1875, lxxii. 85.

Thrombi are frequently stratified, in consequence of the successive deposition of new layers of blood-corpuscles and fibrin upon a pre-existing thrombus. Circulating blood is therefore necessary for the stratification, and such thrombi are likely to be mixed in color. Unstratified thrombi are usually white or red, the former largely composed of agglomerated white blood-corpuscles so moulded and situated as to prevent a stagnation of blood in their vicinity, while the red thrombus is rarely stratified, since its formation demands a stoppage of the blood-current. Stratification is intimately connected with the enlargement or growth of the thrombus, which takes place from the surface exposed to the flowing blood, and which is greater or less according to the seat of the thrombus.

Thrombi are usually divided into those from compression, dilatation, traumatism, and marasmus; in all of which groups an abnormal condition of the endothelium is to be met with.

Thrombi from compression are frequently formed in veins, in the vicinity of growing tumors. Their presence is most constant when the vein is compressed between a resistant surface, especially bone, and the tumor. A compression of the smaller blood-vessels within an organ, as the liver or kidney, may take place in consequence of chronic interstitial inflammation, or the growth of cancerous or other malignant tumors in such organs. The production of this form of thrombus is sought for in the treatment of certain aneurisms by direct pressure, the resulting stagnation of blood being followed by a coagulation within the aneurismal sac.

Thrombi from dilatation are met with both in dilated arteries and veins. In aneurism and varix a slowing of the blood-current is present, and the intima of the diseased region is frequently in such an abnormal condition that a clotting of the blood readily takes place. The shape and situation of the dilatation are of importance in promoting the formation of the thrombus; the more pedunculate and the more voluminous the sac the more certain is the thrombosis.

Traumatic thrombi result from a direct injury to the vessel. This may be mechanical, as in the application of ligatures for the obliteration of vessels, the tearing of the veins during childbirth, and the infliction of wounds of every variety. The injury may likewise be chemical, from the action of caustics; somewhat analogous to which, are the effects of heat and cold. Allied to the traumatic thrombi are those which arise [p. 59] from acute inflammation of the intima extending from wounds or inflammatory processes in the vicinity of blood-vessels.

Marantic thrombi are those whose origin is attributable to that enfeebled condition of the body known as marasmus. This represents a weakening of the several functions, especially the circulation, respiration, and locomotion. Such may take place in disease or old age; and it is important to bear in mind those diseases in which marasmus is likely to arise, as thrombosis often proves a complication of such affections. Protracted fevers, as typhus and typhoid, puerperal diseases, the disturbances following surgical operations, chronic wasting diseases, as the tuberculous and scrofulous affections, are all likely to be accompanied by thrombosis. Stagnation of the blood, as well as alterations of the intima, is an important local condition in this variety of thrombosis, which is usually valvular or parietal at the outset, and may be both arterial and venous. Such thrombi are likely to become continued and to serve as a frequent source of embolism.

Thrombi are also divided into primitive, or autochthonous, and secondary varieties. The primitive thrombus is one which owes its local origin to conditions existing at the place of its formation and attachment. The secondary variety demands for its existence a primitive thrombus, whose place of development is remote in time and seat, and from which a part has been transferred to serve as the nucleus for the secondary formation.

The continued thrombus is often confounded with the secondary variety. Continuance is rather a quality of all thrombi, and is essentially growth, whether by lamellation or agglomeration. Such continued thrombi are extended in the course of the circulation, usually by a conical end, which is pointed toward the heart in the case of venous thrombi, but away from this organ when the thrombi are arterial.

Parietal and obstructing thrombi form another subdivision. The former arise from a limited part of the wall of the heart or blood-vessel, and project into its cavity. They are always in contact with flowing blood, and are white or mixed in color and primitive. They may attain a considerable size, and may eventually become obstructing thrombi. The latter are so called when they are of sufficient size to cause a considerable or total obstruction to the current of blood. In the last case the vascular canal is wholly filled by the thrombus. The shape of the older parietal forms is usually globular or pedunculate, owing to the growth in all directions except at the place of attachment; the obstructing thrombi are elongated.

Thrombi are also characterized by consistency and relative absence of moisture. A thrombus is brittle and dry as compared with a clot. In distinguishing between the two, difficulty arises only in the case of a thrombus which may have formed within a few hours before death. Post-mortem clots are moist, elastic, readily withdrawn from blood-vessels, and have a smooth and lustrous surface. Their color is either red, gray, grayish-yellow, or yellow, and is very often mixed. The lighter colors are due to causes which favor the precipitation of red blood-corpuscles before actual clotting takes place, or which occasion an increase of the white blood-corpuscles in fibrin. The thrombus becomes adherent to the vessel wall within a few hours, after its formation, in the case of the red thrombus, and at once, in the case of the white variety. A clot is never adherent, although it may seem so from its entanglement between the trabeculæ and [p. 60]tendons of the heart and the cavernous framework of venous sinuses. Such apparent adhesions are easily recognized by the smooth, shining, intact intima which is disclosed after the removal of a clot.

The thrombus not only tends to become enlarged by further depositions of material from the blood, but it also tends to become diminished in size from the contractile properties of its fibrinous constituent. Moisture is forced from the thrombus in consequence of this shrinkage, and its dryness is increased by subsequent absorption through the wall to which it adheres.

The changes eventually taking place in the thrombus are known as organization, calcification, and softening.

Organization is the transformation of the thrombus into a mass of fibrous tissue. This is accomplished, according to the researches of Baumgarten,[21]by an outgrowth of endothelium from the intima of the vessel, the thrombus being absorbed as the growth of tissue advances. In the case of a thrombus due to the ligation of a vessel, a granulation-tissue also makes its way into the thrombus between the ruptured coats, and the new-formed fibrous tissue which replaces the thrombus becomes vascularized through this granulation-tissue. The vascularization of thrombi surrounded by unbroken walls is most likely to result from the extension into the thickened intima of new-formed branches of the vasa vasorum. Cohnheim claims that the organization of the thrombus may take place solely through the entrance of migratory cells, without any active participation of elements of the vascular wall. The canal is thus obstructed or obliterated by a fibrous tissue, which is pigmented or not, as the pre-existing thrombus contained red blood-corpuscles or not. These, when present, become transformed into granular or crystalline hæmatoidin, which may remain as a permanent constituent of the new-formed tissue.

[21] *Die sogenannte Organisation der Thrombus*, Leipzig, 1877.

Even when the thrombus is completely obstructing at the outset, it is not necessary that a total obliteration of the vessel should result from its organization. It not rarely happens, either before or after the thrombus has yielded to the fibrous growth, in consequence of the shrinkage of the fibrin of the thrombus or of the contraction of the fibrous tissue replacing it, that gaps arise which become communicating canals. Through these the blood flows, and the vessel thus becomes only obstructed, not obliterated. The sieve-like tissue thus formed is spoken of as the result of a cavernous or sinus-like transformation of the thrombus. The length of time necessary for the removal of the thrombus and its replacement by fibrous tissue varies considerably. A vascularized granulation-tissue may be present within a week, and in the course of a month the thrombus may have been wholly removed, or a period of months may elapse and the thrombus and granulation-tissue still be present side by side.

The calcification of a thrombus takes place when the latter becomes impregnated with salts of calcium and magnesium. The condition may be present in thrombi which are exposed to a rapidly-flowing arterial stream, as well as in those which lie in venous pockets outside the course of the direct current of blood. The well-known phlebolites are examples of the latter variety. A calcified thrombus may be intimately united to the vascular wall, the results of calcification and organization being associated. Calcification and, in particular, organization represent favorable [p. 61]events in the history of thrombosis, as through their occurrence the process comes to an end, and disturbances, either local or remote, are prevented.

The softening of the thrombus, on the contrary, is always a source of danger. This is partly due to the nature of the products of the softening, whether bland or septic, and partly to the mechanical disturbances produced by the transfer of portions of the softened thrombus to remote parts of the body. All thrombi may become softened. When the process of organization advances normally, the softened parts are absorbed as rapidly as the formation of vascularized fibrous tissue progresses. If this formation is checked or stopped, the process of disintegration still continues. White corpuscles undergo fatty degeneration; red corpuscles give up their coloring matter and become converted, like the fibrin, into granules, and there results a granular detritus. This is present as a viscid, semi-fluid material, either red, gray, or yellow, according to the color of the thrombus. This simple softening is to be regarded as essentially chemical in character, and begins at the oldest portion of the thrombus and advances toward the periphery. Its products are capable of absorption without the production of serious disturbances, and are usually prevented from direct entrance into the blood-vessel containing the thrombus by the continuation of the latter from new coagulation or deposition upon its surface. The thrombus is thus extended as the softening progresses.

When the thrombus is comparatively free from red blood-corpuscles, the softened product, in consequence of its yellowish color, opacity, and viscidity, resembles pus. The so-called encysted abscesses projecting into the cavity of the heart, from its wall, are parietal and globular thrombi, in the interior of which softening has occurred. This form of softening is called simple or bland, as it is free from any evidence of local suppuration, inflammation, or general constitutional disturbance attributable to an absorption of poisonous material.

Septic softening is accompanied by general evidences of a blood-poisoning, and by the local phenomena of purulent inflammation. A suppurative thrombo-phlebitis or arteritis, occurs; that is, an acute inflammation of the wall of the vessel, corresponding in its origin to the seat of the thrombus, and characterized by the formation of pus. In the earliest stage the softened thrombus need not present products differing in appearance from those occurring in simple softening, but their effect is manifested by a rapidly-advancing inflammation of the vascular wall and by the evidence of septicæmia. Inoculation with such material produces a group of symptoms classified under the head of blood-poisoning.

Cohnheim lays special stress upon the presence of micrococci in the softened material, and it is generally agreed that the virulence of septic softening is connected with, if not due to, the presence of microbia. A septic softening may be induced by besmearing, with septic material, the outside of a blood-vessel containing a thrombus, and this form of softening is usually associated with those conditions favoring this relation. Such are the gangrenous wounds following surgical operations, the putrid inflammatory processes affecting the uterine wall after childbirth, the offensive inflammations of the middle ear, and the like. It is possible for a septic softening to occur independently of such contiguous or continuous relations with the surfaces of the body. It is considered, [p. 62]however, that the micrococci present in a softened thrombus must have obtained admission from without through one of the surfaces of the body, mucous or cutaneous, or through undiscovered abrasions of even intact surfaces of peculiar structure, as the alveolar wall or the intestinal mucous membrane. The thrombus is regarded as affording a favorable soil for the growth and activity of the organism.

The mechanical effect of a thrombus varies according to the venous or arterial seat of the same. Venous thrombi, as they are continued toward the heart, tend to become completely obstructing thrombi. In most parts of the body the venous anastomoses are so numerous that the obstruction of a vein is readily compensated for through the collateral venous circulation. When such a compensation is prevented by an extension of the thrombus from branch to branch, and finally to the trunk, an accumulation of blood in the peripheral veins must result. The remote parts become swollen, from the distension of the vessels with blood and the transudation of liquid, and eventually solid material from the blood. Venous thrombosis thus leads to oedema, and even hemorrhage. The more rapidly the obstructing thrombus extends, the earlier and more extreme is the oedema likely to become, while the slower the advance of the thrombus, the more favorable is the opportunity for an enlargement of the collateral vessels through which a sufficient flow of blood is permitted to check oedema and preserve nutrition.

Local mechanical disturbances from arterial thrombi are scarcely perceptible till obstruction is produced, and the results of arterial obstruction will be mentioned in detail in connection with the phenomena of embolism. Cardiac thrombi may occasion local disturbances from interfering with the action of the valves of the heart. Those thrombi which are attached to the valves, especially when calcified, may produce inflammation and aneurism of the opposed wall of the heart, by friction. The most frequent mechanical disturbance from the non-obstructing parietal thrombi of the heart and arteries results from the detachment of fragments and their transfer as emboli to remote parts of the body.

An embolus is a foreign body in a blood-vessel, usually too large to pass through the smallest capillaries, and the disturbances resulting from its presence are included under the term embolism. Although most emboli are detached portions of thrombi, any foreign body of suitable size may become an embolus. Such are tissues, as the pulmonary elastic fibres, fragments of diseased valves of the heart and of the intima of arteries, or portions of tumors growing into vascular canals. Others are globules of oil entering the torn veins when fat-tissue becomes crushed, or air-bubbles admitted through veins either wounded by instruments or opened after parturition by the dislodgment of their obstructing thrombi. Still others are granules of pigment derived from the coloring-matter of the blood, as in melanæmia, or introduced from without, as india-ink and cinnabar. The echinococcus has been found as an embolus, and it is highly probable that the cysticercus, the trichina, and other animal parasites may be disseminated as emboli over the body.

Vegetable parasites, like the bacterium and aspergillus, have also been included in the list, although the disturbances resulting from their presence are less due to mechanical obstruction than to colonization and growth. The experimenter uses the most various objects as emboli—bits[p. 63]of wood, rubber, and glass, globules of mercury, fragments of tissue, etc. Emboli are to be regarded as of arterial or venous origin. The arterial emboli are carried toward the capillaries, while venous emboli are carried toward the heart. The effect of both is partly or wholly mechanical, and partly due to the specific properties of the constituents.

The mechanical effect of an embolus is manifested by the obstruction it offers to the circulation, and the degree of the obstruction depends upon the size, shape, and density of the embolus and the nature and size of the vessel obstructed. An embolus may be so large as to be unable to pass through the valvular orifices of the heart. A long and narrow embolus might pass through a vessel which would not admit one which was short and thick. A jagged and dense embolus, by repeated blows or prolonged and forcible contact, might cause a weakening or rupture of the wall of a vessel, and thus produce an aneurism. Certain vessels (the terminal arteries of Cohnheim) furnish the sole supply of arterial blood to a district, and when they are obstructed, the results, to be mentioned later, differ widely from those taking place where free vascular anastomoses exist. When a trunk bifurcates, the larger branch usually receives the embolus.

Venous emboli are those which approach the heart by the peripheral veins of the body or the pulmonary veins, and the liver by the radicles of the portal vein. Emboli from the veins of the body are carried through the right side of the heart, if not so large as to be stopped at the tricuspid or pulmonary opening. As they enter the latter, they are carried along its course under the influence of gravity and the direction and force of the current, which are determined by the direction and relative size of the bifurcations of the artery, the right primary branch being larger than the left. Eventually, a point of the artery is reached whose diameter is less than that of the embolus, and the latter is stopped. This point usually corresponds with a place of bifurcation, and the embolus frequently rides the wall separating the branches.

Emboli from the radicles of the portal vein owe their most frequent origin to thrombi associated with inflammatory processes in the intestine, especially of the cæcum and vermiform appendage, to inflammatory processes in the spleen and obstruction to the flow of blood through the splenic artery, or to inflammatory changes proceeding from the kidneys. Such venous emboli are carried toward the heart, but are stopped on the way by the intrahepatic branches of the portal vein.

Arterial emboli are those which enter the left side of the heart from the lungs, which arise in the left ventricle or auricle, which may pass through an open foramen ovale from the right auricle, or which arise from the arterial wall. They are carried along the course of the arterial circulation, and are distributed over the different regions and organs of the body. Usually following the more direct course of the circulation, they are more likely to enter the abdominal aorta than to be carried toward the brain or upper extremities. Embolism of the carotids, especially of the left carotid, is more likely to ensue than embolism of the subclavians. Embolism of the coronary arteries is rare, while embolism of the splenic artery, the left renal and left iliac arteries, is comparatively common, and in the order mentioned.

When an embolus is found, or embolism suspected, the source is always[p. 64]to be searched for in those regions from which the affected part receives its blood. The source of arterial and portal emboli is usually found with ease, while the pulmonary embolus may come from so wide a region, the body-veins, that much time may be spent before its place of origin is discovered. An appreciation of the laws of the transfer of emboli renders such a discovery almost certain.

When the embolus reaches a point beyond which it cannot pass, the resulting disturbance depends essentially, as shown by Cohnheim, upon the presence or absence of arterial anastomoses beyond the place of obstruction. He gives the name terminal arteries to those which have no anastomosing arterial branches. These are met with in the spleen, kidneys, lungs, brain, and retina. If the obstructed artery is not terminal, the embolus may produce no further disturbance, the collateral supply of blood through the anastomoses sufficing for the nutrition and function of the part. If, however, the vessel is a terminal artery, and the embolus is completely obstructing, the supply of arterial blood must be wholly cut off from the region beyond the seat of obstruction.

If the embolus does not completely obstruct at once, it soon becomes sufficiently large for this result to ensue in consequence of a secondary coagulation. The rider assumes legs extending into the arterial branches beyond the place of obstruction, and a body which extends backward in the course of the circulation to the nearest branch. The result of the total obstruction of the vessel is to cut off the admission of arterial blood, producing a local anæmia. The contraction of the elastic tissues of the part propels toward the capillaries a certain quantity of the blood in the vessels beyond the point of obstruction, till this force becomes neutralized by the blood-pressure in the vessels surrounding the obstructed region. The anæmic part may subsequently become engorged with blood; it may die, a region of anæmic necrosis resulting, or the dead portion may become softened.

The engorgement of the obstructed territory has received the name of hemorrhagic infarction. A solid, wedge-shaped mass of a reddish-brown color is present, whose shape is due to the arborescent branching of the terminal arteries. According to Cohnheim, the engorgement of the region with blood takes place from venous regurgitation into the obstructed part, till the intravenous pressure is overcome by the resistance of the tissues in the region affected. The capillaries and larger vessels thus become distended, and an escape of liquid and solid constituents of the blood takes place. If the veins are provided with valves, or the venous regurgitant current is opposed by gravity, the hemorrhagic infarction is prevented or greatly impeded.

Litten,[22] on the contrary, who has furnished a recent contribution to this subject, claims that the hemorrhagic results of embolism are not accomplished through venous regurgitation, unless increased venous tension is produced by coughing, vomiting, and like efforts. His experiments lead him to maintain that arterial blood from surrounding tissues is supplied to the obstructed region through the anastomosing capillaries. The force is not sufficient to drive the blood through the capillaries into the veins beyond, but an accumulation takes place in the capillaries, which become dilated and distended. The escape of blood-corpuscles and [p. 65]serum then takes place, the more freely, as Weigert[23] suggests, the larger and more numerous are the pre-existing spaces in the organ. Hence the infarction becomes the most characteristically developed in such organs as the lungs and spleen. Causes which obstruct the venous flow, as well as those which increase the arterial tension, promote the hemorrhagic infarction.

[22] *Untersuchungen über den hemorrhagischen Infarct., etc.*, Berlin, 1879.

[23] *Virchow's Archiv*, 1878, lxxii. 250.

A necrosis of the part whose direct arterial supply is cut off takes place when the structure of the organ affected is such that the admission of arterial blood is wholly interfered with. This is the case in the heart and kidneys, and to a less extent in the spleen. The opportunity is presented for the diffusion of a fibrinogenous fluid, lymph or blood-serum, through the cells of the organ which contains the other essentials for coagulation, and the dead part presents the characteristics attributed by Weigert[24] to death from clotting of the protoplasm, coagulative or ischæmic necrosis.

[24] *Ibid.*, 1880, lxxix. 87.

Embolism of the cerebral arteries produces softening of the brain, not a hemorrhagic infarction or a yellowish necrosis. Weigert attributes this result, on the one hand, to the absence in the brain of abundant cells from which are to be had the ferment and fibrino-plastic material necessary for coagulation, and, on the other, to the closure of the spaces into which blood might collect by the rapid swelling of the tissues from the exuded lymph.

The hemorrhagic results of embolism are also met with in obstruction of branches of the mesenteric artery, which is considered by Litten, at least from its function and in connection with its sluggish current, to correspond with a terminal artery.

If the patient outlives these more mechanical results of embolism, the local changes taking place are those tending to remove the extravasated blood or the dead tissues. The embolus has become an obstructing thrombus, and its removal is accomplished in the manner already stated in connection with the subject of thrombosis. The wedge-shaped nodule of hemorrhagic infarction becomes decolorized through the absorption, in part, of the blood-pigment. That portion which is not absorbed remains at the site of the original lesion as granular or crystalline blood-pigment. A granulation-tissue is formed at the periphery, which extends into the infarcted region, very much as the endothelial and vascularized growth extends into a thrombus. Eventually, a patch of cicatricial tissue remains as the sole indication of the previous disturbance. This termination is rather suggested for the hemorrhagic infarctions of the lungs. The results are more apparent and more easily demonstrated in the case of the anæmic necroses, and the somewhat irregular depressions with wedge-shaped scars, seen upon the surface of the spleen or kidneys, call attention to the probable nature of the process giving rise to these results. A source of embolism must also be associated, that these scars may be regarded as of embolic origin. The embolic softenings of the brain are likewise represented in after years by losses of substance. The superficial, yellow patches or localized oedematous blebs, with corresponding atrophy of the convolutions beneath, call attention to a nutritive disturbance, as do cyst-like cavities in the deeper parts of the brain. Here, too, a source of embolism must be found, that [p. 66]the local destruction of tissue may be attributed to embolic obstruction of vascular territories.

When the embolus arises from a septic thrombus, the results differ from those above described. The embolus then carries not only mechanical possibilities, but also a virulent action. The latter is manifested by the rapid production of local inflammatory disturbances, as circumscribed abscesses and gangrenous destruction of tissue. Since emboli are frequently lodged near the surfaces of organs, a septic pleurisy, pericarditis, or peritonitis is the usual result of the dissemination of the virus contained in the embolus. This virus is similar in character to that found in septic softening of the thrombus, and, like it, is intimately connected with the presence of microbia. Whether the latter are specific in character, as maintained by Klebs and others, or whether they are to be included among those associated with putrefactive processes, still remains an open question.

The symptoms of thrombosis obviously depend upon the resulting obstruction to the circulation of blood, and in the case of primitive thrombi are gradual in their occurrence. The degree of mechanical obstruction is determined by the nature of the thrombus, whether parietal or obstructing, and by that of the vessel, whether provided with anastomoses sufficient to permit a compensatory collateral circulation or not. In the former case, if the thrombus is small and deep-seated, there may be no symptoms to indicate its presence. When the collateral circulation is insufficient to remove the blood from a region whose efferent venous trunk is completely filled with a thrombus, the phenomena of stagnation are produced. The part becomes oedematous, and red blood-corpuscles escape from the distended vessel. If the obstructed vein is superficial, the seat of the thrombus is indicated by the resistance and sensitiveness of the part. Characteristic disturbances of function are associated with thrombosis of the various organs of the body. If the cerebral sinuses are affected, mental disturbances arise; if a cardiac thrombosis is present, it is frequently accompanied by irregularity and feebleness of the heart. When the portal and renal veins are obstructed, functional disturbances arise in the parts from which they receive their blood.

The symptoms of embolism, like those of arterial thrombosis, are primarily due to anæmia. Suddenness is their characteristic in embolism, while they are gradual and progressive in the case of thrombosis. An embolic anæmia is complete or incomplete according to the terminal or anastomosing character of the obstructed vessel. The effect of the anæmia is to stop or check the function of the part, and varies according to the size and situation of the vessel. Hemiplegia, or perhaps aphasia or other evidence of localized disturbance, follows central embolism; angina pectoris, with a disturbed cardiac action, results from embolism of the coronary artery. Sudden suffocative symptoms, with open air-passages, suggest embolism of the larger branches of the pulmonary artery. A considerable hæmaturia often excites suspicion of an embolism of the renal artery, the hemorrhage coming from the vessels in the neighborhood of the obstructed region. Embolism of a large artery of an extremity is often localized by the sensation of a blow at the part, to be followed by absent pulsation, pallor, and coldness of the region beyond the place of obstruction.

[p. 67]The symptoms of the subsequent effects of thrombosis and embolism are to be inferred from what has already been stated with regard to the nature of the possible lesions. To enter into their detailed consideration would demand more space than is permitted, and would modify an established sequence or necessitate a repetition, which is undesirable in a systematic treatise.

Effusions.

The various fluids of the body are derived from without, and admitted into the blood-vessels. The physiological transudation through the walls of these vessels, in the main modified serum, becomes lymph as it appears in the several lymph-spaces. From the latter the transuded fluid either returns through the lymph-vessels to the blood-current or makes its appearance upon surfaces as secretions. These are variously modified as they pass through the specific cells of glands or as they are met with in the several closed cavities of the body.

The transudations thus occurring may vary in quantity within certain limits, the latter being somewhat indefinite, owing to the difficulties in the way of exactly measuring the fluid transuded. The greater part of this transudation is represented by the quantity of lymph flowing through the main lymph-trunk, and of the secretion from the glandular surfaces of a given region of the body; but that transuded fluid is not included which may return to the blood-vessels without being carried into the general lymph-current or secreted from a gland. Such a direct return may be considered to take place whenever the pressure upon the outside of the vessel wall is greater than that within the latter, or when the chemical composition of the fluids on the two sides of the filter permits endosmosis as well as exosmosis. This varying relation in the direction of the current through the vessel wall is likely to be of frequent, if not constant, occurrence in connection with the physiological processes taking place throughout the body.

The undue accumulation of the transudation in the various closed cavities of the body is known as dropsy, and the fluid present is regarded as an effusion or an exudation. These terms are often applied somewhat vaguely, now being used as synonymous, again as representing different conditions of the transudation, which are attributed to the varying conditions of its accumulation.

Exudation is more generally used when an inflammatory process is the cause of the increased transudation, while effusion is more strictly associated with causes other than inflammatory. In the present consideration this etiological distinction will be maintained.

To appreciate the conditions under which pathological accumulations of fluid, whether effusions or exudations, may arise, it is desirable to bear in mind the essential conditions which prevail in the occurrence of transudation, since the former are likewise chiefly derived from the blood and are transuded through the walls of its vessels. These conditions are largely dependent upon the laws governing the diffusion of substances through an animal membrane, the vascular wall representing the filter. As a living membrane its relation is dependent upon vital as well as [p. 68]physical conditions, and the former produce certain important modifications in the physical process of filtration.

The transudation through the vessels takes place chiefly through those with the thinnest walls, the capillaries, although it is probable that a certain degree of transudation may also occur through the walls of the smallest veins. The causes which are instrumental in promoting the circulation of the blood—viz. the contraction and dilatation of the heart, the contraction of the arteries, the inspiratory action of the thorax, and muscular movements throughout the body—are also essential in producing the flow of lymph; and the existence of pressure upon the hæmic side of the filter is the first feature of importance in occasioning the transudation. The constant removal of the transudation from the outer side results from the pressure being less in this position.

At the same time, an increase in the quantity of blood in the vessels is not necessarily productive of any considerable increase in the fluid transuded. Cohnheim calls attention to the experiments of Worm Müller, which show that a plethoric condition may readily be produced by the injection of quantities of blood into the circulation of animals, the amount of which cannot exceed twice the volume of the animal's blood without producing death. Although a temporary increase of the blood-pressure results, a return to the normal quickly follows. This is permitted by the propulsion of the excess of blood into the capillaries and veins, which become consequently distended, especially those of the abdominal organs. There is no increased transudation corresponding with the quantity of fluid introduced, nor is there any considerable distension of the blood-vessels of the skin, subcutaneous or intermuscular connective tissue. Such experiments show no permanent increase in the blood-pressure within the large veins if there is no obstruction to the admission of venous blood into the heart, presumably owing to their capacity for considerable distension.

Although experiments show that a simple plethora with great distension of the capillaries of the abdominal organs occasions no considerable increase of transudation, a different result follows a hydræmic plethora[25] induced by the injection of immense quantities of salt water into the blood-current—often six times as much liquid as the animal had blood. Here, too, the arterial blood-pressure shows no permanent increase, nor does that within the large veins become perceptibly increased till enormous quantities of fluid are injected. The blood flows through the vessels with increased rapidity in consequence of the diminished friction of the diluted blood, and an increased transudation begins at once. The various glands, salivary and gastro-intestinal, kidneys and liver, secrete more copiously, and the flow of a dilute lymph from the thoracic duct becomes greatly increased, while that from the cervical lymphatics becomes moderately accelerated. The lymph from the extremities, however, is no greater in quantity than that flowing from an animal in a perfectly normal condition. The localization of the increased transudation from the blood-vessels is further characterized by the abundant accumulation of watery fluid in all the abdominal organs and abdominal cavity, in the salivary glands and surrounding connective tissue, while elsewhere in the body the organs and tissues are almost invariably in the same condition with [p. 69]regard to moisture as are those of a healthy animal under normal circumstances.

[25] Cohnheim and Lichtheim, *Virchow's Archiv*, 1877, lxix. 106.

The importance of these experiments with reference to the causes of the transudation of fluid from the blood is obvious. The pressure upon the walls of the blood-vessels cannot become sufficiently increased to be accompanied with augmented transudation until limits are reached which are beyond the possibilities of occurrence in the human body. When such limits are attained in animals, the increased pressure, however great it may be, does not suffice to produce a general transudation, but one limited to the vessels of those parts of the body whose normal function is connected with too abundant transudation of fluid. A simple hydræmic condition of brief duration has been proven, by experiment, insufficient to give rise to increased transudation, neither increased secretion nor increased flow of lymph taking place. The inference from these experiments is that an increased transudation is more dependent upon conditions of the filter than upon those of blood-pressure. The absence of any observable changes in the filter leads to the assumption of an increased permeability, of physiological occurrence in certain parts of the body, as the chief feature in the occurrence of increased transudations.

Dropsy arises when the transudation is accumulated. As dropsical accumulations are transudations from the blood, essentially blood-serum with a diminished percentage of albumen, and as such blood-serum is practically lymph from its presence in the lymph-vessels, dropsical effusions are to be regarded as stagnant lymph. Such stagnations may be present in the small lymph-spaces within the connective tissue, or in the larger lymph-sacs, as the peritoneal, pleural, pericardial, and scrotal cavities. In like manner, the stagnation may take place in the cavities of joints and in those of the brain and cord, although the latter represent functional rather than structural lymph-canals.

The term oedema is applied to the accumulation in the connective-tissue lymph-spaces in general, while the term anasarca is confined to those cases where the subcutaneous lymph-spaces are concerned. The accumulation in the great lymph-cavities is known as ascites when peritoneal, hydrothorax when pleural, hydropericardium when pericardial, hydrocele when in the cavity of the tunica vaginalis, hydrocephalus if within the ventricles of the brain, and hydromyelocele when within the central canal of the spinal cord.

The accumulation of dropsical effusions may be considered as possibly resulting from an obstruction to the channels through which the transudation should flow, or from insufficient force to overcome normal obstructions, or from an abnormally increased transudation.

Lymph-channels are frequently obstructed, but no appreciable diffused retention of lymph results unless the thoracic duct is obstructed. This rare affection is followed by enormous distension of the thoracic and abdominal portions of the parts beyond the stenosis. Ascites and hydrothorax may follow, but not necessarily any considerable oedema of the peripheral parts of the body. As a result of the distension of the thoracic duct, rupture is not unlikely to take place, and the effused fluid contains chyle.[26]

[26] Quincke, *Deutsches Archiv für Klin. Med.*, 1875, xvi. 121.

[p. 70]That the obstruction is not followed by oedema is attributable to the innumerable anastomoses between the lymph-spaces, and also to the probability that a part of the transuded fluid returns to the blood-vessels when the obstruction is impassable.

The forces necessary to promote the flow of lymph have already been mentioned, and their entire removal is inconsistent with life. A diminution of their activity is more likely to result in a diminished flow of lymph than its accumulation, although a slowing of the lymph-current may represent a favoring element in the accumulation of an increased transudation.

The occurrence of dropsy with unobstructed lymph-channels, and in the presence of efficient agencies in promoting the flow of lymph, indicates the importance of an increased transudation as the chief element in the occurrence of a dropsical accumulation. An increased transudation, with resulting oedema, is readily produced by preventing the flow of blood from a part, and may be directly observed with the microscope. Cohnheim states that after a sudden venous obstruction, in case an efficient collateral circulation does not interfere, the capillaries and small veins become distended with stagnant blood and appear as masses of red blood-corpuscles. This distension results from the continuance of the arterial flow into the capillaries of the obstructed region under a pressure which is only neutralized by the resistance of the tissues and the transudation from the capillaries. Sotnitschewsky[27] shows that a concurrent paralysis of the vaso-motor nerves, as claimed by Ranvier, is unnecessary. The transudation through the capillary wall is increased, the flow of lymph from the part is accelerated, and oedema arises when the transudation is so much augmented that the calibre of the lymph-vessels is insufficient for its removal; and the greater this insufficiency the greater is the oedema. With the continuance of the arterial flow and intravenous resistance, red blood-corpuscles are forced through the filter, and form an important constituent of the effusion from venous stagnation.

[27] *Virchow's Archiv*, 1879, lxxvii. 85.

Although the existence of an increased pressure upon the capillary wall is obvious from the experiment referred to, there is no increased arterial pressure—rather a diminution—and the important element in occasioning the increased permeability of the capillary wall is the obstruction to the outflow of venous blood from the oedematous region. In consequence of the latter the arterial flow is followed by increased transudation.

Dropsies resulting from venous obstruction, as well as those following an obstruction of the thoracic duct or its branches, or of the several lymphatics of a part, are classified as mechanical dropsies. That from venous obstruction is the most frequent, and its seat may lie in the course of venous trunks or in the heart, lungs, or liver. The venous obstruction must be so situated that the stagnant blood is unable to find a ready escape through collateral branches. The more sudden and complete it is, the more likely is the effusion to contain considerable numbers of red blood-corpuscles.

In addition to the element of venous stagnation in producing increased transudation, the condition of the filter is of importance. The occurrence of oedema in chronic diseases, especially of the kidneys, and in those attended with protracted suppuration, continued hemorrhage, and the [p. 71] rapid growth of tumors, has usually been attributed to the watery condition of the blood, with a diminution of the albumen. Cohnheim, however, suggests that the condition of the vessel wall is of more importance than the contents as the immediate cause of the increased transudation. The more or less protracted action of various agents—temperature, insufficient oxygen, and diminished albumen—is likely to so modify the condition of the endothelium as to favor an increased permeability of the wall. Experiments show that a simple acute hydræmia produces no increased transudation, and that a chronic hydræmia, if connected with dropsy, is likely to be influential by increasing the permeability of the wall. Even in those cases where a hydræmia and an oedema co-exist, the localization of the latter is favored by obvious disturbances of the function of the capillary walls, as in case of the cutaneous oedema after scarlatina. In like manner, a feeble heart, favoring venous stagnation, and gravitation are of importance, as general causes, in promoting dropsy in hydræmic conditions.

The possibility of the occurrence of oedema through nervous influence is not to be denied. The localized and fleeting oedema of urticaria and erythema, the swollen lip and tongue in connection with digestive disturbances, are not to be explained by the two main factors of oedema—viz. venous stagnation and increased permeability of the vascular walls. Cohnheim refers to the rapid occurrence of oedema of the tongue as a result of irritation of the lingual nerve, and oedema is known to occur rapidly in cases of acute myelitis. A similar result follows the experimental destruction of the spinal cord, although the mechanism of its production is not apparent.

Dropsies are subdivided, as regards their distribution, into general and local forms. The causes producing the two varieties are essentially those already described. The causes of all local dropsies are not always to be regarded as the same. Regions which are the seat of mechanical dropsies are often affected by inflammation, with abundant serous exudation—the so-called inflammatory dropsy. The properties of the effusion and exudation are quite different, the former having a small percentage of albumen, but few leucocytes, with a corresponding absence of fibrin, and few or many red blood-corpuscles. The exudation, on the contrary, is highly albuminous, though less so than the blood-plasma; it contains numerous leucocytes and much fibrin; under ordinary circumstances there are but few red blood-corpuscles.

The local dropsies are often characterized by special terms. Hydrops ex vacuo is applied to the collections of fluid found in closed cavities with unyielding walls, as the cranium and thorax, or to the recurrence of fluid in cavities from which the same has been rapidly removed, in the absence of inflammatory disturbances. Collateral oedema is usually applied to the association of oedema with inflammatory disturbances, and represents an extension of the inflammatory process to the region concerned. Oedema of the glottis and circumscribed oedema of the lung are instances. The term hypostatic oedema is often used to designate the association of oedema and inflammation, the former caused by the latter, and to indicate the effect of gravitation in the localization of oedema from the general causes already mentioned.

Another localized oedema of interest, from its frequent occurrence and[p. 72]importance, is oedema of the lungs, often taking place toward the end of life, at times quite suddenly. This form has usually been attributed to increased transudation from arterial congestion or venous stagnation. The former view is directly refuted by the experiments of Welch,[28] who offers the explanation now accepted. With the obliteration of three-fourths of the arterial supply to the lungs of the animals experimented upon, no oedema resulted from the assumed collateral fluxion into the branches of the pulmonary artery which were left open. The obliteration of the same area of venous distribution was necessary before the occurrence of oedema. Oedema of the lungs was further found to result from a ligature of the aorta near the heart. The comparative frequency of oedema of the lungs in man, and the rarity of such extreme mechanical disturbances as those produced experimentally, led Welch to paralyze the left ventricle. The conditions as regards the pulmonary circulation then corresponded with those mentioned as causes for oedema from venous obstruction. The continued action of the right ventricle forced blood into the pulmonary capillaries, where it was compelled to accumulate in consequence of the inability of the left ventricle to receive and expel it. Welch consequently regards the immediate cause of this form of pulmonary oedema as a predominant weakness of the left ventricle. A weak heart does not suffice for the production of the oedema, since this condition is not found when both ventricles are alike enfeebled.

[28] *Virchow's Archiv*, 1878, lxxii. 375.

Degenerations.

The degenerations represent disturbances in the nutrition of the tissues of the body, in consequence of which their functions become impaired, if not destroyed. The latter result obviously attends the death of cells, which may occur in the course of the degeneration. The processes concerned are called necrobiotic by Virchow, as they represent vital processes leading to death. Although in many of them the cell is decaying during their continuance, its recovery is possible with the disappearance of the conditions which have transformed physiological into pathological processes. The degenerations affect intercellular substance as well as cells, and are called metamorphoses, infiltrations, or degenerations, as a transformation of normal into abnormal material, or the addition of extraneous substances, or the functional impairment of the part assumes the greatest prominence.

Cloudy Swelling, Albuminoid Infiltration, Granular Degeneration, Parenchymatous Degeneration.

Of the various modifications in the appearance of cells under pathological conditions, there is none, perhaps, more commonly met with than that known by the above terms. A granular appearance may be regarded as an essential characteristic of protoplasm, and is an attribute of cells of epithelial origin as well as of those which belong to other groups of tissues. The abundance of granules present in a normal cell depends largely upon its shape, size, and situation. These granules present various[p. 73]relations to chemical agents, some being soluble in alcohol and ether, others in acids and alkalies, and many of them, especially those met with in the form of degeneration now being considered, show from the various reactions that they are of the nature of albumen. Since their exact composition, in all instances, is undetermined, they are called albuminoid, and when in excess the cell is considered to be infiltrated with these granules, and the organ presents the appearances regarded as characteristic of an albuminoid infiltration. A granular cell becomes much more granular when it is thus infiltrated, and it is therefore a matter of difficulty to recognize from the appearance of certain single cells, as those of the liver or kidney, whether or not the number of granules present is abnormally increased. When, however, a large number of cells of any given organ contain more than the normal quantity of these albuminoid granules, the appearance of the organ becomes modified. In extreme cases the latter is swollen, doughy in consistency, with ill-defined structural details, and in all instances presents an opaque appearance. The term cloudy swelling is thus purely descriptive, and was applied by Virchow to designate the optical appearances of the condition in question. The granules, which disappear on the addition of acids and alkalies, are apparently either added to the cell or result from a precipitation within the same.

Frequently associated with these albuminoid granules are others, distinctly recognizable as globules of fat. An apparent increase of nuclei is often observed, and in certain organs, as the kidneys, the cells seem less coherent than is normally the case. The study of this condition in the kidneys is further of interest as indicating that the border-line between a parenchymatous degeneration and a parenchymatous inflammation is purely arbitrary. From similar exciting causes there may be associated, with the described alterations of the epithelial lining of the tubes, the exudation of albumen, the formation of casts, the desquamation of epithelium, and the presence of leucocytes within the tubules.

When the macroscopic changes are of moderate degree, and the disturbance of function relatively slight, while the concurrent alterations elsewhere, from the simultaneous action of the same cause, are predominant and characteristic of the disease, the condition is conveniently regarded as a degeneration occurring in the course of the latter, rather than an inflammation. The latter term, on the contrary, is to be applied when the granular infiltration of the cells is associated with other evidences of an inflammatory exudation, and when the pathological disturbances are to be directly attributed to the parenchymatous changes.

It is customary to speak of cloudy swelling as a nutritive change, and the condition may be induced by those causes which interfere with the nutrition of parts or of the whole of an organ. Many authorities regard this granular or parenchymatous degeneration as closely allied to fatty degeneration, since many of the causes which produce the one occasion the other. The former is often spoken of as an earlier stage of the latter, from the frequent association of the albuminoid granules with numerous globules of fat as a result of the more prolonged or more intense action of a given cause.

Organs which give evidence of a granular degeneration contain, as a rule, a diminished quantity of blood. This feature is usually attributed to the pressure of the swollen cells upon capillary blood-vessels. The [p. 74]anæmic organ obviously becomes still more cloudy, gray, and opaque in appearance from the diminished quantity or impoverished quality of the blood.

The granular degenerations of the heart, liver, and kidneys, as a whole, usually occur simultaneously, and afford a most important means for the post-mortem recognition of the infective diseases. The condition is therefore to be looked for in the exanthemata, especially in small-pox and scarlet fever, also in erysipelas, septicæmia in its manifold forms, diphtheria, typhoid and typhus fevers, cerebro-spinal meningitis, etc. A common feature in all these cases is the occurrence of fever, and it has been claimed that this element is the cause of the degeneration. In opposition to this view is the well-known fact of its presence in afebrile cases of poisoning from carbonic oxide, and its absence in certain cases of pneumonia and exposure to high temperatures.

The universal occurrence of cloudy swelling in fatal cases of the affections above mentioned leads to the inference of its presence in those instances terminating in recovery without obvious permanent impairment of the organs and tissues concerned. It is therefore agreed that the process may terminate in resolution—*i.e.* in a disappearance of the excess of granular material. On the other hand, its association, under circumstances, with fatty degeneration suggests as extremely probable that the latter condition may represent a result of the albuminoid infiltration. Even if this more serious issue exists, the possibilities are still at hand for an absorption of the degenerated material and a restitution of the destroyed protoplasm. The effect upon the individual is evidently determined by the persistence and dissemination of the condition, which, in turn, are controlled by the immediate cause and the peculiarities of the individual acted upon.

Fatty Metamorphosis, Fatty Degeneration, and Fatty Infiltration.

The fat which is present within the body under physiological conditions owes its origin primarily to the food taken. A diet which is abundantly fatty furnishes a direct source for much of the fat which appears accumulated in the various organs and tissues. Although it may now appear that such a statement needs but little confirmation, it is not long since the opinion prevailed that nearly all the fat in the body came from the hydrocarbons of the food. This seemed all the more plausible as the herbivora readily accumulated fat, although their diet might contain this element in very small quantities. Hofmann[29] made a decisive experiment with reference to the origin of fat from fatty food by feeding a dog, made lean by starvation, with bacon in abundance, but with little meat. In the course of a few days the greater part of the fat introduced was deposited within the tissues of the animal. Other experimenters have arrived at a similar result, and it can no longer be questioned that fat, accumulated within the body, owes its origin chiefly to the absorption of fat from the food taken.

[29] *Zeitschrift für Biologie*, 1872, viii. 153.

Another source for the fat of the body has long been suggested—namely, the albuminates of the food. In the admirable article on the formation of fat by Voit,[30] from which most of the information herein [p. 75]presented is derived, it is claimed that he and Pettenkofer were the first to prove the origin of fat in the body, under normal conditions, from albumen. This proof was an inference, however, although presenting a high degree of probability. Valuable evidence in the same direction was furnished by Kemmerich, who found that the milk of a cow during a certain period held more fat than was contained in the food; Subbotin and Voit have shown that more milk is secreted the richer the diet in albumen. Still other observers have furnished more decisive proof that fat is formed from albuminates.

[30] *Hermann's Handbuch der Physiologie*, 1881, vi. 1, 235.

Two sources for fat in the body under physiological conditions are thus recognized: 1, the free fat in the food; 2, the fat derived from the decomposition of the albuminates of the food.

Voit admits the possibility of the hydrocarbons serving as a third source, although this possibility is unnecessary in most cases. Should instances arise, however, where other sources for fat are found insufficient, the hydrocarbons must be regarded as filling the gap.

Fat which is taken into the body is considered to be either consumed or stored. That which is stored is chiefly accumulated in the great reservoirs—viz. the subcutaneous and perinephritic fat tissue, the mesentery, omentum, and bone-marrow—although it may be found elsewhere, in the fluids and tissues of the body. This accumulation serves as a source to be drawn from in case of need, and is called upon where the easily-decomposed soluble albumen is disposed of by the functional activity of the cells. An acting muscle demands food for its work, and consumes first the soluble albumen, then the fat. An excessive waste of fat is delayed by the decomposition of hydrocarbons, but the demands may become so great that albumen, fat, and hydrocarbons are consumed more rapidly and constantly than they can be supplied. It being, therefore, admitted that fat is formed from the albuminates, as well as from the fat of the food, the question readily presents itself whether fat may not be formed from the fixed albuminates of the body, especially from those contained within its cells.

It is well known that in the secretion of sebum the superficial cells of the sebaceous follicles contain fat in great quantity, while the deeper layers are comparatively free from any appearances indicative of the presence of fat. It is further admitted that when pus is retained for a time the individual corpuscles contain fat-drops in quantity and become transformed into fatty granular corpuscles. Eventually, the pus is transformed into a detritus in which fat-drops are found in great number.

Similar appearances may be present in the protoplasm of muscular tissue, the cells of the liver, kidneys, and gastric glands, when poisonous doses of phosphorus or arsenic are given. The occurrence of an acute fatty metamorphosis of the cells of various organs in new-born children has repeatedly been observed. The presence of fat in various organs of the body in pernicious anæmia, and in the heart in connection with stenosis of the coronary artery, is universally recognized. The abuse of alcohol, long-continued obstruction to the flow of venous blood, exposure to high temperatures, are all known to be conditions in connection with which fat-drops are found in the various cells of the body. The effects of poisoning with phosphorus and arsenic are of special importance, as showing that the abundance of fat present in the cells represents a result of the degeneration of these cells, [p. 76]since it takes place when the animal is deprived of food. Although there is an evident destruction of albumen, there is also a diminished elimination of carbonic acid and admission of oxygen. These facts are explicable on the ground that the fat present is not consumed, and the accumulation in the cells is evidence of this lack of consumption. The fat is not simply stored, as none is taken in, nor is any food received from which fat might be formed. Its presence, therefore, must be regarded as due to degeneration.

Since fat may be formed in the body as a result of the metamorphosis of cell-protoplasm, it is desirable to ascertain whether there are any means by which stored fat may be distinguished from that present as the result of a degeneration of the cell. The term fatty infiltration has been used to indicate the presence of stored fat, the latter being regarded as simply taken into the cell and retained for a longer or shorter time, without any necessary interference with other functions possessed by the cell.

In fatty degeneration, on the contrary, it is considered that the quantity of fat present indicates a corresponding diminution in the albuminates of the cell, and is connected with a diminution in the function of the latter, all the greater the more abundant the fat.

It is found that in fatty infiltration, as a rule, the fat is present in large drops, the size of the cell being increased in proportion to the quantity of fat present. Although there may be several drops present, they tend to run together, as is suggested by their different size, varying proximity, and the constant presence of a considerable quantity of protoplasm. In organs, on the contrary, whose function is seriously, even fatally, impaired, the fat, as a rule, assumes rather a granular form. Many minute fat-drops are present, and the cell is not particularly, if at all, increased in size. The more abundant the fat the less the protoplasm. Appearances are met with indicating a transition between cells with few fat-granules and those with many.

If the morphological appearances of fatty infiltration and of fatty degeneration were constant, there would obviously be little or no difficulty in determining the nature of the process manifested by the presence of fat. The exceptions occur both in fatty infiltration and fatty degeneration. In the cells of the liver of an animal poisoned with phosphorus fat makes its appearance in large drops, while in the heart and kidneys of the same animal the fat is present in a granular form.

During absorption from the intestine in the process of digestion fat is present in the epithelium in a finely granular form. When digestion is completed fat is no longer met with in these cells. The presence of large or small drops, therefore, cannot be regarded as a sufficient test of the origin of the fat. It is of equal, if not greater, importance to bear in mind the organ concerned.

In the heart, liver, kidneys, and gastric glands, as well as elsewhere, with the exception, perhaps, of the mammary gland, the presence of many small fat-drops in the cells indicates a degeneration of its protoplasm. The presence of large fat-drops, on the contrary, in the organs and tissues, with the exception of the liver, indicates an infiltration. Large fat-drops, then, may be present in the cells of the liver as the result of an infiltration or of a degeneration. In order to form a satisfactory opinion of the [p. 77]nature of the appearances in the liver in doubtful cases, it is important to note the condition of those organs which may be simultaneously in a state of fatty degeneration.

The accumulation of fat under physiological conditions is obviously brought about, on the one hand, by those causes which permit a free introduction, absorption, and deposition, and, on the other, by those which check its oxidation or elimination with the secretions of the body, as the bile, in which it may be present to a considerable extent. A diet rich in fat, or in albuminates readily converted into fat, offers a favorable element for the absorption of fat by the healthy individual. If the organism demands but little of this fat for oxidation, as in the case of the sedentary person, an accumulation is likely to occur. This may become so considerable that obesity results. Tissues in which normally but little fat is accumulated may become infiltrated to a large extent. The intermuscular fibrous tissue thus becomes loaded, and the activity, as well as the nutrition, of the muscles is impaired. This accumulation may be manifested not only in the voluntary muscles, but in the heart as well, which may present abundant sub-pericardial and sub-endocardial fat, the myocardium also being interlarded with streaks of fat, the so-called fatty infiltration of the heart. The abdominal walls may become thickened to the extent of a couple of inches, and the mesentery, omentum, perinephritic tissue, and liver may become enormously increased in weight from the mass of accumulated fat.

This infiltration of fat may take place under pathological as well as physiological conditions. It is apparent that those causes which check oxidation are likely also to prevent the consumption of fat, and it is well known that the destructive processes in the lung, grouped under the term pulmonary consumption, accomplish this result. Something more, however, is necessary than the obliteration of pulmonary blood-vessels and the destruction of an aërating surface. There may be, as in emphysema of the lung, a diminished respiratory and vascular surface, yet evidences of fatty infiltration, particularly of the liver, are wanting. It seems probable that the constant anæmia, with the loss of the blood-corpuscles, of pulmonary phthisis is an important additional factor in checking oxidation in this disease. This factor, it is needless to say, is not a necessary occurrence in pulmonary emphysema.

Litten[31] has shown that when certain animals are exposed to high temperatures the appearances of fatty infiltration and degeneration are present in various organs of the body. He attributes the fatty degeneration to a direct poisoning of the red blood-corpuscles and a resulting diminution of the oxidizing processes.

[31] *Virchow's Archiv*, 1877, lxx. 10.

It is universally admitted that in chronic alcoholism a fatty liver is frequently met with, even in the absence of those chronic interstitial tissue-changes usually characterized under the name cirrhosis. Alcohol is known to check the reception of oxygen and the elimination of carbonic acid, and, whatever other disturbance of cell-activity it may produce, its effect in favoring the accumulation of fat is directly attributable, in part at least, to this disturbance of oxidation.

In those conditions known as cachexiæ, the constant accompaniment of progressive and wasting diseases, as cancer, leucæmia, chronic dysentery,[p. 78]etc., a fatty infiltration, particularly of the liver, is a frequent accompaniment. A cachexia is dependent upon a complex series of processes, many of which tend to check oxidation, and in this respect is to be grouped with the conditions previously mentioned. That the associated fatty infiltration is intimately connected with the deficient oxidation is not to be doubted, although the agents producing this deficiency may vary in detail.

The causes which favor fatty degeneration are numerous, and the result represents one of the most serious conditions which can affect an organ. As oxidation represents the chief means of normally disposing of fat, so, pathologically, deficient oxidation favors the retention of fat due to degeneration. Were a constant renewal of protoplasm to take place, the degenerated fat might be displaced into the circulation or retained within the cell. If the latter event should occur, the result would be apparent as an infiltration, owing to the increased size of the cell, although the condition giving rise to the presence of the fat is a degenerative process. The importance of impairment of nutrition as the chief cause for fatty degeneration is thus obvious. It may readily be produced, experimentally, by measures which check the flow of blood to a part. The same measures necessarily prevent the presence of abundant oxygen, as fewer red blood-corpuscles are presented.

Fatty degeneration resulting from impaired nutrition is apparent in the heart in consequence of stenosis of its coronary arteries, in the kidneys as a result of interstitial processes obstructing the capillary circulation, in the brain from obliterative processes in the arteries at the base or within the organ, and in blood-vessels from the effect of age.

The cause of fatty degeneration may be general as well as local. In poisoning from phosphorus and arsenic the appearances in most of the organs indicate an actual destruction of protoplasm. Analysis of the secretions confirms this inference, as the production of urea is largely increased. Furthermore, there is less oxygen taken in and less carbonic acid eliminated. As has been previously stated, these conditions may be present in the starving animal. The fatty degeneration is thus easily explained as a metamorphosis of cell-protoplasm, and the deficient oxidation of the fat calls direct attention to its accumulation rather than elimination.

In acute yellow atrophy of the liver and in cases of severe jaundice fatty degenerations are constantly met with. That the origin and accumulation of fat in these affections is also due to rapid tissue-metamorphosis and checked oxidation is highly probable. Although the elimination of urea diminishes rather than increases, as shown by Schultzen and Riess, there are other links in the chain of retrograde changes, as the appearance of leucin and tyrosin, indicative of the extensive destruction of albuminates.

It is unnecessary in a work of the present character to call attention to all the possible circumstances under which fat is present in the body as the result of degeneration. Mention may be made of the acute parenchymatous (fatty) degeneration of new-born children, of the results of excessive bleeding, and of pernicious anæmia otherwise occasioned. The fatty degeneration of the uterus after parturition, of paralyzed muscles, and of tumors, the atrophic fatty degeneration of the liver in chronic [p. 79]passive congestion (nutmeg liver), are all well-known examples. To these may be added the fatty degenerations associated with amyloid and interstitial processes. It is apparent that in most of these instances the common features of rapid tissue-metamorphosis and deficient oxidation are present, and, being present, offer a ready explanation for the appearance of the fat.

The clinical importance of fatty metamorphosis requires consideration in connection with the description of the diseases in which its occurrence is a constant feature. As the presence of fat in cells is not necessarily pathological, so an interference with the function of the cell is not invariably implied by its presence. When its existence is suggestive of a local destruction of albuminates, a diminution of cell-activity is a necessary consequence. Such diminished activity must produce different results as the cells are those of muscles, of vessels, or of glandular organs.

Even if fat is found in cells under conditions favoring such a suggestion, it does not follow that the destruction of the cell must result. Not only is it possible that the fat may be reserved for eventual oxidation, and its place in the protoplasm be filled by normal constituents, but it is also possible that the fat may be eliminated, as such, from the body. The latter event is made apparent by the experiments of numerous observers referred to by Cohnheim, who have found free fat in the urine after its introduction into the venous current.

Cheesy Metamorphosis, Cheesy Degeneration, Caseation.

Virchow introduced the term cheesy metamorphosis, tyrosis, to designate the process resulting in the incomplete absorption of pus and the production of apparently similar changes in certain other occasional constituents of the body. The characteristic cheesy appearances were regarded as due to the inspissation of the material concerned, in consequence of the absorption of its fluid. With this inspissation there was frequently associated a partial fatty degeneration, and the cheesy matter represented dead material, which might undergo further changes, of which softening and calcification were the more important.

Inflammatory products, as pus and fibrin, were especially prone to become thus transformed, as well as other relatively transitory materials of new formation—viz. tubercle and parts of various tumors. The type of the cheesy metamorphosis was found in the enlarged lymphatic glands, commonly called scrofulous.

The importance of a clear understanding of the cheesy metamorphosis is now a matter of history. It is merely necessary to allude to the fact that these cheesy products were formerly regarded as indicative of the presence of tubercle, and were the tubercles. Tuberculization and the cheesy condition were synonymous terms, and their indiscriminate use led to much confusion with reference to the nature of tubercle.

Quite recently Weigert[32] has called attention to the conditions present in necrosis resulting from the intermediate stoppage of the blood-current in a part. The effect is manifested, under favoring circumstances, by a cheesy appearance of the affected region, to which the terms decolorized hemorrhagic infarction, anæmic or ischæmic necrosis, have been applied.[p. 80]Weigert lays stress upon the existence of a coagulation of the protoplasm of the cells, with an early disappearance of the nuclei, as the essential feature of this form of necrosis, the conditions present being regarded as analogous to those met with in the coagulation of the blood. The term coagulative necrosis has consequently been introduced by Cohnheim to represent the process first fully described in detail by Weigert. The optical and physical properties of the ischæmic or coagulative necroses of tissue are often manifested as cheesy appearances, although the term coagulative necrosis includes conditions which do not present a suggestion of cheese. It is thus apparent that cheesy appearances may result in two ways: 1, by the inspissation of material in a state of partial fatty degeneration; 2, by a coagulation of the constituents of cells whose blood-supply is suddenly and completely cut off. In the more restricted sense these caseous appearances are regarded as indicative of a cheesy metamorphosis which arises by the former of these methods. Cheesy appearances, on the contrary, dependent upon the sudden death of a part, indicate an ischæmic or coagulative necrosis.

[32] *Virchow's Archiv*, 1880, lxxix. 87.

Whatever may be the origin of the cheesy condition, the material presenting this appearance is liable to further changes, known as softening and calcification. The former event results from the soaking of the dead part with liquid, in consequence of which a detritus results. The softening usually begins at the oldest part of the cheesy mass, and advances toward the periphery. The sanatory evacuation of the emulsive detritus is permitted when a surface continuous with that of the external surface of the body is reached, as instanced by the escape of softened cheesy material from the lungs through a bronchus. The possibility of the complete removal of the dead mass is thus at hand, and an eventual obliteration of the resulting cavity may take place by an adhesive inflammation of its walls.

The complete absorption of the cheesy material of an ischæmic necrosis may occur by the extension into the latter of a granulation-tissue from the periphery. Whenever cheesy appearances are found on surfaces, as the degenerated tubercles of mucous membranes or the circumscribed necroses in diphtheritic inflammation or in typhoid fever, healing may be accomplished by their detachment as sloughs, a clean ulcer being left. Cheesy material is frequently encapsulated—*i.e.* imbedded in a layer of dense connective tissue, a condition which indicates a local cessation of the process through which the cheesy appearances arose. The same may be said of the infiltration of the cheesy mass with earthy salts—calcification—an event which will again be referred to in connection with the consideration of the general subject.

Hyaline Degeneration, Fibrinous Degeneration, Croupous Metamorphosis.
Certain of the conditions now regarded as indicative of a coagulative necrosis or a hyaline degeneration were previously described by Wagner as the result of a croupous or fibrinous metamorphosis. According to this observer, the cell-contents were transformed, under certain circumstances, into a substance resembling externally clotted fibrin. The formation of croupous and diphtheritic membranes, especially of the larynx, pharynx, and trachea, was thus explained, also the hyaline casts of the kidney.

[p. 81]The results of this metamorphosis presented a hyaline appearance under the microscope, and the term hyaline degeneration is now applied more especially to indicate the production of microscopic changes, while the hyaline appearances visible to the eye are rather included under mucous, colloid, or amyloid metamorphoses.

The limitations in the use of the term hyaline degeneration are but ill defined. On the one hand, there is included the transformation of muscular tissue, first discovered by Zenker; on the other, the various changes described by Recklinghausen and others, among which are embraced the results of Wagner's croupous metamorphosis. As the hyaline appearances are a frequent result of coagulative necrosis, these terms are frequently used to indicate the same condition, according as the optical or etiological features are uppermost in the mind of the observer.

The hyaline or waxy degeneration of muscular fibre described by Zenker represents a metamorphosis of the protoplasm of striated muscle in particular, although the fusiform cells of the muscular coat of the stomach and intestine may present a similar transformation.

The microscopic appearances are more characteristic than those visible to the naked eye. To the latter the muscle appears paler, more translucent, and homogeneous, and proves to be more brittle than normal. The muscular fibres are found with the microscope to be swollen, irregular in outline, the myosin transformed into flaky, glistening masses, without evidence of the normal transverse striation. These appearances have given rise to the term waxy degeneration, which suggests a possibility of confusion with the earlier recognized waxy degeneration of organs, due to the presence of amyloid material. The waxy transformation of muscular fibre, however, does not present the reaction with iodine characteristic of amyloid substance. The degeneration of the muscle is usually regarded as the result of a coagulation of the myosin, and it is claimed by Cohnheim that the latter takes place only in dead muscle, either during the life of the individual or as a post-mortem appearance.

The hyaline degeneration of muscular fibre is found in certain febrile diseases, as typhoid and typhus fevers, scarlatina, variola, and cerebro-spinal meningitis. It may also be met with when a muscle has been exposed to violence, as in the insane who have been placed under mechanical restraint. It has further been found in the vicinity of tumors, especially where muscles have been invaded by their growth. Cohnheim and Weil describe a similar condition in the tongue of frogs after ligature of the lingual artery.

The pathological importance of the above-mentioned degeneration of muscle is most prominent in cases of typhoid fever. The occurrence in this disease of the hæmatoma or blood-tumor of the rectus abdominis is thus explained, the degenerated muscle and its contained blood-vessels being ruptured. The muscles of the thigh and the diaphragm frequently undergo this degeneration; the change is more rarely met with in other muscles of the body.

Recklinghausen regards a hyaline substance, hyalin, as a normal constituent of cell-protoplasm which escapes in drops when the cell dies. Its presence indicates a diminution in the vitality of the cell from various causes. Under the microscope it appears as a sharply defined, highly refractive meshwork, enclosing spaces of irregular shape and size, in[p. 82]which are frequently found nuclei, more rarely cells or granules. Langhans has described this appearance as channelled fibrin. It has been met with in the placenta, diphtheritic membranes, blood-vessels, tubercles, and gummata.

The latest contribution to the history and nature of this form of degeneration has been furnished by Vallat,[33] from whose article many of the above data have been obtained.

[33] *Virchow's Archiv*, 1882, lxxxix. 193.

Mucous Degeneration, Mucous Metamorphosis, Mucous Softening.

Of the various degenerations presenting a colloid—*i.e.* gelatinous—condition, the mucous variety is one of the most striking. Its gross appearances may not differ materially from those to be described under the head of colloid degeneration, but the diagnostic characteristic of the change is to be found in the presence of mucin. The presence of this substance is readily detected by the addition of acetic acid to mucus, the effect being a fibrillated appearance of the latter, the fibres presenting a more or less parallel distribution. This fibrillation of mucus is regarded as the result of a coagulation of its mucin, previously held in solution by an alkali. Mucin is thus present in the body as a normal constituent, and, in the secretions from mucous membranes, owes its origin to the existence of epithelial cells, whether these represent gland-cells, as in the case of the muciparous glands of the bronchial mucous membranes, or whether they are superficial cells, as those of the gastric and intestinal mucous membranes.

In the origin of mucus as a secretion from glands Heidenhain[34] claims that a destruction of gland-cells accompanies the continuance of the secretion. At the outset, however, the mucin escapes from the cells, the latter remaining relatively intact. With the persistence of the secretion there results a destruction and a new formation of the muciparous cells. In the pathological production of mucus from mucous membranes, as in catarrh, there is no reason to doubt that the persistence of an irritation is the cause of abundant mucus, and that the latter is dependent upon the rapid formation and destruction of epithelial cells.

[34] *Hermann's Handbuch der Physiologie*, 1880, v. 64.

The origin of mucus from epithelial cells under physiological and pathological conditions being apparent, it readily follows that the epithelioid cells of tumors might be supposed to be liable to a similar metamorphosis. It is well known that cancerous tumors, especially those of the stomach and large intestine, are frequently met with, which present an abundant gelatinous material, more or less completely filling the spongy, fibrous meshwork. These are the alveolar, gelatinous, or colloid cancers.

The gelatinous or colloid material often gives the reaction of mucin, and the microscopic appearances of the tumor show that the jelly-like substance lies in that part of the tumor which corresponds with the position of the epithelioid cells. The latter are found in various stages of degeneration, the appearances being similar to those observed in the mucous degeneration of true epithelium.

The prevailing theory of the origin of cancer from epithelial structures[p. 83]readily suggests an explanation for the frequency of the mucous variety of cancer in connection with those parts from which mucus normally arises from the degeneration of the epithelium.

The mucous metamorphosis affects connective tissues as well as epithelium. The Whartonian jelly of the umbilical cord and the vitreous humor of the eye are known, through the investigations of Virchow, to owe their gelatinous condition to the presence of mucin. The latter lies in the intercellular substance; that is, between the cells. The appearance of these indicates no degenerative process, but the presence of mucin is obviously an essential constituent of the tissue. Whether this mucin represents a transformation of the gelatin of the intercellular substance, or a secretion from the fixed cells, or a metamorphosis of the migratory cells of the tissue, is not known. In mucous tissue, however, there is present mucin, wholly independent of any epithelial degeneration. Mucous tissue is present in the eye as a normal constituent of the adult, and in the umbilical cord as a normal constituent of the infant at full term. It is also abundantly met with in the subcutaneous and intermuscular tissues of the foetus. Its pathological occurrence in the adult as a circumscribed tumor, the myxoma, may also be mentioned.

A gelatinous substance containing mucin is found in the adult independent of the mucous tissue, but obviously arising from a transformation of intercellular substance. The most striking example of this occurrence is the cystoid softening of cartilage, especially of the costal cartilages of old people, the basis substance being transformed into a fluid containing mucin. A similar metamorphosis is of frequent occurrence in the intervertebral disks and in the destruction of cartilage in acute and chronic inflammations of the joints. The intercellular substance of cartilaginous tumors also becomes softened and converted into a liquid containing mucin.

In osteomalacia and in the absorption of bone the mucous degeneration of the bone-cartilage plays an important part. The lime salts are first set free, and the cartilage then undergoes a mucous degeneration; the product is either absorbed or remains as a liquid within cavities of large or small size. The mucous metamorphoses of fibrous and fat-tissues, likewise of bone-marrow, are well recognized instances of the occurrence of a mucous transformation of the intercellular substance of connective tissues. Finally, clotted fibrin, so often met with as the product of the inflammation of serous surfaces, may undergo a mucous metamorphosis, and, thus transformed, offer a suitable material for absorption.

Colloid Degeneration, Colloid Metamorphosis.

Laennec used the term colloid in a descriptive sense to indicate a gelatinous appearance, and for a long time its use was thus restricted. As the colloid appearances were found to differ in their chemical reaction, their distribution, and their pathological importance, and as the term was further extended to include appearances seen with the microscope, it obviously became necessary to subdivide the colloid series of changes according to the observed differences. Its use is now limited to those gelatinous conditions or appearances due to the presence of a fixed albuminate, homogeneous or finely granular, translucent, colorless or pale[p. 84]yellow, of varying consistency, which does not become fibrillated on the addition of acetic acid, and which does not change in color when acted upon by iodine. This albuminate is considered in most instances to represent the result of a transformation, a metamorphosis of cells, and is associated with an impairment of their function—a degeneration which is progressive, and leads, sometimes, to the destruction of the organ, as occurs in certain instances of colloid degeneration of the thyroid body. Usually, the process is limited, affecting particular parts rather than the whole of an organ. The reaction presented by a solution of sodium albuminate in the presence of neutral salts leads to the view that colloid material may represent a coagulation of an albuminous substance or substances under favoring conditions. The presence of colloid masses in the kidney thus meets with a plausible explanation.

The place of its typical occurrence is the thyroid body in certain cases of goitre, and it is early met with as a homogeneous substance replacing the granular cell-protoplasm. With its increase the latter disappears, and the entire cell is transformed into a homogeneous sphere. At times the colloid substance may be seen to project from the surface of the cell as a pale rounded clump. The aggregation of these clumps results in the presence of masses of various size, in which may be found granules of fat or pigment and crystals of cholesterin, which are accidental, not essential. Colloid masses are sometimes met with—in lymphatic glands, for instance—as concretions, mulberry-like aggregations of stratified colloid bodies, which may be infiltrated with earthy salts. Colloid material may eventually become liquefied, transformed into a sodium albuminate; and the presence of cysts in certain varieties of goitre is thus explained. The coexistence in the kidney of colloid accumulations and watery cysts has led to the view that the latter may, under certain circumstances, result from the former through the liquefaction of the colloid material. The same view is held with regard to the origin of cysts frequently met with in the choroid plexuses.

The colloid metamorphosis of cells is also to be found in the epithelium of mucous membranes and their glands, in the prostate, suprarenal capsule, sebaceous glands of the skin, and in the cells of certain tumors.

Amyloid Degeneration, Amyloid Infiltration, Waxy Degeneration, Lardaceous Degeneration.

The colloid appearances due to the amyloid degeneration of cells are of the greatest clinical importance from their frequent occurrence and the gravity of the symptoms connected with their presence. In amyloid degeneration there is the transformation of the cell-protoplasm into an albuminous material different from other albuminates found in the body. This transformation is at the expense of the functional activity of the cell, and the latter becomes inert. Amyloid degeneration represents no mere substitution, but an addition, since the affected tissue is increased in volume. The albuminate was called amyloid by Virchow in consequence of its color-reaction with iodine. Its method of origin is wholly unknown, never being found in the circulating fluids nor in articles of food. It is met with chiefly in the cell, although its presence in the intercellular substance of old people is recognized, and its occurrence in [p. 85]the midst of the thrombotic deposition on inflamed valves and in the results of inflammatory processes is also recorded.

At present the question is under discussion whether the amyloid degeneration may affect cells of the most varied character, or whether it is limited to those of connective tissues. Eberth[35] maintains that in all cases the amyloid disturbance is seated in the connective tissue. Kyber,[36] the latest investigator, in opposition to this view maintains that this affection is not limited to the connective tissue, but may also be seated in the parenchymatous cells of organs. Whether the one of these views is to exclude the other, or whether both are not correct, remains for future investigation to decide.

[35] *Virchow's Archiv*, 1880, lxxx. 138; 1881, lxxxiv.
[36] *Ibid.*, 1880, lxxxi. 7, 111.

Wherever the amyloid material may be situated, the result is a transformation of the cells into a homogeneous, glistening, colorless material, which occupies more space than the original cell, and, when abundant, is accompanied with a loss of the primitive details of the cell-structure. This material is recognized by the color it presents when acted upon by iodine alone, by iodine and sulphuric acid, or by methyl-aniline. The first produces a reddish-brown color, the second a blue, and the last a violet or purple color. These reactions are all characteristic, and the first is of special value in the macroscopic recognition of the process, while the last two are of special importance in the microscopic recognition of the earlier stages of the affection.

With the advance of the degeneration and its dissemination, the organ affected presents, in the diseased portions, pale-gray, glistening, translucent patches, and becomes increased in size and density in proportion to the quantity of amyloid material present. The change appears primarily in the vessel wall or outside the same, and there results a diminution in the calibre of the vessels, with a lessened quantity of blood in the organ.

From the homogeneous and translucent appearance of the surface and the increased density of the tissues the resemblance to bacon or wax is suggested, and the terms lardaceous, bacony, or waxy degeneration have been applied. Notable differences in degree and seat occur in connection with the organs diseased. In the spleen, for example, the change may be limited to the arteries of the Malpighian bodies and their immediate surroundings. To this condition the term sago spleen is applied, the enlarged, rounded, translucent, and projecting bodies suggesting granules of boiled sago. The appearances of the diseased part are further affected by the association of other conditions, as the presence of fat or pigment. When fat is present, it is often to be regarded as a result of the gradual and progressive increase in the obstruction to the circulation of blood in the organ.

Although so little is known of the immediate cause of amyloid degeneration, its distribution in the various organs of the body is fully ascertained, as well as certain of the conditions which are likely to be followed by its presence. It is known to occur as a localized process in cartilage, in the conjunctiva, in certain tumors, cardiac thrombi, scars, retained inflammatory products, and renal casts. The causes of this localized appearance are wholly obscure, and little or no general inconvenience results. Its presence, however, on a large scale and in various parts of [p. 86]the body at the same time, is met with under such circumstances as indicate a distinct etiological relation. An appreciation of these circumstances is of importance, since their existence demands an investigation as to the probable presence of the degeneration. The organs thus affected are the spleen, liver, kidneys, and intestine. It is to their disturbance of function that the pathological importance of amyloid degeneration is to be especially attributed.

Other organs which may sometimes be affected are the lymphatic glands, pancreas, suprarenal capsules, omentum, uterus, bladder, prostate gland, heart, and thyroid body. In the case of a general diffused infiltration these organs are variously degenerated, now some, and again others, showing a more extensive alteration, while few or many may be simultaneously diseased. The longer the process has continued, the greater the degree of the disturbance and the larger the number of the organs infiltrated. Although, in general, a period of months and years may be demanded for these extensive changes, very serious disturbances may arise within a short time, and Cohnheim[37] records several cases which suggest that widely diffused amyloid degeneration may occur within a few months—in one instance in less than four months.

[37] *Virchow's Archiv*, 1872, liv. 271.

All that is at present known with regard to the etiology of this process applies to certain general diseases with which in the course of time it is likely to be associated. These have one element in common, that of chronicity, and are likewise the occasion of a progressive wasting of the body. Of these affections, that which holds the first place is chronic pulmonary consumption, especially that form in which extensive destruction of the lungs and ulcers of the intestine are present. Another disease whose effects are in like manner to be regarded as general is syphilis, and in the later stages of this disease amyloid degeneration is likely to occur, and often to represent by its resulting disturbances the immediate cause of death. Again, chronic suppurative processes, especially those due to disease of the bones and joints, are a frequent antecedent of amyloid degeneration. Finally, the process has been found in connection with leucæmia, chronic intermittent fever, rickets, gout, and certain malignant tumors. This last group, however, is one in whose sequence the degeneration is to be regarded as exceptional.

The clinical importance of this process is due to the resulting disturbances in the function of such important organs as the liver and intestines, the spleen and lymphatic glands, and the kidneys. The nature of these disturbances obviously demands detailed consideration in connection with the description of the diseases of the respective organs. It may be mentioned here that the infiltration of the walls leads to a narrowing of the calibre of blood-vessels, and thus a diminution in the supply of blood to the part or organ. The resulting impairment of nutrition becomes enhanced from the condition of the blood, which is impoverished from the simultaneous infiltration of the blood-making organs. The nutrition of the individual thus suffers as well as that of the immediately diseased organ. Fatty degeneration and atrophy of the parenchymatous cells of organs like the liver and kidneys is the constant result of long-continued and extensive infiltration of these glands.

Mention is intentionally omitted of the so-called amyloid bodies, [p. 87]corpora amylacea, considered in connection with amyloid degeneration in most text-books on pathology and pathological anatomy. They usually present a different reaction with iodine, their origin has but little in common, their distribution is for the most part unlike, and little or no clinical importance is to be attached to their presence.

Calcification, Ossification, Petrifaction.

When salts previously held in solution are precipitated under abnormal circumstances in the tissues of the body, the part is said to be calcified, ossified, or petrified. Although these terms are often used as equivalent, the last is to be regarded as more general than its predecessors, since it includes the deposition of other than the calcareous salts.

In the pathological ossification, as well as its physiological prototype, the carbonates and phosphates of calcium and magnesium are present in a specially formed tissue of the nature of bone-cartilage, whereas calcification occurs independently of such a new-formed tissue. The deposition of the calcareous salts takes place either in the cells or intercellular substance of living or dead tissues, when the terms calcification or ossification are applied, or as accumulations of various size in tissues or canals, which are known as concretions and calculi.

The immediate causes of the physiological deposition in the formation of bone are so obscure that only more or less probable explanatory theories are advanced, to all of which obvious objections arise. The causes of a pathological precipitation may be regarded as equally hidden. It is apparent, however, that old age usually furnishes the necessary factors. This in part may be due to the feeble nutrition associated with impairment of function in advancing years. In part it may be the result of the numerous opportunities offered in a long life for the occurrence of inflammation, the products of which are frequently infiltrated with calcareous salts. The latter are apparently kept in solution by the action of living cells, for, though presented to all in the fluids of the body, they are precipitated most constantly in dead parts or in the vicinity of those cells whose function is presumably lessened from disease or age. The solvent action of living cells is further demonstrated by the effect of the giant-cells in removing calcium salts from living or dead bone.

The causes of calcification are therefore to be regarded as local, depending upon a destruction or weakening of the cells of a part—conditions which are directly attributable to an interference with nutrition. The deposition of calcium salts thus represents a disorder of nutrition, and may be experimentally produced by agencies which occasion a necrosis of tissues.

Although the immediate causes of the precipitation of the calcium salts must be expressed somewhat vaguely, the places and effects of their accumulation are sufficiently well known, as are the resulting appearances. The presence of these salts in sufficient quantity produces a homogeneous, granular, strongly refractive appearance of the cell or intercellular substance, in addition to a greatly increased resistance to pressure. When muriatic acid is added to the affected part, the salts are dissolved, with the escape of abundant bubbles of gas when a carbonate is present, and with a rapid fading of the glistening appearance, without effervescence, [p. 88]when the salt is a phosphate. After the removal, the cell or intercellular substance is readily recognized, with such modifications in its appearance as may be due to the action of the strong acid. The parts in which this deposition or infiltration has taken place are either relatively normal in appearance or variously altered from disease, and the calcium salts are to be regarded as absorbed from the constituents of the food and deposited, or as taken up and transferred from the bones of the body. That both sources are drawn upon is obvious from the abnormal presence of calcareous material in the soft parts, in connection with increased density of the bones, as well as with a diminution in the density of the latter. The term calcification is more correctly applied to the presence of the salts in normal tissues other than bone, or in the products of disease not simulating bone-cartilage in structure. A pathological ossification is to be considered present when an actual new formation of bone has taken place so limited and so situated as not to suggest a tumor of bone, or when the calcium salts are deposited in a new-formed tissue whose structure stimulates that of bone-cartilage.

Tissues which may become calcified are, in the first instance, the connective tissues, and of these fibrous tissue and cartilage are especially liable. Epithelial, muscle—in particular the unstriped variety—and ganglion-cells may also become calcified. The frequency with which blood-vessels, especially arteries, are affected is such that it is regarded as almost normal in advancing years that calcareous material should be deposited within the vascular walls. A distinction is drawn between an ossification and a calcification of the blood-vessels. The former term should be limited to the osteoid plates so often found as circumscribed thickenings of the aortic intima, and which are obviously new-formed patches of fibrous tissue in which the calcium salts are accumulated. A calcified artery, on the contrary, is one usually of a size varying between that of the common iliac and the temporal arteries, whose wall has become rigid and unyielding, suggestive of a pipe-stem, from the presence of calcareous deposits in the muscular middle coat.

From the frequency with which the osseous plates of the aorta are associated with the fatty and fibrous changes in chronic inflammation of the intima, the so-called atheromatous degeneration of the same, it is customary to speak of the calcified artery at the wrist or temple as an atheromatous artery or as evincing an atheromatous degeneration. The common feature in the aortic changes and in the calcified muscular coat is the element of age. They are frequently, though not necessarily, associated. The one is the result of an inflammatory process productive of a new, fibrous, tissue in which the calcium salts are infiltrated; while the other is due to a deposition of the latter in the normal, pre-existing, muscular elements of the vessel.

Calcification and ossification of blood-vessels are frequent when the latter become dilated, as in aneurisms, whether these occur as circumscribed tumors or as a serpentine elongation and widening of the affected vessel.

Cartilage is also a tissue which presents a double relation to calcareous deposition. On the one hand, there may exist an ossification resulting from the extension of a growth of bone from the perichondrium into the cartilage. The structure of this bone presents all the details found in[p. 89]normal bone—lacunæ, lamellæ, and marrow-spaces. On the other hand, a section of the cartilage, especially the costal cartilages, may contain opaque, gray, or grayish-yellow patches, grating under the knife, which are wholly due to the presence of calcium salts in the hyaline intercellular substance of the cartilage. This calcification of the cartilage, which may also involve the capsules of the cells, is frequently associated with an ossification, although this relation is in no way essential.

Calcification of the placenta, of the fibrous framework of the lungs, of the mucous membrane of the stomach, or of the atrophied glomeruli of the kidney, are well-recognized instances of the infiltration of calcareous material in normal or atrophied tissues. On the contrary, ossification of the fibrous inflammatory products of the pleura, pericardium, and peritoneum are instances of a pathological bone-formation, analogous in its nature to that met with in the intima of the aorta. The fibrinous and fibrino-cellular products of the inflammation of serous surfaces are favorable positions for the deposition of calcium salts, as are thrombi arising from the walls of blood-vessels. The latter are rather instances of the calcification of dead parts, analogous to the members of the group which includes the formation of calculi and concretions, the calcification of the dead foetus in abdominal parturition, of cheesy lymphatic glands, and of cheesy material in the lungs and elsewhere. Finally, there remains the calcification of tumors of the most varied nature, the salts being present either in living or dead parts of the tumor.

Instances of the deposition in the tissues of other than calcareous salts are abundantly met with in gout. In this disease cartilage, ligaments, and tendons, bone-marrow, muscle, the endocardium and aorta, the membranes of the brain and spinal cord, the skin and kidneys, may contain deposits of acicular crystals and amorphous granules. Although these deposits are largely composed of sodium urate, calcium urate may be present with other salts, as sodium chloride and calcareous compounds. According to Ebstein,[38] the earthy salts in gout are deposited in necrotic patches of previously diseased tissue. The local conditions are therefore analogous to those concerned in the formation of chalky concretions.

[38] *Die Natur und Behandlung der Gicht*, Wiesbaden, 1882, 45.

Concretions and calculi are collections of earthy salts, the former lying within tissues, the latter being present in canals opening externally. Both represent the results of a deposition in and upon organic material, which is often an inflammatory product, at times surrounding a foreign body acting as the exciting cause of the inflammation.

The earthy matter of which the concretion is composed consists mainly of carbonate and phosphate of calcium, while the chemical properties of the calculi often vary in accordance with the nature of the secretion which flows by them. The salivary, pancreatic, intestinal, lachrymal, and prostatic calculi are chiefly formed of calcareous salts. These salts also are an important, if not the chief, constituent of biliary and urinary calculi. In the former pigment, bile acids, and cholesterin may also be present. Urinary calculi are of still more varied composition, containing not only the calcium salts, as the oxalate, phosphate, and carbonate, but also uric acid and the urates of sodium and ammonium, in addition to the ammoniaco-magnesian phosphate.

The infiltration with calcium salts may prove beneficial as well as [p. 90]injurious— beneficial under those circumstances where further changes might prove harmful, as in the softening of cheesy material or the maceration of a dead foetus in the abdominal cavity. The calcification of certain tumors, as the fibro-myoma of the uterus, is equally sanatory, the further growth of the calcified parts being thus checked. The calcification of an aneurismal sac may prove beneficial in strengthening a weakened blood-vessel.

The injurious effects are seen more particularly in case of the calcareous infiltration of the middle coat of arteries. Such vessels become converted into rigid and unyielding tubes at various parts of their course, and the nutrition of peripheral parts becomes correspondingly lessened. Hence, in great measure, the liability of old people to serious inflammatory processes from trivial irritation of peripheral portions of the body, such inflammations often terminating in gangrene.

The calcification and ossification of the cardiac valves and the calcification of attached thrombi, furnish frequent and constant occasion for disturbances in the functions of the heart, resulting in dilatation and hypertrophy, with the sequence of symptoms of chronic valvular endocarditis.

The great clinical importance of the presence of calcium salts in the circulatory apparatus is such that further reference in this place to its results is unnecessary, as its special relations are more important than its general features.

Calculi act as local causes of inflammation, and their presence is likely to be followed by ulceration, abscess, and stenosis, perhaps obliteration, of the smaller canals in which they may lie.

Pigmentation.

The pathological pigmentation of the body results, presumably, from the metamorphosis of the coloring matter of the blood or from the introduction from without of pigments insoluble in the fluids of the body. The former of these methods has recently been studied by Langhans[39] and Cordua,[40] and the present views of this subject are chiefly due to their observations, as well as to the earlier investigations of Virchow and others.

[39] *Virchow's Archiv,* 1870, xlix. 66.

[40] *Ueber Resorptionsmechanismus von Blutergüssen,* Berlin, 1877.

The hæmoglobin contained in red blood-corpuscles is considered to be composed of a coloring matter, hæmatin, combined with an albuminate, globulin. When blood is removed from the body the hæmoglobin is readily separated from the corpuscles by various agents, and is then dissolved in the plasma, which becomes lac-colored. This solubility of the hæmoglobin is of importance in connection with the absorption of extravasated blood. During the time necessary for this process to take place, observable changes are apparent in the color of the affected part when its seat is superficial, especially cutaneous. These changes in color are largely dependent upon the modifications undergone by the hæmoglobin.

It is well known that a yellowish discoloration of the general surface frequently takes place when extensive internal hemorrhages have occurred, constituting a form of jaundice (hæmatogenous) attributed to the presence of the coloring matter of the blood. As yet there has been no satisfactory chemical analysis of this diffused pigment, which if not hæmatin must be regarded as its derivative, although a coexistent increase of the urobilin in the urine has been observed. The association of the stained skin and urine, [p. 91]in the absence of causes favoring an absorption of bile-pigment, leads to the inference that the abnormal discoloration is due to the absorption into the circulating fluids of the body of a pigment dissolved out of the extravasated red blood-corpuscles. This view is confirmed by the microscopic examination of the latter, which discloses the presence of pale, shadowy, round outlines enclosing faintly granular material, which are regarded as decolorized red corpuscles. In the course of a few days glistening crystals and granules of a yellowish-red color make their appearance in the midst of the unabsorbed blood. The crystals are usually oblique rhombic prisms, varying in size from the larger symmetrical shapes to the more minute, apparently granular, forms. Acicular crystals are also to be met with, more yellow than red in color, and are sometimes present in great abundance, although they may be wholly absent. Virchow has applied the term hæmatoidin to these crystals. Owing to the resemblance in the chemical reactions of solutions of hæmatoidin and of the biliary coloring matter, bilirubin, and to the similar crystalline forms of the latter, it has been maintained that the two are identical. Late investigations indicate that solutions of crystals with the appearances of hæmatoidin are not invariably alike in their reaction. A solution of these in chloroform may become decolorized when acted upon by a dilute alkali, or it may not be thus altered. Bilirubin presents the former relation, while chloroform solutions of the coloring matter of the yelk of egg and of the corpus luteum, called lutein or hæmolutein, are not decolorized by an alkali. Although the crystalline forms of hæmatoidin and bilirubin are not to be distinguished, it is not to be conceded that the two substances are identical. As Maly,[41] the latest writer on this subject, states, the term hæmatoidin is merely indicative of a microscopical picture. Although the identity of the coloring matter of the blood and of the bile is not admitted, the intimate relation of the two is not only suggested by the similarity of crystalline form, but by the relation determined between urobilin, bilirubin, and hæmoglobin. Urobilin is the coloring matter extracted from the urine in fever by Jaffé, and it has since been obtained from bilirubin by Maly,[42] who has given it the name of hydrobilirubin. This hydrobilirubin has also been derived from hæmoglobin. According to Maly, this genetic relation between the coloring matter of the blood and bile, shown in the production of hydrobilirubin, is the only chemical evidence of the connection of the two pigments.

[41] *Hermann's Handbuch der Physiologie*, 1880, vii. 155.

[42] *Op. cit.*, 161.

Hæmatoidin is to be regarded not only as directly derived from solutions of hæmoglobin, but as originating through the medium of indifferent cells. Langhans claims that this pigment is formed within movable cells which accumulate in great numbers in the vicinity of the blood-clot, and, in virtue of their amoeboid properties, take into themselves the extravasated corpuscles, entire or in fragments. The indifferent cell may become enlarged into a giant-cell, and then contain numbers of whole or disintegrated red corpuscles. In time these colored corpuscles and fragments become smaller, more glistening, and darker-colored, and eventually are transformed into granular or crystalline hæmatoidin. These granules may be set free by the fatty degeneration of the cell, or may be transferred within the cell to distant parts.

[p. 92]The diffusion and absorption of a solution of hæmoglobin, and the formation of crystals of hæmatoidin from the same or through the medium of cells, are supplemented by an apparent inspissation and condensation of the hæmoglobin. The resulting dark-brown pigment may remain at the seat of the hemorrhage indefinitely, and may be accompanied with reddish-brown flakes, which, as shown by Kunkel,[43] are composed of hydrated ferric oxide.

[43] *Virchow's Archiv*, 1880, lxxxi. 381.

Another feature in the absorption of extravasated blood is to be found on examination of the nearest chain of lymphatic glands. These may be seen swollen, of a dark-red color, and homogeneous surface. In density and color, as well as shape, they suggest the small supplementary spleens so frequently met with. These glands owe their change in appearance to the presence of large numbers of unaltered red blood-corpuscles which have entered the lymphatics traversing the region of hemorrhage. Within the lymph-glands they undergo a metamorphosis similar to that taking place at the part from which they were transferred. In the course of weeks or months there remains in the place of extravasation simply pigment, either as crystals or granules. Such pigment may remain for years imbedded within the tissues, or it may become absorbed, no trace of the original disturbance remaining. Its removal may take place presumably through a local solution of the pigment or the transfer of the granules or crystals by means of wandering cells to the nearest lymphatic glands or to the more remote parts of the body. An eventual elimination may occur through the secretions, especially the urine or bile, or there may result a deposition and permanent retention of the granules.

The investigations of Langhans are especially interesting, as suggesting efficient means for the production of pigment by cells whose function is intimately connected with pigmentation, as the cells of the rete Malpighii, of the choroid, and of certain tumors. The observations of Gussenbauer,[44] however, lead to the conclusion earlier advanced by Virchow, that pigment may be produced by the diffusion into cells, outside the vessels, of a solution of the pigment of the blood in the plasma of the latter. A precipitation of this dissolved pigment into granules is considered as eventually taking place.

[44] *Ibid.*, 1875, lxiii. 322.

The method of origin of pigment thus described applies only to those discolorations which are unquestionably due to the metamorphosis of the coloring matter of the blood. Examples are furnished not only by the extravasation of blood on a large scale, but also by the escape of red blood-corpuscles in small numbers. Such an escape takes place from the pulmonary vessels in chronic obstruction to the admission of blood into the left side of the heart. The resulting brown induration of the lungs owes its color to the metamorphosed blood-pigment which is present as hæmatoidin in the interstitial tissue of the lungs, as well as contained within amoeboid cells in the alveolar and bronchial cavities.

It is probable that a similar transformation of hæmoglobin takes place in the spleen and elsewhere in melanæmia. In this condition the black granules of pigment, although differing in color and form from hæmatoidin, contain iron, and have received the name melanin. These granules are either free in the blood or are contained within the white[p. 93]blood-corpuscles. Their origin in the spleen is directly suggested by their frequent presence, often in considerable numbers, in the large, so-called splenic, corpuscles of the blood in the hepatic capillaries. Eventually, the pigment is found at more remote points in the circulation, and becomes fixed in the interstitial tissue of the various organs of the body.

The black pigment of the cells of melanotic tumors, also called melanin, is not to be directly traced to the hæmoglobin. Virchow[45] early called attention to the absence of iron in such pigment. Ferrated and non-ferrated varieties of melanin are thus to be recognized, the term being used in the same way as hæmatoidin, indicative of a microscopical appearance. A still further complication in the composition of melanin is suggested by Kunkel,[46] who has isolated a ferrated pigment from melanotic tumors. It shows, however, with the spectroscope, no relation to hæmatin, bilirubin, or hydrobilirubin. That its nature is similar to the normal pigment of the skin and choroid is suggested by the customary origin of the melanotic tumors in such pigmented tissues, and by the resemblance in appearance and reactions.

[45] *Virchow's Archiv*, 1847, i. 378.
[46] Ziegler, *op. cit.*, 100.

That pigment of the most varied sort may be introduced into the body from without, and may remain indefinitely in the organism, is sufficiently well known from the results of tattooing. What is essential in such cases is, that the pigment shall be finely divided and insoluble in the fluids of the body. The most important of such pigmentations are those taking place through inhalation into the lungs. The reception by this channel of particles of soot is so common that it is most exceptional for the lungs of an adult to be free from the bluish-black discoloration due to this agent. Particles of coal-dust presenting the details of vegetable structure are met with in the lungs of individuals exposed to an atmosphere charged with this material. The worker compelled to inhale the dust of iron eventually accumulates a store of this substance, the quantity of which is essentially dependent upon the length of exposure, the degree of impregnation of the atmosphere, and the insufficient nature of the protectives employed.

Although a large part of the pigmentation under such circumstances is due to the direct presence of the foreign body, the appearances are also partly the result of consequent minute hemorrhages. The coal-dust and the iron-filings are often sharp and jagged fragments, which penetrate the delicate tissues, and the escaping red blood-corpuscles are acted upon by the amoeboid cells in the air-passages, with the consequent formation of hæmatin or hæmatoidin, as are the blood-corpuscles in larger hemorrhages. The inhaled pigment finds its way, either directly or by the agency of amoeboid cells, into the lymphatics and fibrous tissue of the lungs, and remains indefinitely either in the bronchial and pulmonary lymphatic glands or in the interstitial tissue of the lungs.

Attention may be here called to that pigmentation of the skin and deeper-seated parts of the body, especially of the kidneys, known by the term argyria. The long continued internal use of nitrate of silver, in former years so extensively employed, especially in diseases of the nervous system, results in the reduction of the silver and its deposition as minute particles in the tissues. Whether the silver is first reduced in the [p. 94]intestine and then absorbed, or whether it is absorbed as an albuminate and subsequently reduced, still remains an open question.

Although the pathological pigmentations form an extended series of alterations, the clinical importance of the condition may be regarded in many instances as trivial. The pigments resulting from extravasation produce no disturbance of function. The presence of bile-pigment does not account for the symptoms of jaundice. The clinical importance of melanæmia has perhaps been overrated. The earlier observations led directly to the inference that mechanical obstruction to the circulation in various organs might take place. The particles of pigment and the cells containing them were so numerous that this inference seemed quite probable. The evidence is still lacking, however, which proves the existence of definite symptoms and characteristic lesions as the result of the melanæmic condition.

The inhaled foreign bodies, as coal and iron, are productive of greater disturbances, and are well known as efficient causes in the production of chronic pulmonary consumption.

The coal-miner's and scissors-grinder's phthises usually have, as an anatomical basis, catarrhal conditions of the aërating surfaces and interstitial inflammations of the pulmonary connective tissue. Mechanical obstruction to the aëration of the blood may also be present from the extreme quantity of the foreign material in the lungs.

Tuberculosis.

Until the investigations and discoveries of the past few years, the presence of tubercles in the various organs and tissues of the body had been regarded as the essential element of tuberculosis. The evidence to be presented in the following pages will show that the immediate cause of tubercles may produce other lesions as well, and that the presence of a specific virus as the efficient cause of whatever may be the lesion, rather than the existence of tubercles, is to be regarded as the characteristic feature of the disease tuberculosis.

The tendency of the present is to regard the latter term as including the various morbid processes connected with the origin, presence, and growth of a specific, organized virus, their dissemination, metamorphoses, and effects. Whether all those processes in connection with which the virus is found are due to the latter, or whether some may not arise and exist independently of the same, are among the questions whose answer is remote rather than at hand.

As the presence of the cause of tuberculosis is the test demanded by some authorities for the existence of the process, so the anatomical classification has depended upon the existence of the tubercle. The substitution of tubercle for organized virus in the general definition of tuberculosis represents the distinction between the anatomical and the etiological classification of this affection.

A tubercle was originally a small rounded body, a little tuberosity, and at the close of the last century the specific tubercle was distinguished from other rounded nodules.

Till the discovery of Villemin, the recognition of the tubercle was[p. 95]essentially based upon its anatomical characteristics. Previous to the studies of Reinhardt and Virchow these related to appearances, which were attributed to a deposition of material, scrofulous or tuberculous, from the blood or lymph. The idea was eventually maintained that this material formed the basis of a growth or new formation, and Virchow showed that the tubercle was composed of a tissue, of cells and intercellular substance, growing within and from pre-existing tissues. He classified the tubercles among the tumors as circumscribed new formations whose structure resembled that of granulation-tissue. The specific tubercle was, at the outset, minute, smaller than a millet-seed, submiliary, although indefinite numbers of these minute tubercles might be grouped together and form closely massed aggregations. From this agglomeration of single tubercles, and their frequent association with inflammatory products, both of which were prone to early death and transformation into a cheese-like mass, the extensive tubercular infiltrations of organs arose. The latter were regarded as a frequent cause of the wasting disease phthisis, which was either pulmonary, intestinal, or renal according as the lungs, intestine and mesenteric glands, or kidneys were the predominant seat of the tubercular growth.

The histological features of the tubercle were further investigated by Wagner,[47] who described the resemblances and differences of the structure of the tubercle and the lymphatic gland. Schüppel[48] soon after published his monograph, essentially confirming the statements of Wagner. According to these observers, the typical tubercle, as found in lymphatic glands, presents essentially the same peculiarities of structure when seen elsewhere in the body. This structure consists of a non-vascularized network of fibres, in the meshes of which cells are imbedded. The fibrous network resembles the reticulum of a lymphatic gland, and nuclei are often found at those points where the fibres are united. This appearance has suggested that the network is formed of branching and anastomosing cells. Within the meshes are three sorts of cells—viz. giant-cells, epithelioid (endothelioid) cells, and small, round, indifferent cells. One or several giant-cells, each with its abundant nuclei, lie near the centre of the tubercle or are diffused throughout the same. These are usually immediately surrounded by the large epithelioid cells, with one or more nuclei, which are often so numerous as to compose the greater part of the tubercle. The indifferent cells, resembling lymph-corpuscles, occur singly or in groups, distributed throughout the tubercle more abundantly at the periphery, between the cells previously described, and with them completely fill the spaces of the fibrous network.

[47] "Das tuberkelähnliche Lymphadenom," *Archiv der Heilkunde*, 1870, xi. 6; xii. 1.
[48] *Untersuchungen über Lymphdrüsen-Tuberkulose*, 1871.

Although the typical tubercle is thus constituted, the structural features depend somewhat upon its age. It is generally admitted that the freshest tubercles, as found in the external coat of the smaller arteries of the pia mater, are composed of little else than a circumscribed accumulation of small, round cells, without a distinct reticulum. The giant-cells, the epithelioid cells, and the well-characterized reticulum appear as the tubercle increases in age. It is thought probable that the giant-cells represent the agglomeration of the small, round cells in pre-existing cavities, lymphatics, blood-vessels, or secretory canals. The epithelioid cells in like [p. 96]manner are considered to result from the enlargement or fusion of the smaller cells, while the reticulum represents either a secretion from, or a transformation of, the cellular elements of which the tubercle is composed.

The subsequent history of the tubercle is dependent upon its metamorphoses. These are known as cheesy degeneration, calcification, and fibrous transformation.

The absence of blood-vessels, already stated, and the abundantly cellular nature of the growth, with the possible action of micro-organisms, result in a tendency to the early death of the cells and a necrosis of the tubercle. This is the cheesy degeneration, and is regarded as a form of coagulative necrosis, which begins at the centre, advances toward the periphery, and results in the transformation of the gray into a yellow tubercle. This termination in cheesy degeneration likewise affects inflammatory products surrounding the tubercle, and even relatively normal tissues in which numerous tubercles may lie. This cheesy material either softens or becomes infiltrated with lime salts, calcified. The softening of the tubercle results in the formation of a material capable of removal as a discharge from the surfaces of the body or by absorption through the lymphatics and blood-vessels. In the former event ulcers arise upon, and cavities communicate with, the surfaces of the body opening externally.

The cheesy material frequently becomes calcified, thus remaining as a comparatively inert mass. The earthy salts may be diffused throughout a uniformly cheesy basis, or they may be deposited in a partially softened, cheesy menstruum, when a mortar-like material results.

The tubercle becomes fibrous with the diminution in the number of its cells and the increase in the thickness of the reticulum, with the transformation of the latter into a homogeneous hyaline substance. The cornified, horn-like tubercle is one whose size is diminished from the shrinkage of its cells into glistening flakes, without an evident associated cheesy or fatty degeneration.

The intimate relation of scrofula to tuberculosis has been variously expressed from time to time in accordance with the amount and accuracy of the existing knowledge. At the outset the enlargement of the lymphatic glands, especially of the neck, characterized the scrofulous affection. As the enlargements of the glands were found to present intrinsic differences connected with differing clinical histories, only those glands were regarded as scrofulous which presented the cheesy appearances. With the recognition of the cheesy condition of tubercles the latter were identified with the scrofulous gland, from the cheesy condition common to both.

This identification of scrofula and tubercle prevailed till Virchow showed that cheesy material might have a different origin, and maintained that there were cheesy lymphatic glands without tubercle, as well as tuberculous lymphatic glands which might become cheesy. A distinction was thus drawn between scrofula and tuberculosis. The former term was applied to that condition of the individual which favored the retention and cheesy degeneration of inflammatory products, not only in the lymphatic glands, but elsewhere in the body. Tuberculosis, on the contrary, was characterized by the production of tubercles which were often accompanied by retained inflammatory products, both of which were prone to undergo cheesy degeneration.

[p. 97]The frequent association of well-defined tubercles with what were regarded as antecedent scrofulous disturbances also suggested an intimacy of relation between scrofula and tuberculosis. Virchow[49] had always maintained the possibility of regarding tuberculosis as a heteroplastic or metastatic scrofula. The occurrence of cases of tuberculosis without evidence of an antecedent scrofula prevented him from making a more absolute statement of the above relation.

[49] *Die Krankhaften Geschwülste*, 1864-65, ii. 629.

The views with regard to the connection between scrofula and tuberculosis have become essentially modified of late years as a result of the investigations concerning the etiology of tuberculosis.

In 1856, Buhl[50] first published his view, although he had for several years been impressed with the idea, that miliary tuberculosis was an infective disease resulting from the absorption of a specific virus. He based his theory upon the almost constant coexistence of one or several cheesy collections and miliary tubercles. The former were recognized as the remains of previous inflammatory processes, and the tubercles were looked upon as the immediate result of the absorption of this cheesy material. The individual thus infected himself. Buhl[51] claimed that the simultaneous occurrence of tubercles and inflammatory products was the co-effect of the same cause, and that the acute miliary tuberculosis, as a localized process, was merely an inflammation with the development of tubercles. He restricted the term tuberculous inflammation, however, to those forms which necessarily and from the beginning, produced tubercles whose presence was limited to the tissue inflamed. The tuberculous inflammation was regarded as a primary condition, while the acute miliary tuberculosis was a secondary process resulting from infection.

[50] *Lungenentzündung, Tuberkulose und Schwindsucht*, 1872, iii.

[51] *Op. cit.*, 123.

The tuberculous inflammation of this author was largely characterized by those features which, with the exception of the constant presence of tubercles, were recognized by others as attributes of a scrofulous inflammation. At the same time, he objected to the latter term as a substitute, since its use would imply that no other cheesy product than that from a tuberculous inflammation would serve as the origin of tubercles. Buhl strictly maintained that the absorption of any cheesy material, whatsoever its source, might give rise to a general growth of tubercle in the body.

The views of this author were popularized mainly through the teachings of Niemeyer[52] concerning pulmonary consumption. The latter adhered to Virchow's views relating to scrofulous inflammation, but maintained that most consumptives were in imminent danger of becoming tuberculous in accordance with the doctrines of Buhl.

[52] *Klinische Vorträge über die Lungenschwindsucht*, 1867.

The theory of an infectious origin of tuberculosis, advanced from time to time by others, but most forcibly presented and maintained by Buhl, was first demonstrated by Villemin[53] in 1865. This observer showed that certain animals, especially rabbits and guinea-pigs, might be successfully inoculated, beneath the skin, with fragments of gray tubercle, cheesy products, sputum, and blood from cases of phthisis. The development of tubercles took place within three weeks after the [p. 98]inoculation, and became general within four weeks. He also demonstrated that rabbits became tuberculous when inoculated with bits of the tumors occurring in the pearly distemper of cattle.

[53] *Etudes sur la Tuberculose*, Paris, 1868, 528.

Villemin's observations have been repeatedly confirmed and extended; although subjected to the severest criticism and control, their results are so constant that the law of the inoculability of tubercle is almost universally regarded as fixed. Its value as a test is evident from the statement of Cohnheim,[54] who regards as tuberculous only that which produces tuberculosis when transferred to suitable animals. The transfer may be made in various ways. Chauveau and others were successful in producing an intestinal tuberculosis by the introduction of tuberculous material into the intestinal canal of animals, especially the Herbivora. Tappeiner[55]succeeded in producing pulmonary tuberculosis, with or without general tuberculosis, in dogs, by compelling them to breathe air in which were contained minute particles of sputa from tuberculous pulmonary cavities.

[54] *Die Tuberkulose vom Standpunkte der Infections-Lehre*, 1880, 13.

[55] *Virchow's Archiv*, 1878, lxxiv. 393.

The production of a tuberculosis of the iris, as well as of remote organs, by the inoculation of tuberculous material into the anterior chamber of the eye, was an ingenious method devised by Cohnheim and Salomonsen.[56] It permitted the direct observation of the several steps in the process of absorption of the inoculated material and development of the tubercles.

[56] Cohnheim's *Vorlesungen über Allgemeine Pathologie*, 2te Auflage, 1882, i. 707.

The objections to the various experiments above alluded to are based upon the assumption that the results of the inoculation are not tubercles, but inflammatory products resembling tubercles. It is further advocated that the inoculation of indifferent material, as bits of glass or hairs, as well as other foreign substances, will produce the so-called artificial tuberculosis, especially in rabbits and guinea-pigs. It is admitted that these animals readily become tuberculous when exposed to simple inflammatory irritants, the local action of which frequently results in the production of cheesy material. This termination is now regarded as due to faults in the method of experimentation, the animals not being thoroughly protected from the influence of the virus of tuberculosis.

The objection on the ground of structure loses its force in connection with the well known differences in the structure of miliary tubercles in the human body, already mentioned. The tubercles resulting from inoculation often resemble in structure the meningeal tubercles of the brain rather than the type presented by tubercles in lymphatic glands. The development of tubercles in the iris may take place without any permanent inflammatory reaction. The association of evidences of inflammation with the development of the tubercle is therefore unnecessary.

The experiments of Villemin have not only demonstrated the infectious nature of tuberculosis, but have also led to a more accurate knowledge of the relation between tuberculosis and its allied affections, scrofula and pearly distemper.

The anatomical characteristics of scrofula have obviously proved insufficient in determining the relation presented by this affection to tuberculosis. The tendency to cheesy degeneration of its inflammatory[p. 99]products was the feature of chief importance. Villemin showed that portions of a scrofulous (cheesy) gland when inoculated were followed by tuberculosis, and that the inoculation of cheesy material from non-tuberculous or non-scrofulous sources was not followed by this result. The assumption of Buhl, that the absorption of cheesy material, as such, was the cause of tuberculosis, was thus disproved. The frequency with which the inoculation of cheesy material, from what were regarded as scrofulous sources, was followed by tuberculosis, led to more exact studies concerning the anatomical peculiarities of scrofulous inflammation. Köster[57] called attention to the regularity of the occurrence of miliary tubercles in the fungous granulations of the inflamed joints of scrofulous and tuberculous individuals. Wagner[58] and Schüppel[59] discovered that scrofulous glands, in most if not in all instances, were tuberculous glands. The regularity of the presence of tubercles in scrofulous abscesses and ulcers of the skin and in scrofulous caries was shown by Friedländer.[60] This observer likewise called attention to the presence of agglomerated tubercles as the chief constituent of the new formation of lupus. These anatomical discoveries resulted in uniting more closely the affections scrofula and tuberculosis from the histological standpoint, and the union has become more firmly cemented from the etiological investigations.

[57] *Virchow's Archiv*, 1869, xlviii. 95.

[58] *Loc. cit.*

[59] *Op. cit.*

[60] *Volksmann's klinische Vorträge*, 1873, lxiv.

Schüller[61] has shown that the introduction of finely divided material from a scrofulous joint—that is, from one containing tubercles—into the lungs of rabbits was followed by a tuberculosis of the tracheal wound, the lungs, and liver. Similar experiments with reference to the introduction of lupus-tissue produced results suggestive of tubercle, if not actually tuberculous.

[61] *Untersuchungen über die Enstehung und Ursachen der Skrophulösen und Tuberkulösen Gelenkleiden*, 1880.

The intimacy of relation between tuberculosis and pearly distemper is a necessary result of Villemin's[62] experiment, in which the rabbit became tuberculous after inoculation with fragments of the pearly tumor. Gerlach,[63] and especially Schüppel,[64] showed that the structure of the nodules of the pearly distemper is the same as that of the tubercles of man, and that the two diseases are identical from the histological point of view.

[62] *Op. cit.*, 537.
[63] *Virchow's Archiv*, 1870, li. 290.
[64] *Ibid.*, 1872, lvi. 38.

From the anatomical identification and the etiological connection, as shown by Villemin, Gerlach, and Aufrecht, the pearly distemper became designated as a bovine tuberculosis.

The experiments of Villemin were further productive in leading to the discovery by Koch of the bacillus tuberculosis. It was early obvious that certain cheesy material and gray tubercles possessed the infectious qualities, and Villemin[65] maintained that the immediate cause of the latter was a germ introduced from without, which propagated and perpetuated itself in man and certain animals. This view acquired prominence through the investigations of Klebs, who in 1877 claimed to have isolated the micrococci which produced tubercles when injected into animals. Three years later Schüller[66] confirmed the statements of Klebs, and asserted that he had been enabled to obtain infective micrococci by cultivation from [p. 100] miliary tubercles, scrofulous glands and joints, and from the tissue of lupus. Aufrecht[67] found micrococci, single and in chains, and short glistening rods, within tubercles resulting from inoculation with material from pearly tumors. The same organisms were found in tubercles produced by the inoculation of tubercles from man, and he regarded these rod-shaped bodies as the specific element productive of miliary tuberculosis.

[65] *Op. cit.*, 620.
[66] *Op. cit.*, 55.
[67] *Pathologische Mittheilungen*, 1881, p. 43.

The isolation of the virus of tubercle was thus regarded as an open question till the announcement by Koch[68] of the constant presence of a hitherto unknown, characteristic, well defined organism in all tuberculous affections, which, when isolated and introduced into animals, produced tuberculosis, the resulting tubercles likewise containing the organism.

[68] *Berliner klinische Wochenschrift*, 1882, p. 15.

The latter, the bacillus tuberculosis, was to be seen in preparations methodically treated and carefully stained with aniline colors, by all of which, excepting the browns, the bacillus was tinged. It was found in miliary tubercles of the lung, cerebral and intestinal tubercle, cheesy bronchitis and pneumonia, phthisical sputa, scrofulous glands, and fungous inflammation of the joints. It was also seen in the nodules of pearly distemper and in the cheesy masses from the lungs of cattle. It was furthermore met with in the cheesy lymphatic glands of swine, in the tubercular nodules of a fowl, and in the tubercles of guinea-pigs, rabbits, and monkeys. The bacilli were likewise found in the tubercles resulting from the inoculation of animals with tubercular virus from its various sources.

The microphytes were described as very slender rods, varying in length from one-fourth the diameter of a red blood-corpuscle to its entire diameter, and spores were occasionally seen within the rods. In shape and size they resembled the bacilli of leprosy, but the latter were narrower and pointed at the ends. They were found in greatest abundance when the tuberculous process was recent and rapidly advancing, and were present within, as well as between, cells. The younger giant-cells contained them in larger numbers than the older forms. They were present at the periphery of cheesy nodules rather than at the centre.

The bacilli were cultivated through successive generations and required a temperature of between 30° C. and 41° C. (86° F.-105.8° F.) for their development, one of 37° C. or 38° C. (98.6° F. or 100.4° F.) being the most favorable. The crop first became apparent on the tenth day after sowing, and the growth extended through a period of three to four weeks, forming a compact scale. The cultivated bacilli, even propagated through several generations, when inoculated, produced the same positive results as follow the inoculation of fragments of tuberculous material, although animals might be used which are not easily infected with tuberculosis.

Koch's publication was immediately followed by a statement from Baumgarten[69] of his discovery of rod-like bacteria in the tubercles of rabbits resulting from the inoculation with pearly masses, and in the pleural and pericardial tubercles of man. They were made evident by treating the sections for microscopic examination with very dilute solutions of soda or potash.

[69] *Centralblatt für die med. Wissenschaften*, 1882, xv. 257.

[p. 101]The discoveries of Koch thus show that the production of tuberculosis is dependent upon the presence of distinctive bacilli, and that these bacilli are present not only in miliary tubercles, but in scrofulous glands and joints, in cheesy inflammation of the lungs, and in the pearly distemper of animals. The identification of tuberculosis with the pearly distemper and certain scrofulous affections is thus established from the etiological as well as the histological point of view.

As the bacilli are to be regarded as the virus of tuberculosis, so their introduction into the human body is necessary for the production of this disease in man. It is obvious, however, that other factors than the virus are necessary, for not every one exposed to the reception of tubercular bacilli becomes tuberculous. It may well be that scrofula is still to be regarded as that condition of the solids and liquids of the body which offers favorable opportunities for the retention and growth of the bacilli, and thus for the production of tuberculosis. Formad[70] claims that he has discovered structural peculiarities of tissue as a cause for the scrofulous habit, which he regards as synonymous with a predisposition to tuberculosis. These peculiarities are manifested by a narrowness of the lymph-spaces and their partial obliteration by cellular elements. He also maintains that these features are not only of congenital origin, but may be acquired through malnutrition and confinement.

[70] *Studies from the Pathological Lab. of the Univ. of Penna.*, reprint, 1882, xi. 3.

The occurrence of a local, circumscribed tuberculosis in extreme old age, without antecedent or other concurrent evidence of scrofulous disturbances, suggests that favorable opportunities for the development of the tubercular bacillus may arise in advancing years. In like manner, the frequent termination in phthisis of cases of diabetes suggests the likelihood of tuberculous inflammation arising in the absence of any evidence of previous scrofulous or tuberculous disease. The scrofulous condition or constitution, as indicated by vulnerable tissues, with a protracted course of inflammations, and a persistence of their products, with a tendency to cheesy degeneration, may still exist without a sign of tuberculosis. Those who claim that scrofula and tuberculosis are identical must, in the light of Koch's discovery, demonstrate the presence of the bacillus in all scrofulous inflammations, and deny the existence of scrofula apart from indisputable manifestations of the activity of the bacilli of tuberculosis. It may be that such evidence will be presented; until it is collected scrofula and tuberculosis are to be regarded as distinct though often coexistent. The scrofulous person is frequently tuberculous, the tuberculous person is usually scrofulous; the non-scrofulous person, however, may die of tuberculosis, while the individual may be scrofulous without containing tubercle.

The actual inheritance of tuberculosis is very unlikely, although this disease is frequently found in successive generations of a single family. The various members of the family are rather to be regarded as furnishing a suitable soil for the growth of the tubercular bacillus, and their exposure to its seed is favored by the existence of tuberculosis in one or more members of the household. The scrofulous condition is still to be regarded as hereditary as well as acquired, and the scrofulous remain as the class to be especially protected from the reception and effects of the bacilli of tuberculosis.

[p. 102]It is obviously a matter of importance to determine in any given case of phthisis whether bacilli are present or absent. A ready means of ascertaining this fact is offered by the examination of the sputum in cases of pulmonary phthisis, the feces in intestinal phthisis, the urine in renal phthisis, and the aspirated pus in cases of supposed tuberculosis of the joints. Koch has found in examining the sputa from numerous cases of phthisis that the bacilli were present in one-half the number, and that they were absent from the sputa of individuals who were not phthisical. Balmer and Fraentzel[71] have found bacilli in the sputum from one hundred and twenty cases of phthisis, and concluded that the progress of a case of pulmonary tuberculosis might be readily determined from the number and degree of development of the typical bacilli present in the sputum. The more numerous and well-developed bacilli, with distinct and constant spores, were found in the graver cases, which advanced more rapidly. The sputum of the protracted cases contained few, small, and thin bacilli with scanty spores. The presence of fever was associated with numerous bacilli, while its absence was noted in those cases where but few were present.

[71] *Berliner klinische Wochenschrift*, 1882, xlv. 679.

The bacilli are readily detected by means of the staining method devised by Koch. Various modifications have been presented from time to time, of which that of Ehrlich[72] has proved the most satisfactory. The essential features are to obtain a dry, thin layer of a selected portion of the suspected sputum, which is then to be deeply stained with fuchsin or methyl-violet; the excess of color is to be removed with nitric acid, and the preparation is then ready for examination with the microscope. A power of four or five hundred diameters is sufficient for the recognition, and the object should be illuminated with a flood of light through a large diaphragm or an achromatic condenser. The bacillus retains the color notwithstanding its exposure to the acid, and the violet colors are more strongly presented if the preparation is tinted yellow after the action of the acid. If the bacilli are stained red with fuchsin, the background should be made blue. It is important that the reagents should be freshly prepared and filtered, that other bacteria may not obscure the picture, and that all the apparatus employed should be thoroughly clean.

[72] *Allg. med. Centr. Zeitung*, 1882, xxxvii. 458.

A fragment of thick, opaque sputum is to be taken in forceps, placed on a cover-glass, and spread into a thin layer by means of a second cover-glass. The prepared slide is then to be passed slowly through an alcoholic flame, or that of a Bunsen burner, till the layer of sputum is dried. A saturated alcoholic solution of methyl-violet or fuchsin is made and filtered, and added, drop by drop, to a filtered, saturated solution of aniline oil shaken in water. The color is to be added with stirring till an opalescent film forms on the surface of the mixture. The slide containing the dried sputum is to be placed in or on this staining fluid, and allowed to remain for half an hour or less, the application of warmth hastening the process, when it is removed, and the specimen is decolorized in a solution of one part of nitric acid and two parts of water. The preparation is then washed in water, and may be examined directly in water, glycerin, or, after dehydration in alcohol, in oil of cloves. The tinted bacilli are made more prominent by a secondary staining, for a minute or two, of the red (fuchsin) preparation [p. 103]in a concentrated solution of methyl-blue, the violet preparation being secondarily stained in a like solution of aniline-brown. If the preparation is to be permanently preserved, it should be dehydrated in strong alcohol after washing with water, and it may then be treated with oil of cloves and mounted in Canada balsam.

After the observer has become thoroughly familiar with the tubercle bacilli by means of the method of Ehrlich, much time may be saved by following that of Baumgarten.[73] The cover-glass bearing the dried sputum is placed in a very dilute solution of caustic potash (two drops of a 33 per cent. solution in a watch-glass of distilled water) till the layer of sputum becomes transparent. The cover is then placed on a slide moistened with a drop of water, tapped slightly, and examined with the microscope. The bacilli are readily seen, and may be differentiated from other varieties of bacteria, if necessary, by again drying the object and examining it in a drop of a dilute watery solution of aniline-violet or of other preparations of aniline used for staining nuclei. The tubercle bacilli remain unstained, while putrefactive bacteria are tinted.

[73] *Centralblatt für die med. Wissenschaften*, 1882, xxv. 433.

The tubercular products of the invasion of the body by the bacillus tuberculosis are regarded as primary or secondary, according as they are present at that part of the body which directly receives the organisms or as they are dependent upon the transfer of the latter to parts remote from the region of their admission and immediate effects. This differing relation is also expressed by the terms local and general tuberculosis. In the former the bacilli excite the growth of tubercle only at a given part of the body. Their apparent effects may be wholly limited to this region, and it not rarely happens that the same is quite distant from the channels through which the bacilli are admitted. A general tuberculosis occurs when the latter are disseminated over the body, and their effects, especially the production of numerous tubercles, are found at various parts. The dissemination may take place at the time of entrance, or, as is more commonly the case, apparently occurs at some subsequent period, the immediate disturbances being localized at a given portion of the body. The necessary conditions being here offered for the propagation of the bacilli, their sudden distribution in great numbers is afterward permitted when favorable opportunities arise for their absorption. Such conditions are present when the local tubercular growths extend into lymphatics or blood-vessels. The frequency with which scrofulous glands are tuberculous—that is, contain miliary tubercles—is already fully recognized, and a tuberculosis of the lymphatic glands is essentially regional. These glands become affected in consequence of disturbances, the local effects of which may have wholly disappeared, in the region from which they receive their lymph. The cervical glands become permanently enlarged, perhaps tuberculous, in connection with persistent or recurrent inflammatory processes in the tonsils and pharynx, the bronchial glands from similar bronchial or pulmonary affections, and the mesenteric glands from like intestinal disturbances. In such instances, the direct reception of the bacilli into the lymph-current is assumed rather than demonstrated from a knowledge of the possibilities of absorption and an appreciation of the conditions in the glands.

That an actual growth of tubercles from the wall of the intestinal[p. 104]lymphatics may take place has long been known, and Ponfick has recently discovered that tubercles may be found growing from the wall of the thoracic duct. The possibility of the direct admission into the lymph-current of the infective element in tuberculosis is thus apparent, and its indirect entrance into the blood-current is equally obvious. That the bacillus of tubercle may be directly received into the blood-current is likewise evident from the observations of Weigert, who found tubercles growing from the walls of the pulmonary blood-vessels, venous as well as arterial. This discovery of a tuberculosis of the blood-vessels was confirmed by Klebs, who had found a tuberculosis of the azygos veins. The occurrence of multiple miliary tubercles of the pulmonary veins, especially near the place of entrance of smaller branches, has been asserted by Mügge,[74] although appearances similar to those described by him may be met with, due simply to the agglomeration of white blood-corpuscles and their necrosis. Such a condition simulates very closely the miliary tubercle, but is usually analogous to the appearances figured by Virchow,[75] and described by him as one of the phenomena of coagulation. In his observation the white bodies were adherent to the red clots, and were with them drawn from the pulmonary artery.

[74] *Virchow's Archiv*, 1879, lxxvi. 243.
[75] *Die Cellular Pathologie*, 4te Auflage, 1871, 184.

With the admission into the body, and the colonization of the tubercular bacilli, their effects may either be progressive until the death of the individual is occasioned, or, with the cessation of the growth of the bacilli or a possible modification of their noxious properties, recovery may ensue. The history of scrofulous glands, as well as that of circumscribed pulmonary inflammation in scrofulous persons, both presumably of a tuberculous nature, show that the effects of an invasion of the parasites may be overcome.

The regions of the body which are usually the seat of a primary tuberculosis are unquestionably the respiratory and intestinal tracts. With regard to the first of these regions, the one most frequently affected, there can be no doubt that in most instances the inhaled air carries the bacilli or their spores, or both. Their constant presence in the sputum of the frequent cases of tuberculous phthisis suggests a ready means for their escape into the atmosphere. The well recognized infective qualities of the sputum, as demonstrated by the various experiments before the bacillus was discovered, demand the thorough disinfection of phthisical sputa, since these are in all probability the chief source of the dissemination of the disease.

The tuberculosis of the intestine in like manner is to be regarded in the main as the result of an absorption from its surface of the specific agent. An obvious direct means of the approach of the bacilli is offered in the sputum, which, when swallowed, is likely to retain its virulent properties. The frequent coexistence of chronic pulmonary and intestinal tuberculosis is thus most readily explained. To what extent the presence of the bacilli in the pearly distemper of cattle and in the tuberculosis of other edible domesticated animals, as fowls and swine, may lead to an infection of the intestinal wall, still remains an unsolved problem. It is not yet determined at what temperatures the bacilli are destroyed, although their growth takes place only between 30° C. (86° F.) and [p. 105]41° C. (105.8° F.). The inoculation of pearly masses produces tuberculosis in certain animals, yet the effect of cooking in destroying the bacilli and their spores is likely to prove of great importance. Aufrecht's[76] attempts at inoculating rabbits with cooked pearly masses proved unsuccessful. Schottelius[77] publishes an interesting series of observations relating to the prolonged use of meat from cattle affected with the pearly distemper, and shows that after a period of years no disease of the nature of tuberculosis occurred among the one hundred and thirty individuals included in the families concerned. Whatever may be the value of this negative testimony, there is, as yet, no evidence on the other side which satisfactorily determines the point in question—viz. that the flesh of animals affected with pearly distemper produces tuberculosis in the human consumer.

[76] *Op. cit.*, 51.
[77] *Virchow's Archiv*, 1883, xci. 129.

The milk from cows thus diseased has likewise been regarded with suspicion, and the frequency of intestinal tuberculosis among children has been attributed to this source. Although the theoretical possibility of the escape of the bacilli into the milk of cows affected with pearly distemper is obvious, their presence in such milk is first to be demonstrated under conditions which necessitate their origin from the animal. If boiling the infective material for three minutes destroys its virulence, as claimed by Aufrecht, a ready means is offered of destroying the tubercle bacilli which may be present, not only in the milk from animals affected with pearly distemper, but in all milk which has been exposed for a certain time to an atmosphere which may contain the bacilli of tuberculosis. In the light of our present knowledge extreme hygienic precautions are only demanded in those cases where such a congenital or acquired basis (constitution) is present as facilitates the development of tuberculosis.

Morbid Growths.

In a system of practical medicine it is obviously important to include under the head of Morbid Growths not only what is spoken of by the surgeon as a tumor, but also those new formations of tissue which, in virtue of their nature, seat, manner of growth, and retrograde changes, produce an important series of disturbances in the physiological processes of the individual. The surgeon deals essentially with the swelling, which, producing irregularities in the outline of the accessible surfaces of the body, is regarded as an excrescence or outgrowth. It is important for him to realize the nature of this swelling, that he may follow a different treatment for the abscess, the wen, the watery accumulation, or the fleshy mass. The last is the tumor in the limited sense; it is the growth which, though called morbid, becomes so only in consequence of its presence being associated with symptoms whose existence and persistence interfere with the well-being of the possessor.

The physician, on the contrary, is more concerned with the tumor as a growth than as a swelling. The latter element in deeply-seated portions of the body may not be brought to his attention. The growth takes place in such a manner as to be productive of certain symptoms more or less serious, among which swelling is least obvious. The morbid [p. 106]growth to him becomes prominent as it displaces or replaces normal tissues by those newly formed, which may or may not be normal to the part in which the growth is situated. His tumor is therefore a morbid growth, a new formation, a neoplasm or pseudoplasm, rather than a swelling, a bunch, or an excrescence.

In a consideration of the general pathology of morbid growths the first question which suggests itself relates to the method of origin of the tumor. The tendency of the present seeks for a local cause, and the most recent theory, that of Cohnheim, demands an accumulation of dormant embryonal cells as such a cause. Cohnheim supports this view by the experiments of Zahn and Leopold, which show that foetal cartilage transplanted into the tissues of a mature animal may grow so rapidly as to present the characteristics of a cartilaginous tumor, while tissues transferred from the animal after birth do not increase in size, but are usually absorbed.

As the active elements of the growth are cells, and all cells admissibly arise from pre-existing cells, it follows that the primitive cells of a tumor are derived from those resulting from the segmentation of the ovum or are introduced from without. Numerous experiments have been made with a view to the inoculation of tumors, the transplantation of living fragments of the latter to the living tissues of a healthy individual, for the sake of producing a tumor, but hitherto almost invariably without success. The alternative remains that the embryonal cells are those whose derivatives are present in, and form the essential element of, the morbid growth. All tumors may thus be said to have an embryonal origin. As the segmentation of the ovum eventually results in the production of normal tissues and groups of tissues whose structure and function are wholly different, so the possibility of the production of abnormal groupings of tissue with corresponding irregular manifestations of function is obvious.

The cells of the part from which a tumor arises may be regarded as indifferent, those whose limitations of growth, like the early embryonal cells, are only determined by the changes they undergo, or their limits of growth may be already defined in kind, and their like be produced in the formation of the tumor. The origin of a tumor thus presupposes the existence of such indifferent cells, or the presence of those whose limit of transformation has already been reached. The leucocytes of the body, whether found as white blood-corpuscles or lymph-corpuscles, or as the wandering cells of connective tissue, are, as Virchow has indicated, such indifferent cells. Always present and apparently transitory, what they are to become can only be determined from their condition and surroundings at the time of observation. Although their actual transformation into the various cells of a more permanent type is merely a matter of inference in the growth of tumors, the evidence presented by Ziegler[78] leads directly to the conclusion that their presence is necessary to the new formation of tissues whose growth is the result of an inflammatory process. These tissues may occur under such restrictions as permit them to be classified as tumors, and the granulomata, or tumors whose tissue resembles that of the granulations upon the surface of a wound, represent a well defined group in structure as well as method of origin.

[78] *Op. cit.*, 150.

[p. 107]The production of the cells of a tumor from indifferent cells is at present an assumption, based upon the frequent presence of the latter within tumors and in their vicinity; and the obvious objection arises that even if the presence of these cells is admitted as indispensable, it by no means follows that they are directly transformed into the more characteristic cells of the tumor. That they may serve for the nourishment of the amoeboid cells of certain tumors is suggested by the existence of both in morbid growths, and the well-known property of amoeboid corpuscles to take in formed material, even cells, from without.

The origin of tumors from cells whose limits of growth are already defined is rendered probable from the absence, entire or in great part, of indifferent cells from certain tumors, and the direct continuity of the latter with a similar normal tissue of the body. Various tumors show such an intimate relation, and there is no sharply defined border-line between the normal tissue and that which represents the tumor. The occasional presence of islets of well characterized tissue at points more or less remote from the normal position of such tissue at the time of their discovery suggests a feasible source for an eventual tumor. Virchow long ago called attention to isolated nodules of cartilage within bones in the vicinity of epiphyseal cartilages, probably detached from the latter, which might serve as the origin of a cartilaginous tumor in this region. This inclusion of tissue is also suggested by the frequency of certain tumors in certain regions where the developmental conditions are favorable. Lücke[79]mentions the frequency of dermoid cysts near the median line of the head, the vicinity of the eye, and the side of the neck. Such regions are those where fissures exist during foetal life, with normal involutions of the outer germinal layer; which involutions may become irregular, and eventually included or shut in, as the fissures become closed. A similar explanation is offered for the frequent occurrence of cartilaginous tumors at the angle of the jaw, it being thought probable that bits of embryonal cartilage, during the formation of the ear, become included in the salivary glands.

[79] *Volkmann's Sammlung klinischer Vorträge*, xcvii. 819.

In like manner, Cohnheim explains the frequent occurrence of certain epithelial tumors at the orifices of the body—the cervix uteri and the vicinity of the tracheal bifurcation—not through the exposure of these parts to injury, but because they are regions in which embryonal irregularities of development are likely to arise.

That congenital, local peculiarities are an important element in the origin of tumors has already been strongly advocated by Virchow. Not only are children born with tumors, but instances of growths eventually arising from birth-marks, and the occurrence of certain tumors in the same locality in successive generations of the same family, are sufficiently familiar.

Although certain tumors are admitted to be due to congenital peculiarities of tissue, and even to represent atypical growths from embryonal tissue, the theory of such an embryonal origin for all tumors seems unnecessary. The resemblance in symptoms as well as in appearance, and even in structure, of certain tumors to inflammatory products, and their frequent association with these, has led to the suggestion of an irritant as an exciting cause for the tumor, even in the absence of local peculiarities of tissue. [p. 108]It is obvious that were the embryonal theory of origin, as extended by Cohnheim, universally applicable, the growth demands something more than a focus of embryonal cells. An immediate cause for their growth after a dormant period, extending even into old age, is required. Cohnheim finds such in a sufficient supply of blood. He attributes the development or rapid growth of the tumor to this feature, and supports his view by the usual appearance of exostoses when the skeleton is at its period of most vigorous growth, and of dermoid cysts at a time when the formation of the beard indicates active developmental conditions in the outer germinal layer.

The growth of ovarian cystomata at and after puberty, and of these and mammary tumors during pregnancy, are also explained on the ground of a more abundant supply of blood at such periods. He and others find in physiological conditions a source for the abundant blood-supply—that is, the efficient nutrition for the growth of a tumor. The necessity of sufficient nutrition in the development of tumors is universally admitted, and its source may be looked for in pathological as well as physiological conditions.

The existence of an irritant of some sort often seems probable, and, although its absence is more frequently determined than its presence, it is obvious that when present it may be overlooked. Although traumatic irritants of considerable mechanical severity exist in but a small percentage of tumors, their occasional influence in the production of morbid growths is not to be denied. Their action may be explained as producing a congestion or as enfeebling the opposition of physiological tissues to pathological growths. The importance of an irritant as the exciting cause, however its action may take place, is supported not only by the sequence of injuries and tumors, but also by the frequent occurrence of tumors in parts exposed to injury and irritation. Such exposure may result from position, structure, or function. The orifices and prominences of the body, the retained testis in the inguinal canal, are notoriously liable seats of tumors. Soft, friable, and slightly resistant structures, like mucous membranes, are not only the frequent place of origin of tumors, but the most exposed parts of such structures are oftenest affected. The exposure resulting from function is manifest by the relation presented by the periods of greatest functional activity of the growth of tumors in such organs as the mammary gland, uterus, and ovaries.

The importance of an irritant is still further suggested by the association of tumors with inflammation. The growth of tubercles and cancer from serous membranes is frequently accompanied by an acute inflammation of the latter; fibrous tumors and chronic interstitial inflammations often coexist, while elephantiasis is usually preceded by recurrent, erysipelatous inflammation of the skin.

The recent discovery of infective organisms as an exciting cause for many of the members of an entire group of tumors, the granulomata, has resulted in making prominent the etiological rather than the structural features of the tumors concerned.

Local peculiarities of tissue, whether congenital or acquired, are thus regarded as representing the beginnings of the growth. With the multiplication of the cells their transformation may take place or a change in their grouping may arise. The essential condition in the production [p. 109]of the morbid growth is that the formation of the cells should take place at an abnormal time or place and should progress in a normal or abnormal manner.

The growth takes place with greater or less rapidity in one or another direction according to the nature of the tumor and its seat. The more closely the tumor resembles the normal structures of the body, the slower is its growth; the more it differs in composition, the more rapid is its progress. This difference may arise from a predominance of cells over intercellular substance, as in the case of the sarcoma, or it may result from an atypical combination of tissues, as seen in the development of epithelium and connective tissue in cancer.

The seat of the tumor is of importance mainly on account of the vascular supply of a part and the more spongy or yielding nature of certain regions. That the more abundant the nutrition of certain regions of the body, the more favorable the opportunities for growth, may be admitted without question. The spongy nature of tissues implies a predominance of cavities over solid constituents. These cavities are lined by surfaces which represent, on the one hand, the walls of lymph-spaces, on the other the free surfaces of the body exposed to the air, as the mucous or cutaneous surfaces and the pulmonary surface. The rapidity of growth in the direction of the least resistance is amply shown in the projection of tumors above the surface of serous membranes and the frequent presence of fungoid excrescences in various parts of the body.

The growth of tumors extends in all directions, but a distinction has long been drawn between the concentric or interstitial manner of growth and the excentric or infiltrating form. This distinction is based upon the presence of a sharply defined limitation of pathological and normal tissues or upon the absence of such a limitation. Such a distinction is merely of relative importance, as certain tumors may grow in both ways. This is best observed in those bulging superficial tumors whose base is irregularly extended into the continuous healthy tissues.

The concentric variety of growth includes those tumors which have commonly been described as encapsulated, and which are capable of ready enucleation from their surroundings in virtue of a thin layer of loose connective tissue lying between the tumor and the contiguous tissue. Such a capsule represents the matrix, the pia mater, in which lie the blood-vessels going to and coming from the tumor, and is often nothing else than the distended and hyperplastic fibrous tissue remaining after the absorption of the muscular fibres or gland-cells from the tissues surrounding the morbid growth.

The excentric, peripheral, or infiltrating extension of the tumor takes place when the surrounding parts are invaded by the active elements of which the tumor is composed. The amoeboid property of the cells of certain tumors is well known, and the possibility is admissible that the indifferent cells of the body, so often accumulated at the periphery of the growth, become impregnated with a formative function by the constituents of the tumor. Such amoeboid and wandering cells represent a means through which the growth of the tumor may become extended in its vicinity as well as in more remote parts of the body.

The extension in the vicinity may be continuous or the reverse, the latter through the formation of secondary nodules, which may [p. 110]eventually become fused with the primary mass. The continuous growth takes place, as has been more particularly shown by Köster, along the lymph-channels surrounding the tumor, which may become filled, distended, and eventually obliterated by projections from the neoplasm. Both methods of peripheral growth, by secondary nodules and continuous extension, represent an infection of the surrounding tissues, especially if it be admitted that the cells through which the increase is accomplished are direct descendants of the pre-existing cells of the part. Not only does the extension take place through the lymphatic vessels about the tumor, but blood-spaces as well as lymph-spaces may be invaded. Thrombi are then found whose structure is frequently that of the tumor, and whose connection with the same is direct through the perforated wall of the vessel. These features in the growth of tumors lead directly to the consideration of the means by which multiple tumors appear in remote parts of the body after a single tumor has appeared in a given locality, and after the removal of such a primitive growth.

The distinction between primary and secondary tumors is now so obvious that one is inclined to forget that the presence of numerous tumors at various parts of the body was at one time regarded as evidence of the constitutional or dyscrasic nature of the morbid growth. Such a multiplicity seemed to indicate that the blood was charged with the constituents of the tumor, which were deposited at various parts of the body.

Although certain multiple tumors may be present in different localities without an apparent relation between an antecedent and a subsequent growth, such tumors are usually limited to certain systems of the body. Multiple bony tumors are found growing from bones, fibrous and warty tumors from the skin, and fibro-myomata from the uterus. Cohnheim's theory of the embryonal origin of tumors may seem applicable in such cases, but the frequent association of the osteomata with chronic inflammatory conditions, of cutaneous warts and fibrous tumors with local irritative processes, makes such a hypothesis unnecessary.

Those tumors whose multiplicity is of the greatest clinical importance are the rapidly growing forms terminating fatally. Such are those which reappear in the scar after the removal of a cancer, or in the adjoining chain of lymphatic glands or at remote parts of the body. The most satisfactory explanation of their presence, and of the generalization, recurrence, or metastasis of tumors, is derived from what has already been stated with reference to the manner of the growth of the latter.

It is well known from experiments on animals that various living, normal tissues when transplanted to remote parts of the same individual or to other individuals may continue to grow. Cohnheim claims, as has been previously stated, that a distinction is to be drawn in this respect between the tissues of the adult and the foetus, where the genesis of tumors is concerned. This observer, in connection with Maas,[80] has found that the transplanted material (periosteum), although growing for a while, disappears at the end of five weeks, and it is asserted that fragments of tumors, when transferred, suffer a similar fate. Wile,[81] on the contrary,[p. 111]who has experimented with reference to the fate of transplanted tissues and portions of tumors, reports that one hundred days after the transfer of periosteum the lung was found to contain several centres of ossification. He regards the latter as proceeding from the fragments of periosteum introduced into the jugular vein, and his results thus widely differ from those of Cohnheim.

[80] *Virchow's Archiv*, 1877, lxx. 161.

[81] *The Pathogenesis of Secondary Tumors*, reprint from *Philadelphia Med. Times*, July, Aug., and Sept., 1882.

Notwithstanding the numerous experiments which have been made in various parts of the world to excite the growth of transplanted bits from tumors, most of them have terminated unsuccessfully. Although a temporary growth of fragments of tumors has taken place after transplantation, their eventual disappearance has usually occurred. Cohnheim lays stress upon this fact in connection with his theory of the origin of tumors. He considers that the fragments of tissue and tumors disappear in consequence of the inability of the foreign particles to withstand the metamorphosis of physiological tissues. If this opposition is neutralized, the existing germs of tumors become capable of development. Wile, however, found that eight weeks after the introduction of a bit of cancer into the lung of an animal the fragment had increased nearly twice in size. He also refers to the positive experiments of Newinsky,[82] who transplanted a bit of cancer from a dog to the subcutaneous tissue of another, young dog, and found, after five months, not only an ulcerating cutaneous cancer at the place of inoculation, but also a metastatic nodule of the size of a hazel-nut in an axillary lymphatic gland.

[82] *Allgem. medicinische Central-Zeitung*, 1876, lxxi. 875.

For the present consideration it may be borne in mind that fragments of normal (foetal) tissues, as shown by the experiments of Zahn and Leopold, when introduced into the organs of animals, may become enlarged. It is also certain that bits of tumors, after their introduction into the tissues and organs of animals, have become increased in size. What their eventual fate might have been does not appear; and herein lies the weak point of the experiments with reference to the production of secondary tumors. For such experiments to be regarded as crucial it is necessary that a large number of previously healthy animals, after inoculation with fragments of morbid growths, should present in various parts of the body well characterized tumors whose structure should be like that of the particles introduced.

The experiments above referred to are of value in confirming the views concerning the generalization of tumors which have been generally admitted since Virchow's discoveries with regard to the phenomena of embolism.

Tumors are said to become generalized when they appear not only in various systems of the body, but in various organs and tissues. They are found usually in considerable numbers, and with such differences in size, shape, and appearance as to indicate different ages. Such tumors are regarded as arising directly or indirectly from a common source. This source is called the primitive or primary tumor, and its derivatives the secondary tumors. The latter are usually considered as the direct descendants of the former, although their relation may be that of several successive generations.

The primitive tumor in its growth may extend into lymphatics and blood-vessels, as has already been suggested. Such an extension may be [p. 112]so little obvious when the tumor is removed by the surgeon that all diseased tissues are apparently separated from the body. A recurrence of the tumor is said to take place when the growth returns in the cicatrix, frequently in a multiple form. The explanation of such a recurrence is based upon the probable presence, at the time of the operation, of fragments of the tumor within the tissues forming the base and edges of the wound. During and after the healing of the wound their growth is supposed to continue till they become apparent as small tumors. The progress of these recurrent tumors is at times extremely rapid, and they may attain a considerable size in the course of a few weeks. Such nodules are secondary in point of time, although they were actually a part of the primary growth.

Secondary nodules in descent as well as time are those which appear at distant parts, often after the discovery of the primary tumor. Such nodules are regarded as resulting from the transfer of particles of various size from the primitive growth, either through the lymph-vessels or blood-vessels. If the invasion of the body takes place through the former, the fragments may be floated along to the nearest lymphatic gland, where it remains when too large to pass through. If it retains the capacity of growth or of stimulating a like growth, there results a more or less complete transformation of the gland into a morbid tissue like that from which the fragments came. Adjoining lymph-glands may become infected from the first, until eventually an entire series becomes more or less completely transformed into morbid growths. A like invasion of the lymphatic glands may take place through a continuous extension along the lymph-vessels; and it is not rare to find the sub-pleural or sub-peritoneal lymphatics as an elevated meshwork in consequence of the neoplastic growth within them. Such a method of extension may take place when a cancer of the stomach or liver is associated with a cancer of the pleura, the intervening lymphatics of the diaphragm offering a direct and continuous communication.

With the outcropping of a tumor upon a serous surface the possibility of the detachment of particles is at hand. These may become transplanted to the opposed serous surface or may be transferred to the most dependent parts, and there serve as seed for subsequent growth.

The probability of the embolic nature of many secondary tumors was early suggested in the history of embolism. Rapidly growing tumors were known to be capable of perforating the walls of adjacent blood-vessels, especially veins, and to continue growing along the course of such vessels. The possibility of the detachment of portions of these tumors and their transfer along the course of the circulation was an inevitable inference from the results of experimentation with foreign bodies. Cancerous emboli were thus recognized as a possible variety, and their distribution was subject to the same laws as those governing emboli otherwise constituted. Multiple nodules were frequently found in the lungs in connection with tumors growing into the inferior vena cava, while multiple nodules in the liver were usually associated with tumors of the gastro-intestinal canal or other regions whose vessels formed a part of the portal circulation. The readiness with which portions may be detached after death from the soft masses projecting into the interior of veins suggests the ease with which particles may be [p. 113]separated during life. The experiments already referred to show that isolated fragments of tissue serving as emboli may grow in the place of their reception, and it is presumable that the resulting growth takes place under the same conditions as those prevailing at the place from which the embolus started. The question whether the secondary tumor arises from the reproduction of elements transferred from the primitive disease, or whether these excite a characteristic, specific growth of the cells in the place of their retention, may still be regarded as open. The experiments favor the former view, and they alone are capable of satisfactorily determining the point in question.

The secondary nodules, whatever may be their method of origin, present the peculiarities of the primitive growth. If the cells of the latter are pigmented, those of the former show the same peculiarity. If the structure of the primitive tumor contains bone, cartilage, or squamous epithelium, the secondary growths show like characters, though they may be present in the heart or other organs where such tissues are not present as normal constituents. So constant and characteristic is this feature that the structure of the tumor is usually as well displayed in the examination of the secondary as of the primitive nodule. Indeed, the structural peculiarities of the growth may be more characteristically shown in the former in those instances where the primitive tumor has undergone degenerative changes obscuring its histological features.

The tissues of the tumor are subject to the various changes which take place in the normal tissues of the body. Their growth is attended with a multiplication of cells and a formation of intercellular substance. Tumors whose growth is the most rapid are those whose blood-vessels are the most numerous and whose relation to the cells is most intimate. The slower the advance of the tumor, the more permanent is it likely to become, while the more rapid the progress, the more transitory are its elements. The growth may continue, and yet the actual size of the tumor may diminish through the absorption of its degenerated parts. The cells of the neoplasm may undergo fatty degeneration, or they may become cornified. They may undergo the mucous metamorphosis or the amyloid and colloid degenerations. They may take up pigment or they may produce the same. The intercellular substance varies in its character as does that of normal tissues. It may be slimy, homogeneous, or fibrillated. It may contain mucin, chondrin, or gelatin, and may be infiltrated with calcareous salts. Limited necroses with characteristic cheesy appearances are of frequent occurrence.

Tumors may become the seat of inflammatory processes, indicated by suppuration and fever, which may result in abscess or gangrene, or their progress may terminate in the production of scars. Ulceration may occur in consequence of the extension of an inflammatory process to the surface, or it may result in the course of the degenerative softening of a tumor. In both cases the cutaneous or mucous surface is involved and destroyed, and the interior of the tumor being exposed putrefactive processes, with fistulæ and sinuses, arise, the latter favoring the retention of the product and the persistence of the inflammatory process.

Tumors are always pathological, but the resulting disturbances vary within wide limits and are often of a complex character. The familiar distinction between benignant and malignant tumors is based chiefly [p. 114]upon this variance in the nature of the disturbances. Those are benignant which closely resemble the normal structures of the body, increase but slowly, and, if they attain a large size, produce mainly mechanical disturbances. They may prove serious, even fatal, if so seated as to interfere with the function of important parts of the body. Very large and heavy tumors may prove burdensome solely on account of their weight, while others of similar character, elsewhere seated, may interfere with respiration or circulation, and eventually with nutrition. Tumors in exposed situations may become important only in virtue of their liability to injury, while others impede the function of a part or an organ by pressure upon its nerves and vessels or by obstructing its ducts.

The malignant tumors, on the contrary, differ in their structure from the normal tissues of the body. Their growth is rapid and infiltrating rather than slow and concentric. Such tumors usually have a predominance of cells and thin walled blood-vessels. The former may be little else than nuclei enveloped in an easily destructible protoplasm, or they may be composed of multi-nucleated masses of protoplasm, and are then known as giant-cells. The most malignant tumors are those which tend to become generalized as well as to spread locally. They recur locally, and appear in the nearest lymph-glands and at remote parts of the body. The disturbances produced by the malignant tumors depend less upon their mechanical relations than upon their tendency to destroy tissues and disturb functions. With their presence and progress in vital organs there is associated, from their manner of growth, a destruction of the cells of such organs, as the kidneys and liver, the lungs and heart. When they are seated in the spleen and lymphatic glands, a disturbance in the blood-making process must be associated. Their occurrence in the alimentary canal opposes the admission, digestion, and expulsion of its contents, and produces disturbances varying as to the seat and peculiarities of the tumor. The progress of the malignant tumor is often associated with ulceration, watery discharges, and hemorrhage. The frequent coexistence of emaciation, weakness, anæmia, and a yellowish discoloration of the skin forms a group of disturbances which, included under the name "cachexia," have long been prominent as significant of malignant tumors. At the present day this cachexia is regarded rather as the result than the cause of the tumor, whereas formerly the reverse was the case.

The modern classification of tumors is based chiefly on their structure, in part upon their method of origin, and in part upon their cause.

With the observation of the similarity of appearances in the flesh of which the external and internal neoplasms are composed, the suggestion readily presented itself to regard the external tumors and the internal growths as similar in character. External forms, physical characteristics, clinical peculiarities, all proved insufficient as a means of identifying the two, and the step was a short one which led to the minute study of the flesh of the tumor and a comparison of its resemblances and differences. This comparison obviously included a knowledge of the structure and peculiarities of normal tissues. As histological studies advanced, so did the pursuit of pathological histology, and the tumors which were once designated as encephaloid, mastoid, pancreatoid, or nephroid, from real [p. 115]or fancied resemblances to certain organs of the body, became analyzed into their microscopic rather than macroscopic characteristics.

It is unnecessary to say that the modern classification of morbid growths owes its foundation and a large part of its superstructure to Virchow, whose classic work, *Die Krankhaften Geschwülste*, showed the direction which future investigators were to pursue and the nature of the discoveries likely to result.

The tumor represents the result of the growth of a tissue or tissues which are like or resemble those which form the normal constituents of the body. Although a new formation is present, it is composed of tissues lying within the possibilities of the individual. A new formation of feathers, as Virchow suggests, is beyond the productive powers of human tissues, though within those of feathered animals. A goose can produce a tumor containing feathers, not one in which hairs are found; in the human species tumors containing hairs may occur, not those, however, in which feathers are present. Although the cells of the tumors of man may deviate in their appearances from the cells of normal tissues, this deviation is never so extreme that their analogue cannot be met with in some part of the body.

As the normal tissues originate from pre-existing tissues, so the pathological tissues of the tumor grow only from the antecedent tissues. The matrix from which the tumor arises is a normal tissue. There is produced from it, as a neoplasm, either a tissue which follows the type of the maternal tissue, a homologous tumor, or one which deviates in type from that of the matrix, a heterologous growth. Although the latter differs in its composition from that of the matrix, it does not vary essentially from a like tissue to be found elsewhere in the body. It occurs where it does not belong either in place, time, or quantity. The homologous tumor appears rather as a hypertrophy of the tissue from which it arises, and the line between this variety of growth and a simple hypertrophy is often purely arbitrary.

Although tumors, in the more limited sense, are solid, fleshy masses, the new formation of tissues may result in the presence of a tumor within which is a cavity with various contents. Such a cavity is not a mere hole, but has a distinct wall of connective tissue lined with epithelium or endothelium. A distinction is thus drawn between cysts and growths—one which is of daily importance in the practice of medicine—and Virchow's oncology includes the consideration of the two varieties of tumors.

Cystic tumors are subdivided according to the nature of their contents and the method of their origin. One group is composed of clotted blood within cavities resulting from the laceration of tissues or in preformed spaces. If the cyst primarily is merely a rent, the wall becomes thickened in time from a growth of the limiting tissues, and the blood-clot, of which the tumor was chiefly composed, may remain or become absorbed. If the latter event occurs, its place of deposit may become obliterated by a fusion of the walls of the cyst, or may persist from the subsequent addition of serum.

The cystic tumor whose contents are extravasated blood is the hæmatoma, familiar instances of which are met with in the hæmatoma of the dura mater, of muscle, of the vulva, and the polypoid hæmatoma of [p. 116]the uterus. The latter is the long retained and constantly enlarging blood-clot, due to the adherence of portions of the placenta after childbirth.

The second group of cystic tumors has for its contents a more watery fluid, and to this the term hygroma is applied. This watery fluid lies, for the most part, within preformed cavities, and its accumulation is connected with a dilatation of these cavities. Instances are met with in the tumors resulting from the accumulation of fluid in the membranes of the brain or spinal cord, and in the ventricles of the former or in the central canal of the latter. These lead to the congenital cystic tumors of the cranium or spine, with watery contents. The ganglion, the house-maid's knee, as also the hydrocele of the tunica vaginalis, are regarded as hygromata. The hydrocele of the neck and elsewhere in the subcutaneous or intermuscular connective tissue is now removed from the hygromata to the tumors which arise from lymph-vessels. A like transfer of other hygromata might be made in accordance with the prevailing views concerning the cavities in which the watery fluid is accumulated.

A third group of cysts contains material which represents essentially a production from the wall, with a difference of composition dependent upon the nature of the wall. Such cysts give rise to tumors through the retention of their contents, and they are called retention-cysts or retention-tumors. In the wall of the cysts is a gland-tissue, which may line the surface or lie beneath. The glandular structures may be cutaneous, mucous, or represent a part of the great glands of the body, as the liver and kidneys. The atheromatous cyst of the skin, the mucous cysts of the gastro-intestinal mucous membrane, and the ovula Nabothi of the uterus are examples of the retention of secretion within glands. The dropsical dilatations of the antrum, the vermiform appendage, the uterus, the biliary and renal canals furnish instances of tumors resulting from the retention of secretion on a large scale. In the subsequent history of these retention-cysts the secretion may be modified chemically and physically; the cells upon the walls may be transformed from columnar forms into flattened and scale-like varieties. In time, the original secretion frequently becomes a watery fluid, resembling the contents of the hygroma previously mentioned.

This grouping of cysts in contradistinction to fleshy tumors omits the consideration of a series of cystic tumors of enormous size, the multilocular tumors of the ovary. This class represents a more complex form of cystic growth—one whose tendency is toward the reproduction of cysts, to which the term cystoma is applied. The cystoma is the result of an active new formation of epithelium and connective tissue, and is classified as a variety of the epithelial group of tumors.

Morbid growths, as distinguished from cysts, are divided by Virchow into the simple and complex forms. The former consist of a single tissue, the histoid tumors; the latter of several tissues suggesting an organ, the organoid tumors; while still others, in which the number and grouping of tissues is so complex as to simulate systems of the body, even monstrosities, have received the term systematoid or teratoid tumors.

Virchow claimed that the growth of most tumors took place from the connective tissues, and that most of the organoid tumors, especially cancer, arose from the formative action of the connective tissue in the part where [p. 117]it first made its appearance. The structure of cancer suggested an organ, as it consisted of collections of cells resembling epithelium, within spaces or alveoli whose walls were formed of connective tissue. The epithelioid cells of the cancer, as well as the connective-tissue corpuscles, were considered to arise from pre-existing cells of connective tissue.

The first, most important, modification of Virchow's views, which has led to a more rational appreciation of the relation of the various tumors, especially of the epithelial group, to each other, arose in consequence of the investigations of Thiersch and others with regard to the origin of certain cancers. This observer[83] claimed that the epithelioid element of cutaneous cancers arose in all instances from pre-existing epithelium, either of the rete mucosum or cutaneous glands. Similar views were suggested, with various degrees of precision, by other authors concerning certain cancerous tumors elsewhere, but were first applied to all cancers with a more exact formulation by Waldeyer,[84] to whom the prevailing views with regard to the histogenesis of morbid growths are due. According to him, the essential (epithelioid) element of all primitive cancers arises from pre-existing epithelium; consequently, no cancer-cell can arise except in organs where epithelium is normally present.

[83] *Der Epithelial Krebs, namentlich der Haut, etc.*, 1865.

[84] *Virchow's Archiv*, 1867, xli. 470; 1872, lv. 67; *Volkmann's Sammlung klinischer Vorträge*, 1871, xxxiii.

This comprehensive statement was rendered possible by the embryological researches of Remak at the outset, and afterward by those of His and Waldeyer. Remak showed that after differentiation of the cells of the ovum into the several germinal layers, those from one layer could not serve to originate the cells belonging to another layer. The development of normal tissues takes place within the limits defined by this differentiation. Epithelium thus is not derived from connective tissue, nerves, or muscles, nor was the reverse known to occur. To His is due the exact appreciation of the superficial cells of serous membranes, which had been previously called epithelium, and had thus been confounded with the epithelial cells of mucous or cutaneous membranes and of secretory glands. He showed that these cells had a wholly different origin from epithelium, and were simply scale-like cells of fibrous tissue, to which he applied the name endothelium. The latter is now used as the term for the thin, squamous cells of fibrous tissue, whether they are found lining the walls of the great serous cavities or the smaller lymph-spaces, the endocardium, or the inner coat of blood-vessels and lymphatics.

The importance of this distinction is obvious when the occurrence of tumors, called cancers, is observed in parts which contain no epithelium. Aside from the vagueness of the term cancer, as applied clinically, tumors are sometimes met with, even in parts where epithelium normally does not exist, whose structure resembles more or less closely that of cancer as usually recognized. Such tumors are to be regarded as of an endothelial rather than epithelial character, and as such their histogenesis falls under the general laws of the development of tissues.

Waldeyer[85] has suggested that the primitive basis for the development of the genito-urinary tract contains cells which are equivalent in their possibilities of ultimate development to the epithelium of the limiting germinal layers—a suggestion which is of importance in permitting the[p. 118]epithelial tumors of the ovary to be brought under the general embryological laws of development.

[85] *Eierstock und Ei*, 1870.

As the growth of embryonal tissues is so defined that descendants are like their ancestors in all respects, so the development of tissues in the adult is regarded as defined with equal precision. Eberth and Wadsworth[86] have shown that the regeneration of corneal epithelium takes place from pre-existing epithelium. E. Neumann and others claim in like manner the development of muscular tissue from antecedent muscular cells.

[86] *Virchow's Archiv*, 1870, li. 361.

The relation of cancer to epithelial tumors is regarded as similar to that borne by sarcoma to tumors composed of connective tissues. The growth of the epithelial elements into the neighboring parts is through paths determined by pre-existing or new-formed connective tissue. The active element of the cancer lies more especially in its epithelioid cells, and its growth takes place in an atypical rather than a typical manner. Of the various epithelial tumors, there are those like the cutaneous horn or corn, the adenoma or cystoma, whose epithelial growth takes place in accordance with normal methods of production. The epithelioid constituent of the cancer, on the contrary, grows often with great luxuriance and with but little tendency to carry out the normal mutual relations of the epithelium and connective tissue of the part from which it proceeds. The epithelioid masses or sprouts are composed of cells whose relation to each other resembles that of normal epithelium in the absence of an intercellular substance, while the shapes of the cells correspond more or less closely with that of the epithelium in the region from which the tumor arises. The epithelioid cells of cutaneous cancers resemble those of the surface, the rete, or the glands of the skin. Cancers of the stomach or uterus contain epithelioid cells whose shape simulates the varieties in the stomach and uterus. Such resemblances are carried out in the degenerations which the cells of cancer undergo. The horn-like, keratoid, transformation of epidermoid cells in cutaneous cancers, the mucous degeneration of the epithelioid cells of cancers of mucous membranes, are sufficiently familiar. Notwithstanding these resemblances, which are also present in secondary tumors at remote parts of the body, the epithelioid growth advances without limit and without reproducing the normal type. Cancer is therefore defined as an atypical, epithelial new formation.

Sarcoma, on the other hand, whose clinical features correspond so closely with those of cancer, simulates, as shown by Virchow, the connective tissues. It is composed of cells and intercellular substance, both of which may be as varied as are those of the connective tissues. The shape of the cells is as diverse and their contents as various, while their possibilities of degeneration are alike. The cells of the sarcoma are not simply cemented together, as are epithelial cells, but they are separated from each other by an intercellular substance, which corresponds in its appearance and chemical properties with that of mucous, fibrous, cartilaginous, or osseous tissue. The structure of the sarcoma differs from that of these tissues in presenting a predominance of cells over intercellular substance, while the reverse is the characteristic of most varieties of connective tissue. In this predominant cell-formation lies its absence of type, [p. 119]whereas the atypical character of the cancerous growth is manifested rather by the irregular grouping of the cellular masses than by an abundance of cells.

As the original cancer is considered as possible only in parts where epithelium is a normal constituent, so the primitive sarcoma is possible only in parts where connective tissue is present. The apparent great frequency of sarcoma in recent times is thus obviously explained. With an agreement as to its histological characteristics, its possible place of origin is any of the connective tissues of the body, and their presence is universal. In the manner of its growth, its recurrence, and generalization it is subject to the same laws which determine similar events in the history of cancer. Its degenerations are often the same, and its symptoms are due to the action of like causes.

The importance of distinguishing between these atypical tumors is real, in that it is only through the association of causes, symptoms, and results with defined and constant characteristics that a practical knowledge of tumors is to arise. The time-honored distinction between malignant or semi-malignant and benignant growths is always to be sought for, and can only be fully possessed when the natural history of the new formations is known. With an exact appreciation of the structure of a tumor it becomes possible to study its special pathology. From a knowledge of the latter are to be derived those features of importance in determining the relation of morbid growths to other deviations from normal and physiological processes. An immediately practical benefit arises from the Thiersch-Waldeyer modification of Virchow's theory of the origin of tumors, in that it permits with greater ease a more accurate clinical diagnosis. Lücke[87] has been prominent in calling attention to the suggestions thus presented.

[87] *Volkmann's Sammlung klinischer Vorträge*, 1876, xcvii.

The diagnostic value of the theory above-mentioned is rather negative than positive. With rare exceptions, a tumor cannot be epithelial in character if its origin is from an organ or a part in which epithelium is absent. The possible exceptions admit theoretical explanations which present considerable degrees of probability, and are also based upon the existing views of the development of tissues.

A tumor whose origin from the connective tissues is determined partakes of the characteristics of its matrix, and is a connective-tissue tumor. Its development from fibrous tissue is more likely to result in a fibroma; from fat tissue, a lipoma, or a myxoma; from cartilage or bone, a chondroma or osteoma.

Tumors developing at certain periods of life in certain parts of the body are more likely to belong to one than another of the histogenetic groups. Tumors of the connective-tissue series are stated by Lücke as more prevalent before the age of thirty-five years, while those of the epithelial group are more likely to occur after this age, and cancer of the lip is of special frequency in old age. The fibro-myoma is of most frequent occurrence in the uterus, and rarely attains a large size till the approach of the climacteric.

The rapidity of growth of tumors is also associated with their genesis. It has previously been stated that the more rapidly growing tumors are those whose cells are most abundant and in the closest and most [p. 120]intimate relation to blood-vessels. The type of such tumors is the sarcoma with its scanty intercellular substance, while the other (histoid) tumors in the same series, as the fibroma, lipoma, chondroma, etc., are of relatively slow growth. Tumors of the epithelial series are of slow growth, from the constantly increasing distance of the new-formed cells from the vascular connective tissue which provides their nourishment. When, however, the growth of the epithelium advances into the connective tissue, pushing out in all directions and coming in contact with new series of vessels, the opportunities for nutrition are favorable. In like manner, when the new formation concerns the connective-tissue stroma, as well as the epithelial sprouts, vascularization proceeds with the development of the tumor, and favorable conditions for rapid growth are presented. Large epithelial tumors may thus arise within organs, but, as the surfaces are reached, the sources of nourishment become farther removed and the degeneration of the epithelium favors its detachment and the formation of ulcers. Hence the tumors whose advance is associated with ulceration belong rather to the epithelial than the connective-tissue group.

The tendency of the cancerous tumors to become generalized through the lymphatics, and that of sarcomatous growths through the blood-vessels, is admitted as an important feature in the differential diagnosis. Although there are numerous exceptions, the rule is available. Its explanation is based upon the assumed inability of the larger epithelial cells of the cancer to pass through the lymph-glands; being detained, they serve as new centres of growth. The smaller cells of the sarcoma, on the contrary, are permitted a passage through the gland. The numerous and thin walled blood-vessels present in the rapidly growing sarcoma permit an extension of the latter into their interior, and thus a ready opportunity is offered for the formation of emboli.

Another important modification in the classification of tumors has resulted from the recent discoveries regarding the nature and effects of infective agencies. Virchow grouped together under the term granulomata certain growths composed of granulation-tissue occurring in syphilis, lupus, leprosy, and glanders. Their relation to inflammatory processes was very intimate, yet they were recognizable as tumors from their possession of many of the characteristics generally admitted as belonging to such morbid growths. Although at times their presence might be regarded as evidence of an inflammatory disturbance, their frequent appearance independently of general symptoms of the latter was apparent. These tumors, furthermore, were so frequently accompanied by inflammatory products as to suggest a like cause for both. Virchow stated that the recognition of the etiology of these tumors was indispensable to their separate consideration, and laid stress upon the presence of a specific virus, contagious and infectious, in the case of syphilis. His views concerning the etiology of leprosy, though more guarded, yet carried the suggestion of the importance of exact investigation concerning the assumed contagious character of this disease. The contagiousness of glanders was not only admitted, but the similarity of its manner of origin and propagation to the invasion of syphilis was also stated. Not only were the resemblances between glanders and syphilis recognized, but lupus, leprosy, tubercle, and scrofula were also admitted as presenting a similar relation.

[p. 121]The importance of recognizing the etiology of these tumors rather than their anatomy as a basis of classification was strongly urged by Klebs,[88]who proposed the term infective tumors for the group of granulomata, including syphilis, lupus, leprosy, and glanders; and for tubercle, scrofula and the pearly distemper of animals, which Virchow had classified as lymphomata. This group has been still further extended by the addition of the lymphomata occurring in typhoid fever, scarlet fever, and diphtheria. Ponfick[89] has recently added the disease actinomycosis to the series, and Cohnheim suggests that certain of the lympho-sarcomata may be similarly classified.

[88] *Prager Vierteljahrschrift*, 1875, cxxvi. 116.
[89] *Die Actinomykose des Menschen*, 1882.

The growths thus included have a common element of structure—the granulation-tissue, with its possible disappearance through absorption or its transformation into an abscess or dense fibrous tissue. Such features are those common to the granulation-tissue resulting from ordinary inflammation. Their essential characteristic, however, lies in the etiology of this granulation-tissue, and for many members of the group the cause has been discovered to be microscopic organisms. The constant presence of these is determined in sufficient numbers, in such distribution, and in such relation, as to explain the nature and occurrence of the tumors.

The evidence recorded is not equally full and exact for all members of this group. Neisser[90] has discovered the bacillus of leprosy, and the discovery by Koch[91] of the bacillus of tuberculosis, scrofula, and pearly distemper has already been referred to. Schütz and Löffler[92] have lately announced their isolation of the micro-organism causing glanders, and Bollinger[93] discovered the fungus whose presence is necessary for the existence of actinomycosis.

[90] *Virchow's Archiv*, 1881, lxxxiv. 514.
[91] See page 99.
[92] *Deutsche medicinische Wochenschrift*, 1882, lii. 707.
[93] *Centralblatt für die med. Wissenschaften*, 1877, xxvii.

In the above affections the organisms are to be regarded as the characteristic active agent in producing the phenomena of the disease in which they occur. The presence of micro-organisms in syphilis, typhoid fever, scarlet fever, and diphtheria is admitted, yet their absolute identification and constant presence as a cause of the various manifestations of the respective diseases still remains to be proved.

The classification of tumors herewith presented is essentially that of Virchow, with such extensions and modifications as have arisen in consequence of the investigations and discoveries during the twenty years which have elapsed since the delivery of his memorable series of lectures. Cysts are mentioned, as well as growths, from the importance of the former in practical medicine. The frequent simultaneous occurrence of cysts and growths in the same tumor should be mentioned, and the cystic feature is usually indicated as a qualification.

CYSTS.

Cavities, either new formed or pre-existing, with various contents. The latter are blood, liquid other than blood, and gland-secretion or retained secretion. The wall varies in structure in accordance with the method of origin of the cavity.

[p. 122]

Hæmatoma.

A collection of extravasated blood, usually within the tissues. Examples, hæmatoma of the pericranium (periosteum), of the external ear, muscle, dura mater, ovary, broad ligament, vulva, anus, uterus (from retained placenta), hæmatocele, dissecting aneurism.

Hygroma.

A collection of transuded or exuded fluid in pre-existing or new-formed spaces. Examples, hydrocele, hydromeningocele, hydromyelocele, hydrencephalocele, ganglion, inflamed bursa.

Retention-Cyst.

An accumulation of retained secretion in follicles or canals from obstruction to its escape. Examples, atheroma and comedo of the skin, mucous cysts of the gastro-intestinal mucous membrane, ovula Nabothi, and cystic polypus of the uterus; retention-cyst of the antrum, vermiform appendage, gall-bladder, and bile-ducts; dropsical dilatation of the ovarian follicles, Fallopian tube, uterus (hydrometra), parovarium (cyst of the broad ligament); hydronephrosis and multilocular cystic kidney, spermatocele, ranula, galactocele.

The growths are classified according to the tissues of which they are chiefly composed and from which they originate, and according to their etiology. There are consequently the connective-tissue group; that of tissues of higher function, as muscle, nerve, and vessels; and the epithelial group, in which the new formation of epithelium is the essential feature. The teratoid group comprises a more complex massing of tissues, representing a combination of those derived from all the germinal layers of the embryo. The infective group includes those tumors whose structure is closely allied to that of the products of inflammation, but whose origin is the direct result of the introduction from without of a microphyte.

CONNECTIVE-TISSUE GROUP.

Each member mainly composed of a more or less typical growth of a connective tissue:

Myxoma,
Lipoma,
Glioma,
Chondroma,
Fibroma   (including   papilloma   and   melanoma),
Osteoma.

To these are added tumors composed of an atypical growth of a connective tissue, chiefly manifested by a predominance of cells:

Endothelioma,
Sarcoma.

The sarcoma includes as many varieties as there are tissues in this group, hence,

Myxosarcoma,
Liposarcoma,
Gliosarcoma,
Chondrosarcoma,
Fibrosarcoma,   melanosarcoma,
Osteosarcoma.

[p. 123]

GROUP OF TISSUES OF HIGHER FUNCTION.

Myoma, of striped (rhabdomyoma) and smooth (leiomyoma) muscular tissue,
Neuroma,   of   nerve   tissue,
Angioma,   of   blood-vessels,
Lymphangioma,   of   lymphatics,
Lymphoma (?), of lymph-gland tissue.

EPITHELIAL GROUP.

Epidermis:
Callus,
Corn,
Keratosis,
Horn,
Onychoma.

Epithelium of mucous membranes or glands:
Struma (?),
Adenoma,
Cystoma.

In the above varieties the growth of epithelium is more or less typical, a simple hyperplasia, either alone or combined with the new formation of fibrous tissue. Only the last three members of the series are tumors in the limited sense.

CANCER.

Cancer remains as an epithelial tumor, representing the atypical growth of cells resembling epidermis or the epithelium of glands and mucous membranes, extending into parts where epithelium is not found as a normal constituent. A new formation of connective tissue is usually associated with that of the epithelial cells.

Numerous varieties of cancer are described, according to the physical and structural peculiarities of the tumor. The scirrhus and encephaloid of the earlier writers are now transformed into fibrous and medullary cancer. This change in name is due to the stress laid upon the predominance of the fibrous stroma as the usual cause for the hard, dense, scirrhous cancer, while an abundance of epithelioid cells in relatively large alveoli is present in the encephaloid, marrow-like, medullary variety.

When the growth takes place from the skin or mucous membranes, the surface frequently presents numerous and usually arborescent papillæ or villi. The papillary cancers of the skin and the villous cancers of mucous membranes are thus distinguished.

Cancerous growths of the skin and transitional membranes, often called epithelioma or cancroid, usually contain epithelioid cells resembling epidermis, and are therefore designated as epidermoid or pavement-celled cancer. The alveolar contents of certain cutaneous cancers are cells resembling those of the deeper layers of the rete mucosum, while those of other cancers of the skin resemble rather the epithelium of sweat-glands. Growths of the former character extend laterally, ulcerate early, and are known as superficial cutaneous cancer. They form one of the varieties of the so-called rodent ulcer. Cutaneous cancers, simulating in their structure a reproduction of the epithelium of sweat-glands, represent a variety of glandular cancer. The latter term is applied to cancerous growths which arise in glandular organs, with suggested resemblances of their cells to the gland-cells of the respective organ. [p. 124]Cylindrical-celled cancer is frequently met with in those parts of which a cylindrical epithelium is a normal constituent.

The degenerations of the epithelioid cells and stroma suggest qualifying terms. The mucous and colloid cancers are those whose alveolar contents or stroma have undergone a mucous or colloid degeneration. The keratoid cancer is one which presents the horn-like transformation of its epidermoid cells. The melanotic cancer contains abundant pigment, melanin, within its cells.

These differences in the structure and appearance of the tumor are frequently associated with certain modifications of growth and clinical properties. The epidermoid cancers are less likely to recur after early removal; the medullary cancers are of rapid growth and prone to ulceration; while the fibrous or scirrhous forms are of extreme slowness of growth. In general, however, the pathological importance of cancerous tumors is essentially the same wherever the seat and whatever the peculiarities of structure.

TERATOID GROUP.

Includes those tumors, usually of congenital origin and apparent at birth, composed of connective tissue, epithelium, nerves, muscle, and vessels. These tissues are often so grouped together as to suggest systems of the body and parts of an individual. Cysts are often present which simulate cavities found in the body, whether of normal or pathological origin.

In this group are the dermoid cysts with their various contents, epidermis, sebum, hair, teeth, and bone. The solid teratomata, with all varieties of connective tissue, as fibrous tissue, fat tissue, cartilage, bone, neuroglia, in addition to nerves, muscle, and vessels. Squamous, cylindrical, and ciliated epithelium may be present and line cavities, at times tubular, whose walls are formed of skin or mucous membrane. Other tumors of this group are commonly included under monstrosities, and comprise the varieties of duplication of parts of the body, of which the extreme instances are such double monstrosities as the Siamese Twins, Ritta and Christina, the Spanish Cavalier, and the like.

INFECTIVE GROUP.

The chief characteristic is the cause, micro-organisms, which, introduced into the body, produce, through their dissemination and development, multiple growths of tissue like those resulting from persistent inflammation. As their structure corresponds with the productive results of inflammation, and their cause is analogous to the infective causes of inflammation, these morbid growths are closely allied to inflammatory disturbances. Their classification among tumors is desirable, as they represent circumscribed growths whose appearance, persistence, and effects closely resemble those characteristics of the morbid growths, in the limited sense, in which the new formation of tissue occupies a wider range:

Granuloma of tuberculosis, scrofula, leprosy, glanders, actinomycosis, syphilis, lupus. *Lymphoma* of diphtheria, scarlet fever, typhoid fever.

[p. 125]

GENERAL ETIOLOGY, MEDICAL DIAGNOSIS, AND PROGNOSIS.
BY HENRY HARTSHORNE, M.D.

ETIOLOGY.

Recognizing pathology as simply morbid physiology—that is, the study of the body and its functions in states of disorder from morbid conditions—how these morbid conditions are produced is the complex question to be answered by Etiology.

Nor is this question (or series of questions) by any means only of speculative or theoretical importance. It is, indeed, eminently practical. What a difference, for example, there must be in the diagnosis, prognosis, and treatment of an attack of inflammation of the eye, in accordance with its causation by ordinary conditional influences (taking cold), by a particle of steel imbedded in the cornea, or by syphilis! How great the difference between the wound made by the teeth of an animal, in one case with, and in another without, the presence of rabies in its system! Take the instance of what we call fever: at a certain stage it is almost the same in half a dozen diseases. By the causation, when known, of this common congeries of symptoms we judge of the essential nature of the malady, and so of its proper treatment.

It is a maxim in philosophy that every event or effect must have at least two causes. In medical etiology we often find many causes conspiring to produce one effect. These may be, and commonly have been, grouped together under two heads; as, 1, predisposing, and 2, exciting, causes. But under each of these may come a number of agencies contributing toward the production or modification of disease. Thus, of predisposing causes we may enumerate inherited constitution, habits of life, previous attacks of disease, atmosphere, and other immediate surroundings. Exciting causes—say, of an attack of apoplexy—may be, in the same case, mental shock, a stooping posture, an over-heated room, etc. One disease is very often the next preceding cause of another. So we speak of the great class of sequelæ of acute or subacute disorders; as, ophthalmia after measles, deafness following scarlet fever, or blindness small-pox, abscesses following typhoid fever, paralysis diphtheria, etc. But this kind of causation is extremely common also in chronic affections. What a train of organic troubles, of kidneys, heart, arteries, brain, and other parts, attend the affection to which we give the name of Bright's disease! How complex the sequence often of valvular disease of the heart, itself in many instances the effect of rheumatic fever, with [p. 126]endocarditis as a local manifestation of that disorder! Hardly any discovery in pathology (or pathogeny, the generation of diseases) of the last half century has been more remarkable and fruitful than that of thrombosis and embolism, with their serious and not rarely fatal consequences, through obstruction of the blood-supply to different organs.

Previous diseases constitute an often overlooked class of factors in predisposing to new attacks, and also in determining their course and results. Of some affections one attack prepares the way for another, as is the case with intermittent fever, convulsions, delirium tremens, and insanity. Just the reverse is true of yellow fever and of all the exanthemata, as scarlet fever, measles, small-pox; likewise of the analogous disorders, mumps and whooping cough. The moot question in this regard concerning syphilis may be left for discussion elsewhere.

Our classification of the causes of disease may be set forth in simple form, thus:

1. Pre-natal causation—viz. hereditary transmission of a proclivity to certain disorders, and also the influence of circumstances acting on either parent at the time of conception or on the mother during gestation.

2. Conditional causation—*i.e.* that belonging to variations of temperature, humidity, etc., affecting individuals.

3. Functional causation—that which is connected with excessive, deficient, or abnormal exercise of any of the functions of the economy.

4. Ingestive causation—*e.g.* bad diet, intemperance, poisoning.

5. Enthetic causation—viz. that of all contagious, endemic, and epidemic diseases. Closely allied to this is epithetic morbid influence—namely, that of the parasites producing certain affections of the skin, as itch, favus, etc.

6. Mechanical causation. The effects of this belong chiefly, though not exclusively, to the domain of surgery.

Pre-natal causation is of immense consequence, and its study takes in the whole scope of the influences of species, race, family, and individual parentage. Darwin's observations and speculations, and those of other evolutionists, have not ignored the field of human life in considering the struggle for existence and the survival of the fittest. If we are obliged to admit that such a struggle and survival do exist for men as well as for animals and for plants, it is nevertheless obvious that either man's reason and will introduce exceptions to the ordinary laws of development and selection in nature, or else a very peculiar standard of fitness must be recognized in the survivals of humanity. Many feeble, inert, deformed, and diseased forms survive and perpetuate offspring through a long series of generations, while strong and admirable ones perish, often even destroying each other.

Leaving this theme, upon which biological science has not yet pronounced its last word, we may inquire, What diseases are reasonably ascribed to hereditary transmission? First, it must be remarked that seldom is a disease actually received directly from a parent. Putting aside a few asserted instances of variola and allied or analogous affections in utero, congenital constitutional syphilis and (more rarely) scrofulosis seem to afford almost the only examples of this. Nearly always it is a predisposition merely that is inherited. This, however, may be very strongly marked. Its seat is evidently in that (as yet) occult law or [p. 127]process of individual organic development to whose manifestation we give the name of the constitution. In some families all the men grow bald before forty; in others, scarcely so at eighty. Some may expect deafness in middle life, others blindness in old age, and others, again, have a probability of death from disease of the heart at about fifty or apoplexy at about sixty years of age. Such considerations enter into every examination for life insurance, and they are no less important in our prognostications of the results of diseases in practice.

Speaking more definitely, gout is undoubtedly often hereditary. That is, a healthy childhood may be followed by liability to gout in adult or middle age, even in the absence of direct provocatives to that disorder, but much more frequently when they are present. Gout affords an example of the general fact that inherited proclivity to special diseases shows itself at nearly the same time of life in each generation—scrofula in childhood, phthisis in adolescence or early maturity, gout from thirty to forty, apoplexy after sixty, etc. But exceptions to such rules are not at all rare. Gout also exemplifies another important fact—viz. the occasional modification of the transmitted morbid tendency or "diathesis." Parents who have regular gout—*i.e.* painful attacks of acute inflammation of the smaller joints, followed by deposits of urates, carbonates, etc.—not unfrequently have children who are subject to neuralgia or dyspepsia or modified rheumatic attacks (not sufficiently recognized in practical treatises), to which the name "gouty rheumatism" is most applicable. Again, in one generation there may be a marked tendency to insanity; in the next, to paralysis; in a third, to tubercular meningitis during infancy.[1] Or some of these successions may occur in a reverse order.

[1] For example, in one family known to me the grandmother had paralysis, the mother died insane, and her three children all died of tubercular meningitis.

Constitutional syphilis is undoubtedly often conveyed by inheritance from either parent. Sometimes the impression of this diathesis is so intense as to devitalize the foetus in utero, causing still-birth. Or the manifestations of the disease occur early in infancy, with symptoms like those of the secondary or tertiary affection in the original subject of it. Not often, indeed, is the exhibition, in some manner, of inherited constitutional syphilis delayed beyond the time of childhood.

Scrofulosis is well known to follow in the same family through successive generations, in a manner apparently demonstrative of hereditary derivation. It is true that here we have a problem not without complication. Certain circumstances, as poverty of living, dampness of locality, want of fresh air in houses, etc., promote scrofula in children. Now, are we sure that it is from its parents that each child, exposed to these morbific surroundings, has obtained its disposition to strumous disorders? or may it not be that every time the diathesis is thus originated de novo? It is to be answered that decisive evidence in favor of inheritance is present in a number of cases where the affection occurs so early in infancy as to be almost or quite congenital in its beginnings; and in other instances where removal of the parents into improved localities, and with better living altogether, has not prevented the manifestation of the same tendency in their offspring for two or three generations. The inquiry does not differ very greatly in its nature from that concerning cases of enthetic diseases—*e.g.* cholera, yellow fever, typhoid fever; as to which the [p. 128]succession of cases may be such as to allow hypothetical explanation, either by transmission from one individual to another or by the subjection of all to a common local infection or epidemic influence. But in both sorts of cases crucial instances may, with care, be found which determine at least the general etiological law for each malady.

Pulmonary phthisis has been always considered to be, in a marked degree, a hereditary disease, until, latterly, the hypothesis of a tubercular virus has threatened to displace old views about it. If, however, we accept the classification of cases of pulmonary consumption approved by several leading pathologists, in which a position is provided for non-tubercular phthisis, we may at least place hereditary vulnerability, or proclivity to consumption, in this category, while awaiting the final decision of science upon the real nature and origin of tubercle. My own conviction continues to be positive, that tubercular phthisis is often transmitted by inheritance, in the same sense as other diseases are generally so—namely, by the bestowal upon offspring of a constitution especially liable to the occurrence of the disorder at the time of life when it is generally most apt to appear. The investigations of Villemin, Cohnheim, Schüller, Koch, Baumgarten, and others have given (1882) much prominence to the idea of the possibility of the transplantation of tubercle from one human or animal body to another. Koch's elaborate experiments especially are asserted to have shown the existence of a bacillus tuberculosis, a true, minute vegetative organism, which can be cultivated outside of the body, in a suitable material, at a temperature like that of living blood, and which, when inoculated, produces tubercular disease. The discussion of this subject will occur on a later page as a part of the general topic of the causation of enthetic diseases.

Rickets occupies a much less prominent place in the experience of American practitioners than in that of some countries abroad, and it is therefore less easy here to obtain materials for the study of its etiology. Among those who have had large opportunities for its observation, opinion is divided very much in the manner above referred to. Thus, Wiltshire and Herring assert it to be certainly hereditary; Jenner denies this altogether, while Aitken adopts the ground that predisposing causes are derived from the parents or the nurse, which are so capable of influencing the health of the child as to lead in course of time to the establishment of the disease.

Goitre is manifestly a family disorder to a large extent in certain regions, most familiarly in Alpine valleys in Switzerland. But this local feature takes us back to the same kind of question: Is it the transmission of a specially modified constitution from parents, or the direct action of morbid local influences on the children themselves, that produces bronchocele and its frequent attendant, cretinism? Undoubtedly, goitre often occurs in children of healthy parents brought from another locality into one where the disease is common; and, per contra, goitrous subjects not infrequently recover from the affection when removed for a length of time from the place where it was developed in them. We are, apparently, at least safe in taking here a position like that of Aitken concerning rickets: viz. that predisposing causes are derived from parentage, whereby, more easily than in those of different descent, certain influences will develop goitre or cretinism, or both together.

[p. 129]As to leprosy, there seems no more room for doubt that it is often—nay, generally—hereditary. The obscurity attending its history, however (more than one cutaneous affection having been from time to time classed under the same name), will justify our referring the reader for the particular discussion of its etiology to another part of this work. (See DISEASES OF THE CUTANEOUS SYSTEM.)

Hæmophilia is clearly hereditary in certain families. Immermann asserts it to be even a race-liability in the Jews. "Bleeders" upon occasion of very small wounds of the skin, gums, etc. have been known in several successive generations, including (Börner; Kehrer) women at the time of parturition, who then are apt to have dangerous hemorrhages./

Cancer presents as unmistakable examples of inheritance as any other disease. Paget asserts this to be traceable in one case out of three; Sibley, in one of nine; and Bryant, one of ten cases. De Morgan and others have shown the same thing to be true of non-malignant morbid growths. But, as Paget has remarked, when other local disease or deformity is inherited, it usually involves in the offspring the same tissue, often the same part of the body, as in the parent, but the transmitted cancerous tendency may show itself anywhere: "Cancer of the breast in the parent is marked as cancer of the lip in the offspring. The cancer of the cheek in the parent becomes cancer of the bone in the child. There is in these cases absolutely no relation at all of place or texture."

Cataract is believed by good authorities to be promoted by hereditary tendency. It is of the nature of a degeneration. Possibly, in a greatly-prolonged decay of all the organs with age, all eyes tend to become cataractous from structural alteration of the crystalline lens. Under observation a quite different rate of degenerative change takes place among the organs of the body in different individuals and families. Thus, the lens becomes opaque in some at an age when the hearing continues good and the muscles retain considerable vigor, while in members of other families the eyes remain in a sound condition at a time when other organs and powers have failed. Congenital cataract appears to be altogether independent of any proclivity transmitted from parents in the nature of an inheritance.

Affections of the nervous system very often show hereditary descent. Neuralgia prevails strongly in certain families. Particularly, that form of cephalalgia called sick headache is apt to appear, in the periodical form, through several generations. Apoplexy and paralysis are prone to occur at nearly the same time of life under the transmission of like constitutions by parentage. Still more often this has been observed of epilepsy and hysteria, and, most of all the neuroses, in insanity. Monomania and melancholia have been in a great number of instances traced to generative succession—sometimes, especially suicidal monomania, through four or five generations. Predisposition to intemperance, methomania, is also a terrible inheritance in some families. Although the production of this malady requires the provocative of indulgence in the use of alcohol for its development, yet the facility with which this result occurs under the same circumstances in different families is too marked to leave room for doubt of its hereditary nature.

Less certainly, but with much probability, we may assign parental endowment as one of the factors in the causation of organic disease of [p. 130]the heart, arteries, liver, and kidneys, as well as of angina pectoris, asthma, croup, dyspepsia, and hemorrhoids.

Is a special proclivity to any of the group of enthetic febrile diseases ever inherited? Dr. George B. Wood believed this to be the case with enteric or typhoid fever. Few others have shared this opinion, but it is not impossible that it has a basis of truth.

Reference has been made already to the difference between periodical malarial fevers (intermittent, etc.) and yellow fever, in that an attack of the latter does, and one of the former does not, protect the individual, usually, from liability to the disease on exposure to its cause. Does this protection extend to offspring of parents who have been "acclimatized" to yellow fever? Facts on this point are not easy to obtain. While, however, there appears to be no proof that a single generation can ever suffice to outgrow (so to speak) liability to this disease, it is well known that creoles in Louisiana and the West Indies are less susceptible to it than recent white residents, and that the negroes are much less so, as a race, than the whites. Furthermore, negroes whose ancestors have long been domesticated in our Southern States appear to re-acquire susceptibility to yellow fever in a degree more nearly like that of white people than is observed in natives of Western Africa imported within one or two generations.

As to autumnal malarial fevers (remittent, intermittent), the black race exhibits a sort of race-acclimatization, giving negroes, both in Africa and in America, a much less degree of liability than is common to all races of European descent.

How far any similar modification may occur in the course of generations in regard to susceptibility to small-pox and allied diseases remains at present a matter of speculation. Some authors insist that there must be at least a kind of natural selection, according to which a great epidemic of variola, destroying the lives of many of those most predisposed to suffer from it, will leave the remaining population less likely to be attacked by it. The endeavor has even been made to explain away in this manner much of the diminution of mortality from small-pox commonly credited to vaccination. But the statistics of the ravages of variola in different countries before and after the introduction of vaccination show that, while we cannot deny that some alternation (of generations respectively more and less susceptible) may occur, no such law can compare in influence with that of vaccination in the protection of individuals subjected to it. Indeed, the argument may be inverted; thus: if in the days before Jenner small-pox itself weeded out the persons most liable to it, or in some way prepared a partial family- or race-protection, such a protection ought to be gradually conferred upon a whole population through universal and persistent vaccination carried on for several generations.

Is it possible for one hereditary constitution or diathesis to become, in transmission, not only modified, but transmuted, into another? Some of the older pathologists imagined this to be the case with syphilis, to whose past influence upon parents and ancestors they traced the origin of scrofula. But no sufficient ground for such a pathogeny can be ascertained. All that appears to be left after scrutiny of the facts is, that syphilis is a depressing and perverting agency, and so may join with [p. 131]other depressing causes in preparing the way for the engendering of scrofulosis.

A few points still remain to be briefly mentioned in connection with the hereditary conveyance of proclivity to disease. One or several members of a family will often pass through life without any manifestation of such transmission, while others, their brothers or sisters, give marked evidence of it. Sometimes a whole generation may be passed over, and yet the predisposition may be abundantly shown in that next following. This is closely similar to atavism, as it is called in zoology and general biology, according to which traits occurring under admixture or variation of animal or vegetable stocks may be absent in the immediate offspring of a couple, but reappear in their next succeeding descendants, or even a still later reversion may take place. Such instances are not rare, and they need to be considered in the proper study of the influence of parentage, intermarriage, etc. upon health and disease.

A practical question of much importance (belonging, however, rather to sanitary than to medical science) is, how far confirmation or modification of hereditary proclivities may occur through the effect of the conditions of marriage upon offspring. Consanguineous marriages have been, time out of mind, held to be very objectionable. The question has been much discussed whether the ground of sanitary objection is properly against such marriages as per se injurious to offspring, or whether the bad effect consists merely in reduplicating and intensifying family constitutional taints. It would not be in place here to go into this controversy. My own conclusion is, that a natural law of sexual polarity or affinity exists, according to which, in all the higher organisms, reproduction is most normal and gives the best results when a considerable genetic difference (within the limits of species) exists between parents. While, however, this is probable, but difficult to demonstrate, it appears to be certain that when a father and mother both possess morbid constitutional predispositions (say, to phthisis, insanity, or gout), their children will be at least twice as likely to suffer from the same as if only one parent were so endowed. Whether or not, then, the marriage of two perfectly healthy first-cousins may be expected (as several statisticians aver to have been shown) to be attended by defects of health in their progeny, the union of such relations when their common progenitors were in marked degree consumptive, or scrofulous, or liable to insanity, epilepsy, etc., has attached to it so unfavorable a prognosis for offspring as to be rightly forbidden. Moreover, so few families possess an absolutely faultless health-record that the chances of increasing existing morbid traits by intermarriages are quite sufficient to justify the commonly held objection against them.

We must allude very briefly to the influence of conditions affecting conception and gestation upon the health of offspring. Intemperance in parents has, in many instances, been known to promote convulsions, infantile or epileptic, and other cerebral or nervous disorders in children, besides a general feebleness of constitution. Even intoxication at the time of procreation has been asserted to mark a similar difference between one child and another of the same parents.

All are familiar with the (no doubt often quite imaginary) accounts of the effect on infants in utero of powerful sensory or mental impressions upon the mother during gestation. Abortion has, unquestionably, been [p. 132]often produced by violent nervous shocks. Without deciding the question whether "monsters" are ever developed in correspondence with particular experiences of the mother, we may hold it to be clear that all depressing and disturbing agencies may interfere with the process of nutrition of the foetus, and thus develop mental anomalies, and that constitutional impairments may thus be greatly promoted.

All inherited predispositions, it is important to remember, are aggravated, and each proclivity changed to actuality, by those influences which in individuals tend to like effects upon health. Such become exciting causes of various diseases. If these be constantly avoided, and all the surroundings and the mode of life of the individual be maintained in a manner most favorable to health, the hereditary tendency may remain inert through a long lifetime. Every physician must have seen this in scores of instances. The application of the principle through special precepts belongs to personal hygiene. But no physician can rightly ignore the study of this subject, or omit the utilization of his acquaintance with it by preventive advice to members of the families under his professional care.

Our last remark in connection with pre-natal causation must be upon the effects of circumstances and modes of living on masses of men, especially in large cities and populous countries. Something has been said already of race-acclimatization by which there may be acquired a lessened susceptibility to certain endemic fevers.[2] Almost a reverse action is exhibited in the gradual lowering of vital energy under what has been called the "great-town system." While those having all the comforts of life and avoiding excesses may manifest but little of this deterioration, it is very observable in that mass of men, women, and children who become the subjects of medical charities. Closeness and uncleanliness of living, with more or less exposure to dampness and extremes either of heat or cold, with intemperance and syphilis, are the main causes of this general constitutional impairment. So important is it that it should never be forgotten, not only in our estimate of the causation of diseases, but in our anticipation of their results, and also in our adaptation of measures of treatment, medical and surgical, to different classes of patients. All that it is allowable here to suggest in this regard may be summed up (although very imperfectly) in the word hospitalism.

[2] It is important (but not before remarked in this article) that cholera does not appear to allow of any such diminution of liability to it among the natives of the country in which it is endemic.

Conditional causation has been, to a certain extent, included under what has been above said, as it is the action, in part at least, of surrounding conditions, that establishes a family- or race-proclivity and inheritance. But we must say something more about the direct action of conditions upon individuals.

Man, although organized with great delicacy of structure, is capable, by the use of his intelligence, of adapting himself to a wider variety of external conditions than any other animal. He is the only truly cosmopolitan being on the earth. From the remote Arctic regions to the hottest tropical climates there are tribes whose ancestors have dwelt for centuries in the same localities. Not that no unfavorable influence attends these extremes. The Esquimaux are stunted, the Southern Hindoo and [p. 133] Central African are enfeebled and degenerate, partly from climate. But with man's numerous protective devices, great cold and great heat only exceptionally affect individual health. Freezing to death follows unusual exposures; the loss of an extremity by sphacelus from congelation is more often met with; heat-stroke also is tolerably frequent; and the influence of heat in producing cholera infantum in some large cities is very important; but much the most common kind of conditional morbid causation is produced either by sudden changes of temperature or by diversity of exposure of different parts of the body. These are the two usual modes of "taking cold." When dampness accompanies a relatively low temperature, such an effect is much more apt to follow than in a cold dry atmosphere.

Actual cold-stroke, the analogue of heat-stroke, may sometimes happen. I once saw such a case in a previously healthy boy twelve years of age, who, after standing for an hour in his night-shirt on a cold winter night, became almost immediately ill, fell into a comatose state, and died in about thirty-six hours.

A simple rationale may be discerned for the phenomena of catching cold. When, for example, a draught of air blows for a time upon the back of a person at rest (especially one who has just before used active exertion), the local refrigerant impression induces constriction of the superficial blood-vessels. Hence follow two effects: one, the repulsion of blood in undue amount toward interior organs; the other, diminution, perhaps arrest, of excretion from the skin of the exposed portion of the body, and consequent retention of some effete material, promoting esotoxæmia.[3] If, then, there be in the body any weak organ—that is, one whose circulation is partially impeded or whose nutritive and functional activity is low—it suffers first and most from the impulsion of blood from the surface. Congestion, irritation, and inflammation may follow, and we have an attack of pneumonia, pleurisy, bronchitis, or some phlegmasia.

[3] That is, blood-poisoning, originating within the body itself; exotoxæmia being that which is enthetic—*i.e.* resulting from a poison derived from without.

Excessive heat with dryness, as under the blasts of the Simoon or the Harmattan of Arabia or Northern Africa (apart from insolation, sunstroke, or heat-stroke), may sometimes parch the body even to a fatal degree. Much more common is the combination of high temperature with humidity. This has a relaxing effect, promoting indolence of temperament and predisposing to disorders of a catarrhal nature, especially of the digestive organs, such as were called fluxes by the older writers.

Cold climates are well known to present the greatest number of cases of acute and chronic affections of organs of the respiratory system; warm and hot climates, those of the stomach, liver, spleen, and bowels. But we must recollect what various complications belong to climate. Two important factors, especially, must be kept in view in comparing the causation of diseases in colder and warmer countries—namely, the difference in the articles of food partaken of in each, and the external sources of enthetic disorders; *e.g.* endemic and epidemic fevers, etc.

With humidity must be considered variations in atmospheric pressure. Physicists have long known that while watery vapor, by itself, is heavier than air which is perfectly dry, moist air is lighter than air containing [p. 134]little or no moisture. Hence the barometer falls as the quantity of atmospheric moisture approaches saturation. Other causes, however, also affect barometric pressure. With the same degree of humidity, cold air is denser and heavier than warm air, and by its contraction lowering the "column" of atmosphere—the temperature of which is reduced—a flow toward the upper part of the column increases the actual mass of air pressing upon a particular place. Elevation of a locality above the general level of the earth reduces atmospheric pressure, sensibly as well as measurably. So "the difficult air of the iced mountain-top" has become proverbial.

These variations are familiar, though all their effects upon human health have been by no means, as yet, fully studied. Most difficult to determine and analyze are the influences of changes of pressure, chiefly hygrometric, upon the course of diseases and upon the result of severe surgical operations. Among the few important series of observations bearing on this topic have been those of Dr. S. Weir Mitchell on neuralgia,[4] and Dr. Addinell Hewson on the prognosis of major operations,[5] in connection with the state of the weather. The former ascertained a marked relation between the approach of a wave of low barometric pressure and attacks of irregularly periodic neuralgia; the latter proved, by the statistics of the Pennsylvania Hospital for a number of years, that the most favorable time for amputations or other capital operations is when the barometer is high, or at least on the ascent.

[4] *American Journal of Medical Sciences*, April, 1877, p. 305.
[5] *Pennsylvania Hospital Reports*, 1868.

Electrical atmospheric states and vicissitudes have, quite probably, a practical consequence beyond what is usually ascribed to them in connection with health and disease. But their effects are so difficult to disentangle from those of other meteorological causes that we must be content at present without attempting their exact specification. The same observation may be made with reference to ozone.

Elevation of site has importance, not only in regard to climatic hygiene, but also to its therapeutic use, particularly in the treatment of phthisis, goitre, and some affections of the nervous system. But in our brief and general survey of Etiology this topic must be left without discussion, since no disorder appears to be traceable to elevation alone, beyond the temporary prostration on exertion, with hemorrhages from the nose, lungs, etc., often produced in those who climb to great mountain-heights or ascend rapidly in balloons. It has been shown by ample experience that considerable populations may live in ordinary health through long periods at altitudes more than 10,000 feet above the level of the ocean.

Depression below the surface of the earth has never become a part of human experience beyond the limit of a few hundred feet. Miners living underground in a few places in Europe have been found to exhibit comparatively feeble health, but the privation of sunlight, the confined atmosphere, and the dampness of such unnatural abodes will suffice to account for these effects.

Under functional causation of disease we may include all excessive, deficient, or abnormal exercise of any of the organs of the body. To simple excess may be ascribed the scrivener's or bank-officer's paralysis of the muscles of the hand used in continuous writing; brain [p. 135]exhaustion from mental labor or anxiety, unrelieved by sufficient sleep; and sexual impotence, temporary or lasting (or sometimes even general paralysis), from inordinate sexual or sensual indulgence.

Deficiency of functional exercise is observed to produce disability, as when the muscles of a limb, for instance, are for a long time restrained from use. Surgeons meet with this inconvenience (unless assiduously guarded against) when a fractured limb is kept long at rest in a fixed position. Atrophy of the mammæ in single women of retired lives is common; atrophy of the testicles in unmarried men much less so. These changes, however, are physiological, not pathological; upon alteration of conditions—*e.g.* marriage—the atrophy will disappear altogether.

Abnormal functional action as a cause of morbid results is seen when the eyes are injured by reading, writing, or doing any delicate work in a bad light; for instance, late twilight. Also, in a secondary or accessory manner, when a near-sighted person, having the action of the muscles of convergence in excess of his accommodation, or a long-sighted (hyperopic) person, whose accommodation is in excess of convergence, suffers from asthenopia, perhaps with headache, distress, nausea, etc. Another example of abnormal functional exercise and its effects is that of self-abuse, where the unnatural mechanical imitation of the physiological act of sexual coition induces disturbances of the nervous and circulatory systems, besides debility from excess.

Ingestive causation is a sufficiently fit designation for all errors of diet, as well as misuse of medicines, and poisoning. Starvation or inanition belongs to the same category by negation. Gluttony and intemperance are major members in the ingestive series, while haste in taking food, without mastication, and the use of heavy bread, unripe fruit, and other indigestible articles, account for many cases of dyspepsia and some of colic, cholera morbus, diarrhoea, etc. With young children, especially, no more frequently acting cause of disorder exists than dietetic mismanagement, most of all during the period of dentition, and earlier, when, from absence or insufficiency of mother's milk, they have to be artificially fed. Then the supply of good fresh cow's, goat's, or ass's milk may carry them well through infancy, while a regimen of arrowroot or gum-arabic and water, or stale, half sour milk, may either starve or sicken them to death. On the subject of poisons and of misuse of medicines we have no occasion here to make special remark. Only it may be mentioned that the possibility of either is always to be remembered by the physician in making up his mind in regard to the origin of symptoms observed.

Enthetic causation is a large subject, including all origination of disease by the introduction of morbid materials from without the body.[6] Medical opinion has generally accepted, and facts fully sustain, the recognition of three groups of enthetic disorders, viz.: those which are personally contagious; such as are locally epidemic; and epidemic diseases. Of the first group it will suffice to mention, as an example, syphilis; of the second, intermittent fever; of the third, influenza.

[6] Simon has proposed the term exopathic to indicate the origin of such maladies; autopathic disorders being those which originate within the body itself.

Were all maladies whose causation is evidently of external origin capable of the same clear discrimination as these, we should have no difficulty with the present topic. But, in fact, no subject connected with [p. 136]the history of disease has become surrounded by more intricate controversy. Many times the same facts are, or appear to be, explicable in two or three different ways. What some hold to be proofs of contagion from person to person, others are ready to account for by the subjection of a number of persons or of a whole community to either a common local or a widespread migrating (epidemic) influence. It is sometimes impossible, in the nature of things, to obtain an absolute demonstration of the truth of one or another of these theories without such experiments upon human beings as are impracticable.

While endeavoring to ascertain the limits of our present knowledge upon these questions, let us first notice what are the most positive facts concerning them, some of which are common to the whole group or class of what have been, since Liebig, often called zymotic,[7] but latterly more often enthetic, diseases.

[7] The term zymotic has, with many authors, fallen into disrepute, chiefly because Liebig's hypothesis concerning the chemico-physical action of ferments, as well as of contagia, has lost ground in comparison with the vital or disease-germ theory. Yet the analogy between fermentation, putrefaction, and the action of a virus on an animal organism persists; whatever may be the theory of their explanation, something appears to be common or similar in all these processes.

These diseases may be enumerated as follows:

1. *Only produced by contact or inoculation.*

Primary Syphilis,
Gonorrhoea,
Vaccinia,
Hydrophobia.

2. *Contagious also by atmospheric transmission through short distances.*

Variola,
Varioloid,
Varicella,

Measles,
Diphtheria,
Scarlatina,
Rötheln,
Mumps,
Whooping Cough,
Typhus,
Relapsing Fever.

3. *Endemic, occasionally epidemic.*

Malarial Fevers (Intermittent, Remittent, and Pernicious Fever), Dengue, Yellow Fever.

4. *Other zymotic or enthetic diseases.*

Influenza,
Cerebro-spinal Fever,
Erysipelas,
Puerperal Fever,
Tropical Dysentery,
Typhoid Fever,
Cholera,
Plague.

As all observers are agreed in regard to the personal transmission of the first named of these series (variola, etc.), we need to give attention here only to the other groups; except merely to say that the easily demonstrable existence of a morbid material (virus) in the instances of primary syphilis, gonorrhoea, variola, and vaccinia presents a very cogent analogical argument for the presumption that all clearly contagious (even [p. 137]though non-eruptive) maladies, such as mumps and whooping cough, must also have a morbid material as their essential cause; and also in favor of the supposition that a morbid material may probably be the "causa sine quâ non" of each of the other maladies which are known to be endemic or epidemic. A few theorists only have argued in favor of any other view than this. Sir James Murray and Dr. Craig of Scotland, and Dr. S. Littell of Philadelphia, have sustained an electrical hypothesis, and Oldham and others have advocated one connected with changes of bodily temperature, or ozone, etc., for the origination of certain endemic and epidemic diseases. But all the facts point toward the existence of material causes, specific for each of these disorders, and many observations and much ingenuity of reasoning have been brought to bear upon the question as to their intimate nature.

Are these materiæ morborum merely inorganic elements or compounds entering human bodies and acting there as chemical poisons? Against such a supposition we have, as almost decisive objections, not only the absence, under the most searching analysis, of any chemical peculiarity in the air of malarious or otherwise infected regions, but also the clinging of many endemic and epidemic causes (as known by their effects) to particular localities, notwithstanding the recognized law of the diffusion of gases which must antagonize such concentration. Therefore, we may rule out, as highly improbable at least, the hypothesis of the inorganic gaseous nature of malaria, as well as of the essential causes of yellow fever, cholera, plague, and the other analogous diseases.

By the once general use of the term zymotic, there is suggested a line of thought which has been quite prevalent since the prominence of Liebig's teachings in chemical physiology, until recently. That great chemist did not imagine that a true zymosis or fermentation occurs under the action of a virus upon the human economy. His thought was more clearly expressed, in the phraseology of the late Dr. Snow of London, as the theory of continuous molecular change. Its most striking physical instance or analogue is the extension of flame from a burning body to combustible matter within its reach. Sugar formation from starch by diastase, and the change of albumen into peptone by pepsin, are familiar examples, in organic materials, of the propagation of molecular movement in special directions and with characteristic results.[8] It does not seem to be more than a short step from these to the processes which we study in fermentation, putrefaction, septicæmia, and the multiplication of small-pox contagion, from the smallest inoculation, in the human body.[9]

[8] In anticipation of the argument concerning the necessity of the action of minute living organisms to produce fermentation, putrefaction, and specific diseases, emphasis may be here laid upon the fact that the above named changes, and many others like them, are produced, in the absence of such organisms, by chemical agents formed in the body, or even (as when sulphuric acid changes starch to sugar) by inorganic substances. Pasteur considers that the yeast-cell secretes a sort of diastase which changes starch or cane-sugar into glucose, on which the cell then lives, decomposing the glucose into alcohol, carbonic acid, etc. Koch and others now assert that a bacillus produces the souring of milk, and another the butyric acid fermentation.

[9] The assertion of some advocates of the "germ theory of disease," that only living organisms reproduce their kind, loses weight as an argument in view of the natural history of small-pox and analogous diseases; unless it be proved that every particle of contagious matter is (at one time at least) a living organism.

But here comes in a new hypothetical factor, introduced by the aid of [p. 138]the microscope, although anticipated conjecturally before actual discoveries in this field were made certain. So prominent is this subject in the discussions of the present time, under the expression "the germ theory of disease," that we are justified in giving attention to it here somewhat at length.

Stahl proposed a purely chemical theory of fermentation early in the seventeenth century. Not much later Hauptmann suggested the probable causation of epidemic diseases by minute living organisms. Linnæus[10]revived this hypothesis in the eighteenth century. These two topics of inquiry, with the intermediate one of putrefaction, then received much attention, at first apart, but afterward with recognition of their analogies. When Fabroni, Cagniard de la Tour, Schwann, and Kützing had, with the aid of the microscope, made familiar the life-history of the yeast-fungus[11](Saccharomyces cerevisiæ), more close consideration still was given to these remarkable changes in organic materials and forms, dead and living.

[10] Linnæus accepted the asserted observation by Rolander of acari in the stools in dysentery. The great naturalist deviated somewhat here from his usual carefulness and accuracy, as that observation was not afterward verified.

[11] Lëuwenhoek, however, had observed and described it in 1680.

Starting from the physical basis of inorganic chemistry, Liebig followed the series up from the so-called catalytic[12] action by which the presence of a substance, itself apparently unchanged, induces reaction between two or more other bodies, to those which occur within plants and animals, as examples of vital chemistry. Such is the influence of diastase or invertin, which in the seeds of plants brings on the conversion of starch into sugar and of cane-sugar into glucose and levulose. Such is the agency of ptyalin in the saliva, of pepsin in the gastric juice, and of pancreatin or trypsin in the secretion of the pancreas, in the processes of digestion. From these it appears to be an easy transition to those changes which occur in organic matter no longer living, as in the fermentation of vegetable juices and the putrefaction of animal tissues.[13] Liebig endeavored to explain these also in the same manner as the chemico-vital processes; and he then went farther to apply the same generalization to the propagation of disease, by what is called virus, in the instances of contagious, endemic, and epidemic maladies.

[12] The idea expressed by this term was especially favored by Berzelius and Mitscherlich.

[13] It is noticeable, however, although generally forgotten, that the one set of changes and assimilations (namely, those of digestion) are formative actions of life, and the others destructive, in the direction of, or subsequent to, death.

But, meanwhile, observation and speculation gave almost equal prominence to the importance of minute living organisms in the apparent instigation of all these evidently analogous changes of fermentation, putrefaction, suppuration, septicæmia (Piorry, 1835), infection, and contagion.

Upon this side the leading investigator for many years has been Pasteur. As long ago, however, as 1813 Astier, and in 1840 Henle of Berlin, and near the same time Sir Henry Holland of London and Dr. J. K. Mitchell of Philadelphia, gave expression to opinions of a similar kind, based upon many important facts before very much overlooked. By exact experimentation, moreover, Schwann, Helmholtz, Schroeder, and Dusch ascertained that the agent or agents causative of fermentation and putrefaction can be detained by heated tubes, by animal membranes, [p. 139]and by cotton wool, anticipating the later observations of Pasteur,[14] Tyndall, Chauveau, and others to the same or similar effect. These results of experiments are commonly understood to prove the particulate character of the agents so studied. What may be called an era in the practical application of etiological inquiry dates from the introduction by Lister (about 1860) of the principles of antiseptic surgery, based upon the theory that disease-germs, derived from the atmosphere or other external sources, are the essential causes of suppuration, septicæmia, pyæmia, gangrene, etc. following injuries or operations.

[14] Pasteur's experiments with long-drawn bent tubes had especial significance.

So far from this inquiry being yet terminated, while experiments and observations have become more and more numerous and elaborate, opinions continue to differ; and we must yet await the time when, by successively excluding, one after another, all the sources of error, a truly scientific conclusion may be obtained.

Roughly speaking, it may be said that parties in the debate are chiefly ranged upon two sides—those who favor the probability that only chemical, not vital, action is to be traced in fermentation, putrefaction, suppuration, infection, and contagion; and those who regard minute organisms, discovered or undiscovered, as causative of, and indispensable to, all these processes.

Without intention of injustice to other able investigators, the principal names so far associated with the former of these views may be thus mentioned: Panum (1856), Robin, Bergmann, Liebig, Colin, Lebert, Vulpian, Onimus, B. W. Richardson,[15] Beale,[16] Senator, Rosenberger, Hiller, Nægeli, Schottelius, Harley, Jacobi, Curtis, and Sattherthwaite. Of those maintaining, in some form and with more or less positiveness, the disease-germ theory, the most conspicuous, especially as observers, have been Tuchs (1848), Royer (1850), Davaine, Branell, Pollender, Pasteur, Tyndall, Lister, Mayrhofer, Ortel, Letzerich, Nassiloff, Hueter, Toussaint, Hansen, Salisbury, Klob, Hallier, Basch, Virchow, Neisser, Eberth, Tommasi Crudeli, Klebs, Talamon, Schüller, Tappeiner, Cohnheim, Koch, Baumgarten, Buchner, Aufrecht, Birch-Hirschfeld, Greenfield, and Ogston. Besides these the elaborate studies of microphytes by Cohn, and those of Coze and Feltz, Waldeyer, Recklinghausen, and others upon septic poisoning, have been of acknowledged importance; and the experimental labors of Burdon Sanderson in England, and Sternberg,[17] H. C. Wood, and Formad in the United States (under the auspices of the National Board of Health), possess great value. But the scientific caution of these last inquirers, like that of Magnin, has prevented them from formulating, as yet, positive and final opinions upon the subject. It is not saying too much to assert nearly the same of [p. 140]several of those mentioned above, as inclining to one or the other side of the controversy.[18]

[15] Dr. Richardson has long contended for the doctrine first proposed by Panum, that a peculiar chemical agent, (called by Bergmann *sepsin*) is the cause of blood-poisoning from virulent absorption or inoculation. Latterly, attention has been called by Selmi and other observers to the existence of complex compounds called *ptomaïnes* in decomposing animal substances—*e.g.* the human body after death—these having considerable resemblance in their toxic action to the poisonous vegetable alkaloids.

[16] Opposed at least to the ordinary form of the germ theory of disease.

[17] Sternberg's observations and experiments (following those of Pasteur) with the inoculation of animals with saliva, proving that even when taken from perfectly healthy men this may be fatally poisonous to animals, possess remarkable interest. They do not seem, however, to be decisive either way in regard to the germ theory of infection.

[18] Billroth and Cohnheim are among those who have changed their opinions on this subject after prolonged investigation.

It would appear, then, that the data for a final conclusion have not yet been made certain. Several hypotheses are conceivable, and capable, each, of plausible support:

1. The purely chemical theory of Liebig, Gerhardt, Bergmann, Snow of London, and B. W. Richardson.

2. The bioplastic hypothesis of Beale, according to which germinal matter may be detached from a living body and planted, while yet retaining vitality, upon another, and there may undergo changes more or less morbid, and destructive of the body by which it has been received. This theory of migrating or transplanted bioplasts has received very little support besides that of its distinguished author.

3. That the minute organisms discovered so constantly upon diseased parts of plants and animals (*e.g.* ergot of rye, *Peronospora infestans* of potato-rot, *Botrytis Bassiana* of silk-worm muscardine, *Panhistophyton* of silk-worm pebrine, *Empusa muscæ* of the fly, *Achorion, Tricophyton, Oidium*, and *Leptothrix* of human affections of the skin and mucous membranes) are incidental or accidental only[19]—acting, as R. Owen observes, [p. 141]most commonly as natural scavengers in the consumption of effete organic material; but that they may become noxious under two sorts of circumstances—viz. when their numbers are enormously increased, as is known to be the case with trichinæ in the human body, and also when they are brought in considerable number into contact with bodies already diseased, or at least suffering under depression of vital energy.

[19] This possibility has not been as yet altogether ruled out in regard to Koch's *Bacillus tuberculosis;* concerning which active discussion has been going on during the past year or two (1882-83). A very large number of observers confirm the statement that the bacilli are found in most specimens of tubercle. Several, also, have repeated with success Koch's inoculation experiments, in which tubercle appeared to be propagated by carefully isolated bacilli. But many facts still stand in the way of the conclusion that the bacillus is the causa sine quâ non of tuberculosis. First, examples of the production of phthisis by apparent contagion or infection are few. Although Dr. C. T. Williams found bacilli in the air of the wards of the Hospital for Consumptives at Brompton, yet of the experience of that hospital Dr. Vincent Edwards, for seventeen years its resident medical officer, reports as follows: "Of fifty-nine resident medical assistants who lived in the hospital an average of six months each, only two are dead, and these not from phthisis. Three of the living are said to have phthisis. The chaplain and the matron had each lived there for over sixteen years. Very many nurses had been in residence for periods varying from months to several years. The head-nurses," says the writer, "sleep each in a room containing fifty patients. Two head-nurses only are known to have died—one from apoplexy; the other head-nurse was here seven months, was unhappily married, and some time afterward died of phthisis. Of the nurses now in residence, one has been here twenty-four years, two twelve years, one eight years, one seven years, one six and a half years, and one five years. No under-nurse, as far as I am aware, has died of phthisis. All the physicians who have attended the in-and-out patients during the past seventeen years are living, except two, who did not die from phthisis."

Against the inoculation and inhalation experiments of Villemin, Tappeiner, Koch, Wilson Fox, and others, by which the specific character of tubercle has been said to be proved, must be placed those of Sanderson, Foulis, Papillon, Lebert, Waldenburg, Schottelius, Wood and Formad, Robinson, and others, by which tubercles have been induced by the injection, inoculation, or inhalation of various non-tubercular materials. In answer to the argument from these, it is asserted by Koch and his supporters that "there is no anatomical or morphological characteristic of tubercle," its only sufficient test being its inoculability. This is almost begging the question; at all events, it leaves it, for the present, unsettled. Moreover, tubercular deposits do not always contain bacilli, as has been shown by Spina, Sternberg, Formad, Prudden (*N.Y. Medical Record*, April 14 and June 16, 1883). The last named made, in one well marked case, six hundred and ninety-five sections from ninety-nine tubercles in different portions of a tuberculous pleura, all of Koch's precautions being observed in the examination. Belfield (*Lectures on Micro-Organisms and Disease*) admits the possibility that tuberculosis may be produced by either of several causes. It has, at least, not yet been demonstrated that the tubercular tissue is more than a nidus or favorable "culture-ground" for the bacilli, or that, in the presence of a constitutional predisposition, they may not merely promote a more rapid destruction of the invaded organs or tissues.

4. That such organisms are the essential and direct causes of enthetic maladies by invading the human and other living bodies as parasites, consuming and disorganizing their tissues, blood corpuscles,[20] etc. Pasteur considers the abstraction of oxygen an important part of their action.

[20] Against this view stands especially the objection that, as Cohn, Burdon Sanderson, and others have fully shown, bacteria and other Schizomycetæ obtain their nitrogen, not from organized tissues, but from ammonia, and their carbon and hydrogen from the results of decomposition in organic tissues. (See B. Sanderson, in *Brit. Med. Journal*, Jan. 16, 1875.) Pasteur has regarded the relation of these organisms to oxygen as important; some of them requiring it for their existence (ærobic), and others not (anærobic). He has defined fermentation as "life without free oxygen."

5. That these microbes, microphytes, or mycrozymes act not as parasites, but as poison-producers, secreting a sort of ferment which is the specific morbid material (Virchow); or, when multiplying in excess of their food-material, they may die, and their dead bodies, like other decaying organic matter, may become poisonous. This possibility, although not distinctly suggested (so far as I know) hitherto, appears to me to be not unworthy of consideration. That the numbers of micro-organisms present have some important relation to morbid conditions has long since been inferred from familiar facts.

6. That they are not generators, but carriers, of disease-producing poisons; their vitality giving to the latter a continuance of existence and capacity of accumulation and transportation not otherwise possible.

Briefly, the following is a summary of the most generally accepted classification of those microscopic organisms[21] whose rôle in the causation of diseases is now under discussion; chiefly following Cohn and Klebs:

Orders: Hyphomycetæ, Algæ, Schizomycetæ.

Hyphomycetæ, *genera:* Achorion, Tricophyton, Oidium.

Algæ, *genera:* Sarcina, Leptothrix.

Schizomycetæ, or Bacteria, *genera:* Micrococcus, Rod-bacterium, Bacillus, Spirillum.[22]

[21] For further details concerning these the reader is referred to the works of Magnin, Belfield, and Gradle on *The Bacteria*, and on the *Germ Theory of Disease*.

[22] Cohn also separates vibrio and spirochæte as genera distinct from spirillum. They may, however, be regarded rather as species of that genus. Some recent authors included bacterium and bacillus under one genus, bacillus; against which simplification there seems to

FIG. 1.

Micrococci: *a*, zoogloea form; *b*, micrococcus from urine, in rosary chain; *c*, rosary chain from spoiled solution of sugar of milk (Cohn).

be no valid objection.

Micrococci (Sphærobacteria of Cohn) are asserted (under certain conditions) by Letzerich, Wood, and Formad[23] to be causative of diphtheria; Ogston has found them in ordinary pus; Rindfleisch, Recklinghausen, Waldeyer, Birch-Hirschfeld, and others report them to be always present in the abscesses of pyæmia; Buhl, Waldeyer, and Wagner state their occurrence in intestinal mycosis; Eberth, Köster, Maier, Burkhardt, and Osler, in ulcerative endocarditis; Orth, Lukomsky, Fehleisen, and Loeffler, in erysipelas; Coats and Stephen in pyelo-nephritis; Friedländer, in pneumonia; Eklund (*Plax scindens*) in scarlet fever; Keating[24] and [p. 142]Le Bel, in measles; Leyden and Gaudier, in cerebro-spinal meningitis; Carmona del Valle, in yellow fever; Prior, in dysentery; Gaffky, Leistikow, Bokai, and Bockhardt, in gonorrhoea;[25] besides other similar observations by numerous writers.

[23] *Bulletin of National Board of Health*, Supplement No. 17, Jan. 21, 1882.

[24] *The Medical News*, Philadelphia, July 29, 1882.

[25] Sternberg's careful experimentation seems to show the identity of Neisser's gonococcus with the Micrococcus ureæ, commonly found in decomposing urine.

Bacterium termo is regarded by leading authorities as the special ferment or causative agent of putrefaction[26] (Billroth, Cohn).

FIG. 2.

Bacteria: *a*, zoogloea of *Bacterium termo;* *b*, pellicle of bacteria from surface of beer; *c*,*Bacterium lineola*, free; *d*, zoogloea form of *B. lineola*.

[26] Others have referred putrefaction to vibriones, less precisely described.

Bacillus includes, hypothetically at least, several species; as Bacillus subtilis, the innocent hay-fungus; Bacillus anthracis, the microbe of malignant pustule (anthrax, milzbrand, charbon) and the splenic fever of sheep; Bacillus typhosus (Klebs, Eberth, Meyer) of typhoid fever; Bacillus lepræ (Hansen, Neisser, Cornil, Koebner) of leprosy;[27] Bacillus malariæ, reported as having been demonstrated[28] by Klebs and Tommasi Crudeli, Marchand, Ceri, and Ziehl; Bacillus tuberculosis (Koch, Baumgarten, 1882); the bacillus of malignant oedema (Gaffky, Brieger, Ehrlich); that of syphilis (Aufrecht, Birch-Hirschfeld,[29] Morrison); of glanders (Loeffler, Schuetz, Israel, Bouchard); of pertussis (Burger); besides the Actinomycosis of Israel, Ponfick,[30] Bollinger, and others. Koch has very recently (1883) been reported to have discovered in Egypt the bacillus of cholera.

[27] Dr. H. D. Schmidt of New Orleans, an experienced pathologist, reported (*Chicago Medical Journal and Examiner*, April, 1882) that critical examination of numerous specimens of tissues from three cases of leprosy under his care failed to verify the existence of bacilli as characteristic of that disease.

[28] Not certainly, however, as shown by Sternberg (*Bulletin of Nat. Board of Health*, Supplement No. 14, July 23, 1881). Dr. Salisbury of Ohio in 1866 made a series of observations, on the basis of which he asserted the discovery of a genus of malarial microphytes, which he referred to the family of *Palmellæ*.

The oval and spherical organisms described by Richard and Laveran as found in the blood of malarial patients resembled micrococci rather than bacilli.

[29] More recently described by him as micrococci.

[30] *Die Actinomykose*, 1881.

FIG. 3.

Bacillus malariæ of Klebs and Tommasi Crudeli.

FIG. 4.

Bacteria from gelatin solution, inoculated from swamp-mud, X 1500 (Sternberg).

FIG. 5.

Vibrios in gelatin culture-fluid, X 1000 (Sternberg).

FIG. 6.

Protococcus from slides exposed over swamp-mud, X 400 (Sternberg).

FIG. 7.

Bacilli from swamp-mud, X 1000 (Sternberg).

FIG. 8.

Bacilli from septicæmic rabbit, X 1000 (Sternberg).

FIG. 9.

Bacilli from human saliva, X 1000 (Sternberg).

FIG. 10.

Bacillus anthracis (Sternberg).

FIG. 11.

Bacillus tuberculosis, within and outside of pus-corpuscles (Sternberg).

Spirillum (Spirochæta of Ehrenberg) has its best ascertained example in the minute forms first observed by Obermeier, and afterward by many other observers, in the blood of patients suffering with relapsing fever. They have been found present in the blood only during the febrile paroxysm, disappearing in the intermission and through convalescence.

Hastening to close our consideration of this subject, we may note, without much argument, a few of the points of difficulty needing yet to be more fully illuminated by [p. 143]careful observation before any form of the germ theory can take its place as an established doctrine in etiology:

1. The absence of the characters belonging to definite organisms[31] in the easily-studied virus of small-pox and vaccinia stands, a priori, against the probability of such organisms being essential to the causation of other enthetic diseases.

[31] The particulate character of variolous and vaccine virus has been already alluded to, as asserted to have been shown by Chauveau and others. Yet it is not absolutely demonstrated that filtration may not produce an important chemical alteration in some kinds of highly unstable organic material subjected to it. Cohn figures a Micrococcus vacciniæ in his article on Bacteria (*Microscopical Journal*, vol. xiii., N. S., pl. v., Fig. 2). Beale denies (*Microscope in Medicine*, 4th ed.) the existence of any organisms in vaccine virus. Lugginbuhl, Weigert, Klebs, Pohl-Pincus, and others have asserted their existence, but, especially in the absence of any successful culture experiments, it does not seem to be proved.

2. Analogy in nature, showing the commonly beneficial action of nutritive processes in re-appropriating the products of organic decay on a large or on a small scale, makes the scavenger theory of the general function of minute cryptogamic organisms more probable, per se, than that which holds many of them to be destructive parasites or poison-producers in the bodies which they may inhabit. Few well known parasites are capable of causing death in higher animals or in man.

3. These microbes are among the minutest objects which can be studied under the microscope. Bacteria average about 1/9000 of an inch in their longest diameter; micrococci and spores (Dauersporen, Billroth) are yet smaller. Much care, therefore, as well as skill, must be exercised in making observations upon them.[32] Huxley asserted a few [p. 144]years ago that a distinguished English pathologist had mistaken for movements of minute living organisms the "Brownian movements" seen in the particles of many not living substances under a high magnifying power. One observer, at least,[33] considers that the forms designated as bacteria and micrococci, etc. are either forms of coagulated fibrin or granules from morbidly-altered blood-corpuscles (zoogloea of Billroth, Wood, Formad, and others). Koch denies the validity of the observation of organisms in tubercle by Klebs and Schüller, while insisting upon his own demonstration of a bacillus tuberculosis. Authorities must, by mutual confirmation or correction, remove these obscurities.

[32] A very interesting discovery was made by Tyndall, to the effect that while one boiling of a liquid would sterilize it for the time by destroying all the bacteria present, their spores might still retain vitality and be afterward developed. By repeated exposure to a boiling temperature, taking these spores in their developing stage, they were destroyed, and complete sterilization was effected.

[33] R. Gregg, *N.Y. Med. Record*, Feb. 11, 1882. Sternberg, however, has replied to him (*N.Y. Med. Record*, April 8, 1882, p. 368). The latter admits a doubt as to whether the granules seen within the leucocytes by Wood and Formad in diphtheritic material, and believed by them to be micrococci, are such, or are merely granules formed or set free by disorganization of protoplasm within the leucocytes. This uncertainty well illustrates the difficulty of these investigations.

A chemical test much relied upon is, that bacteria resist the action of acids and alkalies, which destroy granular material of animal origin; also, that all these organisms are deeply stained by aniline dyes and by hæmatoxylin. The most decisive test, however, is cultivation in a liquid sterilized by heat. Koch prefers a process of dry culture for the bacillus of tubercle.

Gradle (*Lectures on the Germ Theory of Disease*, Chicago, 1883, p. 28) says that the absolute criterion of the life of bacteria is their power of multiplication.

4. Bacteria and micrococci have been abundantly discovered (Kolaczck; J. G. Richardson) in healthy bodies upon the various mucous membranes and in the blood. The correctness of such observations has been denied, but, so far at least as the mucous membranes are concerned, it has been well established by Nothnagel, Sternberg, and others. Bacteria have sometimes been found in countless numbers in fecal discharges.

5. Bacteria become most numerous in materials of a septic or infectious character after their period of toxic intensity has passed by.

6. Suppuration can be produced (Uskoff, Orthmann) without the presence of minute organisms of any kind. Bacteria have been found [p. 145]under Lister's antiseptic dressings without suppuration following. Paul Bert destroyed all the microbes in a septic liquid, and yet found it to retain its poisonous quality. Rosenberger (1881) has made similar observations.

Panum, Coze, and Seltz, Bergmann and Schmiedeberg, Hiller, Vulpian, Rosenberger, Clementi, Thin, and Dreyer have, by various elaborate investigations, proved that fatal septic poisoning can be produced in animals by the products of organic decomposition, without the presence of living organisms. Zweifel's experiments seem to have shown that normal blood, when deprived of oxygen, in the absence of micro-organisms, may acquire septic properties.

As stated by Belfield,[34] many experiments by Schmidt, Edelberg, Köhler, Nencki, and others, have shown that septicæmia may be induced by the injection into the blood of free fibrin ferment and other substances, in the absence of minute organisms. To such an affection some authors now give the name sapræmia, to distinguish it from bacterial infective disorders.

[34] *Lectures on the Relation of Micro-organisms to Disease*, 1883.

Griffini ascertained that mixed saliva, filtered through porous plates, and thus containing no microbes, will still produce septicæmia in animals, when subcutaneously injected. Colin (1876) has denied the conclusiveness of the experiments of Chauveau, which have been held to prove the particulate nature of variolous and vaccine virus. Moreover, it is well known that eggs with shells unbroken are tainted when placed near others which are unsound.

7. While Klebs and Koch maintain the definite specificity of each minute microphytic organism, Nægeli and Billroth assert their mutual convertibility. Burdon Sanderson avers[35] that "the influence of environment on organisms such as bacteria is so great that it seems as if it were paramount." Buchner, Grawitz, Greenfield, Pasteur, Wernich, Thorne, Willems, Law, Wood, and Formad report experiments making it appear that modification by culture is possible with bacilli and micrococci, converting an innocent into a malignant parasitic organism, or a death-producing microbe into one capable only of causing [p. 146]a transitory and not dangerous local affection; which nevertheless secures to the animal thus treated immunity when subsequently exposed to the deadly infection. Most interesting have been the successes with such culture-inoculations obtained by Buchner, Greenfield, and Pasteur with anthrax in sheep; by Pasteur also in chicken cholera; and by Willems and Law[36] with the lung-plague of cattle.

[35] *Brit. Med. Journal*, Jan. 16, 1875.

[36] *N.Y. Med. Record*, June 18, 1881, p. 679. Exposure to the air for a considerable period seems to be the agency chiefly relied upon for what may be called the dynamic modification of these microphytes. When cultivated in the depth of a liquid, so that air is excluded, they are supposed to acquire a habit of obtaining oxygen by decomposing organic substances, and thus act destructively upon the cell-elements of living bodies. Analogous

differences have long since been observed in the study of fermentation between surface and sedimentary yeast.

In none of these cases is there reported any morphological change whatever in the bacillus (Grawitz) or micrococcus (Wood and Formad); the change in the effects noted, and, in the case of the micrococci of malignant diphtheria, the acquired capacity of reproduction through several generations, are all.

8. The immunity against subsequent attacks on exposure (similar to the protection given by vaccination) continues to be without full explanation upon any theory. But it is especially difficult to reconcile it with the hypothesis of the infection being caused by, and dependent upon, the presence of peculiar microphytes. Why should not these, whether as parasites or as poisons, always produce the same effects?

9. The view entertained by Thorne, Wood, and Formad, that a common benignant affection, such as ordinary sore throat, may be converted into a violent infectious disease— *e.g.* malignant diphtheria—by modification of innocent micrococci into those with lethal characters, through local or bodily conditions, is sufficiently contravened by the great frequency of such conditions compared with the decided relative rarity of such malignant epidemics or endemics.

10. Throughout all the investigations which have been, and are likely to be, conducted, there remains the extreme difficulty, if not impossibility, of total separation between the microbes themselves and the matter of the vehicle in which they exist—the membrane, urine, blood, virus, artificial culture-material, or whatever it may be. All the effects ascribable to the disease germs may be, with no more difficulty, attributed to the toxic action [p. 147]of a portion, however minute, of the soil in which they have lived, whose modifications must be concomitant with those which they undergo. It appears necessary, therefore, at the present time, to regard this whole question as still undecided, with a predominance of probability, however, in favor of the view that these minute organisms, or some of them, have a direct and important relation of some kind to the causation of specific endemic, epidemic, and contagious diseases. Altogether, the strongest arguments are on the side of the view that the micrococci, bacilli, etc. cause diseases, not as parasites, living upon their victims, but as poison-producers infecting them.[37] The germ theory continues to be in the position of a probable hypothesis, not in that of an established doctrine of etiological science.

[37] This comports much the best with the general natural history of parasites on the one hand, and of venoms, ptomaïnes, etc. on the other. Gautier, Ogston, and others have expressed the opinion that microphytes may produce ptomaïnes.

Practically, the result is nearly the same as if it were altogether settled, since it is admitted on all sides that the presence of microphytes (bacteria, micrococci, spirilla) coincides with those conditions under which originate several of the most malignant diseases. Measures which prevent the appearance or promote the destruction of these minute organisms are at least often, and to a great degree, preventive, if not curative, of such disorders; and the glory of Jenner's discovery, by which the ravages of small-pox have been made (potentially at least) controllable, seems not unlikely to be paralleled by the achievements of Pasteur and others in a similar preventive mastery over other maladies of men and animals. There is, therefore, no branch of inquiry in connection with medical science more worthy of being assiduously encouraged and extended. The present may almost be said to be, in the history of medicine, an era of myco-pathology.

For an exhaustive study of Etiology attention would now have to be given to the modifying influences affecting the occurrence and character of diseases in connection with age, sex, and temperament. But, as neither of these is ever, per se, causative of any malady, and they merely determine some modification of the action of morbid causes when these occur, want of space must be our justification for leaving them to be considered, in this work, in connection with the special causation of the different[p. 148]diseases which will be hereafter described. A larger treatment of our present subject belongs rather to hygiene than to practical medicine.

MEDICAL DIAGNOSIS.

For the purposes of the medical practitioner all professional studies unite to the end of furnishing preparation for the diagnosis and treatment of diseases. At the bedside the cardinal questions are, How does the present condition of our patient differ from health? and, What ought we to do to bring about his recovery?

Diagnosis involves three main directions of inquiry: 1, as to the general bodily state of the patient; 2, morbid changes in particular organs, tissues, or functions; 3, as to what name properly designates the disorder, according to accepted nomenclature.

Pathology can never be out of view in connection with either the theoretical or the practical study of diagnosis. But it is most closely regarded when the last of these questions is before us, since the names of diseases generally have a more or less distinct reference to their pathological nature. Yet clinical observation always suggests the early use of provisional terms for recognized groupings of morbid phenomena; and sometimes these clinical designations remain for a long time in use because of the imperfection of pathology.

We ascertain, in practice, the nature of a given case, first, by considering its symptoms. These are those obvious evidences of deviation from health which the patient himself is aware of, or which the physician readily discerns or elicits by simple inquiry or examination.

Secondly, taking the clue furnished by symptoms, a closer inspection is made, with the intent of finding what is the actual state of important organs, as the heart, lungs, liver, spleen, kidneys, and alimentary canal.

Lastly, when these means fail to remove all obscurity, or when special scientific investigation is practicable, instruments of precision are employed, as the thermometer, sphygmograph, ophthalmoscope, æsthesiometer, or aspirator; or by the microscope and chemical analyses still more minute examination is made into the particulars of the morbid processes present and their results.

We may subdivide diagnosis, then, into: 1, symptomatology; 2, organoscopy or physical diagnosis; 3, instrumental diagnosis.

Symptomatology.

Semeiology (from [Greek: sêmeion], a sign) is a term much in use, with essentially the same meaning as symptomatology, but less conveniently distinctive, since it does not so well indicate the contrast between obvious signs, or symptoms, and those more recondite, obtained by the methods of physical diagnosis.

Signs of disease cannot be recognized as such except by one who is[p. 149]familiar with the appearances, actions, and manifestations which belong to health. Nor can they be understood, so as to infer what they mean, without knowledge of normal physiology on the one hand, and, on the other, of the natural history of diseases. Physiology constitutes the etymological grammar, symptomatology the vocabulary, and diagnosis the syntax of practical medicine. Just as grammatical knowledge will not enable any one to read or speak a language without acquaintance with its words, so clinical observation is necessary to the physician over and above all the knowledge he may have of physiology and pathology. He must learn to know diseases by sight, or at least by personal contact and observation.

Every one has, of course, a general familiarity with the state and actions of his own and other bodies in health, yet a more exact knowledge of the movements of respiration, circulation, secretion, etc., as well as the form, size, and relative location of all the organs of the body, is needed. Physiology and medical anatomy furnish such information. The more thorough this knowledge is appropriated, the better fitted the student is for practical diagnosis. For its application, however, cultivation of all the perceptive powers is very important. Some men have a genius for quick and clear discernment of symptoms and for their interpretation, as well as for that of physical signs. But all can much improve their senses, and their sagacity in using them, by experience. For this, if for no other reason, scientific training, in field or laboratory studies, affords the best introduction to the work of the medical student and physician. The traits most needed for success in diagnosis are exactness and comprehensiveness. First, to be sure precisely what each sign is that comes under observation; next, to overlook no existing symptoms or physical signs; and, last, so to combine them into a mental map, diagram, or picture, as to make a coherent and rational whole. This nosogram may then be compared with the descriptions of standard authorities, to find its place (if it has one) in technical classification. First, however, ascertain the thing, the morbid state or combination of states; afterward the name, or morbid species, when practicable. It is always to be remembered that complication of diseases, or at least the existence of some irregular manifestations along with those which are characteristic, is more common than the occurrence of purely typical cases. The portraits of most diseases in the books are averages, like the composite class-photographs of Douglas Galton. Not nearly every case will correspond with such an average in all respects. Moreover, so great is the possible variety of alterations among the different organs of the body that the chances of two instances of disease being precisely alike in every particular are hardly greater than those in favor of every move being the same in two games of chess with the same opening.

In an essay like the present it is not easy to decide upon the best manner of treating the subject before us. Too much or too little may be said. With advanced readers the whole history of symptoms and physical signs might be left to the special discussions occurring in articles upon different diseases. But it may be taken for granted that those who consult the present work will do so either at a comparatively early stage of their studies or when time has made desirable a renewal of what may have been once known and then forgotten. Since, then, it is impossible [p. 150]to anticipate what may be the exact needs of either class, a somewhat elementary statement of main facts appears justifiable here.

Following the natural method, we may suppose a call to visit a patient. Arriving in his presence, the first question (mostly left out of view and rarely expressed) may be, Is it a case of real or only imaginary indisposition? Army medical officers, more than most others, can appreciate the possibility of this inquiry sometimes disposing of the whole case.

Supposing it to be real, is it an illness or an accident or other injury? Is it severe or of trifling account? Acute or chronic? We observe the position of the patient, lying quietly in bed, sitting up, or walking restlessly about the room. Then the countenance is observed—pale or flushed, tranquil or excited in expression. We feel the forehead, touch the cheek and hand. Is the skin hot or cold, dry or moist? The pulse is felt; the breathing also is counted.

Of the patient himself or of another (in serious acute cases better of his care-taker, in another apartment) we ask questions whose answers give us the general history of the case. When not before known these should include his antecedent personal history, even extending to that of the family, as far as can be learned. What tendencies have they, or has he or she, shown by previous attacks and their results?

So we come to the present attack: When did it begin, and how? What have been its prominent symptoms since? Questions are then to be put concerning the heat of the body, appetite, complaint of pain, sleep, movement of the bowels, discharge of urine: in the female, menstruation; if married, pregnancy or parturition, how often and when occurring last. Thus the practitioner is enabled to get a clue to the diagnosis, to be followed out through his own observation and closer examination. If the patient be a child and the attack be acute and febrile, an early question must be as to its having passed or not through the different diseases of childhood—viz. the exanthemata, mumps, and whooping cough, and also what exposure to any of these it may have been recently subjected to.

Going farther into particulars, let us review some of the possible developments obtained in the above questioning of symptoms.

When lying in bed the decubitus may be significant, as, upon the back with the knees drawn up in peritonitis; with the hands pressing the abdomen in colic; tossing to and fro in the delirium of fever or of early cerebral inflammation; on one side constantly in acute inflammation of the liver or in pleurisy. Or the patient may be obliged to be propped in a sitting posture (orthopnoea) from heart-disease, asthma, or ascites, or leaning forward upon the back of a chair or a pillow with aneurism of the aorta. More remarkable still may be the subsultus tendinum of low fever, the opisthotonos of tetanus, the respiratory spasms of hydrophobia, or the clonic movements of epileptic, hysterical, or occasional convulsions.

In the face we see pallor in syncope and in anæmia in any of its varieties and with varied associations; a general redness in some cases of apoplexy and in remittent fever; flushing of the forehead and eyes especially in yellow fever; dusky redness in typhus, and a more purple hue in typhoid fever; yellowness in jaundice, in some cases of remittent and in most of yellow fever; sallowness in cancer; a bright central glow upon each cheek in early pneumonia or the hectic of phthisis; a blue or ashen appearance in the collapse of cholera, and blackish-blue in [p. 151]cyanosis or carbonic acid poisoning; bronzed in Addison's disease; puffy about the eyelids in Bright's disease; the surface swollen, yet resistant to the touch, in myxoedema. The eyes (one or both) glare prominently in exophthalmic goitre; squint in advanced cerebro-meningitis; roll to and fro often in the prostration of cholera infantum and in convulsions; are clear and bright in phthisis; yellowish in hepatic disorder; dull and clouded in low fevers; without expression in imbecility and general paralysis.

Contraction of the pupil is observed in inflammation of the retina or of the brain, narcotism from opium (until near death) or eserine, or apoplectic effusion near the pons varolii. Dilatation of the pupil is seen in most cases of hydrocephalus and of apoplexy; in nerve-blindness (amaurosis), glaucoma, cataract, and narcotism from atropia, duboisia, or hydrocyanic acid. Inactivity of the pupil (Argyll Robertson) under changes of light and darkness is common in locomotor ataxia. Different states of the two pupils under the same light show disorder, either ophthalmic or cerebral in site, or may indicate pressure on the cervical sympathetic ganglia, as from aortic aneurism.

In elderly persons we ought always to look for the arcus senilis, which is a sign of a tendency to fatty degeneration. It is a ring, or part of a ring, with ill-defined edges, best seen by lifting or depressing an eyelid, at the junction of the cornea and sclerotic coat of the eye. In some quite healthy old persons there may be seen at the same junction a clearly-defined circular line of calcareous nature. This must be distinguished from the true fatty arcus senilis.

Of the face we may also notice the pinched nose, hollow eyes, and falling jaw of the facies Hippocratica, presaging death; the square forehead of the rickety child (not common in this country); ulcers on the forehead, scars at the mouth-corners, or copper-colored eruptions in syphilis; the full, flabby lips of scrofula. In peritonitis or gastritis the mouth is apt to be drawn up with a peculiar expression of suffering and nausea. Very striking is the characteristic one-sided appearance in facial palsy, from lesion of the seventh nerve. There may be a smile, a frown, or other expression on the sound side of the face, while the paralyzed side is quite immovable. As the seventh nerve (portio dura) supplies the orbicularis muscles, its paralysis (so often temporary) may cause inability to close the eye upon the affected side. Ptosis, or inability to open the eye, involving the levator palpebræ, which is innervated by the third nerve (motor oculi) is more significant of cerebral lesion.

Even the ears may have language, as when their lobes are full and glistening red in the gouty diathesis, or wrinkled in prolonged cachexiæ, or when they are running with discharges in the struma (scrofula) of childhood. The hair becomes dry and lustreless in phthisis, and falls out during convalescence from many acute diseases.

If we look at the gums in a case of lead-poisoning, we may expect to find a blue line along their edges. Scurvy is betokened by a swollen, spongy, and easily-bleeding state of the gums. Many scorbutic cases, however, lack this so-called pathognomonic feature. It may be remarked, by the way, that absolutely pathognomonic signs of particular diseases, never absent and exclusively seen in them, are very few. Albuminuria, for example, is not always present in Bright's disease, and is [p. 152]also met with in a number of other affections. Sugar in the urine may follow inhalation of chloroform or an attack of cholera, as well as diabetes mellitus. Rice-water discharges may be absent in the collapse of cholera, and patients may die with yellow fever without black vomit. Still, these symptoms have great diagnostic value, and, taken with others associated with them, may often enable us to attain to a diagnosis of much importance.

Perfect teeth in an adult in this country are rather the exception than the rule. In the notched incisors of inherited syphilis, however, there is something quite distinctive. The notches in Hutchinson's teeth are vertical, not horizontal.

Old as medicine is the examination of the tongue in disease. It may be protruded with difficulty, as in low fevers, in apoplexy, and in cerebral paralysis (bulbar sclerosis, glosso-labio-pharyngeal paralysis) or thrust to one (the paralyzed) side in hemiplegia. It is pallid in anæmia; yellow in bilious disorder; red in glossitis (then swollen also), in scarlet fever, and in gastritis; furred in indigestion, gastro-hepatic catarrh, and the early stage of various febrile attacks; dry, brown, cracked, or fissured in typhus or typhoid fevers and in the typhoid state of malarial remittent fever; bare of epithelium in advancing phthisis and in imperfect convalescence from severe acute diseases. Coldness of the tongue is one of the worst signs in the collapse of cholera.

As we examine the throat internally we look for signs of faucial inflammation in redness and swelling, with or without enlargement of the tonsils, or relaxation and elongation of the uvula, or ulceration, or the gray or brown membranous deposit of diphtheria. In the mouth of a child we may find the little white vesicular patches called aphthæ, the curd-like exudations of thrush, or possibly the much worse grayish ulcerations of cancrum oris, or the rarer ashen sloughs of gangrene of the mouth.

Outside of the throat we must remember the significance of glandular swellings or scars of suppurated glands in children; nor overlook, if present, stiffness of the muscles, or torticollis, or goitrous enlargement of the thyroid gland. Observation should be made also of the site of the carotid artery on each side, and of the jugular veins, since aortic regurgitation may be indicated by violent action of those arteries or tricuspid regurgitation by pulsation of the veins in the neck.

Long before vaso-motor physiology had any place in science the pulse was known to afford valuable indications in disease. Either of the accessible arteries will answer instead of the radial; its convenience merely makes the wrist the common place of comparison. By careful examination of the pulse something may be learned of several of the factors concerned in its production. These factors are—1, the muscular force of the walls of the heart; 2, the state of the cardiac valves; 3, the muscularity of the arteries; 4, the elasticity of the arterial coats; 5, the state of the capillary circulation; 6, the qualities of the blood; 7, the condition of the nervous system as to excitability or apathy.

A feeble heart must induce a feeble pulse. Moderate debility may be attended by slowness of the pulse, but usually a weak circulation is marked by frequent, small beats, like the vibrations of a short pendulum. A strong heart-beat (other things being equal) is relatively slow, with a proportionate pause after the second sound.

[p. 153]Valvular lesions produce various effects upon the pulse. Most notable are the irregularity connected often with mitral insufficiency and the jerking pulse (Corrigan) of aortic regurgitation.

Believing, as the present writer does, in the existence of a true arterial systole following and supplementing the ventricular contraction,[38] it must be urged that a vigorous muscularity in the arteries promotes strength in the pulse—not by resistance, but by auxiliary propulsion of the blood. Another condition altogether is tonic, spasmodic contraction of the arteries. This is not often met with pure and simple, but a measure of it is seen in the corded or wiry pulse of acute enteritis or peritonitis.

[38] This view, although advocated by Sir Charles Bell, Legros and Onimus, Hermann of Zurich, and others, is opposed to the most prevailing vaso-motor physiology. Several complications and some contradictions in pathological discussion at the present time would be cleared up by the abandonment of the now commonly-held stopcock theory of arterial function, which has really nothing whatever to support it except the misinterpretation of some experiments upon arteries made many years since.

Deficient elasticity of the arteries is not easily separated in observation from muscular relaxation. When arteries undergo degeneration (atheromatous, fatty, or calcareous), their middle coat suffers the deterioration of both elastic and muscular tissues, these being substituted by materials either more or less yielding, and always less resilient, than the natural fabric of the vessels.

The influence of the condition of the capillary circulation upon that of the arterial system and the heart is manifest in inflammations. By reflex excitation the arteries are made to contract actively and impel the blood more forcibly than in the normal state toward the centre of impeded nutrition (stasis). This has been abundantly proved by the comparison of the amount of blood flowing through the arteries of a sound limb and those of its fellow, when the latter is the seat of a violent acute inflammation.

Blood-states also affect the pulse by the differences in direct stimulation to which the heart and arteries are subjected according to the qualities and composition of the blood. It is probable that the fever-pulse of typhus, typhoid, the exanthemata, septicæmia, and pyæmia has its origin in morbid conditions of the blood, acting in a twofold manner—directly upon the heart and arteries themselves, and mediately through the vaso-motor ganglia.

Lastly, the nervous system stands in an important relation to the action of the heart and arteries, and thus to the pulse. In a nervous, excitable person, changes in the rate of the pulse may take place, with slight significance, which in a different constitution might be of serious import.

To understand the language of the pulse care must be taken in several respects:

1. Both wrists should be felt. Sometimes there is an abnormal variation in the course of the main radial trunk which may pass over the thumb. Again, an aneurism may cause a great difference between the two radial pulses, or, possibly, an embolus may occlude one of the radial vessels, annulling its pulsation.

2. Other arteries also, especially the carotids, should be examined—in all obscure cases at least. Visibly beating, distended, and tortuous temporal arteries are occasionally met with. They are not pathognomonic of any one malady, although often referred to the gouty diathesis. They [p. 154]may attend irregular malarial attacks, or may be connected simply with a hyperæmic state of the brain.

3. The heart's impulse should always be compared with the arterial pulsation. The former may be strong and regular, while the latter is small, feeble, or intermittent. Something must then be wrong, either in the aortic valves or in the arterial system.

5. On account of possible nervous agitation, the pulse should usually be examined more than once, during each visit to the patient.

6. Sex, age, position of the body, and time of day must all be taken account of. In men the average rate of the pulse is between 65 and 75 per minute; in women, between 70 and 80. The pulse-rate of early infancy varies from 100 to 120, and is very easily hurried. That of old persons is commonly between 60 and 70, until, at a very advanced age, with debility, its frequency may be increased, especially upon exertion. Lying down, we find the slowest pulse; sitting, somewhat more rapid; and most so in the standing position. In health the time of day makes no constant difference apart from the effects of food and exercise. In disorders attended by fever there are important changes to be regularly observed. Excepting the variable paroxysms of remittent and intermittent, which are a law unto themselves, in febrile affections the pulse may be expected to be slowest in the morning and most excited in the early part of the night. A diminution of this difference is a favorable sign. Sleep generally slows the pulse decidedly. The ordinary statement is, that the pulse is always slower during sleep, but I have several times found that in states of exhaustion without fever it may be considerably more rapid while the patient is asleep. Nothing is more sure to increase the strength and rapidity of the pulse than high temperature.

7. Very important is the relation between the pulse and respiration. Normally, four pulsations occur to each respiratory act. In pulmonary affections, while the circulation is often disturbed pari passu with the breathing, it may be quite otherwise. Great acceleration of the rate of breathing, with little increase in the rapidity of the pulse, should lead us to suspect disease involving the respiratory organs. Conversely, a much hurried or otherwise perturbed pulse, with little or no change in the breathing, points toward the heart as either functionally or organically the seat of disorder.

Let us further consider, briefly, the kinds of pulse to be met with and interpreted in practice.

A natural pulse is always, per se, a good sign. Yet in the history of a disease usually so well marked as yellow fever some fatal cases have been recorded (walking cases) in which the pulse, almost to the last, was natural.

Strength of the pulse, to a certain degree, belongs to it normally. But this is often exaggerated, and we may have the strong, hard, full, perhaps bounding, pulse of an inflammatory affection (of the brain, for example, or of the joints in acute rheumatism) in a person of vigor. A bounding pulse often accompanies mere palpitation of the heart, whose source may be the sympathetic influence of indigestion or nervousness. A similar pulse is apt to be constantly present in hypertrophy of the heart. In this case it is made more forcible as well as more rapid by [p. 155]active exertion; while palpitation, without organic trouble, is usually diminished by moderately active exercise.

A full pulse is not always strong, nor is a small pulse necessarily weak. Mention has been made already of the tense, corded pulse met with in acute peritonitis, and sometimes in enteritis. Gastric inflammation, with nausea, may exhibit a depressed pulse, weak and but little accelerated. Under still other circumstances we may find a full pulse which is soft, easily compressible, even gaseous. Most frequently a feeble pulse is rapid, and a very rapid pulse is weak. Slowness, in marked degree, attends apoplexy, opium narcotism, and fracture of the skull compressing the brain. Functional disturbance of the heart may occasionally exceed in effect these causes of retardation. I have met, under such circumstances, with a pulse of 20 in the minute; one of 18 has been recorded. A few apparently healthy persons have habitually a pulse with but 40 or 50 beats in the minute.

Quickness in each beat may occur, while a long interval makes the rate per minute slow. The jerking pulse of aortic regurgitation is the most remarkable example of this. Galabin asserts that without imperfection of the valves of the aorta a decidedly abrupt pulse may attend great lowering of arterial tension. Something of the same kind may be noticed in the temporarily excited pulse of very nervous subjects under agitation.

Dicrotism, or reduplication of the pulse-beat, is not uncommon in typhus and typhoid fever. Here relaxation of the heart as well as of the blood-vessels appears to allow a momentary interruption in the succession of the arterial upon the cardiac systole.[39]

[39] An exceptional phenomenon, noticed by a few observers, is the recurrent pulse; *i.e.* a pulsation felt below the finger, whose pressure interrupts the flow of blood through an artery. It may be explained by supposing unusual fulness of the vessels (local, if not general) with, at the same time, relaxation of their walls; bearing in mind, also, the manner of anastomosis of the radial and ulnar branches which favors recurrence.

Intermittence and irregularity of the pulse are not exactly the same thing. Occasional intermittence may be merely a nervous symptom or a muscular twitch of the heart, like the twitches now and then occurring without significance in voluntary muscles. Persistent intermittence, with feebleness of the pulsations (these being generally somewhat rapid), is among the signs of dilatation of the heart.

It is possible for intermittence of the radial pulse to accompany regularity in the heart-beat. This usually results from narrowing (stenosis) of the aortic valvular outlet from the left ventricle. Only a certain number of impulses fairly reach the more distant arteries. This symptom may result also from fatty degeneration of the heart.

Absence of pulse in one radial vessel, while it is present in the other, shows the presence of an obstacle to the circulation on one side, which may be an aneurism, or an embolus plugging the artery.

Irregularity of the pulse, a total derangement of its rhythm, while not often important in young children, is a serious symptom at other times of life. In one disease most common in childhood, acute hydrocephalus, the pulse in the first stage is apt to be hard and rapid, in the middle stage slow and tolerably full, in the third rapid, feeble, and often irregular. Mitral disease frequently presents considerable irregularity of the pulse; and so does dilatation, even without mitral lesion. Brain trouble, especially late in life, whether structural or functional, may produce the [p. 156]same symptom. B. W. Richardson has pointed this out as one of the effects of the excessive use of tobacco, even in young persons.

The pulse of continued, relapsing, and remittent fevers is, during the febrile exacerbation, rapid (100 to 120); in the earlier part of the attack full, but only moderately hard, or even soft and yielding. As the attack passes its height and critical defervescence occurs, the pulse grows slower, unless great prostration has supervened; in which case it increases in rapidity, while it fails more and more in fulness and resistance.

The pulse of the moribund state is nearly always small, very rapid (130-150), and thready, without force or fulness. It may become imperceptible before death. A pulse of 140 beats in the minute is always alarming; if much beyond that rate the case is desperate. A pulse of more than 150 beats in the minute is very difficult to count accurately.

Exophthalmic goitre is attended characteristically by a full, somewhat rapid, and bounding pulse, the cardiac impulse being also proportionately violent and extended. Exercise much increases this hyper-pulsation.

Pulsation of the jugular veins is ordinarily explained by tricuspid regurgitation, a portion of the blood being sent back to the vena cava with an impulse reaching to the jugulars. In some instances, however, as the writer has repeatedly observed, jugular pulsation takes place without any abnormality in the action or condition of the heart, from a local inflammation (as tonsillitis) causing a marked exaggeration of the muscular contractility resident in the larger veins.

Retardation of the flow of blood through the veins is manifest during the collapse of epidemic cholera. On pressing the blood back in a vein upon the hand, for example, and then lifting the finger, instead of the movement being, as in health, too swift to be seen, it is so slow as to be easily followed.

Capillary movement may be estimated in a similar manner. If it be very sluggish, pressure upon the cheek, forehead, or hand will cause a pallor which remains for some seconds, instead of disappearing at once when the pressure is withdrawn. This is, it may be noticed, entirely different from the pitting upon pressure, without much if any change of color, in local oedema or general anasarcous effusion. The tache méningitique of Trousseau is a pink or rose-red line left for a time after drawing the finger across the forehead or abdomen in cases of acute hydrocephalus (tubercular meningitis).

Respiration must be watched carefully in all cases of disease. Normally, in the adult, while at rest, from 16 to 18 respiratory movements occur in each minute. The number is somewhat greater in women, and is considerably increased in children, at birth being about 40 in the minute. Men breathe most by the diaphragm; in women there is a greater lifting of the ribs. In either sex a disorder attended by pain in breathing may modify this proportion. If pleurisy, for example, be present, the ribs will be but slightly lifted, abdominal breathing taking predominance. When peritonitis makes every movement of the abdomen painful, costal respiration is maintained almost alone. Likewise, a unilateral pleurisy or pneumonia will check the respiration on the affected side, with an increased movement on the sound side. This difference is less manifest to the eye than to the ear in auscultation. In all febrile [p. 157]affections respiration is hurried proportionately with the pulse, unless some complicating local disorder disturbs the relation.

Dyspnoea may be produced by many different causes, whose possibility must be remembered in its interpretation as a means of diagnosis. In asthma violent efforts are made to compel the entrance of air into the lungs by the intercostal muscles and diaphragm, aided by all the accessory muscles of respiration, including the sterno-cleido-mastoid and others of the neck. Expansion of the nostrils may occur in sympathy with these efforts. Yet the amount of resistance may be shown by a partial sinking-in of the lower ribs, as well as by the patient's distress. These last signs are sometimes very marked in the collapse of one or both lungs now and then occurring in whooping cough.

Croup induces a similar struggle for breath, although the obstruction is differently located. Early in the croupal attack a hoarse sound may accompany each inspiration and expiration. Later, when the danger to life from apnoea becomes more imminent, a hissing or whistling sound succeeds. This last-mentioned kind of sound results temporarily, also, from the spasmodic obstruction to breathing in laryngismus stridulus.

Besides the affections of the lungs which impede respiration (as pneumonia, hydrothorax, etc.), we may have dyspnoea induced by extra-pulmonary causes, such as dilatation of the heart, aneurism of the aorta, mediastinal cancer, pleuritic effusion; also by abdominal dropsy, extreme elephantiasis, etc. Mention need hardly be made here of respiratory obstruction from defective or injurious qualities of the air, threatening or producing asphyxia.

Sighing respiration takes place in heart disease not infrequently. A peculiar modification of the breathing movements has been associated especially with fatty degeneration of the heart. From the distinguished authors who first described it this is called the Cheyne-Stokes respiration. Intervals of suspension of breathing occur, after which short, shallow inspirations begin, and gradually increase for a time in depth; then they grow shorter and shallower again, until apnoea is reached. Such a cycle may occupy from half a minute to a minute and a half, with from fifteen to thirty increasing and decreasing respirations in all. It has been shown by several observers that this type of respiration is not peculiar to fatty degeneration of the heart. It has been met with in cases of cardiac dilatation, aortic atheroma, cerebral hemorrhage, tubercular meningitis, and uræmia.

Sometimes a kind of dyspnoea common in advanced disease of the heart, especially in mitral lesion with dilatation, has been confounded with this. Here the breathing is constantly labored (orthopnoea); but the patient from time to time dozes off into an imperfect sleep, in which the breathing almost entirely ceases. Then he is awakened with a start of distress, perhaps out of a painful dream. This succession of dozing apnoea and waking dyspnoea belongs to a late stage of heart disease, and usually ends in death.

Stertorous respiration is familiar in apoplectic coma, as well as in that of brain compression from injury or from opium or alcoholic narcotism. In uræmic coma true stertor is less apt to be observed; sometimes the respiration in this condition has a hissing sound.

Along with the movements of respiration we may notice that the breath [p. 158]is hot and has a heavy odor in the early stages of all febrile disorders. Disagreeable breath is common, however, in persons not ill, from bad teeth or from indigestion. It is worst of all, putrid, in gangrene of the lung. Certain cases of chronic or subacute bronchitis (as well as of ozæna) also have very offensive breath. Coldness of the breath is a very bad sign; it is observed sometimes before death in the collapse of cholera.

Hiccough (singultus) is a spasmodic affection of the diaphragm. It is innocent, though annoying, in most cases, resulting from indigestion or from nervous disorder; in children, occasionally, from long crying. When it takes place in cases of general prostration it betokens threatening depression or exhaustion of vital energy.

The voice is mostly altered by serious disease. It may be feeble and whispering, from debility; hoarse, from laryngeal inflammation and tumefaction; thick, from cerebral oppression; lost (aphonia), in some cases of chronic laryngitis and in paralysis of the vocal muscles. The manner of articulating words is often changed in disorders of the nervous system. A marked example of this is the monotonous scanning speech of cerebro-spinal sclerosis.

Cough is an extremely variable symptom, always to be understood in connection with the attendant circumstances. Usually, however, the character of the cough itself is more or less distinctive. A dry, hard cough may be merely sympathetic or nervous, or it may belong to the first stage of acute bronchitis. A hacking cough, with little expectoration, is not infrequently observed for a time in incipient phthisis. Pneumonia has, if any, a short and rather sharp cough. Progressing bronchitis is recognized by the deepening and greater or less loosening of the cough. In advanced phthisis there are distressing spells of deep, laborious coughing, especially in the night or in the morning after sleep. Croup is known (whether sporadic or in the form of laryngeal diphtheria) by the barking cough of the early stage and its whistling character toward the fatal end. Nearly the same sort of hissing or whistling sound in breathing has been mentioned already as occurring in laryngismus stridulus. Paroxysms of coughing, with or without whooping, are pathognomonic of pertussis.

Expectoration often affords important signs. Briefly, it may suffice to say here that it is mucous, whitish, or colorless in early bronchitis; more or less yellowish and muco-purulent in severe and protracted bronchitis; rusty, from admingling of the coloring matter of blood, in pneumonia, early and middle stages; bloody and muco-purulent in early and of heavy roundish (nummular) masses in late pulmonary phthisis; putrid, rotten, in gangrene of the lung.

Continuing our survey of obvious symptoms, we must now take account of the conditions of the general surface of the body. Temperature is of great consequence. Most precisely determinable by the thermometer, the touch, when educated, will give very useful indications of its changes. It is difficult, and not commonly desirable, to separate variations of moisture from those of temperature. Reserving for another place the special consideration of medical thermometry, it may be here said that the skin is hot and dry in the typical condition of fever, whatever its special associations. Heat and moisture of the skin are more often met with together in the fever of acute articular rheumatism than in any other[p. 159]affection. As a rule, perspiration lessens febrile heat. Copious (colliquative) sweating is habitual in many wasting diseases, notable in pulmonary phthisis. It is then a sign of great general relaxation of the system.

Coldness of the surface attends prostration, either from temporary collapse or from positive exhaustion. The skin is perceptibly cold in the algid stage of cholera. It may be so in very severe cases of sporadic cholera morbus. In the chill of intermittent, while the patient has the subjective sensation of coldness, his temperature is seldom reduced, and is often higher than natural, although lower than during the febrile exacerbation.

The color of the skin is pallid in anæmia, phthisis, dropsy, etc., and in syncope; ashen or livid in cholera collapse and in the cold stage of pernicious malarial fever; yellow in jaundice, remittent, and yellow fever; sallow in chlorosis, cancer, and chronic dyspepsia; purple, almost black (especially the lips and ends of the fingers), in asphyxia; dark, as if stained with ink, after long use of nitrate of silver; bronzed in Addison's disease; bright red in scarlet fever, etc. The eruptions of this and other exanthemata, and of the different cutaneous diseases, will be best considered in the special articles treating them of in this work.

Odor is perceptible and peculiar (though not easily described) in some bad cases of typhus fever and of small-pox; less often in aggravated chlorosis. Lunatics and paralytics (especially when assembled together in institutions) often give off a noticeable smell. Most distinct, however, is the cadaverous odor, sometimes perceptible for hours before death. Corroborative of this, in summer, is the flocking of flies around the bed of a dying patient. In a hospital ward this selection amongst a number of patients may be quite observable.

Emphysema, from the presence of air in the connective tissue under the skin, is rarely met with except as the consequence of an injury or of local gangrene.

Oedema is local watery effusion, which may have various causes and significance. Anasarca must have a general causation, either connected with the state of the blood or with disorder of the heart, kidneys, or liver, or of more than one of those organs at once. Pitting on pressure is the sign of watery effusion. Soft crackling under the touch distinguishes emphysema. A firm enlargement of the surface of the face and upper part of the body occurs in myxoedema.

Swellings of all kind must be carefully observed, and their nature inquired into— whether they be inflammatory or other chronic enlargements of joints, tumors, fibrous, fatty, or cancerous, aneurisms, hernial protrusions, or of any other character. In protracted disease of the liver (cirrhosis) it is not uncommon to find the superficial abdominal veins dilated and tortuous.

Abdominal enlargement may result from adipose accumulation (obesity), distension of the bowels with wind (meteorism), ascites, ovarian cysts, cancerous or other tumors, aneurism of the aorta, abscess, retention of urine, or pregnancy. By the methods of physical diagnosis, along with careful inquiry into the history of each case, we are to make out the distinctions amongst these different conditions.

Emaciation always marks either defect of nutrition or morbid excess of tissue-waste. It is counterfeited in the sudden collapse of malignant[p. 160]cholera, and exaggerated in appearance during the analogous condition of cholera infantum. On recovery from these states, especially the latter, roundness and fulness of the face and limbs may return much too soon for the actual restoration of fat and flesh. A young child may be plump and chubby to-day, seemingly wasted with acute illness to-morrow, and, if soon relieved, the next day almost as rotund as ever.

Continued diarrhoea, phthisis pulmonalis, mesenteric disease, cancer, and aneurism of the aorta are among the most frequent causes of great emaciation. Sometimes, as in progressive pernicious anæmia, we are struck with the comparatively slight degree of wasting of the body while the disease is advancing toward death.

In myxoedema there is a swelling or general enlargement, especially of the upper portions of the trunk. This is not anasarcous, but depends upon a morbid change in the connective tissue throughout the body.

Articular enlargements may be (particularly in the knee in children) scrofulous, or gouty (in the smaller joints), rheumatic, with evidences of inflammation, acute or chronic; or, what is not well named, rheumatoid arthritis. In this last affection there is a gradual swelling and stiffening, with but little inflammation, of several, sometimes all, the joints of the extremities. Locomotor ataxia is in some cases attended by a degenerative alteration in one or more of the larger joints.

The limbs may furnish to the eye many expressive signs of disease or disability. In the listlessness of one arm and hand, while the other can perform various movements, we see reason to suspect hemiplegia. If the fingers are rigidly contracted, as well as powerless, we have this diagnosis confirmed, whether the rigidity be early or late in its stage. We must then look for a similar condition of the lower extremity on the same side. Paraplegia and general paralysis have their more extended (bilateral) indications in like manner. Characteristic also are the wrist-drop, from paralysis of the extensors of the hand, in lead-palsy; weakness or incapacity of the flexors and extensors in writer's cramp; the hand fixed helplessly in the position for writing in paralysis agitans (advanced stage); the main en griffe, with shrunken muscles and drawn tendons, of progressive muscular atrophy (wasting palsy). In the legs at first and chiefly, but in time also in the arms, increase of bulk with loss of power in the muscles shows the existence of pseudo-hypertrophic muscular paralysis.

Gouty fingers have their joints not only swollen, but distorted by deposits of urates and carbonates. Clubbed finger-ends, in the adult, are seen mostly, with incurvation of the nails, in advancing consumption. The nails are sometimes striated after attacks of gout, the lines disappearing gradually during the interval. In many acute diseases, transverse ridges are noticeable on the nails, marking the date when their growth was arrested and subsequently resumed. These are specially remarkable after attacks of relapsing fever.

A tendency to dropsical effusion is generally first shown, besides a puffiness of the face, in the feet and ankles, the shoe or slipper marking off the enlargement above its margin. Often this has no other cause than debility, with a watery condition of the blood. Varicose veins, with old and resultant ulcers, are also among the possible things to be found in examination of the legs and feet.

[p. 161]Movements of the hands are incessant and jerking in chorea; perpetually trembling in delirium tremens, and often in one arm and hand only, in paralysis agitans; with tremor, seen in voluntary motions alone, in multiple cerebro-spinal sclerosis. More unusual is the rhythmical closing and opening of the hand, successively, of athetosis.

In the walk of patients able to be upon their feet there may be much significance. A hemiplegic subject will circumduct the feeble limb after the other; one suffering with paraplegia will shuffle the feet slowly along the floor; the hysterical paralytic drags the lame limb behind the other; the patient with spastic spinal paralysis rises on his toes in walking, with his legs held close together; the shaking paralytic rather trots forward, with the body bent; and the subject of locomotor ataxia lifts his feet and kicks out forward or sideways, then bringing down the heels with a stamp at each step. In progressive muscular atrophy and advanced pseudo-hypertrophic muscular paralysis a waddling or rolling gait is seen. Choreic patients are very irregular in their walk, as in all other movements. Hip disease (coxalgia) shows itself in a child by its lifting the pelvis and limb of the affected side and bending the knee, so as to touch only the toes to the ground. Club-foot and other deformities require no description in this place.

Sensibility of the extremities and of other parts of the surface of the body needs to be examined into, with all its possible variations (hyperæsthesia, anæsthesia, analgesiæ, etc.), especially when the nervous apparatus is for any reason supposed to be involved. Motions of an unusual character must likewise be carefully noticed. "Westphal's symptom" is regarded as having considerable diagnostic value. It is otherwise called the tendon-reflex, with its modifications. When a person in health is seated with one leg crossed over the other or with the legs dangling over the edge of a high bench or table, and a sudden blow is struck upon the tendon of the patella, the leg and foot will be spontaneously jerked forward. In locomotor ataxia, even from an early period, this tendon-reflex is abolished. In spastic spinal paralysis (lateral spinal sclerosis) it is exaggerated. Quite analogous to this is the ankle-clonus. This is obtained by firmly flexing the foot and then tapping sharply upon the tendo Achillis.

The foot is then involuntarily extended and flexed several times in succession. There is more doubt in regard to the associations of this symptom than as to the knee movement, but it has been clinically shown to be exaggerated in spastic spinal paralysis.

At our first acquaintance with a case of disease, while making inquiry into its nature, the genital organs must not be forgotten. Not that we need always make examination of them, but any pointing in symptoms toward them must be borne in mind, so as to guide us in or toward further procedures in diagnosis. In making, in obscure cases, a diagnosis by exclusion, we are sometimes driven to a scrutiny of the genital system.

We have now, however incompletely, touched upon the greater number of obvious signs or symptoms which a view of a patient would furnish without making minute inquiry of himself or others concerning his or their knowledge of the illness. Such are the objective signs of disease, which must be still more exactly and extensively discerned and understood by means of the processes of physical and instrumental diagnosis. [p. 162]But the subjective symptoms also, and all those observed and described by the patient and his or her friends, must receive very careful attention. Much practical skill may be shown by the kind of questions asked and the use made of the answers given.

First, as to the alimentary apparatus:

Taste is very commonly altered in disease, being sour in indigestion, bitter in disorders of the liver, saltish in hæmoptysis, rotten in gangrene of the lungs.

Dryness of the mouth is the rule in fevers. Sometimes the saliva is viscid and adherent. Increased flow or salivation was formerly frequent in practice under large doses of mercurials. Jaborandi or its alkaloid pilocarpin will generally produce it. Iodide of potassium occasionally has the same effect in less degree.

Loss of appetite nearly always attends serious diseases of any kind. Excessive craving for food (bulimia) is rare. Tapeworm accounts for it in some instances. Desire for strange articles of food, as slate-pencils, ashes, etc., is met with in some instances of chlorosis and of hysteria. A return of natural appetite is one of the best signs toward the close of any acute attack of illness.

Thirst is seldom absent in fever. It is also usually present in the state of collapse, as from cholera, pernicious intermittent, or the shock of severe (especially railroad) injuries.

Dysphagia or difficulty of swallowing may result from simple debility, as in the moribund state; inflammation of the fauces, tonsils, or pharynx; stricture of the oesophagus; obstruction by a foreign body or by a cancerous or aneurismal tumor; retro-pharyngeal abscess; paralysis of the muscles of the throat, such as sometimes follows diphtheria. Soreness of the throat is present in some, but not in all of these examples of dysphagia, being most marked in the inflammatory condition of pharyngitis, tonsillitis, scarlet fever, and diphtheria. Ulceration of the throat should always be carefully looked for, and if present investigated to ascertain whether it is simple, diphtheritic, or syphilitic. We must be careful not to mistake a mere local accumulation of mucus, or aphthous vesicle, or the curd-like formation of thrush or muguet, either for ulceration or pseudo-membranous deposit. Aphthæ and thrush are most frequently met with in children, though small aphthous ulcers frequently appear toward the close of wasting, and especially cancerous, affections. If there be a doubt, pass a moistened hair pencil lightly over the apparent deposit, or allow the patient to gargle the throat with water, and then re-inspect it.

Many causes may produce nausea and vomiting, which almost always occur together; that is, vomiting rarely takes place without previous nausea, although the latter may exist without the former. In the manner of vomiting there are some differences more or less characteristic, as the distressing retching of sea-sickness and of tartar emetic or other irritant poisoning, and the spasmodic out-spurting of rice-water fluid in malignant cholera. The matter vomited is often very important in diagnosis. In mere indigestion the food taken is apt to come up, and the same may happen in flatulent colic. When the liver is involved, as in bilious colic, bile also is ejected. Nothing peculiar exists in the ejecta of morning sickness in pregnancy. The ejecta contain mucus in gastritis, blood in ulcer and in cancer of the stomach, stercoraceous [p. 163]material in obstruction of the bowels, black vomit in bad cases of yellow fever. Hysterical vomiting sometimes closely imitates the latter in appearance.

Other affections attended by vomiting are cholera morbus, remittent fever, brain disease, Bright's disease of the kidney, etc.

Spitting blood may be either hæmatemesis or hæmoptysis proper. If the former, nausea generally precedes the ejection of the blood by vomiting, and it is apt to be mingled with food partly digested. It is coughed up, bright red and frothy usually, when coming from the lungs or bronchial tubes. But blood may proceed from the gums or throat, or may run back through the posterior nares from the nose, and then it gives alarm by seeming to proceed from the chest. It is necessary to inquire very particularly into all such possibilities in every case of hemorrhage.

Between vomiting of blood from ulcer and from cancer of the stomach we have mostly these distinctions: in ulcer it follows soon after taking food, in cancer (this being generally at the pylorus), an hour or more after eating; ulcer is attended also by tenderness on pressure at a certain spot over the stomach, without tumor; cancer presents a tumor, with much less marked tenderness on pressure. By aid of the microscope in examination of the matter vomited this diagnosis may be completed.

Constipation is an exceedingly frequent symptom under many and diverse circumstances. Pathologically, we account for it in several ways: 1, torpor of the muscular coat of the intestinal canal; 2, deficiency of secretion in the glands of the bowels and in the liver; 3, imperfect innervation of the abdominal organs; 4, mechanical obstruction, as by a foreign body, intussusception, strangulated hernia, cancerous or other tumor, stricture of the rectum, etc. Dyspeptic persons are ordinarily constipated. So are almost all patients at the beginning of attacks of measles, scarlet fever, small-pox, and other acute febrile maladies. Typhoid fever is scarcely an exception to this; although the bowels in that affection become loose after a few days, they seldom are so at the very beginning of the attack. Sea-sickness is commonly accompanied by total or nearly total inaction of the bowels, the secretion of the intestinal glands being almost null, often for many days together. Torpor of the brain is sometimes attended by marked constipation. The latter may be a contributing cause of the former, as in certain severe cases of scarlet fever, in which threatening coma may be relieved by active purgation. We must not, however, occupy space here by attempting to enumerate the many conditions under which constipation may present itself as a symptom.

Almost as various are the associations of the opposite state of the bowels, diarrhoea. Excessive or abnormally frequent discharges from the bowels may be either fecal, bilious, mucous, membranous, purulent, bloody, fatty, or watery, and they may occur with or without pain and straining (tenesmus).

If, with frequent disposition to pass something, only small quantities of bloody mucus escape, with pain and bearing down, we recognize dysentery. When, instead, a large quantity of colorless fluid, with or without floating flakes (rice-water), comes from the bowels at short intervals, with vomiting of the same sort of material, we suspect epidemic cholera, and must inquire for corroborative or corrective indications in[p. 164]reference to that suspicion. Very bad cases of cholera morbus also may, at a late stage, present this symptom. So may exceptional cases of pernicious malarial fever. The diarrhoea of typhoid fever exhibits usually liquid stools of a brownish color (gutter-water passages). Occasionally, hemorrhage from the bowels adds to the danger of this fever, as well as to that of malarial remittent fever. In phthisis pulmonalis, at a late stage, colliquative diarrhoea, like colliquative perspirations, shows the breaking up of the system by excessive waste. Very foul, offensive discharges from the bowels may always be understood as showing that in the alimentary canal, whether originating there or in the blood, morbid changes have been going on. The indication is to promote the elimination of such material as soon and as thoroughly as possible.

Clayey stools show absence or deficiency of bile in the intestines, whether from its non-secretion by the liver or from obstruction to its entrance by a gall-stone in the common gall-duct. Green stools are not uncommon in sick children. The cause of the color has been much disputed. Probably it depends chiefly on a modification of the bile-pigment, with some admixture of altered blood. When mercurials have been taken sulphide of mercury may give a green color to the discharges.

Blood, nearly or quite unmixed, coming from the bowels, may have its origin in internal hemorrhoids, intestinal ulceration, cancer of the rectum, intussusception, rupture of an aneurism, typhoid or yellow fever, or vicarious menstruation.

Pus is discharged per anum in cases of dysenteric or other ulceration of the bowel; also when an abscess occurring in any part of the abdomen (most frequently hepatic) opens into the intestine. Pseudo-membranous discharges, shreds or other fragments of fibrinous material, appear sometimes in what may be called diphtheritic dysentery. Tubular casts are occasionally seen (diarrhoea tubularis), which, however, are most likely to consist of thickened and accumulated mucus. Fatty discharges from the bowels are rare. Authors report observation of them in cases of disease of the liver or pancreas, as well as in phthisis, typhoid fever, diabetes mellitus, cholera, and tubercular enteritis of children.

Lientery is the term applied when imperfectly changed food appears in the stools. It shows, of course, great deficiency in the process of digestion.

Urination affords symptoms often of extreme consequence in disease. Suppression of urine is one of the most alarming of signs; an approximation to it only is likely to be met with in cholera, a late stage of scarlet fever, typhus or typhoid fever, in acute yellow atrophy of the liver, and in advanced kidney disease. Careful examination of the abdomen, by inspection, palpation, and percussion, as well as by inquiry of attendants, is needful in all cases of fever or other disorders with delirium or stupor, to ascertain the presence or absence of retention of urine. Dysuria—*i.e.*difficult urination, strangury—may have several causes. Cantharides, absorbed from a blister, may produce it temporarily. The more continuous states which cause it are—stricture of the urethra, enlargement of the prostate gland, and calculus in the bladder. In stricture, when the patient can pass water, it is apt to be in a twisted stream. Dribbling often occurs when the prostate is enlarged. When a stone is present the [p. 165]stream may flow naturally for a time and then suddenly cease from obstruction at the outlet of the bladder. Enuresis, incontinence of urine, is often very troublesome in children; its diagnosis presents no difficulty.

Diabetes properly means simply excessive flow of urine. It may be attended by no change in the secretion except dilution of its solids (diabetes insipidus), as in certain nervous cases or after very large imbibition of fluids. More serious is diabetes mellitus, in which large amounts of sugar are found in the urine.

Variations in the quantity and in the composition and solid ingredients of the urine, as ascertained by aid of chemical analysis and the microscope, will be fully considered in other portions in this work.

Menstruation in the female requires scrutiny in every case of deviation from health. Its abnormities will be elsewhere treated of. The subject of the signs of pregnancy belongs of course to treatises on Obstetrics.

Pain is one of the most important of the signs of disease. We must always examine its character, location, and associations. As to character, that of pleurisy is sharp and cutting, increased by deep breathing or coughing. In pneumonia and in myalgia it is dull or aching. Rheumatic joints or muscles suffer a gnawing, tearing pain. In neuralgia it is darting, shooting, lancinating; and the last of these expressions is often applied to the pains of cancer. Griping pains occur in colic, and bearing-down pains in dysentery, as well as in the second stage of labor. Besides these varieties we have the pulsating pain of an acute external inflammation, as of the hand, especially before suppuration has occurred; the burning and smarting of erysipelas; and the stinging, nettling sensations (formication) of urticaria.

Tenderness on pressure is significant either of local inflammation, whose other signs are then to be discerned, or of non-inflammatory hyperæsthesia. The origin of the latter may require careful examination of various organs for its discovery. If pain is relieved by pressure, we may be sure of the absence of severe acute local inflammation.

Not infrequently the seat of disease may be at some distance from that of pain, as in the familiar instances of pain at the top of the head in uterine derangement; in the glans penis from calculus in the bladder; in the knee from hip-joint disease; under the shoulder-blade in liver disorder; about the heart or between the shoulders from dyspepsia.

Anæsthesia, loss of sensibility, has much value as a symptom in neurotic affections, as paralysis, etc. Its discussion will find place in connection with diseases of the Nervous System in other portions of this work.

As an example of the diversified associations of pain, cephalalgia (headache) may be mentioned as having at least the following possible causes: congestion of the brain, neuralgia, rheumatism of the scalp, uterine irritation, disease of the kidneys, early stage of remittent, typhoid, or yellow fever, alcoholic intoxication, chronic disease of the brain.

Abdominal pain may, in like manner, be traced, in different cases, to many morbid conditions, such as flatulent colic, lead colic, neuralgia or rheumatism of the bowels, intestinal obstruction, dysentery, passage of a gall-stone or of a nephritic calculus through one or the other duct[p. 166]respectively; cancer, aneurism of the aorta, caries of the spine; in the female, dysmenorrhoea, metralgia or ovaralgia—*i.e.* neuralgia of the uterus or ovaries.

Similar diversity in the origins of pain might, but for want of space, be pointed out in morbid states of the contents of the chest and of other parts of the body.

Subjective symptoms often affect the special senses.

Taste and touch have been already referred to. Of sight we may have photophobia, connected with exaggerated sensibility of the retina or of the brain; muscæ volitantes, specks, rings, or chains of spots from floating semi-opaque particles in the vitreous humor; diplopia, double vision; hemiopia, seeing only half of an object at a time; amblyopia, indistinctness of vision of all objects.

Hearing is affected, besides all possible degrees of deafness, with the subjective sensations of ringing, whistling, or roaring sounds—tinnitus aurium. One form of this (as I conclude from observation in my own ears) depends upon spasmodic vibration of the tensor tympani or stapedius muscle. Sometimes the seat of the sensation is in the auditory nervous apparatus proper. It has, not seldom, a marked connection with brain-exhaustion. An attack of Menière's disease (labyrinthine vertigo) is often preceded by it. No constant signification, however, can be attached to aural tinnitus. Large doses of quinine or of salicylic acid will occasion it in many patients.

Very briefly, deafness may be here disposed of by mentioning that, in greater or less degree, it may be produced by accumulated wax in the ear; obstruction of the Eustachian tube; thickness of the membrana tympani; perforation of that membrane; mucus or pus in the middle ear; disease of the ossicles of the ear; paralysis of the auditory nerve; typhus or typhoid fever; excessive doses of quinine or salicylic acid.

Vertigo is chiefly of two kinds, dizziness or giddiness (swimming in the head), and reeling vertigo, or a disposition to fall or turn to one side or the other. Giddiness is produced by running or whirling many times in a circle, or, in some persons, by swinging rapidly or sailing. Reeling vertigo is mostly observed in connection with disorder of the brain or of the labyrinth of the ear (Menière's disease). Dizziness, with nausea, is common as a symptom of cholæmia (cholesteræmia of Flint) in what is popularly called a bilious attack.

Delirium is present in many acute disorders, and not infrequently at a late stage in pulmonary phthisis. Its special study will be taken up in connection with the special articles upon these affections.

Coma, or stupor, is met with chiefly in the following morbid states: severe typhus or typhoid fevers; malignant scarlet fever; small-pox; rarely in measles; pernicious malarial fever; uræmia; apoplexy; opiate narcotism, or that from chloral or alcoholic intoxication; asphyxia from inhaling carbonic acid gas, ether, chloroform, etc.; fracture of the skull with compression of the brain.

For an account of aphasia and other morbid psychological manifestations the reader is referred to the articles on Aphasia, Insanity, Hysteria, etc. in this work.

Physical and Instrumental Diagnosis will be treated in connection with those diseases in which they have special importance.

[p. 167]

PROGNOSIS.

The elements of medical prognosis are essentially involved in diagnosis. Our ability to anticipate the mode of progress, duration, termination, and results of any case of illness depends upon our knowledge—1, of the nature of the malady, with its tendencies toward death, self-limitation, or indefinite continuance; 2, the soundness or imperfection of the patient's constitution, with or without special predispositions or the consequences of previous ailments; 3, the present state of his system as to the performance of the general functions, his strength, and vital resistance or persistence; 4, the probable modifying influences of medical treatment, and also those of situation, surroundings, and nursing— *i.e.* the care of those attending to the patient during the absence of the physician and having the duty of carrying out his directions.

1. As to the nature of the malady. While every sickness must be supposed to encroach somewhat upon the vital energy of its subject, very few diseases (leaving aside deadly poisons and surgical injuries) are, ab initio, certainly fatal. Hydrophobia (rabies canina) has been, until latterly, regarded as incurable, and always mortal within a few days or a week or two. A few cases have, during the last few years, been reported as cured, but the diagnosis of these continues to be somewhat doubtful.

Cancer exhibits a tendency to extend its destructive malnutrition so as to render death inevitable unless it can be removed early and completely, or unless the morbid process can be arrested in some manner not yet known. Remedies, such as condurango and Chian turpentine, which furnished hope of such an effect, have, after prolonged trial, been abandoned as not justifying the confidence of the profession.

Tubercular phthisis was once considered to be almost necessarily a fatal disease, although with a very indefinite period of duration. Under improved hygienic management, with mild palliatives and recuperative medication, a not inconsiderable minority of cases now end in recovery. This term may be properly applied when, with cicatrization of a cavity or cavities in the lungs, no more tubercle is deposited and lung-substance enough is left for good respiration, even although the structurally changed portions of pulmonary tissue do not undergo entire repair.

Tubercular meningitis is a nearly always incurable affection. Yet a few instances of lasting recovery have been reported where the diagnosis was as certain as it can be in that disease in the absence of post-mortem examination. A child attended by myself, in whom the symptoms had been of the most unfavorable kind, became apparently quite well, and continued so for a month. Then it was attacked suddenly with convulsions, which were almost unremitting until it died within a day or two.

Gangrene of the lung is very seldom recovered from, but, unless the diagnosis from examination of putrescent sputa has been at fault, there have been cases in which, with the limited destruction of the affected lung, it was not fatal.

Pseudo-membranous croup destroys life in the majority, but not in nearly all the cases of its occurrence. It is most likely to end in death when distinctly a part of an attack of epidemic or endemic diphtheria.

[p. 168]Valvular heart lesions were formerly regarded as incurable, in the sense of restoration of the normal condition and action of the valves impaired, yet not incompatible with years of life. This restoration certainly very seldom takes place. But the experience of many close observers leads to caution in anticipation of necessary and permanent disability of the heart because of murmurs, or even functional disturbances, seeming to prove either aortic or mitral insufficiency or stenosis.

Aneurism of the aorta is very seldom recovered from, but, besides a variable duration, whose period can almost never be anticipated with exactness, there appear to have been some cases of disappearance, or at least prolonged quiescence, of the tumor and of its morbid effects.

Yellow atrophy of the liver is one of the disorders most rarely ending otherwise than in death.

With a course altogether indefinite in time, there appears to be a tendency to exhaust vital energy, without self-limitation, in the different forms of organic degeneration, such as fatty heart, Addison's disease, chronic Bright's disease, diabetes mellitus, cirrhosis, and amyloid degeneration of the liver, etc. The same may be said also of the different forms of cerebral and spinal sclerosis, of pernicious anæmia, and of myxoedema.

Lastly, it is an exception to a very general rule of fatality when a case of trichinosis, with well-marked abdominal, muscular, and general symptoms, ends otherwise than in death within a few weeks.

Self-limitation is familiar in the natural history of typhus and typhoid fever, relapsing fever, yellow fever, cholera, diphtheria, whooping cough, mumps, small-pox, varicella, scarlet fever, and measles. In the sense of a definite duration of each paroxysm intermittent and remittent fevers are self-limited. Are they so also in tending toward recovery, without curative treatment within a certain time? This has been asserted, and in the case of remittent there is evidence that spontaneous cures do sometimes happen. Some observers aver that ague tends toward cessation of the chills after six, eight, or ten weeks. The obstinacy of the attacks in many instances under anti-periodic medication seems to make it probable that spontaneous recovery from intermittent hardly belongs to the typical natural history of the disease.

Whether the term self-limited can or cannot with propriety be applied to pneumonia and other acute inflammations, as pericarditis, etc., has been a mooted question. If it be so, it appears to the writer to be true in a different meaning of the word self-limitation from that in which it is applied to variola or typhoid fever. Yet some nosologists deny this distinction, and regard pneumonia as strictly a lung fever. Some of the facts supporting this view belong to the history of pneumonia as complicating malarial fever; *e.g.* in the winter fever of some parts of our Southern States. It must be admitted, however, that the inflammatory process, though morbid, is generally eliminative or corrective of a disturbing cause which produced it, and, unless that cause is continued or repeated in action, a limitation belongs to the succession of stages, ending either in resolution or in adhesions, serous accumulation, suppuration, or gangrene.

2. It is not necessary to dwell here upon the significance in prognosis of the patient's original constitution and hereditary or acquired[p. 169]predispositions, or on that of results left by previous attacks of illness. These are all obviously of importance. In a member of a family predisposed to consumption a bronchial attack following exposure may be much more dangerous than in others. So also a cause of mental agitation may produce insanity in a person who inherits a tendency thereto or who has before had an attack of mental derangement, while it would be innocuous to another who has no such proclivity. A second or third attack of delirium tremens is much more dangerous to life than a first attack. On the other hand, if yellow fever occurs at all in a patient who has before had it, the course of the disease is apt to be milder than usual. The most striking example of the influence of previous disease is seen in the comparative mildness of varioloid—*i.e.* small-pox modified by the system having been placed under the action of the vaccine virus.

3. Most important of all data in prognosis are, in most cases, the indications of the present state of the patient's system as to the performance of the organic functions, his sum of energy, and vital resistance and persistence. Especially must these indications be regarded comparatively; that is, ascertaining whether, in a period of weeks, days, or, sometimes hours (in malignant cholera even of minutes), the patient's general condition has been and is gaining or losing in the evidences of strength and healthy function of the great organs.

Every student of clinical medicine must become acquainted, as soon as possible, at the bedside, with these tokens and evidences, which make almost the alphabet of practice: What is a good, a doubtful, and a bad pulse? How does a patient breathe when moribund from simple exhaustion, and how does such respiration differ from the toil and struggle of asthma or the stertor of narcotism? Why does a glance suffice to make known to a surgeon the state of collapse after a railroad accident, or to a physician that of cholera or pernicious intermittent? What is the impression given to the finger upon the skin by intense fever, and what by the relaxation which precedes death? These and many other such questions are to be answered fully to each student only by the use of his own senses, with such interpretation as is to be obtained by the careful comparison of cases, with the aid of books and didactic instruction.

To a well-trained eye and hand a look and a touch will often suffice to make known the commencement of convalescence or of the precipitous decline toward death. Yet a wise physician will be very cautious in acting upon even seemingly obvious prognostications.

Changes may be going on in important organs whose effects have hardly yet begun to show themselves, and which may after a while materially alter the aspect of the case. Particularly near the beginning of an attack of enthetic disease, such as scarlet fever, small-pox, typhus or typhoid fever, the physician should beware of too confidently forecasting the progress of the case for better or for worse. In nothing, probably, is the prudence of a practitioner more often or more severely tested than in his answers to inquiries made concerning prognosis.

4. Anticipation of the modifying action of remedies is undoubtedly a proper factor in our estimate of the probable result of any case of illness. Few diseases, however, are as yet so subject to control by specific medication as to allow certainty in such expectations. In a first attack of ague we may look with much confidence toward the speedy cure of our[p. 170]patient under quinia. In one who has had chills all winter even this confidence may need qualification. A sufferer with syphilitic rheumatism may generally be promised relief under the use of iodide of potassium, or one afflicted with scabies under the application of sulphur ointment. We seldom have misgivings about our ability to give relief in colic, constipation, or diarrhoea. Yet the first two of these may prove to be symptoms of intestinal obstruction resisting treatment, and the last may depend upon chronic ulceration of the bowel, giving it unexpected continuance. In all such instances careful and (when practicable) accurate diagnosis must precede prognosis; our estimate of the action of remedies becomes then a secondary, although often a valuable, part of the calculation of the probabilities of the case.

Prognosis in particular diseases involves the consideration not only of those signs of the general vital condition to which we have just been giving attention, but also of such as are more or less peculiar to each disorder. To a certain extent these signs may be grouped. We may refer to good and bad signs in pulmonary, cardiac, intestinal, renal, cerebral, and febrile affections respectively. Still, there will be for each malady, if it really has a distinctive character, some tokens which experience shows to be specially indicative of favorable or unfavorable progress and results.

Let us notice some of these as examples.

In pneumonia the best signs are the lowering of a high temperature, reduction of the number of respirations to 20 or 25 in the minute, expectoration of sputa less and less tinged with red or brown, and gradual reduction of the region of dulness on percussion. Worst, in the same disease, are an axillary temperature over 106°, respirations 40 or more per minute, with delirium, and expectoration becoming more abundant, grayish, and purulent; also with continued dulness on percussion and abundant mucous râles on auscultation.

In croup the best sign is, after a hoarse, dry, barking cough and dyspnoea, a soft, liquid râle, heard in the larynx and trachea during respiration or coughing. Worst, in croup, is a steadily or paroxysmally increasing difficulty of breathing, with a dry hissing or whistling sound of respiration and cough succeeding the barking sounds of the earlier stage.

In phthisis pulmonalis among the best signs are the patient's increasing in weight, coughing and expectorating less, ceasing to have hectic and night sweats. These may give renewed hope, even before much change is discernible in the physical signs. Of bad omen are intense hectic fever, incessant cough with abundant nummular sputa, copious perspirations, diarrhoea, breathing growing shorter and shorter, and extreme emaciation and debility.

In all organic affections of the heart an extremely rapid and irregular pulse, with orthopnoea and increasing anasarca, and especially the Cheyne-Stokes respiration (described under DIAGNOSIS), must cause unfavorable expectations.

In obstruction of the bowels the best of all symptoms is, usually, of course, a copious fecal evacuation. Yet a few cases have occurred in which a very large evacuation, delayed by obstruction for a week or two, has been almost immediately followed by collapse and death. The worst signs in cases of obstruction are (besides long-unyielding constipation)[p. 171]stercoraceous vomiting, a small, rapid pulse, and increasing coldness and clamminess of the surface of the body.

In cholera infantum the best signs are cessation of vomiting and purging, the discharges growing more nearly natural, the face becoming less shrunken in aspect, sleep taking the place of coma vigil or waking apathy, and water or milk, when taken, remaining on the stomach. Worst, in the same disease, are incessant rejection of everything swallowed, watery passages from the bowels every half hour or hour, shrinking of the face and body to skin and bone, with an apathetic expression of the open or half-open eyes, the latter rolling often from side to side.

In epidemic cholera good signs are the arrest of vomiting and of rice-water discharges from the bowels, rapid movement of the blood in the veins after removal of momentary pressure, return of natural color and warmth to the skin, with filling up of the pulse at the wrist. Bad signs in cholera are shrinking of the cheeks and of the flesh upon the hands, deepening ashiness or blueness of the skin, coldness and clamminess to the touch, dyspnoea, loss of pulse, incessant vomiting and purging of rice-water stools, constant cramps of the limbs, and suppression of urine.

In acute cerebral meningitis good signs are lessened temperature of the head, quiet sleep without stertor, disappearance of delirium, more natural pulse, and attention to surrounding objects, without disquietude. Bad signs in the same disease are deep stupor, strabismus, convulsions, paralysis, involuntary defecation and urination.

In typhus fever good signs are the pulse becoming slower and fuller, the skin less hot, more soft and moist, the tongue moist and clean, the face losing its dusky flush, and consciousness returning instead of muttering delirium.[40] Bad, in the same fever, are deepening of the flush of the countenance, profound stupor, rapid and feeble pulse, lying on the back and sinking down toward the foot of the bed, with suppression of urine.

[40] Incidentally, it may be mentioned that the return of the pulse to its normal rate is often considerably delayed in convalescence from typhus and typhoid fevers and other protracted diseases. If, then, the temperature is not above 99° F., and is stable from morning to night, the tongue is clean and moist, and appetite begins to appear, we need not be alarmed, although the pulse continues as high as 90 or 100 per minute, in a case attended by positive debility.

In typhoid fever many of the good and bad signs are the same as in typhus, belonging to closely similar general conditions. But in typhoid fever we observe also as favorable signs the lessening of tympanites, more nearly natural fecal stools, and the absence of tenderness in any part of the abdomen. As unfavorable, increase of tympanites and diarrhoea, sometimes large hemorrhages from the bowels; worst of all, at a late stage, sudden increase of abdominal distension, with dulness on percussion, coldness of the skin, great rapidity and feebleness of the pulse following perforation of the bowel, resulting usually in fatal peritonitis.

In scarlet fever, measles, and small-pox it is a favorable sign for the eruption to come out well at the usual time; its sudden recession threatens malignancy. In small-pox a confluent eruption marks a dangerous case, and so does the occurrence of distinct pustules in the throat. Early in scarlet fever stupor is very threatening, though not necessarily mortal. Late in the same disease bloody urine, or, worse yet, suppression of urine, may well cause alarm.

In all children's diseases the early occurrence of convulsions shows a[p. 172]severe but not always a dangerous attack. The late occurrence of convulsions is commonly much more serious in its significance.[41]Convulsions are always of vastly less importance, prognostically, in children than in adolescents or adults. Yet they are always serious signs. While recovered from in the large majority of cases, they may at any time be fatal.

[41] Yet I saw a case of acute cerebro-meningitis, in a girl ten years of age, in which a violent convulsion occurred on about the sixth day of the disease, and was followed by convalescence.

These enumerations, selected as examples merely, might be much farther extended but that the special prognosis of each disease will be fully set forth in the several articles upon them in the body of this work. Those now given may suffice for the illustration of the method and general principles by which the physician must be guided in his anticipation of the progress and result of cases of disease. The caution may be repeated, to observe great care in forming a conclusion in regard to prognosis in every instance, and still more in expressing it, unless in the presence of very clear and positive evidence.

[p. 173]

HYGIENE.
BY JOHN S. BILLINGS, M.D.

The purpose of this paper is to indicate some of the ways in which hygiene, both private and public, is connected with the duties of the general practitioner, and to give some information as to modern methods of investigation and work in preventive medicine.

While the business of the physician is more especially the care of the sick with reference to the cure of disease, or, where that is beyond his power, as is too frequently the case, to relieve suffering and secure temporary ease for his patient, he is nevertheless often called upon to answer questions as to the causes of disease, and the best means of avoiding or destroying these causes. Not only does diagnosis often turn upon considerations of etiology, but a very considerable part of the treatment of actual disease must be hygienic in the broader sense of the word. The prescription or the surgical operation must not only be supplemented by advice as to residence, clothing, food, exercise, etc., but must, in many cases, be merely supplementary to such advice, which indicates the really essential method of treatment; and the giving this advice then becomes the most important part of the physician's work, although not usually recognized as such by his patients. The chief value of the prescription is, in fact, often to methodize the mode of life of the patient and to remind him at frequently recurring intervals of the regimen which has been ordered with it.

The physician has also certain duties in relation to the public at large, as well as to his individual patients, and these duties become more numerous and important as the density of population increases, so that in the large cities of most civilized countries he finds himself, nolens volens, in almost daily contact with legally constituted authorities in the shape of registrars, health officers, coroners, etc., and is not infrequently summoned before the courts as a supposed expert in matters connected with the public health.

Moreover, the physician who has become eminent in his profession is, in many cases the adviser, and, so far as professional subjects are concerned, to a great extent the guide, of those who legislate for, or execute the laws of, not only his own city or county, but his state and the nation; and he must to a corresponding degree be held responsible for the position which he takes and the advice which he gives in regard to public health matters. This is true whether his attitude on these subjects [p. 174]be active or passive, for his silence will be taken to mean that there is no necessity for action or change.

The limits of this paper do not permit the presentation of proofs and illustrations of these somewhat dogmatic assertions, but it is believed that they will meet with general assent from medical men without formal and detailed argument, and that it is unnecessary here to urge the interest or importance of practical hygiene upon the medical profession, or to enlarge upon the desirability that the practitioner, as well as the professional sanitarian, should be familiar with the conclusions of modern science and technology with regard to it.

In the minds of many intelligent and thoughtful physicians there is, no doubt, a feeling of unformulated distrust as to the real possibilities or probabilities of improving the health and diminishing the mortality of the community at large; and this feeling is in part due to the exaggerated claims and emotional exhortations of some advocates of hygiene. A careful and unprejudiced survey of what has been accomplished by sanitary measures will, however, largely dissipate this distrust.

The natural term of the life of man is fixed by the physiologist at about one hundred years, which is nearly in accordance with the law indicated by Flourens, that the period of life of an animal is about five times that required to perfect the development of its skeleton and unite the epiphyses with the shafts of the long bones. The actual average duration of human life is less than half this, but there is satisfactory evidence that it has increased in civilized countries. The ancient estimate is expressed in David's declaration, that "the days of a man are threescore years and ten, and if by reason of strength they be fourscore years, yet is their strength labor and sorrow." Kolb, a cautious and learned statistician, concluded, from his studies, that while the maximum age reached by man has not materially changed for many centuries, the number of persons who now survive infancy and of those who reach a ripe old age has decidedly increased; and this opinion is sustained by Mr. Lewis, the secretary of the Chamber of Life Insurance of New York, who points out that while civilization largely interferes with the laws of evolution by survivorship, it aids by economizing the waste which occurs in its absence. "Under natural selection, when variations in capacity arise, thousands of them are wasted where one is secured, fixed, and transmitted. But human society economizes much of this waste, fastens upon and improves an immensely larger proportion of the capacities lavishly produced by Nature, and thus concentrates forces which would otherwise spread their operation over countless ages."[1]

[1] "Influence of Civilization on the Duration of Life," *Reports Am. Pub. Health Ass'n*, N.Y., 1877, vol. iii. p. 173.

We have, however, no record of the duration of life in ancient Greece and Rome, and it is quite possible that it was greater than in Western Europe during the Middle Ages, which formed a period of retrogression in a sanitary point of view. The Jew, the Greek, and the Roman, prior to the Christian era, were probably cleaner in person and in dwellings than the people of the time when dirt became the odor of sanctity.

In the absence of reliable data for this country, it is impossible to speak with certainty of the results of attempts made here to prevent disease and death. Each sex, race, and age has its own rate of mortality, [p. 175]and until this rate is determined we can only guess as to whether good work is being done or not.

We can never hope to diminish the total number of deaths which will occur in long periods, say two hundred years, but we may rationally try to prolong the average duration of life, to diminish infant mortality, and to secure greater comfort and better health for individuals and for the community at large.

The reader must remember that only a mere outline of the subject can be presented here; the details would require several volumes, and the tendency to specialization in this, as in other branches, is so great that it is hardly to be expected that any one man shall have either the theoretical or the practical knowledge necessary for covering the entire field. There are certain things in relation to hygiene which every physician should know; there are many other things with regard to which it is sufficient if he knows where to find full and reliable information when he needs it. With this preface we will pass at once to our subject, which may be conveniently divided as follows:

Causes of disease, means of discovery, and prevention.

I. Personal hygiene in its relations to the practice of medicine.

II. Public hygiene in its relations to physicians.

I. Causes of Disease, Means of Discovery, and Prevention.

Although the origin of disease has from the earliest times been the subject of study by medical men, the physician has not heretofore, usually, been called upon to investigate the causes of disease in particular localities, until the occurrence of sickness in that locality has called attention to the matter. The education of the public as to the importance of sanitary work has, however, recently made great progress, and it is now not unusual to ask the opinion of the family physician as to the healthfulness of a given locality or house. The question may be presented in three different ways: First. In a given case of disease, what is the probable cause? Second. Given the presence of a known or suspected cause of disease, what are the best means of avoiding or destroying it? Third. In the absence of cases of disease, to determine whether causes of disease are probably present, and if so, what causes.

The word "cause" is here used in its widest sense, including not only what are commonly called predisposing and exciting causes, but also those conditions which aggravate or continue the disease. These causes may be roughly classed as follows: Heredity; impure air; impure water; climate; habitations; occupation; food; intemperance of various kinds; clothing; errors in exercise; sexual errors; parasites; contagia; expectant attention and other mental causes, including worry, etc. In most cases two or more of these classes of causes are combined in action for the production of a given case or outbreak of disease, and when we refer any disease to a single factor, what is meant usually is, not that this is the sole and exclusive cause, but that it is the most prominent one.

Bearing this in mind, let us consider briefly some of the causes above mentioned.

I. HEREDITY.—That the child inherits from its parents its physical [p. 176]type, including color, stature, physiognomy, temperament, and certain peculiarities of structure or arrangement of internal organs, is well known. This hereditary influence is stronger from the immediate than from the remote ancestry, although the curious phenomena of atavism sometimes form exceptions to this rule. The hereditary causes of disease can be guarded against when known. Theoretically, by preventing generation on the part of persons who are unfit to produce offspring; practically, to a certain extent, by taking special precautions against these causes and their effects in the individual, particularly at those ages in which these influences seem to have their greatest force. The most important of these hereditary diseases are syphilis, consumption, scrofula, cancer, gout, certain skin diseases, insanity, and criminal tendencies of various kinds.

The physician's advice is rarely asked with regard to the propriety, from a sanitary point of view, of a proposed marriage, nor is it often taken when given, unless, indeed, it happens to correspond with the wishes of the recipient; nevertheless, he is occasionally in a position to exert influence in such a matter, and when this is the case the following general rules may be borne in mind: 1. No marriage should occur between persons having the same hereditary tendency to disease; and this is especially important in marriages between relatives. 2. A girl should not marry under the age of twenty. 3. A person affected with hereditary or well-marked constitutional syphilis, or having a strong consumptive taint, or tendency to mental unsoundness, should not marry at all.

The precautions to be taken in individual cases in which there is a known hereditary predisposition to certain diseases will probably be indicated in the articles upon those special diseases. The most important of these, from the sanitary point of view, are consumption and gout, partly because of their frequency, partly because of the undoubted power which a proper regimen, applied in time, has in controlling them. The pain in gout has often an excellent sanitary effect; it is an inducement to temperance much stronger than any amount of good advice.

The influence of heredity in producing abnormities of refraction and accommodation of the eye, and the importance of detecting these early and giving them proper treatment, have not hitherto received, from the general practitioner, the attention which they deserve. Children of parents affected with astigmatism, ametropia, etc. should be carefully examined before being placed at school, and if necessary fitted with proper glasses.

The heredity of idiosyncrasies as to certain articles of food or certain drugs must also be borne in mind by the physician, for, although implicit confidence is not always to be placed in the statement of a patient that he cannot take a certain medicine, yet a knowledge of the facts will occasionally save the prescriber from some awkward mistakes.

The importance of bearing in mind the family peculiarities is best appreciated by the old family doctor who has had two or three generations pass under his hands: he knows, for example, that in one family he may expect brain complications, in another lung troubles, and that what would be grave symptoms in one house are of comparatively small import in another. Unfortunately, the greater part of this kind of knowledge has not yet been formulated, and each physician has to acquire it for himself; but he will find the process of acquisition greatly facilitated if in all cases in a new family he makes it a rule to learn something of the medical [p. 177]history of the parents, and he will find intelligent laymen quick to appreciate his inquiries in this direction.

The importance of taking into account hereditary influences is well illustrated by the care which is taken to obtain information with regard to them in well-conducted life insurance companies. The medical examiners of such companies have their attention specially called to this matter, and the following extract from a manual of instructions shows how it is regarded from a business point of view: "If consumption is found to have occurred in the family of the applicant, he is to be regarded not insurable under the following circumstances, viz.:

	YEARS OF AGE.
If in both parents, not insurable until	40
If in one parent, not insurable until (Except for ten-year endowments, then 20 years.)	30
If in two members (not parents)	35
If in one member (brother or sister) (Except for ten-year endowments, when peculiarly favorable.)"	20

If apoplexy, paralysis, or heart disease is found to have occurred in any two members of the applicant's family, he is to be regarded as insurable only upon the endowment plan, the term of insurance to expire prior to his reaching the age of fifty years. If insanity shall have so occurred (in two members), a provisionary clause is essential, and is attached to the policy by the company.

II. IMPURE AIR.—The dangers of impure air, water, and food depend largely upon the fact that through these media may be introduced into the body particles of organic matter, living or dead, which tend to produce disease in the recipient. The parasites are types of this mode of disease-production, and these blend with the contagia of the specific diseases in such a way that it is not easy to draw the distinction in all cases. There are also certain poisonous gases and inorganic compounds which may occasionally be present in air or water to such an extent as to produce disease; but as a rule the gaseous impurities of the air are offensive to the smell rather than dangerous, as will be seen when we come to consider the effluvium nuisances.

The subject of ventilation, for the purpose of procuring an adequate supply of pure air, is one of so much importance, and one upon which the physician is so liable to be called for practical advice, that it seems proper to state briefly the general principles which should govern investigations into, or recommendations upon, this subject.

The impurities of air which are to be disposed of by ventilation are for the most part derived from the human body, chiefly from respiration, and these only will be considered here. In some cases it is necessary to make special provision for the products of combustion from gas, etc., but as a rule this is rather for the purpose of regulation of temperature than anything else. The impurities of air due to the presence of human beings consist mainly of carbonic acid, ammonia, sulphuretted hydrogen, and sulphide of ammonium, and of various organic compounds, mostly in the form of minute particles of organic matter of uncertain structure, but extremely prone to decomposition. It is usual to estimate the degree of impurity by the amount of carbonic acid present, and this leads many persons to suppose that the carbonic acid is in itself the chief and most dangerous impurity. This gas is, however, not perceptible to the senses,[p. 178]nor is it injurious to health, unless present in much greater proportion than that in which it will be found in the most crowded habitations or assembly-rooms. Its importance in questions of ventilation depends upon the fact that its increase in a room beyond the amount present in the outer air may usually be taken to be in direct proportion to the amount of the really dangerous and offensive impurities present, and that the amount of carbonic acid can be ascertained by chemical tests with comparative ease and rapidity; which is not the case with regard to the organic matter. The carbonic acid is therefore taken as the measure of the impurity, although it is not itself the impurity of which we are most anxious to be free.

To decide as to whether a room is well ventilated or not, some standard of permissible impurity must be fixed, and this standard is now usually taken to be, in a room occupied by human beings, that condition of air which produces in a person having a normal sense of smell, and who enters from the fresh air, a faint sensation of an odor very slightly musty and unpleasant. Upon testing the air of such a room, it will be found that the amount of carbonic acid impurity present—that is, the excess of this acid over the amount in the external air—will be between 2 and 3 parts in 10,000.

As the amount of carbonic acid in normal air varies from 2 to 5 parts in 10,000 in different places, and in the same place at different times, it is better to look to the carbonic acid impurity as above defined rather than to the total amount of the acid found present, if strict accuracy is desired; but usually the statement of Dr. Parkes is correct, that the organic impurity of the air is not perceptible to the senses until the total carbonic acid rises to the proportion of 6 parts in 10,000 volumes. When the carbonic acid reaches 9 parts in 10,000 the air is close, and when it exceeds 1 part in 1000 the air is usually decidedly unpleasant. If we take 2 parts in 10,000 as the permissible maximum of carbonic acid impurity, it follows that the amount of fresh air which must be supplied and thoroughly distributed for each person per hour is 3000 cubic feet. If 3 parts per 10,000 be taken as the permissible maximum (which is the standard of Pettenkofer), the amount of air per head per hour must be 2000 cubic feet. While it is impossible, as Dr. Parkes remarks, to show by direct evidence that the impurity indicated by 7, 8, or even 10, parts of carbonic acid per 10,000 is injurious to health, it is advisable to accept his standard, because it is a simple one, and can be practically applied without special apparatus or technical skill, and because there is evidence of the injury to health which continued exposure to air impure, by this standard, ultimately produces.

Keeping this standard in view, the physician may be called on for an opinion as to whether the ventilation of a given building is satisfactory or as to the merits of a proposed plan for ventilation. The first is a question of fact: What are the effects produced upon the inmates? Are there unpleasant odors in the building or not? What percentage of carbonic impurity is present? What is the number of cubic feet of air per head that is introduced and removed per hour? And what is the character of the fresh-air supply as to purity? Does it come from the cellar, or from other rooms, or from a foul area? Air-currents can usually be best investigated by the fumes of nascent muriate of ammonia produced by [p. 179]exposing a cylinder of common blotting-paper, moistened with dilute hydrochloric acid, to the vapors coming from a crumpled fragment of the same paper moistened with common aqua ammonia and placed within the cylinder. The process for carbonic acid determination is simple, and can be learned in three hours in a laboratory under a skilful teacher. It does not seem worth while to describe it here. The determination of the amount of air passing through a given register, flue, or chimney in a given time is to be made by the use of an anemometer, an instrument which registers the velocity of the current of air passing through it.

In judging of the merits of a plan of ventilation the following points should be remembered: The defect in most plans for ventilation is in the air-supply. Many people suppose that they have made all necessary provision for ventilation if they have put in tubes or openings for the escape of foul air, forgetting that these outlets will have no effect if corresponding inlets are not provided. Examine, first of all, therefore, the ducts, flues, and openings proposed for the fresh-air supply, with reference to their size and position and the amount of air to be furnished by them. These will almost invariably be found to be too small. The proper size of flues and registers for a given room is ascertained by dividing the number of cubic feet of air to be supplied per second by the velocity in feet per second which the air is to have in the flue or opening, bearing in mind that it is much better that these flues and registers shall be too large than too small, since it is easy to reduce their capacity, but, in most cases, impossible to increase it. When the fresh-air register is so situated that the current of air from it is liable to strike upon the person of an occupant of the room, the velocity of this current should not exceed 1½ feet per second if unpleasant draughts are to be avoided; and it will usually be found best that the velocity of the air in the flue shall not exceed 6 feet per second, except in the case of very large flues, where the element of friction becomes of comparatively small importance. In the great majority of cases the amount of air to be supplied depends upon the number of persons, and not on the cubic space; but in exceptional instances, where the amount of cubic space is very large in proportion to the number of persons, and the heating is effected by warm air, it may require more air to keep the room at a comfortable temperature than is necessary for the supply of the occupants. The cubic space is also relatively much more important in rooms which are to be occupied but a short time continuously, and can then be thoroughly aired, than it is in rooms constantly occupied.

The methods of calculation can be best illustrated by one or two examples. What should be the number and size of flues and registers for fresh-air supply for a hospital ward to contain 24 beds, the ward being a rectangular pavilion with windows on opposite sides? In this case the room is constantly occupied, and the supply of air should be 1 cubic foot per head per second, or, in all, 24 cubic feet per second. The velocity of current at the registers should not exceed 3 feet per second—better only 2. This will require from 8 to 12 square feet of clear opening in the registers. If we allow four on each side of the room, each register must have at least 1 square foot of clear opening. The velocity of the air in the flues supplying these registers should not exceed 4 feet per second, and therefore the area of each flue should be about 9 by 12 [p. 180]inches. Suppose the same question be asked with regard to a school-room to contain 48 pupils. In this case the room will not be occupied more than two hours at a time. The air-supply desirable may be put down at 35 cubic feet per head per minute, or 28 cubic feet per second for the whole. The velocity in the flues may be put, as before, at 4 feet per second; hence we need 7 square feet area of flue, or seven flues, each having 1 square foot of area. It is safe to say that there are not twenty school-houses in the United States which have fresh-air flues of sufficient area; the deficiency is made up, for the most part, by leakage of the outer air through cracks around windows and directly through the wall, and also by the passage of air from the central hall into the room, this last air coming from the cellar or basement.

The velocity of the air at the foul-air registers and in the foul-air ducts may be greater than in the fresh-air flues, since there is no danger of its causing draughts, and hence there is no truth in the common notion that the outlets should be larger than the inlets to allow for the expansion of heated air. It is important that the velocity of the current in the outlet shaft or chimney should be at least 8 feet per second at the point where it escapes into the outer air; and if the outlets be too large for the inlets, the result may be that some of the foul-air flues will work backward and become inlets. The plan of making everything a little larger than is necessary is not a safe one as regards chimney-flues and outlet shafts.

The merits of a plan of ventilation depend not only on the amount of air introduced, but on its distribution. The test for distribution is chemical analysis of samples taken in different parts of the room and at different levels. A very good idea of the direction taken by the incoming air can also be obtained by the use of fumes of nascent muriate of ammonia, as above described. In considering the distribution which will probably take place in a given plan, care should be taken not to fall into the common error of supposing that because pure carbonic acid gas is heavier than air, therefore the carbonic acid derived from respiration sinks to the floor, and that special provision should be made to remove it at that point. The law of the diffusion of gases effectually prevents this separation and sinking of the carbonic acid from the mixture of gases expired, and it will be found to be present in about equal proportions in all parts of an inhabited room.

The methods of introducing and distributing fresh air depend to a great extent upon the methods of heating employed; and it is necessary to remember that while good ventilation is a very desirable thing, satisfactory heating is, in cold weather, still more desirable, and must be attained even if the ventilation is interfered with for that purpose. The principal difficulty in the way of securing good ventilation is its cost. In a cold climate satisfactory heating, good ventilation, and cheapness are not compatible; it is comparatively easy to obtain any two of them, but impossible to have the three together. This fact should be fully understood and realized by the physician, for its comprehension will save much time in considering the merits of various patent ventilators and ventilating appliances, which, according to their inventors, produce good ventilation at no expense beyond that of the original cost of the apparatus; which is practically about the same as a claim to have discovered perpetual motion. Patent ventilators are usually cowls to be placed upon the top of outlet[p. 181]flues. I know of none which are superior to the common Emerson Ventilator, on which there is now no patent. In cold weather the air must be warmed to secure comfort; it must be changed to secure ventilation. The changing of the air carries off heat, the loss of which must be supplied by fuel, which fuel costs money. The greater the ventilation, the more rapid the change and the more heat required. It is therefore quite possible to judge somewhat of the merits of a heating and ventilating apparatus—for example, of a school-house—from the amount of fuel consumed; but the conclusion will be precisely the reverse of that drawn by the average trustee, since it will be, that within certain limits the less fuel required the less satisfactory the apparatus.

The evil effects of insufficient ventilation, although very certain and very serious, are not immediate, or such as to attract attention at first, except in very aggravated cases with excessive over-crowding. The power of the organism to adjust itself to surrounding circumstances is very great, and perhaps as great in regard to the endurance of foul air as anything else. Yet this power is greater in seeming than in reality, for at last such air produces disease and shortens life. Its effects are manifested in diseases of the respiratory organs, acute and chronic, and it is now generally admitted that the undue prevalence of phthisis in troops is due to the foul air of the barrack-rooms.

Some persons are much more susceptible than others to the effects of impure air, and will suffer from headache, languor, loss of appetite, etc. where others would experience little inconvenience. Children thus susceptible dread the school-room as ordinarily constructed and ventilated, and their discomfort should be taken into account and guarded against.

Thus far, reference has been made only to those impurities of air due to respiration and lights; in other words, the necessary impurities found in human habitations. The impurities due to sewer gases will be referred to hereafter; they should be prevented absolutely, and not provided for by ventilation. One of the most difficult problems presented to the physician is to determine whether the effluvia from a given locality are injurious to health, and if so, to what extent. These effluvia may be due to certain occupations or manufactures, or they may result from the disposal of excreta, from obstructed drainage giving rise to swamps and the collection of decaying organic matter, and in other ways. The best definition of the term "injurious to health" in this connection is perhaps that suggested by Dr. Ballard—*i.e.* that exposure to the offensive effluvia causes bodily discomfort or other functional disturbance, continuing or recurring as the exposure continues or recurs, and tending by continuance or repetition to create an appreciable impairment of general health and strength, to render those exposed more liable than others to attacks of disease, and more apt to suffer severely when attacked, and, in the more serious forms, to the direct production of the disease and the shortening of life.

The group of symptoms due to offensive effluvia is, as Dr. Ballard remarks, a tolerably constant one, and consists of loss of appetite, nausea, headache, giddiness, faintness, and a general sense of depression, with, in some cases, vomiting and diarrhoea. But it is usually impossible to prove by statistics that these phenomena are due to a given effluvium complained of, for those who suffer from it are usually exposed to other causes of ill-health, such as poverty, overcrowding, collection of filth, etc.; and, on the [p. 182]other hand, many of those exposed to the effluvium seem to suffer very little, if at all, from their surroundings. And so true is this, that in the carefully prepared report upon effluvium nuisances recently issued by Dr. Ballard,[2] it will be found that as a rule no attempt is made to prove that the effluvia from any particular branch of industry are injurious to health; the test practically applied is that they produce offensive odors.

[2] *Report in respect of the Inquiry as to Effluvium Nuisances arising in connection with various Manufacturing and other branches of Industry.* By Dr. Ballard, London. Her Majesty's Stationery Office, 1882, 8vo.

The legal view of this subject is given in the various decisions as to what should be considered a nuisance, the essence of which is the use of one's own property in such a way as to inflict damage upon, and injure the rights of, another. If a man collects on his own premises, for his own use, any material, such as water or filth, he is bound to retain it within his own premises or to let none of it escape in such a way as to damage others; and this holds good as regards gases, vapors, and odors. The decision of Mansfield, in the case of Rex *vs.* White, is often quoted approvingly by jurists, viz.: "It is not necessary that the smell be unwholesome; it is enough if it renders the enjoyment of life uncomfortable." But, practically, the question as to whether the discomfort produced is sufficient to produce ill-health will be the one upon which the physician is called to give evidence, and the one also upon which he will find it most difficult to obtain data sufficient to enable him to form a positive opinion.

III. IMPURE WATER.—Of all the various preventable or removable causes of disease to which the attention of the physician engaged in practice in the small towns and rural districts is directed, it will usually be found that the water-supply is the most important, because it is in these localities that it is most liable to become contaminated in such a way as to produce sickness.

All water used for drinking purposes is impure in the chemical sense, since it contains some inorganic matters or salts, and in most cases organic matter also. It is difficult to define precisely what should be considered an impure water in a sanitary sense, and the best we can do is to indicate probabilities in the absence of positive evidence of the production of disease by the suspected water. So far as inorganic impurities are concerned, the most important, from the sanitary point of view, are the salts of lead, magnesia, and lime, but in this country these are so rarely the cause of disease that they hardly require special notice. The physician should, however, bear in mind possibilities of lead-poisoning in some obscure cases which he will meet.

The diseases due to impure water are certain specific fevers, diarrhoeal diseases, and some affections due to parasites which find entrance to the body through this medium. The water-supply is to be suspected in case of prevalence of diarrhoeal disease in a community, and especially if the outbreak is sudden and affect a number of persons and families. Sudden outbreaks of cholera, typhoid fever, or malarial fever, confined to a limited locality, should lead to careful examination of the water-supply. The impurity in water which causes these diseases is supposed to be either organic or the product of organic life, and at present the prevailing opinion is that the really dangerous impurities consist of minute living organisms or [p. 183]germs. It is usual to estimate the impurity of water by the amount of organic matter present, but it is evident that this alone can give no positive information, since by this standard milk and soup would be very dangerous. Much depends upon the character of the organic matter, whether it is derived from the animal or vegetable kingdom—whether it is in a state of fermentation or putrefaction, etc. etc.; but the presence of specific germs in it is the most important part of all, and at the same time the most difficult to ascertain. Nitrogenous organic matter in a state of decomposition is dangerous, yet it does not always produce disease, even when ingested in comparatively large quantity, as in case of "high" game or tainted meat; and it is easy to find instances where water strongly polluted with sewage has been used for a considerable period without producing marked ill effects. It is, however, so extremely probable as to be for practical purposes certain, that water contaminated with the discharges from persons suffering from certain diseases will produce similar diseases in those who drink it, and there is also enough evidence that water containing filth of various kinds either produces or promotes disease to warrant much more attention to this subject than has heretofore been bestowed upon it.

The chemical examination of a suspected water is by no means a simple process, and in most cases had better be referred to an expert in such matters. It is highly desirable, however, that the physician should have sufficient technical knowledge to be able to make a rough analysis at least, if for no other reason than that he may be able to appreciate the results reported by the chemist. As a rule, when a water is so polluted with decomposing organic matter as to be positively dangerous it will have an unpleasant odor, which is best developed by half filling a quart bottle with the water to be examined and shaking it thoroughly. The so-called simple and ready methods which are from time to time advocated in the newspapers, such as the addition of sugar to the suspected water and allowing fermentation to take place, the use of tannin as a precipitant, or the decolorization of a solution of potassium permanganate, are really of very little value and should not be relied upon. In the hands of an expert the best simple method of determining the quality of a water is by evaporation of a known quantity and the ignition of the solid residue. From the amount of the total residue, the quantity left after ignition, the amount of blackening produced, and the odor, a very fair opinion can be formed as to the amount of organic matter present, and whether it is of animal or vegetable origin.

It is not within the province of this paper to describe the methods used by chemists in water analysis, of which the principal are known as the Franklin and Armstrong, the Wanklyn, and the permanganate methods. A careful examination of these methods has recently been made under the direction of the National Board of Health, and a preliminary note of the results, prepared by Professor Mallet, has been published in the *Bulletin*. From this it appears that the chief value of chemical analysis is, first, the verification of gross pollution, which will usually be detected by the appearance and smell of the water; and, second, in periodical examination of a water-supply to detect changes from the normal or usual character of the water, which may be taken to have a certain local standard of purity. Special importance is attached to the careful determination of [p. 184]nitrates and nitrites in water to be used for drinking, these being the results of oxidation of organic matters, and therefore giving evidence of previous contamination.

Prof. Mallet concludes that "there are no sound grounds on which to establish such general standards of purity as have been proposed, looking to exact amounts of organic carbon or nitrogen, albuminoid ammonia, oxygen of permanganate consumed, etc., as permissible or not. Distinctions drawn by the application of such standards are arbitrary and may be misleading." While this is perfectly true, considered from the standpoint of scientific precision, it does not sufficiently take into account the value of probabilities in these matters, considered as motives to action. It is perfectly true that there can be no fixed standard—that a water which the chemist would report as relatively pure might be much more apt to produce disease than one which he would pronounce impure—but it is nevertheless true that from the results of chemical analysis, taken in connection with evidence as to the source and history of the water, an opinion can be formed as to the danger from its use which is sufficiently reliable to be acted upon in the absence of positive evidence, such as the production of disease.

In many cases the matter must be doubtful, and Prof. Mallet truly says that it will not do in all such cases to forbid the use of the water, for it often happens that this should not be done unless it is absolutely necessary; but there are many other cases in which there is very little doubt, and where action should be governed by the probabilities.

The microscopical examination of suspected waters sometimes gives decided indication as to the nature of the impurities; and it may be that hereafter, in connection with physiological tests, it will become of even more importance than the chemical. To determine the presence of organisms in a sample of water the best method known at present is to kill and coagulate them by means of osmic acid or chloride of platinum, and allow them to subside. This method is of course inapplicable if it be desired to use them for either culture- or inoculation-tests.

Chemists have no uniform system of reporting the results of their analyses, some using grains per gallon, U.S. or Imperial as may be, and others parts per hundred thousand or per million of the water. It is therefore difficult to appreciate the value of the figures as given by them. The following, in parts per 100,000, will enable the practitioner to form a general estimate of the character of analytical reports; but the opinion in individual cases is so modified by the coincident amounts of chlorine, ammonia, nitrous and nitric acids, that the experienced sanitarian only is qualified to put on the results an estimate which shall be in accordance with our present knowledge of such matter:

Upland Surface-Waters.

All owable.	Doubt ful.	Im pure.

Total organic elements	to .4	.4 to .6	Over .6
Oxygen required	to .3	.3 to .4	Over .4
Albuminoid ammonia	to .015	.015 to .025	Over .025

All Other Waters.

Total organic elements	to .2	.2 to .4	Over .4
Oxygen required	to .15	.15 to .2	Over .2
Albuminoid ammonia	to .010	.010 to .015	Over .015

[p. 185]In connection with impure water should be mentioned impure ice. Ice is purer than the water from which it forms, but if cut on a foul pond it will itself be foul, and the vitality of some microscopic organisms is not destroyed by their being frozen, as is shown by the fact that samples from the centre of blocks of ice will inoculate sterilized infusions with the germs of putrefaction, precisely as the water of which the ice is composed would have done before it was frozen. Disease has been traced to impure ice, and it may be that it is more frequently due to this cause than has heretofore been supposed; at all events, it is well to bear the possibility in mind.

The subject of impure water will be further considered in speaking of habitations.

IV. CLIMATE.—The literature of the effects of different climates upon the human body is very extensive, following the general rule that the less positive or precise knowledge there is upon a given subject the more will be written about it. Of all animals, man seems to adapt himself most readily to the extremes of climate; and, although it is commonly supposed that a tropical climate is injurious to those coming from cooler regions, yet it has been found that where he takes the same precautions to ensure cleanliness, pure water and air, and proper food, the European does not have a higher rate of mortality in Algeria or in the East or West Indies than he does at home, if the effects of cholera and yellow fever be excepted.

Dr. Parkes defines the effect of climate upon the human body to be "the sum of the influences which are connected with the solar agencies, the soil, the air, or the water of a place;" in other words, he makes it nearly equivalent to the locality or the environment. By "climate" we understand, commonly, the sum of meteorological influences, the most important of which, as regards health, are temperature, humidity, and wind. The effects of temperature in producing disease are often confounded with the effects of change of temperature, which last is perhaps the more important of the two, and should be specially borne in mind in advising climato-therapy for chronic or wasting diseases.

The influence of climate in causing disease, although well known for over two thousand years, has not led to much effort to avoid or prevent effects which are accepted as inevitable by the great majority. It is true that in the effort to secure physical comfort by houses, clothing, artificial heat, and the like, much hygienic work has been done, and the steadily increasing tendency on the part of all who can afford it to seek rest and comfort at the seaside or in the mountains during hot weather is no doubt due, in part, to the fact that experience has shown that the money expended in thus securing health and strength is a good investment. It is unfortunate that "health resorts," so called, do not always prove to be such: they become fashionable, overcrowded; the arrangements for the disposal of excreta are cheap makeshifts, leading to soil- and water-pollution, until finally an epidemic of diarrhoea or typhoid fever occurs, with the usual results.

The consideration of climate as a therapeutic agent belongs with the articles relating to the several diseases to which it is applicable. The great desideratum wherewith to place this subject upon a scientific and practical basis is a system of reliable returns of the deaths, and if possible of [p. 186]certain diseases, throughout the country, and especially at those points most in vogue as health resorts.

V. HABITATIONS.—That a man's health depends very much on the character, condition, and location of his dwelling-place is now so generally admitted that in many cases where a physician is called in he will be asked whether he thinks the disease has been caused by any peculiarity about the house or the bedroom of the patient. And a careful examination will usually discover in one of them several evils to be remedied, although their connection with the case in hand may be very doubtful. There are very few homes properly constructed from a sanitary point of view; and, although we may not agree with Dr. Wilson, that "the modern prison is in all sanitary essentials the best existing type of what a healthy dwelling ought to be," it is nevertheless certain that the health of the inmates is much more carefully consulted in planning a penitentiary than it usually is in planning a college, a hotel, or a dwelling-house. Matters are gradually improving in this respect: the worst of the tenement-house rookeries and fever-nests in most of our large cities have been improved or abolished, and our wealthier citizens are beginning to pay some attention to their house-drainage as well as to the pattern of their mantelpieces. But the great majority of men are still careless and negligent as to the sanitary condition of their homes, and probably two physicians out of three live in houses in which numerous defects would be pointed out by a sanitary engineer—defects of which they are themselves more or less aware. The majority of people in our large cities under existing conditions cannot afford to have healthy houses, and the great causes of the excessive mortality, and brevity of life, in all such cities, are poverty and overcrowding, the latter resulting from the former. The problem as to the best mode of improving the sanitary condition of the tenement-house population does not, however, come before the practising physician for special consideration, and need not be considered here. Nor is the physician liable to be consulted with regard to the sufficiency, from a sanitary point of view, of the plan of a house yet to be built, although he will occasionally be asked as to the healthfulness of a proposed site. The questions which he will be asked are such as the following: "Is the cause of this particular case of disease in the house, or connected with it? and if so, what is it?"—"Do you think this is a healthy house?"—"Is the location a healthy one?"—"Is it necessary that I should give up this house to preserve the lives and health of my children?" While it is, of course, often impossible to answer with precision such questions as these, an answer of some kind must be given; and this should not be a mere random guess, but based on a deliberate estimate of the probabilities in the case. The healthfulness of a house is to be judged of, in part, from its history, if it be possible to obtain any; in part, from such facts as can be discovered by a careful examination of the premises and vicinity. The sanitary history of a house is the history of the diseases and deaths which have occurred in it, together with a set of plans showing the precise location and character of the house-drainage and of its fresh-air supply. Such a record is in most cases, unfortunately, not attainable, although to a person proposing to buy or rent a house it would often be quite as important as a record of title. In a well-organized health-office it should be possible to ascertain the number and causes of the deaths which have [p. 187]occurred in any given house or square in the city, and also the character and location of its drainage and sewer connections. Such records are especially valuable in an investigation of an outbreak of disease in a community.

The sanitary inspection of a house includes the site and the building itself. The character of the site is mainly determined by its dryness, by the presence or absence of organic matter in the soil, and by its porosity taken in connection with the character of the vicinity. One-third of the volume of some soils consists of air, and all dry soils and rocks contain a much larger quantity of air than is commonly supposed. The influence of soil upon health is exerted mainly through the media of water and air, but it also affects temperature and vegetation, being an important factor in climate. Residence on a damp soil has a tendency to produce diseases of the lungs, and especially phthisis; but how it does this is unknown, though it would be easy to construct a plausible theory in connection with the supposed causation of phthisis by a bacillus. The practical point for the physician is, that the prevalence of phthisis in a locality, even if it be so limited as to comprise but a single house, should cause suspicion and investigation as to the character of the soil-drainage. Soil-moisture is also an important factor in the development of periodical fevers, and the effect of thorough drainage in diminishing malaria is now generally understood.

It sometimes becomes an important question as to the influence which a collection of water, such as a mill-pond or a reservoir, has upon the health of a community, and the physician may be called on for an opinion in such cases where large property interests are involved. The essential points to be borne in mind are—first, that stagnant water and damp soil do not in themselves produce malaria; there is something else necessary, which is commonly designated by the word "germ." Second, that they are in most cases essential conditions for the production of the disease, so that if removed the disease will disappear. Third, that the development of malaria may follow either the rise or fall of the ground water. Fourth, that the condition of the border of the collection of water as to presence of organic matter and moisture is of more importance than the pool itself. And, finally, that each case is a problem by itself, to be determined by the history of the sickness of the vicinity, and that only probabilities can be stated in any case, although these probabilities may be so great as to amount, practically, to certainty. Of the four factors which appear to be essential to the production of the malarial poison—viz. moisture, high temperature, organic matter of vegetable origin, and certain micro-organisms—the first is the one which in any given locality is most under human control; it is the link in the chain of causation which is most easily broken.

The influence of the rise and fall of the soil water in typhoid fever, upon which so much stress is laid by Pettenkofer and others, no doubt exists, acting in some cases through pollution of the drinking water by the subsoil water leaking through a polluted soil; in other cases, perhaps, by air from the soil bearing the unknown germ. The filtering power of soil as regards air is, however, very great, a few inches of sand being sufficient to remove the ordinary germs of putrefaction from air drawn through it, and this for a long period; while, on the [p. 188]contrary, many feet of the same sand will not remove the germs from water passed through it. Usually, as Dr. Parkes remarks, in an examination of soil the immediate local conditions are of more importance than the general geological formation, yet this last, as influencing conformation and the movement of water and air over and through a country, is also important. The practical questions on this point are, what higher ground than the site in question exists in the vicinity? what are the character and direction of the strata between such elevation and the site? and, what sources of soil-pollution exist on the higher level? As to the site itself, is it on made ground? what is the height of the foundation above the subsoil water? and, what precautions have been taken to secure drainage and to cut off communication between the interior of the house and the ground air? Probably a trial excavation or boring may be necessary to determine some of these points.

The level of the subsoil water should be at least five feet below the foundations, although it is often impossible to obtain this. At all times when the temperature of the house is higher than that of the external air—*i.e.* during a large part of the year and nearly every night—there is a strong and constant aspirating force at work to draw into the house, through the cellar floor and walls, all gases and vapors contained in the adjoining soil. If this soil contains a large proportion of organic matter, as is often the case in filled-in ground in cities, or if there be a leaky cesspool or sewer or gas-pipe under or near the house, the ground air passing into the house may be of such a character as to be positively dangerous to its occupants. For this reason it is very undesirable to have a sewer or soil-pipe crossing beneath the site of a house, and when such location is a necessity, as it often is in cities, the soil-pipe should be laid in a cement-lined trench covered with a movable flap, so that it can always be easily inspected and any leaks detected and remedied. Dampness in the cellar or basement of a house is always a sign of danger. The exhalation of gases and vapors from the ground into the house can be to a great extent cut off by a layer of impervious material, such as concrete covered with asphalt, but this layer must cover the sides of the cellar as well as the floor to be thoroughly efficient. If a house have no cellar, the space between the floor and the ground should be thoroughly ventilated; and for this purpose, as well as to secure cleanliness, the floor should be sufficiently elevated to permit of easy access beneath it.

Next to its dryness, the nature and condition of the arrangements for removing excreta and soiled water from a house are of the greatest importance in determining its healthfulness; and in cities it is with regard to the sufficiency of these, including the whole system of house-plumbing and pipe-fitting, that the inquiries of one wishing to determine as to the presence or absence of causes of disease will most frequently be directed. The soil-pipes, etc. of a house are commonly referred to as constituting the system of house-drainage, but it is desirable to use another term, for we need the word "drainage" to describe the removal of surface and subsoil water, and it should be distinguished from "sewerage," which has a different purpose and requirements.

In a properly-arranged system of house sewerage all the pipes, traps, etc. are easily accessible for purposes of inspection, and an examination of them is a comparatively simple matter. This examination is to be [p. 189]made with reference to the following points: 1. Are all the pipes, joints, and connections air-tight? 2. Is the soil-pipe well ventilated, or has it dead ends? 3. Is the communication between the soil-pipe and the street sewer uninterrupted? 4. Are the pipes properly trapped, and is there liability to the removal of water from any of the traps, either by siphonage or evaporation, to such an extent as to break the seal? 5. Is the water-supply of each closet entirely cut off from the main supply to the house by means of a tank or cistern?

In houses as heretofore constructed it is often very difficult to obtain satisfactory information upon these points, because a large part of the soil-pipe and its connections is buried beneath the house or concealed in the walls or floors; in which case the services of a skilled mechanic will usually be necessary to obtain access to the various parts of the system. In a paper of this kind it is of course impossible to go into details as to methods of inspection, or as to what is and what is not satisfactory; but the following are the general principles upon which a judgment as to the merits of a system should be formed, and these should be so clearly understood by every physician that he can be neither persuaded nor frightened into thinking them incorrect by the eloquence of the man with a patent remedy to dispose of. The principal dangers to health from house sewerage are due, first, to the passage of air from the general system of sewers or from a cesspool into the house through the soil-pipe and its connections; second, to the generation of offensive and dangerous gases and organisms in the soil-pipe itself, and the passage of these into the house; third, to leakage of soil-pipe causing contamination of the water-supply either by improper connections of water-pipes with water-closets or slop-hoppers, or by contamination of wells, cisterns, or tanks with sewage or sewer gases.

There is, of course, no such thing as a sewer gas having a definite and distinctive composition, and the nature of the mixture of gases in sewers is constantly varying according to season, temperature, etc. The tendency which sewer air has to cause disease depends in part upon certain gases, in part on minute particles of solid or semi-solid matter which are suspended in the air. In rare instances the sewers also contain illuminating gas, derived from leakage of gas-pipes in the vicinity. These gases produce debility, headache, loss of appetite, etc. As found in sewers and soil-pipes, they are so diluted that they are not absorbed by the water of a trap and given off on the other side to a sufficient extent to produce an evil effect. The air in a soil-pipe which is not ventilated is much more impure than that of the ordinary sewer, since the process of decomposition is constantly going on in the slimy coat which lines the interior of the pipes; and it is for this reason that it is so important to secure thorough ventilation of all the soil-pipes in a building. When this ventilation is secured, the proportion of dangerous gas in the pipes becomes very small, and the amount absorbed by the water in traps is almost inappreciable. The chief danger to life from sewer and soil-pipe air arises from the presence of minute particles of organic matter, dead and living, the so-called germs. Danger to life from these germs cannot be entirely removed by dilution, as can be done with gases. It has been found by the experiments of Dr. Carmichael and Dr. Wernick that an ordinary water-trap entirely prevents the passage of these germs, and that organic putrescible fluid will remain unchanged when exposed only to the air immediately [p.

190]above such a trap. A pin-hole or minute sand-crack in the soil-pipe, or a very slight defect in a joint, is far more dangerous than a trap.

The forms of disease produced by sewer air and its contents are more especially diphtheria, typhoid fever, and ill-defined disorders of the throat and digestive organs. It is possible that the germs of other specific diseases, such as scarlet fever, may be at times transmitted through sewer air, but such transmission must be very rare. While it is true that the germs of the specific diseases are very rarely present in sewer air, the house system of sewerage must be arranged as if they were always present, in order to obtain security. It must also be remembered that a system originally well planned and properly constructed will not always remain so; the pipes will corrode, the joints will become loosened, the valves will become clogged, and whenever alterations or repairs are made there is always danger of injury. Bearing these points in mind, the method of investigating a system can be readily understood.

The first step is to ascertain whether there is a trap outside the house disconnecting the sewer from the house system and permitting inspection. If there is not, the first thing to be done is to make an excavation and open the drain at the proper point for placing such a trap. The next step is to set the water flowing in the various closets and watch the flow at the external trap, or opening, which has been made to ascertain whether there is any obstruction in the pipe within the house. If the sewer is properly arranged for inspection, as has been above suggested, to determine whether there is any leakage from the sewer under the house will be an easy matter; if, however, it is buried beneath the cellar floor, as is usually the case, an excavation should be made along the floor in the line of the pipe, with a view to having it properly arranged, as well as for the purpose of examining the soil. It may also be tested by opening the upright soil-pipes at the farther end of the house-drain at the height of three or four feet above the floor and pouring water into it, having temporarily stopped up the drain at the external trap or opening. If the water remain at a constant level in the upright piece, the sewer is water-tight; if not, the leakage may be ascertained by the rate at which it sinks. Having settled this, the next point is to determine whether all the soil-pipes are air-tight and properly trapped. The test usually applied for this purpose is the pouring of a small quantity of strong oil of peppermint, followed by a dash of hot water, into the top of the soil-pipe, which should always pass through the roof and be freely opened to the outer air. If the odor of the oil is perceptible in the house, it indicates a leak, which must be further sought for. Ether may be used for the same purpose. The smoke test is, however, the best, but it requires a special apparatus which as yet is little used in this country. It is applied by a small machine with a fan, by which the smoke from burning cotton-waste saturated with oil, or of coarse brown paper impregnated with sulphur, can be blown into the pipes; this locates leaks with great precision.

It is not, of course, expected that a physician will personally make the examination necessary to determine whether the plumbing of a house is in good order, but he should be able to make it, if necessary, if for no other purpose than to know whether the inspector employed for the purpose understands his business.

The dangers to health from a properly-constructed system of house[p. 191]sewerage, such as is now generally agreed upon by sanitary engineers, are so very small as to practically amount to nothing, being, in fact, less than those of a well-kept yard privy of a country house, setting aside altogether the question of water pollution. The real difficulties in the way are the expense of such a system, which is considerable, and the finding of skilled and honest workmen to construct it and keep it in repair. Not every one who chooses to style himself a sanitary engineer or a sanitary plumber is to be regarded as such, by any means, but the physician should make it his business to know who are really reliable in this respect, for he will constantly be called in for advice on this point by those who have learned that good plumbing is the only true economy, but who do not feel themselves competent to distinguish between good and bad work. The main points of a satisfactory system are the following.[3]

[3] For further details consult the following: *American Sanitary Engineering*, by E. S. Philbrick, N.Y., 1881; *House-Drainage and Water-Service*, by James C. Bayles, N.Y., 1878; "House-Drainage and Sanitary Plumbing," by W. P. Gerhard, in *Fourth Annual Report State*

Board of Health Rhode Island, 1882; *The Sanitary Engineer*, a weekly journal published at 140 William St., New York City.

    1. All soil- and waste-pipes should be extended up to and through the roof, and be freely open at the top. The extension of the soil-pipe should be full size—*i.e.* from four to six inches in diameter.

    2. There should be a fresh-air inlet in the house sewer just outside the house, and between this inlet and the main sewer should be a trap so arranged as to permit of inspection. This prevents the ventilation of sewers through the soil-pipes. If a perfect system of sewers, uniformity of house-connections, and uniform height of houses could be guaranteed, this inlet and trap would not be so necessary, although even then it would be useful.

    3. Every water-closet, wash-bowl, bath-tub, sink, etc. should have a trap placed as close to it as possible. This trap is desirable, whether the discharge be into the sewer system or not. For example, a kitchen sink, the pipe from which passes to the outer air and discharges there, should be trapped, for this pipe is foul, and if it be untrapped will act as an air-inlet.

    4. The nearer to the soil-pipe that the fixtures can be arranged the better. It is especially desirable to avoid the necessity for long horizontal waste-pipes from stationary waste-bowls and from bath-tubs.

    5. Bell traps, D traps, bottle traps, and mechanical traps are objectionable. The S trap is, upon the whole, the best, but it should be provided with a vent-pipe to prevent siphonage.

    6. The best kind of water-closet for general use is probably some form of what are known as the wash-out closets. They are made in one piece of earthenware, have no machinery inside them, have a quantity of water in the basin into which the excreta drop, and do not require a separate trap beneath them. Each closet must, however, be carefully tested by itself: a very small warp or twist produced in the baking may so interfere with the siphonage as to make it practically worthless, and the basin cannot be altered or repaired. For use in public places some of the hopper closets are very satisfactory, the best which I have examined being the Rhoads Hopper and the Hellyer Hoppers. Where there are no [p. 192]children, and it is certain that the fixtures will be used with reasonable care, valve closets may be used. No form of pan closet can be considered as satisfactory, nor have I found any form of plunger closet that I would specially recommend.

    7. Water-closets should always be flushed from a special tank provided for the purpose, and never direct from the main system of water-pipes. The flush must be large and rapid, and this requires a large supply-pipe, and for many forms of closets a flushing rim. Whatever be the form of closet, it should not be encased in a wooden box or closet, as is usually done, but it should stand freely exposed to light and air. Sanitarians commonly advise that water-closets should be located in outer walls and have an open window for ventilation. Such a position is usually impossible, and is not specially desirable in our climate. The open window acts as an inlet quite as often as it does as an outlet, and the air of the closet is thus swept into the house. The room should be ventilated in such a way that the tendency of the air at the door shall always be from the house into it. This is to be effected by a shaft passing through the room up and through the roof; and it is well to have this shaft take its air-supply from just behind the closet or from beneath the seat. It is best made of galvanized iron, and at a convenient point should be expanded into a lantern and have a gas-jet placed in it. The air-supply for the closet is to be taken at the bottom of the door or through a transom or louvres. Ventilating pipes from a water-closet should never be run into a brick flue. While it is not so important as many writers seem to think that a water-closet should be placed on an outer wall, it is very important that it should be as light as possible, and the placing it in a dark corner in the basement or under the stairs is very objectionable.

    8. No overflow-pipe from any cistern or tank, except the one used for flushing water-closets, should be connected with the soil-pipe or sewer. Trapping such an overflow-pipe does not prevent the danger. The same rule applies to waste-pipes from refrigerators and to the waste-pipes from the safes which are commonly placed beneath fixtures.

9. Grease-traps placed inside a house—for instance, beneath the kitchen sink—are of very doubtful expediency, and if they cannot be placed outside, they had better not be used at all.

In an unsewered city one of the first things to be considered in a sanitary inspection is the manner in which the sewage of the premises is disposed of. The question is, however, by no means superfluous in many sewered cities, for cesspools and vaults are to be found in most of them, and not only in yards, but beneath houses, and houses of the better class. A privy-vault or cesspool beneath a dwelling or near its cellar walls is always to be considered as very dangerous, for it is practically impossible to prevent the passage of gases from it into the interior of the house. A cesspit is a dangerous thing anywhere, even in the country; but in a city it is so dangerous that its existence should not be permitted.

If the water-supply of a house is derived from a well, and there is reason to suspect that this may have been contaminated from a neighboring privy-vault, the first test to be applied to the water is that for the detection of chlorides. If none are present, the water is not polluted. If they are present, the quantity is to be noted, and a peck or two of common salt is then to be thrown into the suspected vault. If repeated [p. 193]examinations of the water show a marked increase in the amount of chlorides present, it may be inferred that the contents of the privy pass to the well. The fact that the water of infected wells and springs is usually much liked and sought for is to a considerable extent due to the presence of these chlorides. Wanklyn recommends the addition of 50 grains of common salt per gallon to drinking water to render it palatable. Popularity of a certain well is therefore a reason for suspecting its purity.

This subject may be dismissed with one caution. Taking the dwelling-houses of a city or town as they come, it will be found on examination that over half of them would be described by a competent inspector as being in a condition which might produce disease. It is therefore more than an even chance that in any case of disease some sanitary defect will be found about the premises quite irrespective of any direct causal connection with the case. Let the physician therefore be cautious in deciding as to such causal connection, and not conclude that because a case of diphtheria or typhoid fever and a leaky soil-pipe occur in the same house, therefore one is the cause of the other. Such cases occur in houses whose sewerage is perfect and in houses which have no sewerage, and it is folly to attribute them exclusively or mainly to sewer gases.

The same caution applies to investigations into the causes of a sudden outbreak of disease in a community where a number of cases occur almost simultaneously or in rapid succession. Such an outbreak may be due to direct contagion, although sometimes very difficult to trace; as, for example, an explosion of small-pox in a community largely unprotected by vaccination, and where, owing to circumstances connected with the first few cases, a large number of persons have been exposed to the cause about the same time. The same applies to an apparently sudden development of yellow fever throughout a city.

Another cause of such outbreaks is a polluted water-supply, as in some epidemics of diarrhoeal disease or of typhoid fever. If the outbreaks of these diseases are pretty sharply localized, and depend upon the fouling of a well or wells, it will usually not be very difficult to trace this cause. If, however, the town has water-supply by means of pipes from a single source, while the outbreak of disease is limited to a part of the town or to a single large building, it will probably be almost impossible to establish any connection between the disease and the drinking water. The possibility of the contamination of a part only of a system of general water-supply by means of the drawing of foul air into the temporarily empty pipes connected directly with a water-closet flush should never be forgotten, for such a case has actually occurred, and the account of its discovery is one of the best pieces of sanitary detective work with which I am acquainted. If the outbreak of typhoid fever cannot be traced directly to the water-supply, the next point to be investigated is the milk, and after that other possible modes of the conveyance of the contagium.

In cases of obscure disease characterized by fever of no definite type, disorder of the digestive organs, headache, malaise, etc., and which seem to be connected with residence in a particular house or in one room in a house, the possibilities of arsenical poisoning from wallpaper or hangings should be remembered, for much useless medication and some real danger will be avoided if this cause be promptly recognized. The effects[p. 194]produced by arsenical dust are very various, and simulate sometimes some of the specific fevers, indigestions, or neuroses in a way that is very puzzling if the true nature of the case is not suspected. The popular notion is that arsenic is found only in greens (more especially in bright greens in wall-papers), whereas in fact it is found not only in dull greens, but in some browns, grays, and dull reds. The test for its presence in quantity sufficient to be a cause of disease is an easy one, and is fully given in any manual of chemistry or toxicology.

VI. OCCUPATION.—While the effects of occupation upon health are no doubt great, they are in many cases so blended with those of condition in life, including habitation, food, and intemperance, that it is very difficult to distinguish them. In attempting to investigate these effects by means of statistics, it is necessary to beware of a fallacy which not unfrequently vitiates the conclusions drawn from otherwise carefully prepared tables intended to show for different occupations either the relative mortality or the average age at death. This fallacy lies in the fact that the number of persons engaged in each business is unknown; that, in this country at least, men often change their occupations; and that certain trades or professions are chiefly carried on by persons of certain ages. This last is perhaps best illustrated by the remark of Dr. Farr, that the fact that the average age at death of second lieutenants is much less than that of major-generals proves nothing with regard to the comparative healthfulness of the two grades. Statistics showing merely the number of a particular class or grade dying in a given time are absolutely worthless, unless the number of the same class or trade living at the same time is also given.

It is also necessary to bear in mind the power of habit and the effects of natural selection, especially when the effects of an unhealthy occupation are immediate and marked upon those unfitted for them. For example, young men, when first employed as scavengers or in sewage-pumping works, usually suffer from disorders of the digestive organs. A certain number find it necessary for their health and comfort to soon leave the business; some acquire protection by passing through an attack of fever; and by this process of selection a class of men are obtained who seem to thrive in the midst of filth and remain unaffected by effluvia which will promptly cause illness in those unaccustomed to them. When men find that, to use a common phrase, they "cannot stand" a particular kind of work, they are apt to give it up and try something else, especially if the effects are prompt and well marked.

Much attention has been given of late years in England, France, and Germany to the means of protecting both the workmen and the neighborhood from the ill effects of dangerous and offensive trades, and the reports of the medical officer of the Privy Council and of the Local Government Board are a mine of information on this subject. It may be truthfully asserted that in those trades in which the special danger is caused by dust of various kinds, or by gases, or by metallic poisons—and these three include the greater number of the dangerous occupations—it is almost always possible to so arrange the work as to make it comparatively healthful and harmless. Overcrowded and unventilated workrooms are responsible for much disease, and when to these is added the risk of metallic poisoning, as is the case with printers, artificial-flower [p. 195]makers, etc., bad results are almost sure to follow. It is curious that so comparatively little ill effect seems to be produced by exposure to great heat, as in stokers, foundry-men, glass-blowers, etc.; but further information is needed on this point as to the real facts in the case. In some occupations the chief evils arise from want of out-door exercise, a subject which will be considered presently. The want of useful or interesting occupation sometimes becomes indirectly the cause of disease among the wealthier classes, and the giving a man or woman something to do is in such cases the best prescription which can be made. This danger is especially apt to occur in the case of an active, energetic man who retires from business, intending to spend the rest of his life in pleasure and in the enjoyment of the fruits of his industry: the preventive or remedy is obvious.

VII. FOOD.—The comfort, energy, usefulness, and moral character of a man depend largely upon his digestion, and this in turn depends largely on what it has to act upon—viz. food. There are, it is true, many men who boast that they can digest anything, and who are really comparatively indifferent as to the kind, or mode of preparation, of the food set before them, so that the quantity be sufficient; but were it not that habit and heredity—which is the family habit—combine with natural selection to adapt men to their food, it is probable that the frying-pan, the pie, and soda-bread would depopulate large portions of this country. As it is, there can be no doubt that fried food swimming in grease, leathery, sodden pie-crust, and heavy bread tend to make life short and the reverse of merry; and when the effect of these is combined, as it often is, with those of malaria, damp soil, and a free use of whiskey, the result is plenty of work for the doctor and very little to pay him with. This state of things is being gradually improved, but in all classes of society and in almost all parts of the country the rule is, that while the raw materials of food are abundant and of excellent quality, the cooking is bad. This is due, in part, to an idea that it is to a certain extent discreditable to a person that he should give much attention to his food, at least so far as its appearance and taste are concerned, and that a man who can plan a good dinner must be more or less of a sensualist and a glutton.

Another popular error is, that a large amount of disease is due to overeating, and that abstemiousness in diet is either certain to secure health, or is, at all events, indispensable for this purpose. Upon this point the reader should consult a capital paper by Dr. Austin Flint on "Food in its relations to personal and public health," which will be found in vol. iii. *Reports American Public Health Association*, N.Y., 1877. After remarking that many of the popular errors about food and diet are relics of old and abandoned medical theories, one of which is embodied in the not uncommon advice that one should always stop eating before the appetite is fully satisfied, and that food should only be taken at regular fixed periods, no matter how hungry one may be, he says: "Physiology, experience, and common sense are alike opposed to these popular notions relating to food. Conditions for perfect health are, first, a sufficient appetite; second, the gratification of normal appetite before the want of food reaches the abnormal degree expressed by hunger; third, the satisfaction of appetite by an adequate quantity of food. These conditions of health are fulfilled by compliance with instructive provisions for[p. 196]alimentation. But, it will be asked, is appetite infallible as a guide in dietetics? Following it as a guide, is food never taken beyond the requirements of health? I answer, It is a reliable guide under normal circumstances. The inevitable circumstances of life are often not altogether normal, although producing no distinct morbid affection. Experience teaches, for example, that in a state of fatigue or exhaustion (which is not a normal state) inconvenience may arise from the full gratification of appetite; that if unusual exertions, mental or physical, are to follow, a hearty meal may occasion disturbance; and other examples might be added. Irrespective of abnormal or disturbing influences, if appetite be not infallible, it is, at all events, more reliable than a rule based on theoretical ideas, popular notions, or on purely physiological data. Moreover, it was evidently not intended that the quantity of food should be accurately adjusted to the needs of the economy. To do this is impossible, and therefore it is necessary to elect between the risk of taking either more or less food than is actually required. Which is to be preferred? Undoubtedly, it is vastly better to incur the risk of taking too much than that of taking too little. Nature provides for a redundancy, but there is no provision against a persistent deficiency. Ex nihilo nihil fit. An ample supply of alimentary principles is indispensable to nutrition; and inasmuch as the supply cannot be made to contain precisely the needed amount of the different alimentary principles, we may say that a superabundance of food is a requirement for health.

"As in appetite we have a guide in respect of the times of taking food and the quantity to be taken, so taste is a guide in respect of the kinds of food required. The discrimination of food with reference to the wants of the system is the evident purpose of the sense of taste, and the enjoyment connected with this sense was designed to afford a security, in addition to appetite, for adequate alimentation.

"Among professional men and those who live sedentary lives the mistake is not uncommon of paying too much attention to the sensations after a meal, and deciding therefrom whether certain articles of food are unhealthy or not. If the man who does this is not already dyspeptic, he will pretty surely become so. The remedies in this case are exercise and attracting the attention to something else."

A physician ought to understand something of cooking, and a short course of practical instruction in what might be dignified as the culinary laboratory would be of more real value to him than some of the branches which are now considered indispensable in the medical curriculum. He should know why oysters are the best thing with which to begin a dinner, and why a cocktail is one of the worst; how to make a salad, or a cup of good coffee, or a perfect consommé; and a number of other things pertaining to gastronomy of which most people are woefully ignorant.

It is not within the scope of this paper to give details with regard to the diet of either the sick or the well, but it seems proper to remark with regard to the feeding of infants, more especially in our large cities in the summer months, that all the various patent preparations for infants' food are more or less pernicious, and should be discountenanced by all medical men. The proper food of an infant is milk—human milk if it can be had, cow's milk if it cannot. If it be remembered that an infant suffers [p. 197]from thirst as well as hunger, and care be taken to give it enough pure cool water to quench this thirst, it will be found that in most cases it will thrive on pure cow's milk.

With regard to adulterations of food, the only form of such adulteration found in this country, which has any special interest from the sanitary point of view, pertains to milk. This adulteration is in most cases the dilution of the milk by water, and this is very common in large cities. The danger from the use of such milk is by no means confined to infants, and it is probable that a larger proportion of the typhoid fever, diphtheria, scarlet fever, cholera infantum, and diarrhoeal diseases in our cities is due either directly or indirectly to the milk-supply than is now even suspected. The possibility of this mode of origin should always be borne in mind in investigating the causation of such affections.

A very large amount of food is now furnished preserved in tin cans, and it is almost invariably of excellent quality. There is a possibility of the contamination of such food by the salts of lead or tin, but such contamination to an extent which is injurious to health must be so extremely rare as to be hardly worth considering. The danger from the entrance of parasites, such as trichinæ, etc., in the food is also extremely small—in fact, is nothing where the food is properly cooked.

Milk has so often been the cause of disease, and is so universally used, that it seems worth while to refer to it again. The special aptitude of milk for absorption of odors has long been known, and of late years it has been clearly proven in a number of instances that milk has been the means of conveying the cause of typhoid fever and of scarlatina. Diphtheria, yellow fever, and intermittent fever have also been supposed to be conveyed by milk. The variety of nutritive principles contained in milk, which makes it so valuable as a food, also gives it the power of sustaining many different sorts of minute organisms, and it perhaps comes as near being a universal culture-fluid as anything yet devised for that purpose. The possibilities of the contamination of milk are so numerous, and especially in the case of that furnished from small establishments, that, in the case of outbreaks of typhoid or diarrhoeal diseases in a town, investigations into causation should always include the milk- as well as the water-supply. Milk from diseased animals is no doubt often used without producing bad results, but its effects in conveying to man the disease known as milk-sickness are well established, and it has also been known to produce symptoms of the contagious aphthæ, or foot-and-mouth disease, in man, when derived from an animal affected with that disease. The only danger in the use of the milk of animals fed upon sewage-grown grass appears to be in the possible contamination of the milk, after it is drawn, by particles of dust in the stable, derived from the food or litter of the animal or from uncleanliness of the exterior of the udder, etc.

VIII. INTEMPERANCE.—Every one knows that alcoholic drinks are the cause of a vast amount of disease, crime, and misery in all civilized countries. No one knows how this is to be prevented, for no one knows how to make the great mass of the people wise and contented. The effects produced by excessive use of alcohol are well known to all physicians, and the remedy is self-evident. I see no use in adding to the heap of useless rubbish which exists in the shape of the great mass of existing[p. 198]popular literature on this subject, and therefore leave the subject to the reader, who is quite sure to know all that is really important on this subject.

IX. CLOTHING.—The hygiene of clothing is also a subject which may be treated summarily in this paper. People wear what they can afford, made according to the prevailing style. Diseases due to insufficient, excessive, or badly-fitting clothing occur most frequently in women and children, and the use of such clothing is for the most part due to poverty or fashion, either of which is beyond the power of the physician to successfully cope with. Here and there, in individual and exceptional cases, he may be able to do a little good by advising against tight lacing, high-heeled shoes, insufficient covering for the chest or legs, etc., and he will find that a knowledge of the peculiarities of the various styles of modern under-clothing will sometimes be very useful. Men are, as a rule, comfortably and sensibly dressed to suit their business and surroundings, and require no advice on this subject.

X. EXERCISE.—The ease and completeness with which the functions of an organ or of an organism are performed depend to a great extent upon the frequency and regularity with which such functions are exercised. Hence comes the importance of bodily exercise for the preservation of health, and every physician meets cases of disease due largely to want of work.

The term "exercise," or "bodily exercise," is commonly used as if it referred only to the muscles, and the amount of exercise which a man should take in a day is stated as equal to a certain number of foot-pounds. The mere giving work to muscles is not, however, exercise in the sanitary sense. A better definition is that of Du Bois Reymond—viz. that "exercise is the frequent repetition of a more or less complicated action of the body with the co-operation of the mind, or of an action of the mind alone, for the purpose of being able to perform such actions better." From this point of view it will be seen that exercise relates quite as much to the nervous system as to the muscles. When, for example, a student takes a walk over ground with which he is familiar, and is at the same time so deeply engaged in thought as to be practically unconscious of what he is doing, only being recalled to himself, it may be, by arriving at his own door, the exercise which he has had is but partial and insufficient. Going to the extreme, we can, as Du Bois Reymond remarks, conceive of a man with muscles individually exercised until they were like those of the Farnese Hercules, and yet who would be unable to walk, much less execute more complicated movements; for the proper co-operation of the muscles, which is effected through the nervous system, is quite as necessary as the force of their contraction.

The amount of exercise which is necessary for health varies with the individual and with age, season, etc., so that it is difficult to state any general rule upon this subject; but if stated in terms of muscular force only, the estimate of Dr. Parkes seems a fair approximation—viz. that every healthy man ought to take daily an amount of exercise equivalent to 150 tons lifted 1 foot, or a walk of about nine miles. The majority of trades and bodily occupations demand at least this amount of work, but in some of them the greater part of the exertion is made only by certain groups of muscles, and they are carried on in crowded and [p. 199]ill-ventilated shops. Such workmen, as well as all who are engaged in sedentary pursuits, require exercise in the open air—exercise which will bring into play the unused muscles and will break the train of thought of the professional man.

One of the most important questions with regard to physical exercise is the extent to, and manner in, which it should be provided for in a proper system of education. One of the latest and most instructive articles on this subject is that by Du Bois Reymond in the "Physiology of Exercise," a translation of which is given in the *Popular Science Monthly* for July and August, 1882. He divides the physical training which is more and more becoming a part of modern systematic education into three classes: The first, the turning, or gymnastics of the Germans; the second, the Swedish system, in which the exercises are limited to very simple though varied movements; and the English system, or rather want of system, consisting largely of athletic games and contests of various kinds. His objection to the Swedish system is that, while it strengthens the muscles, it does not increase the power over composite movements; in other words, it does not exercise the nervous system. Naturally, he prefers the German system to any other, although admitting that the English meets better the demands arising from our structure. "Were the end masterhood in running, jumping, climbing, in dancing, fencing, riding, in swimming, rowing, or skating, then nothing could be more advisable than to practise equally the necessary concatenations in the actions of the ganglion cells, without pausing at the not practically applicable preliminary and intermediate steps of the German turning."

From a sanitary point of view, the gymnasium, as usually located and managed, is by no means equivalent to out-of-door sports and contests, although it is often the best substitute for them. The form of exercise most used by men whose occupation does not involve bodily labor is walking, and next to this riding. Whatever mode be selected, it is very desirable that it should be taken for some other object than that of the mere making muscular exertion, or otherwise it will soon come to be looked upon as an unpleasant task, the time spent upon which is given grudgingly; and it will be partially or wholly abandoned as soon as the immediate discomfort which induced its use has ceased.

It is not an uncommon error among men engaged in mental work to suppose that they can, and ought to, take the same amount of exercise which gives good results in those whose occupations involve physical rather than mental effort, or to think that the more exercise they take the more study or writing they are equal to. This is a grave mistake. Expenditure of brain-tissue is not to be repaired by muscular exertion, but by sleep and food, and exercise in the fresh air sufficient to produce appetite and sufficient weariness to ensure restful sleep is all that is necessary. For a time it is true that the student or writer who has a well-developed body can continue to burn the candle at both ends, and win literary honors while also standing high as an athlete; but this surely leads to physiological bankruptcy in the end.

It is to be remembered that good muscular development is not necessarily synonymous with health, and that strength is not a guarantee against disease. And, while it is true that in this, as in most other matters of individual hygiene, each man must to a great extent be a law to [p. 200]himself, and learn by experience what kind of exercise and how much of it he requires, yet the physician can often supply the motive which was wanting, or check undue effort. Exercise for the sake of health and comfort is not an end, but a means; yet if this means can be made to secure to the patient an end agreeable and pleasant in itself, so much the better.

XI. CONTAGION AND DISINFECTION.—By "contagion" we mean the communication of disease from one person to another, either by direct contact or through some medium, such as air, water, etc. It therefore includes "infection," which is now generally used as a synonym for it. The so-called infective diseases of modern German writers (Infections-Krankheiten) include, besides what are commonly termed in English, contagious diseases, the so-called miasmatic diseases.

The characteristic of a contagious disease is its specificity; that is, the disease transmitted is always the same in its essential characteristics. It does not, however, follow that all cases of the disease are equally liable or have the same power to transmit it; in other words, the degree of virulence of the contagiousness is not an essential characteristic. That the same disease sometimes spreads rapidly and is very fatal, and at other times seems hardly to have any contagious properties and is very mild, has long been noticed, and has been attributed to an unknown something called the medical constitution of the place—the constitution médicale of French writers. The true cause is probably very complex, but in some cases, at all events, it seems to be due to difference in the contagion itself. If we suppose this contagion to be a minute organism, it is easy to form a theory as to the cause of these differences, but there is much careful experimental work to be done before we shall have positive knowledge on this point. The results obtained by Pasteur in attenuating the virus of chicken cholera and splenic fever indicate one line which these experiments will take, and the researches of Koch point out another.

The diseases which spread by contagion until they form epidemics are those which have from the earliest times attracted the most general attention, and which have given rise to organized efforts for prevention—*i.e.* to public hygiene.

They are also the diseases which have given rise to the most bitter controversies among medical men as to the means of their propagation and the best methods of prevention. Plague, cholera, yellow fever, and typhus are those with regard to which this difference of opinion has chiefly occurred—one party considering their chief cause to be contagion, or specific germs derived directly or indirectly from the bodies of the sick; the second party declaring that they are due to filth plus an unknown something, which is variously termed epidemic constitution, pandemic wave, Providence, or x. The great majority of opinions at present is in favor of the view that they are all contagious, but not all, or always, contagious from person to person—that they spread from infected localities, which localities receive their infection from cases of the disease. The best means of dealing with them under ordinary circumstances are now tolerably well understood, and where these means can be commanded—as, for instance, among troops in time of peace—epidemics of these diseases can be stopped with great precision and promptness by isolation and disinfection.

[p. 201]By "isolation" is meant not only the separation of the sick from the well, but the isolation of the infected locality or water-supply until it has been rendered harmless.

By "disinfection" is meant the destruction of the specific causes of disease, and more especially of the infectious or spreading diseases. A disinfectant is not necessarily an antiseptic or a deodorant, nor are these last necessarily disinfectants. The best practical antiseptic for sanitary purposes is cleanliness; the best disinfectants are heat, bichloride of mercury, sulphate of iron, chloride of zinc, sulphurous acid, chlorine, sunlight, and pure air, and, for yellow fever, cold. With our present very imperfect knowledge of the nature of specific causes of disease which we wish to destroy, we have no means of determining the presence of these causes in or on an article of clothing or of furniture, or in a room or other locality, except by the production of their specific effects on man or by inductive reasoning; in other words, we can only say that it is more or less probable that such causes are present. This makes it necessary, or at least expedient, to employ disinfectants in many cases where the presence of such causes is doubtful. The practical difficulties are, first, to bring the disinfecting agent into such relation with the causes of disease that it can act upon them, and act upon all of them; second, to avoid unnecessary destruction or injury of things which should be preserved. The majority of the causes of disease upon which we wish to act by disinfectants are probably minute particles of solid or semi-solid matter which are living, and may be conveniently designated by the word *"germs."* In the presence of moisture the destruction of the vitality of these germs can be effected with comparative ease and rapidity, but when they have become dried, or, as in the case of the bacilli, are in the form of spores, it is a more difficult matter.

To illustrate the methods to be pursued and the precautions to be taken, let us suppose the physician to be called on for directions as to the management of a case of scarlatina, the object being to prevent its spread. The first thing to be done is to get the patient in a room by himself, and to leave nothing in this room which is not necessary. Remove the carpet, curtains, and all stuffed or upholstered furniture. Let the nursing be done, as far as possible, by one person only, and do not allow others, and especially children, to enter the room, no matter if they have had the disease. The danger of contagion depends upon particles coming from the skin and mucous membranes. All excreta, and more especially the sputa or discharges from the mouth or nose, are to be treated as dangerous. The excreta should be received in vessels containing a solution of sulphate of iron, one and a half pounds to the gallon. All clothing, towels, bed-linen, handkerchiefs, napkins, etc. should be placed in a solution composed of four ounces of sulphate of zinc and two ounces of common salt to the gallon of water as soon as they are not needed for further use. Especial care should be taken that none of these articles are removed from the room while dry, and while they are in the room, and before they have been moistened, they should not be shaken or disturbed more than is absolutely necessary. If for any reason the zinc solution above referred to is not at hand—which should very rarely be the case—the clothing, etc. should be placed in a bucket, tub, or boiler containing enough scalding water to entirely cover them, and be removed [p. 202]from the room in this vessel. All such articles should be boiled at least one hour.

No sweeping or dusting in the ordinary way is to be done in the room; dust and dirt are to be removed by damp cloths, which are to be treated like the bedding and clothing. The great object is to prevent as far as possible the production of dust in the atmosphere of the room. The entire body of the patient, including head, face, and limbs, should be kept thoroughly anointed with camphorated oil, vaseline, or some similar substance, and especial care should be taken in this respect during the period of convalescence so long as any roughness or desquamation of the skin continues. No toys or books which it is desired to preserve should be allowed to remain in the room, and under no circumstances should books or toys be borrowed to amuse the child if they are to be returned. The best way to disinfect such articles is to burn them in the room.

When the patient is fully convalescent and all desquamation has ceased, cleanse him thoroughly with a warm bath and soap for four successive days. If at the end of that time no roughness of the skin remains, he may be dressed in clean clothes and taken from the room, for he is no longer a source of danger. The room itself and the furniture are then to be thoroughly cleansed and disinfected. The ceiling and walls, if of ordinary hard finish, are to be scraped and whitewashed. All woodwork should be rubbed with damp cloths and the floor well scrubbed. Care should be taken to remove all dust from the ledges over windows and doors. All the cloths used in this cleansing process are to be burned.

If these directions have been carefully carried out, there is no need for further disinfection. But if upholstered furniture has been allowed to remain in the room, or other articles which cannot be burned or scrubbed or soaked in the zinc solution, it may be desirable to attempt to disinfect the whole room and its contents by means of chlorine or sulphurous acid gases. Of these, sulphurous acid gas is the cheapest, and upon the whole the best, but it must be used in large quantity, and for a longer time than is customary, if it is to be relied upon. For this purpose all openings into the room should be closed, and pillows, mattrasses, upholstered furniture, and articles which cannot be treated with the zinc solution should be opened, so that they may be exposed throughout to the fumes. The sulphur should be burned in an iron pan or pot, placed in a tub containing water or upon a large surface of sand. About 18 ounces of roll sulphur should be used to each 1000 cubic feet of space, and after twenty-four hours 12 ounces more should be burned and the room be then closed for twenty-four hours longer, after which it may be opened and aired. In case of death the body should at once be wrapped in a sheet thoroughly soaked with the chloride of zinc solution, and either be placed in an air-tight coffin at once or be buried without delay. The funeral should be strictly private, and the sheet referred to should not be disturbed or the body exposed to view.

The cases most liable to spread the disease are those in which the attack is very light and the child is not confined to its bed. It is desirable that children in a house in which there are cases of scarlet fever should not be allowed to attend school or mingle with other children who have not had the disease.

With regard to disinfectants, it may be well to note that none of the[p. 203]various patent disinfectants are superior to bichloride of mercury, chloride of zinc, sulphate of iron, chlorine, and sulphurous acid; very few are equal to them, and none cost so little. As a gaseous disinfectant for rooms, etc. chlorine is superior to sulphurous acid, but it has the disadvantage of injuring metals, is not so easily applied, and is more costly. It will destroy the vitality of the spores of the bacilli more rapidly and certainly than sulphurous acid, which last, to make sure work, must be exhibited for a much longer period than is customary. I should not feel confident as to the thorough disinfection by sulphurous acid of the hold of an infected ship unless the fumes had been applied for sixty hours. Carbolic acid as ordinarily used is an antiseptic rather than a disinfectant. Its vapor in a sick room is absolutely useless. When applied in strong solution it is effective, for a time at least, but as thus used it is expensive, its odor is unpleasant to many, and masks the odors from putrefying substances and excreta, etc., thus preventing the warning which these odors would give. Its use is in many cases very much like removing the rattle from the rattlesnake.

The suggestions made above for limiting the spread of scarlatina from a case to be treated in the residence of the patient apply—with certain modifications for each form of disease, which will readily suggest themselves to the physician—to all the affections due to portable contagia.

Among the poorer classes, however, it will often be found impossible to obtain the separate room and service and the constant intelligent care which are necessary to ensure the desired result; and in such a case the patient should be removed to a hospital, for his own sake as well as for that of the community. The utility of small hospitals for infectious diseases is by no means generally understood, and very few of our small cities and towns are provided with anything of the sort. If the subject is urged on the authorities of a place, the reply will be that it is an unnecessary expense, that the people would not go to it, and that such an institution is in itself a source of danger. The facts are, that such a hospital costs very little, and is the cheapest insurance against epidemics which a town can have; if it is kept clean and comfortable, the people will use it freely, and if properly managed it does not offer the slightest danger to the vicinity. This question will be further discussed in the last section of this paper.

The principles of isolation as applied to a single case as indicated above may also be applied to infected localities in case of epidemics. When taken in time, all diseases which depend upon particulate contagia for their origin can be stamped out by isolation and disinfection. Unfortunately, to effect this promptly and successfully requires money, labor, and the co-operation of the well in the vicinity; which last it is usually impossible to obtain voluntarily or to compel sufficiently to secure the desired results. A question which sometimes arises in case of epidemics, and with regard to the necessity for which physicians will be consulted, relates to the closure of the public schools. It is certain that the assemblage of children in schools exerts a powerful influence on the spread of such diseases as scarlet fever, diphtheria, and whooping cough. On the other hand, the closure of the schools infringes upon the rights of a large number of the community, and if long continued, as it sometimes must be to be really efficacious, inflicts upon them [p. 204]a permanent loss. It is, moreover, a confession on the part of the authorities of inability to induce or compel what must always be a comparatively small part of the community to take the proper precautions. It is never justifiable to close schools on account of small-pox, and where there is a competent health authority supported by the influence of the medical profession, it must be a very exceptional set of circumstances which justifies their closure for diphtheria or scarlatina.

It is not deemed expedient here to discuss the vexed question of quarantine. It is more important against yellow fever than any other disease, because every day of delay of the entrance of the disease which it secures lessens largely the subsequent mortality, since the duration of the disease is limited by frost. This is not the case with cholera, and the mere keeping this disease out of a place for a few weeks does not diminish its ravages when it has once gained an entrance. To rely altogether on quarantine, either maritime or inland, to keep yellow fever, cholera, or any other disease out of this country is a far greater mistake than to neglect it altogether. The practical way to isolate and quarantine is to get as close to the affected spot as possible. Precautions at Havana for yellow fever, or at Hamburg for cholera, are far more useful to the United States than the same amount of work at our own ports can possibly be; really good work in this direction must be not only national, but international.

XII. MENTAL CAUSES OF DISEASE.—A man may give too much attention to his health and the means for its preservation, and the doing so is both a sign and a cause of disease—probably oftener the former than the latter, except in cases of psychological epidemics. The power of expectant attention, especially if accompanied by belief or fear, to produce derangement of function in the nervous system, and through this to affect the circulatory and digestive systems, is well known to medical men. The effects of an undue amount of brain-work, and especially of the anxiety and worry which often accompany this when it is specially directed to the acquiring of wealth, fame, or power, are also familiar to physicians in our large cities. The analogies between mental and physical exertion are close in some respects, and especially as to the effects of over-exertion in a limited time under the influence of excitement.

The danger from simple mental work, such as study, when there is no excitement from a contest, is small, and depends mainly on lack of physical exercise and consequent disorder of the digestive organs. The risk of producing what Fothergill calls "physiological bankruptcy" is greatest in the youth studying for a prize, the speculator, the man who feels responsibility which he knows he probably cannot meet. The danger of injury from overwork under excitement is a very real one in many of our schools, and, while the evil results are most apparent in girls of the middle and upper classes, the boys and the young men also suffer. The system of pass examinations, in which the standing of the pupil is to be determined, not from the average results of his daily recitations, but from a single examination at the end of the year, produces the greatest risks to health; and this is especially the case where the ambition and pride of the children are stimulated by competition for prizes, medals, etc. Such systems of grading by a single final examination should not be used in ordinary schools, and for some pupils there will always be a risk to health connected with them even when they are of age. No doubt the stimulus of[p. 205]competition is useful with the majority of children as well as of adults, but with some of them it is pretty sure to go too far.

The symptoms produced by undue mental strain are familiar to all physicians, and there is usually little difficulty in tracing the effect to the cause when attention has been directed to the matter; in fact, the patient himself usually knows very well the cause of his troubles. The remedy is, of course, rest—but that does not mean idleness. In speaking of occupation, allusion has been made to the fact that the physician must at times advise his patient as to the adoption of some pursuit, and in cases of this kind such advice is also useful.

The effects of mental strain are often mingled with, and aggravated by, those of stimulants which have been used to spur the flagging energies. Alcohol, tobacco, opium, or coffee used in this way finally increase the very discomforts which at first they relieved.

II. Personal Hygiene in its Relations to the Practice of Medicine.

In the preceding section have been indicated briefly some of the principal causes of disease and the methods for their investigation or removal. We have now to consider some of the practical applications which may be made of the laws of etiology and prevention of disease in the treatment of the sick. While the removal of the cause of illness by no means always effects a cure, yet the importance of a knowledge of this cause as an aid to diagnosis, prognosis, and therapeutics is so evident as to require no proof.

To discuss with anything like completeness the practical applications of what would be commonly considered as hygienic rules in the treatment of disease would be to write a treatise on nursing, and would also include a large part of the practice of medicine, for regimen is the more important half of practical therapeutics. The hygienic requirements peculiar to each disease will be pointed out by the writers upon special subjects, and I shall only venture upon one or two general remarks in addition to the hints already given in speaking of the several causes.

In the acute stages of disease the sensations—or, if the term be preferred, the instincts—of the patient are usually the best guide to his regimen so far as they go. In most cases he desires quiet, shade, but not absolute darkness, and little or no food, although there is often a craving for drinks, especially of a cooling character. In the specific fevers which have a tolerably definite period and course it is important to keep up the nourishment even during the period of anorexia, in order to provide against the debility which is to follow. This nourishment is best given in the form of drink, and very frequently fresh milk is the type of what is required. The old notion that whatever a sick man desired must be hurtful, and therefore that the fever patient must be kept hot and refused cool water, has now almost entirely passed away.

In convalescence from acute disease and in many chronic cases, the sensations of the patient are not to be trusted as a guide in the choice of food. In such diseases as yellow fever and typhoid fever to allow the convalescent to follow the dictates of his appetite is to run great risk of a fatal result. In other cases the patient really has no wish in the matter, but it [p. 206]will often be found that one who can think of nothing which he desires to eat, and who will even refuse a dish which he has requested and been thinking about, will eat with enjoyment some unexpected dainty when presented at the right moment and properly served as a skilled nurse knows how to do. The manner of serving the food, independent of its cooking, is not a matter of such small importance that the physician can afford to overlook it, and he will succeed best as a practitioner who best appreciates the influence which cracked goblet, a chipped saucer, a soiled napkin, or, on the other hand, a hot plate or a touch of color in the shape of a leaf or flower, may have upon the capricious appetite of the sick. In ordering diet for convalescence it is not an uncommon error to select only those articles which are agreeable to the physician himself, forgetting the old proverb, that what is one man's meat may be another man's poison, and also that it is above all things desirable to avoid monotony. One doctor always orders chicken, another eggs, a third a mutton-chop, etc. The practice in this respect has probably been unduly influenced by the reports of Beaumont of the results of his observations on Alexis St. Martin, and we still find that the relative digestibility of various articles of food is estimated according to the scale laid down in these reports, with no allowance for individual peculiarities, previous habits, mode of cooking, etc. The secret of success in the diet of convalescence lies mainly in the simplicity of the individual dishes, in varying the different meals, in the manner of serving, and in carefully observing the effects on the sick person, and being guided by the results.

To promote appetite and digestion, and to secure refreshing sleep, one of the most important things is fresh air, but in many houses a sick person will obtain but a very limited allowance of this if the physician does not give special attention to the matter. Except in cases of contagious disease, the rules for managing which have been given in a previous section (p. 201), as soon as a patient is sufficiently recovered to be moved for a short time into another room his bedroom should be thoroughly aired and cleansed, and this should be done morning and evening thereafter.

In treating cases of contagious disease the question often arises as to means of individual prophylaxis to be used by those who must be exposed to the effects of the infected locality or of the presence of the sick. The attempts which have been made to secure this individual protection in the midst of an epidemic have been numerous and varied, ranging from the use of the "vinegar of the four thieves" of the Middle Ages to the employment of the sulphites and chlorates to make the blood unsuited to the growth and multiplication of the supposed germs, or of cotton-wool respirators to strain the infected air, or of supposed specifics for particular diseases, as belladonna for scarlet fever and vaccination against small-pox. As yet, there is little or no satisfactory evidence as to the value of individual precautions against those diseases whose contagion is conveyed through the air, small-pox alone excepted, but in case of diphtheria in one member of a family of children it might be well to try the use of chlorate of potash internally, combined with the local application of the tincture of the chloride of iron, as suggested by E. M. Hunt. The question is one to be investigated by careful observation and experiment; and, though it is improbable that any definite results will be obtained except in those diseases which are communicable to animals, and therefore [p. 207]susceptible of direct experiment, still, it is possible that some advance may be made. In rare and exceptional cases—as, for instance, in exploring a crowded, filthy, and intensely infected typhus-fever nest, as a tenement-house, or an infected yellow-fever ship—it may be worth while for the physician or inspector who is unprotected by a previous attack of these diseases to make use of a cotton-wool respirator, which is readily extemporized, and belongs to that exceedingly valuable and popular class of remedies which, "if they do no good, can do no harm." In epidemics of typhus, cholera, or yellow fever one of the most valuable prophylactics is to have a mind so occupied with other matters that it pays little or no attention to the danger, while in case of small-pox fear of the disease is indirectly the best prophylactic, since it leads to careful vaccination.

This branch of the subject is closed with the remark that it would be well if physicians, and especially the younger ones, gave more attention to the preservation of their own health than many of them do. The possession of a medical diploma does not prevent the evil effects of irregular and hurried meals, insufficient sleep, exposure to inclement weather, and lack of systematic and sufficient exercise; and too much tobacco, sometimes too much alcohol, and in exceptional cases too much study and literary work, so often combine with anxiety about individual patients or with pecuniary worries to damage the digestion and nervous system of the young practitioner that the wonder is that so many survive the ordeal. And, in fact, the mortality among physicians under the age of thirty is higher than that of any other profession during the same period of life.

III. Public Hygiene in its Relations to Physicians.

An important difference between man and animals is found in the extent to which he will sacrifice a present pleasure or convenience to secure a future good or to avoid a future evil. The savage will do this to only a very limited extent—little more, in fact, than the beaver or the squirrel—and the lesson is learned but slowly and by sad experience. This is especially the case as regards matters affecting health. When a man begins to take special precautions as to his diet or exercise, having in view rather his future health than his present comfort and tastes, he has in most cases already begun to suffer from the effects of his imprudence, and does not commence a hygienic course of life as a perfectly sound and healthy person. The same is true for a community. It will not usually submit to the burden of taxation necessary to secure drains and sewers or a proper registration of vital statistics, nor to the cost and inconvenience of the machinery necessary to limit the spread of contagious diseases, until the neglect of these things has resulted in such an amount of disease and death as to forcibly call attention to the matter. The result is, that the burden is far heavier than it would have been had the work been undertaken in proper season, and individuals may find it to their interest to leave the place and settle elsewhere rather than remain and meet their proportion of the expense.

When a state or municipality has so far advanced in civilization as to consider it desirable to take measures to protect the public health by preventing individuals from polluting the air or water liable to be used by[p. 208]their neighbors, etc., the services of the medical profession are always called upon. The foundation of public hygiene is information as to the occurrence of certain forms of disease, the cause of which can be referred with more or less precision to a certain limited locality. This information may be very imperfect, consisting of little more than rumor and opinions as to the existence of an undue amount of sickness or mortality in a certain place, or it may consist of precise reports setting forth the number of deaths from each cause, the proportion of each of these to the population by age, sex, occupation, etc., and of the whole to births—constituting what is commonly called the "vital statistics of a place"—and also of reports of the occurrence of certain preventable diseases; and between these two the information may be of various degrees of completeness, but, whatever there be, it is for the most part obtained either directly or indirectly from medical men. The reliability and completeness of the information thus obtained by the state determines to a great extent the direction and character of the work done in destroying or preventing the causes of disease, and it is also an important means of increasing our knowledge with regard to the nature of these causes.

The character of this information depends largely upon the character of the physicians who furnish it. In a large part of the country medicine is legally in the position of any common occupation; that is, the term "physician" is defined as applied to "any one who publicly announces himself to be a practitioner of this art, and undertakes to treat the sick either for or without reward." Under such circumstances there can be no guarantee that all who call themselves physicians are properly qualified or competent to furnish reliable information for registration purposes, and, as a matter of fact, a large number are not so qualified. It is for this reason that there is such a close connection between public health authorities, registration of vital statistics, and the registration of those physicians whose certificates as to causes of deaths, etc. will be accepted by the state; and hence the nature of the public health organization of a state and the personnel of its officials are matters of great importance to physicians. On the other hand, the efficiency of a public health service depends very largely upon the relations which it holds with, and the light in which it is regarded by, the medical profession. A health officer who is distrusted and disliked by the physicians of his district cannot effect much unless he can overcome this feeling, and his tenure of office must always be very insecure.

The official relations of the practitioner with the health authorities are usually confined to the subjects of registration of vital statistics and of checking the spread of contagious diseases. The most marked exception to this rule is furnished by the States of Alabama and North and South Carolina, in which the State Medical Society is the State Board of Health, having been given legislative powers and the right of selecting the health officers. The most complete organization of this kind is that of the State of Alabama, where by the act of 1875 the Medical Association of the State was constituted the State Board of Health, and the county medical societies in affiliation with the State Society were made county boards of health, to be under the general direction of the State Board. These county boards at first had advisory powers only, and were to be conducted without expense to the State or the county, except that the competent legal[p. 209]authorities of any county might invest the county board with such powers and duties for the promotion of the public health as might be mutually agreed on; but in such case the right to elect or appoint those employed in sanitary administration is reserved to the board of health, while all questions relating to salaries, appropriations, and expenditures shall be reserved to the legal authorities. It was further provided "that no board of health, or advisory or executive medical body of any name or kind for the exercise of public health functions, shall be established by authority of law in any county-town or city of this State except such as are contemplated by the provisions of this act, the object of this prohibition being to secure a uniform system of sanitary supervision throughout the State." By an act of 1881 the county board is directed to elect a health officer, who is to keep a register of the births, deaths, and cases of pestilential or infectious diseases occurring in the county, and furnish to physicians, free of charge, reliable vaccine—to obtain information as to the sanitary condition of his county, etc. etc. It will be seen that this plan of organization is an attempt to overcome the practical difficulties in the way of obtaining from physicians the information necessary for the registration of vital statistics and the work of preventing the spread of infectious diseases.

While the great majority of physicians are willing to furnish the information as to the cause of death, etc. which is necessary for a useful registration, there are always some who either neglect or refuse to do so; and if the law be made compulsory, it provokes hostility unless compensation is furnished, while as regards the requiring physicians to furnish information as to the existence of contagious diseases, this always rouses opposition on the part of a certain number of medical men, even if payment for such notification is provided. And while this opposition is no doubt in many cases due to improper motives, such as personal hostility to the existing authorities, party politics, or a desire for notoriety, its strength nevertheless rests upon the fact that it is unjust for the state to compel the services of any man or class of men without furnishing compensation. The advocates of health and registration laws are thus placed between Scylla and Charybdis: if they propose compensation, which involves appropriations from the public treasury, the law cannot be passed; if there is no compensation allowed, complete results cannot be obtained.

The Alabama law makes compulsory the furnishing by physicians of information relating to births, deaths, and infectious diseases, and gives compensation—not in money, but by allowing the medical profession to have the sole management of the matter and to choose the health officers to whom they are to report; in other words, they are allowed to tax themselves. The result in Alabama is yet doubtful. If competent and faithful health officers and registrars can be obtained without paying them a fair compensation, it will be contrary to experience; and if these officers receive a salary, it will be strange if the positions do not become the reward of partisan political work.

It should be noted that the requiring a physician to report the births occurring in his practice stands on a very different basis from the requiring him to report the cause of death, since there is no special necessity for the former. It requires no expert knowledge to report a birth, and the duty should obviously devolve on the householder.

[p. 210]In those States in which by law only properly qualified medical men, as determined by examination, have the right to practice, to hold medical office, or to furnish medical certificates, the State certainly is entitled to require of all physicians thus registered and authoritatively recommended to the people as competent, that they shall furnish, free of charge, certificates of the cause of death in those cases where they are cognizant of such cause.

States and municipalities often demand much more than this; as, for instance, that the medical man shall fill out the whole certificate, including age, nativity, nativity of parents, etc., and that he shall furnish the information to the registrar. In some cases it is provided that any physician having attended a person during his last illness shall furnish the certificate: this would apply to cases where the physician may not have seen the case for weeks before death.

While it is most convenient to have the certificate of cause of death upon the same form which contains the data necessary to identify the individual, the certificate should be distinct from the latter, and the duty of making the return to the registrar should devolve on the householder or undertaker, and not on the physician. On the other hand, it is easy for the physician to be hypercritical in these matters: his certificate is to be considered rather as a statement of opinion than as a statement of facts within his personal knowledge, precisely as he would certify as to his own age and birthplace.

The compulsory notification of infectious diseases to the health authorities is a matter presenting much greater difficulties than that of certificates as to causes of death. The state has no right to require such notification from the physician without giving some quid pro quo, and it is not expedient to make it compulsory, even with payment, except from physicians employed by the state or municipality, to furnish gratuitous medical attendance to the poor. The state has the right to require such information from the parent or householder, and it has also the right to require the physician to notify the parent or householder as soon as he recognizes the existence of such infectious disease. It is extremely desirable that the health authorities of a city should receive promptly, and direct from physicians, notification of the occurrence of such diseases, and there will usually be no difficulty in obtaining this if the health officer has tact and discretion and the city is prepared to do its duty. This duty is not confined to registering the information or placarding the house, nor will it be properly performed by merely removing the sick person to a hospital and disinfecting the premises. If the case occur in a family which can secure its proper isolation, and the attending physician certifies that it is so isolated and makes himself responsible for its management (for which responsibility he should be paid by the patient or his friends), the health officer should not interfere nor do more than furnish a competent person to secure disinfection if required. The employment of a trained nurse known by the health authorities to be competent and reliable would do away with most of the difficulties connected with such cases in the upper and middle classes of society; and such nurses should be registered just as physicians and midwives are.

Where the case cannot be thus isolated and properly cared for, it should be removed to a proper hospital. This presupposes that the city has such a hospital, and if it has not, and is not prepared for such cases, notification[p. 211]is useless. When the city places a house in quarantine so as to interfere with business, it should be for the shortest possible time consistent with securing thorough disinfection of the premises, and the city should bear not only the cost of such disinfection, but the cost of caring for the persons in the house in an isolated place until no further danger is to be apprehended for them. When the city undertakes to pay all expenses for isolation and disinfection of such cases, it has the right to require that all such cases shall be so treated, leaving it to private parties to meet the cost in case they prefer not to use the buildings and apparatus provided by the city for that purpose. And when the city does its duty in this respect, it will be found that physicians and the people will do theirs, with rare exceptions.

When a city becomes very unhealthy the usual policy is to conceal the fact as much as possible, and to attribute the mortality to some other than the real cause. The influence of the mercantile part of the community is in such a case strongly exerted on the daily press and on the health authorities to produce such representations of the condition of things as will tend to allay apprehensions on the part of their customers. The healthfulness of a place is usually estimated from its mortality reports, but the reliability of these is by no means always what it should be. Yellow fever is called typho-malarial or pernicious fever, typhoid is reported as diarrhoea or malarial fever, etc. etc., and great stress is laid upon what is called the sanitary condition of the place, which is declared to be excellent.

Unfortunately, this phrase, "sanitary condition," means different things at different times. When the mortality is low, sanitary condition means the healthfulness of a place; when it is high, it means the cleanliness of a place. To a certain extent physicians are responsible for the truth of the statistical returns, not so much in relation to the number as to the causes of deaths; but none save those who have practised in a city liable to epidemics can realize the enormous pressure which is brought to bear on medical men to induce them to aid in or wink at concealing the true state of the case. Of course, this ostrich-like policy is in the long run an exceedingly unwise one, but neither the average householder nor community can be expected at present to pursue any other, except under pressure.

There are many questions as to the best form of public health organization, and the powers and duties which should be conferred upon it, which can only be properly answered by taking into consideration the circumstances in each case. In a large city the health officers must have great powers if they are to be really efficient. They have to contend with ignorance, custom, and self-interest, and their action must in many cases be prompt and unrestricted if it is to be efficacious. They must sometimes be in conflict with wealthy and powerful corporations, whose interests are opposed to the reforms which they urge, and although their business is to protect the most important interest of the community at large— *i.e.* its health—against the interests of individuals, yet these last are much more immediately concerned, and are, naturally, so active that they are often, although few in number, able to defeat any attempt to interfere with their occupations.

It not unfrequently happens that a health board may have all the power[p. 212]necessary, so far as the laws are concerned, and yet may be able to accomplish little for want of funds to pay the inspectors and other officials whose services are necessary. For a city, a health officer usually does better work than a board of health: his responsibility is more direct, and he has stronger motives to do good work, than a board. Of course, a poor health officer is less efficient than a good board of health, but the general rule is as above stated. The problems of hygiene require special knowledge, and the man who is to deal with them requires special training. The folly of treating diseases by their names with popular or patent remedies is not greater than that of the attempt to make a healthy house or city by men who are not architects or engineers or physicians, or who have only the information possessed by the average architect or engineer or physician. And, of all professional or educated men, the physician especially should recognize his own ignorance. When he is asked what one should take for dyspepsia or pneumonia his answer is, "Take the advice of a physician;" and so when he is asked how the plumbing of a house should be arranged, how a hospital should be ventilated, how a city should be sewered, how a marsh should be dealt with or a water-supply provided, he should reply, "Get expert advice and supervision, and be prepared to pay the amount necessary to secure it." It is the special duty of the physician to exert his influence to secure properly constituted sanitary authorities for his own locality, his State, and for the nation, and to support these against the hostility which they must inevitably arouse if they are efficient. And he should do this, not blindly and as a partisan, but intelligently and with due consideration of all the important interests involved.

The body of educated physicians in a community forms the tribunal by which the work of sanitary officials is to be judged, and they cannot judge wisely unless they appreciate the difficulties with which health officials have to contend. If a city has an incompetent or dishonest board of health, the medical profession of that city are to a certain extent responsible for it; if a competent, energetic, and faithful sanitary officer is crippled and harassed or forced out of office because he is on the wrong side of politics, or because in the legitimate and proper exercise of his functions he has come in conflict with the interests of powerful and wealthy individuals or corporations, it is the duty of medical men to support him, and to do this actively and promptly. And I take great pleasure in being able to say, as the result of somewhat extended observation, that, as a rule, the physicians of this country do cheerfully and promptly co-operate with the sanitary authorities where such exist, and are the first to try to have them properly organized and given the necessary means and powers to do effective work.

[p. 213]

DRAINAGE AND SEWERAGE IN THEIR HYGIENIC RELATIONS.
BY GEO. E. WARING, JR.

For reasons, sometimes sound and sometimes fanciful, the drainage question often presents itself to the medical practitioner as an annoying if not as a serious one. It is not necessary for the physician to make himself an adept in the art of sanitary drainage, but he can properly meet neither the demands of nervous patients nor the exigencies of sometimes serious situations without having an intelligent general idea concerning it. Not only to prescribe improvement, but frequently to allay ill-grounded apprehension, he should be able to address himself, intelligently and promptly, at least to the few simple problems presented in connection with ordinary houses. I use the expression "ill-grounded apprehension," not because the drainage in and about houses is generally tolerably good, for it is not, but because the race seems to have so inured itself to certain grave defects in plumbing-work that one may reasonably hesitate, and look elsewhere for the occasion of diseases before accusing the imperfect sanitary appliances of an average house.

Anything like a treatise on the technical details of house-drainage would be quite out of place here. There are note-books easily accessible to such physicians as care to make a thorough study of the subject. It does seem worth while, however, to pass in careful review, in a work of this character, the various conditions of interior and exterior drainage upon which a physician is frequently called to pass judgment.

The perfect drainage of a house, like the perfect drainage of a town, implies the immediate and complete removal, to a point well beyond its limits, of all waste matters which are a proper subject of water-carriage; such a thorough ventilation of the channel which these matters have traversed as to reduce to a minimum the production of deleterious gases arising from the decomposition of the film with which they may have soiled the walls of their conduit; and adequate provision for the absolute and permanent exclusion from the atmosphere within the house of the air of the pipe or sewer. This is a brief and simple statement of the fundamental and absolute requirements of all good drainage. It is founded on the one grand object which governs all improvement of this character: the prevention of decomposition of refuse matters anywhere in house or town.

Practically, it is safe to say that these conditions are never complete, and that instances of perfect work are so exceptional as to need no[p. 214]consideration here. We have to assume, substantially in every case that is presented, that we are dealing with defective work, ordinarily with work that is very seriously defective. Most houses have been built by contractors, and the plumbing is perhaps the item of the whole structure that it is considered easiest and safest to scamp or to neglect. Even where the motive of economy has had no controlling influence, the drainage has almost invariably been planned by a plumber who has learned his trade and conceived his ideas in the performance of work which was done at a time when no one realized the serious consequences of its being improperly done. The absence of interior ventilation, leaky joints, ill-arranged connections between the various plumbing appliances and the main outlet from the house, pipes and traps so large that an ordinary current is powerless to keep them clean, defects of form, defects of material, and defects of construction, are met with on every hand. This general statement is of itself sufficient to show how hopeless it is for the average physician to prescribe the manner in which the drainage of a house should be constructed or remodelled.

If we view the question solely with reference to its bearing on the causation of disease, we enter a field where neither the sanitarian nor the physician is ever sure of his footing. The precise relation between bad drainage and ill-health no man knows. Certain diseases are undoubtedly traceable to conditions of air or of drinking-water due to the improper disposal of organic wastes, but the extent and exact bearing of these influences are still greatly a matter of conjecture. It is, however, undoubtedly safe to assume—and the assumption is supported by ample general observation, if not by precisely ascertained facts— that whether we are considering serious diseases or the slighter ailments, every argument leads to the enforcement of the most strenuous requirements of cleanliness. Through all the ages no one has disputed, and no one has improved upon, the simple sanitary formula, "Pure air, pure water, and a pure soil." We may safely wait until the enthusiastic investigators now engaged with the subject shall have adduced the testimony of positive facts, if we will in the mean time adhere strictly to the requirements of Hippocrates' prescription. The physician will surely not go wrong if he treats all obvious defects of drainage as positive evils, and insists upon their complete reformation.

Not to confine ourselves to houses which are provided with the ordinary modern plumbing-works, but to include all collateral branches of the subject, we have to consider the following conditions:

I. THE REMOVAL OF HUMAN EXCREMENT:

(*a*) By water-carriage in houses provided with modern plumbing;

(*b*) By some form of dry conservancy;

(*c*) By the fiendish privy-vault which prevails so generally, save in the larger cities.

II. THE REMOVAL OF LIQUID HOUSEHOLD WASTES:

(*a*) By delivery to public sewers;

(*b*) By irrigation disposal;

(*c*) By delivery into cesspools.

Incidentally to the above there must be considered the influences of the ultimate disposal of all household waste, whether by the public sewer or the private house-drain.

[p. 215]I. THE REMOVAL OF HUMAN EXCREMENT.—We are too apt to judge of the power for mischief of any waste matter by its original offensiveness, and the world at large regards the solid and liquid exuviæ of the human body as the most dangerous material with which it has to deal. Doubtless it is so under certain exceptional circumstances. If impregnated with the infective principle of cholera or of typhoid fever, for example, its influence for evil may be widespread and active, but in the absence of such infection these substances offer a less serious problem, and, as their offensiveness causes them to be more carefully avoided, their evil influence is less, and is less widely disseminated, than is that of the comparatively inoffensive wastes of the kitchen-sink. This is a consideration important to be borne in mind. Nothing is more common than the expression of the opinion that the wastes of a population are offensive and dangerous in proportion to the degree to which excrementitious matter is allowed to flow away with its general drainage. The fact is, that the drainage from a house or from a town, if reasonably diluted with water, is very slightly offensive until it has passed through a considerable degree of decomposition. The outflow of a perfectly sewered town, where the whole community uses water-closets, is less offensive than the neglected back-yard drain of an average New England farm-house. The trouble begins with the condition of putridity. Fecal matter and urine are somewhat quicker than the other wastes of the house to enter into putrefaction, but the difference is only one of degree, and the latter rapidly overtakes the former in the foulness of its condition; so that where a house is provided with two cesspools, one for water-closet matter and the other for kitchen waste, it is quite impossible to determine from the character of their contents which is which; therefore examinations of the drainage of a house should by no means be confined to the manner in which its excrementitious matters are disposed of. Setting aside, in this connection, the peculiar liability of these matters to become the seat of specific infections, it is fair to assume that equally complete and cleanly arrangements are needed for all else that flows to waste, as for the discharges of the water-closet. The purpose of these remarks is of course not to belittle the importance of proper care in the disposal of human excreta, but to prevent the giving of an undue importance to this branch of the subject, with too light treatment of the very serious difficulties presented by the others.

(*a*) Modern conveniences may fairly be said to be the bane of modern society, or at least of such of its members as have the questionable good fortune to be housed within the same four walls with every device that a misguided talent for invention has led the American mechanic to provide for the comfort and convenience of the occupant. Properly regulated, there is no element of modern house-building more conducive to health than such a system of plumbing as brings within reasonable limits the labor of supplying abundant water at every point in the house, and obviates the need for exposure and removes the temptation to neglect and postponement attending the use of out-of-door houses of convenience. The spigot and the water-closet are the two essential sanitary agents which the plumber offers to us. The bath may be replaced by the sponge, the stationary wash-basin may be, and generally should be, replaced by the bowl and pitcher of our fathers, but there is no sufficient [p. 216]substitute for an ample supply of water on each floor of the house and for a cleanly water-closet placed within doors. The evil that the plumber has inflicted upon the race is due very largely to his not having held his hand when he had fairly provided for our reasonable requirements. When he fills our bedrooms with stationary basins, connects our refrigerators with the sewer, provides twenty outlets for water which had better reach the drain through less than half that number, and incidentally underlays all our floors with pipes, every foot of which is a possible source of danger, he turns what ought to be a blessing into what is too often an unmitigated curse.

It will not be easy to convert persons who have become accustomed to the universal diffusion of plumbing-works throughout the house to a belief that their best sanitary interest, and, perhaps hardly less, the best requirements of refinement, point to the abandonment of what is practically superfluous in the way of wash-bowls, bidets, foot-baths, sitz-baths, urinals, etc.; but one who has given careful attention to the subject cannot hesitate to recommend that in a house which is "strictly first class" it would be the part of wisdom to reduce by at least three-fourths the openings which lead to the soil-pipe and drain and sewer, and to concentrate upon the remaining fourth the flushing effect of wastes which are now so widely distributed. Strenuous effort is being made, not only by those who write and talk in the interest of the plumber and manufacturer, but by many who honestly believe that the good the plumber has to give us cannot be given with too free a hand, to prove that so long as they are properly constructed and properly arranged we may use plumbing appliances at every point in the house with the utmost freedom and with a minimum of danger. The minimum of danger, and often more than the minimum, does, however, exist. It exists, perhaps, in a constantly increasing degree with every extension of the work, and it can only be the part of wisdom to insist, so far as advice can have influence, on the reduction of all these appliances to the least requirements of reasonable comfort and economy of labor. My own advice would be, in all cases, to permit the use of no wash-bowl or bath or other vessel at a greater distance than a few feet from a vertical soil-pipe, and not to permit their use in any case in bedrooms or in closets opening only into bedrooms.

At the risk of seeming extravagant, I would say that the stationary wash-bowl as ordinarily used is one of the most uncleanly of modern household appliances. Long experience in the inspection of houses and in the examination of waste- and drain-pipes has led me to the belief that servants, by no means rarely, use these vessels as the most convenient means of voiding and cleansing chamber utensils. Their overflow-pipes are coated with soap and with the exuviæ of the skin to a degree which makes them usually the seat of an offensive decomposition. Their plugs and chains are almost invariably foul, and those devices which provide for closing the outlets by valves or plugs, somewhat removed from the strainers at the bottom of the bowl, bring the water in which the face is washed into an interchanging communication with a considerable length of foul and uncleanable waste-pipe—a communication that is made active by the bubbling of the contained air as the pipe fills with water. The labor of filling pitchers from a spigot on the same [p. 217]floor, and the labor of emptying chamber-slops into a water-closet on the same floor, are not to be considered as compared with the greater cleanliness and the greater sanitary security that such an arrangement ensures. There is no serious objection to the placing of wash-basins and baths in the same apartment with the water-closet, or elsewhere immediately adjoining the soil-pipe; but it certainly cannot be disputed that the extension of the drainage system by horizontal lead pipes to remote points is altogether and wholly to be condemned.

However, the question more immediately at hand is that of the disposal of human excreta by the use of water-closets; and it is the water-closet that first attracts the attention of one who is called upon to examine the sanitary condition of the work. There are several radical defects in water-closets, which are so widespread and which have become so familiar to the world at large as to attract less attention than they deserve. For example, it is a radical defect of a water-closet to be tightly encased in carpentry. Nearly all the water-closets now in use have a somewhat complicated mechanism about their bowls. They consist in part of earthenware and in part of iron, generally with an unstable connection between the two. More often than not they overflow or drip or leak, and whatever may escape from them, whether foul air or foul water, is confined within an unventilated space, but a space which is still not absolutely excluded from the atmosphere of the house. The removal of the "riser" or vertical board under the front of the seat will usually disclose at once a condition that suggests at least the need for thorough ventilation. It also discloses in some cases a complication of machinery and pipes and levers and chains which makes a thorough dusting and cleansing of the space difficult, even were it accessible. There are water-closets which are essentially good in their construction and working, which it is important to protect by a "riser," but this "riser" should never be of close work. It should at least be freely perforated with large holes, or, better still, be made with slats or blinds, so that there may be the freest possible circulation of air under the seat. If there is an entire absence of machinery, so that the whole space may be left open, being well finished with tiles or hard wood or other suitable material, it is better that it should be unenclosed and that the seat should be hung on hinges, so that it may be turned back, exposing the whole space to easy cleansing. It is better too, in all cases, that the ventilation should not even be interfered with by a cover over the seat, the freest possible exposure to the air being of great importance.

A very large majority of the water-closets in use throughout the world are either very imperfectly flushed "hoppers," which are generally foul and which are often defective in their traps, or that worst of all forms, known as the "pan" closet, where a slight depth of water is held in the bowl by a hinged pan closing over its outlet. This pan swings in an iron chamber under the bowl, which is entirely cut off from ventilation, which is generally foul with adhering fecal matter, and which as an abomination has no equal in the whole range of plumbing appliances. The closet of which it forms a part has everything to condemn it, and only its cheapness and its apparent cleanliness, and the habit of the world in its use, to commend it. If flushed, as it usually is, by a valve on the supply-pipe, it is rarely flushed adequately, and its use not seldom leads to an indraft [p. 218]of foul air (or worse) into the main water-supply system of the house. Such closets may be easily inspected as to their condition by shutting off the water-supply, opening the pan, and lowering a candle into the container below. Such an inspection will almost invariably disclose an extremely and dangerously filthy condition. Yet the worst part of the container, that which never receives an adequate flush, is even then concealed from view by the pan being thrown back against it. The nose will here be a good adjunct to the eye, and the odor escaping from this filthy interior chamber will generally afford convincing testimony of the impropriety of allowing such a vessel to remain in use.

It is a rule almost without exception that closets, except perhaps on the first floor of the house, which are flushed by valves connected with the bowls, are to be condemned. However good or however bad the state of a closet thus supplied with water, its condition will always be improved by giving it a copious flush from an elevated cistern delivering never less than two and a half gallons of water at each use, and delivering it through a pipe so large and so direct as to secure a thorough cleansing at every discharge.

It would be out of place here to enter into a detailed description of the various closets which are and which are not to be recommended for use. So far as the physician's inspection is concerned, it is perhaps sufficient to say that wherever an odor, however slight, can be perceived, and wherever a fouling of the interior surfaces of the closets or of the spaces under the seat can be detected by the eye, radical reformation is necessary. The only safety with a water-closet, as with any other vessel connected with the drainage of the house, is to secure an immediate and complete washing away of all foul matter of every kind. Where this result is not attained, it should be insisted upon. This much lies within the province of the medical attendant; the manner in which it shall be secured is not necessarily for him to decide.

One other branch of this subject is worthy of attention. The cleanliness and freedom from offence of the water-closet or of a waste-pipe or drain is in proportion to the frequency with which it is used and to the abundance of the discharge of water through it. A dozen closets used by a dozen persons will be quite likely all to be offensive. If the dozen persons all used only one closet—not a pan closet—the frequency with which its trapping water is removed and the frequency with which its walls are washed would secure its tolerable condition, even if not of the best construction. In this case, as in all others, simplicity should be the controlling principle.

(*b*) Dry conservancy next after water-carriage is the best and safest system for the removal of human excreta. By dry conservancy is meant the admixture of dry earth, ashes, or similar material with the matters to be disinfected and absorbed. Theoretically, the effect of such admixture is entirely satisfactory; under very careful and intelligent regulation it is practically so. It has been proved, however, by much experience that under ordinary circumstances—that is, where no greater care is given than is ordinarily given to a water-closet or to a common privy—the dry conservancy system is open to serious objections, though always an improvement on the cruder privy-vault. The theory of the effect of a sufficient admixture of earth or ashes with urine and fecal matter is, that by the [p. 219]admission of air thus secured to every part of the material there is a complete oxidation of their organic constituents, similar to, though slower in its operation than, actual combustion in an active fire. In isolated houses and in hospitals, factories, and other buildings not provided with sewerage facilities, there is no question that the earth-closet or the ash-closet affords the best available means for disposal, if we except a system, to be described hereafter, for the distribution of water-carried wastes over or under the surface of suitable ground.

Incidentally—and this is of special interest to the physician—the use of dry earth or of dry ashes in the close-stool of the sick chamber effects not only an immediate and complete deodorization, but without doubt a complete disinfection as well. A quart of dry earth at the bottom of the vessel to receive the deposits, and rather more than a quart with which immediately to cover them, constitutes a means of relief always available and always efficient.

Where the house is provided only with an old-fashioned out-of-door privy the greatest relief and the most complete security may be given at little cost by filling the vault, and placing under the seat a movable box to receive the mixture of fecal matter and of the absorbent material, which, if it is desired to avoid the simple patented appliances made for the purpose, may be kept in a box or barrel in the apartment and thrown down after each use of the closet with the hand-scoop. The objections to the common privy are so obvious, so universal, and so well understood that the practical value of such a means of relief should be appreciated without argument.

(*c*) Privy-vaults are the sole reliance for the disposal of fecal matter, and often of chamber-slops, of probably 95 per cent. of the population of this country, and of Europe as well. It is curious, in examining the recommendations of public health officers and the requirements of local boards of health, to observe the uniformity with which this most important subject is passed over with the prescription that the vault shall be tight, sometimes that it shall be vaulted over, and sometimes that it shall not be within a certain small number of feet of a boundary-line or of a drinking-water well. These prescriptions are most absurd. It is safe to say, that of the millions of privy-vaults in this country not more than hundreds are really tight; that a still smaller number are so vaulted over as to prevent the free exhalation of the gases of decomposition; that those which are so vaulted over are in all respects of worse sanitary effect than those which have freer communication with the air, and that their possibilities of evil reach many times farther than the limits of distance usually required to intervene between them and the well or the neighboring property. In view of the universality of their use and of the completeness with which modern communities are inured to their presence, it seems almost hopeless to attempt to secure a proper realization of their great defects. They are always the seat of the foulest, and even of the most dangerous, decomposition. They taint not only the air and the soil, but the water of the soil which goes so often to feed our sources of drinking-water, and their local stench is of itself sufficient to sicken all who have not by daily and lifelong habit become accustomed to it. Taking the country at large—farm houses and village houses as well as the dwellings of cities—it is not too much to say that the best sanitary service that [p. 220]can be rendered by those interested in the removal of causes of ill-health would be in securing the abolition of these barbarous domestic appliances. In many ways the cesspool is as bad as the vault, but in some respects the vault is facile princeps as a public and private nuisance of the most annoying and dangerous character. Wherever a public or private sewer is available, wherever disposal by irrigation is possible, and wherever even the crudest attention can be secured for an automatic or simpler earth-closet, the strongest effort should be directed to the absolute inhibition of the common privy-vault.

II. THE REMOVAL OF LIQUID HOUSEHOLD WASTES.—As has been stated above, the liquid household wastes are of much more serious consequence from a sanitary point of view, as compared with excrementitious matters, than the public has been wont to suppose. These, owing to the large amount of water which they contain, are beyond the reach of any system of dry conservancy. They consist almost invariably of a flood of water containing but a small percentage of refuse food, urine, soap, filth of the laundry, grease—everything, in fact, except fecal matter and the coarser garbage and ashes—constituting the waste of the household. Where water-closets are used fecal matter is generally added to the flow, but its relative quantity is small, and its presence or absence does not seriously affect the problem of disposal.

In a house provided with abundant, generally superabundant, plumbing appliances, with a large consumption of water, the whole apparatus is constructed on the theory that all manner of filth is to be taken up by running water and carried well without the house. Where this theoretical end is completely attained there exists a condition of drainage rarely met with and little to be criticised. Unfortunately, the theoretical excellence is rarely secured. Running water confined within a narrow channel, and so compelled to move with force sufficient to give an energetic scouring to the walls of its conduit, may be trusted to carry with it or to drive before it pretty nearly all foreign matter that may have been contributed to it, but the moment this vigorous current is checked, that moment the tendency to excessive deposit begins. It is checked in practice in various ways:

First. By too great a diameter of the pipe: a volume of discharge requiring a velocity of 4 feet per second in a pipe 1 inch in diameter would have a velocity of only 1 foot per second in a channel 2 inches in diameter, and of less than 6 inches per second in a channel 3 inches in diameter. Ordinarily, except as the deposits are removed by decomposition (always objectionable), the deposited matters accumulate and reduce the original bore to the diameter which will secure a cleansing flow. It is the part of wisdom to provide only this bore at the outset or not greatly to exceed it, and it is one of the earliest recommendations of an experienced sanitary engineer to reduce the size of too large bores where they exist.

Second. By the use of traps larger than the pipes leading to them and from them, thus increasing the natural tendency of all traps to stagnation and deposit.

Third. By the use of vertical waste-pipes, which are almost universal, and which are very often necessary. The velocity of a current measured along the axis of the pipe is less if the direction is vertical than if it is laid on [p. 221]a steep slope, because of the tendency of liquids flowing through vertical pipes, which they do not fill, to adhere to the walls and to travel with a rotary movement. I have seen vertical soil-pipes furred with excrement to a thickness of nearly three-eighths of an inch; I have never seen a corresponding deposit in a pipe of good slope where the current was direct. This latter point is rather one of curious interest than of practical value—certainly from the physician's point of view. Even in original construction it is rarely possible to give soil-pipes other than a practically vertical course as they pass from one story to the next. Indeed, the physician need not trouble himself to consider the question of the size or of the direction of this main channel. He will often find occasion to criticise the use of unduly large waste-pipes from single vessels; as, for example, two-inch pipes leading from bath-tubs; two and a half-inch pipes leading from laundry-tubs; and three-inch pipes leading from kitchen-sinks. Where reconstruction is to be undertaken, he may with advantage exert himself to secure in these lateral waste-pipes a diameter never exceeding one and a half inches, and from kitchen- and pantry-sinks, whose outflow is loaded with grease, preferably not exceeding the diameter of one and a half inches, with traps of even a little less size. Where several vessels lead into the same waste-pipe these small diameters may increase the tendency to the emptying of the traps by siphonage, but if proper mechanical traps are used for baths, wash-bowls, and laundry-tubs, and if ample flushing appliances are connected with kitchen- and pantry-sinks, the temporary removal of the trapping-water by siphonage may generally be disregarded. It will seldom happen that the removal of water will be so complete as to prevent the satisfactory closing of the mechanical valve by capillarity, even if it fails, in itself, to make a perfectly tight fit.

A favorite recent requirement of theoretical sanitarians, and one which has perhaps for business reasons been eagerly accepted by the plumbing trade, is what is called the "back" ventilation of traps; that is, the carrying of a vent-pipe from every trap in the house to a point above the roof. In my judgment, there is more to condemn than there is to commend this practice, for I believe that the more rapid emptying of traps by evaporation where they are not constantly supplied by frequent use, the dangers of accident to lead pipe, which is generally used for ventilating purposes, and the misapplication of a large outlay which might better be applied in other directions, constitute convincing arguments against this favorite new method of preserving the integrity of the water-seal. There are a number of traps which are closed by floating balls, or by balls bearing upon the outlet, which seem to be quite satisfactory and efficient. The worst waste-pipes, by far, are those of kitchen- and pantry-sinks which pass a large amount of hot grease. This soon cools sufficiently to congeal, and it attaches itself to the walls of the pipe, where it does congeal until the bore is reduced to what is barely sufficient to furnish the necessary limited water-way. Grease-traps of various forms have been invented with a view to retaining this obstructing material. After much experience with all of them that have been in general use, I have become convinced that the only satisfactory way to avoid the difficulty in question is to retain the outflow of the sink until a certain considerable quantity has accumulated, and until its grease has entirely [p. 222]congealed, then to discharge the whole volume rapidly through a pipe of small calibre. This may be done with Carson's grease-trap by throwing in a pail of water to start a siphon action when the vessel has become filled to its overflow-point. It is more simply accomplished by a device of my own, wherein the whole outflow is retained by a plug at the bottom of a large vessel working after the manner of the plug of a wash-basin, until it is filled to the level of the sink, and then opening the outlet for its sudden discharge.

Good workmanship is as important as, if not indeed more important than, good arrangement. It seems a very simple proposition to say that all waste-pipes, whose office it is to carry foul liquids out of the house, should be made tight in material and in joint. It is a remarkable fact, however, that leaky joints in soil-pipes and in drains are by no means rare. Probably there are few houses, very few, in which they do not occur. The soil-pipe is put together by inserting the small end of each section into the bell at the top of the section below it, practically like putting the outlet of one funnel into the larger upper portion of another. There may be abundant space for leakage at every joint from the top to the bottom of the house, without there being the least show of the leakage of water. The foul air within the pipe may escape freely through a dozen openings, while the heavier liquid flow takes its easiest and most direct course downward from the point of one pipe through the bell of the one below. When we come to the horizontal run of the soil-pipe in the basement, if an imperfection of the joint occurs on the lower side there is an obvious drip, which continues at least until closed by rust. Similar imperfections in other parts of the joint would not be so manifested. It has recently been demonstrated that there is no safety in the construction of soil-pipes short of that absolute assurance which can be secured only by an efficient test. Plugging all the outlets of the soil-pipe and filling it with water, the slightest leak will be exposed.

However defective may be the condition of an iron soil-pipe, vertical or horizontal, it is perfection itself compared with the usual state of a drain laid under the cellar floor; and here is a point where the least experienced inspector of house drainage cannot be mistaken. Under all circumstances, at least in all work hitherto executed, he should demand as absolutely necessary that the drains under the cellar floor be removed, that the earth which has been fouled by the leakage of its joints and its breaks shall be taken out to the clean untainted soil below, and refilled with well-rammed pure earth or with concrete, the drainage being carried through a properly-jointed iron pipe above the pavement, and preferably with a fall from the ceiling of the cellar to near the floor at the point of outlet—in full sight for the whole distance. It sometimes happens that the necessity for using laundry-tubs or other vessels in the cellar makes the retention of an underground course imperative. When retained, the drain should be of heavy cast iron with most securely leaded joints tested under a head of several feet. When found to be tight and secure, it should not be, as ordinarily recommended, left in an open channel covered with boards or flags and surrounded by a vermin-breeding, unventilated and uninspected space, but closely and completely imbedded in the best hydraulic cement mortar. Its careful testing before this [p. 223]enclosure is of course the only condition under which the work can be permitted.

Tightness of all waste-pipes being secured, the next point in order is their proper ventilation. A good deal has been said, and little has been proved, about the different effects on the human system of the gases of decomposition which have been produced in the absence of a sufficient circulation of air, and those produced where the ventilation and dilution are more complete. The probabilities of the case are, of course, entirely in favor of the latter condition, and it is accepted by all sanitarians as an axiom that all water-ways and all vessels in which organic decomposition, even the decomposition of adhering slime, takes place, should be ventilated as thoroughly as possible. Until about ten years ago nearly all waste-pipes were tightly closed at the top, and were shut from the sewer by a trap at the foot, allowing absolutely no communication between the outer air and the atmosphere of the pipe except as fresh air might be carried in through the water-seals of the traps at each end. At about that time it was becoming the general custom in the better class of work to carry a small vent-pipe, often only one inch in diameter, rarely more than two inches in diameter, through the roof of the house, closing it at the top and perforating it with a few inefficient holes. This had undoubtedly the effect of relieving the pressure on the atmosphere of the pipe caused by the filling of unventilated sewers with tide-water or storm-water, or by a sudden increase of temperature from the admission of hot water. Later, it was accepted as a universal rule, and it became a quite general practice, to carry the soil-pipe above the roof with its full diameter, providing its summit with some form of ventilating cowl. All this constituted not ventilation, but venting. Real ventilation was introduced only with the very recent improvement of admitting fresh air at the foot of the soil-pipe, so as to make a complete circulation from one end to the other—a circulation sufficient to produce, by the diffusion of gases, a very fair ventilation of lateral waste-pipes of moderate length. It is now coming to be understood that ventilating cowls, of whatever form, are an obstruction to the movement of air in the absence of wind, and that, as what is needed is never a vigorous current, but always a living one, these cowls had better be dispensed with. We have learned, too, that the most efficient means for increasing the flow of air through the top is to increase its diameter at the top, enlarging the highest length of a four-inch pipe, for example, to a diameter of six inches. With this arrangement, and with a foot-ventilation four inches in diameter opening at a point where it can never be obstructed by rubbish or by snow, there will be secured a condition perhaps more efficient in improving the condition of an imperfectly drained house than any other one thing that may be done.

I have sketched above, in a very hurried manner, the main outline of a system of house-drainage which may be accepted or which may be recommended by a physician with confidence of securing a good result. To go more into detail in technical matters would be out of place in a paper of this character. Before leaving this subject, however, it is important to call attention to the fact that what is recognized in our houses as sewer gas is in far greater degree the product of decomposition taking place within the house-drains themselves than the product [p. 224]of decomposition in the distant sewer forced into the house through its connecting drain. It is emphatically a case of the beam in our own eye as compared with the mote in the eye of our neighbor. It is a rule which has exceptions, but they are few, that the contained air of the house-pipes is far worse than the contained air of the sewer; and the conviction is growing that the use of a trap to the main drain between the house and the public sewer is more often objectionable than advantageous. Such a trap always tends to check the flow of the drain and to induce deposits whose decomposition is objectionable. Wherever the abandonment of the trap is anything like universal the considerable ventilation of the sewer thereby secured brings its atmosphere to a condition which makes it not objectionable, and generally useful, as a source of movement in the air of the interior drain- and soil-pipe.

(*a*) Public sewers are more or less good or bad entirely according to their character and condition. As a rule, a well-flushed sewer which is used for no other purpose than the removal of foul waste, built on what is called the separate system, and automatically flushed at least daily, may be considered to be, if well laid and tightly jointed, absolutely safe. A public sewer of large size and of irregular construction, receiving not only household wastes, but the wash of streets as well, may be regarded at least as an object of grave suspicion. These general statements may be so far qualified by the character of the sewers of each class as to run very nearly together; that is to say, separate sewers, with leaky joints, irregular grades, defective alignment, insufficient flushing, and inadequate restriction as to the matters they are to receive, will be an intolerable and dangerous nuisance; on the other hand, a large brick sewer built in the best manner and of the best material, with sufficient fall and sufficient supply to maintain itself in a cleanly condition, is free from the serious drawbacks which usually attach to sewers of this class.

With sewerage as with house-drainage it is not worth while to attempt here to give anything like detailed directions for inspection and for reformation. It will suffice to call attention to this one broad and general rule: Every sewer or drain having for its object the removal of putrescible organic matters must be so arranged as to maintain itself in a condition of practically absolute cleanliness, without, as in the case of storm-water sewers, waiting for the flushing effect of storms, which often come only at long intervals, during which the worst condition of decomposition may be established. Whether the sewer be intended for drainage only or for both drainage- and storm-water, if it contains at any time deposits of any kind, it is defective—more or less so, of course, according to the extent and duration of the accumulation.

Although it should be rigidly insisted upon in every case that the sewer should maintain itself free from deposits, there will still be, unavoidably, a certain amount of foul gas produced by the decomposition of the matters coating its walls, and in order to dilute and to remove this, and perhaps in order to modify their original character, the most thorough ventilation is necessary.

Any sewer or other drain which at any time gives forth the odor of putrid decomposition is in bad condition and should be at once rendered inoffensive. So far as I know, there is no exception to this rule. I have met no conditions in towns of any size where absolute self-cleansing may [p. 225]not be secured. It is worth while, however, to repeat here the statement made above, that sewer gas, in so far as it is a serious factor in connection with the drainage of houses, is the product of the interior pipes of the house much more frequently than of the public sewer in the street.

(*b*) The disposal of liquid wastes by irrigation, so far as this method is applied to the outflow of public sewers, is not of especial interest here, but an important modification has been made of the system of irrigation which is of the greatest consequence in considering the sanitary improvement of isolated country-houses, of hospitals, prisons, etc., and of houses in towns about which there is a small amount of available land. The process which has been found best suited to the purpose is the invention of the Rev. Henry Moule, the inventor of the earth-closet. He found it a serious drawback to the dry-earth system that it was incapable of taking care of the liquid wastes of the house. He devised a method of conducting the liquid into very shallow drains made with open-jointed agricultural drain-tiles, so porous in their character as to allow the liquid carried by them to escape at the joints into the soil, and thus get the benefit of its purifying qualities without the unsightly and often offensive process of allowing the liquid to flow over the surface. The first use made of this system was about 1866. Since that time its use has extended very considerably both here and in England, and many improvements have been made in its details, so that it may now be accepted as entirely satisfactory.

The process in its best development, as applied to the drainage of single houses, may be thus described, many of the appliances used being the subject of patents: The outflow from the house is delivered into a settling-basin or grease-trap of sufficient size to still the flow, to cause solids to settle to the bottom, and grease and other light matters to float at the top. The outlet from this basin is through a pipe having its inlet at some distance below its overflow-point; that is, at the level of the comparatively clarified liquid, below the grease and above the sediment. The outflow passes into another vessel known as a flush-tank, where it accumulates until it reaches the summit of a self-acting siphon. This height being reached, any considerable addition to the flow sets the siphon in action, and the whole contents of the flush-tank are discharged with rapidity into the drain beyond. The discharge completed, air is automatically admitted to the siphon, and no further flow can take place until the flush-tank has again been filled. The drain, of iron or vitrified pipes tightly joined, is continued to the edge of the ground prepared for purification. It here delivers into a series of open-jointed agricultural tiles, laid with their bottoms not more than ten inches below the surface of the ground. The total length of these tile-drains is regulated according to the discharging capacity of the flush-tank, with a view to their becoming entirely filled at each discharge. Within a short time after the flow has ceased the liquid has all left the pipes and entered the soil, its impurities being retained and its filtered water settling away into the porous or artificially drained ground below. During the interval between the discharges of the flush-tank, a day or more, the process of purification (oxidation) of the retained impurities goes on in the soil, and its thorough aëration prepares it to purify the next discharge. This method of [p. 226]disposal is now employed in connection with hundreds of houses, and its use, which has in some cases continued for a dozen years, is constantly increasing. Its application implies a certain amount of fall, but this amount need not be great. The discharging height of the tank need not be more than twelve inches. The main outlet need not fall more rapidly than at the rate of 1 to 300, and the absorption-drains ought not to fall more rapidly than at the rate of 1 to 600. If the tank can be built on the top of the ground, an average surface fall of 1 to 400 can usually be made to meet all the requirements. Where waste matters are to be removed from cellars and basements below the level of the ground, a greater fall is necessary, or the wastes which are there collected must be thrown to the tank by pumping or otherwise.

Where there is a bit of grass-land a little removed from the house (and from sight), it answers a perfectly satisfactory purpose to dispense with the absorption-drains and to deliver the main outlet directly on to the surface of the ground. The effect in both cases is entirely different from what it would be were the flow of the drains not regulated by the use of the flush-tank. The moment we have a constant slight discharge, either on the surface of the ground or into the absorption-drains, we establish a condition of constant saturation which leads to the over-fouling of a small area, which is rarely if ever purified by aëration. For an intermittent discharge some form of flush-tank is an absolute necessity. It is often found in practice, where the flow from the house is considerable, that the discharge of the house-drains into the settling-basin produces such an agitation of its contents as to set in motion and to carry into the flush-tank bits of paper partly macerated, grease, etc. This has been met by a recent improvement, which consists in building a transverse wall in the settling-basin, which checks the current from the house-drain and causes the flow from the house side of the wall to pass over its top in a thin small current which does not materially agitate the contents of that part of the basin from which the outflow pipe is fed.

(*c*) The cesspool is still the chief reliance of the world at large. There is nothing to be said in its favor save what may be based on the old adage that "what is out of sight is out of mind." There is everything to be said in its condemnation, whether we regard its contents as a great mass of putrefying and infecting filth, as the source of oozings which travel through crevices of rocks, through layers of gravel, through seams in clay, or through lighter soils into and under cellars and into drinking-water wells and defectively constructed cisterns, or as an ever-active gas-retort supplying the pipes of the house with the foulest products of putrefaction. It is in all respects and under all circumstances a curse, unless placed far away from the possibility of tainting the air we breathe or the soil over which we live, or from which we or others take our drinking-water, and even then it had better be abandoned.

The simple drainage of the soil involves a question of the greatest importance. If the ground under the house or about it is at any time, unless perhaps immediately after heavy rains, saturated with moisture, we have to apprehend a condition of insalubrity more or less serious in proportion to the degree of saturation and the degree of foulness with which this is associated. The drainage requirements of land outside of the house are less easily determined, but it requires nothing more than a casual[p. 227]examination of the cellar in ordinarily wet weather to determine whether or not an improvement of its soil-water drainage is necessary. If it is at such times wet, or even persistently damp, thorough drainage is demanded; and it is only necessary to say that this should be secured by some process which can under no circumstances bring the air of the cellar into communication with the air of a sewer or foul drain.

I have purposely abstained in the foregoing remarks from invading the province of the physician or the physiologist by discussing the influence of bad drainage on the health of those living subject to it. It may safely be assumed that physicians who care enough about the subject to interest themselves in investigating the condition of local or general drainage have convictions concerning it which could not be strengthened by the opinion of one belonging to another profession. The assumption is also confidently made that no intelligent medical man will hesitate for a moment to accept the dictum that the site of the house must be dry, and that it and its neighborhood must be entirely exempt from the influence of foul organic decomposition.

[p. 229]

GENERAL DISEASES.
FROM SPECIAL MORBID AGENTS OPERATING FROM WITHOUT.

SIMPLE CONTINUED FEVER.	DIPHTHERIA.
TYPHOID FEVER.	CHOLERA.
TYPHUS FEVER.	PLAGUE.
RELAPSING FEVER.	LEPROSY.
VARIOLA.	EPIDEMIC CEREBRO-SPINAL MENINGITIS.
VACCINIA.	PERTUSSIS.
VARICELLA.	INFLUENZA.
SCARLET FEVER.	DENGUE.
RUBEOLA.	RABIES AND HYDROPHOBIA.
RÖTHELN.	GLANDERS AND FARCY.
MALARIAL FEVERS.	MALIGNANT PUSTULE.
PAROTITIS.	PYÆMIA AND SEPTICÆMIA.
ERYSIPELAS.	PUERPERAL FEVER.
YELLOW FEVER.	BERIBERI.

SIMPLE CONTINUED FEVER.
BY JAMES H. HUTCHINSON, M.D.

DEFINITION.—A continued, non-contagious fever, varying in duration from one to twelve days, and in temperate climates almost invariably ending in recovery. It may arise from any non-specific cause capable of producing a temporary derangement of one or more of the important functions of the body, is generally easily distinguished from the other continued fevers by the absence of the characteristic symptoms of these diseases, and presents in fatal cases no specific lesions.

SYNONYMS.—Synocha, vel Synochus Simplex, Febricula, Ephemera or Ephemeral Fever, Irritative Fever, Ardent Continued Fever, Sun Fever.

HISTORY.—Much difference of opinion continues to prevail, even at the present time, in regard to the existence of a simple continued fever, which, on the one hand, occurs independently of local inflammations or traumatic causes, and, on the other, is distinct from typhoid, typhus, and relapsing fevers; many observers contending that the condition to which this name is given is only a mild or modified form of one or other of the graver varieties of continued fever, from which the characteristic symptoms are absent. Prominently among modern writers, Dr. Tweedie[1] has taken this view of the subject, for, after reviewing the arguments for and against the recognition of simple continued fever as a distinct disease, he asserts that there is not sufficient evidence to justify us in encumbering our nosology with a doubtful novelty. If, however, there is room for doubt as to its right to a place in the list of diseases, there is certainly no good reason for characterizing it as a novelty, since it has been referred to, according to Murchison,[2] by many authors from the time of Hippocrates down to the present day, who not only separate it from the graver forms of fever, and give a very accurate description of its symptoms, but seem to have been perfectly familiar with the causes which give rise to it, and to have had very correct notions as to its proper management. Thus, Riverius[3] was aware of the existence of two forms of simple fever—the ephemeral, which lasts, as its name implies, only a single day, and the Synochus Simplex, arising from the same causes, but in which the fever continues for from four to seven days. Strother[4] and Ball[5] also allude to this fever in terms that leave no doubt upon the mind but that they distinguished it clearly from other forms of continued fever. Among more recent writers who have made this distinction may be mentioned Lyons,[6] Jenner,[7] G. B. Wood,[8] Flint,[9] Murchison,[10] and J. C. Wilson.[11] Indeed, the weight of authority is decidedly on the side of those who claim for it a recognition as a distinct and separate disease.

[1] *Lectures on the Continued Fevers.*

[2] *A Treatise on the Continued Fevers of Great Britain*, London, 1873.

[3] *The Practice of Physick, being chiefly a Translation of the Works of Lazarus Riverius*, London, 1678.

[4] *A Critical Essay on Fever*, 1718.

[5] *A Treatise on Fevers*, London, 1758.

[6] *A Treatise on Fever*, London, 1861.

[7] *Medical Times*, March 22, 1851.

[8] *A Treatise on the Practice of Medicine*, Philadelphia, 1855.

[9] *A Treatise on the Principles and Practice of Medicine*, Philadelphia, 1868.

[10] *Ibid.*

[11] *A Treatise on the Continued Fevers*, New York, 1881.

Unquestionably, many cases which have been classed under the head of simple continued fever, are really mild or abortive cases of typhoid or typhus fever, in which, in consequence of partial protection on the part of the patient, the characteristic symptoms of these diseases have not been developed. Such cases are seen in numbers during epidemics of these diseases. But, making due allowance for this source of error, there yet remain many cases which cannot be thus explained. Moreover, the disease occurs at times when no such epidemics exist. It may, therefore, be safely assumed that there is such a fever, and that, consequently, it must be accorded full recognition.

CAUSES.—Any non-specific cause which is capable of producing a profound derangement of one or more of the important functions of the body may give rise to simple continued fever. It may follow, therefore, upon excesses of the table, extreme mental or bodily fatigue, exposure to the direct rays of the sun, or to great heat or cold, or upon the suppression of a secretion. One of its most frequent causes is over-exertion in warm weather. James C. Wilson has called attention to its frequent occurrence as a consequence of the combined influence of the excitement, the physical exhaustion, and the exposure to the direct rays of the mid-day sun which are attendant upon surf-bathing. It is often due in young children to the irritation involved in the process of teething or to that caused by the presence of worms in the alimentary canal. Wood taught that it might also sometimes occur during the prevalence of contagious diseases as an effect of the epidemic influence in those who were partially protected by a previous attack of the disease, or from some other cause, but it is more probable that cases arising under these circumstances are either mild cases of the prevalent disease or else are attributable to fatigue from nursing or to over-anxiety. The disease is more common in the young than in the old, and in children than in adults—probably from the greater impressionability of the nervous systems of the latter.

The causes of the ardent continued fever of the tropics, which is usually recognized as a form of simple continued fever, do not differ materially, except in degree, from those of the simpler forms of the disease; but exposure to the direct rays of the sun would seem to be especially prone to give rise to the disease in those who are unaccustomed to the heat of a tropical climate. Robust young Europeans lately arrived in a warm country are, it is said, peculiarly liable to suffer from it.[12] It is most common in those parts of India which do not experience much of the benefit of the monsoon rains, and whose hot season is not tempered by regular breezes from the sea. It is hence more frequently met with [p. 233]in inland districts in which the temperature is high, but in which malaria-generating conditions are absent.

[12] Morehead, *Clinical Researches on Diseases in India*, London, 1856; also Twining, *Clinical Illustrations of the More Important Diseases of Bengal*, Calcutta, 1835.

SYMPTOMS AND COURSE.—Simple continued fever occurs in this country only as a sporadic disease, and almost invariably ends in recovery; in tropical climates, however, it may prevail epidemically, and sometimes presents symptoms of a very grave character. In its mildest form it not infrequently runs its course in a few hours, and is rarely prolonged much beyond twenty-four, and is hence called ephemera. It then usually begins somewhat abruptly with a chill, but in a few instances this is preceded by feelings of languor and weariness. Febrile reaction is soon established, and is generally well marked; the pulse is quick and full, the temperature rises rapidly, and the face is flushed. The tongue is coated with a whitish fur, the urine is scanty and high-colored, and the bowels are constipated. Other symptoms are excessive thirst, headache, restlessness, and sleeplessness, or, on the other hand, a tendency to somnolence. Vomiting is not common except in those cases which follow upon an error of diet, but there is generally some nausea and anorexia. Muscular pains are also occasionally present, and may give rise to a good deal of distress. The subsidence of these symptoms is often quite as abrupt as their onset, the crisis being frequently marked by a copious perspiration.

In other cases, however, the fever is more prolonged, and the symptoms, although not differing in kind, are apt to be more severe than those above detailed. The pulse is often full, hard, and bounding; the headache throbbing or darting in character; the tendency to somnolence increases, or gives place to delirium; and the pyrexia is more marked. Frequently an eruption of herpes is observed upon the lips and upon other parts of the face, from which circumstance the disease is sometimes called herpetic fever. Davasse[13] also observed in a few cases pale bluish spots, not elevated above the surface and not disappearing under pressure, which are identical with the tâches bleuâtres sometimes seen in typhoid fever and other diseases, and therefore have no diagnostic value. In this form the duration of the disease may be from four to ten or twelve days. The defervescence is usually less rapid than the rise in temperature, and is generally accompanied by a free perspiration, diarrhoea, a copious deposit of urates in the urine, or less frequently by hemorrhage from the uterus or rectum,[14] or from the nose, mouth, or urethra. This constitutes the synocha or inflammatory fever of the older writers. In children in whom there is no reason to suspect malarial poisoning the disease sometimes assumes a remittent form, and then constitutes a variety of the infantile remittent fever of authors—a name, however, which, it must be remembered, has been made to include a great many distinct diseases.[15]

[13] Quoted by Murchison.

[14] Murchison.

[15] Lyons.

When the disease occurs in individuals who are broken down in health from any cause[16]—as, for instance, previous illness, deficient food, long-continued anxiety, or great fatigue—it not infrequently presents symptoms of an asthenic character. The febrile reaction is then less intense, and the pulse feebler and more frequent, than in the variety just described. The duration of the disease in this form is also generally longer. Murchison has proposed for it the name of simple asthenic fever.

[16] Wood.

Under the name of ardent continued fever, Indian medical writers have described a variety of the disease which is frequently met with in tropical[p. 234]countries, and which is usually much more severe than the varieties already referred to. In addition to the symptoms presented by these, Morehead[17] says that there is often intolerance of light and sound, contracted and subsequently dilated pupils, ringing noises in the ears, anxious respiration, pains in the limbs and loins, and a sense of oppression at the epigastrium. The bowels are sometimes confined; at others vitiated bilious discharges take place. The tongue is white, often with florid edges, and the urine scanty and high-colored. At the end of from forty-eight to sixty hours the febrile phenomena may subside, the skin become cold, and death take place from exhaustion and sudden collapse. In some cases the symptoms of cerebral disturbance are greater in degree, and in these coma may soon supervene upon delirium. Convulsions, epileptiform in character, with relaxation of the sphincters and suppression of urine, also frequently occur, and occasionally cerebral hemorrhage. In other cases the symptoms of gastritis are more prominent, or jaundice may appear and aggravate the disease.

[17] *Clinical Researches on Disease in India*, London, 1856. See also "Croonian Lectures," by Sir Joseph Fayrer, *Brit. Med. Jour.*, April 29, 1882.

Symptoms closely resembling those just described are occasionally met with in this country in patients who have been exposed for some time to the direct rays of the summer sun, but who have escaped a sunstroke. Indeed, a few writers have been so much impressed with the general resemblance which this latter condition bears to the fevers that they have insisted upon including it in this group, and have given it the name of thermic or heat fever. This view of the pathology of sunstroke has, however, never been generally accepted.

One of the most characteristic symptoms of the disease in all its forms is the rapid rise of temperature, which may in ephemera be as great as from four to seven degrees in the course of a few hours, and which may be followed in a few hours more by an equally abrupt defervescence. When the fever is more prolonged, although the temperature rises rapidly, it may not attain its greatest elevation for from forty to sixty hours after the onset of the symptoms, and its fall will be more gradual than in the preceding variety. Unfortunately, there are no reliable thermometric records of ardent continued fever. The urine is usually scanty and high-colored during the height of the fever, especially in the severer forms of the disease. Its specific gravity is high, and it contains a large amount of solids, especially of urea. With the fall of the temperature it rapidly increases in quantity, and is very apt to let fall a copious lateritious sediment on cooling. According to Parkes,[18] who closely observed six cases with the view of determining this question, albuminuria does not occur at any stage of the disease. Convalescence is usually rapid, and is not liable to be interrupted by the occurrence of sequelæ.

[18] *The Composition of the Urine*, by Edmund A. Parkes, M.D., London, 1860.

DIAGNOSIS.—The diagnosis in those cases of simple continued fever in which the connection between the disease and some one of the conditions which have been referred to above as capable of exciting it has been distinctly made out, presents little difficulty. It is otherwise, however, when this relationship is not apparent. Indeed, the symptoms of the disease so closely resemble those of an abortive or mild attack of typhoid or typhus fever, in which the characteristic eruption is wanting, that the[p. 235]physician may sometimes remain in doubt as to the nature of the disease he has been called upon to treat, even after the recovery of the patient. This difficulty will of course be especially likely to present itself during the epidemic prevalence of these diseases. Simple continued fever may, however, generally be distinguished from either of the latter by the much greater severity of its initial symptoms, and particularly by the rapid rise of temperature—a rise of from four to seven degrees in the course of a few hours—which does not take place in these fevers, but which, it must be remembered, may occur in erysipelas, measles, pneumonia, and some other diseases. The absence of a characteristic eruption, although it would not render it certain, would be in favor of the diagnosis of simple continued fever, as would also the absence of diarrhoea in cases in which there was difficulty in deciding between this disease and typhoid fever. On the other hand, Murchison regards the presence of an herpetic eruption on the lips as almost pathognomonic of simple continued fever; but in this country such an eruption is not an infrequent attendant upon fevers of malarial origin, and many observers attach great importance to it in the diagnosis of these diseases.

Simple continued fever is not likely to be mistaken for relapsing fever, except during epidemics of the latter disease. It may be discriminated from relapsing fever, the first paroxysm of which it closely resembles, by the absence of severe articular pains, of tenderness in the epigastric zone, of enlargement of the liver and spleen, and of jaundice. It may be mistaken for tubercular meningitis, especially in those cases in which the nervous symptoms are more than usually prominent, or in which a hereditary predisposition to tuberculosis exists; but its true nature may generally be recognized by its more abrupt commencement, and by the absence of the constant vomiting, screaming fits, strabismus, and paralysis so characteristic of the latter disease.

It is scarcely necessary to add that a local inflammation or a traumatic cause may give rise to symptoms simulating those of simple continued fever, and that the diagnosis of this disease must be uncertain until these conditions have been positively ascertained to be absent, or, if present, until they have been proved to be complications, and not the causes of the disease.

PROGNOSIS.—The prognosis of this disease, as it is met with in this country, is favorable. Indeed, when uncomplicated it may be said to end invariably in recovery, except in the aged and feeble, in whom, when it occurs during the great heat of the summer season, it is apt to assume the asthenic form, and to be accompanied by symptoms of a grave character. The ardent continued fever of the tropics, on the other hand, not infrequently terminates fatally, or may leave the sufferer from it a chronic invalid for life, which is frequently shortened by obscure cerebral or meningeal changes, which give rise to irritability, impaired memory, epilepsy, headache, mania, partial or complete paraplegia, or blindness.[19]

[19] Sir Joseph Fayrer, K.C.S.I., M.D., F.R.S., *Brit. Med. Jour.*, April 29, 1881, p. 607.

ANATOMICAL LESIONS.—Death so rarely occurs in this latitude from simple continued fever that the opportunities for making post-mortem examinations do not often occur. There are, however, a sufficient number of such examinations on record to show that the disease gives [p. 236]rise to no specific lesions. According to Murchison and Martin,[20] inspection in fatal cases of ardent continued fever usually reveals the presence of great congestion of all the internal organs and of the sinuses of the brain and pia mater, of an increased amount of intracranial fluid, and occasionally of an effusion into the abdominal cavity, and more rarely into the thoracic cavity.

[20] *The Influence of Tropical Climates on European Constitutions*, by James Ranald Martin, F.R.S., London, 1856.

TREATMENT.—In the milder forms of the disease little or no treatment is required—a fact which seems to have been recognized and acted upon long ago, since Strother remarks that the cure of it is so easy that physicians are seldom consulted about such patients. An emetic when the attack has been caused by excesses of the table, and there is reason to believe that there is undigested food in the stomach, a purgative when constipation exists, and cooling drinks, the effervescing draught or some other saline diaphoretic, are usually the only remedies that are called for. In cases in which the febrile action is more intense and prolonged, in addition to the use of these remedies an effort should be made to reduce the heat of the skin and the frequency of the pulse by sponging with cold water and by the administration of digitalis and aconite. The headache which is often a distressing symptom may usually be relieved by the application of evaporating lotions, and restlessness quieted by the bromides. Subsequently, quinia may be given with advantage. The patient should be restricted to liquid diet during the continuance of fever.

In the asthenic form quinia and the mineral acids, nutritious food, and very frequently alcoholic stimulants, must be given from the beginning. In the treatment of the ardent continued fever of the tropics the cold affusion or the cold bath, with quinia, would appear to be indicated, but Morehead and other Indian physicians advise the use of evacuants with copious and repeated venesections, cupping, and leeches, aided by tartar emetic, till all local determination and the chief urgent symptoms are removed; and Murchison expresses the belief, founded on his own observations, that life is often sacrificed by adopting less active measures.

[p. 237]

TYPHOID FEVER.
BY JAMES H. HUTCHINSON, M.D.

DEFINITION.—An endemic infectious fever, usually lasting between three and four weeks, and associated with constant lesions of the solitary and agminate glands of the ileum, and with enlargement of the spleen and mesenteric glands. Its invasion is usually gradual and often insidious. Sometimes the only symptoms present in the beginning are a feeling of lassitude, some gastric derangement, and a slight elevation of temperature; at others there are slight rigors or chilly sensations, headache, epistaxis, diarrhoea, and pain in the abdomen. The principal symptoms of the fully-formed disease are a febrile movement possessing certain characters, headache passing into delirium and stupor, diarrhoea associated with ochrey-yellow stools, tympanites, pain and gurgling in the right iliac fossa, a red and furred tongue, which later often becomes dry, brown, and fissured; a frequent pulse; an eruption of rose-colored spots, occurring about the seventh or eighth day, slightly elevated above the surface, disappearing under pressure, and coming out in successive crops, each spot lasting about three days; prostration not marked in the beginning, but rapidly increasing; and occasionally deafness, sweats, and intestinal hemorrhages. When recovery takes place, the convalescence is usually tedious, and may sometimes be protracted by the occurrence of one or more relapses.

SYNONYMS.—The following are a few of the many names which have been given to the disease at different times. Most of them have ceased to be applied to it, and only three or four of them are at present in general use: Febris Mesenterica, 1696; Slow Nervous Fever, 1735; Febricula or Little Fever, 1740; Typhus Nervosus, 1760; Miliary Fever, 1760; Typhus Mitior, 1769; Synochus, 1769; Common Continued Fever, 1816; Gastro-Enterite, 1816; Entero-Mesenteric Fever, 1820; Abdominal and Darm Typhus, 1820; Typhus Fever of New England, 1824; Dothienterie, 1826; Enterite-folliculeuse, 1835; Infantile Remittent Fever, 1836; Enterite Septicémique, 1841; Mucous Fever, 1844; Enteric Fever, 1846; Intestinal Fever, 1856; Ileo-Typhus, 1857; Pythogenic Fever, 1858; Mountain Fever, 1870.

NAME.—It has been objected to the name "typhoid fever" as a designation for this disease that it tends to perpetuate among the laity the mistaken impression that typhoid fever is only a modified typhus fever, and also that the word typhoid has been generally applied to a condition of system which is common to a great many different diseases, [p. 238]and which is not of necessity present in this. In spite of these objections, and although it must be admitted that they are not without force, I prefer to retain the name typhoid fever, and for the following reasons: 1st. It was the name given to the disease by Louis, to whom we owe the first full and accurate description of it. 2d. It is the name by which it is best known to the profession, not only in this country but abroad. 3d. No other name has been proposed for it which is not quite as much open to criticism. Thus the term enteric fever, originally suggested by the late George B. Wood, and adopted by the London College of Physicians in its *Nomenclature of Diseases*, is objectionable because it brings into undue prominence the intestinal lesions and implies that they are the cause of the fever. The same objection may be urged against the name "intestinal fever," proposed by Budd. The name "pythogenic fever" rests upon a theory of the disease which has never been proven, and is regarded by most observers as untenable. Under these circumstances even the influence of its distinguished proposer, the late Dr. Murchison, has been insufficient to secure its adoption by the profession at large.

HISTORY.—Certain passages in the writings of Hippocrates have been appealed to by Murchison and other physicians in support of the opinion that typhoid fever was a disease of at least occasional occurrence in ancient times; but, although from the nature of its causes it is probable that it has occurred in all ages and wherever men have congregated in towns and villages, the descriptions given by the Father of Medicine in the passages alluded to are not sufficiently full to render it at all certain that typhoid fever had ever come under his observation. Indeed, there is no author of an earlier date than Spigelius[1] whose writings furnish any positive evidence that he ever met with the disease. Spigelius, however, in spite of the doubt thrown upon his observation by Hirsch,[2] would seem to have had opportunities for examining the bodies of those who had died of it, since he gives an account of several autopsies, in which he says that the small intestine was inflamed and that that part of it next to the cæcum and colon was frequently sphacelated. Panarolus[3] also says that the intestines had the appearance of being cauterized ("apparebant tanquam exusta") in some cases observed by him in Rome a little later in the same century. Willis[4] would certainly appear to have been familiar with two forms of fever, which, from the description he gives of them, could have been nothing else but typhoid and typhus fevers. Sydenham[5] also described a fever in which the prominent symptoms were diarrhoea, vomiting, delirium, a tendency to coma, and epistaxis, and which was distinguishable from the febris pestilens by the absence of a petechial eruption. Baglivi[6] of Rome in the latter part of the seventeenth century described the hæmitritæus of previous writers [p. 239]under the title of febris mesenterica, and maintained that it was always accompanied by and dependent on inflammation of the intestines and enlargement of the mesenteric glands. A similar observation was made soon after by Hoffmann,[7] and by Lancisi[8] in 1718. The latter seems to have fully recognized the characteristics of the eruption, for he says that it consisted of "elevated papules which disappeared completely on pressure." In 1759, Huxham described, under the title "slow, nervous fever," a disease which there can be no doubt was typhoid fever. He moreover pointed out very clearly the distinctions between this disease and another to which he gave the name of "putrid, malignant, petechial fever," and which was unquestionably typhus. Sir Richard Manningham[9] also described typhoid fever under the title of "febricula, or little fever." In the preface of his work he calls attention to its insidious origin, and to the fact that its gravity was often underrated at its commencement, "till, at length, more conspicuous and very terrible symptoms arise, and then the Physician is sent for in the greatest hurry, and happy for the Patient if the Symptoms, which are most obvious, do not, at this Time, mislead the Physician to the Neglect of the little latent Fever, the true Cause of these violent Symptoms." About the same time Morgagni[10] described certain post-mortem examinations in which the lesions of the intestines were evidently those of typhoid fever. Other authors, whose works bear evidence that they were familiar with the symptoms or lesions of typhoid fever, are Riedel, Roederer and Wagler, Stoll, Rutty, Sarcone, Pepe, Fasano, Mayer, Wrenholt, Sutton, Bateman, Muir, Edmonstone, Prost, Petit and Serres, Cruveilhier, Lerminier, and Andral.

[1] *De Febre Semitertiana*, Frankf., 1624; Op. Om., Amsterdam, 1745. Quoted by Murchison.
[2] *Handbuch der Historisch-Geographischen Pathologie*, von Dr. August Hirsch, Stuttgart, 1881.
[3] *Observat. Med. Pentecostæ; Romæ*, 1652. Quoted by Murchison.
[4] *Dr. Willis's Practice of Physick*, translated by Samuel Pordage, London, 1684.
[5] *The Works of Thomas Sydenham, M.D., on Acute and Chronic Diseases*, with a Variety of Annotations by George Wallis, M.D., London, 1788.
[6] *Opera Omnia Medico-practica et Anatomica*, Paris, 1788.
[7] *Opera Omnia Physico-Medico*, 1699. Quoted by Murchison.
[8] *Opera Omnia*, Geneva, 1718.
[9] *The Symptoms, Nature, etc. of the Febricula or Little Fever*, London, 1746.
[10] Quoted by Hirsch.

To Bretonneau[11] of Tours appears to belong the credit of having first distinctly pointed out the association between certain symptoms and the lesions of the solitary and agminated glands of the ileum. He regarded the disease of the intestinal glands as inflammatory, and therefore gave to it the name "dothienenterie" or "dothienenterite" (from [Greek: dothiên], a tumor, and [Greek: enteron], intestine), but, unlike Prost, fully recognized the fact that there was no necessary relation between the extent of the intestinal lesions and the gravity of the febrile symptoms. Hirsch, however, claims this honor for Pommer, whose little work on *Sporadic Typhus* he thinks has not received the consideration its merits deserve. Louis, to whom for his careful study of typhoid fever we owe a large debt of gratitude, was also fully aware of the lesions of the intestinal glands which occur in this disease.

[11] Quoted by Trousseau, *Archives Générales*, 1826.

The progress in pathology which observers were making was temporarily impeded about this time by the fact that while typhoid fever was of frequent occurrence in Paris, typhus fever was comparatively rarely met with and had not been epidemic there for several years. Bretonneau, Louis,[12] Chomel, and indeed the greater number of contemporary French physicians, therefore fell into the error of supposing that the fever which was then common in England was identical with that which they were describing, while the English physicians of the period, with but few exceptions, contended with equal strenuousness that there was but one form of continued fever, and that this was very seldom associated with disease of the intestines. In the second edition of his work Louis abandoned his former opinion, and admitted that the typhus fever of the English was a very different disease from that which formed the subject of his treatise; but the confusion which existed in England in regard to this disease was not completely dispelled until the appearance in 1849 and the following two years of several papers on this subject by Sir William Jenner,[13] in which it was conclusively demonstrated that typhoid and typhus fevers were separate and distinct diseases. In Germany, however, the non-identity of these diseases was recognized as early as 1810. Murchison says that the names by which they are still generally known in that country, typhus exanthematicus and typhus abdominalis, were given to them not long after.

[12] *Researches Anatomiques, Pathologiques et Therapeutiques sur la Maladie connue sur les Noms de gastro-entente, etc.*, par P. C. A. Louis, Paris, 1829.
[13] *Med. Chir. Trans.*, vol. xxxiii.; *Edinburgh Monthly Jour. of Med. Sci.*, vols. ix. and x., 1849-50; and *Med. Times*, vols. xx., xxi., xxii., xxxiii., 1849-51.

The contributions made by American physicians to the knowledge of typhoid fever have been both numerous and important. In 1824 it was described by Nathan Smith[14] under the name of typhus fever of New England, and in 1833, E. Hale, Jr.,[15] of Boston, published in the *Medical Magazine* for December an account of three dissections of persons considered by him to have died of the disease. In reference to these cases, Bartlett[16] says that if the diagnosis could be looked upon as certain and positive they would constitute the first published examples of intestinal lesion in New England. In February, 1835, William S. Gerhard of Philadelphia, who was then under the impression that the two diseases were identical, reported two cases under the name of typhus fever, the symptoms and post-mortem appearances of which he showed differed in no respect from those he had been accustomed to see in the cases of typhoid fever he had observed with Louis during his studies in Paris. The year after Gerhard had, however, the opportunity of observing an epidemic of true typhus fever, and was at once struck with the difference between the symptoms of the cases which then fell under his care and of those he had seen in Paris. In an admirable paper which appeared in the numbers of the *American Journal of the Medical Sciences* for February and August, 1837, he points out very clearly the differential diagnosis between the two diseases. He particularly insisted on the marked difference between the petechial eruption of typhus and the rose-colored eruption of typhoid fever. He showed that the latter disease was invariably associated with enlargement and ulceration of Peyer's patches and with enlargement of the mesenteric glands, and that these conditions were never presented in the former. He also fully recognized the fact that typhus fever was eminently contagious, while, on the other hand, he was fully aware that typhoid fever was not contagious under ordinary circumstances, "although in some epidemics," he says, "we have strong reason to believe it becomes so." The appearance of this paper marks an epoch in the history of typhoid fever. Murchison, when speaking of it, says that to Gerhard, and Pennock (who was associated with Gerhard in his observations) certainly [p. 241]belongs the credit of first clearly establishing the most important points of distinction between this disease and typhus fever, and M. Valleix alludes to it in terms equally complimentary. It is undoubtedly owing to it, more than to any other cause, that the differential diagnosis of these two diseases was perfectly understood by the great body of the profession in this country long before the question of the relation which they bore to each other was definitely settled in Great Britain,[17] or even in France.

[14] *Medical and Surgical Memoirs*, Baltimore, 1831.

[15] *Observations on the Typhoid Fever of New England*, Boston, 1839.

[16] *The History, Diagnosis, and Treatment of the Fevers of the United States*, 1842.

[17] The honor of having first clearly pointed out the distinguishing characters of typhoid and typhus fevers has been recently claimed for Sir William Jenner, but, as we have seen above, his papers on this subject were not published until thirteen years after that of Gerhard.

Bartlett gave in the *Medical Magazine*, June, 1835, a short account of the entero-mesenteric alterations in five cases of unequivocal typhoid fever, which alterations, he said, corresponded exactly to those described by Louis. In the same year, James Jackson, Jr., of Boston, published an account of the intestinal lesions observed by him in cases during the years 1830, 1833, and 1834; and again in a *Report of Typhoid Fever*, communicated to the Massachusetts Medical Society in June, 1838, says that the alterations of Peyer's patches had been noticed at the Massachusetts General Hospital previous to 1833 in cases which were carefully examined. In 1840, Shattuck of Boston published in the *American Medical Examiner* an account of some cases of typhoid and typhus fever which he had observed at the London Fever Hospital during the previous year. In this paper, which had been already communicated to the Medical Society of Observation of Paris, and which had unquestionably exerted a marked influence upon medical thought there, he pointed out very fully the distinguishing characteristics of each disease. In 1842, Dr. Bartlett issued the first edition of his work on *The History, Diagnosis, and Treatment of the Fevers of the United States*, which contains very full descriptions of both of these diseases, and of the means by which they may be distinguished from each other. Since then there have been numerous additions in this country to the literature of typhoid fever, among the most important of which may be mentioned the chapter on the disease in the respective works on *The Practice of Medicine* by Professors Wood and Flint, the article on typho-malarial fever in the *Transactions* of the International Medical Congress of 1876, and the article in the work on *The Continued Fevers*, by James C. Wilson. Abroad, the medical press has been no less active. Within the last twenty or thirty years Jaccoud and Trousseau in France, Liebermeister and Hirsch in Germany, and Tweedie and Cayley in England, have all made important additions to our knowledge of the disease. To the late Dr. Murchison[18] of London, however, is justly due the honor of having produced the best treatise on typhoid fever in any language, and the writer cheerfully acknowledges that he has drawn largely upon it for the material of the present article.

[18] *A Treatise on Continued Fevers*, London, 1873.

GEOGRAPHICAL DISTRIBUTION.—Although it will be generally admitted that the conditions of civilization favor the occurrence and extension of typhoid fever, yet there is abundant evidence that they are not absolutely necessary to its production, as there is no country, whether civilized or not, of the diseases of which we have any knowledge, in which it has not occasionally made its appearance, being met with in every variety of climate. It is endemic in North America, attacking alike the inhabitants [p. 242]of Greenland and British America and those of Mexico. In our own country it prevails from time to time in every State of the Union, committing its ravages as well among the rocks and hills of New England as in the more fertile valleys of the West and South. In many of the newly-settled portions of our country malarial fevers are, as is well known, exceedingly rife. In proportion, however, as towns and cities spring up, and as the land is properly drained, they diminish in frequency, and are gradually replaced, to a certain extent at least, by typhoid fever; but the influences which produced them retain for a long time enough of power to stamp their impress upon all other diseases. In large portions of the Western and Southern States typhoid fever is therefore rarely uncomplicated, and is much more likely to assume the form which will be fully described later as typho-malarial fever.

Typhoid fever has also occurred frequently in Central America and the West India Islands. It has prevailed from time to time in the states of South America, and occasionally assumed in some of them—as, for instance, Brazil and Chili—an epidemic form.

Typhoid fever is endemic in the British Isles, but, according to Murchison, is most common in England, more common in Ireland than in Scotland, and in Scotland more common on the west than on the east coast. It also exists as an endemic disease in every country of the continent of Europe, from Sweden and Norway on the north to Turkey on the south, and in some of them—as, for instance, France and Germany—would seem to be of much more frequent occurrence than in this country, or even in England. Medical literature is also not deficient in evidence that it has prevailed at various times in all the different countries of Asia and Africa and in Australia. Morehead asserted in the first edition of his *Clinical Researches on Diseases in India* that India enjoyed an absolute immunity from typhoid fever, but in the second edition of this work he acknowledged that a larger experience had led him to change his opinion on this point. Moreover, the writings of Annesley, Twining, and other Indian authors furnish convincing proof that the disease is by no means unknown in that country. Indeed, even the relative immunity from it which it has been claimed that tropical and subtropical countries possess has been found, upon a fuller study of the diseases of these countries, not to exist to anything like the degree that was formerly supposed.

The occasional occurrence of typhoid fever in islands separated from the main land by a considerable distance—as, for instance, the island of Norfolk,[19] which is situated in the Pacific Ocean four hundred miles west of South America—is an interesting fact, and one which, with the present limits to our knowledge on the subject, it is impossible to explain satisfactorily.

[19] Metcalfe, *Brit. Med. Jour.*, Nov., 1880.

The ETIOLOGY of typhoid fever may be considered under the heads of—1, predisposing, 2, exciting causes.

1. PREDISPOSING CAUSES.—All observers agree that the predisposition to typhoid fever is greater in childhood and early adult life than after thirty years of age. Thus, Murchison states that during twenty-three years nearly one-half the admissions to the London Fever Hospital were of patients between fifteen and twenty-five years of age, and that in more than a fourth, the patients were under fifteen years. On the other hand, [p. 243]in less than a seventh were they over thirty, and in only one in seventy-one did their ages exceed fifty. Taking these facts in connection with the circumstance that the entire population of England and Wales in 1861 was 12,481,323 persons under thirty years of age and 7,584,901 above thirty, it follows, he says, that persons under thirty are more than four times as liable to enteric fever as persons over thirty. Jackson found that the average age of the patients in two hundred and ninety-one cases observed at the Massachusetts General Hospital was a little over twenty-two years, the average age in the fatal cases being somewhat greater than in those in which recovery took place. Liebermeister, from an analysis of a large

number of cases treated at the hospital in Basle, has arrived at the same conclusion. No age, however, enjoys a complete immunity from the disease. Manzini[20] has recorded a case in which lesions of Peyer's patches similar to those of typhoid fever were found in a seventh-month foetus which died within half an hour after its birth. Cases are also on record in which death has occurred from this disease in the first few weeks of life. I have myself observed several cases in young children at the Children's Hospital in Philadelphia. The probability is, that it is of even more frequent occurrence in children than is generally supposed, as this class of patients is not often admitted into general hospitals, and as from the absence of some of its characteristic symptoms when it occurs in the very young the nature of the disease is often unrecognized.

[20] Quoted by Murchison.

On the other hand, the disease occurs not infrequently in advanced life: 83 cases out of 5911 were observed at the London Fever Hospital in persons over fifty, 27 in persons over sixty, and in 2 the age was seventy-five. In a case recorded by D'Arcy the age of the patient was eighty-six, and in one reported by Hamernyk it was ninety.[21] Bartlett long ago contended that the disease was not so rare as was generally supposed among people over forty years of age; and there is really no good reason to believe that the susceptibility to the causes of the disease in an unprotected person diminishes with advancing years, the immunity from this disease which elderly people appear to enjoy being probably due to the fact that, as the disease is not uncommon in early life, they are in many instances protected by having already passed through an attack.

[21] Quoted by Murchison.

The mean age of the male patients treated at the London Fever Hospital was slightly in excess of that of the female, but in the cases analyzed by Jackson the reverse of this was observed.

The statistics of all general hospitals, with very few exceptions, show a greater or less preponderance of males over females among the typhoid fever patients treated in them. According to Murchison, of 5988 cases admitted into the London Fever Hospital during twenty-three years, 3001 were males and 2987 were females. Of 891 cases admitted into the Glasgow Infirmary during twelve years, 527 were males and 364 females. Liebermeister states that 1297 male typhoid patients and 751 female were treated in the hospital at Basle from 1865 to 1870. Occasionally, the difference is even greater than is indicated by these figures. Thus, of 138 cases observed by Louis, all but 32 occurred in males. When, however, we consider that the proportion of men who apply for admission to hospitals when sick is much larger than that of women, we should hesitate before accepting these statistics as proof that the former [p. 244]are more liable to be attacked by typhoid fever than the latter. Indeed, the opinion which Murchison expresses is generally accepted as correct by authors, that neither sex is more likely than the other to contract the disease. Liebermeister asserts that pregnant and puerperal women and those who are nursing infants enjoy a relative immunity. On the other hand, Nathan Smith says that while the sexes are equally liable to it, more women are cut off by it than men, in consequence of its appearance during pregnancy or soon after parturition.

It was long ago pointed out by certain French observers that newcomers are much more liable to be attacked by typhoid fever than persons who have lived for some time in an infected locality. In 129 cases examined with reference to this point by Louis, the patients in 73 had not resided in Paris more than ten months, and in 102 not more than twenty months. Bartlett noticed that during an epidemic in Lowell which he had the opportunity of observing the disease attacked the recent residents in much larger proportion than the old. Liebermeister also calls attention to this peculiarity of the disease. Murchison's experience in reference to this point has been somewhat similar, for he found upon examination of the records of the London Fever Hospital that 21.84 per cent. of the patients admitted there for typhoid fever had been residents of London for less than two years. Almost all of these patients came, he says, from the provinces of England, and were in good health and comfortable circumstances at the date of their arrival in London and for some time after. Moreover, a large proportion of them were first attacked within a few weeks after changing their residence from one part of London to another. He also refers to instances in which successive visitors at the same house at intervals of months, or even years, have been seized shortly after their arrival with typhoid fever or with diarrhoea, from which the ordinary occupants were exempt. These facts indicate with sufficient clearness that habitual exposure to the causes of the disease confers, to a certain extent at least, an immunity from their effects, just as it does in the various forms of disease arising from malaria. It is not unlikely, as has been suggested by Wilson,[22] that one of the causes of the frequency of typhoid fever in the early autumn in our American cities among well-to-do people is to be formed in the circumstance that during an absence of two months or more in the mountains or by the sea they have to some extent lost the immunity acquired by habitual exposure to sewer emanations, and return to the atmosphere of the city unprotected.

[22] The occurrence of typhoid fever in the early fall among persons who have spent the summer out of town is, however, susceptible of another explanation. In many instances they have returned to houses which have been not only unoccupied, but closed, during several months, and which, in consequence of the more or less complete evaporation of the water in the traps of the drain-pipes, have been thoroughly permeated by sewer gas.

There is no evidence that any particular occupation acts as a predisposing cause of typhoid fever. Among the 621 patients treated at the Pennsylvania Hospital during the last ten years, were representatives of every branch of industry, and the same fact has been observed at every general hospital, not only in this country, but abroad. There is also no reason to believe that the station in life of itself exerts much influence in predisposing to the disease. The rich suffer equally with the poor. It would appear, indeed, that since the recent general introduction of ill-ventilated water-closets and stationary washstands into the houses of the [p. 245]better classes the liability of the former to suffer from the disease is greater than that of the latter.

Persons recovering from an illness or in an infirm condition of health do not appear to be more liable than others to be attacked by typhoid fever. Among the many patients who have fallen under my care only a very few were in ill-health at the time of their seizure. The same fact has been noticed by Murchison and other observers. Indeed, Liebermeister goes so far as to say that typhoid fever attacks by preference strong and healthy persons, while it avoids those suffering with chronic ailments. That this latter class of patients enjoys no immunity from the disease when exposed to its causes is shown by a fact which he himself records. During his service at the hospital at Basle from 1865 to 1871 several of the patients in the medical and surgical wards were attacked by typhoid fever, the cases being especially numerous in two rooms which were situated one directly over the other. Upon investigation it was found that a wooden pipe which extended from the sewer to the roof ran by both of these rooms. The sewer at the point where this pipe ran into it was of faulty construction, and was turned at a right angle, so that the refuse matter collected there. Since this source of infection was made known repeated cleansings, washings, and disinfections have been followed by satisfactory improvement, and Liebermeister believes that if the sewer were entirely altered the infection would disappear.

It would seem only natural that intemperance, by diminishing the powers of resistance in the individual, would increase his liability to contract typhoid fever, but there is no proof that it does so. Few of the patients who have come under my care were intemperate, and still fewer were broken down by this cause. There is also no evidence that grief, fear, or any other depressing emotion is a predisposing cause of the disease, and the same may be said of bodily fatigue and overcrowding. On the other hand, much importance has been attached by writers to idiosyncrasy as a predisposing cause of typhoid fever. What the peculiarities of constitution are which increase the liability to the disease are not definitely known, but there can be no question that it occurs much more frequently, and is much more fatal, in some families than in others.

Typhoid fever occurs with the greatest frequency in this country, as it does with very few exceptions elsewhere, during the latter half of summer and the early part of autumn. Indeed, its greater prevalence at this season than at other times has given to it the name of "autumnal" and "fall fever," by which it is popularly known in many sections of this country as well as of England. On the other hand, the disease is usually at its minimum in May and June. The number of cases, however, does not usually immediately diminish upon the onset of cold weather. On the contrary, R. D. Cleemann,[23] from a comparison of the mortality returns of Philadelphia for a period of ten years, observed that after diminishing in November they not infrequently underwent a marked increase in December. Of 621 cases treated at the Pennsylvania Hospital during the last ten years, 89 were admitted during spring, 259 during summer, 182 during autumn, and 91 during winter. Of 5988 cases treated at the London Fever Hospital,[24] 759 were admitted in the [p. 246]spring, 1490 in summer, 2461 in autumn, and 1278 in winter. Of the whole number, 27.7 per cent. were admitted in the two months of October and November, and in April and May only 7.3 per cent. Hirsch[25] has published statistics which do not differ materially from these. He also mentions the interesting fact that in Rio Janeiro the maximum of the disease occurs in the months from March to June, or, in other words, in the season which in that latitude corresponds to our autumn. There are, however, some exceptions to the general rule of the greater prevalence of the disease during the autumn. Bartlett, who was aware of its greater frequency at that time, refers to an extensive and fatal epidemic which occurred in the city of Lowell in Massachusetts during the winter and early spring; and similar visitations have been observed in other places.

[23] *Transactions of the College of Physicians of Philadelphia*, 3d S. vol. iii.
[24] Murchison.
[25] *Handbuch der Historisch-Geographischen Pathologie*, Stuttgart, 1881.

Most authors agree with the statement made by Murchison, that typhoid fever is unusually prevalent after summers remarkable for their dryness and high temperature, and that it is unusually rare in summers and autumns which are wet and cold. Certainly, the severest epidemic of the disease which has been observed in Philadelphia in several years occurred in the year 1876, during and after a summer of exceptionally high temperature, and one characterized by a decidedly diminished rainfall. Still, there can be no question that the increased prevalence of the disease at this time was due, in part at least, to the crowded condition of the city consequent upon the Centennial Exhibition. In 1872, although the mean of the summer temperature was slightly higher than that of 1876, the disease did not prevail in an epidemic form. This may be explained by the fact that the rainfall of the summer months of this year was decidedly greater than the average. Hirsch, however, attaches much less importance to temperature as a factor in the production of typhoid fever than most other authors. He says that he has found, from a comparison of a large number of epidemics, that the disease occurs almost as often in cool as in hot summers, in cold as in warm autumns, and in mild as in severe winters. Murchison, moreover, admits that mere dryness of the atmosphere is not conducive to an increase of typhoid fever. On the contrary, he says, warm, damp weather, when drains are most offensive, is often followed by an outbreak of the disease.

The relation which temperature and moisture bear to the causation of typhoid fever is therefore not definitely ascertained. It is certain, however, that the largest number of cases does not occur at the period of the greatest heat, but is usually not observed until from six weeks to two months afterward, and the minimum is not reached until about the same length of time after that of the most intense cold. This difference in time Murchison explains by the hypothesis that the cause of the disease is exaggerated or only called into action by the protracted heat of summer and autumn, and that it requires the protracted cold of winter and spring to impair its activity or to destroy it. On the other hand, Liebermeister, who believes that the breeding-places of typhoid fever lie deep in the earth, holds that the time is consumed in the penetration of the changes of temperature to the place where the typhoid poison is elaborated, in the development of the poison without the human body, and in the period of incubation. In some places the maximum of the disease is observed earlier in the year than in others. In Berlin, for [p. 247]instance, the largest number of fatal cases occurs in October, while in Munich it does not occur until February. This depends, he thinks, upon the difference in the distance beneath the earth's surface of these breeding-places in different localities, and the deeper they are the longer, he says, will it be before they are affected by the heat of summer or the cold of winter, since the changes of the temperature of the air are followed by corresponding changes in the temperature of the earth more and more slowly the deeper we go beneath the surface.

Buhl and Pettenkofer have, as the result of a series of observations carried on in Munich over a number of years, reached the conclusion that an intimate relation exists between the variations in the degree of prevalence of typhoid fever and the rise and fall of water in the soil. When the springs were low they found that there was a marked increase in the number of cases; when, on the other hand, they were high, there was just as decided a diminution. Out of this fact they have evolved the theory that the cause of typhoid fever lies deep in the soil, and has the power of multiplying itself there, and that this property is very much increased when the water-level sinks, and the upper layers of the earth are consequently exposed to the air. It is, on the contrary, diminished when the water-level rises and the earth is again saturated with moisture. It is unquestionably true, as has already been stated, that it is principally after hot and dry weather, when the springs are of course low, that typhoid fever is most prevalent, and that it very frequently subsides after the occurrence of very heavy rains; but it is not necessary to adopt the theory of Buhl and Pettenkofer to explain these facts. It seems quite as probable that the increased prevalence of the disease after dry weather is due, as suggested by Buchanan and Liebermeister, to the greater amount of solid matter which is then suspended in the water of the springs. A larger proportion of the germs of the disease, if there should be any present in the soil, will therefore be contained in any given quantity of the drinking-water. The theory fails to account, as pointed out by Murchison, for the connection which is frequently observed between defective house-drainage and outbreaks of typhoid fever, occurring irrespectively of any variations in the subsoil water. And, moreover, outbreaks of the disease have occurred under precisely opposite circumstances, as the outbreak at Terling in 1867, recorded by Thorne,[26] which was coincident with a rise in the subsoil water after drought.

[26] Quoted by Murchison.

It is believed in many parts of our country that there is an antagonism between typhoid fever and the various forms of malarial fever, and it is unquestionably true that in many districts in which the latter were formerly prevalent they have ceased to be frequent, and have been replaced apparently by the former. In the cultivation of the soil the causes of malarial fever disappear, or at least become less potent. On the other hand, the increase of population and the neglect of all sanitary laws in the building of towns, and the construction of sewers with their house connections, seem to favor the occurrence of typhoid fever. But there is no real antagonism between the diseases. During the recent Civil War typhoid fever was not infrequently developed in soldiers suffering from malarial disease. Indeed, so frequent was it to have the manifestations of the two diseases in the same individual that many observers at that [p. 248]time supposed they had a new disease to deal with, to which they gave the name of typho-malarial fever.

2. EXCITING CAUSES.—Much diversity of opinion has existed in times past and to a certain extent continues to exist, in regard to the contagiousness of typhoid fever. In the early part of this century there was quite a number of good observers, including Nathan Smith in this country, and Bretonneau and Gendron of Château du Loir in France, who held the opinion it was an eminently contagious disease. Indeed, Smith went so far as to say that its contagiousness was as fully demonstrated as that of measles, small-pox, or any other disease universally admitted to be contagious. This was also the opinion of William Budd, who maintained that the contagious nature of typhoid fever was the master truth in its history. The late Sir Thomas Watson was also a warm supporter of the same view. At the present time, however, the large majority of physicians, whose opportunities for observation give weight to their opinions, do not regard the disease as contagious in the strict sense of the word. During the past twenty-four years I have been almost uninterruptedly connected with large general hospitals, and during that time have had a large number of cases of typhoid fever under my care, and a still larger number more or less under my observation. During all this time I have never known but one case to originate within a hospital, and that occurred in a servant whose duties did not bring her in immediate contact with the sick. Murchison's experience with a much larger number of cases has been very similar. In twenty-three years, in which 5988 cases were treated in the London Fever Hospital, only 17 residents contracted the disease, and most of these had no personal contact with the sick. Liebermeister asserts that he has never known a case to originate in a hospital from direct

contagion. When such cases appeared to have occurred, they could generally be traced, he says, to some defective sanitary condition of the hospital.

There are, nevertheless, many facts on record which, unless duly weighed, appear to lend a good deal of support to the theory of the contagiousness of typhoid fever. Among the most important of these are (1) the occurrence in rapid succession of several cases in the same house, and (2) the limited epidemics which occasionally follow the arrival of an infected person into a previously healthy locality. These facts are, however, susceptible of an entirely different explanation.

1. In those instances in which several cases of the disease have occurred in the same house, it not infrequently happens that some defect in its sanitary conditions is detected, or that the drinking-water is found to be impure. The same cause which produced the first case may, therefore, also have produced those which succeeded it. Indeed, the interval between the cases is sometimes so short that for this reason alone, if there were no other, they could scarcely be attributed to contagion. It not infrequently happens that the seizure of one member of a large family is followed on the next day by that of another, and on the third or fourth by that of still another. Now, while it is undoubtedly true that the period of incubation has appeared in some cases to be very short, we know that under ordinary circumstances it is usually about two weeks.

2. The explanation of the second fact is not more difficult, but in order that it may be clear to the reader it will be well to give in detail a few [p. 249]of the instances on record in which the arrival of an individual sick with typhoid fever in a previously healthy locality has been followed by an outbreak of the disease. Nathan Smith refers to two cases of this character. In both of these the disease appeared to be communicated to several individuals by patients who had contracted the disease elsewhere. So little is said in the reports of these cases of the water-supply of the localities in which they occurred, or of the manner of disposing of the discharges of the patients, that they would scarcely now be used as arguments in favor of the contagiousness of the disease. The report of a local epidemic by Austin Flint, Sr., is more satisfactory in this respect, and is as follows: A stranger was detained in a small village near Buffalo by an illness which proved fatal in the course of a few days, and which was recognized as typhoid fever by his attending physicians. Up to this time, it is stated, typhoid fever had never been known in the neighborhood. In the course of a month more than one-half of the population, numbering forty-three, was attacked by the disease, and ten had died. The family of the tavern-keeper at whose house the stranger lodged was the first to suffer, and of the families immediately surrounding the tavern but one wholly escaped, that of a man named Stearns. Upon investigation, it was ascertained that this family alone, of all these families, did not use the well belonging to the tavern, but had its own water-supply. The occurrence of the disease naturally produced great excitement, and Stearns, between whom and the tavern-keeper a quarrel existed, was suspected of having poisoned the well; but an examination of the water showed this suspicion to be unfounded. There can, however, be little doubt that the water of the well, which was in all probability contaminated by the discharges of the stranger, was the means of propagating the disease; for although it is said that the family of Stearns was cut off by the quarrel from all intercourse with that of the tavern-keeper—a fact upon which some stress is laid by Flint—it does not appear that a similar isolation existed as regards the other families affected.[27]

[27] *A Treatise on the Principles and Practice of Medicine*, by Austin Flint, M.D., Philadelphia, 1868.

The manner in which the arrival of a sick person may cause the dissemination of the disease in a previously healthy community is even better shown by the following histories of local outbreaks:[28]

"The water-supply pipes of the town of Over Darwen were leaky, and the soil through which they passed was soaked at one spot by the sewage of a particular house. No harm resulted till a young lady suffering from typhoid fever was brought to this house from a distant place. Within three weeks of her arrival the disease broke out and 1500 persons were attacked. At Nunney a number of houses received their water-supply from a foul brook contaminated by the leakage of a cesspool of one of the houses, but no fever showed itself till a man ill with typhoid came from a distance to this house. In about fourteen days an outbreak of fever took place in all the houses."

[28] Wm. Cayley, M.D., *Brit. Med. Jour.*, March 15, 1880.

There are many other observations which seem to render it certain that the alvine dejections are a most important medium by which typhoid fever is communicated to others; and yet there is no evidence that they possess this power in a fresh condition. They have been repeatedly examined, and even handled, with impunity, and, as has already been stated, it [p. 250]is rare for the disease to be imparted to the immediate attendants upon the sick, or in a well-ventilated hospital to the other patients in the same ward, provided that the discharges are disinfected and removed immediately after being passed, and the bed-linen and clothes of the patient changed whenever they are soiled. The feces must therefore undergo some changes before they become possessed of virulent properties. This appears to be shown conclusively by the following facts: (1) laundresses who wash the soiled clothes of typhoid fever patients not infrequently contract the disease; (2) the occupants of houses connected by ill-trapped drains with sewers into which the discharges of such patients have found their way often suffer severely from the disease; and (3) the use of water polluted by such discharges is, as has already been shown, almost certain to induce the disease in persons not protected by a previous attack.

The following histories of outbreaks of typhoid fever will show clearly how the dejections of patients may be the means of propagating the disease to others:

ILLUSTRATIVE CASES—Lausen[29] is a village lying on the railway between Basle and Olten shortly before coming to the great Hauenstein Tunnel. It is situated in the Jura, in the valley of the Ergolz, and consists of 103 houses with 819 inhabitants. It was remarkably healthy, and resorted to on that account as a place of summer residence. With the exception of six houses it is supplied with water by a spring with two heads which rises above the village at the southern foot of a mountain called the Stockhalder, composed of oolite. The water is received into a well built covered reservoir, and is distributed by wooden pipes to four public fountains, whence it was drawn by the inhabitants. Six houses had an independent supply—five from wells, one from the mill-dam of a paper-factory. On August 7, 1872, ten inhabitants of Lausen, living in different houses, were seized by typhoid fever, and during the next nine days fifty-seven cases occurred, the only houses escaping being those six which were not supplied by the public fountains. The disease continued to spread, and in all 130 persons were attacked, and several children who had been sent to Lausen for the benefit of the fresh air fell ill after their return home. A careful investigation was made into the causes of this epidemic, and a complete explanation was given. Separated from the valley of the Ergolz, in which Lausen lies, by the Stockhalder, the mountain at the foot of which the spring supplying Lausen rises, is a side valley called the Furjust, traversed by a stream, the Furlenbach, which joins the Ergolz just below Lausen, the Stockhalder occupying the fork of the valley. The Furlenthal contains six farm-houses, which were supplied with drinking-water, not from the Furlenbach, but by a spring rising on the opposite side of the valley to the Stockhalder. Now, there was reason to believe that under certain circumstances water from the Furlenbach found its way under the Stockhalder into one of the heads of the fountain supplying Lausen. It was noticed that when the meadows on one side of the Furlenbach were irrigated, which was done periodically, the flow of water into the Lausen spring was increased, rendering it probable that the irrigation water percolated through the superficial strata and found its way under the Stockhalder by subterranean channels in the limestone rock. Moreover, some years before a [p. 251]hole on one occasion formed close to the Furlenbach by the sinking in of the superficial strata, and the stream became diverted into it and disappeared, while shortly afterward the spring of Lausen began to flow much more abundantly. The hole was filled up, and the Furlenbach resumed its usual course. The Furlenbach was unquestionably contaminated by the privies of the adjacent farm-houses; the soil-pits communicated with it. Thus, from time immemorial, whenever the meadows of the Furlenthal were irrigated the contaminated water of the Furlenbach, after percolation through the superficial strata and a long underground course, helped to feed one of the two heads of the fountain supplying Lausen. The natural filtration, however, which it underwent rendered it perfectly bright and clear, and chemical examination showed it to be remarkably free from organic impurities, and Lausen was extremely healthy and free from fever. On June 10th one of the peasants of the Furlenthal fell ill with typhoid fever, the source of which was not clearly made out, and passed through a severe attack with relapses, so that he remained ill all summer; and on July 10th a girl in the same house, and in August a boy, were attacked. Their dejections were certainly, in part, thrown into the Furlenbach; and, moreover, the soil-pit of the privy communicated with the brook. In the middle of July the meadows of the Furlenthal were irrigated as usual for the hay crop, and within three weeks this was followed by the outbreak at Lausen.

[29] William Cayley, M.D., *British Medical Journal*, Mar. 15, 1880.

In order to demonstrate the connection between the water-supply of Lausen and the Furlenbach, the following experiments were performed. The hole mentioned above as having on one occasion diverted the Furlenbach into the presumed subterranean channels under the Stockhalder was cleared out, and 18 cwt. of salt were dissolved in water and poured in, and the stream again diverted into it. The next day salt was found in the spring at Lausen. Fifty pounds of wheat flour were then poured into the hole, and the Furlenbach again diverted into it, but the spring at Lausen remained clear, and no reaction of starch could be obtained, showing that the water must have found its way under the Stockhalder, in part by percolation through the porous strata, and not by distinct channels.

Volz[30] refers to an epidemic which occurred at Gerlachsheim, a village of Germany, some years ago, in which, in the course of three weeks, 52 persons residing on one of the principal streets were attacked by the disease. It was found, upon investigation, that they all got their water from a well which was polluted by the stools of the first patient. A. Pasteur[31] reports an epidemic caused by the contamination of a well by typhoid dejections, and which ceased when the use of the water was discontinued. Niericker[32] also reports an outbreak which was found to be due to a similar pollution of the drinking-water, and which likewise ceased when the water-supply was derived from another source.

[30] *Schmidt's Jahrbuch.*
[31] *Revue méd. de la Suisse*, Mars 15, 1881.
[32] *Schweiz. Corr. Bl.*, ix. 1, 1879.

An outbreak of the disease which occurred in a farm-house situated about eight miles from the city of Philadelphia came under my own observation. The first case occurred in a young girl of sixteen, who, with the exception of an occasional visit to the city, had not been away from her own home for several months before she was [p. 252]taken ill. The disease ran in her a severe course, and eventually terminated fatally. About three weeks afterward four other members of the family were attacked, one of whom died. Two other persons, living in a house on the opposite side of the road, but who were in the habit of drinking water from the same well, also took the disease. There was no other case of typhoid fever in the immediate vicinity, nor had there been for some time. The farm-house is situated in a cup-shaped depression, so that water flowed toward it from all directions. The cellar was constantly filled with water during the winter, and just before the outbreak had contained not only an unusually large quantity, but also a large amount of decaying vegetable matter. The well from which the family drew their drinking-water is situated within a few feet of the kitchen door, and at some distance from the cesspool used by the family, so that there was no reason to believe that there was any communication between the two. The wall of the well was found to be very much loosened by the roots of two trees growing in the immediate vicinity. As the ground was also very much cut up by the burrows of rats, the water used for the various household purposes, and which was habitually thrown into a gutter which ran past the well, found a ready access to it. There would seem to be but little doubt that the first patient contracted the disease in some way during her visits to the city, and that the disease in the other patients arose from their drinking the water of the well which had been polluted by that used in washing her soiled linen.

Ballard[33] has shown very clearly that milk may also be a medium of communication of the disease. He found that an epidemic which occurred in the parish of Islington, London, in 1871 was (1) almost entirely confined to a district comprised within a circle having a radius of not more than a quarter of a mile; (2) that out of 62 families living within this district, who were known to have suffered from typhoid fever, 54 were constantly supplied with milk from a particular dairy, and it was satisfactorily proved that at least three of the remaining eight had occasionally partaken from the same source; and (3) that out of 142 families, comprising all the customers of this dairy, and living not only within the district above specified, but in other parts of the parish, 70, or very nearly one-half, were invaded by typhoid fever within the ten weeks during which the outbreak lasted. Upon a visit to the farm from which the milk came it was ascertained that a member of the dairyman's family had been ill with typhoid fever, and that the water of the well which supplied the family with drinking-water had been polluted by his discharges. Although the dairyman denied that this water had ever been mixed with the milk, he admitted that it had been used to wash the milk-pans. Murchison was also able, in an outbreak which occurred in another district of London, to trace the disease to the same source.

[33] *On a Localized Outbreak of Typhoid Fever in Islington*, London, 1871.

Typhoid fever may be likewise propagated in consequence of the contamination of the atmosphere by the typhoid poison. This may be the result of allowing the undisinfected stools, or linen soiled by them, to remain for some time exposed to the air, or may arise from pollution [p. 253]of the soil from the same cause or from defective sewage. Hermann Schmidt[34] refers to several epidemics breaking out in garrisons which he believed to be due to pollution of the soil. In the citadel of Wurzburg typhoid fever occurred through several years, and persisted in spite of the cutting off of the water-supply, which was believed to be impure. It was finally found that the ground upon which it was built was saturated with all kinds of impurities. Volz refers to outbreaks of the disease from the same cause.

[34] *Die Typhus Epidemie in Fusillier Bat. zu Tübingen in Winter 1876-77, enstanden durch einathmung, giftiger Grundluft*, Tubingen, 1880.

But perhaps the most striking example of this mode of propagation of the disease is that recorded by Budd,[35] and is as follows: Two adjacent cottages, which for the sake of convenience may be designated as Nos. 1 and 2, had a privy in common, which was in the form of a lean-to against the gable end of No. 2. Through this privy there flowed with very feeble current a small stream which formed the natural drain for it. Having already performed this office for some twenty or thirty other houses higher up its course, the stream had acquired all the character of a common sewer before reaching the cottages in question. About a quarter of a mile farther on it acted as a drain for a privy, common as before, for two other cottages, Nos. 3 and 4. Notwithstanding the condition of the stream, which was so foul that it was said that the stink from it was often enough "to knock a man down," no evil result appeared to have occurred until a man living in No. 1 contracted typhoid fever—elsewhere, it was believed. As a matter of course, all his discharges were thrown into the common privy. In this way for more than a fortnight the stream which passed through it was daily fed with the specific excreta from the diseased intestines of the patient. No further cases occurred until the latter end of the third week or the beginning of the fourth week, when several persons were simultaneously attacked by the same fever in all four cottages. From first to last, the outbreak was confined to these four cottages, and there was no other case of typhoid fever at this time in the neighborhood.

[35] *Typhoid Fever: Its Nature, Mode of Spreading, and Prevention*, by William Budd, M.D., F.R.S., London, 1873.

The mattrass used by typhoid-fever patients, their bed-linen and clothes, have each been the medium by which the disease has been communicated to others. This is, as has already been pointed out, unquestionably due to the fact that these articles are generally soiled by their discharges, and that time has been allowed for the latter to acquire infective properties. It seems not improbable that the few cases in which the disease appears to have been contracted from the dead body may be explained in the same way. The statistics of the London Fever Hospital show that laundresses are more liable to contract typhoid fever than the immediate attendants upon the sick. This liability is greatest in those cases in which the bed-linen and clothes of patients are not immediately disinfected after use. According to Budd, the sputa in cases of typhoid fever where bronchitis is excessive may sometimes contain the germs of the disease, and mentioned a case in which he believed they were the means by which the disease was propagated.

The question naturally arises here, whether this is the only way in [p. 254]which the disease can originate. This is a subject which has given rise to a good deal of controversy, and therefore demands some consideration at our hands. On the one hand, it is argued that typhoid fever never occurs in the absence of the specific poison or germ of the disease, and that this is contained principally, if not wholly, in the alvine dejections. On the other hand, it is contended that it may, and often does, originate spontaneously, and that all that is necessary to produce it is the presence of decomposing fecal or other organic matter, and the consequent contamination of the food, drink, or atmosphere. Both of these views have found able advocates. Among the upholders of the latter view is Murchison, who cites the histories of several outbreaks of typhoid fever which occurred in localities which had not been visited by it for many years, and which, after a careful investigation of all the circumstances attending them, he was forced to conclude had no connection with any previous case of the disease, and could only be explained by admitting that it might occasionally have an independent origin. Among the more remarkable of these outbreaks is the following, which we give in Murchison's own words:

"In August, 1829, 20 out of 22 boys at a school at Clapham within three hours were seized with fever, vomiting, purging, and excessive prostration. One other boy, aged three, had been attacked with similar symptoms two days before, and had died comatose in twenty-three hours; another boy, aged five, died in twenty-five hours; all the rest recovered. Suspicions were entertained that they had been poisoned, and a rigorous investigation ensued. The only cause which could be discovered was, that a drain at the back of the house, which had been choked up for many years, had been opened two days before the first case of illness, cleared out, and its contents spread over a garden adjoining the boys' playground. A most offensive effluvium escaped from the drain, and the boys had watched the workmen cleaning it out. This was considered to be the cause of the disease by Latham and Chambers, and by others who investigated the matter, and also by Sir Thomas Watson. The morbid appearances in the two fatal cases were described as like those of the common fevers of this country. Peyer's patches and the solitary glands of the small and large intestines were enlarged like 'condylomatous elevations,' and in one case the mucous membrane over them was slightly ulcerated. The mesenteric glands were enlarged and congested."

"A remarkable instance of a circumscribed outbreak of fever was recorded by Sir R. Christison in 1846. It occurred in an isolated farm-house in the thinly-peopled county of Peebles, N.B. Every one of the fifteen residents was seized with fever, and three died. Many of the servants who worked during the day at the farm were also affected, but none communicated the disease to their families who did not visit the farm. There was no evidence that the disease was imported from without, and the only explanation of the outbreak was, that the drains and sewers were found all closed and obstructed with the accumulated filth proceeding from the privies and farm-yard, the effluvia from which was very offensive."

"About Easter, 1848, a formidable outbreak of fever occurred in the Westminster School and the Abbey Cloisters, and for some days there [p. 255]was a panic in the neighborhood respecting the 'Westminster fever.' No case of fever had occurred in the Abbey Cloisters for three years, and there was no evidence of its having been imported. Within little more than eleven days it affected thirty-six persons, all of the better class, and in three instances it proved fatal. Shortly before its first appearance there occurred two or three days of peculiarly hot weather, and a disagreeable stench, so powerful as to induce nausea, was complained of in the houses in question. It was found that the disease followed very exactly in its course the line of a foul and neglected private sewer or immense cesspool, in which fecal matter had been accumulating for years without any exit, and into which the contents of several small cesspools had been pumped immediately before the outbreak of fever. This elongated cesspool communicated by direct openings with the drains of all the houses in which it occurred; the only exception was that of several boys, who lived in a house at a little distance, but who were in the habit of playing every day in a yard in which there were several gully-holes opening into the foul drain."

The following cases would seem, however, to furnish stronger evidence in favor of the occasional spontaneous origin of typhoid fever than any of those referred to by

Murchison. The first is recorded by P. Herbert Metcalfe,[36] and occurred in Norfolk Island in the Pacific Ocean, 400 miles from the nearest inhabited land. The patient was a gentleman who had come from England four months previously. To Metcalfe's certain knowledge, there had been no typhoid fever on the island for fifteen months. Three years previously a man is reported to have died of it, and in 1868 there had been an epidemic of fever, but he could not ascertain of what kind. Upon inquiry, he found that his patient had been drinking water from a well which had the reputation of being unclean, and that he was the only person who had done so. He also found that at a distance of seven feet there was an open sewer, and that just opposite to the well much of the sewage-water became so stagnant as to form an offensive cesspool. The well was cleaned out, and at the bottom of it were found four feet of stinking sewage mud, the skeleton of a duck, a pig's jaw, etc. The well was so situated that had there been any typhoid fever previously to this case the water could not have been contaminated by the specific poison, as the above-named sewer only conveyed water from the kitchen, which is a building detached from the dwelling-houses of the mission, and is far from and on a higher level than the open closets in use.

[36] *British Medical Journal*, Nov. 6, 1880.

In the second case, which is reported by R. Bruce Low,[37] Medical Officer of Health, Helmsley, Yorkshire, occurred in a lad who had not been away from his home for months. No stranger had visited his house, and there was no fever in the district, the last case having occurred eight months previously in a sequestered valley eight miles away. The patient's habits and those of his family were revoltingly dirty. The garden privy was in bad repair, the filth level with the seat, and the smell from it very offensive. Thirty years before there had been five cases of slow typhus in the house. In his remarks on this case Low says: "This case did not owe its origin to direct infection, and the question naturally arises, was this a case originating de novo, or had the poison [p. 256]been due to infection in some way or another from the cases which occurred thirty years previously?"

[37] *Brit. Med. Jour.*, 1880.

There can be but little doubt that in many of the cases cited by Murchison as instances of the spontaneous origin of typhoid fever there was an introduction of the germs of the disease from without. At all events, the evidence to the contrary is by no means convincing. For example, in the account of the outbreak at the Westminster School it is expressly stated that "the contents of several small cesspools had been pumped before the outbreak of the fever" into the large cesspool, the emanations from which it was believed had caused the fever. It does not seem that it was positively ascertained that none of these small cesspools had been used by a typhoid-fever patient, or that typhoid stools had not found their way into them in some other way. Moreover, in diseases generally admitted to be contagious it is not always possible to ascertain positively the source of infection in a particular instance. But after the elimination of all doubtful cases there yet remains a certain number in which it is reasonably certain that there has been no recent importation of the typhoid-fever germs, as in the case which is reported by Metcalfe and which occurred on Norfolk Island, and in that recorded by Low. The assumption does not seem an unwarranted one that in these cases the poison of the disease, which had been present before in a latent condition, had been suddenly called into activity by favoring influences. The following observation of Von Gietl[38] shows the length of time typhoid-fever stools may retain their infective properties: "To a village free from typhoid an inhabitant returned suffering from the disease, which he had acquired at a distant place. His evacuations were buried in a dunghill. Some weeks later five persons, who were employed in removing dung from this heap, were attacked by typhoid fever; their alvine discharges were again buried deeply in the same heap, and nine months later one of two men who were employed in the complete removal of the dung was attacked and died." If we assume—and there is no reason to doubt that this point was fully investigated by Von Gietl—that the patient in the latter case had not been otherwise exposed to the causes of the disease, the observation shows that the stools in typhoid fever retain their virulence for nine months. If for nine months, why may they not do so for a much longer period—for as many years, for example? No probability is violated by this hypothesis. On the contrary, it is in full accordance with what we know of some of the lower forms of life, and will serve to explain many outbreaks of the disease which would otherwise be inexplicable—for example, the outbreak at Clapham referred to by Murchison. Admitting that the disease in this instance was really typhoid fever—and this has been denied by some observers, among whom is Sir Thomas Watson—the assumption does not seem an unwarrantable one that the germs of typhoid fever had been present in this choked-up drain long before it was cleared, but that in consequence of their exclusion from the air their infecting power was at a minimum. It was, on the contrary, much increased when the contents of the drain were exposed to the vivifying influence of the atmosphere.

[38] Quoted by Cayley, *Brit. Med. Jour.*, Mar. 15, 1880.

On the other hand, it is alleged that an individual may be exposed to the direct emanations of sewers or of foul privies, or even drink water[p. 257]contaminated by leakage from them, without contracting typhoid fever, so long as they do not contain the specific germ of the disease. Every physician in large practice, either in the city or country, can call to mind instances in which the air of houses or the water-supply has been polluted in this way, and yet no typhoid fever has occurred. Let, however, the specific cause of the disease be introduced from without, and this immunity almost invariably disappears. There is no reason to believe that the contamination of the water used by the family which suffered in the outbreak of the disease which has been already referred to as having come under my own observation last year was of recent origin. On the contrary, there was evidence to the contrary, and yet no disease occurred until it was imported by a member of the family who was in the habit of making frequent visits to the city. Even more strongly corroborative of this view is the history of the epidemic reported by Ballard, in which milk was the medium of communication. The water which had been used with impunity to wash the milk-pans, or perhaps to dilute the milk, became a source of danger only after the occurrence of the disease in the family of the dairyman.

Several epidemics of typhoid fever have been recently reported in which the disease appears to have been caused by the use of the flesh of diseased animals or of meat in a condition of putrefaction. In some of these the symptoms were rather those of irritant poisoning than of typhoid fever, and consisted principally in violent vomiting and purging coming on very shortly after the ingestion of the unwholesome food. There yet remains a certain number in which the symptoms cannot be thus explained.[39] One of the most remarkable of these occurred in 1878 at a festival which was held at Kloten, a place about seven miles north of Zurich, of which the following is a condensed description: Out of 690 persons who sat down to the collation, 290 were taken ill; 378 other persons, who did not attend the festival, but who partook of the meat provided for it, were also affected. In addition these, 49 secondary cases occurred—*i.e.* of persons who subsequently became affected without having eaten of the meat. All other sources of infection could be certainly excluded, as Kloten was quite free from typhoid fever at the time, and as it was clearly shown that the water was not the cause of the outbreak. All the visitors at the festival who ate no meat escaped, as did also several persons who drank wine to excess and subsequently vomited. The period of incubation was short, as in other epidemics arising from the same cause. Some of the people were ill on the second day, with loss of appetite, nausea, headache, pain and swelling of the belly, and slight fever. These cases were slight, and generally ended in recovery. The greater number were affected between the fifth and ninth days. The symptoms in these cases, which usually ran a rapid course, and generally ended in recovery, were chills, fever, diarrhoea, great prostration, frequently violent delirium, and also profuse intestinal hemorrhage. The rose-colored eruption was present in almost all of them, and in a few the tâches bleuâtres were detected. On post-mortem[p. 258]examination the characteristic appearances of typhoid fever were found. With regard to the meat supplied, the following facts were ascertained: Forty-two pounds of veal were furnished by a butcher at Seebach, taken from a calf which appears to have been at the point of death when it received the coup de grace from the hands of the butcher. All the flesh of the animal was sent to supply the festival at Kloten, but the liver was eaten by an inhabitant of Seebach, and he was attacked by typhoid fever. The brain was sent to the parsonage at Seebach, and all the household became affected by the same disease. It was also ascertained that another of the calves was diseased. The veal from this calf had been kept fourteen days, and was in a decomposed state. All the meat was placed together in the meat-receptacle of the inn at which the festival was held. This receptacle was in a horribly filthy state, and Cayley thinks there can be no doubt that the putrefying flesh of this last calf, together with the state of the receptacle, would rapidly excite decomposition in the whole supply.

[39] *On Some Points in the Pathology and Treatment of Typhoid Fever*, by William Cayley, London, 1880; also Prof. Huguenin, *Schmidt's Jahrbuch*, from *Schweiz. Corr. Bl.*, viii. 15, 1878; Carl Walder, *Schmidt's Jahrbuch*, from *Berl. klin. Wochenschr.*, xv. 39, 40, 1878; George R. Shattuck, M.D., Supplement to *Ziemssen's Cyclopædia*, New York, 1881.

Geissler, it is true, doubts whether the epidemic above described was really typhoid fever, and points out that the symptoms occurred too soon after the ingestion of the diseased meat, and reached their full development too rapidly. The cases were also accompanied by more pain in the abdomen than is generally met with in typhoid fever. The proportion of recoveries also appears to have been unusually large. Unquestionably, the patients in the Kloten epidemic were in a large number of instances simply suffering from the action of an irritant poison; but the presence of the characteristic lesions of typhoid fever in some of the fatal cases renders it certain that this disease also existed in the village at the same time.

In the report of this epidemic it is not stated that either of the calves which furnished a part of the meat for the entertainment were suffering from typhoid fever at the time they were slaughtered. It is now known positively that this animal is liable to be attacked by this disease, and a certain number of cases are on record in which the eating of the flesh of such animals has been followed by typhoid fever.[40] That it does not oftener occur from this cause is probably due to the fact that a certain time must elapse before the flesh of such an animal acquires infective properties, and that it is usually used as food before this has been allowed to pass.

[40] *Medical Times and Gazette*, Feb. 8, 1879, p. 149, from *Berl. klin. Wochenschrift*, No. 39, 1878.

Ludwig Letzench[41] asserts that he has produced some of the intestinal appearances of typhoid fever, as well as a high degree of pyrexia, in rabbits by the subcutaneous injection of the sputa and stools of typhoid fever patients.

[41] *Arch. f. exper. Pathol. u. Pharmak.*, 1878 and 1881.

THE BACILLUS TYPHOSUS.—From what has preceded, it will be seen that the writer is disposed to range himself with those who hold that the exciting cause of typhoid fever is an organized germ, or, in other words, a contagium vivum. Although this view cannot be regarded as positively proven as yet, it has recently received some support through the investigations of Klebs, Eberth of Zurich, and others,[42] who believe that they [p. 259]have found in the bodies of those who have died of typhoid fever a micro-organism peculiar to that disease.

[42] Klebs (*Philadelphia Medical Times*, Dec. 3, 1881, from *Archiv für experimentelle Pathologie und Pharmakologie*, Bd. xiii. H. 5 and 6) claims that he has proved "that there exists in typhoid fever a separate and distinct bacillus—the *Bacillus typhosus;* that it undergoes certain transformations, consisting at first of little rods and small fine threads, containing a spore in the centre and often at the end, which spores divide off and form new bacilli. It later assumes a larger thread-like form, twisted at the end, and frequently taking a beautiful spiral shape; that the bacilli are observed first in the masses of epithelial cells which accumulate in the alimentary tract or in the air-passages; that they later penetrate the tissues, and are carried along by the blood-vessels and the lymphatics, and form a large network among the tissues they invade; that, under a certain procedure, which never causes this same staining in any other living organism or tissue, they appear of a blue color; that they are found only in enteric fever, in which disease every part of the human body is the seat of masses of these bacilli, their quantity corresponding exactly with the severity of the symptoms; and that they produce, when carried into the system of animals, exactly the same disease with the same morbid alterations as in men." He says, further, that "the Bacillus typhosus enters the system by the respiratory passages and by the alimentary canal. This is the cause that in some cases of typhoid fever almost no abdominal symptoms are present, but a low form of pneumonia,

developing from the very beginning, so that the lung seems alone to bear the brunt of the disease." He has found these bacilli in greatest numbers in Peyer's patches.

Eberth (*British Medical Journal*, Nov. 26, 1881, from *Virchow's Archiv*, Bd. lxxxi. and lxxxiii.) has shown that in typhoid fever the intestinal mucous membrane, the mesenteric glands, and the spleen contain rod bacteria, differing, as he believes, from organisms found in the body in other conditions (among others in phthisis with extensive ulceration of the intestinal mucous membrane). In seventeen cases of typhoid these bacilli were found in six and wanting in eleven. In the six cases the number of bacilli were in inverse proportion to the duration of the disease. They were not found in the spleen in the cases of the longest duration, and only scantily in the mesenteric glands. These bacilli appear not to differ in shape and size from the ordinary rod bacteria, but Eberth believes that they differ from them in their small capacity for taking on the staining of hæmatoxylon, methyl-violet, and Bismarck brown.

Wernich's views (*Vjhrschr. f. Off. Geshpfl.*, xiii. 4, p. 513, 1881) in regard to the nature of the Bacillus typhosus differ from those held by the two authors just quoted. He regards the specific Bacillus typhosus as nothing but the ordinary Bacillus subtilis of the large intestines, which under certain circumstances acquires the power to accommodate itself to the small intestines, to undergo a higher development and to become the exciting cause of disease.

PERIOD OF INCUBATION.—The conditions under which typhoid fever occurs in large cities render it difficult, if not impossible, to arrive at a definite conclusion as to its period of incubation. Occasionally, however, the time which has intervened between the exposure to the cause and the invasion of the disease may be ascertained with precision in the outbreaks which occur in small towns or in isolated country-houses. Under these circumstances it has been found to vary within very wide limits. In the three cases related by Griesinger the attack began the day after exposure to the infection, and in the outbreak at the school at Clapham, referred to by Murchison, twenty out of twenty-two boys were seized with the disease within four days of exposure to the causes. Other instances of a similar character are on record. In cases like the above the rapidity with which the attack follows upon exposure to the cause is no doubt due to the intensity of the poison—a view which is to a certain extent at least supported by the fact that the invasion of the disease under these circumstances is very apt to be abrupt; the attack being often ushered in with vomiting and purging or with grave cerebral symptoms. Sometimes, indeed, the gastro-intestinal symptoms have been so violent as to have given rise to suspicions of criminal or accidental poisoning. In the majority of cases, however, the period of incubation is probably very much longer than in those above referred to. In the outbreak which recently occurred in a farm-house about seven miles distant from[p. 260]Philadelphia, the history of which has already been given in detail, the second case began three weeks after the first, the other six following in rapid succession. In the celebrated epidemic which occurred at Lausen in Switzerland in 1872, and which is referred to by Cayley,[43] the first ten patients were attacked within three weeks of the time when the contamination of the spring which supplied the village must have taken place, and these ten cases were followed in the course of nine days by fifty-seven others. In the town of Over Darwen 1500 persons were seized with typhoid fever within three weeks after a patient suffering from this disease was brought to a particular house, the sewage of which was allowed to soak into the ground through which the water-supply pipes of the town passed, and at a point at which they were leaky. Lothholz observed in an epidemic which occurred in the neighborhood of Jena that the average period of incubation was three weeks, the shortest period eighteen days, the longest twenty-eight days. Haegler found in three cases produced by contaminated water a period of at least three weeks.[44] There are, however, epidemics on record in which the period of incubation was under two weeks, as, for instance, that of Basle, referred to by Liebermeister, in which a few persons were attacked who had only been in the city from seven to fourteen days. Cayley also refers to localized outbreaks of the disease, as those of Calne and Nunney, in which persons were attacked within fourteen days of their exposure to the cause. C. J. C. Muller of Posen[45] says that the average period of incubation of the disease is fourteen days; that it may be not more than ten days, or, on the other hand, as long as from three to four weeks; and that he has known a case in which it was thirty-four days. Murchison believed that it was most commonly about two weeks, and William Budd arrived at the conclusion, from the observation of a large number of cases, that it varied from ten to fourteen days.

[43] *Brit. Med. Jour.*, Mar. 15, 1880.
[44] *Ziemssen's Cyclopædia*, vol. i.
[45] *Neue Beiträge zur Aetologie des Unterleibs-Typhus*, Posen, 1878.

From this review of the opinions of various authors the conclusion would seem to be justifiable that the period of incubation in typhoid fever is usually between two and three weeks, but that in many cases it does not exceed ten days, and in rare instances has unquestionably been very much less. On the other hand, there are authentic cases on record in which it is said to have reached, or even exceeded, twenty-eight days. Unfortunately, we do not possess any reliable data with which to decide the question whether it is shorter or longer when the poison is imbibed with the ingesta than when it is inhaled. It would seem, however, that there is a difference in the susceptibility of different individuals to the poison of this disease, in many persons a single exposure to the cause being sufficient to induce an attack, while in others the disease is contracted only after repeated exposure.

MORBID ANATOMY.—As a thorough knowledge of the morbid anatomy of typhoid fever is absolutely necessary to a correct understanding of its pathology, it seems to me better to deviate from the order usually observed in systematic treatises and to proceed at once to a description of the former, rather than to defer it, as it is usual to do, until after the symptomatology of the disease has been discussed.

Rigor mortis is generally more marked and more prolonged than after[p. 261]typhus. Emaciation is often extreme in cases in which death has taken place after the third week, especially if they have been attended by much diarrhoea and fever. No traces of the characteristic rose-colored eruption are found after death, no matter how profuse it may have been during life. Sudamina, on the other hand, persist, and discolorations of the dependent portions from settling of blood are always present in the dead body.

The lesions of typhoid fever may be divided into two classes. The first class includes certain changes in the glands of Peyer, the solitary glands of the intestines, the spleen, and other lymphatic structures of the body. These changes, which consist essentially in a medullary infiltration of these glands, will be minutely described presently. They are peculiar to the disease, and are just as characteristic of it as the condition of the lungs and their membranes found in pneumonia and pleurisy are characteristic of those diseases. They are usually most developed in grave cases, but occasionally they are slight and but little marked in cases in which the general symptoms were severe. They therefore cannot be regarded as the sole cause of the latter. It is more probable that they are themselves the results of the local action of the typhoid poison, and bear somewhat of the same relation to typhoid fever that the eruption in small-pox does to that disease. The second class is made up of lesions which are met with not only in this disease, but in other diseases accompanied by high fever, and are therefore unquestionably the result of the general process. They consist essentially of parenchymatous degenerations of various organs and tissues, and are generally more marked in typhoid fever because the pyrexia is not only of high grade, but also of longer duration than in other diseases.

We shall first consider the lesions peculiar to typhoid fever. Among the most important of these are the changes which occur in the agminated and solitary glands of the intestines. These have been usually described as passing through four stages, as follows: (1) the stage of medullary infiltration; (2) the stage of softening or sloughing; (3) the stage of ulceration; (4) the stage of cicatrization. These stages are said to last almost a week, and correspond to certain definite periods of the disease, but it is not uncommon to find in the same intestine glands in two or more of these stages. Indeed, the same gland may sometimes be found ulcerating at one side while cicatrization is going on at the other.

In the first stage the agminated glands are enlarged, each patch preserving its oblong shape, and being flattened on the surface and elevated from half a line to two lines above the surrounding mucous membrane, from which it is separated by an abrupt border, and which it may in a few cases overhang like a fungous growth. The solitary follicles are also swollen, and may vary in size from a hempseed to a split pea. In very severe cases all the glands may be more or less involved, but in mild cases the changes may be limited to three or four of the patches of Peyer, although the solitary glands rarely wholly escape. It is uncommon also for the latter to be alone affected, but a few such cases have been reported. In these the mucous membrane appears to be studded with pustules, and hence Cruveilhier designated this variety as the forme pustuleuse. The mucous membrane covering the affected glands is reddish-green in color, and that in their immediate vicinity is [p. 262]often injected. The changes above described occur early in the disease—Murchison has seen them in two cases in which death took place at the end of the first day—and they are often well marked at the end of the third or fourth day. They are usually limited to the glands in the lower part of the ileum, the agminated glands being often found perfectly healthy four feet above the ileo-cæcal valve. In mild cases, indeed, the lesions may be confined to those nearest to this valve. So, too, the changes in the solitary glands may be confined to the last twelve inches of the smaller intestine, but this is by no means universally the case, for these glands are not only often found enlarged higher up in the small intestine, but also occasionally in the cæcum. The agminated glands are sometimes found enlarged in the bodies of those who have died of measles and of some other diseases, but the degree of enlargement is rarely as great as in typhoid fever, and the further changes presently to be described are never found except in the latter disease.

Under the microscope the medullary infiltration upon which the enlargement of the glands depends is found to be due to proliferation of the cellular elements. In the case of the agminated glands this proliferation may be limited to the follicles or it may extend to the intercellular tissue, and even to the adjacent mucous membrane. In the former case the patches have a reticulated aspect; they are soft and but little elevated. These are the plaques molles of Louis and the plaques reticulées of Chomel. In the latter they are harder, smoother, and more elevated. To this variety Louis has given the name of plaques dures, Chomel that of plaques gauffrées. The morbid process is also very apt to extend from the solitary follicles to the surrounding mucous membrane.

In a large number of the glands in many cases, and probably in all of them in the abortive form of the disease, the changes never advance beyond the first stage, a restoration to their normal condition taking place by colliquative softening.[46] The morbid material upon which their enlargement depends breaks down into an oily débris which is gradually absorbed. This retrograde process takes place faster in the follicles than in the interfollicular tissue, and, as pigment is very apt to be deposited in the depressions thus formed, the patches acquire an appearance which has been compared to that of a recently shaven beard. This appearance is met with, however, in other diseases, and is therefore not peculiar to typhoid fever.

[46] Rindfleisch, *Pathological Histology*, Sydenham Society Translation, vol. i. p. 441.

The description of the changes in these glands in the subsequent stages of the disease which follows is taken mainly from Rindfleisch's work on *Pathological Histology*.

In the stage of necrosis small portions of single Peyerian patches, varying in size from that of a lentil to from three-quarters of an inch to an inch and a quarter in diameter, assume a yellowish-white, opaque tint instead of their former reddish and translucent aspect, gradually become separated from the surrounding tissue by a sharp line of demarcation, and then pass into a state of cheesy necrosis. Here and there the same changes are observed to have taken place in the solitary glands. When once this has occurred, recovery can only take place by expulsion of the necrosed parts and consequent ulceration. Necrosis of the glands [p. 263]probably rarely occurs before the beginning of the second week, but it has occasionally been observed much earlier. Murchison reports cases in which he saw it as early as the first and second days. The process usually involves the mucous membrane only, but it may extend to the muscular and even to the peritoneal coats.

In the third stage the dead parts are gradually thrown off, the process of separation usually occupying several days. At first an increased degree of congestion, followed by suppuration, is observed at the edges of the sloughs, which before their complete detachment may often acquire a yellow, green, or brown color from the imbibition of bile. The ulcers which result correspond in size and form with the sloughs. They are, therefore, in the case of the agminated glands elliptical in shape, with their long diameter corresponding to the axis of the intestine. Their edges are swollen and overhanging, and their floor is generally formed by the deepest layer of the submucous connective tissue. They sometimes penetrate much more deeply, and may even extend to the peritoneal coat, and thus give rise to perforation of the bowel. The ulcers which result from sloughing of the solitary glands are, as a rule, small and round. Murchison says that ulceration may also be produced in the following way: The mucous membrane becomes softened, and one or more superficial abrasions appear on the surface of the diseased patch, which extend and unite into one large ulcer, and this ulcer proceeds to various depths through the coats of the bowel, and even to completed perforation, but Rindfleisch and other recent German writers do not allude to this process.

The fourth stage, or that of cicatrization, usually commences with the beginning of the fourth week. The swelling of the edges of the ulcers gradually diminishes, and they become adherent to the tissues beneath. The floor of the ulcers covers itself with delicate granulations, which in course of time are converted into connective tissue. This is ultimately coated with epithelium, but neither the villi nor the glands of the mucous membrane are ever reproduced. The resulting cicatrices may be recognized by the affected parts of the bowel being thin and more translucent than in health, and may retain these characters after the lapse of several years. They never give rise to contraction of the bowel. The time occupied in the cicatrization of each ulcer is said to be about two weeks. It occasionally happens that while cicatrization is taking place at one end of the ulcer the process of necrosis and ulceration is still going on at the other, so that two or more ulcers may occasionally run together. This form of ulcer may often retard recovery, and may sometimes end in perforation of the bowel, even after convalescence seems to have been established.

The color and consistence of the mucous membrane of the cæcum and colon are in a large proportion of cases normal. In a few the membrane is paler than in health, and in others it is of an ash-gray color. It is also sometimes injected and softened. The solitary glands are frequently enlarged and ulcerated, like those of the ileum. In the former case the mucous membranes of the large intestine throughout its whole extent, but especially that of the cæcum and of the part of the colon adjacent to it, is studded with minute elevations about a line in diameter. When ulceration has occurred the ulcers are generally round [p. 264]and small, but they may occasionally be oval and of considerable size. In the latter case their long diameter will correspond in direction with that of the circular fibres of the intestine. Murchison has known them to measure fully an inch and a half in length. The colon is generally found much distended with flatus.

Enlargement of the mesenteric glands from cellular hyperplasia and hypertrophy of the connective tissue is constantly associated with the morbid changes of the intestines just described. This enlargement varies in different cases. In some the glands are not larger than a pea or bean; in others they are said to have reached the size of a hen's egg. It is always more marked in the glands which lie in the angle between the lower end of the ileum and the cæcum, and usually bears some proportion to the intensity of the local disease; but it is not to be regarded merely as a result of the local irritation, as it has been observed in parts of the mesentery corresponding to perfectly healthy portions of the intestine, and as the meso-colic glands have been involved in cases in which the colon was free from disease. It has, moreover, been observed in cases in which death has occurred very early in the disease, and there can therefore be little doubt that it is as much the result of the infective process as the infiltration of Peyer's patches. In addition to being enlarged, if death has taken place before the end of the second week the glands are hyperæmic and of a purplish color. Later than this, when the sloughs become detached from Peyer's patches, the swelling of the glands diminishes; they lose their color and become pale, and if convalescence ensues they return finally to their former healthy condition. Still, Murchison has seen them shrivelled and pale or bluish for some time after convalescence. In other cases the substance of the glands softens, with the formation of a puriform liquid. If the softening only involves a small part of the glandular structure, restoration to health may take place through the absorption of this liquid. If it is more extensive, the whole of the glands may break down into this puriform liquid, which, when the patient recovers, undergoes caseous and finally calcareous degeneration. Occasionally, a gland in this condition is the cause of death from rupture and extravasation of its contents into the cavity of the peritoneum.

The glands in the fissure of the liver, the gastric, lumbar, inguinal glands, and indeed all the lymphatic glands in the body, have occasionally been found swollen and congested, but their enlargement cannot be classed among the specific lesions of the disease, but is merely the result of a local irritation. Thus, Jenner says that in the case of extensive ulceration of the oesophagus which came under his observation there was marked enlargement of the oesophageal glands. Liebermeister says that the lymphatic follicles which surround the glands at the root of the tongue and in the tonsils are often affected in the same way as the glands. In most cases after a time the swelling disappears, but sometimes softening and rupture take place.

The spleen is almost invariably found to be increased in volume and to have undergone changes in consistence and color. The degree of enlargement and the other changes vary of course with the stage of the disease at which death has occurred. The enlargement occurs with less frequency in elderly than in young people, and is most marked at the height [p. 265]of the disease, the organ being then often twice or three times its normal size, and in some cases, it is said, even larger. Later, and especially during convalescence, the enlargement has generally very much diminished. During the first ten days of the disease the spleen is generally tense and firm, engorged with blood, and dark red in color. Between the tenth and thirtieth days its appearance remains the same, but the organ is found to be soft and friable. During convalescence it becomes paler and firmer again, and is often so shrunken in size that its capsule is relaxed and wrinkled. Hemorrhagic infarctions are often met with. These sometimes soften and break down into a puriform liquid, which may sometimes cause peritonitis by rupture into the peritoneal cavity. Rupture of the spleen is also said to have occurred from mechanical violence. These changes are due in part to variations in the amount of blood, and in part to a medullary infiltration of Malpighian corpuscles similar to that which takes place in Peyer's patches and the glands of the mesentery.

LESIONS WHICH ARE NOT PECULIAR TO TYPHOID FEVER, BUT ARE OF MORE OR LESS FREQUENT OCCURRENCE.—The mucous membrane of the pharynx and oesophagus may present a perfectly healthy appearance, but occasionally it is congested and the seat of ulcerations which are for the most part superficial. Sometimes, however, they have been found to extend to the muscular coat, but they have never been known to penetrate all the coats of these organs. Jenner refers to one case in which there was extensive ulceration of the oesophagus, but usually the number of ulcers is not large. In a few cases the mucous membrane of the pharynx is coated with diphtheritic false membrane, and the submucous tissue is infiltrated with serum and pus (Murchison).

The stomach and the upper part of the intestinal tract present no lesions which are at all peculiar to typhoid fever. In a certain number of cases congestion, softening, and even superficial ulceration, of the mucous membrane of the stomach, and less frequently of that of the duodenum, have been found. The mucous membrane of the jejunum and of the upper part of the ileum is not usually much reddened, and may be even paler than in health. In cases which have been protracted it may be of an ashy-gray or slate color. The contents of this part of the intestinal tract, which is rarely much distended by flatus, do not differ materially in appearance or consistence from the matter which generally composes the typhoid stool. The bowels may, of course, be found filled with blood in cases in which a recent hemorrhage has taken place. Invaginations of the small intestines, unaccompanied by any evidences of inflammation, are occasionally met with in the bodies of those who have died of typhoid fever. They are produced, there is good reason to believe, during the death agony, but are not peculiar to this disease, as they occur in many other diseases.

Enlargement of the liver has been found in only a few cases after death from typhoid fever. Softening is more common, but even this is not a frequent result of the disease, for it was absent in 41 out of 73 cases examined with special reference to this point by Louis, Jenner, and Murchison. The organ is occasionally hyperæmic, and darker in color than in health, but it is oftener pale or normal in appearance. Even, however, where it appears to be perfectly healthy to the unassisted eye, [p. 266]the microscope shows that its cells are very granular and filled with oil-globules which often render the nucleus indistinct or completely conceal it. When death has taken place at an advanced stage of the disease many of the cells are found to be completely broken down into a granular detritus. These changes are usually proportional to the degree of pyrexia which has been present during life. Rarer lesions of the liver are pyæmic deposits, embolism, abscess, and emphysema.

The mucous membrane of the gall-bladder has been found to be the seat of ulcers by Jenner and numerous other observers. It also occasionally presents the evidences of catarrhal or diphtheritic inflammation. The gall-bladder usually contains a pale watery liquid of a less density than bile. When, however, inflammation of its lining membrane has existed, its contents are mixed with pus and shreds of false membrane.

The mucous membrane of the larynx is sometimes found to have been the seat of catarrhal or diphtheritic inflammation, and sometimes also of ulceration. Jenner says that in typhoid fever laryngitis independent of pharyngitis is extremely rare, but the German writers express a different opinion. Griesinger estimated that laryngeal ulcers were present in one-fifth of the fatal cases. Hoffmann found them twenty-eight times in two hundred and fifty autopsies, and that the ulcers had extended to and involved the cartilages in twenty-two out of the twenty-eight cases. They are most commonly found in the posterior wall of the larynx, and may involve the vocal cords. These are often discovered after death in cases in which their existence was not suspected during life. They were formerly supposed to be the result of typhoid infiltration of the laryngeal glands, but careful investigation has shown that they are the consequence of diphtheritic inflammation of the mucous membranes. Inflammation and ulceration of the trachea are comparatively rare. Hypostatic congestion and infarction of the lungs are not uncommonly found after death from typhoid fever, and less frequently the lesions of pneumonia. Evidences of recent pleurisy are also discovered in a few cases. Acute miliary tuberculosis of the lungs is more often met with as a sequela than as a complication.

The changes in the brain and its membranes caused by typhoid fever are few and unimportant, even in cases attended by severe nervous symptoms. Those most frequently found are adhesions of the dura mater to the inner surface of the cranium, injection or oedema of the pia mater, congestive oedema, and sometimes softening of the brain and effusion at the base of the brain. The microscopic changes do not appear to have been carefully studied. Liebermeister says that the gray substance of the cortical portion of the brain and of the interior is sometimes of a rather yellowish-brown color, and that he noticed besides diffuse yellow and blackish-brown spots in different places, particularly in the corpus striatum and thalamus opticus. In such places, he says, the microscope shows a diffuse yellow coloration, a deposit of small brown pigment-granules, and also, especially in the optic thalamus and corpus striatum, the ganglion-cells thickly crowded with brownish or blackish pigment-granules in such numbers as to conceal the outlines of many of the cells. These changes Hoffmann,[47] who has specially studied them, is inclined to place by the side of the parenchymatous degeneration of other organs. [p. 267]The ganglion-cells of the sympathetic ganglia are said by Virchow also to contain an unusual amount of pigment.

[47] Quoted by Murchison.

The muscles are frequently the seat of marked changes in typhoid fever. Their macroscopic appearances vary with the stage of the disease at which they are examined. When death takes place in the first or second week they are usually dark red or reddish-brown in color, and very dry. If it is delayed until later, they "present a peculiar fawn or yellow tint permeating the ordinary red in patches and veins not unlike the appearance of veined marble." Their consistence is also so much diminished that the finger may be readily passed through them. Occasionally, pseudo-abscesses and hemorrhages into the muscular sheath are found, and Dauvé and B. Ball[48] report cases in which, in addition to these changes, rupture of muscles had occurred. Zenker, who was the first to call attention to them, ranged the changes seen under the microscope under two heads: (1) granular or fatty degeneration; (2) waxy degeneration. In the first variety the transverse striæ disappear and the sarcolemma appears filled with finely granular matter. In the second variety the striated muscles become, as it were, pervaded by a coagulating material which sets, and in contracting breaks up the fibres into great numbers of short waxy-looking lumps, not unlike a certain variety of casts of the tubuli recti of the kidneys. When recovery takes place the affected fibre is believed to be regenerated by a cell-growth within the sarcolemma. These changes occur in most fevers, as typhus, small-pox, scarlet fever, and are attributed by authors generally to the hyperpyrexia which is a frequent accompaniment of these diseases. Hayem, however, asserts that he has found them well marked in cases not characterized by a high temperature, and that, on the other hand, they are sometimes absent in cases where this has been present. The waxy form of degeneration may affect all the striped muscles, but is oftenest seen in the muscles of the abdominal walls, the adductors of the thigh, the muscles of the diaphragm, and tongue.

[48] *L'Union Médicale*, 1866, quoted by *Biennial Retrospect of Medicine and Surgery and their Allied Sciences*, for 1865-66.

The heart, in common with the other muscles of the body, suffers from both the forms of degeneration above described, but the granular form appears to be more common than the waxy. In protracted cases it is usually much softened, and when thrown upon a plate no longer retains its form. It has usually lost its normal color and acquired the tint described by the French as feuille morte (faded leaf). Upon minute examination the degeneration is found to have taken place in patches, the diseased fibres being found alongside of others which have scarcely undergone any alteration. These patches are especially common in the papillary muscles of the mitral valve—a fact which explains the occasional presence of systolic murmurs in typhoid fever. In addition to the microscopic appearances of the muscles already described, Hayem[49] has observed in his examinations of the heart a cellular infiltration of the connective tissue and a proliferation of the muscle nuclei. These changes are sufficient in his opinion to establish the existence of myocarditis. The same observer thinks he has also found evidences of the frequent occurrence of endoarteritis in the multiplication of the cellular elements [p. 268]of the internal coat of the small arteries, which he has discovered under the microscope.

[49] *Leçons cliniques sur les Manifestations cardiaques de la Fievre typhoide*, Paris, 1875.

Some discrepancy of opinion exists in regard to the condition of the blood in typhoid fever. Trousseau, for instance, speaks of it as being profoundly altered and in a state of dissolution; Liebermeister says that at the height of the disease the blood is very dark-colored, and that after coagulation it presents a small and soft clot; and Murchison, that a dark, liquid condition of the blood is rarer than in typhus, and that fine white coagula are more common. Harley too has frequently found firm colorless clots of fibrin in the heart and roots of the great vessels in subjects dead in the third week of the disease. Forget concludes from an examination "of one hundred and twenty-three specimens of blood derived from patients in all stages of the disease that an appreciable alteration of the blood in the several periods of enteric fever cannot be accepted as a general fact; that the blood is rarely altered in the first period; that the alteration is more marked in proportion as the disease is more advanced; that the alteration is not always in proportion to the gravity of the disease."[50] I have myself seen the disorganization of the blood as complete in severe cases of typhoid fever which have rapidly proved fatal as in cases of diphtheria or of other malignant diseases. On the other hand, in protracted cases and during convalescence the blood is often thin and watery.

[50] Quoted by Harley, Reynolds's *System of Medicine*, vol. i.

The kidneys are sometimes engorged with blood, sometimes pale and flabby. Under the microscope the appearances are similar to those just described as occurring in the liver, and it is therefore unnecessary to refer to them more fully here. As a rule, the epithelium becomes granular earlier and to a marked degree in the cortical than in the tubular portion. The absence of albuminuria must not always be accepted as proof of a healthy condition of the kidneys, as this symptom has been wholly wanting in cases in which the organs have been extensively diseased.

Analogous changes have also been observed in the salivary glands and pancreas, except that, according to Hoffmann, a cellular proliferation precedes the degenerative process.

CLINICAL DESCRIPTION.—The invasion of the disease is usually so gradual that it is often impossible to obtain from patients exact information as to the time of the beginning of their illness. Among those who present themselves for treatment at the

Pennsylvania Hospital it is not uncommon to find that many have suffered for several days, it may be as long as a week, or even longer, before taking to their beds, from vague feelings of discomfort, from headache more or less intense, aching pains in the back or limbs, or from sensations of chilliness alternating with flashes of heat. In other cases derangements of the digestive system are more prominent, such as nausea, or even vomiting, diarrhoea, or irritability of the bowels. Notwithstanding these symptoms, and the indisposition to exertion engendered by them, they have frequently continued to follow their usual avocations up to the time of their application at the hospital for admission. There is generally, however, no difficulty in recognizing at once the nature of their disease. Upon examination the pulse is found to be frequent, the respiration accelerated, the tongue furred, the skin hot and dry, and the abdomen tympanitic.

[p. 269]Among patients whose position in life enables them to pay greater attention to trifling symptoms than those who are compelled to seek hospital relief, opportunity is frequently afforded to the physician to study the disease at a period less remote from its commencement. The symptoms it presents when seen as early as the second day are generally of a very indefinite character. There may be a feeling of malaise, headache with a tendency to giddiness, pain in the back and limbs, a slightly coated tongue, thirst, and anorexia. The patient may complain of chilly sensations alternating with flashes of heat, but it will rarely be found that the attack has commenced with a decided chill. Diarrhoea may also be present at this time, or may not supervene until later. Even in cases in which it is absent the bowels will generally act inordinately after the administration of a gentle purgative. Occasionally, the attack begins with vomiting, but this is not, in my experience, a frequent mode of commencement. If the visit be made in the morning, the febrile symptoms will be little marked, the pulse being only slightly accelerated and the temperature being rarely more than from a half to a degree above the normal. In the evening, however, the thermometer usually indicates a greater elevation of temperature.

At subsequent visits the same symptoms are presented. It will be observed, however, that the fever is decidedly remittent in character, the evening temperature being always from a degree to a degree and a half higher than that of the morning, while the temperature of each succeeding day is a little higher than that of the day which preceded it. The patient is restless and wakeful at night, or sleep, when obtained, is unrefreshing and disturbed by dreams. He grows dull and slightly deaf, and although able to answer questions intelligently when roused, does so with an effort, and soon after lapses into his former condition. Although obviously growing weaker every day, it is sometimes difficult to get him to take to his bed. The diarrhoea continues and increases in severity; the stools become watery in character and ochrey-yellow in color; they may exceed six, or even twelve, in the twenty-four hours. Epistaxis either consisting of a few drops of blood only, or so profuse as to endanger life, may also occur during the first week. Examination of the abdomen toward the middle or close of the first week will almost always reveal the existence of tympany and of tenderness and gurgling in the right iliac fossa, and very frequently also of slight enlargement of the spleen. The urine at this stage of the disease is dense, scanty, and of high color. The tongue too will be observed to be more heavily coated than at first, and to be dryish, the fur being disposed on the middle of the dorsum of the organ, while the tip and edges are free from it and abnormally red in color. Usually, toward the close of the first week, the pulse will be found to be between 100 and 120 in frequency. It often, however, does not attain this frequency, and in some cases does not exceed 50 throughout the whole of the attack. At the same time, the thermometer generally indicates a temperature of from 102° to 104°, and in bad cases even one much higher than the latter.

These symptoms are not pathognomonic, but Murchison regards their existence in a young person as warranting the suspicion that he is suffering from this disease. About this time, however, or, to speak more accurately, usually from the seventh to the twelfth day, a new symptom occurs [p. 270]which is more characteristic. This is an eruption of isolated rose-colored spots, the tâches roses lenticulaires of Louis, occurring principally upon the surface of the abdomen, but not infrequently seen also upon the chest, back, limbs, and even, according to some authors, upon the face. They are round in shape, with a well-defined margin, usually about a line in diameter, but sometimes considerably larger, slightly elevated above the surface, and disappearing upon pressure, but returning when the pressure is removed. They can almost always be found at this stage of the disease if diligently sought for.

If the disease tends to run a severe course, all the symptoms become aggravated toward the end of the second week. The tongue grows dry and brown, the pulse more frequent, feeble, and markedly reduplicated in character, the diarrhoea still more severe, and the fever higher than before, with little or no tendency to remit in the morning. The nervous symptoms also come into prominence. The headache may grow more violent or may be replaced by increased dulness, which may sometimes be so decided as to render it difficult to fully rouse the patient. At other times delirium is a prominent symptom. This may only occur at night, but not infrequently is observed during the daytime as well. It is usually more active in character than that which accompanies typhus. Trembling of the tongue and of the limbs is not uncommon at this time. The urine becomes more abundant, paler, and less dense than before. Even in cases characterized by symptoms as severe as those above detailed some improvement is, however, often observed to take place between the fourteenth and twenty-first days. The morning remission becomes more decided, the evening temperature less high than that of the preceding day; the stools lessen in number, and gradually assume a more healthy appearance; the pulse diminishes in frequency and gains in force; the tongue becomes moist, and shows a tendency to throw off its fur; the trembling grows less marked; the dulness and delirium lessen; and the patient falls into a refreshing sleep. In other cases, in many of which recovery eventually takes place, there is at this time, instead of an improvement, a still further aggravation of the symptoms. The pulse becomes more feeble and frequent; the tongue is not only excessively dry and brown, but shrivelled and fissured; the lips and teeth are encrusted with sordes; the stools contain shreds of membrane, and often blood; the subsultus tendinum increases; carphololgia, or picking at the bed-clothes, occurs. The prostration becomes so extreme that the patient frequently slips down in bed from sheer weakness. The active delirium of the previous stage is replaced by the low muttering form, or the patient lies upon his back with his eyes half closed in a semi-unconscious condition, from which he is with difficulty aroused, and which may deepen into coma. Occasionally, however, the active delirium continues, and is associated with an obstinate wakefulness; the urine and feces are passed involuntarily, or, with an apparent incontinence of the former, there may be retention, which is very apt to be overlooked. If these symptoms continue for any length of time, bed-sores may form not only over the sacrum, but on other parts subject to pressure, and the patient, worn out by long-continued suffering, dies from exhaustion.

Occasionally, in the midst of these symptoms, and sometimes even in cases in which the condition is not so alarming, prostration approaching[p. 271]collapse, without obvious cause, suddenly supervenes. The pulse becomes a mere thread, the surface is bathed in a clammy sweat, and the temperature is found to have fallen from four to seven degrees, and in some cases even more. These symptoms almost always indicate that intestinal hemorrhage has taken place, and are followed by the discharge of blood either in the course of a few hours or not until a day or two subsequently. If the hemorrhage be moderate in amount, and does not recur, reaction usually takes place in a short time; but if, on the other hand, it is profuse or frequently repeated, death may occur, either immediately or later, as the result of the exhaustion it has induced. Very much the same set of symptoms attend the occurrence of perforation of the bowel, an accident which is also liable to happen in the course of typhoid fever, but which may generally be distinguished from intestinal hemorrhage by its being accompanied by a sharp pain in the abdomen, which is frequently so severe as to cause the patient to cry out, by its not being attended with the same reduction of temperature, and by the absence of blood in the discharges. In a day or two all doubt will be set at rest, if the case be one of perforation, by the occurrence of general peritonitis.

A fatal termination is by no means the usual result, even in cases in which the disease has assumed its worst features. Indeed, it may be said that there is no condition in typhoid fever so grave that recovery from it is impossible. Many authors would make perforation of the bowel an exception to this general rule, but there are observations on record which would seem to show that this accident is not invariably fatal. Even in cases in which the patient has lain helplessly on his back in a semi-unconscious or comatose condition, passing his discharges under him, the physician will often be gratified to find at one of his visits some evidence of improvement, trifling as it will probably be. It may be only a slight change of position, an inconsiderable fall of temperature, or a scarcely appreciable moistening of the tongue; but these changes, insignificant as they apparently are, are sufficient to indicate to the practised eye of the observant physician the approach of convalescence. Next day there will be a still further reduction of temperature, a more decided moistening of the tongue, a sensible diminution of the nervous symptoms, and a reduction in the frequency of pulse. In this condition, however, as may be readily imagined, convalescence may be retarded by numerous accidents, and life may hang trembling in the balance for several days, or even weeks, before it is fully established. It is not necessary to recount here the various steps by which a return to health is reached, as they are essentially the same as those which mark the convalescence of the less severe variety of the disease, and have already been fully referred to in the description of that form.

But even after the establishment of convalescence, and after the patient has been free from fever for several days, febrile attacks lasting for a day or two, or even longer, may occur as the consequence of very slight causes, such as undue excitement, or fatigue of any kind, or the immoderate indulgence of the appetite, which in this condition frequently needs to be restrained. These attacks are usually spoken of as recrudescences of fever, and do not differ materially from attacks of irritative fever occurring under other circumstances. They usually subside under appropriate treatment with the removal of their cause, but leave the patient somewhat [p. 272]weaker than they found him. In other cases, it may be a week or ten days after the fall of the temperature to the normal, and frequently at a time when all danger seems to have been passed, a true relapse of the disease occurs. In this, of course, all the symptoms of the primary attack are reproduced, including even the eruption of rose-colored spots. The temperature usually, however, attains the maximum more rapidly, and the duration of the fever is generally shorter, than that of the original attack. A second relapse is also not very uncommon, and even a third may occur. Various complications and sequelæ also occur in the course of typhoid fever, which will be referred to fully hereafter.

Another form of the disease, which it may be well to allude to briefly here before closing the general description of the disease, is the abortive form. In this variety the attack begins and runs its course up to a certain point, including often even the occurrence of the eruption, as it does in the majority of cases; but at a period which varies between the seventh and fourteenth day the symptoms suddenly subside and the patient rapidly convalesces. In some cases it may be difficult to distinguish this form from an attack of simple continued fever, and, in fact, in cases in which the eruption is absent it will be impossible, unless other cases of typhoid fever have occurred in the same house or family, or unless the patient has been unmistakably exposed to the influences under which the disease arises.

In a few cases the disease begins abruptly with a chill, intense headache, or with gastro-intestinal symptoms, which have in rare instances been so violent as to have suggested to the mind of the attending physician the possibility of corrosive poisoning. This, according to Chomel, is the most frequent mode of commencement, but his experience on this point is opposed to that of the great majority of observers.

I shall now proceed to describe in detail some of the most important of the symptoms presented by the disease.

Even in the beginning of an attack of typhoid fever the face has a listless and languid expression, although the eyes are usually bright and the pupils dilated. In mild cases no further alteration of the physiognomy than this may be noticeable throughout the whole course of the disease, but in bad cases, when the typhoid condition is fully developed, the expression becomes dull and heavy. There is, however, never the general suffusion of the face seen in typhus. On the contrary, the face is often pallid, or there is at most a circumscribed flush on one or both cheeks, which is most marked during the exacerbations of fever or after the administration of food and stimulants. During convalescence the effects of the long illness are fully visible in the face.

Prostration, or loss of muscular strength, is present from the beginning in a large number of cases of typhoid fever, but is generally not so marked in the early stages as in typhus fever. It is usually most intense in grave cases, but to this rule there are numerous exceptions. It is not rare to find patients, in whom the other symptoms are severe, able to sit up in bed, and even to rise to stool, throughout the attack. Bartlett records a case in which the patient did not confine herself to bed until the occurrence of perforation, and I have had under my care a man who, supposing he was suffering only from a slight diarrhoea, performed the duties [p. 273]of a nurse in a military hospital until two days before his death, although the autopsy showed very extensive ulceration of the intestine. Several cases have come under my care in the second week in which patients have walked a considerable distance to make application for admission to a hospital. Generally, however, the prostration becomes extreme in the third and fourth weeks of bad cases, the patient lying helplessly on his back, and frequently slipping down in bed from sheer weakness.

Epistaxis may occur at any stage of typhoid fever, but is most common in the forming stage. Observers differ in opinion in regard to its frequency. Murchison noted it in only 15 of 58 cases, and gives it as his belief that it is more common in France than in England or this country. Flint found that it had occurred in 21 only of 73 cases, and Jenner in 5 of 15 fatal cases. On the other hand, Bartlett says that it is quite a common symptom, and Wood and Gerhard, from the frequency with which they had met with it in the beginning of the disease, were accustomed to regard its presence as of importance in a diagnostic point of view. Part of this divergence of opinion is probably due to the fact that it is usually small in amount, and therefore very apt to be overlooked. I have in many cases, after having been told there had been no epistaxis, found the evidence of it upon the fingers or bed-clothes of the patient. It may, however, be so profuse as to endanger life and render necessary the use of the tampon. Except in the latter case it is without influence upon the course of the disease.

The skin may be almost constantly dry as well as warm throughout the whole course of the fever in a small proportion of severe cases. But, on the whole, perspiration occurs with greater frequency in typhoid fever than in any other acute disease, unless it be rheumatism. It takes place most commonly at night after the evening exacerbation, or in the morning when the patient awakes from sleep, but it is not very rare to find the skin clammy at other times. The sweating is usually general, but in a few cases it is local only. When colliquative, it is frequently exhausting, and is then a grave symptom. It is sometimes prolonged into convalescence, when it is not only annoying, but in consequence of the prostration it induces may sometimes retard the restoration to health.

I have never been able to satisfy myself that any peculiar odor is given off by the skin in typhoid fever, and most observers make a similar statement. Chomel, however, asserted that the perspiration has a strong acid odor, and Bartlett agreed with Nathan Smith in thinking that typhoid fever patients exhale a peculiar odor, not pungent and ammoniacal, like that of typhus, but "of a semi-cadaverous and musty character," which is especially noticeable during the later stages of severe and fatal cases.

The eruption is one of the most characteristic symptoms of the disease. Indeed, in many cases, without it the diagnosis would be impossible. It is rarely absent in a well-developed case. Murchison says that it was noted in 4606 cases only out of 5988 admitted into the London Fever Hospital in twenty-three years, but admits that it would probably have been found in some of the others if it had been properly looked for. Wood says that he has seldom met with cases in which it was absent. It is oftener absent in children than adults—a circumstance which makes the diagnosis of the disease in the former often a matter of great difficulty. It consists of isolated rose-colored spots, slightly elevated above [p. 274]the surface, circular in form or nearly so, having well-defined margins, usually about a line in diameter, but sometimes varying from half a line to two and even three lines in diameter, and disappearing on pressure, to return when the pressure is removed. They are generally first observed some time between the seventh and fourteenth days, but cases are on record, especially in children, in which they are said to have appeared much earlier, and others in which they could not be discovered until the twentieth day. In the latter cases, however, it is not improbable they had really been present at an earlier period, but had escaped detection. The eruption occurs in crops at intervals of three or four days, each spot lasting from three to five days, and the whole duration of the eruption being usually from ten to twenty, and varying of course with the severity of the attack. It may continue to appear as late as the twentieth day, and in cases of relapses very much later. Spots are sometimes seen on the abdomen or elsewhere after the subsidence of fever, and whenever seen indicate that the diseased process is not at an end. They are usually scattered over the lower part of the front of the chest and the abdomen, but are also not infrequently met with upon the back, and if they are not found upon the abdomen, the patient should be gently turned upon his side and this part of his body carefully examined. When very abundant they are often also seen upon the extremities, and occasionally even upon the face. Wood has seen them abundant on the upper and inner part of the thigh, and confined to that place. When tardy in making their appearance, they may often be brought out by application of a mustard plaster or by that of heat in any form; and it is probably, therefore, owing in large measure to the warmth of the bed that they are often so fully developed upon the back. In number they may vary from two or three to several hundred. In one case Murchison counted one thousand, and in three cases which came under my care in the winter of 1881-82 the body was so thickly covered by spots of an unusually large size that when I first saw the patients I directed them to be isolated under the fear that the disease would prove to be typhus fever. When very numerous the edges of two or three of the spots may run together, giving the eruption an irregular character. No relation between the copiousness of the eruption and the severity of the disease has ever been proved to exist. While the prevailing impression, therefore, that cases in which the eruption is freely developed are apt to be of a mild character, is true in many instances, it is by no means so in all. The three cases above referred to all ran a severe course, and one of them proved fatal. The spots disappear after death, and are rarely converted into petechiæ, but in bad cases I have seen purpura spots, and even vibices, developed independently of them. Sometimes the appearance of the eruption is preceded for a day or two by a delicate scarlet rash, which Tweedie says resembles roseola and has been mistaken for scarlet fever.

Sudamina, so called from their resemblance to sweat-drops, also occur not infrequently in this disease. They are minute vesicles, often not larger than a pin's head, but sometimes two lines in diameter, and occasionally, in cases in which two or three have coalesced, much larger. They usually contain at first a clear serum, which may, however, subsequently become turbid, and when very minute must, in consequence of [p. 275]their transparency, be viewed obliquely to be seen. Frequently, when they cannot be distinguished by the eye, they are readily detected by the touch. They rarely occur before the twelfth day, and often not before the close of the third week. Their most usual seat is the neck, the folds of the axillæ, and the groin, but there is no part of the body except the face in which they may not occur. They are most frequently seen in those cases attended by profuse sweating, and are by no means peculiar to typhoid fever, but are met with in other diseases—as, for instance, acute rheumatism—which are attended by this symptom. They are generally followed by branny desquamation of the cuticle in the position they have occupied.

Spots of a delicate blue tint—the "taches bleuâtres" of French writers—are sometimes observed on the skin in cases of enteric fever. They must be of infrequent occurrence in this country, for, although I have looked carefully for them in every case that has come under my care, I have rarely been able to detect them. According to Murchison, "they are of an irregularly rounded form and from three to eight lines in diameter. They are not in the least elevated above the skin, nor affected by pressure, even at their first appearance. They have a uniform tint throughout their extent, and they never pass through the successive stages observed in the spots of typhus. Two or three of them are sometimes confluent. They are most common on the abdomen, back, and thighs." They are said in some cases to be distributed along the course of the small cutaneous veins, and to occur most frequently in cases which are mild. They are met with in other diseases, and usually precede in appearance the characteristic eruption of typhoid fever.

The hair is very apt to fall out after an attack of typhoid fever. The nails suffer in their nutrition in common with other parts of the body—a fact which may be recognized by the peculiar markings which are found upon them after recovery, and to which attention has been particularly drawn by Morris Longstreth in a paper in the *Transactions* of the College of Physicians of Philadelphia, vol. iii., 3d Series.

The circulation is usually accelerated from the beginning of an attack of typhoid fever. The degree of acceleration is commonly proportioned to the severity of the other symptoms, and especially to the elevation of the temperature, and is generally more marked in the evening than in the morning. It is subject, however, to numerous variations, not only in different cases, but even in the same case from day to day, and even from hour to hour. Murchison refers to a case in which the pulse sank to 37, and never exceeded 56 during the fever, although it rose to 66 during the convalescence. I have never had the opportunity myself of observing such an infrequent pulse in the febrile period of the disease, but have had cases under my care in which the pulse often fell below 60, and in which it never exceeded 80 until after the commencement of convalescence. A comparatively infrequent pulse may coexist with a high temperature. Thus, for example, a pulse of 80 was noted in one of my cases at the same time that the thermometer showed that the temperature was 105°, and on another occasion in the same case the pulse was 82 and the temperature $104\frac{1}{2}°$. As a rule, the pulse is more frequent in cases which terminate fatally than in those which end in recovery; but to this rule there are numerous exceptions. In eight of Louis's cases it never [p. 276]went above 90, and in some of my own it did not reach 100 on more than one or two occasions. On the other hand, in mild cases the pulse may be exceedingly frequent, reaching, and even exceeding in many cases, 120. When the disease is prolonged and the prostration is extreme, a pulse of from 140 to 150 is not uncommon. In the majority of cases which have come under my care the pulse has varied in frequency from 80 to 120. In some cases the range has been between these two figures, in others it has been very much less.

During convalescence the pulse usually gradually diminishes in frequency, and may sometimes fall below the normal standard. I have known it in a few instances to fall to 38, and have often met with pulses ranging between 40 and 60 at this period. In other cases, on the contrary, the pulse continues frequent during convalescence, or readily becomes so after a slight exertion or excitement of any kind. A slow pulse during convalescence has been in my experience most frequent in men whose health previous to the attack was good, and a frequent pulse in women and delicate men. If the convalescence is retarded by a complication, the pulse will maintain its frequency until this is removed.

The pulse will of course present other changes than those above referred to. It is in the beginning firm and full, but after the first week becomes small and compressible, and acquires the peculiarity known as reduplication. Sometimes, when this is not well developed, it will be rendered quite distinct by elevating the patient's arm. Irregularity or intermission of the pulse, although not commonly observed in this disease, occasionally occurs. The heart's action will also be observed to grow feeble in the course of severe cases, and its first sound indistinct, but neither of these changes is as marked in typhoid as in typhus fever. Hayem asserts that in a certain number of cases a systolic bellows murmur, with its point of greatest intensity at the apex, is heard during the course or at the close of the second week. This murmur is sometimes soft in the beginning, but becomes harsh and intense later, or may have these characters from the start to such a degree as to give the impression that endocarditis exists. During convalescence an anæmic murmur is not infrequently present.

The respiratory movements are accelerated in typhoid fever, as they are in all febrile conditions, independently of any disease of the lungs, and their frequency is generally proportional to that of the pulse. In looking over my records of cases I find that the former are less liable to fluctuate from day to day than the pulse, and that when the latter becomes abnormally infrequent they do not sink below the standard of health. In several cases of which I have notes the respiration was from 20 to 28, while the pulse was below 60, and in a case referred to by Murchison the pulse was 42 at the same time that the respirations, although no pulmonary lesion could be discovered, were 48. The respiration is often, as in the case just alluded to, very much accelerated when the most careful examination of the chest will not lead to the detection of any disease there. This is sometimes the consequence of very great tympanites, which, by interfering with the descent of the diaphragm, gives rise to dyspnoea, but it may also occur as a purely nervous phenomenon. The air expired by patients has been examined, and has [p. 277]been found sometimes, in the later stages of the disease, to contain ammonia.

Bronchitis is so common an accompaniment of typhoid fever that auscultation rarely fails to reveal its presence in some form or other. In some cases there may be only slight harshness of the respiratory murmur at the base of the chest, but in a large number of cases the auscultatory signs will be sonorous, sibilant, and mucous râles. The last named may be so numerous that I have known the disease in the beginning mistaken for acute bronchitis, and even acute phthisis, by accomplished diagnosticians.

Headache is one of the most constant symptoms of typhoid fever. Bartlett says that it is rarely absent, Louis found it in all but 7 of 133 cases, and Jackson noted it in nearly all his cases. It is often the first symptom of which the patient complains, and, when not present at the beginning of the attack, makes its appearance soon after. It is almost as common, although less severe, in mild cases as in grave ones. It sometimes persists throughout the attack, but oftener subsides at the close of the first week or toward the middle of the second, or the patient may cease to complain of it in consequence of the dulness which is very apt to supervene. It is usually referred to the forehead and temples, but may extend over the whole head. It is usually dull and heavy, but in a few cases is throbbing. It is said by authors rarely to be severe, but I have known it so intense and acute as to cause the disease at its commencement to be mistaken for meningitis, and Jackson asserted that it is sometimes so severe that local bloodletting, and even venesection, had to be employed for its relief. It would appear to be as common in children as adults.

The headache is sometimes accompanied by vertigo and dizziness, and even by retraction of the head. Distressing pains in the back and limbs may also occur, and in rare cases even contraction of the hands and feet.

In the beginning of an attack of typhoid fever the patient usually suffers from wakefulness and restlessness at night, and it occasionally happens that the wakefulness becomes a distressing symptom. But in a great many cases, sooner or later in the course of the disease, drowsiness supervenes. In mild cases this symptom is late in making its appearance, and is generally slight and evanescent, but in grave cases it may come on as early as the eighth day, and when once present may gradually become more profound until it deepens at last into unconsciousness. It usually persists until the occurrence of death or of convalescence, but may alternate with periods of delirium, the delirium being more frequent at night and the somnolence by day. It is as frequent in children as in adults. Occasionally, the wakefulness of the earlier stage may reappear at the beginning of the third week, and coexist with muttering delirium, or occasionally with delirium of a more violent character. It then constitutes a most unfavorable symptom, the patient frequently passing several days and nights in incessant agitation, and sinking finally from exhaustion due to want of sleep.

Some degree of mental hebetude is rarely absent, even in the mildest cases of typhoid fever, and is usually among its earliest symptoms. It may, however, be absent occasionally in cases which run a severe course. It exhibits itself in the beginning in an indisposition to be disturbed, a slight inability to fix the thoughts, or a loss of memory. Generally, the [p. 278]patient will be able at first, by an effort, to rouse himself from this apathy, but the moment he relaxes this effort will lapse into his former condition. As the disease progresses the hebetude becomes more profound and is overcome with greater difficulty. In mild cases it may continue until the occurrence of convalescence, but in grave cases it is soon lost in delirium. This is one of the commonest symptoms of the disease. If I should rely solely upon my own experience, I should say that it was rare for any but the mildest cases to run their course without its occurring at some time or other. Louis found, however, that it was absent in 32 cases, 8 of which were fatal, out of 134 cases, and Murchison in 33 cases, 3 of which ended in death, out of 100 cases. In 8 of these fatal cases death was due to perforation—a fact which would seem to show, as suggested by James C. Wilson, that this symptom is not dependent upon the intensity of the local disease alone. The delirium of course varies with the severity of the other symptoms, and especially with the intensity of the fever. In its mildest form it consists of a slight confusion of ideas, which is readily dissipated by fixing the patient's attention, and is most apt to occur in the night or when he first wakes up from sleep. In other cases it is much more marked; occasionally it is violent and noisy; the patient may talk wildly and incoherently, he may break out into a paroxysm of screaming, or, possessed with a sudden terror, he may leave his bed and attempt to rush from the room or to jump from the window. Later in the course of the disease the active delirium subsides, and low muttering delirium takes its place. The latter may go on until convalescence occurs, or the patient may gradually fall into a comatose condition, which very often ends in death.

The delusions from which the patient suffers are various. I have known in two instances a perfectly pure young girl call loudly for her baby, which she accused her mother and sister of keeping from her. Very frequently patients insist that they are in a strange place, and beg piteously to be taken to their home and friends; occasionally, in grave cases, the patient declares that there is nothing the matter with him. This Louis was accustomed to regard as a bad symptom, having never known recovery to take place after it. Delirium generally first makes its appearance some time in the course of the second week, but occasionally the invasion of the disease is marked by maniacal excitement. I have known delirium to occur on the second or third day. Louis records two cases in which it was present during the first night, and Bristowe[51] one in which it was noted on the fourth night. It is sometimes so prominent a symptom in the beginning of an attack that the patient has at first been supposed to be affected with acute mania. M. Motet[52] indeed refers to a case in which a man was actually admitted into an insane asylum before the true nature of his disease became known. On the other hand, delirium may not occur until much later in the disease—sometimes not before the close of the third or even the fourth week, when it may suddenly make its appearance when least expected. I have known it to be present in a marked degree during a relapse when it had been wholly wanting in the primary attack.

[51] *Trans. Path. Soc. Lond.*, vol. xiii.

[52] *Archiv. gén. de Méd.*, 1868, quoted by Murchison.

During convalescence, especially in cases in which there has been much[p. 279]mental disturbance during the febrile period, the intellect may be weak, and continues so in some cases even after recovery in other respects is complete; but it is rarely permanently impaired. Insanity may also occur during the convalescence or after recovery, but it is usually under these circumstances amenable to treatment. In some cases the moral sense appears to be weakened after an attack, as in the case reported by Nathan Smith, in which a young man of previously good habits developed thieving propensities after his recovery.

Hyperæsthesia of the skin exists, according to Murchison, in about 5 per cent. of the cases, and may occur at any stage of the disease. It is chiefly observed in the abdomen and lower extremities, and is more frequently met with in women and children than in adult males. In a case which was partially under my care during the past summer the slightest touch made the patient, a boy of fifteen years, cry out with pain, and the administration of an enema gave him excruciating agony. Occasionally, the tenderness over the abdomen is so great that it is sometimes difficult to distinguish it from that due to peritonitis, except by the coexistence of hyperæsthesia in other parts of the body. It is very often associated with spinal tenderness, and sometimes with other spinal symptoms. Murchison does not regard it as a formidable symptom.

Cutaneous anæsthesia may also occur, but it is certainly less common in the earlier stages than hyperæsthesia. Rilliet and Barthez look upon it as of grave diagnostic import when it occurs in children.

Muscular tremor is also a common symptom of typhoid fever. A little tremulousness of the tongue when protruded may often be detected before the close of the first week. A little later the hands will be observed to tremble when held up, and still later twitching of the tendons at the wrist may be appreciable while the pulse is being felt. When muttering delirium supervenes this subsultus tendinum becomes constant, and extends to other parts of the body. The hands of the patient are frequently then in constant motion, either picking at the bed-clothes—a very unfavorable symptom—or moving in an objectless manner through the air. This condition presents many points of resemblance to that often seen in delirium tremens, and is said to come on earlier and to be more marked in those who are addicted to the abuse of alcoholic liquors. Hiccough is occasionally observed toward the close of grave cases, and is justly regarded as a bad symptom.

Spasmodic contraction of various groups of muscles is occasionally observed in severe cases, but is less frequent than muscular tremor, and in my experience is generally met with in the earliest period of the disease. The muscles of the extremities, especially those of the legs, are oftenest affected, but I have known the head as rigidly retracted as in tubercular meningitis, and have seen cases in which strabismus has been an early symptom. Murchison has had patients under his care who have suffered from constriction of the pharynx to such an extent that they could not swallow. He also reports cases in which trismus and spasm of the glottis have been present. General convulsions are not common, but occasionally do occur. Although a very grave symptom, they are not invariably fatal. Recovery took place in one of two cases which came under my own observation, and in four of the six recorded by Murchison. They are not always associated with an albuminous [p. 280]condition of the urine. In neither of my cases was there albuminuria, and in only one of the four of Murchison's cases in which the urine was examined was it present. In one of my cases—the fatal one—the convulsions seemed to have been induced by giving the patient improper food; in the other no cause could be discovered.

Ringing or buzzing noises in the ears are present in the early stage of the disease in a large proportion of the cases, and may sometimes persist until the disease is well advanced. Usually, however, after a few days they subside and give place to deafness. This is a very common symptom, and may either affect both ears or be limited to one. In the former case it is probably generally due to the blunted perceptions of the patient, although in a few instances it may be caused, as suggested by Trousseau, by inflammation of the Eustachian tube. When only one ear is affected the deafness is of more serious import, as it is then dependent upon the presence of local inflammation, which may possibly extend to the meninges. It is, as a rule, most marked in the severest cases. Unless there has been a local inflammation it is not followed by permanent impairment of the hearing. It has even been regarded by some observers as a favorable symptom, but this opinion does not appear to rest upon a more substantial basis than the observation of Louis, that the most profound deafness adds nothing to the gravity of the prognosis.

Imperfect or perverted vision occasionally occurs in the course of typhoid fever. In a case which was recently under my care, and which has already been referred to in another connection, there was double vision associated with strabismus. Sometimes haziness of vision, and sometimes even visual illusions, are observed. Bartlett and Murchison have often known intolerance of light present in cases characterized by active febrile excitement. As a general rule, the pupils are widely dilated and the conjunctiva pearly white—a condition which is in marked contrast with what is seen in typhus fever. When, however, stupor supervenes in bad cases, the pupils are frequently as much contracted and the conjunctivæ as much injected as in the latter disease. In a few cases unequal dilatation of the pupils has been noticed. Trousseau was accustomed in his clinical lectures to call attention to the frequency with which sloughing of the cornea occurred in the condition known as coma vigil, in which the patient lies with his eyes wide open. He attributed this accident to the fact that the eye in this condition is not kept constantly moist by the occasional closure of the eyelids, and hence, as its innervation is also impaired, is especially prone to take on ulcerative inflammation. In other cases there is a free secretion of viscid matter, which often glues the eyelids together.

The sense of taste is often lost or perverted. This is partly due to impaired innervation of the tongue and palate, and partly to the thick deposits which usually cover the mucous membrane of these organs.

FIG. 12.

Chart of typical range of temperature in typhoid fever, after Wunderlich.

Frequent observations of the temperature in typhoid fever not merely give most important information in a diagnostic and prognostic point of view, but also often furnish valuable indications for treatment. From a close study of a large number of cases, Wunderlich and other physicians have discovered that the pyrexia has certain characters which distinguish it from other fevers, and which, being present in a case in which the other symptoms are obscure or ill defined, will often enable us to recognize [p. 281]its true nature. The pyrexia may be divided into three periods, each having its own peculiarities. It is usually said that each period lasts about a week, but in severe cases the second and third periods extend over a longer time than this, and the occurrence of a complication or of any other disturbing influence will have its effect in producing either a prolongation of any one or more of these periods, and especially of the last two, or an unwonted elevation or fall of temperature. During the first period there is a progressive rise of temperature, but the rise is never so abrupt as in typhus or in many of the phlegmasiæ. As there are morning remissions, ranging from a degree to two degrees in extent, corresponding to the morning fall in the daily variations of temperature, the tracing upon the temperature chart will be a zigzag line, each evening temperature being from a degree and a half to two degrees higher than that of the preceding evening, while the same difference will be observed in the morning temperature. The temperature ought, therefore, never in an uncomplicated case to be much over 100° on the first evening or 102° on the second. A temperature of 104° at any time during the first or second day will consequently exclude typhoid fever from the diagnosis. From six to eight days are usually occupied before the maximum is reached. I have seen it attained as early as the fourth day in mild cases, and, on the other hand, not until much later in severe ones. It is usually 104° or 105°, but will of course vary with the gravity of the other symptoms. The temperature rarely rises higher than 106° at this period. On the other hand, I have known cases in which it never exceeded 103° during their whole course. It would therefore be wrong to exclude typhoid fever from the diagnosis, as Wunderlich does, if this temperature is not reached by the sixth, or at latest the eighth, day.

In the next period the temperature usually ceases to rise, but has a tendency to oscillate about the maximum temperature of the previous period as a fixed point, occasionally not quite reaching it, at other times rising a little above it. The morning remissions, too, become less decided. In other words, the fever now becomes continuous. This period, although usually lasting about a week, may extend over more than two weeks, even in the absence of complications, in cases which run a severe course, and when it is prolonged from this cause the temperature may again show a tendency to rise, and may even attain an elevation considerably above that of the preceding period. The prognosis in all such cases in which the temperature rises after the middle of the second week is grave. Temperatures of 108°, and even of 110.3°, have been noted at this time. Death invariably follows such high temperatures as these, but before death actually occurs a considerable fall of temperature very often takes place. Wunderlich has also called attention to the fact that it is not uncommon for a sudden and temporary remission of temperature to take place at this stage, varying from one degree to two degrees and a half, which may last from ten to twelve hours, and which usually has occurred in his experience from the sixteenth to the eighteenth day. Toward the close of the second period the morning remissions will be observed to be more decided, while the evening temperature remains about the same as before. The beginning of the third period is indicated by a diminution of the evening exacerbation, while the morning remissions become still more marked. The diminution is progressive, but slow, the [p. 282]temperature each evening falling short by from half a degree to a degree of the point it reached the preceding evening. The morning remissions, on the other hand, each day become greater, a fall of three and a half degrees being not uncommon. The lysis, therefore, occupies usually a longer time than was required by the pyrexia in reaching its maximum. Toward the close of this period the morning temperatures may be normal, as even subnormal, while an elevation of temperature may continue to take place in the evening. Occasionally, however, an abrupt defervescence takes place. The duration of this period will be very much prolonged if complications are present or if the intestinal ulcers are slow in healing. I have known it to last for more than three weeks. During convalescence the temperature is frequently subnormal even in the evening, but the slightest cause is often sufficient to produce a considerable though temporary elevation of temperature. I have known the temperature in one case to rise from 99° F. to 105.6° in a few hours in

consequence of an indiscretion in diet, and in another from 100° to 104° from the suffering and excitement caused by a severe attack of toothache. Indiscretions in diet are a fruitful source of these recrudescences of fever. The fever of the third period has all the characters of an irritative fever, and is probably kept up by the irritation arising from the intestinal ulcers. On the other hand, that of the first two periods is due to the action of the specific poison upon the nervous system and the other tissues of the body, and corresponds exactly with the primary fever of the eruptive diseases.
[p. 283]

FIG. 13.

Chart showing recrudescence of fever from indiscretion of diet.

The febrile movement, however, rarely follows a perfectly typical course, and I consequently find, in looking over the temperature sheets of a large number of cases, very few which bear, except during the first period, anything more than a general resemblance to the chart which [p. 284]Wunderlich has prepared as typical. A very slight cause will exercise, as has already been said, a disturbing influence upon the course of the fever, and serious complications or accidents will of course produce a still more marked effect. An intestinal hemorrhage, for example, will cause a rapid and decided fall of temperature. I have often known it to fall from 104° to the normal temperature, or even below it. This depression, unless the bleeding continues and the case ends fatally in the course of a few hours, is only temporary, the temperature rising within twenty-four hours to its former height, and sometimes even beyond it. A free epistaxis or a copious diarrhoea will in the same way cause a fall of the temperature, but it is rarely so marked as in the preceding case. The same effect is produced by the administration of large doses of quinia or by the application of cold water either in the form of the bath, the douche, or any other form, to the surface of the body. On the other hand, the occurrence of a complication will cause a rise of temperature, often considerably above the maximum of the first period.

FIG. 14.

Chart showing fall of temperature from intestinal hemorrhage in typhoid fever.

The thermometer should be used at least twice daily. In this country it is generally introduced into the axilla, and less frequently into the mouth, for the purpose of making an observation. In other countries it is not infrequently inserted into the rectum, and even into the vagina. The best hours for making the thermometric observations are eight in the morning and eight in the evening, since it has been ascertained from [p. 285]frequent observations that the daily remissions are more marked between the hours of 6 and 8 A.M., and that the temperature usually reaches its maximum some time between those of 7 and 12 P.M.

Loss of appetite is, except in mild cases, one of the earliest symptoms of the disease, and usually persists as long as the fever lasts. It is sometimes accompanied by positive loathing for food, but generally there is no great difficulty in persuading the patient to take the necessary amount of nourishment. During convalescence the appetite returns, and is occasionally immoderate, so that it is frequently necessary to curb it lest harm should be done by over indulgence.

Thirst, usually proportionate to the degree of fever, is also present in the beginning of the fever. Later, when the patient sinks into a semi-unconscious condition and becomes insensible to the wants of the system, he will cease to call for water, although it is still urgently needed.

Nausea and vomiting sometimes occur at the beginning of the disease, but they have not been such frequent symptoms in my experience as they would appear to have been in that of Murchison, who says that they are of such common occurrence that the patient is often supposed at first to be suffering merely from a bilious attack. He does not regard them, when occurring at this stage, as serious symptoms. Indeed, he expresses the belief that the subsequent course of the disease is sometimes favorably modified by them. They may also occur later in the disease, and are then of grave import, as they are not infrequently the consequence of peritonitis. Louis regarded vomiting as a grave symptom, but it is probable it occurred in the cases from which he makes his deductions late in the course of the disease. It may sometimes occur during convalescence, and may then interfere very materially with the proper nutrition of the patient. The matter vomited usually consists of a greenish bilious fluid, with the food last taken. In some cases blood has been thrown up.

The tongue at the beginning of an attack of typhoid fever is usually moist and coated with a thin white fur, and in mild cases may retain these characters until the close. Even in some cases which terminate fatally in the course of the second week, the tongue, with the exception of being less moist than in health, may present no marked deviation from this appearance. Generally, however, as the disease progresses, and sometimes as early as the tenth day, it becomes dry and brownish, and is protruded with a tremulous motion. Still later it tends to cover itself with a thick brown coating. This coating is disposed principally along the middle of the organ, leaving uncovered the edges and tip, which are very apt to be unnaturally red in color. The bare portion at the tip is often rudely triangular in shape—a point which is regarded as of some importance in the diagnosis of the disease by Da Costa. In bad cases, during the course of the third week the tongue is frequently crossed by cracks and fissures, which are the cause of much discomfort to the patient, and when deep may bleed and leave behind them scars which are recognizable during the remainder of his life. In other cases the tongue is dry, brown, and shrivelled, or covered with a tenacious, viscid secretion which renders it difficult to protrude it.

In favorable cases, as convalescence approaches the tongue regains by degrees its normal appearance. At first the only noticeable change may [p. 286]be that the organ is a little less dry than before. In a few days it will be observed to have become moist and to be gradually throwing off its coating. The process is, however, a slow one, and one, moreover, subject to frequent interruption. Very often, when it seems nearly completed it will be suddenly arrested, and the tongue become dry and brown. Sometimes, instead of cleaning itself gradually, the tongue throws off its coating in large flakes, leaving the mucous membrane red and shining, as if deprived of its papillary structure. Wood was accustomed to teach that if the tongue when thus cleaned remained moist convalescence might be expected, but would always be tedious. This is an observation the correctness of which I have had abundant opportunity to confirm. If anything happens, however, to interfere with the progress of convalescence, it not infrequently becomes dry and coats itself over again. When the restoration to health is retarded by the continuance of diarrhoea or by the occurrence of any intercurrent affection, the tongue will often become pale and flabby and be the seat of superficial ulcerations or of aphthous exudations.

The mucous membrane of the posterior fauces is also often red and dry and covered with a glutinous secretion, which often materially interferes with swallowing. The lips and teeth are in bad cases encrusted with sordes, and the former are dry and cracked, and bleed readily when picked.

Meteorism or tympanites is observed in the greater number of cases of typhoid fever, having been noted by Murchison in 79 out of 100 cases, and by Hale in 130 out of 179 cases, and in only 43 of the remainder of his cases is it expressly stated to have been absent. My own experience leads me to believe that it is present in even a larger proportion of cases; in fact, that it is rarely absent. It is, as a rule, later in making its appearance than the other abdominal symptoms, showing itself usually about the end of the first or the beginning of the second week. It is generally most marked in grave cases, especially those attended by severe diarrhoea, but I have seen it highly developed in cases in which the symptom was not present at all or but little developed. It may vary, moreover, frequently in degree at different times in the same case, but when once present generally persists until convalescence is established or death occurs. When extreme, it may give rise to distressing dyspnoea by preventing the descent of the diaphragm.

The meteorism is usually preceded and accompanied by gurgling and tenderness on pressure in the right iliac fossa. The former of these symptoms is most marked in cases in which diarrhoea exists, and is caused by the presence of liquid and gas in the lower part of the ileum. The tenderness is unquestionably due to the presence of ulcers in the same part of the bowel. There is also occasionally pain in the region of the umbilicus, but this is a much less frequent symptom.

Enlargement of the spleen was noted by Hale as being present in some of the cases which he has described. It is a frequent symptom of the disease, and may be generally demonstrated by percussion in the course of the second week. It has not, however, often happened to me to be able to feel the organ enlarged through the abdominal walls, as Murchison asserts he has been able to do. Indeed, tympanites is usually present in a sufficient degree to render this difficult. The enlargement [p. 287]occurs more frequently in persons under thirty years of age than in those over it.

Diarrhoea is one of the most frequent symptoms of the disease, especially in severe cases, and there are very few mild cases in which it does not occur at some period of their course. Louis noted it in all but three of his fatal cases, Murchison in 93 out of 100, and M. Barth in 96 out of 101. It varies in different cases in severity, in duration, and in the time at which it appears. It may be one of the earliest symptoms, presenting itself frequently on the first day, and often being the only one which occasions uneasiness to the patient or his physician. At other times its appearance may be postponed until the end of the first week, or even until the patient is apparently entering on convalescence. It may be mild in the beginning and become more severe as the disease progresses, or after having been at first acute may cease spontaneously in a few days to occasion any uneasiness. In degree it may vary from two stools to three or four, or even twenty, in the course of the twenty-four hours. It is absent in a few cases, but in many even of these cases the bowels will be found to act inordinately after a very moderate dose of purgative medicine. I have known, for instance, the administration of a single teaspoonful of castor oil to be followed by five or six stools in an adult. Constipation does, however, actually exist in a certain number of cases. Murchison has known the bowels in cases in which a relapse has occurred to be constipated in the primary attack and relaxed in the relapse. There is no relation between the severity of the diarrhoea and the extent of the local lesion. Although oftenest met with in mild cases, constipation has existed in cases in which perforation of the bowel or intestinal hemorrhage has occurred during life, or very extensive lesions been found after death.

The stools are fetid and ammoniacal, and are alkaline in reaction, instead of acid as in health. They are usually liquid and of the color of yellow ochre. Murchison says that they separate, on standing, into two layers—a supernatant fluid and a flaky sediment—but that, occasionally, instead of being watery they are pultaceous, frothy, and fermenting, and so light as to float in water. I have myself often seen the appearance which Bartlett compares to that of new cider. They may contain blood, and when they do, occasionally present the appearance of coffee-grounds. They are not infrequently, in grave cases, passed involuntarily.

Intestinal hemorrhage is fortunately not a frequent symptom of typhoid fever. It may occur as early as the fifth or sixth day, but is more common after the middle of the second week or in the third or fourth week. In 60 cases observed by Murchison in which the hemorrhage exceeded six ounces it began during the second week (mostly toward its close) in 8; during the third week in 28; during the fourth in 17; during the fifth in 1; during the sixth in 3; during the seventh in 1; and during the eighth week in 1; while in one case the date of its occurrence is not noted. In the cases observed by Liebermeister and Griesinger, 113 in all, the bleeding took place in a much larger proportion of cases at an early period of the disease, occurring in as many as 43 in the second week, and in only 27 during the third. In 7 cases in which I had the opportunity of observing it in patients under my own care it occurred on the seventeenth day in 1; on the twenty-third day in 1; during the [p. 288]third week in 2; during the fifth week in 2; and on the fifth day of a relapse in 1. There may be a single hemorrhage, or the bleeding may be repeated one or more times. In 5 of my cases there was a second hemorrhage, and in 2 of them a third; and in several of Murchison's cases it recurred at varying intervals after its first appearance.

When the bleeding occurs early in the disease it is usually insignificant in amount, and is due either to extreme congestion of the mucous membrane of the intestine, giving rise to rupture of the capillaries, or to disintegration of the blood, allowing its ready passage through the walls of the vessels. In the latter case it usually coexists with petechiæ or a hemorrhage from some other part of the body, as, for instance, epistaxis or hematuria. After the middle of the second week the hemorrhage is generally the result of the laying open of a small artery, either by the detachment of a slough from one of the glands of Peyer or by the involvement of its walls in the ulcerative process. It is then often profuse, and may even reach several pints in quantity. Murchison has, however, seen profuse hemorrhage at such an early stage of the disease that it was impossible that ulceration could have taken place. The blood is not always voided immediately after a hemorrhage has taken place; it may be retained for some days. Indeed, if the amount be large the patient may die within a few hours of its occurrence without any appearance of blood externally. This is, however, rare; it is more usual for the hemorrhage to be repeated before death takes place, but the occurrence of the bleeding may be suspected in such cases by the abrupt fall of temperature, sometimes below the normal standard, and by the extreme prostration and pallor which come on suddenly without other assignable cause. The depression of the temperature does not continue long. It generally reaches its former elevation, or even exceeds it, in the course of twenty-four hours.

There would appear to be a slight difference in the frequency with which intestinal hemorrhage occurs in different times and at different places. Murchison noted it in 58 cases of 1564, or 3.77 per cent.; Louis in 8 cases of 134, or 5.9 per cent.; Liebermeister in 127 cases of 1743, or 7.3 per cent.; Griesinger in 32 cases of 600, or 5.3 per cent.; and I have noted it 7 times in 81 cases, or in about 8.5 per cent. Liebermeister makes it twice as frequent in women as in men. It seems to be much less common in children than in adults, for in 252 patients under fifteen years of age observed by Taupin, Rilliet, and Barthez it occurred in 1 only. There is considerable diversity of opinion among observers in regard to the importance of this symptom. Murchison lost 32 of his 60 cases. In 11 of the 32 fatal cases the immediate cause of death was peritonitis; in 14 of the remaining 21 cases the patients died within three days of the bleeding, and in 8 of the 14 within a few hours. Of Liebermeister's 127 cases 49, and of Griesinger's 32 cases 10, terminated fatally; 3 of my own cases ended in death, but none of them until several days had elapsed after the bleeding. In the face of facts such as these there have not been wanting authors to assert that the effect of the hemorrhage was sometimes beneficial. Chief among these are the celebrated Irish physician Graves and his devoted admirer Trousseau. There may occasionally be a slight subsidence of the nervous symptoms upon the occurrence of a hemorrhage, consequent upon the reduction of temperature [p. 289]which usually accompanies it, but this relief is only temporary, and procured at too great expense to be really of service to the patient.

The bleeding is most frequently observed in bad cases. All the cases which were under my care in which it occurred were of great severity from the very start. In 18 of Murchison's 60 cases the antecedent symptoms were mild. In 3 of my cases there was severe diarrhoea. In 2 of the other cases, 1 of which was fatal, the bowels were constipated, and in another one, also fatal, they were slightly loose. In 8 of Murchison's cases, 6 of which were fatal, the bowels had been constipated up to the time of its occurrence. The blood, if voided immediately after its escape into the intestines, is generally fluid and bright red in color. When retained for a day or two it is passed in dark clots, and if retained longer than this it is usually mixed with fecal matter when discharged from the bowels, and gives the stools a tarry appearance and consistence, which is not always recognized by inexperienced attendants as due to blood.

It has been asserted that intestinal hemorrhage has become more frequent since the introduction of the cold-water treatment, but Liebermeister shows this to be an error, for he has found that of 861 cases treated before the introduction of this treatment, 72, or 8.4 per cent., had intestinal hemorrhage, but that of 882 cases treated since its introduction hemorrhage occurred in 55, or in 6.2 per cent. Other methods of treatment have also been charged with inducing a tendency to hemorrhage, but probably not upon more substantial grounds than the above.

The occurrence of perforation may be suspected when the patient is suddenly seized with acute pain in the abdomen, accompanied by symptoms of collapse and occasionally by rigors. The fall of temperature is often considerable. Liebermeister refers to one case in which it was as much as 5½°, or from 104° to 98½°. Very soon the abdomen becomes tender on pressure, and, if it were not so before, hard and tympanitic; the pulse grows frequent, small, and sometimes almost imperceptible; the breathing is thoracic; the physiognomy expresses great suffering; the features are contracted, and the face is bathed in profuse perspiration. Nausea and vomiting come on soon after inflammation has commenced, and rapidly exhaust the patient. The decubitus is dorsal, and the legs are generally drawn up so as to relax the abdominal muscles. Prostration rapidly increases until death puts an end to the patient's sufferings. Occasionally, the symptoms are more obscure. Pain and rigors may both be wanting, and nothing but the extreme prostration, the frequent and feeble pulse, and the distended condition of the abdomen will indicate the gravity of the danger. This is not infrequently the case in delirious patients. Death may take place during the collapse, but this is rare. It more frequently takes place on the second or third day; on the other hand, it may be postponed until much later. Liebermeister and Murchison refer to cases in which there was an interval of two or three weeks between the first symptom of perforation and the fatal result.

Perforation of the intestine was formerly regarded as an inevitably fatal accident, but this view is no longer entertained. I have had under my observation cases in which all the symptoms of this accident were present, and in which recovery took place. In some of these cases there [p. 290]may have been an error of diagnosis, but all of them will not admit of this explanation. Moreover, cases of a similar character have been reported by physicians whose skill in diagnosis is universally recognized. Thus, Murchison reports six such cases, Tweedie two, and Wood one. Liebermeister and Bristowe[53] also both say that recovery is possible. This view is sustained by the results of certain autopsies. In one of these, reported by Buhl,[54] a perforation was found completely closed by adhesions to the mesentery, and in others reported by Murchison partial adhesion had taken place between the edges of the perforation and the abdominal walls or to an adjoining coil of intestine. Occasionally, the inflammation excited by the perforation may be circumscribed and terminate in an abscess, which may permit recovery by discharging itself into the bowel or externally. At other times, however, it ruptures into the peritoneal cavity, when death speedily ensues.

[53] *Transactions of the Pathological Society of London*, vol. xi. p. 115.
[54] Cited by Murchison.

Perforation is, fortunately, not a frequent accident in typhoid fever. It was the cause of death in 20 only of 250 fatal cases collected by Hoffmann. It occurred, according to Liebermeister, in only 26 cases, 3 of which ended in recovery, in more than 2000 cases observed at the hospital at Basle. Murchison observed it 48 times in 1580 cases, Griesinger 14 times in 118 cases, and Flint twice in 73 cases. Murchison found that in a total of 1721 autopsies, the details of which were collected from various sources, it was the cause of death in 196, or 11.38 per cent. It would appear to be rather more common on the continent of Europe than in England or in this country. Perforation is much more frequently met with in men than in women. The patients were men in 15 of 21 of Liebermeister's cases, in 51 of 73 of Murchison's, and in 72 of 106 cases collected by Näcke. It is rarer in children than in adults. Rilliet, Barthez, and Taupin met with it only three times in 232 children under treatment. Murchison has, however, had a fatal case in a child of five years of age. It is also not common after forty years of age, but does occasionally occur, although the contrary has been asserted.

Perforation is most likely to happen during or after the third week of the disease, but it has been met with as early as the eighth day, as in a case reported by Peacock. On the other hand, in three cases cited by Morin[55] it did not occur until the seventy-second, seventy-sixth, and one hundred and tenth day, respectively. Instances are on record in which it has taken place after the patient was supposed to be thoroughly convalescent and had returned to his occupation. When it occurs early it is due to the separation of a slough. After the middle or end of the third week it is probably always the result of the extension of the ulcerative process to the peritoneal coat. In a large proportion of cases the perforation has been preceded by symptoms of great gravity, such as severe diarrhoea, great tympany and tenderness of the abdomen, and intestinal hemorrhage, but in a certain number of instances the cases in which it has occurred have been of a mild character, the patient in many of them not considering himself sick enough to take to his bed or even to abstain from his daily labor. After death the perforating ulcer has been found to be the only one.

[55] Quoted by Murchison.

The most frequent causes of perforation are the irritation arising from [p. 291] indigestible and unsuitable food, distension of the bowels by feces or gas, vomiting, and movements on the part of the patient. Liebermeister calls attention to the frequency with which ascarides are found in the intestines of those who die of perforation, and is inclined to think they may have something to do with causing it. Morin[56] reports a case in which the perforation appeared to be caused by the administration of an enema.

[56] Quoted by Murchison.

For our knowledge of the changes in the composition of the urine we are largely indebted to Parkes and certain German observers. As the disease generally begins insidiously, the condition of the urine before the attack and during the first two or three days has not been ascertained with certainty. During the latter part of the first week the amount of water is greatly diminished, occasionally falling to one-fourth or one-sixth of the usual quantity. In the second and third weeks it increases, and at the end of the fourth week may again be normal. The amount may, however, vary from day to day, but its variations do not stand in close relation to those of the febrile heat; that is, the thermometer may mark one day 104°, and the next day 100°, while the amount of urine remains the same. Still, when the temperature begins to fall permanently it increases at once, or, according to Thierfelder, two or three days after. The specific gravity is usually high in almost all cases in which the urine is scanty, and may be as high 1038. With the establishment of convalescence the specific gravity often diminishes before the water begins to increase. In other words, the lessening of the solids of the urine frequently takes place prior to the increase of the water.

The reaction of the urine is very acid in the beginning, but the acidity is not due to an increased secretion of acid, but simply to concentration. Later it may become alkaline, and even ammoniacal. The color of the urine is darker than in health during the early part of the febrile period. This is due partly to concentration, and partly to increased disintegration of the blood-corpuscles, which is a consequence of the fever.

The quantity of urea is augmented during the fever, and especially during the first week, when the water and chlorides of sodium are most diminished. As a general rule, the higher the temperature the greater the amount of urea. It may, however, be very much diminished during the presence of inflammatory complications. On the other hand, it is not affected by diarrhoea. Uric acid is uniformly increased, the amount of increase being relatively greater than that of the urea; it is often doubled, and sometimes the increase is even more than this. This increase takes place, according to Zimmer, up to the fourteenth day. It diminishes after this, and during convalescence may fall below the normal amount. Copious deposits of urates may occur at any time in the course of the disease. The chloride of sodium is usually diminished in amount. This diminution is partly due to a less amount of this salt being taken with the food, and partly to the fact that large quantities of it pass away with the stools. As the diminution cannot always be fully accounted for in this way, it would appear that it is also stored up in the body during the fever. In cases in which sweating and purging are absent the sulphuric acid is increased in amount. The phosphoric acid is at first slightly diminished, but later undergoes an increase. The hippuric acid is also diminished.

[p. 292] Parkes found albumen in the urine in 7 out of 21 cases. In 5 of these it was temporary, and entirely disappeared before the patients left the hospital. Becquerel found it in 8 out of 38 cases, Andral in only 4 out of 34 cases. Griesinger found it commonly, though it was usually temporary. He met with only four or five cases in which it was never present. Kerchensteiner found albumen in a fourth part of the severe cases. Brattler noticed it in 9 out of 23 cases. I have very frequently found it myself, but it has always been in my cases a temporary phenomenon. Desquamative nephritis may occur occasionally in the course of typhoid fever, and give rise to the appearance of a large amount of albumen in the urine, and also occasionally of blood. Renal epithelia and casts are sometimes seen in cases in which there is albuminuria, but usually soon disappear. Zimmermann asserts that in all but very slight cases casts may be found even when no albumen can be detected. The statement is probably too general, but there is no doubt of the occasional presence of casts under these circumstances. Bladder epithelia and pus-cells are seen in a few cases in small quantities, but decided cystitis is rare, unless it has ensued upon retention of urine. Sugar has not been found except in the urine of diabetic patients, who may have happened to contract typhoid fever. In these patients the sugar diminishes, and is sometimes wholly absent during the continuance of the fever. Leucin and tyrosin have been found by Frerichs, but at present no observations have been made as to the frequency or import of their occurrence.

In many cases, when the prostration is extreme, the urine is passed involuntarily, but in some of these cases the incontinence of the urine is only apparent, and is really the result of over-distension of the bladder. This is a condition which is very apt to be overlooked, and I have known paralysis of the bladder to result in consequence of this neglect, and to continue sometimes after convalescence has been established.

COMPLICATIONS AND SEQUELÆ.—Although cerebral symptoms are among the commonest manifestations of the disturbing effects produced in the economy by the typhoid fever poison, they are almost always independent of inflammation of the brain and its membranes. In a few cases, however, the lesions of meningitis have been found after death. In some of these it has come on without assignable cause, in others it has been the consequence of pyæmia, of tubercles, or of the extension of inflammation from the petrous portion of the temporal bone. Occasionally, during convalescence, some impairment of the intellect is observed. This may consist in simply some loss of memory or childishness of manner. At other times delusions of a mild form are present, or else the patient is liable to attacks of acute mania, sometimes violent, coming on suddenly and without fever. In a few instances the moral sense seems to have been perverted, as in the case reported by Dr. Nathan Smith, already referred to, in which a young man of previously good character developed a propensity to steal after his attack. Recovery with the re-establishment of the physical health almost occurs in these cases. Murchison says he knows of no case in which this condition has been permanent. On the other hand, Dr. C. M. Campbell,[57] who had the opportunity of observing an attack of typhoid fever among some insane patients [p. 293]at the Durham County Asylum, reports that the mental state was in no case injuriously affected by the disease, but, on the contrary, underwent a marked improvement in several of the cases. Indeed, in two of the cases, in which the prognosis had become very unfavorable, mental recovery began during the attack of fever.

[57] *The Journal of Mental Science*, July, 1882.

Paralysis, muscular tremors, and chorea are also occasionally observed after attacks of typhoid fever. According to Murchison, paralysis does not supervene until several weeks after the commencement of convalescence. It may last for several weeks or months, but recovery in the majority of instances eventually takes place. According to Nothnägel,[58] the most common form is paraplegia, but it may also take the form of hemiplegia, strabismus, paralysis of the portio dura, motor paralysis of individual spinal nerves, such as the ulnar or peroneal, or local anæsthesia. On the other hand, neuralgias and disturbances of sensation are not common sequelæ of typhoid fever.

[58] Cited by Murchison. See also article by Paget, *St. Bartholomew's Hospital Report*, vol. xii.

Degeneration of the muscular tissue of the heart is probably present in some degree in every case of typhoid fever, being, of course, most marked in the severest cases. There would seem, however, to be no special tendency to disease of its valves or membranes. Arterial thrombosis or embolism, giving rise to gangrene of the part supplied by the obstructed artery, is of occasional occurrence. Patry,[59] Hayem,[60] Trousseau,[61] and others report or refer to several cases in which gangrene of the leg, hand, or cheek was observed, and among others a case in which sphacelus depending upon obstruction of the carotid artery, the result, as Patry thought, of arteritis, commenced in the left ear, and extended from there to the forehead and cheek.[62] A. Martin[63] reports the case of a woman who expelled from the vagina a fetid-smelling structure of cylindrical form, which proved to be the cervix of the uterus, with the upper part of the vagina, and in whom menstruation was not re-established until after the performance of an operation. Spillmann[64] has also called attention to the occurrence of gangrene of the vagina and vulva in cases of typhoid fever.[p. 294]This complication is generally met with toward the end of the febrile period.

[59] *Archives générales de Médicine*, 1863, vol. i. pp. 129-549.
[60] *Loc. cit.*
[61] *Clinique médicale.*
[62] Since the above was written Barié has called attention in the *Revue de Médicine*, Jan. and Feb., 1884, to the frequency with which acute inflammation of the arteries occurs as a sequel of typhoid fever. The author, whose investigations were limited to the larger arteries, found that the vessels generally implicated are in the order of their frequency, the posterior tibial, the femoral, and the dorsal artery of the foot. The affection is usually unilateral, appears during convalescence or when the patient leaves his bed, and occurs just as often after light as after severe cases. He distinguishes two varieties: 1, acute obliterating arteritis, and, 2, acute parietal arteritis. The first variety is characterized by embryonal infiltration of all the tissues, by disappearance of the smoothness of the intima, which becomes uneven and granular, and by the formation of a secondary thrombus, and almost invariably terminates in dry gangrene. The second is merely an inflammation without such a clot, and always terminates in recovery without gangrene.

The symptoms of obliterating arteritis are—pain, more or less sudden in its onset, directly over the course of affected vessels, and increased by pressure, by the erect position, and by walking; diminution, and then absence, of pulsation; swelling of the limb, without oedema or redness; and, later, the appearance of bluish mottling of the surface, and, more rarely, of patches of purpura; lowering of the temperature, with or without troubles of sensibility, such as formication, anæsthesia, etc., and the appearance of a hard and painful cord, due to the formation of the thrombus. In the parietal form the diminution of the pulsations is sometimes preceded by a considerable exaggeration of their amplitude, and, while the temperature on the affected side is usually lowered, it may sometimes be increased.

[63] *Centralblatt f. Gynakol*, 1881.
[64] *Archives générale*, Mars, 1881.

Venous thrombosis, the result of weakness of the heart's action, is more frequently observed. It occurs generally during the convalescence of cases which have run a severe course, and usually affects the veins of the lower extremities. I have seen both the femoral veins obstructed from this cause at the same time. All the cases which have come under my own observation have ended in recovery, and only 2 of 31 collected by Liebermeister terminated fatally. Death occurred in 3 of the 17 cases collected by Murchison, but in none of them was this result attributable to this complication alone. There is, however, always danger of a portion of the thrombus becoming detached and producing embolism of the pulmonary artery.

Pyæmia is said by Murchison and other authors to be an occasional complication, but it is certainly rare in this country. In the milder cases abscesses form during convalescence beneath the skin in different parts of the body. In the more severe cases pus is deposited in the joints or in the internal organs. Albert Robin[65] has reported two cases in which there was suppurative joint affection. In one of these the joints of the fingers and toes, with the sheaths of the corresponding extensor tendons and both knee-joints and one shoulder-joint, were affected. In the other the left knee was filled with pus. In both cases the fever soon assumed an adynamic character.

[65] *Gazette de Paris*, 1881.

Laryngitis may sometimes occur in the course of typhoid fever, and when it assumes the diphtheritic form and runs on to the formation of ulcers is a very serious complication of typhoid fever, as it is not infrequently accompanied by oedema of the glottis and gives rise to the necessity for tracheotomy. It is fortunately, at least in its worst forms, rare in this country. In Germany, judging from the number of cases collected by Hoffmann and Griesinger, it is of more common occurrence. The ulcers are oftener met with in some epidemics than in others. During the winter of 1860-61, which I passed in Vienna, the frequency with which they occurred was the subject of remark among those who were in attendance upon the various clinics.

I have already called attention to the frequency with which bronchitis in some form or other attends upon typhoid fever. When it invades the smaller bronchial tubes it occasionally gives rise to lobular pneumonia or to collapse of some of the lobules of the lung. Lobar pneumonia may also occur in the course of typhoid fever. It was observed 52 times in 1420 cases of typhoid fever under treatment at the Basle hospital from 1865-68. When it comes on late in the disease, especially if the patient is comatose, or even semi-conscious, it may be entirely overlooked, unless the lungs are carefully examined, as it often does not reveal itself to us by any of the ordinary symptoms. It may, however, occur early, and I have known it so prominent in the beginning of an attack that the existence of typhoid fever was not suspected. It sometimes terminates in abscess or gangrene, but is more usually followed by chronic pneumonia, which may eventually either end in recovery or lay the foundation for phthisis. Pleurisy with effusion is also not an uncommon complication. It was observed, according to Liebermeister, at the hospital at Basle 64 [p. 295]times in 1743 cases of fever. It is also a serious complication, as 21 of the 64 cases terminated fatally. Murchison refers to three cases in which it was followed by empyema. Other morbid conditions of the respiratory organs which may occur as complications of typhoid fever are oedema, infarction, hypostatic congestion of the lungs, emphysema, and pneumothorax. Acute miliary tuberculosis is also an occasional complication, but is oftener met with as a sequel. According to Liebermeister, the tendency to pulmonary complications has diminished since the introduction of the cold-water treatment.

Catarrhal or diphtheritic inflammation of the fauces and pharynx occurs in a large number of cases, and frequently gives rise to a great deal of difficulty in swallowing. Indeed, it has been so frequently observed in some epidemics that a few writers have regarded it as a symptom rather than a complication of the disease. Either of the varieties of inflammation may extend through the Eustachian tube to the middle ear and be the cause of deafness, which usually passes off as the inflammation subsides. Occasionally, however, the affection of the middle ear gives rise to perforation of the tympanum or to caries of the petrous portion of the temporal bone.

Murchison says he has known the symptoms of and lesions of dysentery to coexist with those of typhoid fever in several cases, and Liebermeister asserts that diphtheria of the intestinal mucous membrane is an occasional sequel to severe cases, especially when other mucous membranes are the seat of diphtheritic inflammation. In a few instances which have come under his observation it had given rise to perforation of the bowel or to gangrene of the intestinal mucous membrane.

Jaundice occasionally occurs in the course of the disease. I have never happened to see this complication, and am inclined to think it is rare in this country. Liebermeister, however, met with it 6 times in 1420 cases, and Griesinger 10 times in 600 cases. Hoffmann found it in 10 of 250 fatal cases, and Murchison was able to collect 9 cases, all of which but one terminated in death. Several of Griesinger's cases, however, ended in recovery. In a few cases the jaundice may be attributed to catarrh of the biliary ducts, but this solution of the question will not explain those cases in which the feces remain colored throughout. In fatal cases marked degeneration of the liver has been found, which Liebermeister regards as of similar character to that which occurs in acute yellow atrophy. In two of Murchison's cases the liver was small and its secreting cells loaded with oil. In most cases it does not appear until late in the disease, but it has been observed as early as the fifth day.

Abscess of the liver and diphtheritic inflammation of the mucous membrane of the gall-bladder are among the rarer sequelæ of typhoid fever.

Peritonitis is the most serious of all the complications of typhoid fever. Its most common cause is perforation of the bowel, but it may also be due to the extension of inflammation to the peritoneal membrane without ulceration. Liebermeister believes that it is sometimes the result of the typhoid infiltration so frequent in various tissues of the body taking place in the serous membrane. In other cases it arises from the rupture of softened mesenteric glands, of softened [p. 296]infarctions in the spleen, or of the abscesses which are sometimes the consequence of the circumscribed inflammation by which perforation is occasionally prevented from proving immediately fatal. Less frequent causes of it are rupture of the gall-bladder, with the escape of gall-stones into the cavity of the abdomen, abscesses of the ovary, and abscesses in the walls of the urinary bladder. It is said by Murchison to have been in one case the result of a pseudo-abscess in the sheath of the rectus muscle bursting inward.

Swelling of the parotid gland occasionally occurs in typhoid fever, but is much less common than in typhus. It is most frequently met with in bad cases about the end of the third week or later, and generally involves one side only. The swelling is hard and firm in the beginning, and may terminate in resolution or suppuration. I have seen it three times only, twice in my own practice, and once in that of a medical friend. One of my cases was fatal, the other ended in recovery, as did, I believe, the third case. Murchison saw it in only 6 cases, 5 of which were fatal. According to Hoffmann,[66] 16 cases of suppurative parotitis were found at Basle among about 1600 typhoid fever patients, 7 of the 16 ending fatally. Parotitis without suppuration occurred three times. In 15 cases the attack was confined to one side, 9 times to the right and 6 to the left; in 4 it was double. Trousseau[67] looks upon these swellings as a very grave accident, and says that he has scarcely ever seen a case recover in which it has occurred, either in the course of typhoid fever or any other disease. Chomel, on the other hand, is said to have regarded them as critical and auspicious.

[66] Quoted by Liebermeister.
[67] *Clinique médicale de l'Hôtel Dieu*, t. i. 1861.

Menstruation occasionally occurs during typhoid fever, and may be profuse. Bartels,[68] who has investigated the histories of 172 patients in reference to this point, says that the catamenia always appear if the menstrual period falls within the first five days of the fever, and that they do so in two-thirds of the cases if they are expected between the sixth and fourteenth days. On the other hand, menstruation does not occur if the time for it falls in the third week. He says also that the catamenia generally appears about the time they are expected, or later, and very seldom earlier. Liebermeister, on the contrary, says that they often occur prematurely. Other uterine hemorrhages seldom occur, and never in those who have ceased to menstruate or in whom the function has not been established.

[68] *Petersb. Med. Wochenschr.*, 1881.

Suppuration of Bartholini's glands is said by Speilman to have taken place in one case.[69] In the fourth week the patient complained of violent pains in the right nympha, which, upon examination, was found to be swollen. A tumor as large as a nut, which was red and painful on pressure, could also be felt in the vagina.

[69] *Arch. générales*, Mars, 1882.

Pregnancy was formerly thought to confer an entire immunity from typhoid fever, but recent and accurate investigations have shown that if this immunity really exists, it is only relative, not absolute. Gusserow[70] says that the disease is more frequently met with in the first half than in the latter half of pregnancy. Abortion under these circumstances commonly occurs. Gusserow says that it takes place in from 60 [p. 297] to 80 per cent. of the cases. He believes it to be due to the high temperature, which causes the death of the foetus, which is then expelled from the uterus. In a few cases, however, the child is born living. Of Murchison's 14 cases, 10 recovered, and two of the ten patients carried the child, at the fourth and eighth months respectively, throughout the attack. All the others miscarried or aborted, only one of them being delivered of a living child. Out of 18 pregnant women[71] treated in the hospital of Basle for typhoid fever, between the years 1865 and 1868, 15 miscarried or aborted. In the three years following the introduction of the anti-pyretic treatment only five cases of abortion occurred, and but one of these proved fatal. This accident generally happens during the second or third week of the fever. It is always a serious complication, and if it occurs in the first three months of pregnancy it generally gives rise to profuse hemorrhage, which is usually followed by a fall of temperature as marked as that observed in hemorrhage from the intestines. Just as in the latter case, the fall is only temporary, being soon succeeded by a rapid rise of the temperature to its former height, or even beyond it.

[70] *Schmidt's Jahrbuch*, Bd. 193, No. 1, 1880, from *Berl. klin. Wochenschr.*, 1880.
[71] Liebermeister, *loc. cit.*

The danger of bed-sores occurring in typhoid fever is in consequence of the impaired nutrition of the tissues, the length of time the disease lasts, and the great emaciation which usually attends it—greater than in any other acute disease. They constitute a very serious and troublesome complication, and may occur on any part of the body subjected to pressure, but are most frequent over the sacrum and trochanters. Oedema of the lower extremities from feebleness of the circulation is occasionally observed in the convalescence from protracted attacks. Lendel has published a series of 7 cases observed at Rouen, in which the entire body became very oedematous in the second or third week of the attack or during convalescence. In none of the cases was the urine albuminous. All the patients recovered except one, who died of peritonitis. Similar cases have been reported by other observers. Barthez and Rilliet have seen several cases in children.

Periostitis is an occasional sequel. I have seen it in one case only. Sir James Paget,[72] who appears to have met with it in several cases, says that it never occurs in the continuity of the fever, but always when the patient is apparently convalescent, when his temperature is normal and constant, and he is beginning to move about and to grow stronger and stouter. Its most usual seat is the tibia, but it is also met with in the femur, ulna, and parietal bone. Except in one case, Sir James has never seen it in more than one bone in the same person. It is always circumscribed within a space of from one to three inches in extent, and usually subsides without necrosis or other abiding change of structure; but in some cases the patient has remained for some time subject to repeated attacks of pain and swelling of periosteum. In the few cases, he says, in which the periostitis is followed by necrosis the extent of dead bone has always been less than that of the inflammation over it. Murchison, however, refers to two cases of necrosis of the tibia, to one of the temporal bone, and to two in which extensive necrosis of the lower jaw occurred. Gay[73] also reports a case of extensive necrosis of the thigh-bone in a child three years old, following an attack of typhoid fever.

[72] *St. Bartholomew's Hospital Report*, vol. xxi.
[73] *Path. Trans. Lond.*, vol. xx., p. 290.

[p. 298]Very frequently after an attack of typhoid fever the patient evinces a tendency to grow stout, which is either continuous or else is gradually lost after he fully recovers his health. This increase in flesh is not always accompanied by a corresponding gain in physical strength, and he may remain for a long time after convalescence is apparently complete incapacitated for much bodily or mental exertion. Sometimes, on the other hand, the patient, instead of gaining flesh and strength, may continue weak and emaciated, even when he is taking a full amount of nourishment, which he is, however, unable to assimilate. Cases of this kind may terminate in phthisis, but they occasionally prove fatal, without any discoverable lesion after death except an abnormally smooth appearance of the mucous membrane of the ileum and a shrivelled condition of the mesenteric glands.[74]

[74] Murchison.

Patients suffering from typhoid fever may occasionally contract other specific diseases. Murchison has notes of eight cases in which the eruption of this disease coexisted with that of scarlatina, and says that it was not uncommon in the London Fever Hospital for a patient suffering from the former disease to contract the latter. Similar cases are recorded by other observers. Typhoid fever may also be complicated with rubeola, pertussis, diphtheria, variola, and vaccinia. I have repeatedly seen children convalescent from typhoid fever in the hospitals of Paris contract one or other of the eruptive fevers.

VARIETIES.—A great variety of forms of typhoid fever has been described by various authors, but as many of them present few points of difference from the usual form of the disease, it will not be necessary to discuss them at any length. They derive their names from some peculiarity of the mode of seizure, from the prominence of some one symptom or set of symptoms, or from the presence of complications. They are—(1) The adynamic form, in which prostration is marked in the beginning and throughout the attack. (2) The ataxic or nervous form, which is characterized by the predominance of delirium, subsultus tendinum, and other nervous symptoms. (3) The hemorrhagic form, in which there is a special tendency to hemorrhage from the different mucous membranes. (4) The abdominal form, in which the abdominal symptoms, such as diarrhoea and tympanites, are well developed. (5) The thoracic form, so called from the presence of some thoracic complication. (6) The gastric or bilious form, in which the disease is complicated at its commencement by gastro-intestinal catarrh. La forme muqueuse of French authors is probably identical with the above. (7) The acute form, in which the disease begins abruptly and with great violence, and runs a very rapid course, terminating usually in death before the end of the first week or early in the second, before ulceration can have taken place. Delirium is an early and prominent symptom in this form, so that it has sometimes been mistaken for meningitis.

Certain forms of the disease deserve a little fuller consideration. One of the most important of these is the abortive form, in which, as its names implies, the fever is cut short in its course, and in which there is every reason to believe that infiltration of Peyer's glands takes place as usual, but that the subsequent course of the disease is different, the glands undergoing resolution instead of advancing to ulceration. The majority [p. 299]of observers agree that in the beginning there is nothing to distinguish such attacks from those which follow their usual course. Liebermeister and Jaccoud state, however, that their commencement is usually more abrupt than in the ordinary variety, the former asserting that the temperature generally reaches its maximum earlier, and the same opinion is expressed by other authors. They are occasionally characterized by severe symptoms, including a high temperature. In the few cases which have come under my own observation the symptoms have been mild, but they were sufficiently developed to leave no doubt on the mind as to the nature of the disease. In a case which aborted on the twelfth day there were hebetude, diarrhoea, tympany, and rose-colored spots persisting even after the subsidence of the fever. Constipation would appear, however, to be more frequent than diarrhoea in this class of cases. The subsidence of the fever may occur at any time between the seventh and fourteenth days; Griesinger has seen it occur as early as the fifth day. Sometimes the defervescence occurs abruptly, with copious perspiration; at others it is gradual and similar to that which takes place in ordinary attacks. Between the abortive form of typhoid fever and simple continued fever there are, of course, many points of resemblance, but cases of the former may generally be recognized by the presence of this rose-colored eruption and enlargement of the spleen, or, where these are absent, by their occurring in the same house or under the same circumstances as typical cases of the disease.

Liebermeister has called attention in his article on typhoid fever in *Ziemssen's Cyclopædia* to a class of cases which, he thinks, is also caused by the typhoid infection, and of which the prominent feature is the insignificance of the fever or the entire absence of it which characterizes them. Such cases appear to be of frequent occurrence in Basle. Many of them, he says, never show during their entire course any rise of the temperature, or occasionally a slight elevation only, but an enlargement of the spleen could generally be detected, and occasionally an unmistakable rose-colored eruption. The action of the bowels was usually irregular; sometimes there was diarrhoea, and sometimes, on the other hand, obstinate constipation. The other symptoms were prostration, pains throughout the body, often headache, persistent loss of appetite, with more or less swollen and furred tongue, and markedly diminished frequency of the pulse, which disappears with convalescence, while its quality is not appreciably altered. The long duration of an apparently trifling indisposition he considers as especially characteristic. Cayley also refers to cases, and even epidemics, of typhoid fever in which the temperature has been below the normal throughout the whole course of the attack. Strube[75] had the opportunity of observing such an outbreak during the siege of Paris by the Germans in 1870. "In many of the cases," he says, "the temperature throughout was subnormal, and in others never exceeded the normal point. The roseola was usually profuse; the nerve symptoms were of marked severity, and were in inverse ratio to the temperature, consisting of violent delirium alternating with stupor; the duration of the fever was very short, defervescence usually taking place at the end of a fortnight. Of the 23 fatal cases, in 20 death took place during the first fourteen days. The abdominal [p. 300]symptoms were slight, but the characteristic lesions were found on post-mortem examination. All the cases were characterized by great prostration. These cases presented some features which were probably due to this peculiarity of the temperature; thus, the pulse was but little accelerated, seldom exceeding a hundred; the tongue did not become dry and brown; and the enlargement of the spleen was either absent or much less marked than usual. Strube attributed the peculiar features of this epidemic to the depressed condition of the troops; they had been exposed to great hardships on the way to Paris, over-fatigued by forced marches, and very insufficiently supplied with food."

[75] Quoted by Dr. Cayley.

A mild form of the disease has been described by certain authors, in which the symptoms, although not severe, are characteristic, and in which there is therefore, with due care, little danger of making a mistake in diagnosis. It therefore seems an unnecessary refinement to set apart such cases under a separate head.

The latent form, or the typhus ambulatorius of the Germans, is of more importance from the fact that the symptoms are so mild, or that so many of the ordinary symptoms are wanting or masked by those due to complications, that there is great danger of regarding the attack as of little moment. In many cases there is no symptom present but prostration and fever to indicate that the patient is ill, and these may be so slight that he may positively refuse to go to his bed, and may even insist upon pursuing his ordinary avocation, in the midst of which he is often suddenly seized with alarming symptoms, such as violent delirium, intestinal hemorrhage, or, what is more common, those due to perforation of the bowel. Still, even in these cases a careful examination will often disclose the presence of some symptom which had failed before to attract attention, and which will often reveal to us the true nature of the disease. I was myself the subject of such an attack nearly twenty years ago. Supposing that the excessive prostration from which I was suffering was due to overwork at a large army hospital in the neighborhood of Philadelphia, I determined to seek repose in travel and in change of scene. On the eve of doing so I fortunately sent for a medical friend, who, after a thorough investigation of my symptoms, succeeded in finding a few rose-colored spots upon my abdomen. The attack subsequently ran a mild but well-marked course. Occasionally, the symptoms due to a complication so predominate over those arising from the disease itself that they completely mask it. I have known bronchitis so severe as to divert in this way the attention of a skilful diagnostician from the primary disease. When vomiting, together with other symptoms of hepatic derangement, is especially prominent in the beginning of typhoid fever, the mistake is not infrequently made of attributing these symptoms to a "bilious attack."

TYPHO-MALARIAL FEVER.—Under this name, which was originally suggested by J. J. Woodward, Surgeon U.S.A., early in the summer of 1862, as a designation for a class of cases in which the symptoms of typhoid fever are associated with those of remittent, and which was especially common among the soldiers of the United States Army during the late Civil War, are probably included at least two distinct conditions: 1st, remittent fever, in which the disease, on account of the depressing circumstances surrounding the patient, assumes [p. 301]a typhoid form; and, 2d, typhoid fever, occurring in a patient who has also been exposed to malarial influence. This association of diseases is of course not new, or even undescribed before this name was suggested for it. Woodward thinks that he has found enough in the description of Röderer and Wagler to justify him in concluding that the epidemic which occurred at Göttingen in 1762 was really of this character. There would seem also to be no doubt from the descriptions of Dawson[76] and Davis[77] that the fever which decimated the British army in the Walcheren expedition was typhoid fever, modified by the malarial influence to which the soldiers were subjected. The latter of these authors says that the ileum and jejunum in the bodies of those who died of this disease were frequently found interspersed with tubercles, inflamed and ulcerated in different parts.

[76] *Observations on the Walcheren Diseases*, Ipswich, 1810, by G. P. Dawson.
[77] *A Scientific and Popular View of the Fever of Walcheren*, J. B. Davis, London, 1810.

In our own country the occasional association of these two diseases has also long been recognized. Drake describes it under the name of remitto-typhoid, and Dickson seems to have been perfectly familiar with it, for he says that typhoid lesions will sometimes be found in the bodies of those dead of bilious remittent. Levick recognized the presence of the symptoms of both diseases in some patients who were under his care as early as the spring of 1862, and proposed the name of miasmatic typhoid fever for this class of cases in the following June.[78] Meredith Clymer has also frequently met with cases in which the symptoms of the two diseases were coexistent.[79]

[78] *Med. and Surg. Reporter,* June 21, 1862.

[79] *The Science and Practice of Medicine,* by William Aitken, M.D., 3d Amer. ed.; with additions by Meredith Clymer, M.D., Philadelphia, 1872.

As is indicated by the name given to it, the symptoms in this form of typhoid fever are modified by the presence of malarial poisoning. The cases always manifest a decided tendency to periodicity, the evening exacerbations are more decided than in the ordinary form, the remissions are often ushered in with a profuse sweating, gastric and hepatic derangements are more marked, and headache is more severe. There is frequently less mental hebetude or dulness than in ordinary typhoid fever. In some of the cases observed by Levick[80] the symptoms were those of pernicious congestive remittent fever, such as copious serous discharges, not unlike those of Asiatic cholera, colliquative sweats, and other symptoms of exhaustion.

[80] *Amer. Journal of the Med. Sci.,* April, 1864.

TYPHOID FEVER IN CHILDREN.—It was formerly thought that infants and very young children were not often the subjects of typhoid fever, but, so far is this opinion from being correct, it is now known that they are especially liable to suffer from it. The rose-colored eruption is more often wanting in them than in adults, and the fever more apt to assume a distinctly remittent type; and hence, no doubt, the difficulty which is often experienced in diagnosticating this fever from other forms of fever in children. There is no doubt that many cases which have been described by authors under the head of infantile remittent fever are really examples of typhoid fever modified simply by the age of the patient. It may occur in infants not more than six months old, and is not infrequent in [p. 302]children of two or three years of age. Henoch,[81] who has had the opportunity of observing a large number of cases, says that the rise of temperature is commonly more abrupt in children than in adults, and that the disease generally runs its course in a shorter time. The pulse is more frequent, and may be as high as 144 in cases in which the prognosis is not grave. Dicrotism is very rare. Slowness and irregularity of the pulse, like that observed in basillar meningitis, he has never seen. The nervous symptoms are not so pronounced even when the temperature is high, and they bear no relation in severity to the height of the temperature. Diarrhoea in the cases observed by Henoch was often absent during the whole course of the attack, and the stools were often brownish or greenish instead of yellow.

[81] *Charité Ann.,* 1875.

TYPHOID FEVER OF AGED PERSONS.—The modifications which the disease undergoes when it occurs in patients advanced in life are precisely those to be expected from the diminished activity of the processes of life in them, as compared with those of younger persons. The febrile movement is generally prolonged, although of low grade, the temperature rarely rising high, and frequently during convalescence sinking below the normal. The diarrhoea is commonly not so severe, the delirium so violent, or the rose-colored eruption so often present. On the other hand, adynamic symptoms, such as excessive prostration, tremors, subsultus tendinum, and the like, are frequently prominent from the beginning of the attack.

Several authors, among whom may be mentioned Arnat,[82] Hornburger,[83]and Greenhow,[84] have described a renal form of typhoid fever. In this form the urine is blood red in color or like dark broth. It often contains albumen during the first week of this disease, usually hyaline or more or less granular casts, and occasionally red blood-discs, white cells, epithelia of kidneys and bladder, and epithelial detritus. The specific gravity is high, and the quantity is usually diminished. The prominent symptoms are pain in the region of the kidneys, oedema of face, tense and frequent pulse, great prostration, profuse epistaxis, violent delirium, and hyperpyrexia. The temperature may be 105.8°. On the other hand, the intestinal symptoms are less marked. In fatal cases the lesions of intestinal nephritis have been found at the autopsy.

[82] Thesis, *Sur la Fievre typhoide à forme renale.*

[83] *Berlin klin. Wochenschrift,* 1881.

[84] *Transactions of Clinical Society of London,* 1880.

RELAPSES.—Much difference of opinion will be found to exist among authors in regard to the frequency with which relapses occur in typhoid fever, and this difference does not appear to be due to any greater frequency of this accident in some countries than in others, since Liebermeister met with them in 8.6 per cent. of the cases treated at the hospital at Basle, while, according to other German observers quoted by him, they occur in 6.3 per cent. (Gerhardt), in 11 per cent. (Bäumler), and in 3.3 per cent. (Biermer). Murchison noted them in 80 of 2591 cases in the London Fever Hospital, or in 3 per cent., and Maclagan in 13 of 128 cases at Dundee, or in 10 per cent. about. Immermann[85] of Basle says that they occur in 15 per cent. of the cases, and that in very unfavorable years the proportion may be as high as 18 or 19 per cent. Prof. Henoch[86] observed relapses in 16 cases out of 96, or 16.6 per cent. In my own[p. 303]practice they have not been very numerous. I find that in 80 cases of which I have full notes they are recorded five times, or in 6.25 per cent., and I believe this ratio correctly represents the frequency with which they have happened in all the other cases which have come under my care. Part of this difference of opinion is unquestionably attributable to the fact that under the term relapse are sometimes included two distinct conditions: (1) Mere recrudescences of fever, which occur during the stage of defervescence or that of convalescence, and which are provoked by errors of diet, mental or bodily fatigue, or some other irritating cause. They usually last a day or two, and are entirely distinct from (2), true relapses, in which all the characteristic symptoms of the primary attack are reproduced, and which commonly occur some time after the disease has apparently run its course. There is occasionally no distinct apyretic interval between the two attacks, but in by far the greater number of instances the relapse occurs in the second or third week, or even later, after the establishment of convalescence. In 20 cases reported by W. M. Ord and Seymour Taylor[87] the relapse occurred in the third week of the disease in 1; in the fourth week in 5; in the sixth week in 3; in the seventh week in 7; in the eighth week in 3; in the ninth week in 1. James Jackson refers to a case in which the date of the relapse is not given, but in which he was able to detect the rose-colored eruption in the sixty-sixth day[88] from the commencement of the disease. In my five cases the relapse occurred on the seventh, eighth, ninth, eleventh, and twentieth day after the apparent establishment of convalescence. In these cases the duration of the relapse was 11, 13, 17, 20, and 13 days respectively. The highest temperature noted in any of the relapses was 105°, which occurred in two cases. In both of these this temperature had also occurred in the original attacks. In one of the others, however, a temperature of over 104° F. was repeatedly observed in the relapse, while in the primary attack it had never risen above 102°.

[85] *Schweiz. Corr. Bl.*, viii. 1878.

[86] *Charité Ann.*, ii. 1875.

[87] *St. Thomas's Hospital Report*, vol. ix., London, 1879.

[88] Since the above was written I have had under my care a case of typhoid fever in which a third relapse occurred nearly four months after the patient, a woman aged thirty years, was first taken ill. The following is a brief abstract of the history of this remarkable case: The original attack began about Sept. 20, 1883, was of moderate severity, and lasted between three and four weeks. Convalescence, which seems to have been nearly complete, as the patient had left her bed, was interrupted on Nov. 1st by a relapse, during which she was admitted into the Pennsylvania Hospital. This relapse was severe, and before it had entirely run its course was itself interrupted, on Nov. 17th, by an intercurrent relapse, which lasted two weeks. During these two relapses extensive bed-sores formed upon the nates, occasioning more or less irritation and consequent febrile reaction. On Jan. 11, 1884, a third relapse occurred. This relapse was accompanied by diarrhoea, rose-colored spots, tympany, dry and brown tongue, and other characteristic symptoms of typhoid fever, the diagnosis being fully concurred in by my colleague, Dr. Morris Longstreth, who saw the case with me. Convalescence was again interrupted on Feb. 13th by fever, which continued for two weeks, but which possessed none of the characters of typhoid fever, and was clearly due to imprudence on the part of the patient. The patient is now (April 25, 1884) entirely well, and will shortly be discharged from the hospital.

The onset of a relapse is usually much more abrupt than that of the original attack. It is rarely preceded by prodromata. The temperature rises more rapidly and attains its maximum earlier, which may be much greater than in the original attack. In one case under my care it reached 105° on the evening of the first day, and temperatures of 103.5° and 104° on the evening of the second day are not infrequent.

[p. 304]The rose-colored eruption appears earlier. In 38 cases investigated by Murchison with reference to this point, it appeared on the third day in 7; on the fourth in 8; on the fifth in 7; on the sixth in 2; on the seventh in 12; and at a later date in 2. In the case the history of which is given below it was detected on the second day. The delirium also comes on sooner. The relapse is usually less severe, and is of shorter duration, than the primary attack. All my cases terminated in recovery. Occasionally, however, it is much more severe. In one case in which the primary attack was so mild that the patient could scarcely be persuaded to remain in bed, the relapse was so severe that for many days it was uncertain whether the patient would recover. In another intestinal hemorrhages to an alarming extent occurred on two occasions. Moreover, of Murchison's 53 cases, 7 were fatal; in 2 of the cases death was due to perforation; in 2 to peritonitis, induced by infarction of the spleen; and in 1 to abortion; and of Ebstein's 13 cases, 3 were also fatal. Occasionally, a second, and it is said even a third, relapse is noted. In one of Da Costa's cases hemorrhage from the bowels took place during a second relapse.

FIG. 15.

Pulse.

The following histories and temperature charts illustrate the prominent peculiarities of relapses occurring in typhoid fever:

TYPHOID FEVER (with a relapse).—G—— L——, æt. 20, single, seaman, Italian, admitted March 6, 1878; April 30, 1878, left in ward. Patient is unable to speak English. The following history is obtained through an interpreter: His family history is good, and he is naturally a healthy man, never having had any serious illness—no venereal disease, no cough or rheumatism, no intermittent fever, and he has not been in the habit of drinking to excess. His vessel has been lying off Gloucester Point, and two seamen have recently been similarly affected on another vessel anchored near by. For about two weeks he has had malaise, but not until three days ago was he so ill that he was obliged to give up work. He was then taken with cough, chills followed by fever, diarrhoea, headache, and pain in the abdomen. Has had no epistaxis or vomiting.

Upon admission patient has fever, his face is flushed, his tongue coated with a brown fur in the centre, dry, fissured, and red and glossy at the tip and edges. He has hebetude and some delirium, though not very active; he is deaf. His abdomen is somewhat tense and tympanitic, and covered with very numerous rose-colored spots, which disappear momentarily on pressure; they are also distributed over thighs and chest. There seems to be no tenderness on pressure over abdomen, and there is no gurgling felt. Has moderate diarrhoea, having about three stools daily, which are light yellow in color and are loose and fetid. Urine cloudy orange red, acid, 1021. No albumen.

[p. 305]*3.7.* Ord. Ol. Terebinth. gtt. x; Acid. Muriat. dil. gtt. v every two hours, with Quinine gr. viij daily, and restricted diet.

3.8. Tongue not so dry; is better. Whiskey fl. oz. ij.

3.9. Temperature elevated. Ord. to be sponged.

3.10. Has had four stools in the last twenty-four hours. Some sonorous râles over chest posteriorly. Sponging to be repeated when temperature rises.

3.11. There is some subsultus. There are more numerous râles heard over chest posteriorly.

Ord. whiskey fl. oz. v daily; turpentine stupes to chest. His diarrhoea is better; considerable hebetude.

3.12. Tongue is not so dry, and is cleaner. The spots over his body are beginning to assume more the appearance of petechiæ. They are found everywhere on his body. Has had but one stool within the last twenty-four hours.

3.13. He is brighter; skin feels better; tongue cleaner; pulse but 80. Fewer râles heard in chest. No change in his treatment.

3.14. Spots disappearing. Two stools in last twenty-four hours, not so loose in character. Pulse dicrotic.

3.15. There is no tympany. Had one natural stool yesterday. Sudaminæ over abdomen.

3.16. Doing well. Pulse very slow.

3.17. Tongue moist and clean; no diarrhoea.

3.18. No diarrhoea; spots are still to be seen, but are fading every day.

3.20. Takes a little lemon-juice, as the gums are disposed to be a little spongy. Stop turpentine and muriatic acid.

3.25. Bowels somewhat constipated.
Ord. enema of castor oil.

3.26. Stop quinine; give whiskey fl. oz. iij only. Allowed chicken and two eggs daily.
Ord. Tr. Cinch. Co. fl. drachms ij s.t.d.

4.4. Slight chill, headache, and pain in side. Temp. 101°.

4.5. Temp. normal again; as well as before.

4.8. Has been up for a week, and steadily gaining in strength, except the slight attack on the 4th, when to-day, without his having taken any indigestible food, or indeed any reason to which it could be assigned, he was seized with a relapse, his temperature rising to 105°, but being reduced a half degree by sponging.

4.9. Spots have again appeared in great numbers, and they are very large. Last evening his temperature reached 104¾°, and was reduced to 101° by sponging.

4.10. Doing very well; spots are still making their appearance.

4.12. Diarrhoea not at all excessive.

4.15. Spots are very numerous.

4.20. Temperature nearly normal.

4.25. Doing perfectly well; up and about.

4.30. Left in ward, upon completion of my term of service.
[p. 306]

FIG. 16.

Chart of temperature in typhoid fever with relapse.—Original attack.

FIG. 17.

Chart of temperature in typhoid fever with relapse.—Relapse.

ABORTIVE ATTACK, FOLLOWED BY TYPICAL ATTACK.—Thomas Rogers, October 15, born in Philadelphia, assistant nurse. Admitted[p. 307]January 25, 1883; discharged March 26, 1883, cured. Father died of hemorrhage from the lungs; mother living and healthy. Two years ago he sustained a compound fracture of the left leg from a bale of cotton falling on him; otherwise he has always enjoyed good health. For the past three months he has been assisting the nurse in the receiving ward of this hospital. Four days before admission, without unusual exposure, he had a slight chill, and felt cold for several hours. This was followed by fever and a feeling of weakness. He also had slight headache and the bowels were constipated; no epistaxis.

Upon admission patient has a good deal of hebetude, face flushed, temperature 102°, pulse 106, tongue slightly coated, moist. Has slight pain in right lumbar region, but no distension of abdomen. Urine negative.

Ord. quinine gr. viij. daily; liq. ammon. acet. fl. drachms ij. q.q.h.

Jan. 29th. More hebetude; tongue more coated with brownish fur, red at tip; bowels continue costive; opened by an enema.

31st. Is brighter and better. One doubtful rose-colored spot seen on abdomen.

Feb. 4th. The morning temperatures for the past two days have been subnormal and the evening rise is very slight. All the symptoms also indicate the approach of convalescence.

6th. More fever; pulse weaker; functional murmur heard over heart; sudamina out over abdomen. Ord. whiskey fl. oz. ij.

8th. Some fulness of abdomen; had three loose yellowish-colored stools in the last twelve hours.

9th. A few doubtful rose spots out over abdomen and back; sudamina still abundant.

10th. More tympany; numerous rose-colored spots out over abdomen and back; slight epistaxis and bronchitis.

11th. Pulse more feeble; still slight diarrhoea. Increase whiskey to fl. oz. iv.

15th. Has a good deal of hebetude, but no headache; fewer spots; pulse weaker; temperature lower. Increase whiskey to fl. oz. vj.

17th. Temperature high again; most of the spots have disappeared; slight epistaxis and subsultus; no delirium; bowels not open for two days.

20th. Temperature falling; spots disappearing; still fulness of abdomen.

25th. Temperature has been subnormal for several days, and he is doing well; tongue cleaning. Has emaciated a good deal, and is weak.

March 1st. Is convalescent; tongue has lost its redness.

8th. Continues to improve; allowed semi-solid food.

17th. Is now quite well; has gained a good deal in flesh, and is stronger.

[p. 308]

FIG. 18.

Temperature chart of typhoid fever.—Abortive attack, followed by typical attack.

The examination of the bodies of those who have died during a relapse reveals the presence of two sets of lesions in the cicatrizing ulcers of the primary attack and the recent ulcerations of the relapse. The latter are usually less extensive, and are found to be situated at a greater distance from the lower end of the small intestine, than the former, for the reason that the Peyer's patches most remote from the ileo-cæcal valve are least apt to be affected in the primary attack.

No satisfactory explanation of these relapses has as yet been discovered.[p. 309]They occur in patients of both sexes and of all ages with about the same frequency. They have been attributed to errors of diet, mental and bodily fatigue, and the like, but, while we know that causes of this character often provoke recrudescences of fever, and can understand that they may act as exciting causes of a relapse in cases in which the predisposition exists, it does not seem possible that they should by themselves be able to bring back all the characteristic symptoms of a specific disease. It has been maintained by some authors that a relapse indicates that a new infection has taken place; but this hypothesis, even if we admit that it accounts for those cases in which the patient is allowed to remain in the place in which he has acquired the disease, does not explain those in which he is removed during the first attack to a hospital where all the sanitary arrangements are presumably perfect. Griesinger has endeavored to explain relapses occurring in hospitals by suggesting that they may possibly be due to a fresh contagion from other patients with typhoid fever in the same ward; but this explanation is rendered improbable by the fact that relapses have occurred when cases have been thoroughly isolated. As I have already said, during a long connection with the Pennsylvania Hospital I have only known a single case of typhoid fever to originate within its walls, although relapses probably occur in its wards with the same frequency as in other hospitals. To adopt Griesinger's explanation, it would therefore be necessary to assume that a patient just recovered from an attack of the disease is more susceptible to the action of its contagion than patients suffering from other disease; which seems improbable, to say the least. It has also been maintained that relapses are due to the inoculation of the previously healthy Peyer's patches by the typhoid poison which is thrown off with the sloughs from those first affected. Maclagan alleges that relapses are more frequently met with in cases in which constipation is present in the primary attack, a condition which he regards as favorable to absorption; but this is opposed to the experience of almost every one who has paid any attention to the subject. In the cases which have come under my own observation it certainly was not the case, diarrhoea having been present in all of them. It is more likely, as suggested by Liebermeister, that part of the poison remains latent somewhere in the body, not developed, destroyed, nor expelled during the first attack, but brought later into activity by some exciting cause. Da Costa adopts this view, and says that relapses of typhoid fever are not unlike the outbreaks of malarial fever which occur after worry or fatigue and when there has been no chance for a fresh infection. Different plans of treatment have at various times been charged with increasing the predisposition to relapses. This is especially true of the cold-water treatment, and the records at the hospital at Basle show that the proportion of relapses and the number of deaths from them are both increased under the use of cold water. Liebermeister thinks, however, that this does not necessarily prove that this treatment favors the occurrence of relapses, since before the introduction of this plan of treatment many more typhoid fever patients died in the first attack of the disease. Employing those cases only for statistical purposes in which the patients have survived the first attack, he finds that the difference at once disappears, there being 9 per cent. of relapses before the use of cold water, and 10.3 per cent. after its use.

[p. 310]Gerhardt[89] asserts that in cases in which relapses occur the enlargement of the spleen does not diminish during the non-febrile period that intervenes between the original attack and the relapse.

[89] *Ziemssen's Cyclopædia*, vol. i. p. 193.

Da Costa[90] has shown that the appearance of the white line and furrow left by the primary attack, to which attention has already been drawn, may sometimes be of service to us in diagnosis when we see the patient for the first time during the relapse. In a case which was recently under my care their appearance certainly rendered the nature of the previous illness from which the patient had suffered much clearer than it would otherwise have been.

[90] *Transactions of the College of Physicians of Philadelphia*, 3d S., vol. iii.

DURATION.—The mode of invasion of typhoid fever is generally so insidious, and the first symptoms so little pronounced, that the patient, even if free from mental hebetude and confusion at the time when he first comes under the care of a physician, is usually unable to fix with certainty the time of the beginning of his illness. This inability is of course most marked in what are known as walking cases, in which, notwithstanding that the disease is far advanced, the patient continues to pursue his ordinary avocations or at least refuses to go to bed. In a few cases, however, either in consequence of the violence of the first symptoms or from some other cause, opportunity is afforded to the physician of observing the disease from its onset. In many others the date of commencement may be approximately ascertained. The average duration of such cases, if uncomplicated, has been found to be between three and four weeks. According to Bartlett, the average duration of 255 cases at the Massachusetts General Hospital between the years 1824 and 1835, inclusive, was twenty-two days. It was a little less than this in patients under twenty-one years of age, and a little more in those over. As these cases occurred before the introduction into use of the clinical thermometer, and as the commencement of convalescence is fixed in them at the time when the patients were able to take a little solid food, it is possible the fever may have continued in them some time after convalescence was supposed to have been established. Of 200 cases which ended in recovery, and in which Murchison was able to ascertain with precision the date of commencement, the duration was 10 to 14 days in 7 cases, 15 to 21 days in 49 cases, 22 to 28 days in 111 cases, and 29 to 35 days in 33 cases. The mean duration of these 200 cases was 24.3 days, while that of 112 fatal cases was 27.67 days. From the same author we learn that the average stay in hospital of 500 cases which recovered was 31.24 days, and of 100 fatal cases was 16.52 days, while the average duration of the illness before admission in the 600 cases was 10.78 days. During the twenty years from Jan. 1, 1862, to Dec. 31, 1881, 621 cases of typhoid fever, 121 of which were fatal, were admitted into the Pennsylvania Hospital. No notes of many of these cases were taken, and of some of the others the notes are incomplete or inaccessible, so that they cannot, unfortunately, be used for the purpose of determining the duration of the disease. The books of the hospital, however, show the length of time each patient remained in the wards. From these we learn that the average stay of the 500 patients who recovered was 43.5 days, while that of the 121 patients who died was only 8.75 days, and that of these a large number (28) died within [p. 311]48 hours after their admission to the hospital. As a rule, patients are retained at the Pennsylvania Hospital until they are fully able to return to work, while at the English and continental hospitals it is usual to discharge them when they cease to need active treatment. This circumstance probably explains the much greater average duration of the cases admitted to the Pennsylvania Hospital than that of the cases referred to by Murchison. In the abortive form the duration of the disease may not exceed ten days, and there are authors who contend that it may occasionally be very much less.

Death may occur at almost any time in the course of typhoid fever. I have never seen it myself take place before the seventh day. Murchison reports two cases in one of which the disease terminated fatally within twenty-seven hours of its commencement, and in the other on the second day. Instances are more numerous in which death has occurred on the fourth, fifth, or sixth day, but still they are comparatively infrequent, and, as a rule, the fatal termination takes place most frequently during the course of the third week. On the other hand, death may sometimes occur at a very much later period. This is, of course, the case when it occurs during a relapse, but if the fever continues after the third week the patient may sometimes die from exhaustion or from the intercurrence of a complication. Death may also be the result of a sequela long after the disease has run its course.

DIAGNOSIS.—The insidious invasion of typhoid fever, together with the absence of pathognomonic symptoms in the beginning, always renders the diagnosis difficult, and sometimes impossible, during the first week. Still, even at this time the existence of the disease may be suspected if the frequent use of the thermometer reveals from day to day a gradual increase of the fever and the existence of evening exacerbations followed by morning remissions, the temperature rising each evening from a degree to two degrees higher than it had done the preceding evening. If in addition to this character of the pyrexia there are diarrhoea with ochrey-yellow stools or an increased susceptibility to the action of cathartic medicines, epistaxis, enlargement of the spleen, slight fulness of the abdomen, with tenderness and gurgling in the right iliac region, slight hebetude and some confusion of ideas upon awakening, the diagnosis becomes more probable. During the next week the symptoms are usually much more characteristic. The presence of marked abdominal symptoms, together with the eruption of rose-colored spots, will generally render the recognition of the disease at this time an easy matter. There are, however, a few cases in which no rose-colored spots can be found, and in which the abdominal symptoms, if they exist at all, are so little marked that they do not arrest attention. Even in these cases the temperature record, when carefully studied, will often throw a good deal of light upon the nature of the disease. If the febrile movement resembles that usual in typhoid fever, if it has continued for more than a week, if the patient has not been recently exposed to malarial influences, and presents no symptoms of local disease, the diagnosis may still be made with at least an approach to certainty.

The following are the diseases which are most likely to be mistaken for typhoid fever:

Typhus fever has a course which is so essentially different from [p. 312]that of typhoid that in well-marked cases it would scarcely be possible to mistake one for the other. Cases, however, do occur which, in consequence of a very profuse and dark-colored eruption in the latter, or of the existence of abdominal symptoms in the former, present at first a good deal of difficulty in diagnosis. The invasion of the former is more abrupt and its duration shorter than in typhoid fever. The eruption is usually also much more copious, and appears in the former as early as the fourth, fifth, or sixth day, while that of the latter is rarely observed before the seventh day. The fever in the former is much more nearly continued in type than that of the latter. Defervescence occurs in the former by crisis; in the latter, by lysis. The expression of the physiognomy is different in the two diseases. In typhus there is a uniform dusky hue of the face, with injection of the conjunctivæ and contraction of the pupils. In typhoid fever the pupils are often widely dilated, the conjunctivæ clear, and the face pallid, with the exception of a circumscribed flush on each cheek. Diarrhoea is much less frequent in the former than in the latter, and when it does occur is not accompanied by ochrey-yellow stools. Epistaxis, tympanites, pain, and gurgling in the right iliac region, and intestinal hemorrhage, common symptoms in the latter, are very infrequently met with in the former. On the other hand, petechiæ and vibices, which are of almost constant occurrence in the former, are rarely met with in the latter. The circumstances also under which the two diseases are contracted are different. Typhus originates from overcrowding or is due to direct contagion. The origin of typhoid fever is often involved in more obscurity, but it can generally be traced either to a polluted water-supply or to defective drainage.

Relapsing fever, with due care, is not likely to be confounded with typhoid fever. The abrupt commencement of the former, the high fever, lasting for from five to seven days only, and terminating by crisis with a profuse sweat, and the period of complete apyrexia of a week's duration, followed by the relapse in which the temperature rises even higher than in the primary paroxysm, and which also terminates by crisis, form a chain of symptoms which has no counterpart in the latter. The mind in relapsing fever is usually clear, there being none of the hebetude and mental confusion commonly observed in typhoid fever. The rose-colored eruption is, moreover, wanting, and diarrhoea and tympanites are absent. On the other hand, jaundice and tenderness in the epigastric zone are more common than in typhoid fever.

Influenza sometimes, Murchison says, when epidemic, closely simulates typhoid fever, but as the two diseases occur in this country the resemblance between them is not often sufficiently strong to lead the careful observer astray. In both there are fever, prostration, sleeplessness, delirium and sweating, and occasionally deafness, diarrhoea, epistaxis, and a dry red tongue; but the onset of the attack in the former is more abrupt, its duration shorter, and subsequent convalescence more rapid than in typhoid fever. The prostration, too, is more decided in proportion to the degree of fever present. Coryza and bronchial catarrh are much more marked symptoms in the former than in the latter, while hyperæsthesia of the surface, which is present in almost every case of influenza, is only rarely met with in typhoid fever.

Remittent and typhoid fevers often prevail together in the malarious[p. 313]districts of this country, and, as they present many points of resemblance, they are sometimes with difficulty distinguished from each other. They both may begin with nausea and vomiting; abdominal and cerebral symptoms are common to both, and so is enlargement of the spleen. The typhoid state may supervene in either, and in both the febrile movement is remittent in character. In remittent fever, however, the remissions are more marked, and are usually accompanied with more profuse sweating, than in typhoid fever. Jaundice and other symptoms of hepatic derangement are also more common, and the pains in the back and limbs are more frequent and more severe. The effect, too, of quinine in producing a permanent reduction of the temperature, is generally more decided. On the other hand, the rose-colored eruption of typhoid fever is never present in pure remittent fever. Occasionally, in cases of the variety of typhoid fever known as typho-malarial fever, the symptoms of the latter may be so prominent as entirely to mask those of the former. In such cases the discovery of a few rose-colored spots somewhere on the surface will clearly reveal the true nature of the disease.

Epidemic cerebro-spinal meningitis differs from typhoid fever by its more abrupt invasion, by the retraction of the head which rapidly supervenes, and by the appearance a short time afterward upon different parts of the body of petechiæ, which are not likely, even at first, to be mistaken for the rose-colored spots of typhoid fever. The fever has, moreover, no constant character, but is remarkable, on the contrary, for its great irregularity. The duration of the disease is in fatal cases much shorter, death taking place not infrequently within the first week, and occasionally as early as the second or third day. On the other hand, the duration in cases which recover may be even longer than in typhoid fever.

Simple continued fever may readily be mistaken in the beginning for typhoid fever, especially in those cases complicated by diarrhoea, but, as a general rule, the different character of the febrile movement, its more abrupt commencement and termination, and its shorter duration, together with the absence of the rose-colored eruption, will usually serve to distinguish it.

The eruptive fevers are always readily distinguishable at the period of invasion from typhoid fever, and the mistake of confounding them with the latter disease may generally be avoided by a close study of the character of the pyrexia. In the eruptive fevers the temperature rises abruptly, frequently attaining its maximum in the course of twenty-four hours, and sometimes in very much less time. There are also in all of them early symptoms which indicate pretty clearly their true nature, as, for instance, the sore throat of scarlatina, the naso-pulmonary catarrh of measles, and the rachialgia of small-pox. The uncertainty, moreover, is of short duration, as the characteristic eruption appears in all of them before the fourth day.

Acute tuberculosis of the lungs is the condition which in my experience has been the most difficult to distinguish from typhoid fever. Indeed, in some cases which have come under my observation physicians of recognized skill as diagnosticians have been unable to make the discrimination until after the death of the patient. Muscular prostration, a dry brown tongue, delirium, stupor, bronchitic râles, dyspnoea, and even cyanosis, are symptoms frequently met with in both diseases, so that when the [p. 314]rose-colored eruption and enlargement of the spleen happen to be wanting in typhoid fever, or diarrhoea and tympany present in acute tuberculosis, as they may be, the distinction is often impossible. The diagnosis may, however, even in these cases, be sometimes made after a careful study of the temperature range, which in acute tuberculosis is irregular and rarely presents any resemblance to that which is typical of typhoid fever.

Acute tubercular meningitis has also many symptoms in common with typhoid fever, such as high fever, headache, vomiting, delirium, and stupor, but in the former disease the rose-colored eruption, epistaxis, enlargement of the spleen, and intestinal hemorrhage do not occur. Diarrhoea is also rare, and the abdomen, instead of being tympanitic, is flat, and in many cases even scaphoid. The headache, too, is much more acute than in typhoid fever, and is very apt to be associated with retraction of the head. Here, again, the frequent use of the thermometer will yield very important results in diagnosis, as the temperature range in tubercular meningitis is always irregular and does not present any resemblance to that usually observed in typhoid fever.

Several of the inflammations, especially when associated with the typhoid state, have so many symptoms in common with typhoid fever that they may very readily be mistaken for one another by a careless observer. I have known, for instance, the general disease to be entirely overlooked in a case of typhoid fever complicated by pneumonia, and, on the other hand, it has sometimes been supposed to be present in a case of pure typhoid pneumonia. Gastro-enteritis is another disease which is also occasionally confounded with typhoid fever. The diagnosis in these cases will rest principally upon the presence or absence of epistaxis, enlargement of the spleen, tympanites, the rose-colored eruption, and of a temperature range presenting some similarity to that usual in typhoid fever.

Trichiniasis is not likely to give rise to much difficulty in diagnosis, for although vomiting, diarrhoea, and the typhoid state occur in it as well as in typhoid fever, the former disease may usually be recognized by the severe muscular pains and the local oedema which are constant accompaniments of it, and by the absence of the characteristic symptoms of the latter.

PROGNOSIS.—There is no other disease in which the physician should be more careful in making a positive prognosis than in typhoid fever. On the one hand, accidents of a fatal character frequently occur in cases which are apparently progressing favorably, and, on the other, recovery has often taken place after all hope of it had been abandoned. But, although it is impossible to foretell with absolute certainty the result in any particular case, there are certain symptoms which furnish very important indications for prognosis, and the proper appreciation of which will generally enable us to arrive at a correct conclusion as regards the gravity of the disease. Prominent among these is the character of the pyrexia. A fever characterized by high temperature should always give occasion for great anxiety. This is very fully shown by the statistics of the hospital at Basle. Thus of those patients in whom the temperature did not reach 104°, only 9.6 per cent. died; of those in which it reached or exceeded 104°, 29.1 per cent. died; and, finally, of those in whose axilla the temperature rose to or above 105.8°, more than half died. [p. 315]Wunderlich has arrived at very nearly the same conclusions, for he says that the prognosis is very unfavorable when the temperature rises to 106.16°, that the deaths are almost twice as numerous as the recoveries when it rises to 107.06°, and that recoveries are rare when it rises to 107.24°. Murchison has, however, known recovery to follow a temperature of 108°. The highest temperature recorded in any of my cases was 106° F. In this case, which proved fatal, the temperature reached 105° F. five times. In three other cases, in all of which recovery took place, a temperature of 105.5° F. was observed. In twelve cases the temperature reached 105° F. on more than one occasion. Six of these ended fatally; in the others the patients recovered.

The prognosis is more unfavorable in a fever in which the temperature is continuously high, and in which the morning remissions are slight or wanting, than in one in which the daily fluctuations are greater, even though the temperature may reach a higher point during the evening exacerbations in the latter variety than is attained at any time in the former. Occasional remissions, even if produced by quinia or other remedies, are to be regarded as favorable omens, as they indicate that the fever tends to subside. A high morning temperature ought, therefore, to give rise to more alarm than a high evening temperature. The prognosis is grave when the morning temperature rises to 104° or is persistently above 103°. Murchison says that recovery is rare after a morning temperature of 105°. Fiedler[91] saw, with a single exception, all patients die whose temperature in the morning rose to or exceeded 106.25°, while of those whose temperature in the morning rose to 105.44°, if only on one day, more than half died. Any marked deviation from the usual temperature range in the course of the fever is unfavorable. A rapid rise of temperature indicates increased danger: it may be due to the occurrence of a complication or of some other cause acting unfavorably upon the patient. A sudden and decided fall should excite even more alarm, as it is generally the consequence of a free intestinal hemorrhage. A temporary abatement of the fever, with amelioration of the other symptoms, occurring between the tenth and twentieth days, and giving rise to the hope that convalescence is about to commence, but followed by a return of the symptoms in an aggravated form, is also unfavorable. Such cases, according to Chomel, Louis, Bartlett, and Murchison, almost invariably terminate fatally.

[91] Quoted by Liebermeister.

The prognosis is bad in cases in which coma or wild or violent delirium comes on early. A moderate amount of delirium, especially when it occurs only at night or upon wakening in the morning, and is readily dissipated by attracting the patient's attention, or stupor which disappears when he is thoroughly roused, is not unfavorable. Insomnia, subsultus tendinum, carphologia, slipping down in bed, incontinence of the urine or feces, and retention of urine, are all symptoms of bad omen. Rigidity of the limbs is also a bad symptom; Dr. Jackson reports six cases in which this symptom occurred, only one of which recovered. Excessive subsultus is especially unfavorable, as it is generally most marked in cases in which the ulcerations of the intestines are most extensive. Extreme deafness occurs in mild as well as severe cases; it is therefore without significance in prognosis.

[p. 316]In estimating the importance, in a prognostic point of view, of these various nervous symptoms, it is important to bear in mind that a degree of fever which produces no disturbance of the mental functions in a phlegmatic person will give rise to active delirium and other marked cerebral symptoms in a person of an excitable temperament.

A change in the character of the pulse and of the action of the heart is often the earliest indication of the approach of danger in typhoid fever, and both pulse and heart should therefore be carefully examined at every visit. The first change is usually a diminution in the intensity of the first sound of the heart. This is significant, as it is frequently the earliest premonition of cardiac failure, to which a large proportion of the deaths in typhoid fever is due. A pulse of 120 and over, especially if it is at the same time feeble, is also unfavorable. The important part which the frequency of the pulse plays in the prognosis is shown by the following observations made by Liebermeister at the hospital in Basle: Of 63 cases in which the pulse rose to or above 120, 40 were fatal, or nearly two-thirds. Among these 63 were 37 in which it did not rise to 140; of these, 19 were fatal, or about one-half; in 26 it rose above 140; of these, 21, or about four-fifths, were fatal. In 12 patients it rose above 150; of these, 11 died. Of those in which the pulse rose to 160, the only case that ended in recovery was that of a girl twenty-one years old suffering from an imperfectly developed typhoid. Intermittence of the pulse is unfavorable, especially, according to Hayem,[92] when it occurs during the first week of the disease. In convalescence intermittence is not to be regarded as an unfavorable symptom. The prognosis is bad also in those cases in which, with excessive weakness of the pulse, there are other evidences of cardiac failure, as, for instance, congestion of the lungs, cyanosis of the surface, coldness of the extremities. A very frequent pulse is not so unfavorable in a child as in an adult, or in a person of a nervous temperament as in one of a different disposition.

[92] *Loc. cit.*

Other unfavorable symptoms are a dry, brown tongue, excessive tympanites with great abdominal tenderness, severe diarrhoea, vomiting when it occurs late in the disease, intestinal hemorrhage, and colliquative sweats. The delusion sometimes observed in very severe cases, in which the patient declares that he is not ill, is a very bad sign, many authors, and among them Louis, asserting that they have never known recovery to take place after it has been manifested. Peritonitis is a very serious complication, whether due to perforation or to some other cause. Still, it would appear not to be invariably fatal, since recovery has occurred in cases in which all the symptoms of this complication were present.

Favorable symptoms, on the other hand, are a gradual decrease of the temperature with increasing morning remissions, moistening and cleansing of the tongue, a lessening of the delirium, and other nervous symptoms, reappearance of an intelligent expression, recognition by the patient of friends and attendants, and a diminution of the diarrhoea. A copious eruption is also regarded by many as a favorable symptom. Cases in which constipation exists generally do well. Nathan Smith never knew a patient to die whose bowels were constipated throughout the attack.

The death-rate of typhoid fever is found to vary very considerably in different years and in the different seasons of the year, as will be seen [p. 317] from the two following tables. Statistics as to the mortality of the disease to be reliable must therefore be based upon a large number of cases extending over a series of years.

The following table shows the number of cases admitted into the Pennsylvania Hospital during each of the twenty years ending Dec. 31, 1881, and the ratio of mortality among them:

TABLE NO. 1.

YEAR.	Number of cases.	Number of recoveries.	Number of deaths.	Number of deaths within 48 hours of admission.	Average stay in cases ending in recovery.	Average stay in fatal cases.	Percentage of deaths.	Percentage of deaths after deducting cases fatal within 48 hours of admission.
	8	68	2	7	5	8	23.	17.

862	9		1		4¹/3		6	7
863	36	33	3	2	2¹/5³	3¹/3	8.3	2.9
864	43	35	8	1	8¹/2³	8	18.6	16.3
865	36	31	5	1	8¹/2³	5¹/2	13.9	11.4
866	23	17	6	0	5²/3⁴	9	26.0	
867	24	20	4	0	7¹/3³	6¹/2	16.6	
868	27	23	4	0	4³/4⁴	10	14.8	
869	21	16	5	1	5¹/2³	14	23.8	20.0
870	24	19	5	1	7¹/2⁴	11	20.8	17.4
871	32	26	6	1	7³/4³	3¹/2¹	18.8	15.0
872	21	16	5	3	7¹/2³	¹/2⁴	23.8	11.1
873	12	8	4	2	4³	9	33.3	20.0
874	16	12	4	0	4¹/2⁵	³/4⁹	25.0	
875	20	18	2	1	8⁴	¹/2⁴	10.0	5.3
876	30	21	9	2	5¹/2⁴	1¹	30.0	25.0
877	48	34	14	4	8¹/2⁴	2¹/2¹	29.2	22.7
878	8	5	3	0	9⁴	2/3⁵	37.5	
879	17	15	2	0	3¹/3⁵	8	11.8	
880	40	35	5	2	7⁴	0¹/2¹	12.5	8.0
Totals,	621	500	121	28	3¹/2⁴	³/4⁸	19.5	15.7

Out of the 621 cases admitted, 121 were fatal. This gives a death-rate of 19.5 per cent.; but if we deduct the 28 cases in which the patients died within forty-eight hours of their admission, it falls to 15.68 per cent., or about the same ratio as Murchison found to exist among the cases treated at the London Fever Hospital. Other observers have obtained slightly different results. Thus, the mortality was 11.16 per cent. in 197 cases analyzed by Dr. Hale, and 13.5 per cent. in 303 cases collected by Dr. James Jackson. Dr. Cayley[93] found the death-rate of the several hospitals in London to be 17.8 per cent., and Geissler[94] that it was in all the German hospitals 12.8 per cent. in 1877, and 13.5 per cent. in 1878. Flint had 18 deaths in 73 cases, or 24.4 per cent. According to Liebermeister, the ratio of mortality at the hospital at Basle during the twenty-two years from 1843 to 1864, or before the introduction of a [p. 318]systematic anti-pyretic treatment, was 27.3 per cent., and only 8.2 per cent. during the six years immediately following its adoption. As the results obtained at the Pennsylvania Hospital are apparently not so favorable as those reported at some of the continental hospitals, it is only proper to state that a large proportion of the cases were severe, that many of them were far advanced in the disease when admitted, and that very few of the patients were under twenty-one years of age. These are all circumstances which influence very decidedly the prognosis in typhoid fever. In no other city are the laboring classes able to surround themselves with so many comforts as in Philadelphia. This fact, fortunate as it is in the main, often operates to the disadvantage of the patient by enabling his family to indulge for a time the reluctance which it naturally feels to part with a member when sick. In the case of the young this reluctance is so hard to overcome that children with acute affections are rarely brought to hospitals for treatment. There were also special causes for the large mortality in certain years. This was particularly the case in 1862, when a large number of soldiers fresh from the battlefields of Virginia, and suffering from the typho-malarial form of the disease, were admitted into the hospital. Many of them were moribund upon admission, and others, exhausted by the fatigue incident to transportation here and by previous hardships, soon succumbed to the disease.

[93] *Med. Times and Gaz.*, 1880.

[94] *Schmidt's Jahrbuch.*

Table 2 gives the number of cases, with the number of deaths occurring in each season, at the Pennsylvania Hospital during the last twenty years:

TABLE NO. 2.

	Spring.	Summer.	Autumn.	Winter.
Number of cases	89	259	182	91
Recoveries	73	191	163	73
Deaths	16	68	19	18
Percentage of mortality	18.0	26.2	10.4	19.8

It will be seen from this table that the highest death-rate occurred in the summer and the lowest in autumn, while there was only a slight difference between the death-rate of spring and that of winter. Murchison's experience, based on a much larger number of cases, has led him to conclude that while the disease is a little less fatal in autumn, the difference in the mortality at different seasons is very inconsiderable. Chomel believed that the percentage of deaths was highest in France during the winter months, and Bartlett held the same opinion as regards America. Epidemics of great severity have undoubtedly prevailed in winter, as the in Lowell, Mass., referred to by Bartlett, but there can be little doubt that the death-rate is highest in this country during the warm months of the year. Dr. Cleemann[95] found that the monthly average mortality in Philadelphia for the ten years from 1866 to 1875 was highest in August, and next highest in September, confessedly the two months of the year when the heat in this city is most exhausting. I feel very sure I have lost patients with typhoid fever in these months [p. 319]and in July who would probably have recovered if the weather had been cooler. With a temperature often rising above 90° F. at midday, and sometimes for several days at a time never falling below 80°, all radiation of heat from the surface of the body is arrested, and death frequently occurs as the result of hyperpyrexia.

[95] *Transactions of the College of Physicians of Philadelphia*, 3d S., vols. ii. and iii.

The stage of the disease at which efficient treatment is begun has a manifest influence upon the result. This is strikingly shown by some observations of Jackson: 90 cases were admitted into the Massachusetts General Hospital during the first week—of these 7 died, or 1 in 12.85; 139 cases were admitted in the second week—of these 16 died, or 1 in 8.68; 46 cases were admitted in the third week—of these 10 died, or 1 in 4.60; and 21 cases were admitted in the fourth week, and of these 5 died, or 1 in 4.20. Convalescence also occurred much earlier in those who were admitted early.

Murchison found that in a large number of cases the death-rate varied at different ages as follows: Under ten years it was 11.36 per cent.; from ten to fourteen years it was 12.86 per cent.; from fifteen to nineteen years it was 15.48 per cent.; from twenty to twenty-nine years it was 20.46 per cent.; from thirty to thirty-nine years it was 25.90 per cent.; from forty to forty-nine years it was 25 per cent.; and above fifty years it was 34.94 per cent.

According to Liebermeister, among the 1743 patients treated for typhoid fever in the hospital at Basle from 1865 to 1870, inclusive, there were 130 who were more than forty years old; of these 39, or 30 per cent., died, while the mortality among the patients under forty amounted only to 11.8 per cent. Among the cases of typhoid fever in individuals over forty years of age collected by Uhle, more than half proved fatal. According to Friedrich,[96] there were, among 16,084 children treated in the Children's Hospital at Dresden, 275 cases of typhoid fever, of which 31, or not quite 11 per cent., proved fatal. Age, therefore, exercises a positive influence upon the mortality of typhoid fever. Its influence is less decided in this disease than in typhus, in which the death-rate does not reach 4 per cent. until after the age of twenty, when it rapidly rises from 12.34 per cent. until it reaches 57.03 per cent. in patients above fifty years of age. The comparatively slight mortality of typhoid fever among children is probably due to the fact that the temperature is less often continuously high in them than in adults, and that while hyperpyrexia is frequently present, it is generally better borne and less likely to produce paralysis of the heart. Liebermeister says that the only case which he has seen recover after the temperature had repeatedly risen to 107.5° F. was that of a girl fourteen years of age. It is also said that the intestinal lesions are not so severe, and the liability to complications and sequelæ less marked, in children.

[96] Quoted by Liebermeister.

Typhoid fever appears to be a slightly more fatal disease in women than in men, for while in some local epidemics the percentage of deaths is greater among the latter than among the former, the reverse is found to be the case when the records of a large hospital for a number of years are carefully examined. According to Murchison, the mortality at the London Fever Hospital was about 1 per cent. higher among the female than among the male patients, and about the same difference in the death-rate [p. 320]of the two sexes has been reported by continental physicians. A greater disparity even than this has been observed by Liebermeister at the hospital at Basle, where the death-rate for women was 14.8 per cent., and only 12 per cent. for men. Murchison says that this excess of mortality among the former cannot be accounted for by the influence of child-bearing upon the course of the fever, since it is much more decided between the ages of five and fifteen than in the period of child-bearing.

The rich are not only as liable to contract typhoid fever as the poor, but the disease is also quite as fatal among them. Murchison found from the statistics of the London Fever Hospital that the mortality is not greater among the destitute than among the better class of patients, and expresses the opinion that in private practice enteric fever is probably more fatal among the upper classes than among the very poor. Chomel and Forget seem to have reached a similar conclusion.

All authors agree that the prognosis is unfavorable in corpulent persons, not only on account of the diminished power of resistance to disease generally which such persons exhibit, but also because the febrile movement is often intense in them, and the degenerative changes of the muscles and organs of the body which it induces are generally early developed and of high grade. Liebermeister goes so far as to say that even in the case of ill-nourished, anæmic, or chlorotic individuals the chances for life are better than in the corpulent. Murchison has also expressed the opinion that a large, muscular development is likewise an unfavorable element in prognosis, having seen the strong and robust succumb to the disease oftener than the feeble. The mortality from the disease appears to be greater in certain families than in others. This has been ascribed by some writers to peculiarities of constitution, but it may be due to other causes, as, for instance, difference in the intensity of the poison. The disease is also often very fatal among the intemperate, who usually bear the disease badly in consequence of the presence of various degenerations of one or more of the important organs of the body caused by the excessive indulgence in alcoholic stimulants; paralysis of the heart being not an infrequent cause of death among them.

Certain epidemics have been exceedingly fatal, while in others the percentage of deaths has been very small. There can be no doubt that in most of these cases there has been a difference in the virulence of the poison. Recent residence in an infected locality has been shown by Murchison and other writers to have a decided influence in increasing the fatality of the disease. Second attacks are, on the other hand, usually mild. Some diversity of opinion exists among authors in regard to the effect that pregnancy has upon the course of the disease. Murchison believes that it is a far less formidable complication than is usually thought, while Liebermeister, on the contrary, holds a directly opposite opinion. He also regards the prognosis as unfavorable when the disease occurs in childbed or a short time afterward. Individuals with disease of the heart, emphysema, or bronchial catarrh who contract typhoid fever are said to be more liable to paralysis of the heart than others, hence the existence of these diseases materially diminishes their chances of recovery.

TREATMENT.—Inasmuch as the spread and propagation of typhoid fever may be prevented to a great extent, if not entirely, by the [p. 321]employment of judicious sanitary measures, it is proper, before entering upon the discussion of its curative treatment, to devote a few words to the prophylaxis of the disease.

Whether the physician accepts the theory so ably advocated by Murchison, that typhoid fever may arise from exposure to the products of the fermentation of healthy feces, or adopts the view now held by a large number of investigators, that the disease is never generated in the absence of the specific germ, he will admit the great importance of an efficient system of sewerage, with a thorough flushing of the sewers at regular and frequent intervals, for disposing of the fecal discharges of the population of all towns, no matter how inconsiderable in size. No less important is it that the drains of every dwelling should be well constructed and kept in good order. They should be trapped just before they empty into the sewer, and should be provided with the means of thorough ventilation between the trap and the walls of the house by a free communication with the outer air. The soil-pipe should be carried up three or four feet above the top of the house, and every water-closet, bath-tub, stationary washstand, and sink should have its own separate trap, and none of them should be placed in rooms unprovided with a window or with some other sufficient means of ventilation. Physicians should, as sanitarians, urge upon the authorities of all cities and towns the importance of deriving their water-supply from a source unpolluted by sewerage or by any other substances likely to be deleterious to health. They should also see that when water is stored in a tank inside of a house the overflow pipe does not communicate directly with the drain, since if this is allowed to occur the water may very soon become contaminated with sewer gas, and consequently unfit for internal use.

In the case of isolated country-houses and of small villages some other means of disposing of the fecal discharges of the inhabitants than by sewers has to be found. In the great majority of instances no better way presents itself than by the ordinary cesspool. Care should, however, be taken that this is so constructed and situated that there can be no filtration of its contents into wells from which water for drinking is obtained.

As the alvine dejections of the sick are beyond question the medium by which typhoid fever is most frequently communicated to others, the importance of thoroughly disinfecting them before they have acquired the power of imparting the disease cannot well be overestimated. Liebermeister recommends that the bottom of the bed-pan should be strewed, each time before being used, with a layer of sulphate of iron, and that immediately after a passage crude muriatic acid should be poured over the fecal mass, as much as one-third or one-half of the bulk of the latter being used. He also urges, whenever it is practicable, that the contents of the bed-pan should be emptied into trenches dug anew every two days and filled up when discarded, care being of course taken that they are not located anywhere in the vicinity of wells. Murchison seems to prefer carbolic acid to other chemical agents as a means of preventing fecal fermentation. For this purpose the liquid carbolic acid may be diluted with water in the proportion of 1 to 40 to 1 to 20, or it may be mixed with sand or sawdust. I have myself employed as a disinfectant with success the solution of the chlorides sold under the name of Platt's chlorides. As the discharges must in cities, in the great majority of instances, be emptied into [p. 322]water-closets, these should be freely flushed with water after every time they are used; and it is well to impress upon the attendant on the sick the importance of doing this. The bed-linen of the patient and his clothes, if they are soiled by his discharges, should be removed as soon as possible, and subjected to a high degree of heat (248° F.) or soaked in a solution of the chlorides or of carbolic acid for several hours before being washed. If these precautions are observed, cases of typhoid fever may be treated in the wards of general hospitals without danger to the other patients.

In the doubt and obscurity which generally envelop the diagnosis of the disease when the physician is first called upon to treat it, it is impossible to lay down any positive rules for the management of typhoid fever at its commencement. But even in those cases which begin insidiously, if the patient is carefully examined enough of the early symptoms of typhoid fever will be detected to put the physician on his guard. The thermometer will show the existence of fever, which has a tendency to increase at night. There will generally be found to be a little diarrhoea, or at least an increased susceptibility to the action of purgative medicines; perhaps a little tympany and tenderness in the right iliac fossa, and moreover a prostration which is out of all proportion to the other symptoms.

These symptoms, it is true, are not infrequent concomitants of many diseases besides the one under consideration; but when their presence cannot be otherwise satisfactorily explained, especially if they have continued for several days, it is a safe rule in practice to regard the case as one of typhoid fever, and to regulate the treatment accordingly. The patient must be put to bed at once, and not allowed to leave it on any pretext, not even to empty his bladder, after the first week. This is a rule which should be rigidly enforced in every case, no matter how mild the symptoms may be. Its non-observance, either through the neglect of the physician or the ignorance or wilfulness of the patient, has been the cause of some disastrous results; in illustration of which it is only necessary to refer to the frequency with which perforation of the bowel occurs in walking cases of typhoid fever. Perfect quiet should be maintained in the sick room. Visitors should be excluded from it, and the attendants limited in number to those actually necessary to carry out the directions of the physician. All unnecessary talking is to be avoided, and especially conversation carried on in a low tone of voice, which is always annoying to the sick.

There is only one condition under which I should be disposed to break the rule of absolute quiet and rest laid down above, and that is when called upon to treat typhoid fever in the built-up portion of our large cities during the summer season. If the patient were still in the first week of the disease, if his circumstances were sufficiently affluent to enable him to surround himself with every comfort, and if it did not involve a journey of more than a few hours, I should unhesitatingly send him to the sea-coast. I have so often seen cases prove fatal in summer in consequence of the great heat of the city—a heat, too, which is sometimes almost as great at night as in the day-time—that I should feel that I was giving him an additional chance of life by sending him where the heat was, at least occasionally, tempered by cool breezes from the ocean. During the late war numbers of soldiers were frequently sent in the early stages of[p. 323]typhoid fever from the camps in the South to their homes or hospitals in the North, and it is fair to say that they did at least as well as those who remained behind. But when the journey may be accomplished by means of

Pullman cars and the other appliances of modern travel the risk, and even discomfort, it involves to the patient is reduced to the minimum.

As the disease is usually one of long duration, the patient being rarely able to leave his bed under four weeks, and more frequently being obliged to keep it for a much longer time, the sick room should, wherever practicable, be large, airy, and provided with an open fireplace, which is a much more efficient means of securing thorough ventilation than an open window, while it is not liable to the objection sometimes applicable to the latter of causing a direct draught upon the patient. It is well, however, for the physician to remember that the danger from this source is very much exaggerated by the laity, and that patients in the febrile stage of typhoid fever do not readily take cold. Still, the same end may generally be attained without the least risk to the patient by opening a window in an adjoining room. The temperature of the sick room should be steadily maintained at between 65° and 68° F.

The careful regulation of the diet is also a point of great importance in the management of typhoid fever; for in this disease there are not merely the high fever and other exhausting symptoms, speedily inducing excessive prostration, loss of strength, and emaciation, common to many fevers, but there is also the peculiar ulceration of the bowels, which gives rise to danger of its own and demands special consideration in treatment. The food must therefore be not only nourishing, but also readily digestible, and not likely to create irritation in its passage through the intestines. All solid food should therefore be excluded from the dietary of the patient as long as the fever lasts. Indeed, it is better to continue this prohibition even after the subsidence of the fever if rose-colored spots are still to be seen on the abdomen or elsewhere, or if there exists a tendency to diarrhoea or any other symptom indicating that the disease has not fully run its course. Having myself seen some rather disastrous results from a too early return to solid food, I have been accustomed in my own practice to interdict its use until at least two weeks after the beginning of convalescence. Jaccoud also lays much stress upon this point, saying that the early administration of meat always gives rise to fever, to which, from its cause, he gives the name of febris carnis. On the other hand, Flint[97] and Peabody have recently advocated the giving of solid food immediately after the cessation of fever, in the belief that recovery is thereby promoted. Milk as an article of diet is unquestionably to be preferred to all others in typhoid fever. It is open, it is true, to the objection of occasionally forming tough curds in the stomach, but this may generally be prevented by giving the milk in small quantities at a time, diluted with lime-water or barley-water or mixed with some farinaceous substance. No positive general rule can be laid down as to the amount to be given. This will be found to vary not only in different cases, but also in the same case at different times. Indeed, in those cases which begin abruptly with symptoms of gastro-intestinal irritation, if it is forced upon the patient in large quantities it is not only usually rejected, but also causes an aggravation of the symptoms, while after [p. 324]this irritation is allayed it will be digested without difficulty. As a general rule, most adult patients will be able to take from a quart and a half to two quarts of milk daily, given in quantities of from four to six ounces every two or three hours. It should be remembered, however, that if more is taken than can be assimilated it will act as an irritant and increase the diarrhoea. If, therefore, the stools contain undigested milk, the quantity should be diminished. Patients are occasionally met with, but not in as great number as is often asserted, with whom milk habitually disagrees. In these cases it must of course be replaced in whole or in part by some other article of food. Under these circumstances some one of the liquid preparations of beef may be given with advantage, although it may be objected to them also that they sometimes occasion an increase of diarrhoea. Beef-tea or beef-essence, made from the fresh meat whenever this can be obtained, is to be preferred to all others; but when it cannot, that made from the preparations of Johnston or Brand is the best substitute. When the stomach is very irritable, Valentine's meat-juice, in consequence of the smaller bulk in which it is given, often answers an admirable purpose.

[97] *Medical News*, Mch. 29 and Apl. 5, 1884.

Various farinaceous substances, such as farina, corn-starch, and arrowroot, are also occasionally given in typhoid fever, and, although the last named would seem to be indicated in cases in which diarrhoea is a prominent symptom, their tendency to cause flatulence is so great that their use in the acute stage of the fever has not found favor among physicians generally. In convalescence, on the other hand, they are generally perfectly well borne.

The subject of the administration of alcoholic stimulants in typhoid fever may be conveniently considered in this connection. Some difference of opinion exists in regard to the quantity in which they should be given, and indeed in regard to the necessity for their use at all in many cases, as, for instance, in those of young persons whose health and habits had been good previously to the attack. I have myself treated several such cases without alcohol, and have not been able to perceive that their duration was longer and the result less favorable than in cases in which it was given in the usual amount. It is, moreover, not necessary to prescribe it always, even in very severe cases, at the beginning of an attack. When given at this time, it not infrequently does harm by increasing the fever. It should be reserved, therefore, until the action of the heart grows feeble and the first sound becomes indistinct. It is not possible to lay down any general rule as to the amount to be given, even in severe attacks. This will vary in different cases, and to a certain extent will be determined by the effects it produces. If the pulse grows stronger and the delirium diminishes under its use, it is doing good and should be continued; if, on the other hand, there is increase of delirium and restlessness, the quantity should be diminished.

In cases in which only a gentle stimulus is required wine in the form of wine-whey will often be found to meet the indication fully. Generally, however, it will be necessary to have recourse to whiskey or brandy. The choice between these may usually be left to the patient's fancy; brandy is, however, to be preferred in cases in which diarrhoea is a prominent symptom. These stimulants should be given in small quantities frequently repeated. In many cases a dessertspoonful every two or three hours, [p. 325]either diluted with water or, when the stomach is irritable, with carbonic acid water or given in the form of milk punch, will be sufficient. In others a tablespoonful every two hours, or even at shorter intervals, will be required, but it will rarely be necessary to exceed eight ounces a day for more than a few days at a time.

Although the physician will not often be called upon at the present day to encounter and combat the prejudice so common formerly against the free administration of water in the febrile condition, he will frequently find nurses and others not sufficiently alive to the importance of supplying it when the patient, having fallen into the typhoid state, ceases to ask for it. The high temperature which is generally present in this condition, and the rapid combustion of tissue which it causes, make a full supply of liquid an urgent necessity which it is dangerous to disregard. Water is the best of all diuretics, and it is important in this disease, as indeed it is in many others, that the functions of the kidneys should be kept active, so that the products of the combustion of the tissues may be eliminated with their secretion. Care, however, should of course be taken, as pointed out by Da Costa,[98] that water is not given in such quantity that the desire for and capability of digesting food is destroyed by it.

[98] Preface to Wilson's *Treatise on the Continued Fevers*.

In the few cases which begin abruptly with symptoms simulating those of a so-called bilious attack the practitioner will usually content himself with the administration of medicines calculated to allay the irritability of the stomach and bowels. For this purpose I have found the bicarbonate of potassa in solution, to which lemon-juice is added at the moment it is taken, so as to produce an extemporaneous effervescing draught, often an admirable remedy. In other cases I have used with advantage small doses of calomel or blue mass, followed, if necessary, by a gentle saline purge. When the symptoms have occurred soon after a hearty meal, or when there is evidence that the stomach is overloaded, it will occasionally be necessary to have recourse to an emetic. Usually, the indications for treatment at the beginning of an attack are much less definite, and even in the class of cases just referred to they become so after the subsidence of the gastro-intestinal symptoms. Indeed, the treatment in the larger number of cases must be purely symptomatic until the nature of the disease has fully declared itself. The presence of fever will suggest the use of the neutral mixture, effervescing draught, or spirit of Mindererus, combined, if there is decided tendency to evening exacerbations, with sulphate of quinia in full doses. If there is much diarrhoea, Hope's camphor mixture or opium in some other form may be given; if delirium is a prominent symptom, ice or cloths wrung out of cold water should be kept constantly applied to the head.

But even after all doubt in regard to the diagnosis has been dispelled and the existence of typhoid fever has been recognized, the treatment most in favor with physicians is in large measure symptomatic in character. It is true that various specific treatments, to which fuller reference will be made hereafter, have been lately proposed, but the results obtained by them up to the present time where they have been fairly tested are not so favorable as to induce the body of the profession to adopt them to the exclusion of all other methods. It is certain that no remedy or plan of[p. 326]treatment has yet been discovered which has the power of cutting the disease short, although this power has been claimed at different times for several. Thus, at one time quinia in very large doses was believed to possess it, at another venesection, and at another cold baths. But experience has shown that these and other perturbating remedies often do harm, and there is good reason to believe that the apparent good which has followed their use in a comparatively small number of instances may be better explained by supposing that an error of diagnosis has been made than by attributing to them the power of arresting the progress of the disease. Medicines are, however, by no means useless in the treatment of typhoid fever. There is no question that the disease is not only generally conducted to a favorable issue, but that its duration is often materially shortened, by their judicious use. It is evident, however, that the treatment must vary with the severity of the attack. In a few cases it is scarcely necessary to interfere with the course of the disease by the administration of medicines. In others, on the contrary, it is necessary to act promptly and energetically in order to save life.

When called upon to treat typhoid fever, if the case is a mild one with no bad symptoms, such as excessive diarrhoea, delirium, tremors, and the like, and especially if the temperature does not rise higher than 102° F., I am accustomed, after giving minute directions as to the diet and general care of the patient, to prescribe from two to three grains of sulphate of quinia four times daily. No great power in reducing the temperature of the body can, of course, be claimed for these doses, but experience has shown that the impression which they make is useful, and they do not interfere with the administration of the drug in larger quantities should this become necessary. Their action, too, is tonic, and, as they rarely produce cinchonism, the objection often made to the use of larger doses does not apply to them. I am also in the habit of adding to each dose of quinia from ten to fifteen drops of one of the mineral acids. These acids were originally prescribed in typhoid fever under the impression that they neutralized the cause of the disease, which was supposed to be an alkaline poison. Although the results of recent research, which tend to show that the cause of the disease is an organized germ, give no support to this theory, they continue to be used by a large number of physicians of experience. I do not know that any satisfactory explanation of their action in typhoid fever has ever been given. They are certainly tonics, and are therefore indicated, if not in the beginning of the disease, as soon as the strength begins to fail. If, as the disease progresses, the tongue becomes dry and fissured, and if there is much tympany, it will be well to give, in addition to the quinia, ten drops of the oil of turpentine in mucilage every two hours. This was a favorite remedy of the late George B. Wood, the distinguished professor of the Theory and Practice of Medicine in the University of Pennsylvania, who attributed the improvement in the symptoms which generally follows its use to a direct influence of this medicine upon the ulcers in the intestines. Although inclined to believe that the correct explanation of this improvement is its stimulating action upon the circulation and secretions, I fully agree with him in regard to its usefulness in many cases. Under its use I have often seen the dry, fissured, and shrivelled tongue [p. 327]grow moist and throw off its coating much earlier than in all probability it would otherwise have done.

No other than this simple treatment is required in a large number of cases, but even in mild cases symptoms occasionally arise which render necessary some modification of it. It will, however, be more convenient to postpone the discussion of this part of the treatment of typhoid fever until after the treatment of the more serious forms of the disease has been considered.

When typhoid fever assumes a severe type, the success of the physician in the management of the disease will depend largely upon the readiness with which he detects indications for treatment and the promptness with which he meets them. Usually, one of the first symptoms to demand attention is the high temperature. This is not only an early symptom in many bad cases, but may continue throughout the attack; or it may suddenly supervene in cases in which the fever has previously been moderate in degree, and when excessive may be the direct or indirect cause of death. The reduction of the temperature is therefore an indication the importance of which cannot well be overestimated. Fortunately, there are several methods by which this end may be accomplished. It will, however, be necessary for our purpose to consider only two of them in detail: 1, the cold-water treatment; 2, sulphate of quinia in full doses.

The cold-water treatment is not new, since it was practised in the form of cold effusion in the treatment of fevers as long ago as 1787 by Currie of Liverpool, who may be said to have introduced it, and who asserted that it had the power not merely of moderating the symptoms of these diseases, but also, in many cases, of cutting them short. It enjoyed at first a high degree of popularity, which lasted for from twenty to thirty years, but finally fell into disuse, probably in consequence of the exaggerated character of the claims which were made for it by its advocates. Although resorted to from time to time in various parts of the world, the merit of having brought it again into notice seems to be due to Brand of Stettin, who published a work on *The Hydrotherapy of Typhoid Fever* in 1861. Still more recently, the recorded observations of Bartels, Jürgensen, Ziemssen, and Liebermeister in Germany, and of Wilson Fox and others in England, have so far restored the treatment to professional favor that there are few physicians either in this country or abroad who do not occasionally have recourse to it.

The cold-water treatment may be applied in several different ways: 1, the cold bath; 2, the graduated bath; 3, cold affusions; 4, the cold pack; 5, cold sponging; 6, cold compresses; and 7, frictions with ice. They all act in the same manner, and depend for their efficacy upon their power of abstracting heat from the body, and are useful just in proportion as they do this. There is no reason for believing that they have the power to modify the conditions upon which the production of heat depends, but there is, on the other hand, no doubt that under their use distressing and dangerous symptoms, such as coma, stupor, subsultus, and the like, are often much relieved. They probably act, therefore, by diminishing the metamorphosis of the tissues, and the consequent loading of the blood with excrementitious products which the hyperpyrexia has a tendency to promote.

The cold bath is the most effective of all the methods of applying the[p. 328]cold-water treatment. Liebermeister recommends that the bath for an adult should be at the temperature of 68° F., and its duration should be about ten minutes; if, however, the patient shows signs of great weakness, it should not exceed seven. After the bath he should be wrapped up in a dry sheet or light blanket and put back in bed. If the pulse should then show signs of failing, or if there should be shivering or any other evidence of weakness, he should be given a glass of wine or brandy or a dose of some other diffusible stimulus, and bottles containing hot water should be applied to his feet. The process of cooling goes on for some time after the patient's removal from the bath, for while a thermometer placed in the axilla will show that the external temperature is immediately affected by it, the same instrument placed in the rectum will indicate a gradual fall, which will continue in many cases for at least half an hour. Shortly after this the temperature will be observed to rise, and in many cases it will not be more than two hours before it has attained its former height. Liebermeister therefore recommends that the thermometer should be frequently used, and that the baths should be repeated as often as the temperature rises to 103° F. or above it. He has himself given them as often as every two hours, or as many as two hundred during an entire illness, but usually finds that not more than six or eight a day are required. It often requires some persuasion to overcome the repugnance which most patients feel at first for these baths, and the shock of being suddenly immersed in cold water is agreeable to very few. Later, this repugnance, he says, entirely disappears. Intestinal hemorrhage, perforation of the bowel, and great weakness of the heart's action are all contraindications to the use of the cold bath. They are especially to be avoided, according to Liebermeister, when the force of the circulation is so far reduced that the surface of the body is cold while the interior is very hot. On the other hand, the advocates of this plan of treatment contend that the existence of pneumonia or of hypostatic congestion of the lungs is not a sufficient reason for abandoning it, the congestion often disappearing under its use.

The graduated bath possesses some advantages over the cold bath, as its use involves less of a shock to the system. It is therefore more suitable than the latter for nervous and excitable patients, for persons of advanced age or of general feebleness of constitution, or for very young children. In it the temperature of the water, which at the time of the immersion of the patient should be at or above 95° F., is cooled by the gradual addition of cold water until it is reduced to 72°, or below this point. These baths, to produce the same effect as the cold baths, must be of longer duration. They are contraindicated in the same conditions as the latter, but to a less degree.

Although fully willing to admit the good effects of the cold bath in many cases, having been, of course, myself a witness of them, I am indisposed to have recourse to it except in cases of hyperpyrexia of such intensity that death seems imminent and only to be averted by energetic treatment, or in cases in which other antipyretic remedies have failed to reduce the temperature; and for the following reasons: 1. In the first place, it is generally possible to produce a decided effect by the other methods of applying the cold-water treatment, with much less discomfort to the patient. 2. In a private house it is not always practicable to have [p. 329]a bath brought to the bedside of the patient, and in a general hospital to do so often would occasion a good deal of annoyance to the other patients in the same ward, and I have seen ill result from carrying him some distance to the bathroom. But even where the bath is brought directly to his bedside, it involves so much movement, and is sometimes the cause of so much excitement, that its good effects are more than neutralized by its bad.

Cold affusions, while not nearly so efficacious in reducing the temperature of the body as the cold bath, are open to many of the objections which may be urged against the latter mode of treatment. They are, therefore, rarely employed at the present time. Liebermeister, however, thinks that they may sometimes be resorted to with good effect for their brisk stimulating effect on the psychical functions or the respiration.

The cold pack possesses the advantage over the cold bath and cold affusions of involving less movement on the part of the patient and of being less terrifying to children, and may therefore be resorted to in cases in which the latter method of applying the cold-water treatment is contraindicated, as, for instance, in persons of feeble circulation. It is, however, inferior to either of them in its cooling effects, and must be longer applied to produce the same effect. Liebermeister estimates that a course of four consecutive packs, of from ten to twenty minutes' duration apiece, is about equivalent in effect to a cold bath of ten minutes.

Cold sponging is assigned a very low place among the methods of abstracting heat from the body by many writers. It has, however, often been in my hands of much service, and its easy application and the comfort which patients derive from it are certainly strong recommendations in its favor. I have employed it frequently in cases of intestinal hemorrhage, and even in cases of great debility, and have never yet had any reason to repent my having done so. The addition of a little vinegar to the water has seemed to me to increase the effect of the sponging.

Cold compresses, either in the form of cloths wet with cold water or bladders filled with ice, can only produce a local fall of temperature, and therefore, except when applied to the head, can be of little service.

Frictions with ice are a powerful means of depressing the temperature of the body, and may therefore be resorted to in cases of intense hyperpyrexia when for some reason the cold bath cannot be obtained, and when there are no contraindications to the latter.

Liebermeister classes cold drinks, the internal administration of ice, and the injection of cold water among the means of cooling the body in fevers; but it is doubtful if any great reduction of temperature can be brought about by any of these remedies in the quantities in which it would be safe to use them. The first two, and to a less extent the last, meet a very important indication, that of supplying water to the system. Their free use, therefore, forms a very important part of the treatment of typhoid fever.

Luton of Rheims[99] extols the Diæta hydrica in the treatment of typhoid fever. The patient receives absolutely nothing else to drink but water, which is given in large quantities, for from four to six days. No nourishment is given until the beginning of the third week, and first of all milk. If fever returns, the water is given again. Medicines such as [p. 330]quinia and eucalyptus are given in adynamic conditions, which Luton says are rare under this treatment. He believes that the increase of the typhoid germs is prevented by absolute diet and abundant supply of water.

[99] *Journal de thérapie*, Oct., 1880.

Quinia to produce a decided antipyretic effect must be given in large quantities. Murchison says that a dose of from fifteen to twenty grains causes within an hour or two a fall of the temperature, and, to a less extent, of the pulse, which may last from twelve to eighteen hours, and that he has never known any other disagreeable symptoms result from its use than noises in the ears, temporary acceleration and irregularity of the respiration, and occasional vomiting. This quantity will often, however, be found to be insufficient to produce a notable reduction of the fever, and it is therefore necessary occasionally to increase it. Liebermeister usually gives to adults from twenty-two to forty-five grains of the sulphate or the muriate of quinia, and this dose must positively be taken within the space of half an hour, or, at the most, an hour, as it is useless, he says, to expect the full benefit of this dose to appear if the dose is divided and its administration is extended over a longer time. He never repeats it in less than twenty-four hours, and, as a rule, does not give it again under two days. Jürgensen has exceeded the dose of forty-five grains without observing any bad effects from it. When these large doses are taken the fall of the temperature usually begins a few hours after the administration of the medicine, the minimum being reached in from six to twelve hours, and it is usually not until the second day that the temperature attains its former height. It is found in practice that the most decided results are obtained when the medicine is given in the evening, so that the time of its fullest antipyretic effects will coincide with that of the morning remission. When these large doses produce vomiting, as they occasionally will, the quinia must be given by the rectum or hypodermically.

Quinia possesses the great advantage over the cold bath that it may be given in conditions in which it would be dangerous to resort to the latter. The existence of great cardiac weakness, of perforation of the bowel, or of intestinal hemorrhage do not usually constitute contraindications to its use. In my own practice I have not often found it necessary to have recourse to much larger doses than those recommended by Murchison, preferring to repeat them if necessary rather than to give a single dose of even half a drachm.

It will be well, in this connection, to allude briefly to a few other remedies which have been given for their antipyretic effect. One of these is digitalis, which has been administered for this purpose in very large doses. Thus, Liebermeister recommends that from eleven to twenty-two grains should be given in the course of thirty-six hours. I have never used this drug in these doses, and therefore cannot speak of its effects from personal knowledge of them. I have frequently had recourse to it, however, in more moderate doses, and I think with advantage.

Another is sodium salicylate. This remedy has been used largely in England and Germany, and to a less extent in this country. It has been claimed for it that it has the power of destroying the germs of typhoid fever, but Stricker[100] finds it difficult to accord it this property in the face[p. 331]of the fact that he has had three cases of typhoid fever under his observation which occurred in patients just recovered from rheumatism, which had been treated by this drug. My own experience with it in the treatment of this disease is small, but has been unsatisfactory. While it is undoubtedly an antipyretic, the pulse becomes weak and the inspiration less strong under its use. The brain symptoms do not diminish under its use. Indeed, it is said to produce narcotism in some cases. Dr. Jahn[101] and Dr. Jh. Platzer[102] speak more favorably of it, but admit that its administration is occasionally attended by the inconveniences above referred to. The verdict of the profession in regard to it, tersely expressed by one who had given it a fair trial, appears to be that it is a remedy that brings nothing but disappointment to the physician and disaster to the patient.

[100] *Deutsche Milit.-arztl Zeitsch.*, 1877.
[101] *Deutsches Arch. f. klin. Med.*, 1877.
[102] *Bayr. Arztl. Intell. Bl.*, 1877.

Eucalyptus, in the form of the tincture, is also a favorite remedy with many practitioners. Dr. Benj. Bell[103] is in the habit of giving a teaspoonful every three or four hours in a wineglass of water, and asserts that it diminishes the tendency to diarrhoea and the duration of the illness.

[103] *Edin. Med. Jour.*, Aug., 1881.

The different varieties of typhoid fever require slight modifications only of the treatment laid down above. In the typho-malarial form, especially in those cases in which the malarial element predominates, and in which there is a marked tendency to remission, the early administration of quinia in full antiperiodic doses is urgently called for. In some cases which he had the opportunity of observing in the army, A. L. Cox[104] found great advantage from the use of arsenious acid in rather large doses. When the disease attacks elderly people, an early resort to alcoholic stimulants is usually necessary, in consequence of the excessive prostration it induces in them. Henoch and Steffen[105] assert that cold baths are not so well borne in children as in adults. Their influence is transitory only, and their use has sometimes been followed by fatal collapse. In the renal form dry, and in some cases cut, cups should be applied externally and saline diuretics given internally.

[104] *Outlines of the Chief Camp Diseases of the United States Armies*, by Joseph Janvier Woodward, M.D., Philada., 1863.

[105] *Jahrb. f. Korhde*, 1880.

SYMPTOMS REQUIRING SPECIAL TREATMENT.—Vomiting, when it occurs early in the disease, is usually checked by the administration of an emetic and by the application of sinapisms to the epigastrium. The use of emetics is no longer advisable when it occurs after the first week. It is better then to trust to small doses of hydrocyanic or carbolic acid, aromatic spirit of ammonia, or bismuth. It will often be found that lime-water and milk will remain upon the stomach when every other article of food or medicine is rejected. In some severe cases which have been under my care the symptom was permanently relieved by the frequent administration of small quantities of brandy in iced soda-water. When vomiting is a consequence of peritonitis it usually resists every form of treatment.

Diarrhoea, if the number of the stools does not exceed two or three in the course of twenty-four hours, does not need special treatment. When, however, it is more severe, prompt measures should be taken to check it. Under these circumstances laudanum injections have seemed to me to be[p. 332]by far the best remedy. It is not necessary that these injections should always contain a large amount of laudanum or that they should be repeated frequently. In many cases twenty drops once a day will be found to be sufficient, and it is rarely necessary to exceed forty drops twice daily. Opium given by the mouth or in suppository in equivalent quantity does not act with anything like the same efficacy. If the laudanum injections fail to restrain the diarrhoea, it will be well to have recourse, in combination with opium, to the subnitrate of bismuth or the acetate of lead. Nitrate of silver was at one time much employed in the treatment of typhoid fever, especially by the late J. K. Mitchell of this city, but was afterward suffered to fall into neglect. Its use has been recently, to a certain extent, revived in consequence of the recommendation of William Pepper,[106] who claims for it the power of modifying the course of the disease. I have given it in a number of cases, but have never been able to satisfy myself that it possessed this power. I have therefore ceased to prescribe it except in the later stages of the disease, when the symptoms indicate that the intestinal ulcers are in an atonic condition. Under these circumstances it has appeared to me to promote their cicatrization. It is important, however, to remember that diarrhoea is occasionally caused and kept up by more food being given to the patient than he can assimilate, and it is therefore a good rule to examine the stools from time to time to see whether they contain curds of milk or other undigested food. If such is found to be the case, the amount of nourishment should be diminished, and it will be well also to prescribe pepsin either in powder or in solution.

[106] *Philadelphia Medical Times*, Feb. 12, 1881.

Tympanites also occasionally requires treatment, for in addition to interference with the descent of the diaphragm and other discomfort it produces, the distended condition of the bowels directly increases the risk of perforation. It is usually sufficient to employ embrocations or stupes of equal parts of sweet oil and oil of turpentine, or of camphor liniment. If the tympanites coexist with constipation, enemata, either with or without a small quantity of oil of turpentine, may often be used with advantage. If it is extreme, an intestinal tube should be introduced very carefully into the rectum and the gas drawn off. Charcoal has occasionally been administered in this condition with a view of preventing decomposition of the intestinal contents. Tympanites occasionally rapidly supervenes upon the occurrence of perforation, and must then, of course, be treated with due reference to the latter condition.

Intestinal hemorrhage is a symptom which always demands prompt attention, no matter how slight it may seem to be, for it is to be remembered that not only is there a danger of its recurrence, but that the quantity of blood which appears in the stools is by no means a reliable measure of that actually lost, as more blood frequently remains in the intestines than appears externally. In estimating its severity, it is therefore proper to take into consideration the gravity of the other symptoms which attend it, such as the fall of temperature, feebleness of the pulse. In many cases the enforcement of absolute rest, with the administration of cold drink and a small amount of opium to diminish peristaltic action, is all that is needed. In cases in which the symptoms are graver it will be necessary to have recourse to more energetic [p. 333]measures. Under these circumstances the hypodermic injection of from three to five grains of ergotin, repeated if necessary, has seldom in my experience failed to check the hemorrhage. Dilute sulphuric acid, oil of turpentine, and acetate of lead have also proved themselves useful remedies in my hands. The application of ice to the surface of the abdomen has also been said to be attended with good results, but the objections to the use of this remedy in the condition of collapse, which is so apt to accompany profuse intestinal hemorrhage, are so evident that it is unnecessary to discuss them here. Monsel's solution, tannic acid, and various other mineral and vegetable astringents have been recommended for their direct effect upon the bleeding surface, but, even admitting that they can, when administered by the mouth, reach this unaltered or in a sufficient state of concentration to be active, it is evident that they could only do so after the loss of valuable time.

When perforation occurs, it is obvious that the indications for treatment are to preclude the extravasation of the contents of the intestine into the cavity of the peritoneum, and to prevent the peritonitis which is a consequence of this accident from becoming general. Both of these indications are met by the administration of opium, which diminishes, and, if pushed, arrests, the peristaltic action of the intestines. By means of it the bowels may be kept as free from movement as if "placed in splints." A grain of solid opium may be given every hour until a decided effect is produced, or if it is found to disagree with the stomach an equivalent quantity may be given by the rectum, or it may be substituted by morphia administered by the mouth or hypodermically. With the same view, food is to be allowed in small quantities only at a time, and of a character capable of digestion by the stomach. A light poultice, or, if there is much evidence of inflammation, ice should be applied to the abdomen. It has been recommended also, in cases in which the peritonitis has become general, to apply leeches to the abdomen, but few patients in this condition will readily bear the loss of much blood. It is very important not to interfere with the constipation which results from the above treatment, and which it is one of its objects to promote, until all inflammatory symptoms have been absent for at least a week, when a simple enema may be administered. Peritonitis resulting from other causes than perforation of the intestine does not require any modification of the above treatment.

Severe abdominal pain, when it occurs independently of inflammation, is best treated by the application to the abdomen of light poultices, to which two or three teaspoonfuls of laudanum may be added.

Constipation is an occasional symptom, but it rarely calls for active interference. When it is present so early in the course of the disease that the diagnosis is still uncertain, and has continued for several days, it is best to prescribe a small dose of castor oil; a dessertspoonful is generally sufficient. The late Dr. Gerhard was in the habit of giving a tablespoonful of sweet oil in this condition. The inordinate action which frequently follows the administration of these mild purgatives will often dispel all uncertainty as to the nature of the disease we have to do with. When it occurs in a more advanced stage of the disease it is best met by the administration of enemata, which may contain, if there is much tympanites present, a small quantity of oil of turpentine. Under all[p. 334]circumstances it will be well to remember the advice given by Baglivi two centuries ago, to avoid the use of active cathartics in this disease.[107]

[107] "Fuge purgantia tanquam postem," *Opera Omnia Medico-Practica et Anatomica*, Georgii Baglivi, 1788.

The headache which is sometimes a distressing symptom in the beginning of the disease is usually relieved by the application to the head of cloths constantly wet with ice-water or by that of a bladder filled with ice and lard. If it is very severe and does not yield to these remedies, a few leeches applied to the temples often have a very happy effect in moderating the pain. Murchison recommends that the cold affusion should be administered by simply placing the patient's head over a basin at the edge of the bed and pouring water on it from a height of two or three feet. He also says that warm fomentations are to be preferred to cold in aged and infirm persons of feeble circulation. Sleeplessness will often disappear under the use of remedies presented for the relief of the headache and other nervous symptoms. It is occasionally so persistent as to call for special treatment. If it occur early in the disease, it will generally be sufficient to prescribe at bedtime ten grains each of potassium bromide and chloral, repeated once or twice during the night. Later in the disease this combination ceases to produce any effect, besides which chloral cannot be administered with safety after the action of the heart becomes feeble. It is therefore necessary to have recourse to opium in some form or other. There are, it is true, theoretical objections to its use in typhoid fever, such as its interference with digestion and its tendency to lock up the secretions; but these will hardly weigh in the balance against the fact that the patient will die of exhaustion if the insomnia is allowed to continue, and that under certain circumstances opium is the only drug which will procure the needed sleep. The form in which it is given is not a matter of much importance. I prefer the deodorized tincture, twenty or thirty drops, repeated if necessary in an hour or two, but I have seen good results from the solid opium and from the hypodermic injection of morphia. When the insomnia is attended by much tremor and muttering delirium, camphor may be added to the opium, and given throughout the day as well as in the evening. Violent delirium is sometimes also relieved by administration of opium and alcoholic stimulants, and by the application of cold to the head. It is also much lessened by the cold-water treatment. When the delirium is so violent that restraint is necessary, it is better that this should be mechanical than that it should be left wholly in the hands of ignorant and untrained nurses. A folded sheet passed over the chest of the patient and fastened to the sides of the bed is frequently all that is needed. Stupor requires very much the same kind of treatment as that suitable for the other forms of nervous derangement. If it is extreme, counter-irritants should be applied to the nape of the neck and cold to the head. The late Dr. Wood was in the habit of shaving the hair and applying a blister to the scalp of a patient in this condition, and I have seen good in more than one instance result from this treatment. The urine should also be examined, and if the quantity be insufficient diuretics should be given. If it contain albumen or blood, counter-irritants and even cut cups should be applied to the loins. It is also important, if the patient be in this condition, that the physician should not rest satisfied with the nurse's[p. 335]assurance that the urine is passed freely, but should from time to time examine the supra-pubic region himself. It is not infrequently found under these circumstances that there is really retention, and that the wetting of the bed upon which the nurse has based her assurances is really the consequence of the dribbling of urine from an over-distended bladder. I have known of serious results, such as cystitis, paralysis of the bladder, having followed the neglect of this very simple precaution. Convulsions when they occur are to be treated by the application of cold to the head and counter-irritants to other parts of the body.

Epistaxis is rarely so severe as not to yield to the use of simple remedies, such as the application of ice to the forehead or back of the neck, or of styptics locally. In a few cases, however, it is profuse, and it will then be necessary to have recourse to hypodermic injections of ergotin, as in the case of hemorrhage from the intestines, or to plug the nostrils.

TREATMENT OF COMPLICATIONS.—Hypostatic congestion of the lungs, as it is usually the consequence of feeble action of the heart, is best treated by frequently changing the position of the patient, and by remedies calculated to increase the power of the organ, such as alcoholic stimulants, ammonium carbonate, oil of turpentine, and digitalis. Recent German authors, however, regard digitalis as a dangerous remedy when the heart has undergone the granular degeneration peculiar to fevers. It had, therefore, better not be given if the congestion occurs late in the disease. I have myself always found advantage from the application of turpentine stupes to the chest, and occasionally from the application of dry cups. Pneumonia when it occurs as a complication does not render necessary a material modification of the above treatment. It may sometimes be well, if it occur early in a robust subject, to take blood locally, but it can rarely be justifiable to do so by venesection.

Bed-sores may generally be prevented by frequently changing the position of the patient, by scrupulous attention to cleanliness, and by bathing prominent parts of his body with whiskey and alum. These parts should also be protected from pressure by the judicious arrangement of pillows and cushions. When redness or abrasions appear the part should be covered with soap plaster smoothly spread upon kid. This application may be continued even after the formation of sloughs. As soon, however, as these show a tendency to suppurate poultices should be applied, and the resulting ulcer treated as if occurring under other circumstances.

Thrombosis of the femoral vein is best treated by elevating the affected leg and enveloping it with flannel cloths saturated with hot vinegar and water. Thrombosis of other veins is to be treated on the same general principles. When an artery becomes obliterated, whether from embolism or thrombosis, the part which it supplies should be surrounded with cotton wool and every effort made to favor the establishment of the collateral circulation. If sphacelus occurs, it should be treated on general surgical principles.

TREATMENT OF CONVALESCENCE.—The importance of a strict adherence to a liquid diet in the early part of the convalescence of typhoid fever has already been alluded to. The ulcers in the intestines often remain unhealed for some time after the subsidence of the fever, and errors in diet may therefore readily cause recrudescences of fever, if not true relapses.[p. 336]These recrudescences are sometimes produced by very slight causes. I have seen them follow undue mental exercise or worry, or sitting up too early or too long. It is therefore important to guard our patients at this stage of the disease from undue fatigue or excitement of any kind. Medicines calculated to build up the strength and to improve the nutrition are clearly indicated at this time. If the diarrhoea should persist, nitrate or oxide of silver, sulphate of copper, and subnitrate of bismuth in appropriate doses, given with a little opium, will all be found to be useful remedies. When, on the contrary, constipation exists, it is still necessary to avoid the use of drastic cathartics; indeed, even mild laxatives should be given by the mouth only after enemata have failed to produce a movement of the bowel.

SPECIFIC TREATMENT.—The search for a specific remedy in typhoid fever is not new. It is as old as the theory that the disease is generated by a specific cause. The hypothesis that this is an alkaline poison led many years ago to the use of the mineral acids, and it was only after experience had shown that they were without power to cut the disease short, or even to control many of its symptoms, that they ceased in a measure to be prescribed. Calomel also, which was occasionally resorted to formerly for its antiphlogistic effects upon the intestinal lesions, has been lately recommended in Germany in the treatment of typhoid fever on account of its supposed antidotal properties. Seven and a half grains of the drug, and in some cases a much larger dose, are given four times daily on alternate days as soon as the nature of the disease is fully recognized. It is claimed for this treatment that when it is begun early the rate of mortality and the duration of the disease are much less under it than under any other. Its advocates admit, however, that the latter is not always the case—a variety in the action of the medicine which is attributed to a difference in the way in which the poison of the disease has been taken into the body. Salivation is rarely produced by the calomel. The diarrhoea, which is at first increased by it, subsequently diminishes, and the administration of each dose is followed by a decided although temporary reduction of temperature.

A diminution in the rate of mortality is also said to have been obtained by the administration of iodine in typhoid fever, although the results of its use are on the whole less favorable than those of calomel. Liebermeister recommends that three or four drops of a solution of one part of iodine, two parts of iodide of potassium, and ten parts of water should be given every two hours in a glass of water.

	Number treated.	Number died.	Percentage of mortality.
Non-specifically treated	377	69	18.3
Treated with calomel	223	26	11.7
Treated with iodine	239	35	14.6
Total	839	130	15.5

The preceding table, which is taken from Liebermeister's article on typhoid fever in *Ziemssen's Cyclopædia*, is based upon the results of [p. 337] treatment in 839 cases, a part of which were treated with iodine, a part with calomel, and a part with neither, the rest of the treatment being exactly alike in all of them, and consisting in the employment of a partial antipyretic method.

James C. Wilson[108] has recently used with great success in the treatment of typhoid fever the following prescription, which was originally suggested by Roberts Bartholow: Rx. Tinct. Iodinii fl. drachm ij.; Acid. Carbolici liq. fl. drachm j.—M. Of this, one, two, or even three drops is given in a sherry-glassful of ice-water after food every two or three hours during the day and night. In addition to this prescription his patients were given a dose of calomel varying in amount from seven and a half to ten grains, which was repeated on every alternate night until three or four doses had been administered in the course of the first six or eight days. Of sixteen cases so treated, none proved fatal, although eight of them were severe, the temperature reaching or exceeding 104° F. Da Costa[109] has used carbolic acid in this disease, and has found it useful in controlling the diarrhoea and in lowering the temperature, but suggests the use of thymol in doses of from half a grain to one grain as a substitute, on account of its greater acceptability to the stomach. C. G. Rothe[110] recommends a mixture of carbolic acid, tincture of digitalis, tincture of aconite, brandy, and tincture of iodine. Its use causes a decided fall of temperature and diminution in the frequency of the pulse.

[108] *Transactions of the College of Physicians of Philadelphia*, 3d Series, vol. vi., Philadelphia, 1883, p. 221.

[109] *Ibid.*, p. 234.

[110] *Deutsche Med. Wochenschr.*, 1880.

My own experience does not enable me to speak with positiveness of the value of this plan of treatment. Indeed, it has been used in so few cases, to the exclusion of all other remedies, that it is difficult to decide how far the result attained in cases treated by them is due to them, and how far to the other therapeutic means employed. With the testimony of such competent observers as those above named it is only proper that the treatment by iodine and carbolic acid should have a further trial. More caution, it seems to me, is required in the use of calomel. While it is probable that in a few cases the intestinal lesions may be favorably modified by the purgation which it induces, the indiscriminate use of the drug is, I am sure, calculated to do more harm than good.

[p. 338]

TYPHUS FEVER.
BY JAMES H. HUTCHINSON, M.D.

DEFINITION.—Typhus fever is an acute contagious disease, usually occurring epidemically, lasting from ten to twenty days, and characterized, among other symptoms, by an abrupt commencement, great prostration, profound derangement of the nervous system, and a peculiar eruption which appears between the third and eighth days, and which, disappearing at first under pressure, soon becomes persistent, and in severe cases may be converted into and be associated with true petechiæ. When it proves fatal, it generally does so at or near the end of the second week. The lesions found after death are not specific in character, and consist mainly of a marked alteration of the blood, congestions of internal organs, softening of the heart, and atrophy of the brain.

SYNONYMS.—Petechial Typhus, Putrid or Malignant Fever, Camp, Jail, Ship, or Hospital Fever, Spotted Fever, Irish Ague, Contagious Typhus, Brain Fever, Adynamic or Ataxic Fever, Ochlotic Fever, Catarrhal Typhus.

The term typhus was first applied by Sauvages in 1760, and afterward by Cullen, to certain forms of fever, characterized by marked prominence of the nervous symptoms, to distinguish them from another group of cases to which they gave the name synochus, and is derived from the Greek word [Greek: typhos], which literally means smoke, and which is employed in the treatise on internal affections attributed to Hippocrates for a similar purpose. According to Murchison,[1] Hippocrates used the word to define a "confused state of the intellect, with a tendency to stupor." The appellation typhus, therefore, as indicating a very prominent symptom of the disease about to be described, is perhaps the best that could be given to it. It has been generally adopted by the physicians in England and in this country to denote this disease, but on the Continent, and especially in Germany, it is applied also to typhoid fever, the two fevers being usually designated there as typhus petechialis and typhus abdominalis, respectively.

[1] *A Treatise on the Continued Fevers of Great Britain*, by Charles Murchison, M.D., LL.D., F.R.S., etc., second edition, London, 1873.

HISTORY.—As human want and misery and the evils which follow in the train of war have never been wholly absent from the world, and as these are the conditions which are now known to be favorable to the spread, if not to the generation, of typhus fever, it is highly probable that this disease was the cause of some of the epidemics to which allusion is made by the sacred and profane writers of antiquity. Yet their descriptions are too vague to justify us in assuming that such was positively the [p. 339]case. The records of the first fifteen centuries of our own era are similarly wanting in details, for, with the exception of a brief notice of an outbreak of the disease in the monastery of La Cava, near Salerno, in the year 1083, by Corradi[2] it may be said to have been practically undescribed before the year 1546, when Fracastorius[3] published his work, *De Contagionibus et Morbis Contagiosis*. From the description which this distinguished physician gives there of the epidemics which prevailed in Verona in the years 1505 and 1508, there can be no doubt that the disease he had the opportunity of observing was really typhus fever. Not only are the principal symptoms succinctly described, but its contagiousness and tendency to early prostration fully recognized. We learn also, from the same work, that the disease, although previously unknown in Italy, was one with which the physicians of Cyprus and the neighboring islands were perfectly familiar. According to the same authority, it again made its appearance in 1528 in Italy, and from there extended to Germany.

[2] In *Chron. Cavense Annali*, p. 1, 101, quoted in *Handbuch der Historish-Geographischen Pathologie*, von Dr. August Hirsch, Stuttgart, 1881.

[3] Quoted by Murchison.

During the last half of the sixteenth century epidemics of typhus fever would seem to have been of more frequent occurrence than before it, since many of the medical authors of this period not only refer to it very fully, but also give accurate descriptions of the disease. There is also abundant evidence of the same kind that it frequently prevailed epidemically in almost every part of Europe during the seventeenth and eighteenth centuries, following generally in the wake of famine and of war, and often attaining a high degree of virulence in besieged towns. The histories of many of these epidemics are exceedingly interesting, especially those of the so-called Black Assizes which occurred at different times in several of the towns of England, and which derived their name from the fact that the disease was communicated from the prisoners on trial to the judges and other persons in attendance upon the court; but to give these in detail would be beyond the scope of this article. Although many of the authors of these two centuries boldly advocated copious venesection as the only rational method of treating the disease, there was a not inconsiderable number who recognized its essentially typhoid nature, its tendency to early prostration, and the fact that patients suffering from it bear bleeding badly, as fully as is done by physicians of the present day. They were also unquestionably quite aware of the circumstances under which typhus fever generally arises, for in 1735, Browne Langrish[4] wrote that it originated from "the effluvia of human live bodies," and that its principal cause was overcrowding with deficient ventilation, as a result of which "people were made to inhale their own steams;" and a similar opinion was expressed a few years later by Sir John Pringle,[5] J. Carmichael Smyth,[6] and others.

[4] *The Modern Theory and Practice of Physics*, by Browne Langrish, p. 354, London, 1764.
[5] *Observations in Diseases of the Army*, London.
[6] Quoted by Murchison.

Epidemics of typhus fever have frequently occurred in various parts of Europe during the present century, although they have, on the whole, shown a greater tendency than before to confine themselves to the place in which they first appeared. The most severe of these began in 1846, and after committing great ravages in Ireland extended to England, and[p. 340]subsequently to the Continent. The disease proved much more fatal than the sword in the armies of Napoleon in the towns besieged by him in the early part of this century, and was the cause of an immense loss of life in the Russian and French armies in the Crimea after the fall of Sebastopol.

In our own country typhus fever has appeared several times during the present century, but the outbreaks have rarely attained the magnitude of epidemics, such as are seen in Europe, and have usually been distinctly traceable to importation from abroad. It was first met with, according to Wood,[7] in New England in 1807 and in Philadelphia in 1812, continuing to lurk, this author says, in the lanes and alleys of that city until the winter of 1820-21, when, as a student of medicine, he had an opportunity of studying it. Another outbreak of the disease occurred in the same city in 1836, and is the subject of an admirable paper by the late Wm. S. Gerhard.[8] Since then epidemics of moderate severity have repeatedly occurred at different times in several of the American cities, and have been described, among others, by Flint, Da Costa,[9] and Loomis. A large number of cases of typhus fever (1723), with 572 deaths, were reported to the Surgeon-General's office during the late Civil War, but doubt has been thrown upon the correctness of the diagnosis of many of these cases by Clymer[10] and Woodward,[11] and by other army surgeons, who, as the result of their investigations of this subject, have reached the conclusion that typhus did not prevail as an epidemic, however limited, among our soldiers at dépôts for returned prisoners of war. A like immunity from this scourge may be assumed to have been enjoyed by the Confederate forces, since Joseph Jones,[12] one of the most eminent of their medical officers, has stated positively that no case of true typhus fever came under his observation during the war in any army, in any field hospital, general hospital, or military prison, and that the experience of all of his associates whose opinions on this question he was able to obtain, either personally or by letter, was the same. It is therefore most probable that the cases entered upon the sick reports of both armies as typhus fever were in almost every case, if not in all, cases of typhoid fever occurring in scorbutic subjects.

[7] *A Treatise on the Practice of Medicine*, by George B. Wood, M.D., etc., Philada., 1855.

[8] *The American Journal of the Medical Sciences*, February and August, 1837.

[9] *Ibid.*, January, 1866.

[10] *The Science and Practice of Medicine*, by William Aitken, M.D., Edin.; 3d Amer. ed., p. 462, Philadelphia, 1872.

[11] *Camp Diseases of the United States Armies*, by Joseph Janvier Woodward, M.D., Philadelphia, 1863.

[12] *United States Sanitary Commission's Memoirs—Medical*, p. 600, New York, 1867.

From the foregoing sketch of its history it is evident that typhus fever has prevailed from time to time in almost all the countries of Europe. Indeed, it is probable that no one of them has wholly escaped its ravages, while in others—as, for example, Ireland—it has been more or less constantly present until within the last few years, when its visitations have been less frequent as well as less severe. Even in countries which are popularly supposed to enjoy an immunity from it there is evidence of an incontrovertible character that it has occasionally occurred. Such an immunity has been claimed for France, but in the works of Riverius,[13][p. 341]Ambrose Paré,[14] and others will be found descriptions of the disease which leave no doubt upon the mind of their entire familiarity with it; and Hirsch, in his work on *Historico-Geographical Pathology*, is able to give references to several writers who describe outbreaks that have recently occurred there. The disease has also been observed in Iceland. Typhus fever is of much less frequent occurrence in the other divisions of the eastern hemisphere than in Europe. According to Murchison, there are no authentic records of its having been met in Africa, or, with the exception of India, in Asia, such as it is seen in England and Ireland. There are, however, reports of its occurrence in Asia Minor, Syria, Persia, Egypt, Nubia, Tunis, and Algeria, which Hirsch,[15] on the other hand, believes place the occasional presence of this disease in these countries beyond doubt. The same difference of opinion exists between these two distinguished observers in regard to the accounts which have been published of typhus fever occurring in Mexico, Central America, and South America, the latter holding that they are entirely reliable, the former that the cases described in them were really cases of malarial or typhoid fever. The disease has never been met with on the continent of Australia, in New Zealand, or in the valley of the Mississippi and the States bordering on the Pacific Ocean in our own country.

[13] *The Practice of Physick*, being chiefly a Translation of the Works of Lazarus Riverius, London, 1678.

[14] *Traité de la Peste, de la Petite Verolle et Rougeolle*, par Ambrose Paré, Paris, 1568.

[15] *Loc. cit.*

While Hirsch's researches go to show that the tropical zone has not been so wholly exempt from the visitation of typhus fever as some authors have asserted, they establish the fact that it is of much less frequent occurrence there than in the colder portions of the temperate zone, where the modes of life are certainly much more favorable to its extension. Natives of warm climates are as liable to be attacked by it as others upon coming to places where it is prevailing, and in the Philadelphia epidemic of 1836, which Gerhard[16] has described, negroes and mulattoes suffered from it more severely than the whites.

[16] *Loc. cit.*

ETIOLOGY.—The etiology of typhus fever will be best studied under the heads Predisposing and Exciting Causes.

PREDISPOSING CAUSES.—It may be stated, generally, that whatever impairs the health or reduces the strength of an individual, even temporarily, or acts depressingly on his nervous system, predisposes him to typhus fever. But there are among the predisposing causes some which exert a more special influence on its production than others. Among the more powerful of these is the overcrowding of human beings, with deficient ventilation. Indeed, there are some authors who consider that this has been in many cases alone sufficient to occasion the disease; and although this opinion, as it involves the admission that it may be generated de novo, is contested by others, there is great unanimity among authors in attaching great importance to it. Of the patients admitted into the London Fever Hospital with typhus fever, a large proportion came from the more crowded districts of the city. The disease has always been most prevalent in the poorer quarters of Glasgow, Dublin, and Edinburgh, and when epidemic in Philadelphia in 1836 it was confined to a portion of the town which has always been noted for the squalor and misery of its inhabitants. Among those admitted during that year to the Philadelphia Hospital were seven negroes, said by Gerhard to [p. 342]be "the entire population of a cellar." It is probably largely due to the fact that the better social condition of the poor in this country prevents the degree of crowding which often exists in European cities that the disease is comparatively rare here. The effect of overcrowding is of course much increased by want of cleanliness, either of the person or of the clothes.

Poverty, not merely from its own depressing influences, but also from the fact that it leads to overcrowding, is a powerful predisposing cause of typhus fever. Insufficiency of food, which is one of its many consequences, by impairing his nutrition and thus diminishing his vital resistance, renders the individual more susceptible to the action of the specific cause. Gerhard says that of the patients seen by him in 1836 a very small proportion came from the better class of mechanics, and Tweedie[17] and Sir William Jenner[18] state that it is rare to meet with instances of the disease, except in the case of medical practitioners and students, among those in comfortable circumstances. Bateman[19] goes so far as to assert that "deficiency of nutriment is the principal source of epidemic fever;" and there is certainly a remarkable coincidence in time between outbreaks of this fever and seasons of want and distress. But, as Murchison has shown, destitution is not essential to the production of typhus, for the Dundee epidemic of 1865 was due to overcrowding of the town, brought about by the inhabitants of the surrounding country flocking into it in consequence of labor being unusually abundant and wages good.

[17] *Lectures on the Distinctive Character, Pathology, and Treatment of Continued Fevers*, by Alexander Tweedie, M.D., F.R.S., London, 1842; and *Clinical Reports on Fever*, by same author, London, 1830.

[18] *On the Identity or Non-Identity of Typhoid and Typhus Fevers*, by William Jenner, M.D., London, 1880; also *Lancet*, November 15, 1879.

[19] *A Succinct Account of Typhus or Contagious Fever of this Country*, by Thomas Bateman, M.D., F.R.S., London, 1820.

Similar in its action to the above cause is intemperance. Not only is the habitual drunkard more likely to suffer from typhus fever than the temperate man, but a single debauch has been followed by an attack in individuals who had previously resisted the contagion. On the other hand, the most rigid temperance will not afford in all cases a complete immunity from its effects. The debility left by an illness is also a condition favoring the occurrence of an attack of the disease in those who are exposed to its exciting cause. Fatigue of all kinds renders the body less able to resist the causes of disease, and typhus fever is not an exception to the general rule. Overworked nurses are specially liable to contract it. The depressing emotions also favor its occurrence. It has been observed during epidemics that those who exhibit an excessive fear of the contagion are much more likely to suffer from it than the cheerful and courageous.

No age enjoys an immunity from the disease. In fact, it is probable that all ages are equally liable to it. Buchanan[20] has seen it at the London Fever Hospital in an infant a fortnight old and in a man of eighty, and attributes the prevailing opinion that children rarely suffer from it to the fact that they are not often taken to hospitals, but are retained in their own homes for treatment. Gerhard[21] says that no children in the asylum attached to the Philadelphia Hospital were [p. 343]attacked with the disease during the prevalence of the epidemic there, but the distance of the asylum from the wards in which the cases were treated was probably the reason of their escaping. In the few cases which have come under my own observation the patients were young men, varying in age from twenty-five to thirty-five. The sexes also suffer from it equally. In some epidemics there may be a preponderance of one sex over the other, but in others the reverse has been the case.

[20] *A System of Medicine*, edited by J. Russell Reynolds, M.D., F.R.C.P., etc., vol. i., article "Typhus Fever," London, 1866.
[21] *Loc. cit.*

Occupation, except so far as it brings the individual into immediate contact with the sick, as in the case of physicians, nurses, and clergymen, does not predispose to the disease. There would seem also to be no difference in the susceptibility of the different races to the contagion. Acclimatization affords no protection from the disease, as it does in the case of typhoid fever, and change of the habits of life does not appear to exercise any influence upon the liability to it. On the other hand, the susceptibility of different individuals, and of the same individual at different times, varies considerably. Thus, while in many persons a single exposure to the contagion is followed by an attack, in the case of an engineer mentioned by Murchison it did not occur until after fifteen years of continuous service at the London Fever Hospital. A person who has once suffered from typhus fever is not likely to contract it again, but this protection is not complete, as there are a few well-attested instances of a second attack on record.

The disease prevails most frequently during the winter and early spring, principally because the cold weather of these seasons leads to the closing of windows and all other avenues of ventilation, thus intensifying its exciting cause. Still, some epidemics of great severity have occurred in the warmer months of the year, as, for instance, the one described by Gerhard. It is also doubtful if there is any relation between variations in temperature and the amount of moisture in the air and the prevalence of epidemics of typhus fever, although Hirsch regards a low and damp situation as powerfully predisposing to the endemic and epidemic prevalence of the disease. It is usually met with in towns on the sea-coast or on navigable rivers, but it has also been observed frequently in country districts, and even in regions at a considerable elevation above the level of the sea.

EXCITING CAUSE.—The principal if not the only exciting cause of typhus fever is a specific contagion developed in the bodies of the infected and transmitted from them to the healthy by actual contact, by fomites, or through the atmosphere. The nature of this contagion is unknown. A careful study of its peculiarities seems to justify the opinion that it depends upon the presence of a minute organism in the emanations given off by the sick, which is capable of indefinitely multiplying itself in the human body. But this is only an hypothesis, which rests principally upon the analogy between typhus and some other diseases, as, for instance, relapsing fever and diphtheria, in which such a growth is thought to have been discovered, and upon the fact that the contagious principle whatever it may be, is destroyed by a temperature over 204° F.

The evidence in favor of the contagiousness of typhus fever is conclusive, and may be briefly stated as follows: When it breaks out in a community the disease not only attacks those persons who have been subjected to the same influence as the sick—as, for instance, members of [p. 344]their own families, occupants of the same house, etc.—but also those who have come from healthy localities to visit them. In fever hospitals it is rare for any member of the household who has not already had the fever to escape an attack, and the probability of his suffering is in direct proportion to the intimacy of his relations with the patients. Thus, the nurses are far more likely to be attacked than servants whose duties do not take them into the wards, except those employed in the laundry, who are so often affected by it that Murchison says it is difficult to find women who are willing to take the position. The spread of the disease may often be promptly arrested by the complete isolation of the first few cases, while free intercourse between the sick and the well is invariably followed by its extension, not only in the locality in which it first appeared, but to other localities. But the strongest argument in favor of its contagiousness is found in the fact that patients taken into a previously healthy place have frequently become the starting-point of an epidemic. In this way the disease has often been introduced by Irish immigrants into the cities on our seaboard, and even into some of our interior towns.

Actual contact is not necessary for the communication of typhus fever from the sick to the well. The contagion may be transmitted through the atmosphere. How far it will be transmitted in this way will depend upon many circumstances. In a spacious and well-ventilated ward it is probable that the presence of one or two patients with this disease does not seriously endanger the safety of the other patients, and that the only persons who run much risk of contracting it are the physicians and nurses, who are often compelled in the performance of their duties to inhale the emanations from the bodies of the sick. At the Pennsylvania Hospital, where cases of this disease are occasionally admitted, it has been usual to isolate them by placing them in a room a few feet distant only from the dining-room of the men's medical ward and separated from the ward by a short corridor. The steward of the hospital informs me that during his connection with it, which extends over a period of more than sixty years, he has never known the disease to extend to other persons, except on two occasions. One of these was during the epidemic described by Da Costa, when an unusual number of cases was received, and when one resident physician and two nurses contracted the disease. On the other occasion, which happened during my own term of service in the spring of 1881, a young Danish sailor appeared to have taken the disease from two British seamen. As it was ascertained positively that he had not entered the room in which these two seamen were isolated, and as his bed in the ward was one of the farthest removed from the room, and he had not therefore been more or as much exposed to the contagion as the other patients, it was difficult to understand why he alone of all of them should have suffered from it. The explanation was, however, found in the fact that he had been taken over to the women's ward to act as interpreter for a countrywoman who was not known at the time to be suffering from typhus fever, and that he had remained there some time in conversation with her. Murchison and Buchanan both assert also that typhus fever has never extended from the London Fever Hospital to the inmates of adjacent houses, even when it was itself one of a row of houses. If, on the other hand, several patients with typhus fever are placed in a crowded and ill-ventilated ward, the contagion will then be found to have [p. 345]acquired so much more virulence that few of the other patients will escape its effects.

There is also no question that typhus fever may be communicated by fomites. Numerous instances are on record in which the disease has been communicated by the wearing apparel and bed-clothes of patients, and we have already called attention to the frequency with which laundry-women in fever hospitals are attacked by it. The clothes of persons who are themselves free from the disease, but who have been in close attendance upon the sick for some time, are often also the medium of communication. Indeed, Murchison goes so far as to say that men who have not changed their clothes and "who have been living in close, ill-ventilated apartments and on short allowance, may at length have their garments so impregnated with the poison of typhus as to communicate it to others without being themselves the subjects of it," even if they have not been brought in contact with fever patients. The disease was communicated in this way, he thinks, in the famous Black Assize in 1750 by several prisoners to the court that tried them, although they were themselves free from it. On the other hand, with proper precautions there is little danger of the disease being conveyed by physicians to their own families or to other patients.

Some difference of opinion exists as to the stage at which typhus is most contagious. Many authors believe that it is more infectious during convalescence than at any other time, and base this opinion upon the fact that the removal of fever patients to the convalescent ward is very often followed by the occurrence of the disease among its other occupants; but this is probably due, as Murchison suggests, to the patients being allowed at this time to wear their own clothing, which has not been thoroughly disinfected. It is much more likely that the disease is more contagious during the stage when the febrile symptoms are most marked than during either the stage of convalescence or that of invasion. It would appear also, from the observations of Dr. Gerhard and others, that dead bodies do not readily communicate the contagion or that the contagious principle is easily counteracted after death. Still, there are several well-authenticated cases on record in which individuals have unquestionably contracted the disease from dissecting the bodies of patients dead from this cause.

A question of great interest naturally arises here, as to whether or not typhus fever ever occurs except as the consequence of exposure to a previous case of the disease. Is it, in other words, ever generated de novo? Authorities are divided upon this point, many contending that an independent origin is impossible, and others that it may occasionally arise in this way. Among the latter is Murchison, who adduces in support of the position he takes several instances in which poverty, with overcrowding and deficient ventilation, appears to have been the only cause of extensive outbreaks of the disease, as in the case of the Black Assize already alluded to. These cases the opposite party explain by assuming that the germs of the disease are capable of lying dormant for a long time until roused into activity by favoring circumstances. If the disease is caused, as we have shown there is good reason to believe it is, by the presence of a minute organism, this view does not seem to be untenable. Pasteur has demonstrated that the germs of the splenic fever of some of the lower[p. 346]animals may be deprived of their virulence by cultivation in appropriate liquids. If their virulence is diminished under certain circumstances, the assumption does not seem unwarrantable that under others it may be increased, and if we may draw this conclusion in regard to one form of microscopic growth, we may do the same for others; and the hypothesis is therefore not an unreasonable one that the typhus germ needs the atmosphere engendered by overcrowding for it to acquire the power to produce the disease.

PERIOD OF INCUBATION.—The period of incubation of typhus fever appears to vary considerably in length, but is usually about twelve days. In some cases the interval between exposure to the contagion and the occurrence of the first symptoms of the disease is asserted to have been considerably longer, and in one instance as long as thirty-one days; but it is probable that there has been in most, if not in all, of these cases a second exposure which has been overlooked. On the other hand, it is said to have followed at once upon exposure, as in cases reported by Gerhard, in one of which a nurse inhaled the breath of a patient whom he was shaving, and in an hour afterward was taken with cephalalgia and ringing in the ears, which were immediately succeeded by the other symptoms of typhus. In this and other similar cases which are on record it is difficult to exclude the possibility of a previous infection. In a case, however, reported by Murchison there would seem to be no reason to suspect that any such previous infection could have taken place, as the patient, the matron of an orphan asylum where there was no typhus, was taken ill immediately after opening a bundle of clothes which a child had brought with her from a fever hospital, and which had not been thoroughly disinfected.

SYMPTOMATOLOGY.—It will facilitate the study of typhus fever to give, in the first place, as most of the systematic writers on fever have done, a brief clinical sketch of the disease as it ordinarily occurs, and then afterward to consider its leading symptoms in greater detail.

GENERAL DESCRIPTION.—An attack of typhus fever is sometimes preceded for a few days by prodromata, such as a feeling of malaise, indisposition to exertion, pain in the head and limbs, anorexia, and vertigo; but it oftener begins abruptly with a slight chill, or more rarely with a decided rigor. This is followed in a short time by headache, by a marked rise of temperature, and by an increased frequency of pulse and respiration. Nausea is also occasionally present, and less frequently vomiting. The tongue is at first moist and covered with a thin whitish fur, but soon becomes dryish, and its coating is apt to assume a brownish appearance in a day or two. With these symptoms there are loss of appetite, great thirst, constipation, a dull, heavy expression of countenance, a dark, dusky hue of the face, and injection of the conjunctivæ. Mental confusion is early observed, so that, although the patient may be able to answer questions correctly when thoroughly roused, it is readily seen that his mind is working with difficulty. The sleep is very often disturbed by dreams, so that he awakes from it unrefreshed. Prostration and loss of muscular power are so decided from the very beginning of the disease that the patient is obliged usually to take to his bed at once, and it is much rarer to meet with walking cases of the disease than in typhoid fever. The urine is dense, scanty, and high-colored.

[p. 347]Usually, about the fourth day of the disease the characteristic eruption of typhus fever makes its appearance. It consists of numerous spots of irregular form with ill-defined margins and of a dark red or purplish color, occurring singly or in groups, and varying in size from that of a pin's point to two or three lines in diameter. They disappear at first under pressure, but in twenty-four hours become persistent, and in severe cases may be converted later into petechiæ. Besides this eruption there is another which consists of a faint, irregular dusky red, subcuticular mottling. The two eruptions together constitute the mulberry rash of Jenner, and have been variously described by different authors under the name of measly or morbilliform rash.

As the disease advances the prostration becomes greater and the pulse grows weaker. The tongue becomes dry and brown and trembles when protruded. Later, it is so dry and contracted that it can scarcely be put out of the mouth. Sordes collect about the teeth and lips, and the surface exhales a peculiar odor. The headache grows more severe or gives place to delirium, which may at first be active and violent, and then pass into the low and muttering form, or the delirium may be of the latter variety from the start. The sleeplessness of the early stages may continue, and the condition known as coma vigil not infrequently supervenes. The delirium is usually followed by stupor, which is more or less profound in accordance with the severity of the case, and which is accompanied by all the symptoms which characterize the so-called typhoid state, such as subsultus tendinum, picking at the bed-clothes, slipping down in bed, retention or incontinence of urine, and sloughing of the parts exposed to pressure. In this condition the temperature, although usually still considerably above normal, is lower than during the first week of the disease.

Meanwhile, the issue remains in doubt, and may continue uncertain for several days before any improvement in the symptoms can be observed, or, the stupor passing into coma, the case may speedily terminate in death. When death is the result, it usually takes place about the close of the second week or a little later, but it may occur earlier in consequence of the violence of the fever, or, when due to a complication, may be postponed until after the end of the third week. Fortunately, however, recovery is the rule in this disease. The beginning of convalescence is often as abrupt as that of the attack itself. The temperature will often be found to have fallen to the normal or below the normal, the pulse and respiration to have returned to a healthy condition, and all confusion of the intellect to have disappeared in the course of a few hours. Occasionally, however, its approach is more gradual, and a slight fall in temperature and a corresponding improvement in the other symptoms may be observed before it actually occurs. Diarrhoea, an excessive secretion of urine, with a tendency to the deposition of urates, and moderate sweating, often take place simultaneously with the cessation of the fever, and were formerly regarded as critical discharges. The return to health is usually rapid, and very rarely retarded by the occurrence of complications or relapses, as in typhoid fever. The disease itself leaves no tendency to any other disease.

DESCRIPTION OF SPECIAL SYMPTOMS.—The appearance of a patient with typhus fever is pathognomonic, and is often alone sufficient to enable [p. 348]a physician or nurse familiar with it to recognize the disease when brought in contact with it. The surface generally is congested; the face is flushed, and in bad cases dusky red or even livid in hue; the expression is dull and vacant, except during delirium, when it may be wild or even fierce; the conjunctivæ are injected, the eyes watery, and the teeth encrusted with sordes. The skin is generally hot and dry, except toward the close of bad cases, when it may be cool and bathed in a profuse sweat.

The symptoms connected with the nervous system are among the most characteristic of the disease, and of them none is more marked than prostration. It shows itself early, the patient usually taking to his bed immediately after his seizure or within a few days of it. It is much rarer than in typhoid fever to meet with walking cases of typhus, but Buchanan[22] mentions that patients with the rash already out upon them do occasionally present themselves at the out-door department of the London Fever Hospital. It generally increases as the disease progresses, and is often accompanied by a tendency to syncope. It may attain such a degree that the patient is unable to turn himself in bed or to help himself in any way. Among the most distressing sensations which attend this condition of excessive feebleness is a feeling as if he were sinking into the earth with nothing to support him. Headache is also an early symptom. It is often observed among the prodromata of the disease, and when these are absent supervenes directly after the chill. It is usually frontal, but may be diffused. It is generally dull and heavy, but is sometimes acute, and may be accompanied by a tendency to vertigo, increased by sitting up, and by pains in the back and limbs. It becomes more severe with the progress of the disease until the occurrence of delirium, when it is, as a rule, less complained of. With the headache there is generally some dulness of intellect, except in mild cases. This may be slight at first, and may continue so throughout the whole course of the attack, exhibiting itself principally in some confusion as to dates. In more severe cases it is much more marked, and may finally pass into actual stupor. On the other hand, it may be entirely absent, even in severe attacks, as in a case reported by Da Costa and in some cases recently observed by myself. It is usually soon replaced by delirium, which may be low and muttering or wild and noisy, the former being the more common. Delirium is said to occur most frequently among the educated classes and those oppressed with care and anxiety, but is not rare among those who occupy a lower position in the social scale, especially the intemperate. It is, as a rule, most marked at night, and in mild cases may occur only at that time or upon waking in the morning. When the delirium is active the patient may shout and scream, or leave his bed and attempt to throw himself from the window, being endowed apparently for the moment with strength sufficient to enable him to commit these acts of violence. After the paroxysm is over he sinks back in bed exhausted. The confusion of intellect or delirium continues in bad cases until death supervenes or until the establishment of convalescence. Indeed, the mental disturbance does not always end with the latter, and it is not rare for feebleness of intellect to persist for some time after the patient has in other respects regained his usual health, and in a few cases insanity has followed an attack of typhus fever. Among the most[p. 349]formidable of the symptoms of typhus are convulsions, which are fortunately of infrequent occurrence.

[22] *Loc. cit.*

The patient generally suffers from wakefulness, except during the first few days. When sleep is obtained it may be unrefreshing or broken and disturbed by dreams. In other cases the opposite condition of somnolence may be present. Occasionally, after having apparently slept for hours, he may deny having been asleep at all. This condition, which constitutes the coma vigil of Chomel, is entirely distinct from that described by Jenner under the same name, in which the patient lies with his eyes wide open, gazing into vacuity, his mouth only partly closed, his face pale and devoid of expression, and which is invariably fatal. Muscular tremor is more or less present in all cases of the disease, and in bad cases may be a prominent symptom. The disease, when this symptom is marked, especially if there is at the same time low, muttering delirium and a moist skin, presents a considerable degree of resemblance to delirium tremens. There is very often intolerance of light, tinnitus aurium, and loss or perversion of the senses of taste and smell. Deafness is also not uncommon, and is regarded by many authors as a favorable symptom. In bad cases, in addition to subsultus tendinum, there are carphologia, incontinence or retention of the urine, and paralysis of the sphincter ani.

Some discrepancy is found to exist in the statements of different authors in regard to the temperature curves of typhus fever. They all agree, however, in assigning them certain characters, the knowledge of which is often of great assistance in diagnosis. One of these is a rapid rise of temperature immediately after the invasion of the disease. Wunderlich[23]asserts that he has observed a temperature of 104.9° F. on the evening of the first day, and Lebert has found it as high as 106.4° F. on that of the second. Such temperatures, occurring so early in the disease, must be infrequent, as Murchison has never met with them. Usually, the temperature attains its maximum on the third or fourth day. The maximum is about 104° or 105° F. Murchison says it scarcely ever reaches 106°, except in children, in whom it rarely is as high as 107°, but Lebert states that he has known it to be as high as 107.8°. On the other hand, it may never exceed 103°, even in fatal cases. When the maximum is attained early in the disease there may be for several days, or until defervescence takes place, very little variation in the evening temperatures, but, as a general rule, they are slightly less elevated in the second than in the first week. This usually occurs from the tenth to the fourteenth day, but it may be postponed until the eighteenth, or even until much later. In some cases on the day before the crisis a slight fall, and in others a considerable fall with a subsequent rise of temperature, are observed. Defervescence is often very rapid, the temperature falling five or six degrees in the course of twelve hours. A true lysis is rarely observed. The occurrence of a complication in the course of a disease will not only cause a decided rise of temperature and a modification of the temperature curve, but may also postpone defervescence beyond the usual time. Not infrequently the thermometer indicates subnormal morning temperatures with slight evening rises for several days after the crisis, unless complications arise,[p. 350]when fever of the hectic type may occur. A very slight cause will also often produce a considerable, although temporary, elevation of temperature in this condition. The morning remissions are less decided than in typhoid fever, especially in the first week. As a rule, they do not exceed 1°, but Lebert lays stress upon the fact that in the same curve variations from 0.3° to 1.8° and from 0.6° to 2.1° often occur. Cases which terminate fatally are generally characterized by high fever, with absence of the morning remissions, which may continue uninterruptedly through the second and even the third week. During the death-agony there is frequently a rise of temperature of two or more degrees. A very high temperature in the first week is often the forerunner of severe cerebral symptoms in the second, and a fall of temperature unaccompanied by an improvement in the other symptoms is not always indicative of the approach of convalescence.

[23] *On the Temperature in Disease*, New Sydenham Society's translation, London, 1871.

Anorexia is generally present in typhus fever from the beginning of the attack, and may persist until its close. It is not, however, usually attended by the same repugnance for food as in other fevers. Patients can generally be persuaded at first to take nourishment. Indeed, Dr. Gerhard asserts that the negroes who fell under his care in 1832 frequently asked for solid food. Nausea and vomiting are rare symptoms; the latter may occur late in the disease, and then, not infrequently, is caused by irritation of the brain. Thirst is present in all cases. In the later stages of the disease, when the senses are blunted, water may not be asked for, although urgently called for by the condition of the system. The bowels are, as a rule, constipated in this disease. The exceptions to this rule are, however, more numerous than is usually thought. Wood[24] says that he has frequently seen diarrhoea in typhus fever when it occurs in recently-arrived immigrants. Da Costa[25] mentions that it has occurred in several of the cases which have come under his care, and Buchanan[26] says that he has observed it in at least one-third of the patients admitted into the London Fever Hospital in recent years. When there is no diarrhoea the stools are of normal color and consistence. When it exists they are watery and usually dark greenish in color, and never present the peculiar ochrey-yellow appearance seen in typhoid fever. They are said to be alkaline in reaction. Tympanites is rare in typhus fever. It may be present in cases in which there is diarrhoea, and may then be associated with gurgling in the bowels, but rarely attains the degree common in typhoid fever. Gurgling when present is, moreover, not confined to the right ileo-cæcal region, but may be produced in different parts of the abdomen by pressure. There may also be tenderness in the epigastric and hepatic regions, but the enlargement of the spleen so constantly observed in typhoid is generally wholly wanting in this fever.

[24] *Loc. cit.*
[25] *Loc. cit.*
[26] *Loc. cit.*

The tongue in the beginning of the disease is covered with a thin whitish fur and is moist, and may continue so throughout in mild attacks. Generally, however, it soon becomes dryish, and in bad cases absolutely dry, and is tremulous when put out of the mouth, while its coating becomes thicker and brownish, and finally brown, or even black and cracked. It is rare to see the tongue itself fissured as in typhoid fever. Less frequently it remains red, smooth, and glazed throughout the attack. Occasionally the tongue is contracted in bulk, and it may [p. 351]then, in consequence of its dryness and that of the mouth, be impossible to protrude it. Sordes frequently collect about the gums and lips in severe cases.

The pulse is usually increased in frequency in typhus fever, and varies from 100 to 120, but in many cases it never rises above 90, and in very severe cases it may be as high as 150. This increase is observed from the beginning, and generally bears some proportion to the severity of the fever; but toward the close, when the prostration is great, the pulse may continue frequent even after a fall in temperature has taken place, and is always more frequent when the patient is sitting up than when he is lying down. Occasionally, however, a very slow pulse is associated with symptoms of great severity. When this association occurs the prognosis is grave. In the young and robust the pulse may be full and bounding, but it is more often compressible or small and weak. It is not so often dicrotic as in typhoid fever.

There is sometimes, according to Lyons, a singular want of uniformity in the force and volume of the arterial pulse in different parts of the system, and there may be but one pulsation at the wrist for two of the heart. A very sudden fall in the frequency of the pulse without an improvement in the other symptoms is not a favorable indication, as it may be due to impaired innervation or to degenerative changes in the muscular tissue of the heart. Usually the beginning of convalescence is marked by a gradual fall of the pulse. Later it may fall to 50 or below it, and continue slow for some time, just as it does in typhoid fever.

The heart shares in the general enfeeblement of the system. In severe attacks the impulse soon becomes weak and diffused, and may be entirely absent for some time even in cases which eventually terminate in recovery. Stokes long ago called attention to an alteration in the systolic sound of the heart which he taught indicated the urgent necessity for the administration of stimulants. This sound is observed in the progress of the disease to become shorter and less distinct, and finally inaudible, while the second sound is unaffected. This modification of the heart-sounds is always an accompaniment of great prostration. Occasionally the first sound is replaced by a functional murmur.

The characteristic eruption of the disease is generally preceded by the fainter subcuticular mottling already alluded to, and usually appears between the fourth and seventh days, but it has been observed as early as the third day, and, on the other hand, its appearance is said by Wood to have been delayed until the thirteenth. It consists of minute spots with ill-defined margins, varying in size from that of the point of a pin to two or three lines in diameter, irregular in shape, slightly elevated above the skin at first only, and occurring singly or in groups. They are pinkish in color, and disappear readily under pressure when first observed. They may then, as Gerhard and others have pointed out, present a considerable resemblance to the rose-colored spots of typhoid fever. In the course of twenty-four hours they become brownish, and later, when the attack is a severe one, livid in color. In malignant or even severe cases they are frequently converted into true petechiæ. They do not appear in successive crops, but usually require a couple of days for their full development. Their duration is variable. In mild attacks they may disappear in the course of a few days, but in bad cases often [p. 352]persist until after convalescence, and are recognizable after death. They are confined to no part of the body, but appear usually earliest and most abundantly upon the folds of the axilla and upon the abdomen. Occasionally, however, they are first observed upon the wrists, and in some cases are more numerous upon the arms and legs than upon the body. They are rarely found upon the neck and face, but in children the latter may be so much covered by them that the disease may be readily mistaken for measles. They present some resemblance to flea-bites, but the latter may be easily distinguished from them by the minute discoloration in the centre left by the puncture of the insect. The eruption is oftenest wanting in young subjects. It is usually, but not invariably, most copious in severe attacks, but cases have ended fatally in which it was wholly wanting from beginning to end. Its color is also to a certain extent an index of the severity of the attack; the darker and more livid it is, the graver the prognosis. In malignant cases or those complicated by scurvy, in addition to the petechiæ above referred to, purpura spots and vibices are not infrequently observed. Some authors assert that the eruption is followed by a slight desquamation of the cuticle, but this is denied by others. Sudamina occasionally occur, but they are much rarer than in typhoid fever. The blue spots described by the French under the name of tâches bleuâtres are also sometimes met with.

A very disagreeable odor is exhaled from the bodies of typhus-fever patients after the first week. Although readily recognizable by those who have once perceived it, it is difficult to describe. Gerhard spoke of it as pungent, ammoniacal, and offensive, especially in fat, plethoric individuals, and believed that those patients who presented this symptom in the highest degree were most likely to communicate the disease to others. Murchison has also expressed the opinion that the typhus poison is associated with this odoriferous substance. Others have compared the odor to the smell given off by rotten straw, the urine of mice, and various other substances. Wood says that he has often perceived the same odor in badly-ventilated rooms in which a number of people have been shut up together for some time.

The sensibility of the skin in cases in which the stupor is not so great as to render the patients insensible to all external impressions is said by some writers to be much increased.

There is also occasionally so much tenderness in the epigastric region as to give the impression at first to the attendant that there is inflammation of the stomach or liver.

Pulmonary complications are quite frequent in typhus fever, and, as they often come on insidiously and give no evidence of their presence by cough, expectoration, or even more hurried breathing, that is often seen in uncomplicated cases, it is well to make it a rule to examine the chest of every patient with this disease. To do this thoroughly it is not necessary to make him sit up, which, where great prostration exists, is often attended with danger. If he be turned gently upon his side the auscultator will usually have no difficulty in ascertaining the precise condition of his lungs.

The respiration is usually much more frequent in this disease than in health. Even in cases in which there is no disease of the lungs it is often as high as 30, and in cases in which there is such a complication it may be 60. Its frequency is generally proportional to the severity of [p. 353]the fever. On the other hand, in grave cases in which cerebral symptoms are predominant it may be reduced in frequency much below the normal. When coma or profound stupor exists, it may become jerking and spasmodic, or even simulate the stertorous respiration of apoplexy. Bronchitis, if not of such constant occurrence as in typhoid fever, is certainly not rare. It usually occurs early in the attack, and makes itself known by the presence of sonorous and sibilant râles, which give place later to mucous râles. Expectoration is often absent in these cases; where it exists the sputa are either mucous or muco-purulent. In mild cases no further lesion of the lungs occurs. When the attack is more severe hypostatic congestion is very likely to supervene. This is a condition which is often attended with danger, and which frequently, as has been said already, escapes recognition unless the chest be thoroughly examined, when dullness on percussion, feeble respiration, and subcrepitant râles may readily be detected. Occasionally the physical signs indicate the existence of pneumonia. This, when it occurs in the course of this disease, is always of low grade, and is attended by the expectoration of mucus streaked with blood.

The breath of the typhus-fever patient has a very disagreeable odor, not unlike that given off from the body, and is said by Murchison to contain an increased amount of ammonia.

According to Parkes,[27] the changes in the urine are those usual in ordinary pyrexia. During the fever it is generally diminished in quantity, dark in color, and of high specific gravity. It contains an increased amount of urea and of uric acid, the latter of which is not infrequently spontaneously precipitated. Sulphuric acid is also in excess. On the other hand, the chlorides are diminished in amount or entirely absent. This diminution cannot be ascribed to a decrease in the quantity ingested, for when they are administered with the food they are not found to be eliminated by the kidney. The amount of phosphoric acid does not appear to be affected by the disease. The urine is acid in reaction at first, but its acidity soon diminishes, and it may become alkaline toward the close of bad cases. It may also contain albumen, or even blood, the former being present oftenest in cases characterized by high temperature. According to Da Costa, tube-casts are more often present than absent in severe cases. Those seen by this observer were either coated with rather opaque epithelial cells, many of which were finely granular or covered with granules, which, when tested with reagents, were sparingly soluble in acetic acid, and which with very high magnifying powers did not present the round shape of oil, and were probably the urinary salts collected in the tube-casts. The crisis is sometimes marked by a copious deposit of urates. During convalescence the urine is usually increased in quantity, is pale and limpid, and of low specific gravity, and is found to contain the chlorides in gradually increasing quantity.

[27] *The Composition of the Urine, etc.*, by Edmund A. Parkes, M.D., London, 1860.

VARIETIES.—Many of the varieties of typhus fever recognized by authors—as, for example, jail fever, ship fever, camp fever, and hospital fever—really differ in nothing but name and the circumstances under which the disease has arisen. Others are mere modifications of it, due to the predominance of one symptom or of a certain set of symptoms or to the intercurrence of a particular complication, and likewise do not [p. 354]need a full description here. To this latter class belong the inflammatory typhus, the nervous or ataxic typhus, the adynamic typhus, and the ataxo-adynamic typhus of Murchison. The first variety occurs in young and robust subjects, and, it is also said, in persons of the upper class. It is characterized by high fever, intense headache, and active delirium. In the second variety the nervous symptoms, such as delirium, somnolence, stupor, and muscular tremblings, are the most prominent. The most marked feature of the third variety is the excessive prostration, which is shown in the feebleness of the heart's action and the loss of muscular strength and of control over the sphincters. In this form the eruption is dark colored. Purpura spots and vibices also are very apt to appear, and even hemorrhages from the gums, nose, or other parts to occur. In the ataxo-adynamic form the symptoms of the ataxic and those of the adynamic form are found united. In addition to these there are certain other varieties, arising from differences in degree. These differences are sometimes owing to diversities in the constitution and habits of the patient, sometimes to variations in the character of the epidemic, and are sometimes not readily explainable. One of these is the mild form, in which the symptoms are those of moderate fever, and in which the disease may run its course in seven days. In this form the temperature may never rise above 102° F., the eruption be absent or very scanty, and the characteristic stupor or dulness be wholly wanting. Unless complications arise recovery invariably takes place. A walking form of typhus fever, as has already been said, is much rarer than of typhoid, but it does sometimes occur, Dr. Buchanan having often seen the eruption out upon patients who have walked to the London Fever Hospital to seek admission. In this form the disease, however, does not always run a mild course, as alarming prostration is very apt to come on later in its course. Another variety, the abortive form, has been described by authors. In this an individual, in due time after exposure to the contagion, may present all the characteristic symptoms of typhus fever, but the disease, instead of running its usual course, may terminate abruptly with a critical discharge of some kind. This form occurs during epidemics, and is analogous to the abortive attack of scarlet fever or some other diseases which are occasionally met with. On the other hand, a very severe form, the typhus siderans of authors, also sometimes occurs. In this variety the temperature rises rapidly, and soon attains its maximum; there are frequent pulse and respiration, severe headache, and early delirium and stupor. The mortality in this form is very great. Very frequently death takes place so rapidly as often to leave the physician in some doubt as to the nature of the disease in those cases in which exposure to the contagion cannot be positively traced.

COMPLICATIONS AND SEQUELÆ.—The complications of typhus fever often exercise a decided influence upon the course of the disease, for they not only retard convalescence, but are often the immediate cause of death. Their early detection, therefore, becomes a matter of the greatest importance. They will be found to vary in different years, one epidemic being characterized by complications which are entirely wanting in the next. Among the commonest of them are several different conditions of the respiratory organs. Bronchitis, if not quite so frequent as in typhoid fever, occurs in a large number of cases. It may come on at any stage [p. 355]of the disease, either immediately after the beginning of the attack or in its course, or not until convalescence. In cases accompanied by prostration mucus may accumulate in the bronchial tubes, and be the cause of the patient's death by preventing the due aëration of the blood. It would seem to be an especially frequent complication in Ireland, and it is rather surprising that so acute an observer as Graves appears not to have been aware of its real relation to typhus, and speaks of it as if it were a predisposing cause. "Nothing can be more remarkable," he says, "than the facility with which a simple cold, which in England would be perfectly devoid of danger, runs into maculated typhus in Ireland, and that, too, under circumstances quite free from even the suspicion of contagion; in truth, except when fever is epidemic, taking cold is its most usual cause." A much more serious complication than bronchitis is the form of pneumonia already alluded to as liable to occur in the course of typhus. This may often occur so insidiously that it may be considerably advanced before its presence is even suspected; hence the necessity for examining carefully the lungs of every patient with this disease who comes under our care. Generally, however, it makes itself known by giving rise to rapid breathing and great lividity of the surface, but, as has already been said, both of these symptoms may exist in cases in which there is no chest complication. This pneumonia, if it does not immediately prove fatal, may, by becoming chronic, retard the convalescence. It occasionally is followed by gangrene, and sometimes by phthisis, which may then run a very rapid course. Phthisis is, however, a much less frequent sequela of typhus than of typhoid fever. Pleurisy may also complicate typhus fever, but it is much more rarely met with than pneumonia.

Perhaps next in frequency to pneumonia and bronchitis are diseases of the kidneys. These are very serious complications, whether they antedate the fever or have occurred in its course. Careful examination of the urine will generally lead to the discovery of a small amount of albuminuria in bad cases, but this is fortunately, in the majority of them, only temporary. The urine should, however, always be re-examined before the discharge of the patient, as there is good reason to believe that many otherwise inexplicable cases of chronic albuminuria have originated in an attack of typhus. The presence of albumen and of casts in the urine of a patient apparently convalescent from this disease should therefore make us careful in our prognosis as to his future health. The occurrence of diarrhoea may also very seriously affect the patient's chances of recovery. Dysentery has also been observed in certain epidemics in Ireland, and is not infrequent when the disease breaks out in besieged towns or when it occurs in summer. In grave cases or those complicated with scurvy the blood may be so broken down as to escape readily from the vessels. Under these circumstances, in addition to the purpura spots beneath the skin, we may have epistaxis, hæmoptysis, hæmatemesis, intestinal hemorrhage, or hemorrhage from any other part. Erysipelas, too, may be a troublesome complication, for not only does it exhaust the strength, but, when it invades the mucous membrane of the larynx, as it sometimes does, it may prove rapidly fatal by producing oedema of the glottis. Degeneration of the muscular structure of the heart may also take place. This gives rise to a slow and feeble pulse and to a disposition to syncope. Bed-sores are not so frequent as in typhoid fever. They [p. 356]do, however, sometimes occur, as does also gangrene of the toes and of other parts not subjected to pressure.

Less common complications are jaundice, peri- and endo-carditis, meningitis, local and general paralyses, cancrum oris, a diffuse cellular inflammation ending in purulent infiltration, and inflammatory swellings of the glands, or buboes. The salivary glands—and especially the parotid gland—are very apt to be affected by this inflammatory swelling. This occurs rapidly, is very tender, and in most cases soon runs on to suppuration, although it occasionally in children spontaneously subsides. It may occur at any time during the course of the fever, or not until convalescence, and sometimes affects the glands of both sides of the face. These buboes form a connecting link between typhus fever and the Oriental plague, and Murchison says that the distinguished Egyptian physician Clot Bey, on seeing some cases of the former disease complicated with parotid swellings, declared that in Egypt they would be regarded as examples of the latter.

Many of the above-named complications may occur also as sequelæ, and in addition to these we may have pyæmia, giving rise to purulent collections in the joints and phlegmasia alba dolens. The last named is not in itself serious. Its chief danger is from the breaking down of the clot and the subsequent occurrence of embolism.

Menstruation is said not to be uncommon in the early stages of typhus fever, and may be so profuse as to greatly increase the prostration or even to cause death. According to Murchison, miscarriage does not inevitably occur when pregnant women are attacked with the disease, and if it does occur it is not necessarily fatal to either mother or child.

POST-MORTEM APPEARANCES.—Emaciation when death has occurred early in the course of the disease, and is due solely to the violence of the fever, is usually not well marked, but in those cases which have been protracted through the intercurrence of complications it may sometimes reach an extreme degree. Bed-sores, except under the circumstances just mentioned, are also rare. Rigor mortis is generally not well developed, and is of short duration. In a few cases it would seem, however, to have been well marked. The typhus maculæ are persistent after death, and so are any purpura spots and vibices which may have been present during life, but the subcuticular mottling usually disappears. The skin of the dependent portions of the body is discolored by the settling of blood in it, and putrefactive changes are apt to set in rapidly.

The only constant lesion observed is a profound alteration of the blood, which is darker in color and abnormally fluid. If clots are found at all, they are large, soft, and friable. The fibrin is diminished in amount. In the early part of the disease the red blood-corpuscles are said to be slightly increased in number, but later they are diminished, and under the microscope are observed to be crenated and not to form themselves readily into rouleaux. The white corpuscles are increased in number. No accurate chemical examination of the blood appears to have been made. Many of the post-mortem appearances which have been described as characteristics of typhus fever are really the consequence of this abnormal condition of the blood.

The respiratory organs generally present evidences of disease; the lesions of laryngitis, bronchitis, pneumonia, hypostatic congestion of the [p. 357]lungs, and pleurisy have all been observed after death from typhus fever. Usually, the traces of previous inflammation of the larynx are but slight; in a few cases, however, ulceration has been found, but the ulcers are stated to be always minute and superficial. Ulcers are also occasionally found in the bronchi, and frequently indicate by their appearance the pre-existence of a much higher grade of inflammation. The bronchial mucous membrane is, however, oftener merely reddened and softened and covered with a tenacious frothy secretion. True pneumonia is of infrequent occurrence as compared with that of hypostatic congestion of the lungs, but it nevertheless does occur, and may be of either the catarrhal or croupous variety. When pleurisy exists, it is usually accompanied, according to Murchison, by purulent effusion into the pleural cavity. On the other hand, Lebert says the variety of inflammation of the pleura oftenest met with is the plastic. The intestines present no constant lesion. Gerhard says that in fifty examinations there was but in one case, and that doubtful in diagnosis, the slightest deviation from the natural appearance of the glands of Peyer. In a few cases the Peyer's patches have been found more prominent than usual, but not more so than they are in measles and in some other diseases. Lebert alone of recent authors makes a contrary statement. In an epidemic at Breslau, he says, the solitary glands, as well as the patches of Peyer, were the seat of small, isolated, and superficial ulcers, which were usually situated in the vicinity of the ileo-cæcal valve. The mesenteric glands are generally unaffected, but in the Breslau epidemic just referred to they were not infrequently found moderately swollen. In cases in which dysentery has occurred as a complication the characteristic appearances of the disease will of course be observed, as well as those of typhus fever. The spleen is generally softened and slightly enlarged. The enlargement is not, however, always present, as Gerhard found it in one only out of every five or six of the cases which he examined. Extravasations of blood into its structure are occasionally met with. The liver is usually congested, somewhat enlarged, and frequently under the microscope presents the appearances of commencing fatty degeneration. The kidneys often present unmistakable signs of renal disease in the swollen granular and more or less fatty condition of their gland-cells according to the duration of the disease. The muscles are darker in color than in health. Under the microscope they are found to have undergone the peculiar granular or waxy degeneration described by Zenker, and which have been fully referred to in the article on typhoid fever. Extravasations of blood are occasionally found in them, which may soften and form pseudo-abscesses.

Other post-mortem appearances which are met with less frequently than those above detailed are inflammation, and even ulceration, of the mucous membrane, of the bladder, inflammation of the salivary gland, peritonitis, and congestion of the pancreas and of the stomach.

The muscular tissue of the heart is generally softened and easily torn. It is not, however, as stated by some authors, invariably so, for in several cases in which it was examined by Da Costa it had undergone this change in one case only, in which there was no reason to suspect previous disease of the heart. The alteration is similar in kind to that which takes place in the voluntary muscles. An effusion of serum, which may be of a deep-red color from the transudation of the coloring matter of the blood, is[p. 358]sometimes found in the pericardial sac, as are ecchymotic patches upon the surface of the heart. The endocardium may be stained from the imbibition of blood. On the other hand, endo- and peri-carditis are excessively rare.

Notwithstanding the severity of the cerebral symptoms in typhus fever, there are few or no important changes found in the brain or its membranes after death. The sinuses are occasionally filled with dark fluid blood, and the appearances of congestion of the brain are sometimes present. In other cases there may be an increased amount of serum beneath the arachnoid and into the lateral ventricles, but not more than is often seen after death from other causes. Very rarely a slight film of hemorrhage has been found in the cavity of the arachnoid, and sometimes also the evidences of non-inflammatory softening of the brain. Actual inflammation of the meninges has only been detected in a very few cases. There may also be congestion of the spinal membranes, increase of the spinal fluid, and softening of the cord itself. The ganglia of the sympathetic system appear to undergo a form of granular degeneration.

DIAGNOSIS.—The diseases which most closely resemble typhus fever are typhoid fever, measles, meningitis, and typhoid pneumonia.

The circumstances under which typhoid and typhus fever occur are different. Typhoid is never generated by overcrowding, and if contagious at all is much less so than typhus. Prostration occurs much earlier and is usually much more marked in the latter. The eruption in the former does not appear until the eighth day, and comes out in successive crops, and usually disappears under pressure as long as it lasts, and therefore may be easily distinguished from that of the latter. The duration of typhus is from ten to twenty days; that of typhoid is rarely less than twenty-one. Nevertheless, cases are occasionally met with in which it is impossible to arrive at a correct conclusion as to their nature unless some light is thrown upon it by the existence of other and more characteristic cases in the same house or neighborhood. I have recently had under my care a case which eventually proved to be typhoid fever, but which I and many others who saw it at first believed to be typhus in consequence of the presence of an abundant eruption, which did not disappear under pressure, and was finally converted into petechiæ.

The eruption of typhus is sometimes found upon the face, especially in children, and then presents a considerable similarity to that of measles, which, however, usually appears a little earlier. There is, moreover, rarely the same amount of prostration or stupor in the latter disease, which is also attended by coryza and more bronchial catarrh than is often present in the former. The eruptions in the two diseases differ. In measles it is crescentic in shape, and is more elevated than in typhus. It is also brighter in color, disappears under pressure, except in malignant cases, as long as it lasts, and is followed by free desquamation of the cuticle, which is not often observed in typhus. The temperature may be high in the former, but it usually falls upon the sixth day.

In meningitis the headache is much more severe, and does not disappear upon the occurrence of delirium. It may be so severe as to cause the patient to cry out. The senses are painfully acute. There are intolerance of light and sound, and some hypersensitiveness of the surface, [p. 359]strabismus, inequality of the pupils or some other local paralysis, and retraction of the head. Nausea and vomiting are more common than in typhus, while the utter prostration of the latter disease is wholly wanting, and so is of course the characteristic eruption. The tâche meningitique is wanting in the latter, but too much reliance should not be placed upon either the presence or absence of this sign. The diagnosis is only likely to be difficult in those cases of typhus in which the delirium is active. In that form of typhus in which the symptoms simulate those of delirium tremens some difficulty may also be experienced in making a diagnosis, especially if the patient be a drunkard. In delirium tremens it will be remembered, however, that there is little or no elevation of temperature, that the skin is bathed in perspiration, the tongue moist, and the characteristic eruption absent. Typhoid pneumonia can be distinguished from pneumonia complicating typhus fever by the presence of the eruption in the latter.

Other diseases which have occasionally been mistaken for typhus fever are remittent fever, Bright's disease, giving rise to uræmia and purpura. It does not seem likely that even the severest forms of malarial fever should ever present such a resemblance to typhus fever as to make the differential diagnosis a matter of difficulty; but it would appear from the history of the latter disease given by Murchison that such a mistake has occurred in some of the Spanish American countries. The enlargement of the spleen and liver is much less marked than in remittent fever, and the remissions of temperature are much less decided. Uræmia may at times present a good deal of resemblance to the condition often seen in typhus fever after the supervention of coma or stupor, but the history of the case, the absence of fever and of eruption in the former, will generally enable us to distinguish between the two conditions. It should be remembered, however, that Bright's disease may occur in the course of typhus fever. Purpura may generally be recognized by the absence of fever and by the occurrence of hemorrhages from the nose, gums, and bowels.

PROGNOSIS.—The age, habits of life, and previous condition of health, as well as the character of the prevailing epidemic, must all be fully considered before making a prognosis in any special case. The disease usually runs a much milder course in children and young people than in adults past thirty years of age. After this age the mortality progressively increases, and in advanced life it becomes very high, being often as much as 50 per cent. or over. Sex does not of itself exercise much influence upon the course of typhus fever, for, although a few more men than women die of it, this appears to be attributable to the greater prevalence of drinking among the former. Previous intemperance acts unfavorably by producing a degeneration of the tissues of the body, thus rendering the patient less able to withstand the effects of the disease. Drunkards have therefore always furnished a large proportion of the fatal cases. The mortality among patients who are unfortunate enough to take typhus fever as they are convalescing from other diseases is usually also very great. This has often been observed in general hospitals in which cases of fever as well as those of other forms of disease are admitted. Fat, lymphatic, or muscular people more frequently die of it than those of a different conformation. Gerhard found it especially [p. 360]fatal among negroes in the epidemic of 1836, and Buchanan seems to have had a similar experience at the London Fever Hospital. It is a fact noticed by English writers that people of the better class, although seldom attacked by typhus, often suffer severely from it. The mortality is always high among those patients who previously to contracting the disease have been for some time deprived of sufficient food, or have been overworked, or who have been the subjects of mental anxiety, worry, or any other depressing emotion. It is high also among those who in the beginning of the disease have exhausted their strength in the vain effort to resist the disposition to go to bed. The chances of recovery are, on the other hand, very much improved by the removal of patients from crowded, ill-ventilated houses to the wards of a spacious, airy hospital.

Unfavorable symptoms are a profuse dark-colored eruption associated with purpura spots and vibices, general lividity of the surface, great injection of the pupils, and a dusky hue of the countenance; extreme prostration; an excessively frequent and feeble pulse, especially if it is at the same time irregular or intermittent; absence of the cardiac impulse and of the systolic sound; hurried and spasmodic or abnormally slow respiration; great dryness and retraction of the tongue; excessive prominence of the nervous symptoms, such as headache, delirium, whether active or muttering; unequal or pin-hole contraction of the pupils; strabismus or other local paralysis; sleeplessness; muscular tremblings; subsultus tendinum; carphology; protracted hiccough; retention of the urine; relaxation of the sphincters of the bladder and rectum; coma and especially coma vigil, and convulsions; continued high temperature, rising instead of falling after the tenth day, especially if it is associated with coldness of the extremities and of the breath; a profuse perspiration without a general improvement in the symptoms; diminution in the quantity of the urine, or the presence in it of albumen, blood, or casts; vomiting; and diarrhoea. Hope, however, should never be abandoned even in the most unfavorable cases, as recovery has sometimes occurred when the patient seemed almost in articulo mortis. Convulsions are said to be invariably followed by death, and Graves regarded the presence of the pin-hole contraction of the pupils as of very grave import.

Favorable symptoms are—reduction of the frequency of the pulse, a fall of temperature, a diminution of the stupor or a resumption of consciousness, and a return of appetite and of moisture to the tongue. When the patient begins to improve he will often without assistance turn upon his side after having lain for a long time upon his back, and this change of position is sometimes the first indication of the approach of convalescence.

The mortality varies of course in different epidemics. The cases which have come under my own care being too few in number to draw deductions from on this point, I must rely upon the experience of those whose field of observation has been more extended than my own. According to Murchison, out of 18,268 cases of typhus fever admitted into the London Fever Hospital during twenty-three years, 3457 proved fatal, making a mortality of

18.92 per cent., or 1 in 5.28. Deducting 686 cases fatal within forty-eight hours, the mortality falls to 15.76 per cent., or 1 in 6.34. Included among the fatal cases is a large number in which [p. 361]the disease had run its course to a favorable termination, and in which death was really due to sequelæ, such as pneumonia, erysipelas, etc. Moreover, the death-rate in the hospital is greater than in the community, because children, who rarely die of typhus fever, are seldom brought to it; while, on the other hand, it receives a large number of the infirm and aged inmates of the metropolitan workhouses. Making allowance for these sources of fallacy, Murchison believes that the actual mortality of typhus is not more than 10 per cent. In Gerhard's cases the proportion of deaths amongst the black was much greater than amongst the white men; thus, of the whites 1 died in $4^2/3$, of the blacks 1 in $2^{19}/28$. Amongst the women the reverse was true; thus, 1 white woman died in $4^3/5$, but only 1 colored woman in $6½$, nearly. Da Costa lost 6 out of 39 cases. In one of the fatal cases the diagnosis was doubtful; in another there was a great deal of previous disease; in two others death was due to complications—so that there were but two in which the fatal result could fairly be attributed to the disease itself.

TREATMENT.—Typhus fever is an eminently preventible disease. It is therefore proper that the description of its curative treatment should be preceded by a few words in regard to its prophylaxis.

It is still an unsettled question whether or not typhus fever ever occurs de novo, and although the recent discovery by Klebs and others of bacillus peculiar to typhoid fever (the bacillus typhosus), and of special bacilli in other analogous diseases, renders it highly probable that typhus fever has also its own bacillus, and that therefore it is not likely to arise except as the result of infection, it must be admitted that it has often prevailed in localities into which it has not been possible to trace its importation. Under these circumstances it will be well to refer to those conditions which are asserted by some authors to favor its spontaneous generation, especially as these same conditions are certainly known to favor its propagation. It will not be necessary to do this at any great length, as they have all been fully described in discussing the etiology of the disease. The most important of them is the overcrowding of human beings, especially when combined with deficient ventilation, destitution, and want of personal cleanliness. The knowledge of the laws of hygiene is now so universally diffused that this combination of conditions never occurs at the present time to anything like the degree it often existed in the eighteenth century, and consequently epidemics of this disease are not only less frequent, but are also much milder in character, than formerly. Much work, however, still remains for sanitarians in the improvement of the homes of the poor, which even in this country are too often overcrowded and ill-ventilated.

The extension of the disease in a community will almost always be prevented by the prompt isolation of the first few cases. This can often be thoroughly done, if the patient is in easy circumstances, by placing him in an upper room, which should be stripped of its carpets, curtains, and other unnecessary furniture; by cutting off all communication between him and his attendants and the rest of the household; and by the free use of disinfectants. The room should be airy, and to ensure good ventilation a window should be left partly open. This may be done during the febrile stage, even in winter, without the risk of any injury to the patient. Among the poorer classes, however, [p. 362]isolation can rarely be effectually carried out, and it is therefore much better to remove the patient to a hospital. Upon the admission of such a patient to an institution of this character his clothes should be at once disinfected. This may be done by washing the underclothing in a disinfecting fluid, and then exposing them to a free current of air, and by subjecting the outer clothing to a very high temperature in an oven or to the fumes of burning sulphur. Murchison believes that a neglect of this precaution has often been the cause of the extension of the disease to other inmates of the hospital, especially when the patient resumes during his convalescence the same clothing he wore upon admission. If the hospital is a general one, he should be placed, whenever practicable, in a well-ventilated ward by himself or with other patients suffering from the same disease. As this is not always possible, the number of the other occupants of the ward should be reduced and their beds placed as far away as possible from his. As the infectiousness of typhus fever is very much lessened by free ventilation, this precaution is often alone sufficient to prevent its extension to them. It is also well, however, to supplement it by the use of disinfectants. The diffusion of a solution of carbolic acid in the atmosphere of the ward by means of the steam atomizer has not only rendered the odor emanating from the patient less perceptible, but has also appeared to diminish decidedly the risk of infection. As a still further precaution the patient may be sponged with a weak solution of carbolic acid or some other disinfectant. His nurses should be selected, whenever practicable, from among those who have had the disease themselves. They should never sleep in the sick room, lounge about the patient's bed, or inhale his breath. They should be allowed a certain amount of time every day for rest and recreation in the fresh air, and should have a full supply of nourishing food. On the other hand, they should be warned against the danger of over-stimulation, which is often resorted to in the hope of warding off the disease, and should be relieved as far as possible from attendance upon other patients. It may be well here to say that the nursing of a case of typhus fever should never be undertaken by the relatives or friends of the patient, except as a matter of necessity. Not only do the anxiety and distress they naturally feel unnerve them and render them unfit to carry out the directions of the physician, but they can rarely execute the many offices required in the sick room with half the skill of a trained nurse or with so little annoyance to the patient.

Before the patient is allowed to leave his ward he should have a warm bath. If the disease has occurred in a private house, the room which he has occupied should be thoroughly disinfected. This is best done by replastering, repapering, and repainting it. In many cases, however, it will be sufficient to fumigate it with burning sulphur, and then to air it for several days. The bed and bedding should also be disinfected, and, where this cannot be thoroughly done, the latter had better be destroyed.

Of primary importance in the treatment of typhus fever is the regulation of the diet. Although there are no ulcers in the bowels in this as in typhoid fever, and although, consequently, there is not the same imperative necessity in this as in the latter disease to restrict the patient to liquid articles of food, experience has shown that such articles are much more readily digested and assimilated than solids. The diet [p. 363]should consist, therefore, of milk, beef-tea, and chicken or mutton broth. Of all of these, milk is incomparably the best, and it should form, unless the patient manifest an unconquerable repugnance to its use, a large part of the nourishment in every case. Farinaceous articles of food are generally not well borne in this fever, because the diminution in the secretion of the salivary glands which almost always exists prevents their proper digestion. After the third or fourth day nourishment should be given in small quantities at short intervals, as every two hours, every hour, or even every half hour when the prostration is extreme. It should be the aim of the physician to give an adult at least two quarts of milk or their equivalent daily.

It is sometimes necessary to put a delirious patient under some restraint to prevent him from leaving his bed or doing some other act of violence. Frequently a judicious nurse will be able to accomplish this without the use of an undue amount of force, but at other times it will be necessary to have recourse to mechanical means of restraint. Usually, all that is necessary is to pass a folded sheet across the patient's chest, the ends of which are fastened to the sides of his bed.

It is now a universally accepted axiom among physicians that typhus fever is a self-limited disease, and that any attempts to cut it short is worse than useless. Not only do remedies which are employed for this purpose often produce alarming prostration, but there can be no doubt that they have in some cases been the cause of a fatal termination, which under another plan of treatment would have been averted. During the last century it was not uncommon to bleed, and to bleed largely, in the beginning of an attack of typhus fever, but even then there were physicians—as, for instance, O'Connell, Rogers,[28] Pringle,[29] and Rutty[30]—who raised a warning voice against the practice. Sir John Pringle goes so far as to say that "many have recovered without bleeding, but few who have lost much blood." A very similar opinion was also expressed by Baron Larrey in the early part of this century. Indeed, it is very evident that the same difference of opinion existed as to the employment of venesection in the treatment of acute affections when these authors wrote as prevailed in England and this country until within the last thirty years, and that the disastrous results which occasionally follow the abstraction of large amounts of blood from patients affected with fevers and inflammations were as fully recognized then as now by many physicians. This would seem effectually to dispose of the change-of-type-in-disease theory which was generally accepted in the first half of this century as sufficient to explain the fact which could no longer be overlooked that this class of patients did much better under a supporting than a depleting plan of treatment. Purgatives were also at one time freely given for the purpose of arresting the disease, but the results obtained from their use were scarcely less unfavorable, and they are now never employed with this view. The use of quinia in large doses has also been advocated for the same purpose, but experience, while it has shown that it is a valuable remedy, has demonstrated also that it does not possess[p. 364]this power. Exactly the same thing may be said of the cold-water treatment of typhus fever. There is no evidence that it has ever shortened the duration of the disease.

[28] *An Essay on Epidemic Diseases*, p. 60, by Joseph Rogers, M.D., Dublin, 1734.
[29] *Loc. cit.*
[30] *A Chronological History of the Weather and Seasons, and the Prevailing Diseases, in Dublin during the Space of Forty Years*, by John Rutty, M.D., London, 1770.

If the physician is called to a case of typhus fever during the chill, before reaction has taken place, he will of course have recourse to diffusible stimulants and external warmth to aid in the establishment of this process. More frequently he is not sent for until after the chill has been succeeded by fever. His treatment will then, of course, vary with the condition of the patient. If his stomach is loaded with food, an emetic should be administered to him. If the bowels are constipated, a mild cathartic will often be of service, but after the bowels have been once well moved it is generally unnecessary to disturb them further. During the first day or two, while the fever is still moderate in degree, and during the uncertainty which then usually exists as to the diagnosis, it will be sufficient to prescribe the neutral mixture or the spirit of Mindererus in tablespoonful doses every two or three hours. Upon the third day more active remedies will generally be required to reduce the temperature. This is best done by the cold-water treatment in some form or other, or by the internal administration of antipyretic doses of quinia. The manner in which the cold water is to be used and the cases to which it is applicable must be left in a great measure to the judgment of the physician. In the form of the cold affusion it is now rarely resorted to, although Currie[31] obtained most excellent results with it. It is calculated, however, to alarm a timid patient, and it is probably owing largely to this fact that it has fallen into disuse. The cold bath, packing in a cold wet sheet, and sponging with cold water are the more usual means of employing cold in the treatment of typhus fever at the present day. The cold bath is much used in Germany in the treatment of different forms of fever, and even of inflammation. It is also resorted to in this country, but it has never attained the same popularity here as abroad. The best way of using it is as follows: The patient as soon as his temperature rises above 103° F. should be placed in a bath having a temperature between 80° and 90°, and which, whenever practicable, should be brought to his bedside, as when he has to be carried to the bathroom he is sometimes not only alarmed and rendered very nervous by the operation, but may exhaust himself in his struggles to free himself from his attendants. After his immersion cold water should be gradually added until the temperature of the bath is between 60° and 70° F. The length of time he should be allowed to remain in the bath will of course depend upon circumstances. If shivering is produced by it, he should be at once removed from it and thoroughly dried and put back to bed. If no such symptoms are observed, he may be allowed to remain in it longer. As a general rule, a half hour is as long as will be necessary or safe for him to continue immersed at any one time. His temperature will usually continue to fall for some time after his removal from the bath, but in the course of a few hours it will be found to have risen again to 103° or over, when he should have another bath. In this way it may be necessary to repeat the baths from eight to twelve times a day. Some authors recommend that the patient should be placed at once in a bath having a temperature of 50° F., [p. 365]but this method of applying cold possesses no advantage over that above described, and is, like the cold affusion, very apt to excite alarm in the patient. The cold bath is not, however, well borne by all persons, and alarming symptoms, and even fatal collapse, have followed its use in the old and feeble. It is also contraindicated when the skin is covered with a profuse sweat or when the disease is complicated by an internal inflammation. When the means of giving a cold bath are not at hand, the cold pack will often be found a very efficient substitute for it. Sponging with cold water, although not so efficacious in reducing the temperature, has advantages over either of these methods of applying cold. In the first place, it is more agreeable to most patients and less calculated to excite alarm in those who are timid. Again, it may be more frequently repeated, and may be used in cases in which the cold bath is contraindicated. Occasionally alcohol or vinegar may be added with advantage to the water, with the view of increasing its refrigerant effects.

[31] *Medical Reports on the Effects of Water, Cold and Warm, as a Remedy in Fever and Febrile Diseases*, by James Currie, M.D., F.R.S., London, 1805.

When quinia is given for the purpose of reducing the temperature in the treatment of typhus fever, it must be used in large doses, as much as ten or fifteen grains repeated once or twice in the course of twenty-four hours being required for this purpose. When given in these quantities it has the disadvantage of producing deafness and occasionally of increasing the headache. I have therefore contented myself in the cases which have fallen under my own care with giving it in more moderate quantities, in combination with one of the mineral acids, as, for instance, a couple of grains of quinia in solution with from eight to ten drops of dilute muriatic acid, repeated from four to six times a day. The mineral acids were originally recommended in the treatment of typhus fever in the belief that they neutralized the poison which caused the fever, and which was supposed to be ammonia or some of its compounds. Although this theory is now no longer entertained, there can be no doubt that the tendency in this disease to the accumulation of ammonia in the blood is prevented by their administration. Digitalis, aconite, or veratrum viride may also be given in appropriate doses if with a high temperature there coexists great frequency of the pulse. The first-named remedy is especially indicated if there is at the same time diminution of the secretion of urine.

As the disease progresses other symptoms present themselves for treatment. One of the most urgent of these is the prostration. This not only appears early, but is often extreme, and if not met by appropriate remedies will often of itself be sufficient to cause the death of the patient. As soon as it makes itself manifest stimulants must be prescribed. These are, however, not to be resorted to simply because the patient has typhus fever. Many cases do perfectly well without them. In the young and robust it is often unnecessary to have recourse to them. On the other hand, in the old, the feeble, and the intemperate they should be employed early. The rule laid down by Stokes, that they should be administered as soon as the first sound of the heart becomes indistinct and inaudible, may be adopted for our guidance in this respect. At first they should be given tentatively. If the delirium, headache, and other nervous symptoms are increased after their administration, it is best to withhold them. They should be continued, on the other hand, when under their use the delirium ceases or grows milder, the other nervous [p. 366]symptoms subside, and the patient falls into a refreshing sleep. The amount required to prevent fatal prostration will of course vary in each case. I have rarely myself found it necessary to prescribe more than half an ounce of whiskey or brandy every two hours, and frequently a very much smaller quantity has been found sufficient. Cases are, however, reported in which from twenty to twenty-four ounces daily have been given with asserted advantage.

Another symptom which often demands prompt relief is the headache. When not severe, it may be relieved by the application of cold to the head, either in the form of the ice-cap or by means of cloths frequently wrung out of cold water, and by the administration of moderate doses of potassium bromide; but when intense it requires more active treatment for its removal, such as the application of cups to the back of the neck or of leeches to the temples. General bleeding will accomplish the same result, but the good which is done by it is often more than counterbalanced by the prostration it induces. Sleeplessness is also sometimes the cause of a good deal of distress to the patient. When it occurs early in the disease and is caused by the headache, it will generally subside under the use of the remedies which are employed for the relief of the latter symptom; but when it comes on at a later period, it will often require special treatment. There is some doubt as to the propriety of giving opium under these circumstances, but Murchison, Gerhard, and others assert that it may be given not only without injury, but with positive advantage to the patient. Graves was in the habit of combining it with a small quantity of tartar emetic in the condition in which the sleeplessness is associated with active delirium. If, on the other hand, the delirium is of a low muttering character, it should be given with a diffusible stimulant.

In this condition I have often found a pill containing a small quantity each of opium and camphor, frequently repeated, to answer an admirable purpose, not only in procuring for the patient the needed repose, but also in diminishing the restlessness, jactitation, and subsultus tendinum. Opium should, however, not be used at all or used very carefully in cases in which there is congestion of the lungs or disease of the kidneys. The existence of the pin-hole pupil is also a contraindication to its employment. In young and robust patients, if the insomnia is attended by active delirium, chloral in twenty-grain doses, repeated if necessary, may often be given with advantage, but it should never be prescribed in cases in which the action of the heart is feeble. Other remedies which have been recommended in the treatment of this condition are belladonna, hyoscyamus, musk, chloroform, and cannabis indica. Potassium bromide appears to have no power to relieve it. No special modification of the above treatment is needed when delirium occurs independently of sleeplessness and headache. When the stupor is profound, efforts should be made to rouse the patient by the use of counter-irritants to the shaven scalp or to the nape of the neck. Murchison speaks well of the administration of strong coffee under these circumstances. If there is at the same time suppression or diminution of urine, diuretics should be administered in the hope of stimulating the kidneys to increased secretion. Retention of the urine is not an infrequent occurrence in this condition, and the physician ought never, therefore, to accept the assertions of the[p. 367]nurse or friends of the patient that the latter has passed water, but should satisfy himself by an examination in regard to the condition of the bladder at every visit. He will often find that the apparent passage of urine is nothing more than the dribbling due to an over-distension of this organ. Neglect of this precaution has occasionally been the cause of much subsequent distress to the patient, as cystitis is sometimes set up as a consequence of it. In one case which came under my observation, and in which this precaution had been neglected, the patient suffered from incontinence of urine for some time after his recovery from the fever. Thirst is a symptom which is always present and complained of at the beginning of the fever, and usually bears some proportion to the severity of this process. Weak tea, an infusion of cascarilla-bark, and camphor-water have all been recommended by different authors for its relief, but it is probable that no one of them possesses any superiority over water. If the stomach is irritable and water is not retained, small pieces of ice should be allowed to dissolve in the patient's mouth. Later, when the stage of stupor supervenes, it is very important to see that the patient obtains a full supply of water. In this condition he will not call for it, although it is even more urgently required than before.

Vomiting may occur at any time in the course of typhus fever. If it is observed at the very beginning of an attack, an emetic will often arrest it, but when it supervenes at a later period, it is generally of cerebral origin, and will usually subside under the use of the remedies already referred to which are prescribed for the relief of the nervous symptoms. In addition to these, sinapisms may be applied to the epigastrium, and champagne, when the circumstances of the patient will permit it, should be given in the place of whiskey or brandy. When everything is rejected by the stomach, recourse must be had to nutritious enemata. Constipation is to be overcome by gentle purgatives, as the use of powerful cathartics is very apt to be followed by troublesome diarrhoea. If this should come on, it is best treated by small doses of opium in combination with a mineral or vegetable astringent. When these fail, it may sometimes be relieved by a prescription containing sulphuric acid and morphia, and at others by enemata of from twenty to thirty drops of laudanum in warm water. When glandular swelling occurs in the parotid region or in other parts of the body, an effort should be made to promote resolution by painting them with tincture of iodine. Blisters have also been recommended for the same purpose, but they should be used carefully, as in low conditions of the system they are sometimes followed by sloughing of the integuments. If these remedies fail, poultices should be applied. As soon as pus has formed it should be evacuated by one or more free incisions.

Very few attacks of typhus fever run their course without the occurrence of some pulmonary complication. When this is slight it demands no special modification of the previous treatment, and it is sufficient to apply mustard poultices or stimulating liniments to the chest. But in cases of greater gravity, it matters not whether the complication is bronchitis, congestion of the lungs, or pneumonia, a more active treatment is required. Under these circumstances the ammonium carbonate in five-grain doses, given in mucilage of acacia, frequently repeated, or from thirty minims to a teaspoonful of the aromatic spirit of ammonia every[p. 368]two hours, sufficiently diluted, may be prescribed with great advantage. When gangrene supervenes the prognosis is almost hopeless, but an effort should be made to save the patient's life by the administration of potassium chlorate and of an increased amount of stimulus. Murchison also speaks well of the inhalation of tar vapor and of carbolic acid.

As the other complications of typhus are at least of as common occurrence in typhoid fever, it will avoid a good deal of useless repetition to refer the reader to the article on the latter disease for a description of the treatment which they render necessary.

The patient should be kept in bed for some time after the subsidence of fever. Although relapses are rare in this disease, recrudescences of fever not infrequently occur as a consequence of undue exertion in the early part of convalescence. Syncope is also not infrequently produced by the patient's sitting up too soon. The diet should be carefully regulated until the recovery is complete. It should at first consist wholly of liquid or semi-liquid articles of food, but later meat in some digestible form may be allowed. Stimulants are often as urgently demanded at this time as during the fever itself. They should be given as the strength returns in gradually diminishing quantities. The length of time during which it is necessary to continue them will depend in great measure upon the previous habits of the patient. As a general rule, their use should not be abandoned until he is able to leave his bed, and they may often be continued after this with benefit to him. As convalescence progresses it will be well to substitute ale or porter for the brandy or whiskey the patient had previously taken. A return to health will also be promoted by the judicious use of tonics, such as iron, quinia, Huxham's tincture, tincture of nux vomica, the mineral acids, and even cod-liver oil in some cases.

[p. 369]

RELAPSING FEVER.
BY WILLIAM PEPPER, M.D., LL.D.

SYNONYMS.—Febris recidiva, vel recurrens; Fièvre a rechutes; Fièvre recurrente; Typhus icterodes, vel recurrens; Bilious Typhoid Fever; Rückfall's Typhus; Tifo recidivo; Famine Fever, Hunger-pest, Armentyphus, Hunger-typhus, Spirillum Fever.

DEFINITION.—Relapsing fever is an epidemic contagious disease, the specific cause of which is not certainly known, although a peculiar spirillum appears to be constantly present in the blood. It occurs chiefly among the over-crowded and destitute, but may spread widely when introduced among more favorably situated populations. Its invasion is abrupt, and is marked by a distinct chill or rigor, followed quickly by high fever (104° to 106°), with severe headache and pains in the back and limbs. Delirium is comparatively rare. The tongue is heavily coated, and there are epigastric tenderness, vomiting, constipation, and enlargement of the liver and spleen, with frequent jaundice. There is no characteristic eruption. These symptoms cease abruptly from the fifth to the seventh day, with copious sweating; but after an apyretic interval of about a week's duration a relapse occurs similar to the first attack, but of less duration (three to five days). Second, third, or even more numerous relapses may subsequently occur at less regular intervals. One attack does not protect against a second one to the same extent as with other contagious diseases. The mortality is usually small.

HISTORY AND GEOGRAPHICAL DISTRIBUTION.—It is not important to consider here at any length the history of this disease. Allusions to it were made by Strother, 1729, and by Huxham, 1752, but the first reliable account on record is the description of an epidemic in the year 1739 by John Rutty.[1] Relapsing fever undoubtedly occurred at different times and at various places during the next hundred years, although the records of it are scanty, and for the most part imperfect, owing chiefly to the want of a clear recognition of its essential difference from typhus and typhoid fevers.

[1] *A Chronological History of the Weather and Seasons*, etc., London, 1770, pp. 75-90.

During the decade from 1842 to 1852 relapsing fever prevailed in a very active and widespread form. Epidemics occurred in England, Scotland, and Ireland, in various parts of Germany, and it was during this time that it was first observed and described in America. In June, 1844, an emigrant ship from Liverpool came to America with eighteen cases on board, which were taken to the Philadelphia and Pennsylvania [p. 370]Hospitals. In 1848 a few cases were imported by emigrants to New York, and in 1850 to Buffalo in the same way.[2]

[2] See *Fevers, their Diagnosis, Pathology, and Treatment*, Meredith Clymer, Phila., 1846, p. 99; *Clinical Reports on Continued Fever*, A. Flint, Phila., 1855, p. 364; Dubois 1848.

The next great outbreak of relapsing fever began in Odessa in 1863 and lasted until 1872. It prevailed in various parts of Russia, in Germany, France, and Great Britain, and for the first time occurred extensively in the United States, especially in Philadelphia and New York. The present article is based largely on a study of this epidemic as it presented itself in Philadelphia during the years 1869-70, when the writer, in conjunction with the late Edward Rhoads, had the opportunity of observing about two hundred cases, in the wards of the Philadelphia Hospital. An admirable article on the same epidemic appeared from the pen of the late John S. Parry, in the *Amer. Jour. Med. Sciences*, N.S., vol. lx., Oct., 1870, p. 336.

Between the years 1877 and 1880 relapsing fever occurred quite extensively at Bombay, and was there studied by Carter[3] and Lewis; and during 1879-80 it prevailed in Königsberg, an account of which epidemic has been published by Meschede.[4]

[3] *Spirillum Fever*, by H. Vandyke Carter, M.D., London, 1882.

[4] *Virchow's Archiv*, Bd. lxxxvii. p. 393.

The geographical distribution of relapsing fever is seen, therefore, to have been very extensive; and not only has it occurred in the above-mentioned localities, but there have also been less extensive outbreaks in France, India, Egypt, Algeria, South America, and elsewhere.

CAUSES.—In all probability the essential cause of relapsing fever is a specific poison, but we know nothing of its real nature nor of the precise conditions under which it originates. Recent investigations have shown that the spirillum discovered by Obermeier is constantly present during the febrile stages of relapsing fever, but it cannot yet be decided whether this minute organism is the actual cause or only an invariable accompaniment of the disease.

It appears that conditions of destitution, filth, and intemperance amongst an overcrowded population favor the development of the virus, and hence the epidemics have, as a rule, begun in towns, such as Dublin, Glasgow, Odessa, St. Petersburg, Breslau, etc., where such conditions prevail. Great importance has been attached, in particular, to the scarcity of food and to destitution as powerful factors in favoring the production of the disease. Some of its names (hunger-pest, hunger-typhus, famine fever) have been given with reference to this, and in the case of several outbreaks a careful comparison has been made of the decrease of the food-supply and the consequent advance in price of the staple commodities with the development and progress of the disease. Although this is in all probability true of those centres where relapsing fever originates, it has but a partial application to the secondary centres where the disease is imported and develops.

The presence of destitution and filth, enfeebling the vitality of a section of the community, would favor the spread of this as of any other specific fever, but there is considerable evidence to favor the view that the importance of starvation as a cause of the fever has been exaggerated. This was strongly urged by Parry[5] as the result of his study of the[p. 371]Philadelphia epidemic of 1870, and our own more extended observation showed that the vast majority of the patients appeared to be well fed. On the other hand, the influence of overcrowding as favoring the development and spread of relapsing fever has been clearly established by the study of many epidemics, as in the Breslau attack of 1868, reported by Wyss and Bock, where single tenement-houses furnished as many as seventy-one cases; in the Edinburgh epidemic of 1869 and 1870, where Muirhead found the breathing-space allotted to each individual in the affected houses to vary from 250 to 400 cubic feet; and in the Philadelphia epidemic, where the observations of Parry and ourselves showed the presence of an extreme degree of overcrowding in most of the houses where the disease broke out.

[5] *Loc. cit.*, p. 339.

No age is exempt, but neither can it be said that age exerts any influence upon the occurrence or frequency of relapsing fever. Of 1164 cases in the Philadelphia epidemic of 1869-70 in which the age was noted, the result was as follows:

	Males.	Females.
Under 20	149	76
From 20 to 30	220	140
From 30 to 40	143	101
From 40 to 50	135	67
From 50 to 60	60	34
From 60 to 70	20	6
From 70 to 90	6	7
Total	733	431 = 1164

The youngest cases were in children two or three years old; the oldest patients were women over eighty-five years old.

Sex exerts no influence, though, on account of the larger proportion of males likely to be exposed to the specific cause, the results of nearly all epidemics show a preponderance of male patients in the proportion of 33 per cent., 66 per cent., or even 85 per cent. (Meschede).

Nationality does not act as a predisposing cause,[6] except in so far as certain countries may present more frequently than others the conditions favorable for the development of this disease. Of 1170 cases in Philadelphia in which the nativity was noted, 219 were Irish, 61 English, 161 German, 729 American. Of the latter 729, about one-half, or nearly 28 per cent. of the whole number, were negroes, while the negro population of Philadelphia was only about 3.3 per cent. of the total. This excessive proportion of cases among the negroes was undoubtedly due in large part to the fact that in Philadelphia overcrowding is notoriously more common and extreme among them than in any other portion of the population, although it is also likely that they present an excessive susceptibility to the virus of this as of many other specific diseases.

[6] Hirsch's *Geog. and Hist. Pathology*, New Syd. Soc. ed., 1883, vol. i. p. 615.

Attempts have been made to show some connection between the period of the year or the atmospheric conditions and the rise and spread of epidemics of relapsing fever; but, as Murchison clearly showed, these epidemics are wholly independent of such influences. In Philadelphia, of 1176 cases in which the date of occurrence is known, there occurred in September, 1869, 4 cases; December, 1869, 6 cases; January, 1870, 5 cases; February, 1870, 13 cases; March, [p. 372]1870, 124 cases; April, 1870, 209 cases; May, 325 cases; June, 293 cases; July, 115 cases; August, 19 cases; September, 28 cases; October, 15 cases; November, 1 case; December, 2 cases; January, 1881, 2 cases; February, 1 case; March, 2 cases; May, 7 cases; June, 2 cases; September, 2 cases; October, 2 cases.

Occupation exerts no predisposing influence, but in all epidemics the great majority of cases occur among the vagrant classes, who lead a precarious life and commonly sleep in foul, overcrowded lodgings. Murchison noted that in the London epidemics a considerable proportion of cases occurred among recent residents, but he attributed this, correctly, not to any special local cause, but merely to the fact that this floating population is largely of the vagrant type. In Philadelphia a careful inquiry showed that recent residence produced no special predisposing influence, and a study of other epidemics confirms this view.

Contagion is, however, the essential cause of the spread of relapsing fever when the virus has once been developed. It seems clear from the distinct periods and from the widely-separated localities in which different outbreaks of relapsing fever have occurred that its special poison is capable of being called into existence or activity by favoring conditions. Murchison held the belief that it was very intimately connected with, if not generated by, destitution, and, as already stated, much evidence exists to show that the disease is most apt to break out after periods of scarcity; but no just and convincing proof exists that destitution, any more than over-crowding and other depressing influences, can actually engender a specific contagium capable of being transported to great distances and of originating widespread outbreaks of the specific disease among differently situated populations. It appears necessary to assume the existence of some unknown special virus which finds its suitable nidus for development in the conditions attendant on filth and overcrowding, and which attacks with greatest facility the systems of those who are enfeebled by want and depressed by vitiated air. When once this specific poison has been called into active existence, however, there can be no doubt as to the fact that it can be carried by fomites, and that it is given off from the bodies of relapsing-fever patients so as to affect any who may approach. Although a few observers have doubted this contagiousness of relapsing fever, the evidence in its favor is overwhelming. In many epidemics, as in Philadelphia in 1869, its contagiousness is at least as intense as that of typhus fever. A single case may, indeed, be admitted to a healthy family among the better classes or into the wards of a well-ventilated hospital without propagating the disease, although striking cases of contagion are on record where a patient has communicated the disease to all the members of a family favorably situated and living at a distance from any other possible source of contagion. On the other hand, if admitted to an overcrowded and filthy lodging the disease is apt to spread rapidly. Wyss and Bock report seventy-one cases as having occurred in a single lodging-house during the course of the Breslau epidemic of 1868, and in Philadelphia single houses in several instances furnished more than a score of cases, and several short streets more than one hundred cases each.

In the Philadelphia Hospital twenty-three persons lying sick in the wards with other affections contracted relapsing fever from the patients [p. 373]admitted with that disease; two of the visiting staff, five resident physicians, and nine nurses also suffered attacks of varying severity. This corresponds with the general experience of those connected with fever hospitals during the prevalence of relapsing fever.

As in the case of typhus and other contagious diseases, the distance at which relapsing fever can be contracted by direct contagion through the atmosphere is a very short one, not exceeding a few feet at most.

The poison may be carried by fomites. Instances are on record where persons having visited infected districts have conveyed the disease to others at a distance without contracting it themselves.

When rooms which have been occupied by relapsing-fever patients are subsequently occupied by other persons, these are very liable to acquire the disease. Parry relates two remarkable cases in which relapsing fever was transported to a distance by infected clothes; and it has been more than once observed that during epidemics of this disease laundry-women engaged in washing the clothes of fever patients, but without any means of more direct communication with the sick, were frequently attacked (Cormack, Wyss and Bock).

In connection with the etiology of relapsing fever it is necessary to consider the rôle played by a minute organism which has been frequently detected in the blood of patients suffering with this disease. This spiro-bacterium was first observed in relapsing fever by Obermeier[7] in 1873, and has since been identified as a spirillum or spiroechete. The very numerous observations of Obermeier, Albrecht, H. V. Carter, Motschutkoffsky, Koch, Cohen, Holsti, Enke, Meschede, and others leave no doubt that this peculiar parasite does occur at least very frequently in the blood of patients with this disease. The failure to detect it, which has been reported by several good observers, may readily have been due to the extreme delicacy of the organism, or to the neglect of the proper method of preparing the slides of blood for examination, or to delaying the examination of the blood until after death, when it rapidly disappears. Thus no value can be attached to the negative observations of Rhoads and myself, made prior to Obermeier's discovery, since our method of examination was not sufficiently exact.

[7] *Centralbl. f. die med. Wissensch.*, 1873, No. 10.

The following description of the mode of examining the blood, and of the spirillum, is condensed from H. V. Carter's account: It is necessary to employ magnifying powers of not less than 500 diameters. The fresh blood may be examined immediately after obtaining it by pricking the washed finger of the patient. For preservation dried specimens are needed: a very thin layer of fresh blood is evenly spread with the needle over the glass cover, exposed to the weak fumes of a solution of osmic acid, and allowed to dry under protection from dust; the dried film of blood may then be treated with glacial acetic acid or may be stained.

FIG. 19.

Spirillum from the blood in a case of relapsing fever, X 700 (Koch).

The spirillum [See Fig. 19] is a colorless, slender, twisted filament, which when quiescent has a length of 2.66 times the diameter of a blood-disc (1/1500 to 1/500 inch = 0.012 to 0.043 millimetre). When unfolded they become distinctly elongated. They are very narrow (not more than 1/40000 inch), and present four to ten spiral turns; when fresh they are in active movement and unfold in part, becoming wavy or bent. They [p. 374]resist the action of concentrated acetic acid, and are readily stained by certain dyes. In number, five or ten may be visible in a field or they may be too numerous to count. They have not been detected either in the secretions or in the evacuations. Both Koch and Carter have succeeded in cultivating this special form of bacteria outside of the body.

To judge from the observations thus far made on this difficult question, the parasite is found first toward the close of the period of inoculation or soon after the beginning of the fever, or it may be detected throughout the febrile stage; but shortly before the cessation of the fever it quickly disappears, to reappear at the time of the relapse. There would seem, therefore, to be some close connection between the febrile paroxysms and this organism, and it is not remarkable that many observers have concluded that this spirillum is the essential and specific cause of the fever, and that it is impossible to have this disease present without the appearance of the parasite in the blood; nor that the name spirillum fever has been applied to the disease by Carter.

Such conclusions appear to be premature, however, and we prefer to regard the undoubted existence of the spirillum in the blood of relapsing-fever patients as at present only an important aid in diagnosis, and to await the occurrence of other epidemics and the repetition of careful studies upon this organism, both within and without the human system, before venturing to decide whether it is merely one of the phenomena of the disease or whether it is its true cause and specific contagious principle.

It must be added that both Carter and Koch have succeeded in inoculating monkeys with relapsing fever, and Motschutkoffsky[8] of Odessa, who had the opportunity of inoculating a human being, asserts that he succeeded in producing the disease, and found the incubation period to be not less than five nor more than eight days. Carter also gives an interesting table[9] of six instances of inoculation, four of them by cuts while making autopsies, with consequent development of relapsing fever in each instance. Some allowance must be made for the fact that in all the instances of this series there had been exposure to contagion by close communication with fever patients, though this exposure had existed for several months previously without leading to the development of relapsing fever.

[8] *Centralblatt f. d. med. Wissenschaften*, 1876, No. 11, p. 194.
[9] *Op. cit.*, p. 403.

GENERAL CLINICAL DESCRIPTION.—After a period of not less than five or six days from the reception of the contagion the disease begins [p. 375]abruptly with a chill of variable severity, accompanied by headache and aching pains in the back and limbs. The patient feels weak and is often giddy, but is not always obliged to go to bed the first day. Nausea and vomiting are among the earliest symptoms, and distress at the epigastrium, with tenderness, may attend or even precede the chill. Fever quickly follows; the pulse runs up from 110 to 130 in a few hours; the temperature reaches from 103.5° to 106° by the end of twenty-four hours; the pains increase, and there are insomnia and great restlessness; appetite fails; thirst is extreme; the tongue is moist and furred, and the bowels are quiet. During the subsequent six days these symptoms persist. The temperature presents a daily remission at some period of the twenty-four hours amounting to one or two degrees, the maximum reached in fully-developed cases varying from 104° to 108°. The pulse continues very rapid, and not rarely exceeds 140; the respirations are hurried and rapid, and cough attends many cases. Delirium is rare, but insomnia, restlessness, headache, and rheumatic pains in the back and limbs may prove constantly annoying. Appetite is variable, more frequently lost; nausea and vomiting are common; thirst is very troublesome; and the bowels are constipated or loose. No characteristic eruption appears, but sudamina are frequently present, since in a large proportion of cases there is more or less sweating, even during the continuance of high fever. Abdominal pain, tenderness in the epigastrium and hypochondria, and demonstrable enlargement of the liver and spleen are almost invariable. The urine is concentrated and dark or bile-stained. Jaundice is a common symptom, though its frequency varies greatly in different epidemics. The same may be said of epistaxis.

While these symptoms are at their height and the patient is suffering severely the paroxysm suddenly ceases, and in a few hours he is entirely relieved. This remarkable crisis occurs usually at the close of the seventh day, but may occur as early as the third or as late as the fifteenth day. It is attended with a critical discharge, copious sweating being by far the most common, though diarrhoea, free epistaxis, or hemorrhage from some other surface may replace it. The patient feels weak and languid; the temperature and pulse have fallen below the normal, and remain so for a day or two. Soon there is a rapid improvement in the appetite and the appearance of the tongue, and the patient regains strength day by day, and often feels so well that it is difficult to persuade him that he must avoid exertion and exposure. The enlargement of the spleen subsides rapidly, that of the liver more gradually; epigastric tenderness subsides, but in many cases some degree of it persists for several days. This interval or apyretic period lasts about a week, when, again without warning or provocation, the patient relapses, and is seized abruptly with the same set of symptoms which attended the first attack. This relapse does not usually last more than three days (one to five are the limits), and is terminated by a similar crisis, after which a slow convalescence is entered upon, or else after an apyretic interval of some days' duration a second relapse ensues, and this may, in rare cases, be in turn followed by a third, fourth, fifth, or even sixth similar relapse. In addition, it must be noted that many serious complications are liable to occur. The total duration of the disease thus varies from eighteen to ninety days. Convalescence is often tedious, and there are many troublesome sequelæ. [p. 376]The mortality, however, is not great, averaging 5 or 6 per cent. Death may occur suddenly from collapse at the close of the first paroxysm or from heart-clot; it may be produced by exhaustion in protracted cases; or be hastened by any serious complication; or the patient may sink into a typhoid condition, with low delirium, coma, and suppression of urine for several days before the fatal termination.

DETAILED STUDY OF SPECIAL CONDITIONS.—It is usually difficult to determine the period of incubation. In the unique case in which Motschutkoffsky is said to have produced relapsing fever by inoculation the initial symptoms occurred seven days after the inoculation. Wyss and Bock had several good opportunities of determining the minimum period of incubation, and found it to be six days. We may assume that the ordinary period is six to eight days, but that it varies, in accordance with the virulence of the virus or the susceptibility of the system, from four to fourteen days. During this time the patient feels as well as usual, or at most suffers for a day or two from slight malaise, with vague rheumatoid pains, headache, giddiness, and anorexia. In only 13 out of 181 of our cases in which this point is noted was the invasion gradual. Examination of the blood prior to the invasion does not discover any spirilla.

The invasion is usually abrupt and during the daytime; the patient can often fix the very hour of its occurrence, a severe chill attacking him while at work or at meal-time. This is the most common initial symptom (138 out of 168 our cases of sudden invasion); less commonly, obstinate vomiting and nausea or sudden vertigo are the first symptoms (each 8 times out of 168), or violent headache (14 times out of 168), or sharp epigastric pain. Parry also observed that the occurrence of obstinate and profuse vomiting as the initial symptom was especially frequent in children.

The physiognomy is carefully noted in one hundred and seventy of our records. The countenance is often flushed, with watery eyes and anxious, suffering expression. The flush is less dingy and dull than in typhus; the eye is comparatively rarely injected; and the expression is much less dull and stupid than in that disease. In cases where grave nervous symptoms supervene and the typhoid condition is developed the facies assumes all the characteristics of that state.

The livid bronzing of the face, described by Cormack in 1843 and by Carter (Bombay epidemic of 1877), was noticed in a moderate degree in only nine of our cases, and seems to be of infrequent occurrence. When we observed it it seemed due to an admixture of a faint jaundice tinge with a deep flush. Jaundice, as already stated, is of common occurrence, though its frequency varies greatly in different epidemics. It was present in 25 per cent. of our cases, rather more frequently in the negro patients than in whites, and in degree varied from a slight tinge of the conjunctiva and skin to the deepest staining of the entire body. The presence of jaundice in combination with the general features of high fever imparts a most peculiar and alarming appearance to such patients.

With the occurrence of the crisis the flush rapidly subsides and the face becomes pale, or, if the discharges have been profuse, it may appear sunken, haggard, and almost choleraic. Parry described a peculiar puffed, velvety look at this stage, as though the skin had been much thickened and softened at the same time.

[p. 377]There is no characteristic eruption in relapsing fever. In 150 out of 180 cases where the condition of the skin was carefully noted there was no eruption of any kind; in 4 cases there were small roseolar spots, with peculiar subcuticular mottling, which resembled the early stages of typhus eruption, but soon faded away without becoming petechial. A similar eruption was noticed by Murchison in 8 out of 600 cases. It appears from the third to the seventh day of the first paroxysm; it may or may not recur in the relapse, or it may occur then only. Eruptions apparently similar to this have been described by others as quite common in certain epidemics. Carter describes minutely an eruption which was noted in at least 10 per cent. of his Bombay cases, the spots of which were at first small, slightly raised, and pinkish or rose-colored, and which either faded away soon or changed into purplish, more persistent stains. In a valuable report on the Königsberg epidemic of 1879-80,

Meschede[10] remarks that roseola was observed in cases complicated by exanthematic typhus, which prevailed simultaneously, but in no case of uncomplicated relapsing fever. While, however, this suggestion may apply to some few of the cases of eruption observed by others, it is certainly inapplicable to the vast majority of them. We also noticed an eruption of pale-reddish, slightly elevated papules in seven cases. It must be borne in mind that persons of such a low class as are the great majority of relapsing-fever patients would naturally be expected to present a variety of cutaneous eruptions from filth or vermin, and that in consequence some of the appearances above described may have been of such origin. It is certain that the bites of either mosquitoes, fleas, or bedbugs may in this disease be followed by persistent reddish papules passing into petechiæ. Apart from this, however, true petechiæ have been quite common in some epidemics, while very rare in others. Parry saw "small spots of purpura" once only, in a delicate girl; and we did not observe petechiæ once in several hundred cases, many of which had extensive internal ecchymoses. On the other hand, they have been found in as much as 30 per cent. of all cases (314 out of 1000 cases, Smith at Glasgow). They do not appear on any fixed day, but are more common in the first paroxysm than in the relapses; and although sometimes associated with a tendency to hemorrhages from other surfaces, they have been so often observed in cases of ordinary severity that scarce any unfavorable prognostic value can be attached to them.

[10] *Virchow's Arch.*, Bd. lxxxvii., p. 405.

Vibices and extensive ecchymoses of the surface are of much more grave import, and in cases where fatal sinking is threatened they may appear accompanying a purplish lividity of the countenance.

Herpetic eruptions about the mouth or nostrils were observed in 20 out of 181 of our cases in which this point is noted. They appeared usually toward the close of the febrile stage, and their development was found to have value in determining the approach of the crisis. Bärensprung mentions especially the occurrence of herpes labialis in cases of irregular relapsing fever which bore considerable resemblance to typhus. Sudamina are, as might be expected in a disease attended with so much sweating, of quite common occurrence, though much more so in some epidemics than in others, unless searched for with greater care by the one set of observers. Desquamation was noted in 42 out of 181 of our cases, and [p. 378]invariably at the close of the relapse. It was usually confined to the hands and face, and occurred in the form of comparatively small flakes. This is more frequent than has been the case in most epidemics. Murchison quotes a case in which a piece of epidermis ten inches square separated from the body of a lad convalescent from relapsing fever.

A peculiar odor exhaling from patients with relapsing fever has been repeatedly noticed. A description of this unpleasant symptom, given by Kelly, as quoted by Murchison,[11] accords closely with what was frequently manifest in our own cases: "The smell was peculiar, not fetid or heavy, but somewhat like burning straw with a musty odor." Carter, in describing a similar odor in some of his cases, notes that the skin was not in these instances in a particularly foul state.

[11] *Op. cit.*, p. 346.

From what has already been said, it will be anticipated that the variations of the temperature in relapsing fever constitute the most peculiar and characteristic feature of that disease. A careful study of the accompanying charts will convey a more accurate impression than can be given by any description. The temperature begins to rise before the chill is fully developed, and when there is no initial chill the patient may be found within a few hours of the appearance of giddiness and headache with a temperature of 102.5° to 103.5°. Before twenty-four hours have passed it has risen to from 104° to 106°. During the paroxysm the febrile movement is continued, presenting merely a diurnal variation of one to two degrees, sometimes attended with sweating and partial relief of distressing symptoms, the minimum being observed at different hours in different cases, or even in the same case, though more frequently it occurs in the morning.

In a case reported by Parry a chill recurred at the same morning hour on three successive days. Wyss and Bock report some unusual cases in which a brief intermission occurred, with a fall of pulse and temperature to the normal, most frequently on the day before the real termination of the paroxysm. The highest temperature varies from 104.5° to

108.75°; in our cases the highest observed was 107.5°. This occurs, as a rule, on the last day or the day before the last of the initial paroxysm, and Obermeier has observed a sudden rise of four degrees in half an hour just before the crisis. Meschede,[12] however, found the highest temperature on the corresponding days of the first relapse.

[12] *Loc. cit.*

The duration of the primary paroxysm is usually six or seven days; but this is subject to considerable variations, as will be seen from the following table of 160 cases in which the duration was accurately ascertained: Initial paroxysm lasted—2 days in 1 case; 3 days in 2 cases; 4 days in 10 cases; 5 days in 19 cases; 6 days in 40 cases; 7 days in 58 cases; 8 days in 18 cases; 9 days in 2 cases; 10 days in 5 cases; 11 days in 2 cases; 14 days in 2 cases; 15 days in 1 case; and Parry, observing the same epidemic, found the duration of the first paroxysm to vary from 4 to 11 days. It is, however, rare for the duration to exceed ten days unless some complication be present.

[p. 379]

FIG. 20.

Typical case of relapsing fever, with three relapses, terminating in recovery. (From Motschutkoffsky)

With the beginning of the crisis there is a prodigious and sudden fall of temperature, unequalled in any other condition of disease. Within a few hours it may fall six or eight degrees (going down at the rate of 1.5° or 2° an hour); and falls of 12°, 13°, or even 14.4° (Murchison), in the course of twelve hours have been noted. In our own cases the greatest [p. 380]fall was from 107.2° to 95°, or 12.2°; and this is as low a point as is usually reached, though temperatures of 94°, 93°, or even 92°, have repeatedly been observed. Murchison refers to one case in which collapse supervened, where the rectal temperature was 90.6°. In nearly all of our cases a subnormal temperature occurred at the crisis, and lasted for a day or two subsequently, when it gradually rose and remained normal until the relapse, unless some transient complication caused a temporary rise in the interval.

FIG. 21.

Typical case of relapsing fever (Mary Collins, aged 32), terminating in recovery. One relapse, with slight post-critical rise of temperature.

Occasionally, there is no relapse whatever, but convalescence follows [p. 381]the initial paroxysm. This occurred in 10 out of 181 of our cases, and Murchison found that of 2425 cases reported by various authors no relapses occurred in about 30 per cent. Carter describes these under the name of the abortive form, and found them to constitute 23.8 per cent. of all his cases. It is probable, however, that in many cases so regarded either a relapse of very transient duration has been overlooked, or else that an attack of ephemeral fever has been regarded as of specific nature. In ordinary cases the duration of the intermission averages six or seven days, but here, again, considerable variation occurs. In 139 of our cases where its duration could be accurately determined it was as follows:

3 days in 4 cases.	7 days in 64 cases.	11 days in 1 case.
4 days in 3 cases.	8 days in 22 cases.	12 days in 1 case.

5 days in 12 cases.	9 days in 9 cases.	13 days in 1 case.
6 days in 12 cases.	10 days in 9 cases.	20 days in 1 case.

Despite these variations in the duration of the initial paroxysm and of the first intermission, the average date of the occurrence of the relapse in any large series of cases is about the twelfth day from the primary chill.

The relapse is ushered in with the same striking abruptness as the initial attack. The temperature again rises rapidly to 104° or 106°, and then pursues a continuous course resembling ordinarily that of the primary paroxysm. The difference between the maximum of the two paroxysms is rarely more than 1.5° or 2°, though either may be much milder than the other; as a rule, the highest temperature is attained on the last or penultimate day of the first attack. The duration of the relapse averages three or four days, though it may last but a few hours or a single day, and yet exhibit a rise of 5°, 6°, or 7°; or, on the other hand, it may be prolonged to six, seven, or even more days. Lyons, observing the disease in the Crimea, reports some relapses as having lasted twenty-one days, though it is improbable that a greater duration than seven days occurs without the presence of some complication. The relapse usually terminates by crisis, with an abrupt fall to an abnormally low temperature; though we observed at this time, much more frequently than at the close of the first paroxysm, a gradual subsidence of fever, or lysis. Again the patient regains strength and appetite, but in a considerable proportion of cases subsequent relapses ensue. As a rule, the second, third, and later relapses are attended with a febrile movement of shorter duration and of less severity than the first two paroxysms, and are also separated by intermissions of increasing length. Meschede[13] found from a study of 360 cases that the average duration was for the first paroxysm six or seven days; second paroxysm, four or five days; third paroxysm, three or four days; fourth paroxysm, one or two days; fifth paroxysm, one day.

[13] *Loc. cit.*

In a remarkable case given in full below, the duration of the paroxysms and intermissions were as follows:

First paroxysm,	8 days;	first intermission,	9 days.
Second paroxysm,	5 days;	second intermission,	1 day.
Third paroxysm,	1 day;	third intermission,	6 days.
Fourth paroxysm,	6 days;	fourth intermission,	8 days.
Fifth paroxysm,	5 days;	fifth intermission,	9 days.
Sixth paroxysm,	4 days;	sixth intermission,	10 days.
Seventh paroxysm,	3 days;	seventh intermission,	11 days.
Eighth paroxysm,	3 days;	followed by convalescence.	

[p. 382]The proportion of cases in which more than a single relapse occurs appears to vary in different epidemics. Murchison found that in 1500 cases reported by various authors a second relapse occurred 109 times (1 out of 14); a third relapse, 9 times (1 out of 166); and a fourth relapse, once. Of 182 cases noted carefully by ourselves, a second relapse occurred 24 times (1 out of 7½); a third relapse, 5 times (1 out of 36); a fourth relapse, once; and in the above-mentioned case six or seven relapses.

It follows that the total duration of the morbid process varies from the average of about eighteen or twenty days, in cases with a single relapse, to forty, sixty, or even ninety days. Of course the occurrence of complications may lead to very great modifications of the febrile movement and of the total duration of the disease.

There are several additional points about the febrile process requiring mention. In all the paroxysms there is a greater tendency to local or general perspirations than is met with in other continued fevers, and occasionally there are rigors or slight chills about the same hour on several days after the invasion or on the day preceding the crisis. It has been noted also that, even when the temperature is very high, the quality of the heat, as judged by the feeling of the skin, is different from that in typhus fever, and that the peculiar pungent irritating sensation known as calor mordax is rarely marked. But a more important peculiarity is the fact that the extreme temperatures (106°, 107°, or 108°) that are frequently observed in relapsing fever for several days in succession do not appear to involve any great increase of danger, and in particular are not attended with the production of the grave nervous symptoms so often met with in connection with hyperpyrexia in typhus and typhoid, and often regarded as the direct result of the exalted temperature itself. This striking fact is of much interest in its bearing on the theory of hyperpyrexia, and may possibly be explained by some marked difference in the conditions of heat-dispersion in these different diseases.

The pulse in relapsing fever is very rapid, and on the whole the rate corresponds with the movement of the temperature. It usually rises above 110, the limits being 90 and 140, the lower rate being noticed in the milder and uncomplicated cases and in subjects of phlegmatic constitution. The pulse rises rapidly at the invasion, and may reach 120 in the course of a few hours. Its maximum is usually noticed when the temperature is highest, shortly before the crisis; and when this actually begins the pulse may fall with a rapidity as remarkable as that of the decline of the temperature. Thus, within twenty-four hours it may fall from 152 to 80, or in even a shorter time from 140 to 54, or even as low as 48 (Obermeier) or 44 (Muirheid), or even 30 (Stillé). While this great fall is often noted, it is by no means constant. In our own cases it was frequently observed that the critical fall in temperature was not accompanied by a commensurate fall in pulse. Thus, at the close of a very severe initial paroxysm lasting nine days the temperature was 107°, and fell in the course of twenty-four hours to 99°, and in twenty-four hours more to 96°; during the first day of this fall the pulse was from 96 to 100, and during the second it fell to 76.

This want of correspondence was more marked at the close of the [p. 383]relapse than of the primary attack; thus, in a well-marked case, where the maximum temperature (105.4°) occurred eighteen hours before the crisis of relapse, the temperature fell in four hours from 104.4° to 96.2°, while the pulse, which was 130, fell in twelve hours to 108, and in twelve more to 92. In another case, in a man aged twenty, the temperature at the close of the second relapse was 106.4°, with a pulse of only 100; after the crisis, as the temperature fell, the pulse rose to 120, and did not descend until the end of twenty-four hours; and later, at the close of thirty-six hours, the temperature was 98° and the pulse 72, lower than which it did not go. Carter[14] states that in the Bombay epidemic it was invariably the case that the pulse did not decline to an extent corresponding with the temperature.

[14] *Op. cit.*, p. 140.

During the remainder of the intermission the pulse may be normal, or it may continue accelerated in consequence of some irritative condition; as the time for the relapse approaches it frequently again becomes abnormally slow. In either event it is found that any muscular exertion causes marked acceleration of the pulse.

During the paroxysm the character of the pulse is full and bounding, and there is considerable arterial tension. This is well shown in some of the sphygmographic tracings by Carter;[15] while in one of our tracings from the right radial of a man æt. 32, taken on the fourth day of a severe initial paroxysm, the line of ascent is steep and the summit sharp.

During the crisis, and for a day or two thereafter, the pulse may be weak, compressible, and dicrotic, and occasionally irregular.

[15] *Op. cit.*, p. 103.

The sounds of the heart and its impulse are weakened, except possibly during the first few days of the primary paroxysm. Blood-murmurs over the base of the heart and along the great vessels in relapsing fever were first noticed by Stokes, and have been frequently observed in subsequent epidemics. They were found in a large proportion of our cases, not rarely in both paroxysms, and during the early stage of convalescence when anæmia was marked; but during the intermissions they are rarely audible, and when the action of the heart was slow they were replaced by prolongation of the first sound.

It must be further noted that the pulse-rate is not a reliable indication of the danger in this disease, since, just as is the case with the hyperpyrexia, extreme rapidity of pulse may be present when the general symptoms denote no unusual danger, and when the patient ultimately recovers most satisfactorily.

There is a remarkable disproportion and dissimilarity between the cerebral and peripheral nervous phenomena in relapsing fever and those familiar to us in typhus and typhoid fevers. We have seen that patients almost invariably complain of headache. When prodromes are present it is commonly among them, and it may be the initial symptom to usher in each paroxysm. When the attack is fully developed headache is usually very severe, and no symptom is more bitterly complained of. It varies in seat and character. More commonly it is frontal or general; occasionally we found it occipital, and still more rarely it was unilateral, constituting hemicrania. It rarely continues during the relapse. Headache of an equally acute and violent character may be present in typhoid, but the headache of typhus is much more dull and contusive.

[p. 384]The mental condition is only exceptionally affected, a circumstance which greatly increases the patient's perception of his sufferings. Delirium is not present in ordinary cases, even though very severe and attended with hyperpyrexia; or if present is limited to the period immediately preceding the crisis, when there may be violent and noisy delirium of transient character. In some of our cases forcible restraint was necessary under these circumstances.

There are numerous instances on record showing the abruptness with which noisy, demonstrative, or even destructive delirium may appear, and the equal suddenness with which in the course of a few hours, or even of fifteen minutes, the patient may become rational and composed. Such attacks resemble hysteroidal spells, and probably occur more readily in patients of a nervous or hysterical temperament. They were certainly more common when the patients had been of intemperate habits; and, further, we had opportunities of noting that the occurrence of relapses in habitual drunkards who had previously suffered with delirium tremens was apt to develop a form of delirium which was to all appearance of that nature.

Delirium of a different and much more grave type may appear in connection with the symptoms of the typhoid state. In some cases this results from the presence of serious complications which induce a state of great prostration, while in others it is associated with great diminution or entire suppression of urine. The delirium under these circumstances is apt to be low and muttering, with a tendency to pass into stupor or profound coma.

Vertigo is present more frequently and in a more persistent form than in any other febrile disease. It was noticed as among the occasional prodromes, and was especially severe for the first few days of the initial paroxysm, though it often continued throughout this stage and recurred with the relapse. Occasionally it was complained of in the recumbent position, but usually it was excited only by a change of position.

Wakefulness was one of the most distressing symptoms in all cases, and appears to have been noted in all epidemics. Although the severity of the pain in various parts of the body and the absence of blunting of the perceptions would naturally cause much loss of sleep, the degree of the insomnia and the obstinate resistance it offers to the action of anodynes are apparently far in excess of what could thus be accounted for. Parry found that several of his patients could take as much as three grains of opium every second hour throughout the afternoon and night without either inducing sleep or causing contraction of the pupils.

Convulsions are rare and of very grave import. They may occur at the period just preceding crisis, when the nervous irritation is most intense, and are then somewhat less indicative of a fatal result than if occurring in the course of the paroxysm, when they are apt to be associated with extreme prostration of the nervous centres, with a tendency to subsequent fatal coma. No connection has been observed between their occurrence and the presence of albumen in the urine.

General tremor is rare, and was observed only in those of our cases where there had been habitual intemperance, with presumably a tendency to delirium tremens. Muscular rigidity was noticed occasionally, but may have been only apparent, being induced by the hyperæsthesia and[p. 385]soreness which were marked in some cases. The hyperæsthesia which was observed was both cutaneous and muscular, and was attended with tenderness of the body of the muscle, and also of the nerve-trunk supplying it. Meschede speaks of opisthotonos as a rare complication in his cases.

Motor paralysis involving single muscles or groups of muscles is occasionally noticed, as of the deltoid or of one arm (Meschede). Parry observed transient loss of power of the extremities in several cases, chiefly during the intermission or the period of convalescence. In one of our cases temporary hemiplegia occurred, with partial loss of sensation on the affected side.

The bladder and rectum are rarely affected, except in cases where the typhoid state with tendency to coma is present. Disorders of sensation are, however, much more common. When motor palsy occurs the affected part may also be the seat of impaired sensibility, while in a large proportion of all cases numbness of the extremities, with or without a sense of tingling, is complained of; out of 182 cases we noted this symptom in 94, affecting the fingers alone in 62, the feet alone in 6, and all the extremities in 25 cases. Cutaneous hyperæsthesia or partial anæsthesia are also occasionally observed. But the most noteworthy and constant symptom of this class are the pains in the muscles and joints which are bitterly complained of by nearly all patients with relapsing fever. They constitute, indeed, one of the highly characteristic features of the disease, and possess a diagnostic value. They may occur among the rarely present prodromes, but usually they appear with the chill and increase in intensity during the paroxysm; they may persist with even greater severity during the intermission, or, if they have then subsided, recur with the relapse, and may constitute one of the most troublesome hindrances to convalescence. It will thus be seen that in frequency, severity, and persistency they differ widely from the aching pains in the extremities complained of in typhus and other specific fevers. They are one of the most potent causes of the extreme insomnia, and are apt to dwell in the mind of the patient so vividly that he dreads each relapse on this account, and consequently looks back upon his attack of relapsing fever as a terribly painful experience. These pains are usually described as rheumatic in character, and several times patients presenting themselves at the hospital on the second or third day of the initial paroxysm stated that they had inflammatory rheumatism. As a fact, we observed the utmost intensity of these pains in a few cases where the patients were of marked rheumatic diathesis. The nape of the neck, the muscles of the trunk or extremities, or the large or small joints, or lower parts of the spinal region, may be the seat. At times they extend along the course of nerve-trunks. In character they are described as a deep intense aching, with occasional severe or excruciating, sharp, lancinating pains. Pressure or movement increases them. The joints are not red or swollen (though swelling may appear as a sequel), and the pains seemed to us rather to be referred to the joints than to be caused by any local irritation therein. As already stated, there is often tenderness of the body of the muscles, and this was especially marked in many of our cases on pressure along the course of the nerve-trunk.

Murchison suggests that they are due to the circulation in the blood of an[p. 386]abnormal substance, such as uric, lactic, or phosphoric acid; but it appears to us altogether probable that they are rather to be connected with states of congestive irritation of the sheaths of the nerve-trunks (early stage of perineuritis), or possibly in some cases of the spinal membranes also. It is true that they are sometimes shifting in their seat and fluctuating in their severity, but this is not inconsistent with the above suggestion, while the widespread irritative processes found in this remarkable disease, the resemblance of these pains and the frequently attendant numbness and tingling to the sensations caused by other forms of perineuritis, and the occasional development of local palsies of a single muscle or group of muscles, all are in its support.

The special senses are acute, sometimes painfully so. The eyes are watery and occasionally injected, but this latter condition is rare and slight in relapsing as compared with typhus fever. At the crisis and for a few days subsequently wide dilatation of the pupils is not infrequently observed. Dulness of hearing was present during the paroxysm in 14 of our cases, and a few patients complained of tinnitus; but these symptoms are not at all common in the disease, although it will be seen hereafter that affections of the middle ear are among its sequelæ.

Debility is not such a prominent symptom as in typhus and typhoid fevers. Patients manage to drag themselves about for several days during the initial paroxysm with all the symptoms fully developed, and after admission to the hospital will often be able to help themselves, or even to rise from bed, unless prevented by the severe pains or the vertigo. Still, there are many cases, not necessarily of very grave type, in which there is a marked sense of weariness and exhaustion, and of course in all cases of typhoid character the prostration is great. It must constantly be borne in mind that even when the patient feels or seems able to sit up he must on no account be permitted to do so, since the occurrence of sudden and fatal syncope is one of the accidents constantly to be apprehended. It is not only during the pyrexia that this precaution must be enforced; we meet with extreme debility during the intermission in some cases, and syncope has followed exertions made at that period as well as at others.

During the paroxysms the respirations are much accelerated, at times to a greater degree than would correspond with the pulse-rate, while at others extreme rapidity of pulse may be associated with moderate elevation of the rate of respirations.

As examples of the relation between temperature, pulse, and respirations we quote the following from our records of adult cases:

(*a*) Temperature, 108°; pulse, 124; respiration, 40. In the relapse; no chest trouble.

(*b*) Temperature, 107.5°; pulse, 120; respiration, 28; falling to temperature, 96°; pulse, 68; respiration, 18, within twelve hours, during which crisis occurred.

(*c*) Temperature, 107°; pulse, 144; respiration, 31. In the relapse.

(*d*) Temperature, 107°; pulse, 108; respiration, 44. Initial paroxysm; no pulmonary congestion.

Temperature, 106°; pulse, 116; respiration, 28. Relapse; no pulmonary congestion.

Temperature, 97°; pulse, 76; respiration, 24. Critical fall; cough,[p. 387]congestion of lungs posteriorly, and left one relatively dull on percussion, but pneumonia did not develop.

In many epidemics bronchitis, hypostatic congestion, and pneumonia are of rare occurrence, while in others, as in Philadelphia in 1870, they are comparatively frequent and lead to serious respiratory symptoms. While the pyrexia was high there was very frequently an irritative dry cough, with the fine crepitant and subcrepitant râles attending congestion and imperfect expansion of the lungs heard at the middle and lower portions of the chest posteriorly. In numerous instances the râles would disappear entirely after a few full inspirations in the sitting posture, just as in the corresponding condition in typhoid fever. But in a considerable proportion of all the cases (fully 35 per cent.) there was more troublesome bronchial cough, associated with sonorous, sibilant and subcrepitant râles, with mucous or muco-purulent expectoration.

Bronchitis of this character was a source of serious annoyance to many patients. In several cases there was impaired resonance at the lower margins of the lungs posteriorly, with imperfect bronchial respiration, but without the symptoms of fully-developed pneumonia. Such conditions were regarded as due to hypostatic congestion, and proved amenable to treatment. Pneumonia occurred in eleven cases out of 200 recorded with reference to this complication. It will be more fully discussed under the head of Complications. It was attended with the usual physical signs, and gave rise to extremely rapid and labored breathing, especially when associated with painful enlargement of the liver and spleen. In a case of double pneumonia, with enlarged and ruptured spleen, the respirations were from 80 to 90 for two days, the pulse being 130 to 136. It was a very fatal complication, death resulting in all but two instances.

Leyden[16] has shown that though the percentage of carbonic acid in the air expired during the pyrexia is diminished, the total quantity exhaled is increased, the proportion being as 1.5 to 1 in the non-febrile state.

[16] "U. d. Resp. in Fieber," *Deutsch. Arch. f. klin. Med.*, 1870, 536, quoted by Murchison.

Elaborate investigations have been made of the condition of the urine in relapsing fever by numerous observers, and in the Philadelphia epidemic of 1870 we had the great advantage of being assisted by the distinguished chemist, the late Horace B. Hare, who conducted an extensive series of analyses in our cases. In a number of cases quantitative analyses were continued daily throughout the entire course of the disease.

As a rule, the quantity of the urine is comparatively free during the febrile periods, very scanty at the time of crisis, except in the cases where critical discharges of urine occur, and excessive for some days after the crisis.

Still, there were not rare exceptions, especially to the first of these statements. Thus on four successive days of the relapse of a severe case with delirium, but without albumen, and which ultimately recovered, the analysis gave—

Temperature.	Amount in ccm.	Sp. gr.	Urea in Grm.	Na. Cl.
103	400	1024	23.8	2.64
105	300	1025	15.27	1.95
106	500	1024	24.7	4.3
106 to 97	850	1021	24.735	5.525

[p. 388]And in another severe case, also resulting in recovery, the analysis was, for two days preceding the crisis of the initial paroxysm—

Amount.	Sp. gr.	Urea.	Na. Cl.	
500	1014	2.9		Traces of albumen.
650	1014	5.85	1.365	
After the crisis:				
2250	1004	8.9	5.75	No albumen.

And again, in another case at the height of the initial paroxysm, within twenty-four hours of the crisis, no vomiting, purging, or epistaxis being present; temperature 105°; only 500 ccm. was passed of dark reddish colored urine, non-albuminous, and with sp. gr. 1011.

In a fatal case there was total suppression of urine for three days, the catheter drawing off only a few drops of almost pure liquid blood.

When crisis occurs by copious urination the discharges are frequent, large, and of light color and low specific gravity.

The urine of the intermissions is of similar character, and for several days after crisis it is not rare to have 2000 to 2500 ccm. passed. The largest amounts we noted were in a man who recovered, and who passed at the crisis of the relapse and during the following days the amounts here given.

Amount.	Sp. gr.	Urea.	Na. Cl.
1000 ccm.	1010	14.9	2.6
2000 ccm.	1003	20.2	42.8
3550 ccm.	1002	26.625	130.995
2600 ccm.	1002	19.24	27.30
2800 ccm.	1005	24.96	22.66
2500 ccm.	1013	47.25	11.25
2700 ccm.	1014	59.13	7.29

Carter reports a case where the patient continued for two weeks after the relapse to pass 130 oz. of sp. gr. 1002.6.

The amount of urea varies considerably, and is evidently under the influence of complicated conditions. The rule appears to be that it increases during the paroxysms, diminishes during the crisis, increases during the few days following crisis, and then falls off again. These results are stated upon the authority of Murchison, quoting from Pribram and Robitschek, Wyss and Bock, and others. Our own observations, however, while agreeing in the main with these, show that there are numerous and important exceptions, especially to the occurrence of the post-febrile increase in the elimination of urea.

The largest amount of urea excreted in twenty-four hours by any of our patients was 59.13 grammes, or 912 grains, on the sixth day after the end of the relapse, but as much as 74 grammes (1142 grains) have been found.

Deposits of urates were very common in the urine of the paroxysms and of the crisis. The uric acid has been found increased, and so also have the phosphates, crystals of which are frequently found mixed with the urates.

The chlorides diminish during the paroxysms, until just before the crisis their amount is very small, or they may even have disappeared. Immediately after the crisis they reappear slowly or quickly, and even[p. 389]very large amounts may be discharged, as seen in the figures given by Hare's analyses: 2.6 grm. on day of crisis, 42.8 grm. the following day, and the enormous amount of 130.995 grm. on the next day. A copious flow of urine corresponds with great augmentation in the amount of the chlorides.

Bile-pigment was constantly present in jaundiced cases, the amount being proportioned to the depth of the jaundice and the quantity of the urine. Bile-acids have been detected (Carter and Schmidt), and also leucin and tyrosin (Pribram and Robitschek).

Albumen, with or without tube-casts, is not uncommonly found, and traces of sugar have been detected in a few cases. More careful consideration will be given to these under the head of Complications.

The following appearance of the tongue has been repeatedly described, and when present may be regarded as possessing some diagnostic value: The body of the tongue slightly swollen, so as to show the impressions of the teeth, and by the second day the central part of the dorsum covered with a peculiarly white fur, while the edges and a small triangular space at the tip are clean and red. Such a tongue was seen in many cases at the beginning of the Philadelphia epidemic, but later it was present in but a small proportion. We find it specially mentioned in 97 of our recorded cases, or about 50 per cent., the general description being given that it was moist, rather large, with pink, clear edges, and a triangular clear space at the tip, and with heavy white fur in the centre.

Some accurate observers, as Wyss and Bock, did not notice anything peculiar about the tongue, but merely described it as moist and coated with a thick white fur. The tongue often remains moist throughout the case, the coat becoming yellowish, and later brownish. Of course if there is nasal obstruction from epistaxis or catarrh, and the patient breathes through the mouth, the tongue will soon become dry and brown; but in addition, this state of the tongue with sordes on the teeth and lips, appears in a small proportion of cases (3 per cent., Zuelzer; 12 per cent. of our own patients) in conjunction with grave typhoid symptoms.

During the intermissions the tongue clears off quite rapidly, unless marked gastric disturbance persists, but regains its former state as soon as the relapse occurs.

In rare cases the tongue is red and glazed, and Parry and ourselves observed peculiar painful cracks continuing obstinately after the relapse. It is apparent, therefore, that the tongue presents evidences of vitiated secretions, of local catarrh of the buccal mucous membranes, and of the high grade of gastric irritation so constantly attendant on this disease.

As a rule, there is complete anorexia during all of the febrile paroxysm, while in the intermission the appetite soon returns, and is sometimes truly ravenous. We did not, however, observe in any case a voracious appetite during the febrile paroxysms, such as was very often present during the London epidemic of 1843 and the Irish epidemic of 1847, and is particularly mentioned by Murchison.[17]

[17] *Op. cit.*, p. 360.

Thirst is constant and intense, and is excited not only by the high temperature, but by the irritation of the stomach; it may continue through[p. 390]the intermission, when natural appetite and the power of digesting solid food have returned.

Nausea and vomiting are always prominent symptoms, and most especially so in children. In some cases nausea occurs among the prodromes; and occasionally the attack is ushered in by profuse and uncontrollable vomiting instead of by a chill, and the stomach continues entirely non-retentive throughout the paroxysm. Vomiting is not usually so obstinate and severe, however, and with extreme care in feeding and medication it will often be allayed after two or three days. It occasionally recurs profusely immediately before the crisis, as in the case given in full below, where after a violent attack of vomiting the patient fell asleep, and awakened in a profuse sweat.

This symptom was present in 146 out of 182 of our cases, was usually confined to the febrile stages, and was, as a rule, worse in the initial paroxysm.

The matters vomited consist of the ingesta colored with bile, of glairy mucus tinged with bile, or of green bile, sometimes in considerable quantity. Small particles of blood may occasionally be noticed in the matters vomited, and in rare instances true hematemesis occurs. Judging from the frequency with which in fatal cases we find ecchymoses of the gastric mucous membranes with blood-stained mucus in the cavity of the stomach, we should expect black vomit to be more often observed than is the case. Murchison (p. 361) states that it was not noted in any British epidemic except that of 1843, and then it occurred in only a few cases, although it seems to have varied in frequency at different places. Arrott at that time described the symptoms as "quite common" in the fever at Dundee; and W. Reid of Glasgow recorded the case of a girl in the same epidemic who vomited large quantities of clotted blood, and who also had hemorrhages from the bowels and from the ears. It has occasionally been observed in the continental epidemics. It was observed in four of our cases. By all who have observed blood-vomiting in relapsing fever it is recognized as a symptom of almost invariably fatal import. Three of the four cases in which we observed it proved fatal, but one patient, who had copious hematemesis, both at the close of the first relapse and during the second relapse, recovered after a desperate and protracted struggle.

The bowels are not so often constipated as in typhus, and it is not rare for diarrhoea and constipation to alternate, or for the bowels to be loose throughout the paroxysms. They are noted in 181 of our cases as regular in 32, loose in 61, and constipated in 88 instances. Meschede states that diarrhoea was present in nearly one-half the cases of the Königsberg epidemic of 1879, though usually as a late symptom, the early stage being marked by constipation, which in a few cases persisted throughout. The stools may be consistent and dark or thin and bilious, or occasionally, when gastric or intestinal hemorrhage has occurred, they contain black coffee-ground matter. Occasionally, the diarrhoea has a critical character, and occurs at the close either of the initial paroxysm or of the relapse, though it may not entirely substitute sweating. This mode of crisis occurred in two of our cases, but Douglas observed it in 6 out of 33 cases.

The abdomen may appear enlarged, but this is as much the result of the[p. 391]enlargement of the liver and spleen as of gaseous distension, which is rarely present in a high degree. Abdominal pain is almost constant, and may be very severe. It is especially mentioned as having been present in 148 out of 182 of our cases. It commonly extends throughout the epigastrium and both hypochondria, but may be present on one or the other side, while, on the other hand, there may be general abdominal soreness. It is associated with tenderness on pressure, which may be so great as to hinder the movements of the trunk and to render the descent of the diaphragm in breathing painful. This may be the first symptom to usher in the attack, and it occurs at an early stage in most cases. Many of our patients when admitted to the hospital had already been cupped or blistered over the region of the liver or spleen. This distress was greatest in cases attended with jaundice and marked gastric irritation; and Parry reports that in his cases (occurring in the early part of the epidemic which we studied) jaundice was rare (4 out of 37), and abdominal tenderness was not present. It is not difficult to explain its almost universal presence in view of the severe lesions of the substance of the liver and spleen, the distension of their capsules from the acute swelling of the organs, and the implication of the coats of the stomach.

Enlargement of the liver and spleen probably exists to a greater or less degree in every case of relapsing fever without exception. This statement is based on the concurrent testimony of accurate observers in all epidemics and upon the evidence of post-mortem examinations.

The enlargement of the liver can be demonstrated in nearly all instances by careful percussion. It varies greatly in its degree, however; in mild cases it may be slight, while in severe ones the liver may be found extending at least three inches below the margin of the ribs within three or four days from the initial symptom. In our own fatal cases the weight of the liver averaged between four and four and a half pounds.

The spleen enlarges even more rapidly and to a greater degree than the liver. In fact, its enlargement in relapsing fever is greater than in any other acute disease. It may be detected by percussion by the first or second day, and may then continue to rapidly increase until by the fifth or sixth day a large painful mass is readily recognized by palpation and percussion, or even by inspection. The organ often weighs twelve or sixteen ounces, not rarely twenty to twenty-five, and, as an instance of the extreme limit that may be reached, Küttner reports sixty-eight ounces in one case. This enlargement is greatest toward the close of the first or second paroxysm, and subsides quite rapidly in most cases during the intermissions and as convalescence progresses; we have, however, known a moderate degree of enlargement of the spleen to persist for some weeks after the crisis of the last paroxysm.

The occurrence of jaundice in a considerable proportion of cases of relapsing fever is a clinical fact of much interest. Its frequency varies greatly in different epidemics, and even at different stages of the same epidemic. At times it is rarely met with (1 out of 14, 20, or 35 cases), while in other epidemics it is present in 1 out of every 6, 5, or even 4 cases. Of 182 of our own cases jaundice is recorded in 45, or exactly in 1 out of 4. According to our observation, it occurred in a larger proportion of cases among negroes (14 out of 32) than in whites, and [p. 392]Stillé states that it occurred in nearly every such case that came under his observation. When present it usually occurs during the first paroxysm, and may be limited to that stage; or, again, it may be present in each of three or four successive paroxysms in the same case; or, finally, it may first appear in the relapse. As a rule, it subsides speedily after the crisis, though Carter states that in two or three cases the symptom made its first appearance just after the crisis. It varied from the slightest yellow tinge of the conjunctiva to the deepest staining of the whole surface. The urine is discolored in proportion to the intensity of the jaundice, and the serum of a blister will be deeply tinged. It must be carefully noted, however, that the feces are not decolorized, but, as already described, contain fully a normal amount of biliary coloring matter. This fact has been relied on by Murchison and others to prove that the jaundice in relapsing fever is purely dependent on the morbid state of the blood, and is not due to obstruction of the biliary passages; and we are prepared to admit that the element of blood-dyscrasia may play a part in the production of the jaundice. The anatomical evidence, however, given below, renders it probable that in many cases at least the essential cause is to be sought in an obstructed state of the minute gall-ducts of certain areas of the liver. If the main hepatic duct or the common duct were obstructed, there would of course be paleness of the feces, as the bile would be prevented from entering the duodenum. But when a large amount of highly-colored bile is being secreted, as in relapsing fever, it seems clear that the obstruction of a certain number of minute ducts would cause sufficient resorption of the bile to induce jaundice of varying degrees of intensity, while at the same time allowing a flow of bile through the patulous ducts.

Jaundice must be regarded as an unfavorable or even a grave symptom in relapsing fever, but not to the extent that would be the case were it directly connected with the intensity of the blood-dyscrasia. Many of the most violent cases in all epidemics have been unattended with jaundice, while, on the other hand, many cases in which jaundice has been marked "have had not a single symptom that made them differ from ordinary cases excepting the yellowness" (Henderson). It follows, therefore, that the gravity of a certain proportion of the jaundiced cases does not follow directly from the presence of bile in the blood and tissues, but from the lesions of the liver of which the jaundice is a symptom, or from the existence of widespread irritation of many parts of the body. Thus jaundice is present in an unusually large proportion of the cases attended with marked enlargement and tenderness of the liver and spleen, whether vomiting is also present in extreme degree or not. It was noteworthy that it was disproportionately frequent in negroes, and that in these patients the lesions of the liver and spleen were also unusually pronounced. Again, jaundice is present in an unusually large proportion of the cases attended with low delirium, extreme prostration, defective secretion of urine, and the other features of the typhoid state—so much so that such cases have been described by various writers under the name of bilious typhoid fever.

But, as already stated, it is not legitimate to consider the gravity of these cases as the result of the jaundice, but rather that the jaundice is merely a symptom of the widespread irritative lesions, which in such [p. 393]cases not only involve the liver and spleen, but the kidneys, the lungs, the marrow of the bones, the muscle of the heart, and occasionally the membranes or substance of the brain and cord.

The true prognostic value of jaundice in relapsing fever would then seem to be, that of itself it indicates merely an obstructed state of a certain number of minute bile-ducts, but that its presence justifies the apprehension that the local lesions of the liver may become excessively developed, or that there is a tendency to widespread tissue-changes which at a later stage of the disease may lead to the appearance of grave constitutional disturbance of a typhoid type.

Hemorrhage in relapsing fever is not uncommon, and may occur from various surfaces. Epistaxis is, however, the only form which is frequent enough to justify being regarded as a symptom. It usually occurs in from 5 to 15 per cent. of cases of relapsing fever, but in the Philadelphia epidemic it was much more frequent than this, occurring in not less than 83 out of 182 of our cases. It was not more frequent or profuse in grave cases than in those of ordinary severity, and consequently could not be regarded as a reliable indication of the intensity of the blood-dyscrasia. Although ordinarily moderate in amount, it was occasionally so copious and persistent as to require prolonged plugging of the nostrils, and in at least one case contributed chiefly to cause an intense anæmia, which long delayed convalescence. It occurs at all periods of the paroxysms, but more commonly toward the close. In fifteen of our cases extraordinarily profuse epistaxis attended the crisis, and evidently replaced in part the copious sweating by which the paroxysm more commonly terminates.

SYMPTOMS ATTENDING THE CRISIS.—We have already described the aggravation of all the symptoms which immediately precedes the crisis in typical cases of relapsing fever, and the abrupt fall of temperature, and usually of the pulse, that follows. But this extraordinary change is nearly always attended with some profuse critical discharge, of which sweating is by far the most common, though copious epistaxis, metrorrhagia, diarrhoea, or vomiting may also occur, and to a greater or less degree, but seldom entirely, replace the sweating. In 182 cases in which we carefully noted the mode of termination of the paroxysm there was no definite crisis (termination by lysis or gradual and irregular defervescence) in 76; profuse sweating, 89; profuse epistaxis, 15; profuse diarrhoea, 2.

In most epidemics the proportion of true crises is greater than in the above table—a fact dependent upon the unusually severe and complicated form of the disease which we were studying. The beginning of the sweat may be preceded by chilliness or rigors, by extreme and dangerous prostration, or by violent nervous disturbances; or there may be an attack of profuse vomiting, followed by sleep, during which sweating begins. The sweat may be moderate in amount, but is often extraordinarily copious; the patient is literally bathed in it, the bed- and body-clothing is saturated, and we have seen the mattress saturated. It has an acid reaction, but we do not know of any accurate analyses of it. Some writers have attributed to it a characteristic disagreeable odor, but we did not notice any in our cases that could be considered peculiar to this disease.

CONVALESCENCE.—We have already stated the average duration of[p. 394]relapsing fever to be eighteen or twenty days, while the extreme limits are from eighteen to ninety days. Despite the fact, however, that the mortality is in most epidemics only about 5 or 7 per cent.—greatly less, therefore, than in typhus fever—the convalescence from relapsing fever is frequently slow and protracted. The obvious cause is, just as in the case of typhoid fever, the existence of numerous and serious lesions of the solids and the tendency to many troublesome complications and sequelæ. We have, however, seen many instances of rapid recovery of strength and health, even after prolonged attacks with several successive relapses.

The following case is quoted partly on account of the numerous relapses, and the long duration of the sickness:

B. B. Y., medical student, was much exposed to the contagion of relapsing fever in the wards of the Philadelphia Hospital during the spring of 1870, and in May had an attack apparently of this disease, which, however, subsided in four or five days and was followed by no immediate relapse. He continued his attendance at the hospital during the remainder of May and the whole of June; in July took a trip to the South, where there was no relapsing fever prevailing, and after exerting himself for several days during intensely hot weather, he became sleepless and much prostrated. He returned home, and after recovering from the fatigue felt quite well for about a week, until 3 A.M., August 1st, when he was attacked with a severe chill, followed by great insomnia, obstinate vomiting, intense headache, especially in the back of the neck, occasional sweating, violent fever, recurrence of very severe chill the following day at 11 A.M., epigastric and hypochondriac tenderness, decided jaundice, costive bowels, and scanty, high-colored urine. This paroxysm lasted till the morning of August 9th, when severe vomiting took place, followed by sleep, during which crisis occurred by drenching sweat lasting several hours. Appetite and strength soon began to return, though some jaundice persisted, and by August 17th he felt able to drive out a short distance, and retired feeling somewhat fatigued. He awoke with pain in the back of the neck, which continued increasing till 11 A.M., August 18th (second paroxysm), when a severe chill occurred, lasting three hours and followed by the same train of symptoms, including jaundice, which persisted five days, till Aug. 23d, when crisis again occurred by sweating. On the 24th he felt well enough to use slight exercise, which was followed by prostration and by a return of chill (third paroxysm) the next day at 11A.M., with subsequent headache, fever, irregular sweats, etc., lasting but one day. Again felt well until Aug. 30th, when he was attacked (fourth paroxysm) at 11 A.M. with severe chill, lasting three hours, followed by severe paroxysm, lasting six days, till Sept. 5th, when crisis again occurred by sweating. Again felt well for eight days, until Sept. 13th, when the fifth paroxysm occurred, lasting five days, ending Sept. 18th by critical sweating. This was followed by an intermission of nine days, until Sept. 27th, at 11 A.M., when the sixth paroxysm occurred, lasting four days, and less severe than the preceding ones. This was followed by an intermission of ten days, till Oct. 11th, when the seventh paroxysm occurred at the same hour of the day, and lasted three days. He then went sixty miles from home to a fine, pine-bearing district, and enjoyed an intermission of eleven days, when the eighth and [p. 395]last paroxysm occurred at the same hour, and lasted three days, until Oct. 25th. His convalescence was very satisfactory, and he was enabled to resume his studies by the middle of November. No sequelæ occurred. In 1878 Dr. Y., who had been working very steadily with a rapidly-growing practice, was attacked with severe typhoid fever, with grave nervous symptoms and with albumen and tube-casts in the urine, and died on the twelfth day.

It will thus be seen that in this unusually protracted case there were seven distinct relapses, one of which was brief and interrupted one of the regular intermissions, while the rest were all severe.

Duration of 1st paroxysm,	violent,	8 days.	1st intermission,	9 days.
Duration of 2d paroxysm,	violent,	5 days.	2d intermission,	1 day.
Duration of 3d paroxysm,	less violent,	1 day.	3d intermission,	6 days.
Duration of 4th paroxysm,	severe,	6 days.	4th intermission,	8 days.
Duration of 5th paroxysm,	severe,	5 days.	5th intermission,	9 days.
Duration of 6th paroxysm,	less severe,	4 days.	6th intermission,	10 days.
Duration of 7th paroxysm,	less severe,	3 days.	7th intermission,	11 days.
Duration of 8th paroxysm,	mild,	3 days,	followed by convalescence.	

The total duration of the case, which was entirely free from complications, was therefore ninety days.

VARIETIES.—The foregoing clinical description prepares us to appreciate the varieties of relapsing fever that may be said to exist. They consist of—

The abortive form, in which a single paroxysm of variable length and severity occurs, terminating in a critical fall of temperature and usually with some critical discharge, but not followed by any relapse. There can be no doubt of the existence of such cases, although they are not common; and at times the paroxysm is so slight that were it not for the known exposure of the individual to the prevalent epidemic influence, in the absence of any other adequate cause, the case might readily be regarded as one of non-specific febricula. The caution must, however, be borne in mind as to the occurrence of relapses of such extreme shortness of duration (less even than twenty-four hours) as to readily escape notice unless a careful watch be kept for their detection.

The ordinary or typical form, including the cases with one or two relapses, presenting the usual variations in the severity of the symptoms and in the duration of the paroxysms and of the intermissions.

The multiple or protracted form, if it be thought desirable to thus particularize cases presenting an excessive and unusual number of relapses, as three, four, five, six, or even seven.

The grave or subintrant form, which is designed to include the highly congestive form of Cormack and the bilious typhoid of Griesinger and Lebert.

Under another heading (see relations to other diseases, below) we shall give reasons for regarding the bilious typhoid fever of Griesinger and Lebert as merely a form of relapsing fever, with which a certain proportion of cases of true typhoid fever complicated with hepatic catarrh may have been included.

The characteristics of this grave subintrant form are as follows: Jaundice, occasionally absent, but usually present in an intense degree; marked enlargement of the liver and spleen; a tendency to hemorrhage from various mucous surfaces; extreme prostration; defective or suppressed[p. 396]secretion of urine; hypostatic congestion or inflammation of the lungs in a large proportion of cases; dry brownish tongue; low muttering delirium, often passing into stupor or coma; hiccough; imperfect crisis; and a continuance of some morbid phenomena, so that merely a remission occurs to separate the paroxysms; and a high percentage of mortality. The great modification of the intermission which is so highly characteristic of typhoid relapsing fever is doubtless due in chief part to the serious local lesions developed, and seems to justify the name of subintrant as above suggested. The course of such fever is well illustrated by the following case, in which the characters of typhoid relapsing fever were present in the highest degree, death occurring on the fifteenth day:

Charles Hood, colored, æt. 28, of temperate habits, was taken ill on April 5, 1870, after malaise lasting thirty-six hours, with fever, nausea and vomiting, headache, and general aching throughout body; and was admitted to the hospital April 6th. There was already marked jaundice, and epistaxis had occurred; there were also insomnia; wandering delirium; extreme tenderness over the liver and spleen, both of which were enlarged; dryness of tongue, vomiting, and distension of the abdomen. These symptoms continued, his condition becoming daily more aggravated. Restless delirium alternated with heavy sopor. The jaundice grew deeper. Marked digital formication existed, but the arthritic pains were not so severe as in ordinary cases. The tongue was dry and of a red orange color. Profuse epistaxis occurred on the seventh day of the disease, requiring plugging of both anterior and posterior nares, and followed by great prostration. A gradual fall in the temperature occurred during the sixth, seventh, and eighth days, reaching 99° on the latter day. During this decline the delirium ceased and the mind remained merely dull; the jaundice decreased, as did also the tenderness of the hypochondriac zone. The pulse and respirations improved, and diarrhoea ceased. The improvement was but brief; for about eighteen hours he lay apyretic, with cool hands and feet, and with eyes closed and mind dull but free from delirium. Fever then reappeared and with the ascent of the temperature the unfavorable symptoms recurred. The relapse lasted but two days, and was followed by irregular decline of fever till death occurred on the fifteenth day of the disease. Obstinate hiccough appeared on the eleventh day, and continued, accompanied with occasional vomiting on the fourteenth day. Delirium alternating with sopor reappeared. Jaundice again became marked, and again there was extreme tenderness over the liver and spleen. The pulse grew small and feeble, the respirations shallow and labored, with an expiratory moan. Cough began on the twelfth day, and was soon followed by the physical signs of pneumonia of the lower lobe of both lungs. The urine continued free from albumen. The patient sank into deeper coma, and died on the fifteenth day. Post-mortem examination showed highly-developed characteristic lesions of the spleen and liver, with red hepatization of lower lobe of both lungs. There was no affection of the glands of Peyer. The course of the fever is shown in the following tracing (see Fig. 22).

FIG. 22.

From a case of the bilious typhoid or grave subintrant form of relapsing fever.

COMPLICATIONS AND SEQUELÆ.—As would be anticipated from what has been said of the wide range of the symptoms and of the remarkable course of the temperature in relapsing fever, there are many complications and sequelæ liable to occur, and which require special consideration. [p. 397]They may be classified according as they affect the febrile movement, the state of the blood, or one or other of the groups of organs.

We have already described the various irregularities presented by the febrile paroxysms and the intermissions, and no further allusion need be made to mere variations in length, severity, or number of the former. In rare cases, however, a peculiarity is presented, usually in the first intermission, which is difficult of explanation. About twenty-four hours after an apparently complete crisis, with a fall of temperature to a subnormal point, there may be a sudden and rapid rise or rebound of temperature to 104° or 105°, attended with distressing symptoms of high fever, but lasting only twenty-four or forty-eight hours. A good example of this is given in the case described above and Carter[18] cites several examples of it terminating either in recovery or in rapid death. He asserts that examinations of the blood during such post-critical febrile rebounds invariably showed an absence of spirilla, so that in his opinion such fever must be considered non-specific. Their explanation seems difficult, since the pyrexia is too brief to be associated with any local inflammatory complication.

[18] *Op. cit.*, p. 172.

More frequent and serious is the protracted post-critical pyrexia which we have already described as modifying the interval, so as to produce a subintrant type by maintaining continuous though irregular fever until the accession of the relapse, unless cut short by death. This post-critical fever is non-specific, is unattended with spirilla in the blood, and is to be associated with the extensive irritative processes in the liver, spleen, kidneys, lungs, and other parts that are present in these grave and[p. 398]complicated cases. It is to be noted that the course of those paroxysms which terminate in lysis indicates that they may represent a milder type of the above process.

The peculiarities of the delirium, amounting sometimes to maniacal excitement, which attends some cases of relapsing fever, has been fully described.

Less common are the following: mental hebetude, lasting some days or even weeks after the close of the last paroxysm, or, as in a case of Carter's, gradually increasing mental feebleness, terminating in imbecility. In such cases suspicion must arise of the occurrence of some local lesion of the membranes or substance of the brain.

Partial palsy is mentioned by numerous authors as occurring during or shortly after attacks of relapsing fever. Paralysis of one or both deltoids has been noted, the latter by Cormack, who saw it continue ten days after the patient was well in all other respects. Temporary paralysis of the forearm (Douglas) or of the whole arm (Parry, Meschede) has been observed; and Parry also describes loss of power in the legs lasting for one week. In one of our cases temporary loss of power of the left arm and leg occurred, attended with such impairment of sensibility that the woman had to feel for the fingers of the left hand to assure herself of their existence. This loss of power occurred during the initial paroxysm, and gradually passed away, but she was unable to stand alone on the thirty-first day of the disease. In a case reported by Tennent[19] facial palsy was developed six days after the second crisis.

[19] *Glasgow Med. Jour.*, May, 1871, p. 379.

Various explanations have been offered for these local palsies, but, as already stated (see above), it seems probable that they are referable to morbid conditions of the nerve-trunks, or, less commonly, of the spinal cord. It must be noted, however, that in a certain number of autopsies serious intracranial lesions are found, which are evidently the results of the attack of relapsing fever. These consist of abscess of the brain, meningitis, and specially cerebral hemorrhage. This was present in one of our cases, but Carter found copious hemorrhage in no less than 8 out of 54 autopsies, and in 5 others there were minute capillary cerebral hemorrhages. Still, in nearly all the cases of large hemorrhage we have found recorded the effusion was upon the surface of the brain, and this, combined with the absence of true hemiplegia from the forms of paralysis noted in relapsing fever, and the transient character of these palsies, makes it clear that they are not to be explained by any considerable cerebral hemorrhage. On the other hand, however, it must be admitted that an additional possible cause of them is to be found in minute hemorrhage into small areas known to govern the movements of certain groups of muscles. Again, we have had occasion to note the occurrence of both thrombosis and embolism among the lesions of relapsing fever, and it is evident that either of these accidents, if involving a comparatively small branch of a cerebral vessel in certain motor areas, might cause transient paralysis, such as has been described. Nor can we fail to see that, while such symptoms as the delirium, mania, coma, or subsequent mental impairment may receive other explanations, it is possible that they may arise from similar processes of minute hemorrhage, thrombosis, or embolism involving other parts of the brain.

[p. 399]The frequent occurrence of severe rheumatic pains in the muscles and joints during the course of the disease has been dwelt upon (above); but in some cases they persisted during the intermissions and for a considerable time after all other symptoms of disease had passed away. Occasionally they greatly retarded convalescence by interfering with exercise and sleep. These pains were mostly in the legs, and were increased by exercise, and also seemed to be influenced by changes of weather. Patients who suffered thus were also liable, after exposure or in consequence of severe atmospheric changes, to sharp attacks of similar pains elsewhere, and especially in the course of the intercostal nerves. Occasionally violent and persistent headache follows the disease, not improbably associated with changes in the membranes of the brain, although in other cases severe neuralgia occurs in consequence of the anæmia which may remain in an intense degree after the fever. Troublesome numbness and soreness of the soles of the feet and of the palms of the hands, increased by pressure, has been noted as a sequel persisting for several days or weeks.

Affections of the special senses are not rare. The most remarkable among these is the affection of the eyes, which is apt to occur far more frequently in connection with relapsing fever than with typhus or typhoid. The proportion of cases in which this sequel appears varies greatly in different epidemics. In the British epidemics of 1826 and 1843, when this form of post-febrile ophthalmia was first accurately described by Mackenzie of Glasgow, it was very frequent; and it was equally so in Finland in 1867-68, when Estlander[20] again carefully studied it.

[20] "U. Choroiditis nach Febris Recurrens," *Arch. f. Ophth.*, 1869, Bd. xv., Abth. ii., 108.

On the other hand, so far as can be stated in regard to a sequel which may appear after convalescence is far advanced and the patient discharged from medical care, it was very uncommon in the Philadelphia epidemic of 1869-70. This ophthalmia may occur during the course of the fever, but more frequently it begins during convalescence, and even some months after convalescence has been established. It occurs in patients of both sexes and at all ages. Usually it affects but one eye, but both may be attacked simultaneously or consecutively. Patients who were very ill-nourished and debilitated were most apt to present this sequel, and Murchison regards previous starvation as one of its main causes. The exciting cause and true pathology appear obscure as yet, however, and the existence of a neural origin is not improbable. In some cases the ophthalmia has seemed to result directly from exposure to cold. Among our own patients, as already stated, eye symptoms were less common and severe. A careful record of 184 cases was kept in reference to this question. Several patients complained of diplopia during the febrile stage, and one asserted that every object appeared fourfold to him. Conjunctivitis of moderate severity, usually associated with otorrhoea, occurred in about 5 per cent. of our cases; it generally affected only one eye, and occurred in a few instances as late as the third week after the relapse. In a few cases (four) also there was dulness of vision in one eye, noted during the course of the disease and persisting for some time after convalescence began. In only one instance, however, did permanent impairment of vision ensue, and this man had passed through a violent attack of the fever with unusually grave nervous symptoms. [p. 400]It left him with optic neuritis on the right side, which induced partial atrophy of the nerve and great limitation of the field of vision. Meschede reports intraocular affections in 6 cases out of 180 specially examined, though it is not certain that such affections were directly connected with the febrile process. Ocular ecchymosis occurs in a small proportion of cases, especially of the graver types.

Dulness of hearing is not so common in relapsing fever as it is in typhoid. It was present in 14 out of 184 of our cases during the course of the disease, and in a few instances partial or almost complete deafness in one ear persisted after convalescence, owing doubtless to a slight affection of the middle ear. In one case marked deafness appeared suddenly on the day after the termination of the relapse by crisis. Meschede[21] found disease of the middle ear in no less than 8 per cent. of his cases.

[21] *Loc. cit.*

Purulent otorrhoea from one or both ears is of more frequent occurrence, and without any special exciting cause may present itself at any time during the course of the disease or more commonly after the relapse. In the same manner purulent coryza may occur.

The eruptions occasionally present during the fever have been described. Bed-sores from pressure are much less common than in typhus, but are met with in a small proportion of cases. As a rule, they are of moderate size and heal quickly. Superficial gangrene of the lips, nose, and ears has also been noted in rare cases (Zuelzer) in connection with gangrene of the extremities, probably from embolism. The occasional occurrence of painful boils, of abscesses in the cellular tissues (Wyss and Bock), and the more rare occurrence of erysipelas may be mentioned among the sequelæ.

As already stated, the severe pains in the joints and members which so frequently occur during relapsing fever are, as a rule, unattended by any redness or swelling of the joints. In rare cases, however, there is effusion into the joints during the fever, or more commonly there are attacks during convalescence which simulate subacute rheumatic arthritis. Such attacks may last but a few days, but in several of our cases there was painful swelling of the knees, wrists, and fingers which persisted for several weeks after the fever, being attended with slight crepitation on motion, and altogether behaving like subacute rheumatism.

As would be expected from the severity of the fever, the marked disorder of digestion, and the lesions of the spleen and liver in relapsing fever, anæmia is a common sequel. In cases where there has also been free hemorrhage, usually in the form of epistaxis, the anæmia may indeed reach an intense degree.

The cardiac murmurs which have been described as present in a certain proportion of cases are dependent upon the blood-changes, and when the anæmia is extreme these murmurs are also audible over the large veins and the pulmonary artery, and persist after convalescence is fully established.

Oedema of the lower extremities occurs in a considerable number of cases. It is clearly due in part to the anæmia, but the cardiac debility which follows the fever is also largely concerned in its production. It was, indeed, marked in some of our cases where no anæmic murmurs existed, but where there was great nervous and muscular debility. [p. 401]Usually limited to the feet and ankles, it occasionally extended above the knees, and in one case, where great anæmia and debility from fever and over-exertion coexisted, there was oedema of the hands and wrists, with great distension of the legs up to the hips. It is not associated with albuminuria as a rule, and yields readily to treatment and rest, in the course of a few weeks.

Hemorrhages from various surfaces have already been mentioned, and a full account given of epistaxis, which is by far the most common form. Bloody vomiting has been noticed in a small proportion of cases in various epidemics. It varies in amount, but is always attended with great gravity of the attack, and usually is followed by fatal results. It occurred in four of our cases, two of which presented also black stools containing altered blood, and suppression of urine; while in another it occurred at the close of the first relapse, and during the second relapse was copious and repeated. In this case it was attended with alarming symptoms of collapse, from which the patient rallied, and after a desperate struggle recovered.

Blood may also be discharged from the bowels in such large amount as to constitute actual hemorrhage—a symptom of great gravity; or in small quantity and completely altered, so as to impart an inky black color to the stools—a condition not necessarily attended with urgent danger; or, finally, there may be frequent bloody dysenteric stools.

Hemorrhage has also been observed from the uterus, from the kidneys, from the ears, and from the old cicatrix of a syphilitic chancre. Hemorrhage occurred in 87 out of 183 of our cases, or in nearly 50 per cent. It was from the nostrils in 82 cases, from the uterus in 1 case, from the stomach in 4 cases, and from the cicatrix of a chancre in 1 case.

Sudden collapse occurs with such comparative frequency in relapsing fever as to require special attention as one of its complications. It may occur at any period of the disease, but it is most common at the crisis of the first paroxysm or of the relapse. The symptoms are usually those of cardiac failure, with rapid, small, and feeble pulse; shallow and hurried, or slow, labored, and imperfect respiration; coldness of the extremities, while the central temperature may remain elevated; muttering delirium, rapidly passing into unconsciousness. Occasionally almost instantaneous death occurs from syncope induced by some muscular exertion, as standing up or even rising in bed. In other cases the symptoms indicate the development of cardiac thrombosis, and subsequent examination has verified this opinion. In still other cases the symptoms resemble those which occur in extreme hyperpyrexia dependent upon overwhelming and paralysis of the nervous centres. Copious hemorrhage from the stomach and nose may also induce syncope of alarming and even fatal severity. When from the latter cause, reaction may be induced and the patient may ultimately recover, as we saw in a case where after repeated hematemesis the patient sank into profound collapse. In all of its forms, however, this complication is of extreme and imminent danger, and death follows, as a rule, in a few hours. The cases in which it occurs are usually of severe type, occurring in persons who have previously been in poor health or intemperate, or who have been subjected to privation and improper exposure previous to and during the early stages of their attack. Still, collapse may occur in mild cases [p. 402]also, and whatever the type of the disease there may be no special indication of approaching trouble, when the patient rapidly passes into collapse, to be followed by death in a few hours. It occurred in nine of about two hundred cases under our observation. In one it was the result of hemorrhage from the stomach, and ended in recovery; in one, at the close of the initial paroxysm the patient, who was stupid, with muttering delirium, sank into collapse as the temperature rapidly fell from 105° to 97°, and died in a few hours; in one, on the fourth day of the relapse the temperature suddenly fell from 102° to 96°, with free sweating, but suddenly rebounded to 102°, with very rapid, feeble pulse, distinct basic cardiac murmur, constriction of chest, restlessness and delirium, slight convulsions, and death in eight hours; in one, a man at the end of the initial paroxysm, immediately after his admission to the hospital in apparently fair condition, became violently delirious, with bounding pulse, soon grew comatose, and died in one hour; in one, a man who was in feeble condition, on the nineteenth day, with irregular persistent fever (he had splenic abscess), sat up on the edge of the bed, sank back in syncope, and died in less than an hour; in one, a man who did well until the second day of the relapse, when pleuro-pneumonia and pericarditis were developed, died suddenly four days later: there was considerable pericardial effusion; in one, sudden death from syncope or cardiac thrombosis occurred on the twelfth day in a man who had suppurative parotitis and metastatic abscesses of the lungs; in one, sudden collapse and death occurred in one and a half hours at the end of the initial paroxysm; in one, a drunkard with large fatty liver had pyrexia continuing after the initial paroxysm, and on the ninth day, while in a state of hebetude, with mild delirium and a pulse of 112, coma suddenly occurred, and death followed in two hours.

Pericarditis is a rare complication, and is apt to coexist with pleuro-pneumonia. This combination occurred in one of our cases where pleuro-pneumonia and pericarditis were developed on the second day of relapse, and proved fatal by sudden collapse on the fifth day, with the pericardial sac distended with serum and its layers coated with plastic lymph.

Thrombosis of veins, as in phlegmasia alba dolens, occurs much more rarely than after typhoid fever. Arterial embolism, on the other hand, is not uncommon. Murchison[22] reports a case in which gangrene of the left foot from obstruction of the left femoral artery, together with cerebral softening from obstruction of the left middle cerebral artery, occurred in connection with cardiac thrombosis. Zuelzer alludes to similar cases in the St. Petersburg epidemic of 1865-66, where, in addition to the extremities, the nose, ears, and lips became gangrenous. Other examples of embolism are found in lesions of the spleen and kidneys, where infarctions are of frequent occurrence.

[22] *Op. cit.*, p 384.

Heart-clot, or cardiac thrombosis, appears to occur more frequently than in any other acute zymotic disease, with the exception of diphtheria. Even when the occurrence of passive hemorrhages and of ecchymoses of various tissues indicates marked dyscrasia of the blood, there will not rarely be found firm white clots in one or other of the cavities of the heart. These frequently present unmistakable evidences [p. 403]of ante-mortem formation, and, as already stated, there is a certain proportion of the cases of rapid and unexpected death where the fatal result is directly due to cardiac thrombosis, attended with the usual symptoms.

The constant affection of the spleen has been fully described; it is not therefore surprising that both complications and sequelæ arise in connection with it. At times, in cases which ultimately recover, the pain in the splenic region is so violent and continuous, and is attended with so much tenderness over the enlarged organ, that localized peritonitis is undoubtedly present. Occasionally this perisplenitis persists, and in conjunction with the inflammatory changes in the substance of the spleen maintains an irregular fever after the specific pyrexia has run its course. This was noticed in several of our cases, but especially so in a case where, after the initial paroxysm, an irregular fever was kept up, obscuring the relapse, until the nineteenth day, when death occurred suddenly from syncope on rising on the edge of the bed, and where examination showed splenic peritonitis, with a splenic abscess as large as a pigeon's egg.

The enlargement of the spleen usually subsides during the intermission, and disappears speedily or in the course of a few weeks after convalescence is established. Occasionally, however, it persists, and is attended with marked anæmia. In one case, where death occurred from pneumonia, the sequel of relapsing fever, at about the thirtieth day, the spleen weighed twenty-nine ounces; and in another case, where death occurred from gangrenous pleuro-pneumonia, at the fortieth day, the spleen was still enlarged and presented characteristic changes in its pulp. On the other hand, in a case where death occurred on the twelfth day of typhus, occurring forty-four days after recovery from a very bad case of relapsing fever, making it altogether the one hundredth day, none of the lesions of the first disease were discoverable.

Rupture of the spleen occurs occasionally, and is usually attended with sudden pain, collapse, and speedy death. Murchison refers to two examples recorded by Zuelzer and one by Hudson; Petersen reports fifteen cases, in seven of which sudden rupture occurred with speedy death, while in the other eight the rupture followed local softening from infarction, and resulted in death in a few days from purulent peritonitis.

In one of our cases, where death occurred on the sixteenth day, apparently from double pneumonia and heart-clot, it was found that there was a rupture in the enlarged spleen near its upper end, recent plastic peritonitis in the region of the spleen, and a moderate amount of bloody pulpy fluid throughout the peritoneal cavity.

As we have seen, disturbances within the respiratory tract occur with very different frequency in different epidemics. In many they are rare, while in 1870 we noticed cough and other evidences of respiratory trouble in no less than 90 out of 200 cases.

Severe catarrhal laryngitis is a rare and dangerous complication. It did not occur in our cases, but both Begbie and Paterson report cases of it which required tracheotomy, and Wyss and Bock met with ulcerative laryngitis with perichondritis.

Bronchitis of moderate severity, although rare in many epidemics, [p. 404]occurs so frequently in others, as in Philadelphia in 1870, as to rank as a symptom of the disease.

Pneumonia is one of the most fatal complications. The results of our own observations agree with the statements of Jenner and of Carter, that it is the next most common lesion after enlargement of the liver and spleen. On the other hand, Murchison noted it only in 4 or 5 out of 600 cases. It occurred in at least 11 of our cases, 8 of which were fatal; and unquestionably less extensive inflammation was present in other cases which recovered, in view of the marked respiratory disturbances frequently present. Both lungs were involved in 4 cases; of the remainder, the right and left were about equally divided. Out of 23 autopsies, the lesions of pneumonia were found 8 times. The lower lobes were affected in every case. The form of this disease was croupous in 9 cases; in 1 it was that of metastatic suppuration, and in 1 it was more properly described as splenification. The amount of plastic pleurisy associated with it was usually great, and in one case there was also severe pericarditis. In another case the disease advanced to the stage of gangrene of a circumscribed area of the pleura and of the superficial layer of the lung. In only one instance was albuminuria present. In two cases the pneumonia occurred so late in the course of the disease that it might be regarded as a sequel. Death occurred in one of these on the thirtieth day, and in the other (that in which gangrene ensued) it ran a subacute course, and death did not take place until the fortieth day. In the other cases the disease began at the close of the initial paroxysm, during the intermission, or early in the relapse. As would be expected, the sympathetic fever due to this complication modified and obscured the characteristic course of the specific pyrexia.

This rare termination in gangrene has been noted by other observers; in all five or six times. Parry met with a truly remarkable case of double pneumonia, followed by gangrene, and yet resulting in recovery. Jaundice is apt to attend cases of relapsing fever which are complicated with pneumonia.

Pleurisy is an almost constant accompaniment of pneumonia, and frequently occurs in marked degree. It may also be present in cases of severe splenic inflammation. In all probability, localized plastic pleurisy is not infrequent, and may cause some of the severe thoracic pains so frequently present.

Metastatic abscesses of the lung occur occasionally as a result of the profound toxæmia, and are apparently preceded by patches of infarction, which soften in the centre, as in the usual development of pyæmic abscesses. This condition was found in one of our cases in conjunction with suppurative parotitis. It has been included among the instances of pneumonia.

Acute miliary tuberculosis, involving chiefly the lungs and intestinal canal, occurred as a sequel in one case under our observation, and phthisis has been found to follow by other observers (Carter). It is to be expected that if the patient did not so quickly pass from under observation it would be found that an affection so gravely complicating nutrition as does relapsing fever is frequently followed by serious organic disease.

Parotitis is mentioned by so few authors as to show that it is a [p. 405]rare complication in most epidemics, varying from 1 in 600 to 1 in 50 cases. One gland only is affected at a time as a rule, though both may be involved successively. The inflammation begins either during the intermission or the relapse, and may terminate by resolution or by suppuration. Although a painful and severe complication, it is followed by recovery in a considerable proportion of cases. Carter[23] states "that in some degree it was noted in 2 or 3 per cent. of all cases, and nearly as often amongst survivors as in the casualties." It occurred in three of our cases (185); once it underwent resolution; once suppuration occurred in the parotid and in the masseter muscle, with metastatic abscesses in the lungs, and death; and once the patient, who had previously existing amyloid degeneration of liver and spleen without albuminuria, had severe relapsing fever with two relapses, in the first of which parotitis occurred in both glands, successively terminating in suppuration, after which he did well through an apyretic period of six weeks, when sudden high fever appeared, followed by speedy death.

[23] *Op. cit.*, p. 210.

Pharyngitis and tonsillitis of mild grade occur in from 3 to 25 per cent. of the cases in different epidemics.

Hiccough deserves to be ranked among the complications, because it is of frequent occurrence, obstinate and annoying. It occurred in a considerable proportion of our cases, and much more frequently in those who had jaundice. It was often present both in the initial paroxysm and in the relapse, but disappeared soon after the end of the pyrexia. It bore no constant relation to the severity of the vomiting. Not rarely it lasted several days and nights, causing exhaustion and interference with sleep and proving rebellious to treatment. Hypodermic injections of morphia and atropia, chloroform internally, and extremely careful alimentation proved most serviceable.

Hemorrhage from the stomach has already been spoken of (see above).

Diarrhoea, as already stated (see above), occurs much more frequently than in typhus fever, varying from 1 per cent. (Murchison) to 15 per cent. (Scotch epidemics) or 33 per cent. (Philadelphia), or even 50 per cent. (Königsberg). It is usually of moderate severity, but occasionally is so profuse and intractable as to constitute the main cause of death. In some epidemics the attacks of looseness occur almost exclusively after the relapse, but in others the bowels are frequently loose during the febrile stages. In our cases there were not infrequently from three to eight thin, dark, bilious or light yellowish stools daily after the second or third day of the initial paroxysm, and then the looseness would stop during the intermission, probably to recur in the relapse. Occasionally diarrhoea with very frequent liquid stools occurs at the close of one or both of the febrile stages, assuming a critical character, and substituting more or less of the sweating which is the common mode of crisis, although in several such cases quoted by Murchison from Douglas the sweating, despite the critical diarrhoea, was usually profuse. It can scarcely be said that there is any relationship between diarrhoea and vomiting; both are frequently present, and may even be severe and persistent in the same case, though either may be marked while the other is moderate or slight. Abdominal pain and tenderness in the epigastrium and hypochondria are constant symptoms, but when diarrhoea is marked there are apt also to be griping [p. 406]pains and tenderness in the lower segment of the abdomen. When diarrhoea occurs as a sequel, either beginning after the close of the relapse or continuing in cases where the bowels have been loose during pyrexia, it is apt to prove obstinate and intractable, or even to lead to a fatal result.

The character of the stools varies much; usually thin and dark, they may be light yellowish or even whitish. Thus, in a severe case with deep jaundice we observed seven liquid and decidedly whitish stools in twenty-four hours. In such instances there is undoubtedly more or less complete closure of the biliary ducts by plugs of mucus or by swelling of the mucous membrane. On the other hand, the stools may be inky black from admixture with altered blood, or, lastly, they may consist of mucus and blood, in which event the complication assumes the form of actual dysentery and is attended with increased abdominal pain and with tenesmus. Dysentery was, as would be expected, quite frequent in the Indian epidemics studied by Carter.[24] It is usually of moderate severity, but occasionally it runs into gangrenous inflammation, is attended with perforation of the bowel, or is followed by hepatic abscess. In one instance we noticed a peculiarly fetid puriform discharge from the anus, which occurred during the relapse and persisted for several weeks, gradually subsiding, as though from some unhealthy ulceration which slowly healed.

[24] *Op. cit.*, p. 218.

Jaundice is of frequent occurrence, but has been sufficiently discussedabove.

Peritonitis is not rare in its circumscribed form. This statement is based on the comparative frequency with which localized splenic peritonitis, of varying degrees of severity, is found after death in relapsing fever from various causes, and from the great frequency of severe pain and tenderness in the region of the enlarged spleen in favorable cases. In its lesser degrees it may not add materially to the danger of the patient, but in more severe forms, associated with serious splenic lesions, it may run a protracted subacute course and maintain irregular fever.

General peritonitis is, on the other hand, a rare complication, occurring not more than once in several hundred cases. It results from dysenteric perforation of the bowel, from rupture of a splenic abscess, or from rupture of the spleen itself. An example of this latter accident which occurred under our observation has already been given. Speedy death invariably follows, though in the case just referred to the symptoms of peritonitis were totally masked by those of the coexisting double pneumonia, which seemed to be the immediate cause of death.

Suppuration of the mesenteric glands is a rare complication, mentioned especially by Wyss and Bock. As these glands are not usually found enlarged, there being no irritative lesion of the intestines of common occurrence in relapsing fever, it is probable that the collections of pus which have been found were metastatic in origin.

Dyspepsia is not an infrequent sequel, as would necessarily be the case after a disease characterized by so much gastric irritation and by such serious lesions of the liver and spleen. As a consequence, care in diet is often required for a considerable period after the course of the disease has ended; dyspeptic symptoms are frequently complained of, and marked emaciation and anæmia often protract convalescence.

[p. 407]It may be observed that a striking appearance of emaciation is often developed shortly after the crisis of the first paroxysm, or, more particularly, of the relapse. It is partly due to the actual loss of weight during the high pyrexia, but even more to the abrupt transition from a state of extreme febrile turgescence to one of equally extreme relaxation and maceration of the surface.

The amount of urine has been seen (above) to vary greatly in cases distinguished by no special disorder of the kidneys; the extremes in ordinary cases being from twelve or fifteen ounces just before the crisis to from eighty to one hundred and twenty within forty-eight hours after the crisis. Suppression is, however, sometimes noted, and is always a grave symptom, though Parry[25] reports more than one case in which on several successive days there was not more in twenty-four hours than one fluidounce of non-albuminous urine, and in which no symptoms of uræmia occurred, and the sweat had no urinous odor. In one of our fatal cases, with intense jaundice, hematemesis, inky black stools, and oedema of the feet and of the lungs, there was not a drop of urine secreted during the last four days of the initial paroxysm; death occurred on the eighth day, and the kidneys were found intensely engorged, of a deep blackish-blue color, with numerous ecchymoses in the cortex, due to impaction of the convoluted tubules with blood, while the renal epithelium was granular and swollen, and many tubules were filled with epithelial cells and granular matter. At the autopsy the urinary bladder was firmly contracted and contained a very small amount of bloody liquid.

[25] *Op. cit.*

More frequently, incontinence of urine, with or without retention, occurs during the febrile stages—according to our observation, most commonly in cases attended with mental disturbance and tending to a typhoid condition. The symptom was not of very grave significance, however, and after the use of the catheter for a few days the bladder regained its tone.

Albumen is quite frequently present in small amounts during the pyrexia of relapsing fever. Thus, in 18 cases of ordinary severity, which all recovered, and in which the urine was carefully examined daily, a trace of albumen was found in 5; in 2 cases it appeared both in the initial paroxysm and in the relapse, but in all instances its presence was of brief duration. In one of these five cases the albumen appeared at both critical periods, when the amounts of urine in twenty-four hours were respectively 150 ccm. and 250 ccm.; but in the other cases the transient albuminuria coincided with free secretion of urine (1250 ccm., 1850 ccm.). It is probable that were the same careful search to be made in all cases the presence of albumen would be detected in fully 20 to 25 per cent. On the other hand, in fatal cases the occurrence of albuminuria is by no means constant, although undoubtedly it is present in a larger proportion of such cases than of those of ordinary severity.

Our experience does not confirm that of Murchison, who states that he never met with typhoid symptoms in relapsing fever without albuminuria or some other evidence of retarded elimination by the kidneys. In several of our cases where the typhoid state was developed in the highest degree repeated examination of the urine failed to discover albumen.

[p. 408]Most observers have been struck with the comparative immunity of the kidneys from serious disturbance in a disease presenting such complicated morbid processes and widespread lesions as relapsing fever. To show, however, that these organs suffer specially in certain epidemics, it may be mentioned that Obermeier[26] reports having found albumen with tube-casts of various kinds in 32 out of 40 cases of relapsing fever, thus showing that, in the particular epidemic he was studying, catarrhal nephritis was of almost uniform occurrence. It is true that serious interference with the elimination of urea and other nitrogenous matters may occur without the coexistence of albuminuria, so that it is impossible to deny that severe nervous symptoms may result from impaired renal activity even when the urine contains no albumen.

[26] "U. d. wiederkehrende Fieber," *Arch. f. path. Anat. u. klin. Med.*, Bd. xlvii. p. 170.

Attention has already been called to the variations presented in the amounts of urea, but more extended observations are required to show the precise relations of these variations to the graver nervous phenomena. It will be found, we venture to opine, that, while in one group of relapsing-fever cases of grave type, cerebral symptoms are dependent upon the retention and accumulation in the system of urea and other effete nitrogenous products, owing to interference with renal activity from pre-existing organic disease of the kidneys or from an exceptional degree of congestion of those organs, there are other groups where similar typhoid cerebral symptoms are more directly dependent upon the specific toxæmia, upon the hyperpyrexia, upon exhaustion of the nerve-centres by intense peripheral irritation, or upon congestion or other morbid conditions of the nerve-centres themselves.

In all cases where cerebral symptoms manifest themselves in relapsing fever the daily examination of the urine—which here, as in other zymotic diseases, is a duty in all cases—becomes of extreme importance. Three conditions should be borne in mind in such examinations. In the first place, the attack of fever may have occurred in one already the subject of organic kidney disease, and, considering the classes from which the majority of the cases of relapsing fever are drawn, this possibility cannot be of rare occurrence. Out of eighteen post-mortem examinations in which the kidneys were studied with especial care we found positive evidence of pre-existing organic disease four times. In these cases the albuminuria was marked and persistent, though tube-casts were rarely found, and severe cerebral symptoms of typhoid type were prominently present. In another highly interesting case the patient, who had amyloid disease of the liver, spleen, and kidneys, contracted severe relapsing fever; he had increased albuminuria during both febrile stages, suppurative parotitis, but no grave cerebral symptoms, and apparently recovered. After an apyretic period of six weeks, during which the symptoms of the amyloid visceral disease persisted, a sudden and rapidly fatal pyrexia occurred. Unfortunately, the existence of spirillar infection of the blood was not known at the time.

In the second place, the attack of fever may become complicated with acute nephritis from special localization of the poison, as in Obermeier's cases, or from vulnerability of the kidneys. In such cases careful study of the urine should indicate the event, and the prognosis, though grave, is not so hopeless as in the first instance. An interesting example of [p. 409]this occurred under our observation, where the patient, who had apparently an ordinary attack, was seized with acute catarrhal nephritis, with temporary uræmia, during the relapse, but after a dangerous illness recovered without any organic renal disease as a sequel.

In the third place, may be found the more usual and more readily-determined condition of slight and transient albuminuria (with variations in urea excretion) which has already been discussed, and which has no serious prognostic significance.

The following very interesting case deserves special mention: The patient, a man aged thirty-six, was admitted on the fifteenth day of an attack of acute catarrhal nephritis, with slight ascites, marked oedema of the feet and legs, and highly albuminous urine. In the course of ten days the oedema and albuminuria were much diminished, when on the thirteenth day after admission he was attacked with relapsing fever, the ward in which he lay containing a number of persons ill with that disease. The initial paroxysm was severe, but without any grave cerebral symptoms; the urine grew scanty, dark, and bloody, and the oedema increased and invaded the pelvis. Crisis occurred on the fifth day, temperature falling 9°, sweating copious, urine 473 ccm. in twenty-four hours, color of porter, highly albuminous, and depositing blood, renal epithelium, hyaline, granular and epithelial casts, all stained reddish. Two days later, urine 1600 ccm., light colored, with only a small amount of albumen.

A slight and brief relapse (101° for two days) occurred after an interval of four days; a second imperfect relapse (100.5° for three days) after a further interval of six days; and finally, after a further interval of only two days, a violent relapse (temperature rising rapidly to 106°) with crisis (fall of 8° in twelve hours) at close of fifth day. The oedema gradually diminished from the time of the first crisis, did not increase in the relapses, and disappeared completely and finally about ten days after the last relapse. The urine was very free after the first paroxysm, averaging from 2000 to 2300 ccm. During the subsequent febrile periods it did not decrease, and indeed on the second day of the last relapse, with the temperature at 105°, the amount in twenty-four hours was 3200 ccm. Four days subsequently, during crisis, the amount was only 350 ccm.

The albumen disappeared entirely from the urine in two weeks from the close of the last relapse; there had then been no tube-casts for some days, and the patient was discharged entirely well a short time afterward. The treatment consisted of hot vapor-baths, repeated dry cupping over the kidneys, infusion of digitalis with acetate of potash during pyrexia, and Basham's iron mixture in the intermissions. It seemed that the occurrence of the relapsing fever interfered wonderfully little with the recovery from nephritis.

Hematuria is a comparatively rare and very grave complication. It may occur as an additional evidence of the dyscrasia of the blood in connection with hemorrhages from other surfaces, or as in the case we have before referred to or in that reported by Murchison,[27] it results from intense engorgement of the kidneys. In Murchison's case hematuria, with much albumen and tube-casts, occurred in both paroxysms [p. 410]without any uræmic or typhoid symptoms, and was followed by satisfactory recovery.

[27] *Op. cit.*, p. 370.

Sugar is sometimes present in small quantity as a transient symptom; and diabetes has been observed as a sequel.[28]

[28] Tyson, *Phila. Med. Times*, 1871, i. 418.

Metastatic inflammation of the kidneys, with centres of suppuration, was observed by Wyss and Bock.

When menstruation occurs during relapsing fever, as it may do at any time, it is apt to be excessive, and may amount to severe hemorrhage. Crisis has been known to occur in this manner.

The numerous cases reported by various observers of relapsing fever occurring in pregnant women establish the rule that abortion almost invariably occurs, whatever may be the stage of the pregnancy. In a large majority of cases the mother recovers, but the child, if viable, is stillborn or dies in a few hours. Only two of our patients were pregnant women, and the result in each was unusual. In one, the patient, already the mother of several children, was in the fifth month of gestation; the initial paroxysm was severe, with delirium, but no symptoms of abortion occurred; the intermission lasted six days, during which she felt very well; the relapse was also severe, and crisis occurred on the fifth day, the temperature falling below normal, and the case promising to do well; but on the following day there was a sudden rebound of temperature, pulse 140, severe præcordial pain, and death occurred in twenty-four hours, the contents of the uterus being partially expelled during the act of dying. In the other case, a girl of eighteen years, who had aborted at the third month of gestation eight months previously, and who was again three months advanced in pregnancy when attacked with relapsing fever, went safely through a bad attack and carried her baby successfully to full term.

MORBID ANATOMY.—The surface of the body often presents patches of livid discoloration, and jaundice persists in cases where it has been present during life. There is but little appearance of emaciation, except in cases where it has been present before the attack.

When death occurs while the temperature is high the body remains warm an unusual length of time. Thus, in one case where death occurred at 11.30 P.M., the temperature at 12 was 103°, and at 1 A.M. it was 101.6°, that of the room being 73°; at 6 A.M. it remained at 93°, the room being at 73°; between 9 A.M. and 2 P.M. the room was kept at 55°, but the body was still at 82° at the latter hour.

The voluntary muscles are often jaundiced, and in prolonged cases they may be found flabby and having undergone marked granular degeneration. In many cases, however, they remain quite dark and firm. Ecchymoses of the muscular substance are met with occasionally.

In one case, where during life there had been painful swelling of the left parotid region, with fistulous openings on the cheek, and where death occurred on the twelfth day of the disease, the masseter muscle was swollen, with patches of dark, almost black, discoloration from ecchymosis, and was studded throughout with small collections in its substance. The fluid from these contained very numerous cells indistinguishable from leucocytes. The muscular fibrils were friable and granular, and there was multiplication of the nuclei of the sarcolemma.[p. 411]These unusual lesions seemed to have originated in interstitial disintegrating thrombi, with consequent inflammation of the muscle.

The muscle of the heart is more frequently affected, and in the fatal cases our attention was particularly drawn to those lesions. Ponfick[29] has also described them minutely. The degree of change varies from a partial loss of transverse striation, with slight granular appearance, up to a very high degree of granulo-fatty degeneration. The organ is then flabby, its substance pale gray or brownish, either wholly or in streaks, and microscopic examination shows an extreme degree of fatty granular change. It must not be forgotten, however, that many of the subjects of relapsing fever have been leading irregular and dissipated lives, and that in some instances the lesions of fatty degeneration detected in their organs may have been the result of their previous habits.

[29] *Virchow's Archiv. f. path. Anat.*, Bd. lx. Hft. 2, p. 162.

Lesions of the cardiac muscle were most marked in those of our patients who had been intemperate, and in whom fatty degeneration of the viscera (chiefly liver and kidneys) was also found. They were most fully developed in cases where death occurred at a comparatively late period, while in some very severe cases, in which death occurred as early as the fifth day, the cardiac fibre presented merely faintness of striation without actual granular degeneration.

Ponfick in particular notes that the great majority of the bodies he examined were of persons who had been habitual drunkards.

Pericarditis is occasionally present, and is marked by the usual lesions. In a very severe case in which it contributed largely to the production of the fatal result it was associated with pneumonia. In addition to this, effusions of blood beneath the endocardium and pericardium are not rare; and we have seen them quite large and numerous in cases where the muscular fibre was firmly contracted and the cavities contained quite firm decolorized clots.

Thus in our case No. 62, Series C., "the heart was normal in size, with no appearances of previous disease. There were numerous ecchymoses of both layers of the pericardium. The right cavities contained large, firm, yellowish, fibrous clots, forming a cast of the upper part of the ventricle and of the auricle, and extending both into the pulmonary artery and back into the veins, and so firm that by gentle traction a complete cast of these vessels was drawn out. The clot in the pulmonary artery was throughout firm, fibrous, and yellowish. There were numerous ecchymoses of the pleura and of the mucous membranes of the stomach and urinary bladder, hemorrhagic infarctions in the kidneys and lungs, and granulo-fatty degeneration of the cardiac muscle." Death had occurred in this case about the close of the third week, and was preceded by hematemesis and suppression of urine. We must note in this connection the tendency to embolism that exists in this disease.

Especial interest attaches to the condition of the blood in relapsing fever. Usually it presents no abnormal appearance if drawn during life, though in grave cases it may coagulate imperfectly. We have no knowledge of its minute chemical characters, save that in several cases where there was great diminution in the amount of urine, with uræmic symptoms, urea has been found in considerable amount in the blood (Murchison, p. 368). The red globules present no definite or [p. 412]characteristic changes. In some of our examinations they appeared of light color and became crenated very quickly on exposure. On the other hand, the white corpuscles have repeatedly been observed to be increased in number, at times considerably so (Cormack, Thompson, Zuelzer, Carter, Boeckmann, and ourselves), though this change is not regarded as constant or essential. It has, however, a very great interest in connection with the characteristic lesions of the spleen which will be described hereafter. In several cases we observed that many white corpuscles were small and apparently imperfectly developed. Boeckmann[30] concludes that they increase in number during the febrile paroxysm, reaching their highest number at the crisis, and then diminishing gradually to the normal. The red globules are much decreased during the fever, and return to the normal slowly during convalescence.

[30] *Deutsch. Arch. f. klin. Med.*, Sept. 1881, p. 513.

In addition to these changes, various abnormal elements have been observed more or less constantly. By far the most important of these is the spirillum or spirochete of Obermeier, which has been already carefully described. In proportion as this organism has been carefully looked for it has been found constantly, so that the evidence has become very strong in favor of its uniform presence in the blood of relapsing-fever patients during the febrile stage of the disease.

Ponfick in 1874[31] called attention to the occurrence of large granule-cells in the blood in this disease. They are found during life as well as after death, when they exist in largest proportion in the blood of the splenic, hepatic, and portal veins. Their shape is spherical, ovoid, or elongated; the basis of the cells is a delicate, translucent, albuminous substance; and the granules are of a fatty nature, as shown by the action of reagents. These cells have been found by other observers, and the view is generally received that they are derived from the lymphoid elements of the spleen, and perhaps of other portions of the lymphatic system; and Carter, who has studied them carefully, is inclined to think there is some connection between them and the development of the spirillum.

[31] *Centralbl. f. d. med. Wissensch.*, 1874, p. 25.

Ponfick also first described[32] certain other large, irregularly-shaped, pale, granular, nucleated cells, which occur in smaller number in the blood in relapsing fever, and which he regarded as altered endothelium, derived from the lining of the blood-vessels, of the lymphatics, or of the lacunar spaces of the spleen. Occasionally these cells are found with such highly granular contents as to make them closely simulate the large granule-cells described above. These results of Ponfick have been confirmed by other observers.

[32] *Loc. cit.*

In several of our reports of examinations of blood there is mention made of quite abundant, free granular matter—an appearance also observed by Carter. Finally, the latter describes the occurrence of thread-like filaments and of short, rod-like bodies.

There are no characteristic lesions connected with the gastro-intestinal canal. The mucous membrane of the stomach may be normal or merely injected, though where there has been much vomiting, and especially bloody vomiting, there is marked injection, and not rarely ecchymosis and submucous extravasations of blood, with softening of the membrane.[p. 413]These extravasations are usually small, but Cormack reports a case where one-third of the mucous membrane of the stomach was the seat of ecchymosis and extravasation. In one of our own cases the extravasations occupied an area of four inches square.

The small intestines exhibit patches of congestion or ecchymosis less frequently than the stomach, though it is usual to find injection of the mucous membrane, especially of the lower portion, in cases where there has been diarrhoea. Carter, observing the disease in India, found in one-half of all autopsies some amount of congestion, hemorrhage, or inflammation of the ileum. In two instances he found a layer of diphtheritic deposit over the mucous membrane of the lower part of the ileum.

There are no special alterations of the solitary or agminated glands, and ulceration never occurs. Even in cases where the constitutional infection is severe, whether diarrhoea has been present or not, it is noteworthy that there is rarely any swelling of the solitary glands or Peyer's patches, such as is met with in many other acute specific diseases. It was not present in any of our autopsies.

The large intestine in like manner exhibits no characteristic lesions. Patches of congestion and occasionally submucous ecchymoses may be observed, and croupous exudation occurs here somewhat more frequently than in the small intestine.

Wyss and Bock[33] speak of enlargement of the mesenteric and retroperitoneal glands as of frequent occurrence, but we did not observe it, and Murchison states that these glands present no abnormal appearance.

[33] *Op. cit.*, p. 223.

Alterations of vascularity of the brain or its membranes are met with, but they are variable and bear no definite relation to the precedent symptoms. Ecchymoses of the membranes are occasionally observed, and in one of our cases extensive meningeal hemorrhage was found. Murchison reported a case in which embolism of the left femoral artery occurred, and subsequently of the left middle cerebral artery, inducing death. The suggestion may be hazarded that in some of the cases where there is severe delirium ending in stupor and death there has been multiple capillary embolism of the cerebral vessels.

There is occasionally the evidence of catarrhal inflammation of the upper air-passages, and in some epidemics diphtheritic exudation in the pharynx and larynx has been noted (Wyss and Bock); and Ponfick found acute oedema of the glottis in a considerable proportion of the fatal cases at Berlin. The lesions of pleurisy are met with in a small proportion of cases; in our own autopsies this complication was more frequent than in most epidemics.

The lungs may be normal, and Murchison concludes that they are more frequently so than in typhus. Still, they often present congestion or oedema, and subpleural ecchymoses, hemorrhagic infarctions, and pneumonic consolidation are not rare. Lobar pneumonia was present in 33 per cent. of our own autopsies, in 28 per cent. of Carter's, and in 20 per cent. of those conducted by Ponfick. The inflammation usually presents the regular stages, and is associated with a moderate degree of plastic pleurisy; but occasionally, as in one of our cases, it terminates in gangrene. In the instance referred to there was an area of gangrene about three inches square and one inch in depth, involving the pleura and a[p. 414]superficial layer of lung on the antero-lateral aspect of the left lower lobe. In another remarkable instance, already referred to on account of the suppurative inflammation of one masseter muscle, the lungs, which were stained yellow throughout, presented numerous deep purplish patches, which on section altogether resembled the secondary metastatic deposits of pyæmia, with yellowish softening or even puriform centres surrounded by a rim of purplish livid discoloration. Very numerous similar patches, varying from the size of a pea to that of a hazel-nut, and presenting every stage of development, were found throughout both lungs. In a few instances we found the lesions of chronic phthisis, which had, of course, existed before the attack of relapsing fever. The bronchial glands were found swollen and infiltrated in cases where inflammatory processes in the lungs have existed.

Much interest attaches to the state of the genito-urinary organs in relapsing fever, but caution is required to distinguish lesions that have existed prior to the attack from those properly referable to it.

Owing to the intemperate and exposed lives of many of the patients, renal lesions might reasonably be expected in no small proportion. The comparative rarity of albuminuria (see above), even in severe cases, is suggestive of the view that when it is present it may at least sometimes be due to pre-existing lesions aggravated by the acute infectious process, and further that the extreme gravity generally presented by such cases may be in part due to the impaired condition of the kidneys.

The morbid changes most frequently referable to the fever are moderate enlargement and congestion, occasionally very intense so that we find it described in our notes as deep blackish-purple or blue; ecchymoses of the capsule or of the mucous membrane of the pelvis; small hemorrhagic infarctions, usually in the cortex; and cloudy swelling of the glandular cells. Less commonly are found hemorrhagic infarctions, or small embolic patches advanced to various stages of disintegration, even to the formation of small puriform collections. In quite rare cases the lesions of acute nephritis are present, while caution must be used in interpreting other changes occasionally met with, such as pallor with granulo-fatty degeneration or other advanced alterations of the glandular cells, or hyperplasia of the intertubular connective tissue, with or without contraction of the kidneys.

The mucous membrane of the bladder, as already mentioned, may present ecchymoses, or, more rarely, croupous exudation (Wyss and Bock). The urine contained may be bloody, or, as in one of our cases where there had been total suppression of urine for over seventy-two hours before death, there may be but a small amount of almost pure blood, containing a few phosphate crystals, but no tube-casts. In this case there were also ecchymoses of the bladder and of the pelvis of the kidneys, with intense congestion and numerous small hemorrhagic infarctions of the kidneys.

The liver is constantly though variously affected. It is found enlarged in the great majority of cases, especially if death has occurred during the febrile stage. The ordinary degree of enlargement in our cases was from four to four and a half pounds, but in a few instances the liver weighed one hundred or one hundred and two ounces, though in most of these extreme cases the patients had been drunkards, and there was such advanced fatty alteration of the liver as to make it probable that the [p. 415]organ had been diseased previously. These figures correspond with the results of other observers.

In many cases, especially when death occurs early and during the febrile stage, the capsule and substance of the liver are congested, at times intensely so; and when ecchymoses are found elsewhere they are apt to be present here also, appearing as purplish patches dotted over the capsule and extending into the superficial layer of hepatic tissue. Not rarely, however, the liver substance is paler than normal, and presents a yellowish tinge, apart from the decided yellowish staining present in cases attended with jaundice. Carter describes a partial mottled paleness of the liver as having been frequently observed in his cases, the circumscribed pale areas presenting a corresponding localized degeneration of the cells, as though from some local interruption of circulation.

Cloudy swelling and fatty degeneration of the liver-cells are indeed very often present, and in some epidemics with preponderance of bilious symptoms are constantly found (Ponfick). The degree of the cell-alteration varies from a slight granulo-fatty change to an advanced fatty degeneration, even with a marked tendency, in rare cases, to disintegration of the cells, so as to produce lesions analogous to those of acute yellow atrophy (St. Petersburg epidemic).

The whitish deposits described by Küttner as due to albuminous or fibrinous infiltration are probably referable to transformed hemorrhagic infarctions, and the minute puriform collections that have been observed at the centre of the acini (Wyss and Bock) may have been metastatic in origin, or attributable to the disintegration of minute thrombi associated with irritative hyperplasia of the adjacent lymphoid elements. The consistence of the liver varies: when death occurs early and bilious symptoms have not been marked, it may be even firmer than normal, but more frequently it is softer, and it may be relaxed, flabby, and friable.

The condition of the bile-ducts is of great interest in view of the frequency of jaundice as a symptom in relapsing fever, and most authorities unite in saying that they present no lesions capable of explaining it.

The gall-bladder is usually found full of dark bile, but there is no such degree of inspissation, except in rare instances, as could interfere with its passage through the ducts. Murchison quotes the statement of Peacock that in some instances the bile was thick and viscid, so as apparently to cause obstruction, but all observations agree in showing that this is exceptional. The mucous membranes of the larger ducts may present evidences of slight catarrhal inflammation, but in nearly all cases where they have been carefully examined, even when jaundice had been marked, they have been found patulous and free, so that the jaundice cannot be regarded as due to obstruction of the larger ducts save in rare instances (Pastau). In further confirmation of this may be stated the fact that there is no want of bile in the duodenum and feces.

On the other hand, a careful consideration of the lesions of the substance of the liver will show that it would be most improbable that the minute biliary ducts in the areas most affected should escape implication. Münch, who investigated this subject carefully, found that there was a catarrhal state of the fine bile-ducts in every case of relapsing fever with jaundice; and Litten found the smallest ducts plugged with bile-stained pellets of mucus. It would appear, therefore, that in many cases at least [p. 416]the jaundice is really obstructive in its origin, the seat of the obstruction being in the too-rarely examined minute bile-ducts, though further investigation of this interesting question is required.

The clinical bearing of these conditions has been fully discussed in the appropriate section.

The changes in the spleen are constant, and even more remarkable than those in the liver. It is enlarged with rare exceptions, and especially so if death has occurred during the febrile stage. Upon the subsidence of the fever the spleen probably returns to its normal size more rapidly than the liver. The more common extent of the enlargement in our own cases was from ten to eighteen ounces, though we found the spleen in one case weighing twenty-nine and a half ounces and in another forty-four and a half ounces. In neither of the latter instances was there any reason to suspect malarial complication. The most extensive enlargement we have found recorded is sixty-eight ounces in a case reported by Küttner.[34]

[34] *Schmidt's Jahrb.*, 1865, vol. cxxvi.

There is usually a correspondence between the stage and extent of the splenic and hepatic lesions, but this is not invariable, and one or the other organ may present a far higher degree of enlargement or much more intense interstitial changes. It may be mentioned, moreover, that in some unusual cases the lesions of the lungs, such as ecchymoses and hemorrhagic infarctions, may be disproportionately marked as compared with those of either the liver or spleen.

The capsule of the spleen often presents a mottled look, with at times large purplish ecchymoses; it is apt to be more or less opaque, and local peritonitis, with thin layers of plastic exudation often forming friable adhesions with the abdominal wall, may exist.

In one of our cases the capsule presented a small perforation or rupture, with an exudation of plastic lymph over an area of four by six inches, and diffuse peritonitis, with effusion of bloody liquid with shreds of lymph throughout the abdominal cavity. This fatal termination is fortunately rare, but there are several other instances on record. The splenic pulp may retain its consistency and firmness, even in cases that have run a long course; but more frequently it is softened, and may be almost diffluent. The pulp is often swollen, so that when cut it projects above the section. The color is darker than normal, and often is of a deep maroon color. This swelling is due to enlargement of the blood-vessels, associated with great increase of the cellular elements of the pulp and with enlargement of the Malpighian corpuscles.

When death occurred early in the disease we found these bodies grayish or grayish-yellow in color and of the size of hempseed, so that the section very thickly studded with them closely resembled shad-roe, and this stage of the lesion is frequently described in our notes as the shad-roe spleen. Subsequently, the Malpighian bodies enlarge still more, and stand out above the section a line or more in diameter, and of a lighter color; not rarely, several of them come in contact, and thus form a considerable mass of irregular shape, resembling the infarctions described below.[35] It is probable that central softening may occur later in the [p. 417]Malpighian bodies, though we are inclined to regard the puriform collections frequently found as chiefly due to the disintegration of hemorrhagic infarctions or of embolic patches. Of these, hemorrhagic infarctions are by far the most common and present the familiar appearances. They may be quite numerous, superficial, or deep-seated, and of variable shape and size. At first dark reddish, firm, and sharply separated from the surrounding pulp, they grew reddish-yellow or yellowish later, softened in the centre, and eventually were transformed into puriform collections. Doubtless, in a large proportion of cases that recover such infarctions exist and are slowly absorbed. Ponfick has shown that these are venous infarctions, the arterioles leading to them being patulous. True arterial embolism does, however, occur, though much more rarely (Ponfick, Murchison), giving rise to firm, wedge-shaped infarctions at the periphery of the spleen, which may undergo degenerative changes similar to those above described. The resulting abscesses may burst into the peritoneum, pleura, lung, or bowel. The microscopic appearances have been most fully described by Ponfick, our own comparatively meagre observations having accorded entirely with his subsequent accurate description. The cells of the swollen pulp contain red blood-discs and pigment, and some present collections of bright granules. The lymphoid cells of the Malpighian corpuscles are at first in a state of cloudy swelling with multiplication of their nuclei, and later show marked granular fatty degeneration.

[35] Thus, Wyss and Bock describe "multitudes of minute abscesses as large as poppy or hempseed, and containing a single drop of pus."

The lymphatic glands present no lesions, and the pancreas is normal.

The peritoneum is not affected as frequently as other serous membranes in this disease. Superficial ecchymoses are, however, quite common, especially so over the solid viscera; and more rarely effusions of blood have been found in the subperitoneal connective tissue, involving the muscular or glandular tissues beneath. We have already mentioned (above) the occasional occurrence of local peritonitis, most frequently of the splenic capsule, and also the rare accident of diffuse inflammation from rupture of the spleen.

The marrow of the bones was carefully examined by Ponfick, who first called attention to the presence of important changes in relapsing fever, which have since been confirmed by other observers. These changes consist in proliferation and subsequent degeneration of the lymphoid cells of the marrow, with multiplication of the nuclei in the walls of the minute vessels and fatty degeneration of their coats. As a result of these changes, spots of puriform softening may form, chiefly in the cancellous tissue of the extremities of the long bones, with the production of localized necrosis, and possibly with extension of inflammation to the neighboring articular cavity.

Considerable space has been devoted to the detailed consideration of the pathological changes in relapsing fever, partly because we believe the fact has not been sufficiently recognized that the disease is constantly attended with important and characteristic lesions. These consist, in brief, of remarkable changes in the blood; of widespread ecchymoses and infarctions, which not rarely undergo puriform disintegration; of hyperplasia and subsequent degeneration of the Malpighian corpuscles of the spleen, with changes in the cellular elements of the splenic pulp; of cloudy swelling of the gland-cells of the liver and kidneys, with a [p. 418]marked tendency to fatty degeneration; of changes in the marrow of the long bones; and, finally, of granulo-fatty degeneration of the muscles, and especially of the heart.

DIAGNOSIS AND RELATION TO OTHER DISEASES.—The entire question of the diagnosis of relapsing fever is dominated by that of spirillar infection. Before Obermeier's discovery the differential diagnosis of the initial paroxysm, and to a less extent that of the subsequent events of a case of relapsing fever, was attended with considerable difficulty. But if, as now seems established, immediately before and throughout the initial paroxysm and subsequent relapses a characteristic spirillum is to be detected in the blood upon proper examination, while it rapidly disappears after the crisis, it is evident that as soon as a suspicion is aroused as to the possible presence of relapsing fever the question may be settled conclusively by the microscope.

None the less is it important to consider carefully, but briefly, the symptoms by which relapsing fever is to be distinguished from various affections which may simulate it, because even the most experienced observers admit that the spirillum cannot be invariably detected; because it is not yet known that a similar organism may not be found in some other affections; and, finally, because on the outbreak of an epidemic of relapsing fever, especially in America, where its occurrence has hitherto been so rare, there is strong probability that the nature of the early cases will not be even suspected until the relapse occurs.

Typhus fever often prevails in an epidemic form simultaneously with relapsing fever, so that it was inevitable they should have been for a time confused. Their essential non-identity is, however, now too well recognized to require any lengthy demonstration. The following statement of the heads of the argument may therefore suffice.

In typhus there is no characteristic spirillum, and the lesions which are truly characteristic of relapsing fever are totally wanting. There are convincing differences in the symptoms, course, and results of the two diseases. There is no evidence to show that when fever has been imported into a locality by a single case, typhus fever has ever produced other than typhus, or relapsing other than relapsing fever. The two diseases often prevail together, and may coexist in the same house, each preserving its own distinct characteristics; and persons exposed to the double contagion may contract one or the other, or first one and then the other at a shorter or longer interval, so that an attack of either exerts no protective power against the other. It must be noted, however, that in a large majority of such cases of successive contagion it is relapsing fever which has been followed by typhus, while the reverse has been observed much more rarely.

In 1869-70 the two diseases were prevalent in Philadelphia, and the wards of the municipal hospitals constantly contained a considerable number of cases of both. Three instances came under our care in which after recovery from relapsing fever the patient contracted typhus. All of these patients were employed as assistant nurses, and were continuously under observation from the early part of their attack of relapsing fever to the end of the attack of typhus. In one case the interval of health between the close of the relapse and the onset of typhus was forty-four days; in the second it was thirteen days. In both cases the original disease was[p. 419]thoroughly characteristic and the subsequent attack of typhus was typical. In both death followed, and the post-mortem examination verified the above statement. The third patient had severe relapsing fever, from which he recovered and returned to work, though with pains in the legs, shoulders, and forehead. After an interval of apparent health of eleven days he developed a well-marked attack of typhus, which terminated on the twelfth day in recovery. It may be added that although typhus is not of frequent occurrence in any portion of North America, there have been a number of epidemics unattended with a single case presenting the features of relapsing fever.

Between well-marked cases of the two diseases there should be no difficulty in making a prompt diagnosis. Relapsing fever is distinguished from typhus clinically by the severity of the initial chill; the rapid elevation of the pulse and temperature; the comparative infrequency and mildness of cerebral symptoms, despite the intense fever; the severity of the gastric symptoms, nausea and vomiting; the enlargement of the liver and spleen, with marked abdominal pain and soreness; the frequency of jaundice, of epistaxis, and of other hemorrhages, and of anæmic murmurs over the heart and large vessels; obstinate insomnia; vertigo; peculiar rheumatoid pains and perversions of sensation; the frequency of sweating during the high pyrexia; by the occurrence of crisis, subnormal temperature, apyretic interval, and relapse; the rarity of measly eruption and of bed-sores; the frequency of pneumonia, diarrhoea, ophthalmia, oedema, and desquamation as complications and sequelæ; the usual occurrence of abortion in pregnant females; the protracted course of the disease, and its remarkably low mortality despite the severity of the symptoms, except in cases of complicated or typhoid type; and, finally, by the modes in which death occurs. Of course to this must be added the specific result of examination of the blood in relapsing fever.

Doubt will arise only in very rare cases where a measly eruption appears on or before the fifth day of relapsing fever, with headache and mild delirium, but without severe gastric symptoms, epistaxis, or jaundice. If no relapsing fever were prevalent at the time, such a case might well be regarded as one of mild typhus until the crisis and the relapse disclosed its real nature. But if the two diseases were known to be prevalent in the community, examination of the blood would properly be made at once and the diagnosis be established.

The diagnosis between ordinary cases of relapsing fever and typhoid is readily made by the gradual onset and peculiar course of the pyrexia in the latter disease, as well as by the frequency of delirium, of abdominal distension, and of diarrhoea, and by the characteristic eruption. The occurrence of epistaxis, bronchial irritation, and splenic enlargement is common to both, and an eruption of small rose-pink spots has been noted by some observers (Carter, pp. 194, 317). But jaundice, enlargement of the liver, hypochondriac pain and soreness, excessive nausea and vomiting, severe rheumatoid pains, and numbness and tingling of the extremities, are very significant symptoms of relapsing fever. Attention has already been called to the grave type of relapsing fever in which the typhoid state is fully developed, and to the fact that in such cases the pyrexia is often modified, the onset less abrupt, the crisis imperfect, and the interval occupied by an irregular post-critical [p. 420]symptomatic fever. It is altogether probable that such cases have not rarely been regarded as of true typhoid character; and indeed the attempt has been made by Griesinger to establish as a separate and independent affection, under the name of bilious typhoid fever, a group of cases which close examination seems to show to be chiefly composed of grave complicated relapsing fever with a certain proportion of true typhoid fever, complicated with jaundice.

The recognition of the bilious typhoid type of relapsing fever is based upon the history of the case; the mode of onset; the greater severity of the pains, arthritic and abdominal; the early appearance and intensity of the jaundice; the more marked enlargement of the liver and spleen; the marked tendency to hemorrhages from various surfaces; the peculiarities which careful study of the temperature curve will show, especially about the time of crisis; the rarity of eruption; the characteristic spirillum;[36] and the totally different anatomical lesions, which are, unfortunately, often demonstrable, as this form of relapsing fever is fatal in from 33 to 50 per cent. of cases.

[36] As first demonstrated by Motschutkoffsky.

Since the discovery of the spirillar test for relapsing fever it may be said that Griesinger's bilious typhoid must be stricken from medical nosology as an independent affection.

The case of Charles Hood, above, is a good example of the bilious typhoid form which occurred not rarely in the Philadelphia epidemic.

Murchison points out that, owing to the frequent occurrence of jaundice in relapsing fever, this disease has been mistaken for yellow fever by such good observers as Graves, Stokes, and Cormack. Difficulty in diagnosis would be likely to arise only in regard to the bilious typhoid type of relapsing fever, and since its clinical history has become so well known, a mistake is not likely to occur. The geographical distribution of the diseases is widely different. Yellow fever is influenced powerfully by season and temperature, while relapsing fever is independent of both. Negroes are but slightly liable to yellow fever, while relapsing fever attacks them with special violence. Yellow fever is not contagious, but infectious, and second attacks are extremely rare; relapsing fever is one of the most contagious of the zymotic diseases, but one attack does not protect against a subsequent one. The mortality, the anatomical lesions, the course of the pyrexia, the leading clinical symptoms, are all widely distinct in the two affections; and, finally, no spirillum has been found in the blood in yellow fever. Yellow fever is an extremely fatal disease; the ordinary form of relapsing fever has a mortality of 2 to 10 per cent.; the bilious typhoid form, one of 33 to 50 per cent. In yellow fever the spleen is but slightly enlarged, and the liver is pale and softened; in relapsing fever the liver and spleen are greatly enlarged, and there is great tenderness over the hypochondriac region. In yellow fever albuminuria is much more common, and the urine more frequently suppressed, than in relapsing fever.

The sudden onset, the severe headache and pains in the limbs, the vomiting, jaundice, epigastric tenderness, enlargement of the liver and spleen, occasional epistaxis, hematemesis, or hematuria, absence of characteristic eruption, liability to herpes facialis, pneumonia, and diarrhoea; the occasional occurrence of remissions in the pyrexia, and even of more or less fully-developed chills for several successive days during the initial paroxysm or [p. 421]the relapse, suffice to explain the difficulty which may arise in distinguishing the bilious form of relapsing fever from bilious remittent fever. But the latter disease arises exclusively from malaria, and is therefore powerfully influenced by season and locality; is not contagious; does not present anything approaching to the crisis, the apyretic interval, or the abrupt relapse of relapsing fever; presents pigmentary changes in the blood, instead of the spirillum; and lesions of the spleen and liver totally unlike those characteristic of relapsing fever; can be promptly controlled by antiperiodic doses of quinine, and therefore should have a mortality far less than that of the grave form of relapsing fever. It is not necessary to pursue this subject further, but a reference to the temperature charts of Carter[37] or of Litten[38] will show that in some epidemics single paroxysms resembling those of quotidian ague might occur during the interval between the initial paroxysm and the relapse, or a series of two, three, or more such paroxysms of quotidian or tertian type might represent an entire relapse. Such phenomena are wholly uncontrollable by quinia, and are presumably dependent upon irregularities in the specific infection, instead of upon a blending of malaria with the poison of relapsing fever. There is some ground for believing, however, that those who have recently passed through an attack of the latter are highly, perhaps unusually, susceptible to malarial infection, as we have already seen they are liable to contract typhus.

[37] *Op. cit.*
[38] *Deut. Arch. f. klin. Med.*, xlii. 1874.

The chill, the sudden and high fever, the acid sweat, the high-colored urine, the intense pains and soreness, and the occasional murmur over the heart, will in some cases of relapsing fever suggest the idea of severe rheumatic fever, with illy-developed articular inflammation and with a tendency to hyperpyrexia. The urgent danger presented by the latter condition and the necessity for immediate recourse to cold baths and large doses of quinine or of the salicylates, render it highly important that no such error of diagnosis should be made. It will usually be avoided readily by observing that in relapsing fever there are great nausea, repeated vomiting, insomnia, peculiar formication of the extremities, jaundice, early enlargement of the liver and spleen, with abdominal pain and soreness, and a tendency to epistaxis; and, further, that despite the high temperature, cerebral symptoms such as result from rheumatic hyperpyrexia are not threatened, except in grave typhoid cases or just preceding the crisis.

The onset of relapsing fever may suggest forcibly the invasion period of small-pox, with its marked rigors, high fever, lumbar pain, aching in the head and limbs, nausea and vomiting, and if the patient is known to have been exposed to the contagion of both diseases a diagnosis would be impossible until the third day. But such a dilemma can rarely occur, and under ordinary circumstances the patient's antecedents will enable a correct opinion to be formed.

Severe cases of simple febricula with marked gastric disturbance may, as remarked by Jenner, closely simulate relapsing fever; and the same is true of attacks of acute gastro-hepatic catarrh, with severe headache, sharp fever, cholæmic eye, epigastric tenderness, and frequent vomiting. Of course there is no danger under ordinary circumstances of these simple conditions being regarded as relapsing fever, but when the latter is prevalent in epidemic form it is probable that the mistake is frequently made. [p. 422]Although an immediate diagnosis might be possible only by microscopic examination of the blood, the peculiar clinical symptoms of relapsing fever would soon be found wanting, and suitable treatment would bring the simpler affection under control.

Acute yellow atrophy of the liver occurs chiefly in pregnant women, though it is also met with in men and children; but it is so rare that should a case of it come under observation during the prevalence of relapsing fever there is considerable danger that its nature would be overlooked. It resembles relapsing fever in the occurrence of jaundice and other signs of hepatic disorder, of delirium, and of a tendency to hemorrhage from various surfaces. The temperature, however, is more moderate, and does not exhibit the sudden remission of relapsing fever; the liver is usually demonstrably diminished in size; severe nervous disturbances, such as convulsions followed by stupor and then by coma, are more constant; while the occurrence of spirilla in the blood of relapsing fever and of leucin and tyrosin in the urine of acute yellow atrophy serves to distinguish completely the two diseases. Acute yellow atrophy is, moreover, invariably fatal.

With ordinary care there is but little danger that any of the local complications of relapsing fever will so absorb attention as to lead to a neglect of the specific general disease, so that the cerebral symptoms should be readily distinguished from the onset of any acute intracranial affection; the parotitis which occasionally appears early in the disease should not be confounded with idiopathic mumps; and so for other complications. There is far more danger, indeed, lest some of the complications may be overlooked; and this is especially true of pneumonia, one of the most frequent and most important of them all. Its occurrence is the cause of the supervention of grave typhoid symptoms or of the modification of the normal course of the pyrexia in so many cases that nothing but a systematic daily examination of the lungs will avert serious oversights.

MORTALITY AND PROGNOSIS.—The rate of mortality has varied in different epidemics from 2 or 3 to 24 per cent. Murchison shows that out of 2115 cases admitted to the London Fever Hospital during a period of twenty-two years, and embracing two distinct outbreaks, only 39 proved fatal, making 1.84 per cent. mortality. Adding to these the results of Scotch and Irish epidemics, a total of 18,859 cases, with 761 deaths, is reached, giving the rate of mortality for Great Britain as 4.03 per cent. The great Indian epidemics studied by Carter gave 111 deaths out of 616 cases, equal to 18.02 per cent. Recent German epidemics have given from 5 to 10 per cent. The above rates are obtained where all the cases observed during an epidemic are included. If, however, the mortality of the ordinary form of relapsing fever is computed separately from that of the bilious typhoid form, it does not exceed 2 to 5 per cent., whilst the mortality of the latter form rises to from 33 to 50 per cent., or even higher.

In the Philadelphia epidemic, out of a total of 1174 cases there were, as nearly as can be ascertained, 169 deaths, giving a rate of mortality of 14.4 per cent. Taking all the cases admitted to the hospital under our observation, many of which entered at a late period of the disease and not a few when moribund, the mortality was not less than 13 per cent. [p. 423]The mortality among the negroes who were attacked with the disease was considerably greater than among the whites. Finally, if the mortality of the bilious typhus form be considered separately—although from the frequency of jaundice in this epidemic and the numerous gradations of severity presented it is difficult to form a sharply defined group of this character—it was certainly not less than 50 per cent.

The date of death varies with the epidemic, the form of the disease, and the previous condition of vitality of those attacked. Ordinarily, by far the larger proportion of deaths occur during the first relapse or the second interval, but in bilious typhoid cases, presenting grave complications, especially pneumonia or severe hemorrhages at an early date, or in cases occurring in intemperate subjects, or in those previously in impaired health, the mortality is much heavier in the initial paroxysm or the first interval than at later periods.

Youth exerts the same favorable influences upon the result of relapsing fever as it does in the case of typhus and typhoid. Murchison states that of 717 male patients under twenty-five years of age admitted into the London Fever Hospital, not one died, and in most epidemics similar, though not equally marked, results have been noted. In some epidemics the mortality among young children has been considerable. As a rule, the percentage of deaths increases with each decade after thirty years.

Sex does not exert any definite or constant influence upon the mortality. The number of males affected is far greater; they are liable to be exposed to the contagion in its most concentrated form; a larger proportion of them are probably the subjects of intemperance than in the case of females; and thus most statistics agree in making the mortality somewhat greater in the male sex; but, all things being equal, there is no good reason for holding that sex itself has any value in determining the result.

As in other zymotic diseases, the mortality from relapsing fever is highest during the early period of an epidemic, and the type of the disease grows milder as the epidemic declines. Cases of the bilious typhoid form have become notably less frequent during the later stages of some epidemics than at an earlier period.

Marked difference has been observed also as to the action of remedies at different stages of epidemics, the early cases exhibiting an extraordinary resistance to remedies, and especially to anodynes, which passes away later. When typhus and relapsing fevers have prevailed together, and a clear discrimination between the two sets of cases has not been made, it has appeared that the mortality increased as the epidemic advanced, but this apparent exception has been due to the fact that at first the cases of relapsing fever were in the majority, while later those of typhus, the much more fatal disease, preponderated.

Epidemics of relapsing fever prevail at all seasons, but more commonly they are at their height during the colder months of the year. The total mortality will of course correspond, but the actual percentage is not constantly greater during any one season, although it is probable that the greater liability to chest complications during the colder months will render the disease more fatal then.

The gravity of relapsing fever has varied so greatly in different epidemics that it is very difficult to determine what influence upon the mortality [p. 424]has been exerted by mere difference of race. A further source of difficulty is found in estimating the differences in the physical conditions of the poorer classes in the various communities affected. The mortality has been exceptionally high in the Russian and Indian epidemics and in some of the German ones, while in the British epidemics it has uniformly been light. It is interesting to note that in the Philadelphia epidemic, where the great majority of patients were Irish or negroes, the mortality was high, over 14 per cent. The previous condition of the Irish patients must certainly have contrasted favorably with that of the individuals attacked in the

Dublin and Belfast epidemics, so that the difference in result seems attributable only to a greater virulence of the disease. As an ample opportunity was here afforded to judge of the relative severity of relapsing fever in the negro and white races when the cases occurred at the same season, at the same stage of the epidemic, and in individuals living under nearly similar conditions, it may be stated that the conclusion of all who studied the question closely was that the disease was much more severe among negroes, and in particular that they displayed a greater tendency to serious complications and to the bilious typhoid form.

Although the degree and virulence of the infection undoubtedly constitute the most important elements in determining the mortality, the previous health and habits of those attacked with relapsing fever exert an influence upon the result. This is especially true of habitual intemperance, which, by disposing to disease of the liver and kidneys, greatly increases the liability to a fatal result. It has been seen (above), however, that even when acute catarrhal nephritis existed at the time of the attack severe relapsing fever might terminate favorably. Another observation which we made frequently, and which coincides with what is well known in regard to typhoid and typhus, is that improper exertion and exposure during the stage of incubation and immediately after the invasion produced a highly unfavorable effect on the subsequent course of the disease, and seemed in particular to dispose to dangerous or fatal collapse at the critical periods.

Apart from these general considerations, there are many special points to be considered in regard to the prognosis of relapsing fever:

If after the crisis of the invasion there is not rapid and decided improvement, complications should be suspected.

A sharp rebound of temperature quickly following crisis may be followed by speedy death.

Mere elevation of temperature during the invasion and the relapse, even though to an extreme height, is not attended with the danger which even a somewhat lower degree would indicate in other zymotic diseases.

Increased elevation toward the expected time of crisis should arouse anxiety, as sudden and dangerous cerebral symptoms may occur.

Prolonged duration of the pyrexia, or the substitution of irregular gradual defervescence (lysis) for the characteristic crisis often associated with typhoid symptoms as are these conditions, is significant of complications and of danger.

Wild delirium during the pyrexia, or transient active delirium about the time of crisis, is not necessarily unfavorable, but continuous low delirium, with disposition to stupor, is associated with a typhoid tendency and is frequently followed by death. Excessive muscular [p. 425]tremor or convulsions are highly unfavorable, but not necessarily fatal, symptoms.

Cardiac murmurs are not of serious import. The pulse is not usually as rapid in proportion to the temperature as in typhus or typhoid, and an excessively rapid pulse toward the expected time of crisis, especially if associated with feebleness of the heart's action, points to the danger of sudden collapse at or soon after that time. Previous cardiac disease, especially fatty degeneration in habitually intemperate persons, increases this danger. Continued frequency of pulse after the crisis indicates some complication or the danger of some accident.

Cough of a bronchial origin is not a specially unfavorable symptom, but if associated with the physical signs of pneumonia and with marked disturbance of respiration it indicates extreme danger.

Epistaxis, even when copious, often occurs in favorable cases, but hemorrhage from the stomach or the kidneys is usually, though not invariably, followed by death.

An eruption, measly or of pink spots, with or without minute petechiæ, is rare, and usually occurs in severe cases, but is not of specially unfavorable significance unless associated with the typhoid state or with patches of purpura.

Hiccough is a much less unfavorable symptom in relapsing fever than in typhoid or typhus, and vomiting, even frequent and persistent, may occur in cases of ordinary severity.

Enlargement of the liver and spleen indicates special risk only when persistent for some time after the relapse, in connection with persistent irregular fever. Jaundice has no necessarily unfavorable signification, is frequent in ordinary cases in some epidemics, but when it is associated with the other features of the bilious typhoid form the danger is extreme, at least 33 per cent. of such cases proving fatal.

Slight transient albuminuria may exist without special danger, but if associated with evidences of catarrhal nephritis, or if extreme diminution of urine, with or without albuminuria, exists, cerebral symptoms are apt to ensue, with a high degree of danger.

All serious complications—parotitis, erysipelas, dysentery, abortion, pneumonia, and, above all, peritonitis—greatly increase the risk.

It is not possible to determine in what cases the relapse will fail to occur. Motschutkoffsky's statement, that when a slight post-critical rise occurs a relapse will follow, must be applicable only to a limited number of cases.

In all cases at least one relapse must be expected; the patient in the interval must be regarded as still sick, and after the close of the relapse he must still be treated with rigid care until convalescence is permanently established. It must be remembered in hospital practice that many patients enter toward or after the crisis of the first paroxysm, so that caution is needed in estimating the effect of remedies and the period of the disease.

The undue prominence of certain conditions during the course of the disease is apt to be followed by corresponding sequelæ, and emaciation, anæmia, dyspepsia, diarrhoea, dysentery, enlargement of the spleen and rheumatoid pains may then be anticipated. The liability to ophthalmia and affections of the middle ear is not to be forgotten.

[p. 426]CAUSES OF DEATH.—In fatal cases death occurs from exhaustion dependent on the protracted and severe sufferings of the patient; from cerebral symptoms; from hyperpyrexia; from the virulence of the toxæmia; from uræmic poisoning; from sudden collapse; or from some complication, such as hemorrhagic meningitis, hemorrhages, pneumonia, dysentery, rupture of the spleen, peritonitis, or abortion.

TREATMENT.—The indications for treatment presented by regular cases of relapsing fever seem to be—to moderate the pyrexia; to relieve distressing symptoms, especially pain, insomnia, and gastric irritability; to sustain the strength of the system; to prevent or modify the relapses; and to avoid complications and sequelæ.

It is needless to observe that until the nature of the specific cause of relapsing fever is fully determined, whether the spirillum occupy that relation or not, it is impossible to direct our efforts rationally toward its neutralization or elimination. The various remedies which have been employed for these special purposes have no clinical support to recommend them. And while experiment has shown that the activity of the spirillum is readily destroyed by the direct action of various weak solutions, as of quinine, carbolic acid, iodine, and mineral acids, no special curative effect follows the internal administration of these remedies, even in the largest doses consistent with safety. In fact, there can scarcely be any disease in which treatment is less satisfactory or its results more difficult to estimate. The marked difference between various epidemics, and the wide variation presented by the development of individual symptoms in different cases of the same epidemic, fully account for this.

Quinine, as might be expected, has been largely used, in the hope that it might control the pyrexia or prevent the relapse. Murchison[39] quotes a considerable amount of evidence from various sources to show that it does not possess either of these powers. It was administered to a considerable number of our cases, either in small and frequently repeated doses during the pyrexia or the intermission, or else in large doses repeated several times in immediate anticipation of the expected time of the relapse. Thus in some cases three grains of sulphate of quinia were given every two or three hours until tinnitus was produced, and then this was maintained during the remainder of the pyrexia and of the intermission. The amount given daily was from thirty to forty-two grains. It seemed to rather increase the discomfort in the head, and in some cases it aggravated the irritability of the stomach. The pyrexia was certainly not controlled by it. Given in the same manner during the intermission, it was usually well borne, but was not effectual in preventing the relapse. It is true that in some cases the subsequent relapse seemed to be somewhat modified.

[39] *Op. cit.*, p. 408.

Thus in one case 30 grains were given on the 6th of April; 39 grains on the 7th; 39 grains on the 8th; 42 grains on the 9th; and 60 grains on the 10th; the critical fall had occurred during the night of the 7th, and the relapse began on the evening of the 9th, but the rise in temperature was less abrupt than usual, and the relapse lasted less than five days. It was quite severe, however, so that it is doubtful whether the apparent modification was anything more than is frequently observed in cases where no quinine has been administered.

In another case the fall in temperature at the end of the first paroxysm [p. 427]was from 105.5° to 97° on March 26th: 35 to 40 grains of sulphate of quinine were given daily on April 4th, 5th, 6th, 7th, and 8th; the temperature began to rise on the 3d, but the severe pyrexia and the usual symptoms of the relapse were limited to a period of less than thirty-six hours. This is a less common irregularity, and yet does not afford sufficient evidence of the efficiency of quinine. In other cases, however, as already stated, no appreciable effect followed its administration in this manner.

To illustrate the other method of giving quinia, a case may be quoted in which 20-grain doses every three or four hours were given from April 25th to April 29th, so that in four days 575 grains were taken. The initial paroxysm was of average severity, and terminated at the end of the seventh day, April 20th. The quinine did not postpone the relapse, which occurred on April 28th, but was of much less than the usual duration.

In no other case in which these large doses were given was there even as much reason as in the above instance to attribute to quinine any positive influence upon the course of the disease.

In order to demonstrate that the failure of quinine was not dependent upon a want of absorption, Muirhead injected large amounts subcutaneously with no better results.

In conclusion, it may be said that the evidence shows positively that quinine possesses no specific influence whatever upon relapsing fever; that in only occasional cases, if at all, will even enormous doses given during the intermission postpone or modify the subsequent relapse; and that it is not effective in reducing the temperature. In view, therefore, of the usual gastric irritability and tendency to vertigo and headache, which seem to be increased by large doses of quinine, and, further, in view of the small mortality, and of the fact that when death occurs it usually comes from causes over which large doses of quinine could exert no influence, it seems clear that this drug should be prescribed only in tonic doses and only in cases where it is well tolerated by the stomach.

Arsenic was used in a considerable number of our cases with the view of determining if it possessed any power of relieving the severe pains or of influencing the relapse. It was administered in the form of Fowler's solution (Liq. potassii arsenitis), and was given exclusively by the mouth. If given during the intermission, it was well borne in doses of five to ten drops every four or even every three hours, given freely diluted with water and immediately after food. In several cases it quickly induced puffiness about the eyes, but no effect whatever was produced on the pains or on the succeeding relapse. In more than one such case there was an unusually profuse crop of sudamina during the relapse, many of the vesicles breaking and being followed by brownish stains. When given during the pyrexia it aggravated the nausea and vomiting, so that it had to be suspended. In one unfortunate case, indeed, although promptly suspended, the arsenical solution seemed to have assisted in the establishment of vomiting and purging, which proved uncontrollable and contributed greatly to the fatal result. Hypodermic injections of arsenic have been used considerably with no better results. There seems, therefore, to be no reason whatever for any further use of this drug in relapsing fever.

[p. 428]The high pyrexia and the severe rheumatoid pains have naturally suggested the use of salicylic acid and the salicylate of soda. We were not sufficiently aware of their antipyretic properties in 1869-70 to have recourse to them, but in more recent epidemics Unterburger[40] and Riess[41]have found that large doses of the latter substance (one hundred grains or more daily) will reduce the temperature either in the initial paroxysm or in the relapse, but that the disease is not cut short nor are the lesions of the blood or solids prevented.

[40] *Jahrb. f. Kinderheilk.*, v. x., 1876.
[41] *Deutsch. Med. Wochnsch.*, Dec., 1879.

It must be borne in mind here, as in connection with the action of quinine, that apparent modifications of the relapse are to be viewed with great distrust, since such great irregularities therein naturally present themselves. Care must further be taken lest such attempts to reduce the temperature aggravate the irritation of the stomach, and by lessening the power of taking food induce more serious exhaustion than would have resulted from the unchecked pyrexia. The evidence in our possession is not sufficient to justify a positive decision as to the therapeutic value of the salicylates in relapsing fever, but, apparently, they are applicable to only a portion of the cases, and in these are of but limited utility.

The same failure which has followed the use of quinine, of arsenic, and of salicin and the salicylates has attended the effort to prevent the relapse by berberine, benzoate of soda, tincture of eucalyptus, and other reputed antiperiodics.

Digitalis, veratrum viride, and aconite were used by us quite freely as antipyretics. The first two of these were often suspended on account of the irritability of the stomach, and no valuable results followed their use when well tolerated. Aconite in small doses, frequently repeated, as one drop every two hours, seemed to aid in allaying nausea and to exert some slight influence upon the fever. In cases where there was a distinct tendency to heart-failure, digitalis was given freely with advantage.

Cold baths were not used to reduce the temperature in any of the cases under our observation. They have been employed in other epidemics, but, as far as we know, with no other effect than to cause merely temporary lowering of temperature, without any decided relief to the other symptoms and without any apparent influence upon the course of the disease. Frequent spongings with cool water and the application of ice to the head gave only slight and temporary relief.

Simple febrifuge remedies, such as effervescing draught or spirit of nitrous ether with solution of acetate of ammonium, were well received by the stomach, and appeared to promote perspiration and the more free secretion of urine.

Finding all our efforts to control the pyrexia so unsuccessful, recourse was had in a large proportion of our cases to the hyposulphite of soda, given, dissolved in two ounces of water, in doses of twenty grains every two or three hours. In two cases it seemed to increase nausea, and at times it caused some purging, but otherwise it was well borne by the stomach, and, indeed, frequently appeared to aid in controlling vomiting. The records show that this drug was given in only two or three of the fatal cases, so that although the patients who took it regularly presented every grade of severity of the disease, they did well uniformly. It is certain, however, that the hyposulphite of soda exerted no specific effect [p. 429]upon the disease; it did not reduce temperature, it did not prevent or modify the relapses nor relieve the severe pains; it may have promoted more free and healthy secretions, and, by tending to prevent vomiting, may have aided in maintaining nutrition; but, on the whole, it may fairly be doubted whether this remedy merits any more extended trial.

One chief reason of the failure of antipyretics in relapsing fever is to be found in the existence of widespread irritative lesions of the glandular and mucous tissues, which combine with the specific blood-changes in causing and maintaining the high temperature. It is not surprising, therefore, that the remedies which afford the greatest relief in this disease are opiates and sedatives to the gastro-intestinal mucous membrane. Opium, or morphia, must indeed be regarded as the basis of the rational treatment of relapsing fever. It is called for by the insomnia, the severe headache and the pains in various parts of the body, the nausea and vomiting, and the pyrexia. It does not appear to have been as prominent a feature in the treatment of other epidemics as we found it necessary to make it in Philadelphia. Parry[42] used it very freely, chiefly in the form of opium, by the mouth, and found a singular tolerance exhibited by his patients, several of whom took as large a dose as three grains every two hours during the afternoon and night without producing any sleep or even any contraction of the pupils. This resistance to the action of opium was observed chiefly in the early part of the epidemic, and we may add that it was exhibited chiefly when opium was given by the mouth. When morphia was used hypodermically we found that one-fourth of a grain, given at intervals of six to twelve hours, afforded very great relief to the pains, aided and relieved vomiting, and often induced quiet, refreshing sleep. Its use was not contraindicated by jaundice, by cough or pulmonary congestion, or by moderate contraction of the pupils. It was frequently given so as to maintain decided drowsiness throughout the pyrexia. When the pains persisted during the intermission the morphia was continued in smaller doses or at longer intervals. It occasionally happened that when patients were thus kept continuously under opium influence no relapse occurred; but here, as in regard to the action of quinine, it may safely be asserted either that what was regarded as the initial paroxysm was in reality the relapse, or else that the absence of a relapse was a mere irregularity, and in no way to be attributed to the action of the opium. On the other hand, in cases presenting a tendency to the typhoid state, with a disposition to stupor, or where the urine was scanty and albuminous, no opiate was administered.

[42] *Loc. cit.*

We have already stated that in our cases quinine in acid solution was frequently ordered, and it answered very well to add to each dose of this a suitable amount of morphia.

Atropia, in the dose of gr. 1/60 to gr. 1/40, was usually associated with the hypodermic injections of morphia. This was done particularly in cases where the pains were very severe, when the pupils were disposed to be contracted, or when there was continued profuse sweating. In addition to this, atropia was continued without morphia during the intermission in a few cases. The patients proved susceptible to its influence, and dryness of the mouth with dilatation of the pupils was readily [p. 430]produced by gr. 1/60 every six hours. In one case gr. 1/40 every four hours for two days caused delirium, with the usual symptoms of belladonna action, all of which passed away quickly after withdrawal of the drug. But in none of these cases was the relapse influenced in the least.

Other remedies may be used for the relief of the insomnia, which is always one of the most distressing symptoms. Chloral and bromide of potassium have been found serviceable in various epidemics, and some observers have preferred them to opium for the relief of headache and insomnia. They did not prove reliable in the Philadelphia epidemic of 1869-70. Bromide of potassium, even in large doses, produced scarcely any effect, and, while in a few cases chloral in doses of gr. xx. gave positive relief, in the majority of instances 40 grains failed to cause sleep or relieve suffering. It must not be forgotten also that, as there is a special tendency to cardiac failure in this affection, the action of chloral must be closely watched.

In a small series of our cases where muscular pains, hyperæsthesia, and twitching were marked succus conii was given quite freely, but without any apparent benefit.

The condition of the stomach required attention in almost every case. Nausea, vomiting, and epigastric and hypochondriac soreness were the prominent symptoms. Anorexia was usually complete during pyrexia, and not rarely patients were admitted to the hospital who asserted that for one or more days they had not taken any nourishment whatever. Under such circumstances, and in a disease where the tendency to prostration and cardiac failure calls for stimulants and food, it is evident that strict care must be given to the diet. In many cases skimmed milk with lime-water, meat broths, arrowroot, or gruel, could be taken in small amounts at short intervals, and retained. But whenever these are rejected, no attempt should be made to persist in their use, but koumiss, whey, or chicken-water should be substituted, and continued until the stomach grows retentive. Equal care must be paid to the selection of a suitable form of stimulus. It may be proper to employ a mild and relaxing emetic if the patient be seen at the onset of the disease and if there is reason to suspect the presence of indigested food in the stomach, but under any other circumstances there seems no reason for its use in a disease where vomiting is so common and gastric irritability one of the most troublesome symptoms. Nor should purgatives be given save when very positive indications exist for their use.

Constipation is rarely obstinate; the amount of nourishment taken is very small; in a considerable proportion of cases there is diarrhoea, or at least a sensitive state of the bowels; and as a consequence it is preferable in nearly every case to dispense with laxatives entirely, and, if the bowels must be opened by assistance, to administer a simple enema.

When irritability of the stomach is marked, benefit may be derived from very small doses of calomel frequently repeated, as, for example, gr. 1/8 or 1/4 every one or two hours. Subnitrate of bismuth may be used in combination with this or as a substitute for it. In several instances more prompt relief was obtained from nitrate of silver given in the dose of gr. 1/12 every three or four hours, dissolved in thin mucilage of acacia.

Stimulants were remarkably well borne, and their administration in such form as was acceptable to the stomach was clearly of service, [p. 431]even from an early period of the disease. As a rule, whiskey was employed, given in the form of milk punch. By carefully graduating the amount of alcohol, and when necessary diluting the milk freely with lime-water, the stomach usually received it well. If circumstances favored, dry champagne, or brandy or sherry in carbonated water would often prove preferable. The exhausting nature of the disease, the marked tendency to cardiac failure, and the inability to digest an adequate amount of nourishment, all indicate the early use of stimulants. In cases where a tendency to the development of the typhoid state existed alcohol was freely given, even to the extent of sixteen ounces of whiskey in twenty-four hours. Other stimulants were usually given in these cases, such as carbonate of ammonium, especially if pulmonary congestion existed; turpentine, especially if tympany was marked; or Hoffmann's anodyne or spirit of chloroform, if muscular twitchings, hiccough, or insomnia with wandering delirium were prominent symptoms. In all cases of severity the use of tonics and stimulants should be maintained in reduced doses during the intermission and for some days after the final fall of temperature.

It remains to allude briefly to certain special remedies and to certain symptoms requiring special treatment. Formerly, much diversity of opinion existed as to the propriety of venesection or local depletion in relapsing fever, but Murchison concluded, after a careful examination of the evidence, that it had not been shown to be of service; and certainly the disease as it occurred in Philadelphia in 1869-70 presented no indication whatever for even the mildest depletory measures. This corresponds with the recognized plan of treatment in all the specific fevers.

Blisters are not so objectionable in relapsing fever as in either typhus or typhoid, and there are several conditions in which they have been found decidedly useful. In cases where the headache has obstinately resisted cold applications, bromide of potassium, and opiates, a blister to the back of the neck has afforded marked relief, with no unfavorable result. Again, in cases where the vomiting and epigastric distress were severe and obstinate the application of a blister three inches square to the epigastrium is to be recommended.

Chloroform has proved of value for the relief of various symptoms in relapsing fever. As already stated, it was found the most useful remedy for the hiccough which was so troublesome in a number of our cases, and especially in those where jaundice was pronounced. It also seemed serviceable in controlling the peculiar chills which in varying degrees of severity were present in a few cases, recurring at about the same hour on successive days. These rigors or chills were uninfluenced by very large doses of quinine or other antiperiodics, but were apparently controlled by full doses of chloroform given in advance of the expected hour of recurrence.

Jaundice, which, as has been stated, is partly of hæmic origin, but is probably also due in part to obstruction from catarrhal swelling of the mucous membrane of the bile-ducts, is not influenced by mineral acids, and still less should mercurials or purgatives be administered for its relief. It would seem proper, in cases where this symptom is marked, to observe special care in diet and the use of stimulants, and to employ local sedative[p. 432]astringents, such as small doses of nitrate of silver combined with opium and belladonna.

Muscular soreness, pains, and tremor may call for special treatment on account of their severity. The only remedy which has proved useful in relieving the first two of these symptoms is opium, conjoined with the external use of anodynes. Iodide of potassium fails even in doses as large as can be borne, and the same is true of muriate of ammonium and cimicifuga, which we used thoroughly without any effect. In the muscular pains, however, which torment the patient during convalescence, the ammoniated tincture of guaiacum was found of service. Atropia hypodermically and chloroform internally have been found useful for the relief of severe muscular twitchings.

Upon the whole, therefore, it will be seen that in ordinary cases a supporting and expectant plan of treatment is all that is required. Abandoning the idea of forcibly controlling the fever or of preventing the relapse, care should be given in the first place to the diet and to judicious stimulation.

Opium or morphia should be used to control pain, excitement, and insomnia, aided, as far as the latter is concerned, by bromide of potassium or the cautious use of chloral. Cooling drinks should be allowed, cool applications made to the head, and the body should be repeatedly sponged with cooling and disinfecting lotions. If the stomach is retentive, quinine in moderate doses may be given in acid solution, alternating with a simple fever mixture; but if nausea and vomiting are present, the first purpose will be to allay them by the appropriate measures already discussed.

Epistaxis is a frequent symptom, but usually requires no special attention. Occasionally it is profuse, and then should be promptly checked, since serious exhaustion may follow its continuance. If, therefore, mild astringent applications do not arrest it, recourse must be had to the tampon saturated with diluted Monsell's solution.

The urine must be closely watched and frequently analyzed in relapsing fever. In some epidemics serious alterations in this secretion are rare; in others it is not uncommon for the urine to be scanty, and to contain albumen or blood. When this latter condition is presented, especially if at the same time uræmic symptoms exist, dry cups should be applied over the kidneys, to be followed by the use of dry heat, and free perspiration should be promoted by hot-air baths or by the hot wet pack. It is probable that jaborandi given in repeated small doses, so as to avoid any depressing effect on the heart, will be found valuable in such cases. Infusion of digitalis, with spirit of nitrous ether or with acetate of potassium, may also be used with advantage.

Absolute rest must be insisted on throughout the entire period of paroxysm and relapse. The records of every epidemic present instances of sudden death from cardiac syncope following trifling exertions. The patients should therefore be kept strictly quiet in bed from the initial rigor until their strength is fully restored after the relapse. As the danger of collapse is especially great at the time of the critical fall in temperature, the patient should be closely watched as the end of the initial paroxysm and of the relapse approaches. If there is any sudden rise of temperature, with head symptoms due to hyperpyrexia, large doses [p. 433]of quinine, ice to the head, cold spraying, or the cold bath must be promptly used. As sweating begins the body must be covered with a warm blanket and warm stimulating drinks be administered. If any marked tendency to collapse is observed, the subcutaneous injection of strychnia or of ether and digitalis, conjoined with diffusible stimulants internally and hot applications externally, are to be employed immediately. The special remedies required for the various complications and sequelæ have already been sufficiently indicated.

I desire in conclusion to acknowledge the important assistance received from Drs. Geo. S. Gerhard, Louis Starr, Charles Shaffner, and R. G. Curtin, who, under the supervision of my colleague, the late Dr. Edward Rhoads, and myself, recorded the histories of most of the cases which serve as the basis of this article, and also tabulated them for statistical purposes.[43]

[43] Reference must also be made to the interesting observations on spirilla published by Mülhaüser in *Virchow's Archiv* for July 9, 1884, after this article had been printed. His results go to confirm the view that the spirillum of Obermeier is the essential cause of relapsing fever.

[p. 434]

VARIOLA.
BY JAMES NEVINS HYDE, M.D.

Variola is an acute, febrile, contagious, and systemic affection, preceded by an incubative period, characterized by the evolution of symptoms in a relatively determinate order, with a cutaneous efflorescence successively papular, vesicular, and pustular in type, followed by crusting, and terminating either fatally or by complete convalescence, with or without sequelæ in the form of multiple, circumscribed, and superficial cicatrices.

SYNONYMS.—*Lat.*, Variola; *Eng.*, Small-pox; *Fr.*, Petite Vérole; *Ger.*, Pocken; *Ital.*, Vajuolo.

HISTORY.—Small-pox is a disease which, there is reason to believe, was first developed in the earliest ages of which the human family has record. Originating probably in China, India, and the adjacent countries of the Asiatic continent, its extension over Europe and America was, without question, in the line of progress pursued by the advancing centres of traffic and population. The earliest traces of its ravages can be dimly recognized in the descriptions of writers in the middle and latter parts of the sixth century. In the early years of the tenth century, however, a remarkably accurate picture of the disease was drawn by Rhazes, a physician of Bagdad. His treatise, translated by Greenhill for the London Pathological Society,[1] sets forth the views of an Egyptian physician named Ahron, who wrote in the sixth century. After these dates the remarkable political and social changes in Europe, which are to be attributed either directly or remotely to the Crusades, contributed largely to the opportunities for the spread of the disease and to the occurrence later of those decimating epidemics which became veritable scourges. In the last century the resulting mortality in some of the countries of Europe was often equal to the entire population of one of their largest cities. If a modern traveller could find himself transported to the streets of the city of London as they appeared in the early part of the present century, it is probable that no peculiarities of architecture, dress, or behavior would be to him so strikingly conspicuous as the enormous number of pock-marked visages he would encounter among the people at every turn. In the face of all cavil and sophistry, medical science will always count among its greatest triumphs the modifications which variola has undergone since its preventive treatment was established upon a satisfactory basis by the discovery of the immortal Jenner.

[1] *A Treatise on the Small-pox and Measles,* by Abu Becr Mohammed Ibn Zacaríyá Arrází, London, 1848.

The bibliography of the disease is extensive, and the list of authors contributing to the subject is enriched by the names of such men as Boerhaave, Van Swieten, Sauvages, Willan, E. Wagner, Johanny Rendu, Hebra, and, more lately, Kaposi.

ETIOLOGY.—Respecting the etiology of variola, it can scarcely be affirmed that our knowledge has been greatly extended since the date of the experiments of Jenner. There is no historical knowledge of its generation de novo; and the earliest cases of the malady must therefore be classed with the exceedingly rare instances of spontaneous cow-pox which have proved such a boon to the vaccini-culturists. To-day every case of small-pox is justly regarded as having been directly or indirectly transmitted from one or more individuals affected with a similar disorder. It is thus recognized as specifically infectious, contagious, and inoculable, its transmission occurring, first, without contact, by atmospheric conduction of a volatile contagious principle of unknown nature; second, with contact either by (*a*) actual transference of dry or moist infectious secretions deposited upon a susceptible surface, immediately or through the medium of garments, bed-clothing, paper money, and similar material substances; or (*b*) by inoculation of unprotected persons with the pathological product of an infected organism. There is no doubt but that the contagious principle displays its greatest activities in connection with the contents of the lesions undergoing a change from the vesicular to the pustular phases, though from the beginning to the end of the disease it is probable that all the tissues and fluids of the infected body are in various degrees capable of producing the malady in those who are unprotected. Furthermore, whether associated or not with an organic substance, the contagium of the disease is known to preserve the power of reproducing itself for a period lasting for weeks, months, and even a longer time. A field for its activities once secured, there is a period of time during which few if any evidences of its progress are declared, this period being abruptly terminated by distinct and characteristic symptoms. This is known as the period of incubation.

The nature of the contagium in small-pox has been the subject of much speculation, careful investigation, and experiment, the results having established but few facts of any practical value. There is at present no proof that any bacteria, vegetable germs, or other minute organisms foreign to the human body are the essential causes of the disease. It is certain that in health the human body is completely enveloped in a volatile medium emanating from the secretions of the glands of the skin, which can be recognized by some of the keen-scented lower animals when it is wafted through the air at a distance of several hundred feet from a single individual. It is reasonable to conclude that not only in small-pox, but in other contagious and infectious diseases, these emanations possess a pathological character, and become capable of transmitting such maladies from diseased to healthy organisms. Certain also it is that when the subjects of these diseases are crowded together, as in prisons, hospitals and camps, this contagious element gathers an unwonted intensity. By far the larger number of all transmissions of variola occur after inhalation of the infective medium—in other words, by the avenue of the lungs. It is probably for the same reason that the disease spreads more widely and with greater virulence during the cold seasons of the [p. 436]year, in this latitude especially from December to February—a time when the ventilation of inhabited dwelling-houses is usually much less perfect than in warmer weather.

The disease affects individuals of all ages and both sexes, not sparing the foetus in utero, and, in the case of the latter, occurring both with and without previous infection of the mother of the unborn child. Nowhere are its ravages so extensive and followed by such fatal results as among those who have long been unprotected by previous vaccination. Among the debilitated, as also among the very young and the very old, small-pox is liable to be followed by severe complications and a fatal result. Negroes, possibly in consequence of tendencies inherited through generations of unvaccinated ancestors, are particularly prone to the disease. Lastly, there is occasionally noted an individual idiosyncrasy, in consequence of which either a remarkable susceptibility to the disease exists or a no less singular immunity against its encroachment is conferred.

Thus, physicians, much exposed to its influences in the discharge of their professional duties, are known to be relatively exempt, while other individuals, few in number it must be admitted, have either had repeated attacks of the malady itself, or, after each exposure to its contagious principle, a recurrent illness of variable type. In the immense majority of all cases, however, one attack confers immunity upon the sufferer against subsequent invasion of the disease for the remainder of life. Upon a few occasions I have known variola to occur in individuals previously affected with cutaneous diseases, especially the eczematous—a fact which merely suggests that such pre-existing disorder of the integument conferred no immunity against infection.

SYMPTOMATOLOGY.—The earliest symptoms of small-pox may be occasionally recognized during the stage of incubation, which, as described above, embraces a period of from ten to fifteen days, though these limits are not absolutely fixed, since both shorter and longer incubative periods have been at times established. During the interval the patient may appear to enjoy perfect health, or, on the other hand, suffer from an ill-defined malaise, with anorexia, languor, insomnia, and allied symptoms. Close observation of the patient thus affected will often reveal the existence of a peculiar pallor of the face, accompanied by a skin-color which suggests a slight degree of sallowness of the complexion. These rather indeterminate symptoms are naturally most marked toward the completion of the period of incubation.

The latter terminated, the period of invasion follows, and extends from the conclusion of the incubative stage to the moment when the first cutaneous lesions of variola appear upon the surface. The symptoms which characterize the onset of this period of invasion are conspicuous and characteristic. There is often a sharp vespertine rigor or a more or less continuous chilliness, accompanied by sensations of "creeping" over the surface, lasting even for several hours. Meantime, the temperature rises to 103° or 105° F., the pulse running up to 120 or 130 beats per minute. In this febrile condition there is commonly complaint of a characteristic aching in the head and back, intense, scarcely intermittent, and so peculiar as to have frequently furnished a clue to the diagnosis of the approaching malady. These sensations are quite analogous to the substernal and other pains which frequently precede the first explosions [p. 437]of syphilis, and are all, without question, due to the circulation of a poisoned blood, the influence of which is in this manner confessed by the nervous system. In the case of infants and young children the invasion of small-pox is frequently ushered in by delirium and convulsions—symptoms which are to be explained by the facts just named.

This complexus of febrile and nervous symptoms, varying somewhat in intensity and possibly interrupted by sensations of chilliness, may be recognized as continuing on the second and third days of the period of invasion. Meantime, there may be noted a dusky hyperæmia of the pharynx and tonsils, the surface of which may even display elevated points which develop later into papules. In exceptional instances the intensity of the poison is such that the system fails to rally before the violence of the onset, and a fatal result ensues before the characteristic exanthem appears upon the skin.

On the second and third days of the invasion stage of the disease, if they are displayed at all, the variolous rashes appear. Too much attention can scarcely be paid to the importance of their recognition on the part of the diagnostician. Often indeed have practitioners been deceived by their occurrence, having been either completely blinded to the serious nature of the malady in progress, or, as Bartholow[2] has well shown, having supposed that they were dealing with a concurrence of variola and scarlatina or rubeola.

[2] "The Variolous Diseases," *Med. News*, Mar. 4, 1882, p. 232.

Hebra was the first to point out the significance of the rash known as roseola variolosa or erythema variolosa. Occurring at about the dates named above, it is in a few patients pronounced and vivid, even in solitary instances rivalling in severity the exanthem which succeeds it. In others, the majority of all patients in some epidemics, it may be entirely wanting. The writer has certainly observed its most typical development in women who were either menstruating or in the puerperal state. It is said also to be relatively frequent in subjects of a tender age. Kaposi[3] has recognized it in all its manifestations at every age.

[3] Consult the admirable chapter on variola in his treatise, *Path. u. Therap. der Hautkrankt*, Wien, 1882.

It appears in the form of puncta, striæ, or diffuse and uniform blushes covering extensive areas of the integument, livid red, purplish, or brownish-red in hue, paling under pressure, but never leaving upon the skin over which the finger-nail is quickly drawn the characteristic whitish streak by which many practitioners test the scarlatinal rash. The surfaces involved may be either not raised or slightly elevated above the general level of the skin, and are usually circumscribed. The regions chiefly involved have been carefully described by Th. Simon, and are hence sometimes called Simon's triangles. Thus the groin, the internal face of the thighs, and the hypogastric region may be involved at once (femoral triangle of Simon); the surface of the axilla, the pectoral region, and the inner face of the arm (brachial triangle of Simon), as also the extensor faces of the knees and the elbows, the dorsum of the feet, and indeed every portion of the surface of the body.

In the midst of these rash-covered areas may also appear petechial or hemorrhagic, dark-red, pin-head to bean-sized maculæ, which undergo color-changes both in lighter and deeper shades as the invasion period[p. 438]lapses. In lieu of these, however, transient wheals may come and go over the surface, and even the erythema described above may assume an erratic phase and appear in one part only to disappear and recur at another. None of these flash-light warnings of the oncoming exanthem are proportioned to the latter in the matter of extent and intensity of development. They may be followed by grave or mild manifestations of the disease. The subsequent eruption may also be much more abundantly developed in regions where the invasion rashes have not appeared, and the latter completely fade before the former have advanced to occupy the field thus deserted.

The invasion stage of variola commonly occupies three days. Rarely it extends into the fourth, fifth, and even the sixth, day after the premonitory chill and fever.

Upon its subsidence the exanthem of the disease as a rule promptly appears. Simultaneously, the temperature abates, the rapidity of the pulse diminishes, and there is marked amelioration of the general symptoms. The patient, frequently deceived by the completeness of this defervescence, is apt to conclude that he is convalescent from his disorder, and is thus often astonished at the discovery of the exanthem upon the person, usually the face. In other cases, more commonly those of a grave character, there is failure of this defervescence, the febrile symptoms continuing or even increasing in severity.

The eruption first appears in the form of pin-head sized and larger, firm, conical, discrete, coherent or confluent, reddish papules, sometimes accompanied by mild sensations of a pricking or painful character, often exciting no subjective symptoms by which their presence could be declared. To the touch they are characteristically indurated, and suggest the hardness of small shot imbedded in the skin. They appear first and in greatest abundance upon the face and scalp, involving later and progressively the trunk, the extremities, and the palmar and plantar surfaces. It is at this moment that the eruption most resembles that to be recognized in measles (the distinction between the eruptive symptoms of the two diseases will be considered later). At times a reddish areola surrounds each lesion, especially those appearing upon the trunk. All are situated about the orifices of the follicles and glands of the skin.

On the first and second days of the eruption the papular lesions multiply in number, involve an increasingly large area, and individually augment in size; so they appear first upon the head, and are successively presented to the eye upon the lower portions of the body. The older lesions are usually recognized upon the scalp, face, neck, and shoulders; the more recent upon the extremities. By the third day of the eruptive stage there is usually evident at the apex of the older lesions a minute vesicle containing a drop of pellucid serum, which rapidly changes in character and size till a distinct vesicle is formed with cloudy or lactescent contents. Early in their career an apical depression can be seen, which later deepens into a characteristic umbilication. This umbilication in the vesicular stage is somewhat peculiar. It is more than a mere depression of the summit, such as might be made by thrusting a blunt-pointed pin centrally and downward so as to carry the roof-wall before it. It is made clinically most distinct by the fluting or puckering of the peripheral part of the roof-wall, giving the lesion a crenated appearance which is not [p. 439]assumed by any other cutaneous efflorescence of multiple development. It may be regarded as pathognomonic of variola.

The pock is usually mature by the sixth day of the eruption. It is pea-sized and globular in shape; its umbilication has been usually quite removed by the complete filling of its chamber with distinctly purulent contents; it is often surrounded by a halo due to hyperæmia or exudation; and, the total number of individual lesions being then fairly determined, it is often closely set against its fellows, islets of unaffected integument having meantime become fewer and more contracted. The face, covered with this eruption, then exhibits a typical aspect. The entire integument becomes swollen and brawny or oedematous. The eyes are thus closed by the tumid lids, which are separable with difficulty, and this, too, even though they be the seat of comparatively few lesions. The nose, lips, cheeks, and ears are by similar processes deformed and given a most repulsive unsightliness. Mucus and puriform secretions gather and dry about the mucous outlets. The skin of other parts of the body (hands, feet, genitalia, and the entire extremities) is in a similar condition, merely most noticeable in the exposed and disfigured visage.

The fever of maturation or suppuration, or, as it is often called, the secondary fever, is lighted to activity with the onset of the suppurative process. The temperature rises to a point ranging between 101° and 105° F., the pulse-rate simultaneously rising to 100 and even 150 in the minute, varying of course with the age of the patient and the severity of the attack. During its continuance, from the eighth or ninth to the eleventh or twelfth day of the disease, the victim of the malady is in a deplorable and critical condition. The intense grade of cutaneous inflammation, with its resulting subjective sensations of burning pain and tension, the soreness of the mouth (tongue, pharynx, inside of lips, and palate), due to the existence of pus-filled pocks upon the buccal membrane, and, for similar reasons, the dysphagia and irritation of the larynx and tracheal membrane, are all sufficient to account for the general condition. In cases of mild grade the patient lies conscious, but in a stolid apathy, listlessly accepting the services of his attendants. In others there is delirium of low or high grade, often sufficient to demand constant surveillance, lest in consequence the patient do serious injury to himself.

The behavior of the pustules which appear upon the mucous surfaces accessible to the eye is modified somewhat by the heat, moisture, and friction to which these surfaces are exposed. Typical, fully-distended pustules occasionally persist upon the soft palate and the inside of the lips. Soon, however, the macerated roof-wall yields, leaving a reddish floor where the mucous membrane is exposed, denuded of its epithelial layer or covered with a new tender and hyperæmic pellicle. In grave and severe cases these pustular lesions may extend deeply into the mucous tracts, involving the trachea, bronchi, or alimentary canal. In an autopsy made by the writer on the body of a male subject dead of unmodified variola, there was no portion of the alimentary canal from the mouth to the anus which was not studded by thickly-set pustules. The urethra, vagina, vulva, external auditory canal, and conjunctivæ are, in severe cases, similarly involved. According to Kaposi, the tympanum is usually exempt.

The period of desiccation begins usually on the thirteenth or fourteenth[p. 440]day of the disease, and, according to the severity of the previous pathological processes, requires for its completion from one week to a fortnight. Its onset is characterized by a second marked but gradually developed defervescence. With a diurnal temperature successively less elevated above the normal standard there is a corresponding fall of the pulse-rate. As the disease has by this date taxed the vital resources of the system to the utmost limit, the exhaustion resulting may be declared by a pulse which is flagging, weak, and even in the matter of frequency much below the standard of health.

The cutaneous lesions now again undergo a change. Some of the pustules rupture, and their viscid contents, oozing forth, concrete into a yellowish crust which gradually assumes a brownish hue. Others desiccate en masse, the roof-wall first collapsing upon the contents, thus producing an appearance which again suggests umbilication of the lesions. This is sometimes termed a secondary umbilication. The desiccation en masse is doubtless due to the evaporation of a portion of the fluid exuded into the superficial strata of the integument, and the consequent inspissation of the pus. Often the face at this moment is totally concealed by a dense, dry, brownish or even blackish mask, composed of the crusts furnished by numerous individual lesions. At the same time the tumefaction of the skin subsides, and the subjective sensations to which it gave rise gradually disappear. Beneath the crusts cicatrization advances till the former are lessened, and finally, becoming detached, fall in quantity from the surfaces subjected to friction. Beneath them are seen brownish and violaceous blotches, the integument thus stained slowly losing its abnormal color. It is thus seen to be the seat of multiple, slightly depressed, shining scars of a dead white color, which in the course of time lose somewhat of their disfiguring prominence, but which when typically distinct persist for a lifetime. This exfoliation of crusts continues till the skin is completely rid of its pathological products, the process being completed with entire restoration to health about the conclusion of the fourth or fifth week of the disease. Meantime, in favorable cases, convalescence progresses pari passu. The patient has a returning appetite, decadence of symptoms originating in impairment of function of the mucous membranes, and gains in weight till the restoration to sound health is complete.

Such is the history in outline of what may be regarded as a typical form of uncomplicated variola. It should not be forgotten, however, that in different epidemics there are marked differences in the career and manifestations of the malady, and that even among the cases observed in a single locality visited by the disease the same divergence of symptoms is no less conspicuous. This diversity is due to several causes, irrespective of the remarkable modifications displayed in the variolous who have been previously vaccinated. Individual susceptibility is doubtless to be considered in this connection, as also the temperament, bodily vigor, and hygienic surroundings of those who are infected. It is possible also that the intensity of the poison may be subjected to occasional modifications in its transmission from individual to individual. In this way the following types of variola present themselves in clinical forms with divergent features:

CONFLUENT VARIOLA (variola confluens).—This virulent form of [p. 441]small-pox is ushered in by a relatively short incubative period, followed by a severe invasion of the disease. The premonitory chill is violent; the cephalic and lumbar pains are excruciating; the fever, rising to a high grade, 106° to 110° F., with few and slight remissions, scarcely subsides, if at all, with the appearance of the eruption, the latter developing early, and, to borrow an expression from syphilographers, exploding with violence over large areas of the surface of the body. The initial lesions of the exanthem are dense and deeply-set papules, so closely coherent even at this moment that they scarcely leave between them interspaces of sound skin. During the vesiculo-pustular transformation which they promptly undergo on the second day there is a more or less complete coalescence of the elements of the eruption, which circumstance has given this form of the disease its name, confluent variola. This confluence is most conspicuous upon the face and hands, where large flat vesicles run together, form pus-filled bullæ, and finally convert the surface on which they rest into a single, large, many-chambered pustule. All this occurs upon an enormously swollen and inflamed skin, disfiguring every feature of the face and wellnigh obliterating every external distinction between the scalp, nose, eyes, and mouth. Here and there the mass is elevated by the quantity of exuded pus to a more notable projection from the surface. Pustules filled with blood may appear at several points. At others, the suppurative inflammation may be seen to have eroded the derma, which is covered with a diphtheritic membranous exudation similar to that covering the mucous membranes lining the mouth, nose, and ears. Naturally, the skin in its totality often yields to these destructive processes and in large patches falls into gangrene.

The confluence of the lesions is less marked in other parts of the body than the face and hands, yet the entire surface may be covered with a coherent exanthem which becomes elsewhere, in large areas, confluent. The writer has seen patients in whom the head of a pin could not be placed upon an unaffected patch of skin in any portion of the body. The parts subjected to pressure in the reclining posture, such as the back, shoulders, and buttocks, are especially liable to this coalescence of the pustular lesions.

In confluent variola too, as already intimated, the mucous surfaces suffer proportionately. Pasty accumulations of muco-pus and diphtheritic exudation, like macerated chamois leather, cover the tongue, which is often so enormously swollen as to bulge between the teeth and project from the mouth. These exudations line the mouth, pharynx, larynx, and even the bronchi. Beneath these masses the eroded mucous surface is dry, livid red in color, and has a varnished aspect. Gangrene here may lead to necrosis of the cartilages of the larynx. Aphonia is often complete, deglutition impossible, respiration difficult. The stench arising from the patient is intolerably fetid and pervading, and a single exhalation will poison the best-ventilated apartment. The submaxillary and sublingual glands are enlarged and the neighboring lymphatics swollen.

The patient who is plunged into this grave condition is the victim of a fever which is unquestionably septicæmic in character; he has a small, frequent, and often fluttering pulse; his mental condition is betrayed by a delirium of varying grade or he lies comatose. In this state a fatal [p. 442]result is often induced by either exhaustion of the vital forces or an intercurrent malady, such as pleurisy, pneumonia, cardiac inflammation, oedema of the glottis, or an uncontrollable diarrhoea. In yet other cases the patient falls into a typhoid state, and, after surviving for a fortnight or more with a low fever, a broncho-pneumonia, or a diarrhoea, succumbs to an inevitable exhaustion, the surface of his body being yet covered with a dry, blackish, and fetid crust.

The expression of an intense variolous poison is known as hemorrhagic variola; also as purpura variolosa and black pox. A large number of such cases have been designated and treated as black measles, the real nature of the malady having been mistaken.

The law readily observed by the diagnostician of diseases in general must here be recognized. There are no hard and fast lines in nature. Hemorrhagic variola occurs, without question, in different types. At the one extreme are classed the inevitably fatal cases, where the patient sinks smitten by the malady even before the exanthem is developed; at the other are found the cases of confluent variola, not necessarily fatal, in the course of which hemorrhagic lesions appear in variable number, blood either filling the pustules after the latter have arrived at maturity, or forming ab initio purpuric pocks intermingled with the typical lesions of the variolous exanthem. However ill-defined the limits between these classes may be, the symptoms of hemorrhagic variola are sufficiently characteristic to require separate description. According to Kaposi, it occurs in the two following types:

The first form is termed variolic purpura. Its incubative period is brief and distinguished by unusual conditions of malaise and lumbar pain. On the fourth day there is an intense fever with rapid pulse, and this is speedily followed by a deep purplish-red staining of the face, neck, trunk, and extremities, the skin thus affected being slightly tumid and quite dry. Minute maculo-papules can be distinguished here and there over the surface, often closely set together, and presenting the characteristic color described above. At this stage of the disease the eruption greatly suggests an intense rubeolous exanthem, and has been, as a result, repeatedly mistaken for the so-called black measles. But the excruciating pains persist, there is often coincident delirium, and the pin-head sized maculo-papules noted above become lenticular in shape, cease to lose their color under the pressure of the finger, extend peripherally even in a few hours, flatten and become purpuric patches of a bluish-black shade, palm-sized and even larger, covering extensive areas of the integument, new lesions forming in unaffected islets of the skin; conjunctival ecchymoses appear at the angles formed by the lids, and finally encircle the cornea with an annular purplish-black cushion. The mucous surfaces become dry, crack, and bleed where the epithelium is torn, and become covered with offensive crusts. The odor exhaled by the patient is intolerably fetid. He lies stupid as the march to a fatal issue is hourly hastened. Hemorrhages occur from the larynx, bronchial membrane, intestinal surfaces, and even into the parenchyma of the viscera, the muscles, serous membranes, periosteum, and neurilemma. The urine is retained in the bladder; the respirations rapidly increase in frequency; the pulse flutters; and death closes the scene between one and two days after the onset of the malady. In several cases observed by the writer, [p. 443]occurring in infants and children, the entire course of the malady was completed in twelve hours.

In the second and much rarer form of hemorrhagic variola there are the usual unfavorable portents of intense prodromic symptoms. On the fourth day the skin is swollen and indurated in consequence of the development within its structure of numerous firm, roundish, slightly acuminate papules, so thickly set together that it is wellnigh impossible to distinguish between them. These are early in betraying the bluish-black hue significant of hemorrhage into their mass. They multiply in number and increase in size, while their hemorrhagic stains widen and sweep from each as a centre, like the waves that spread from a pebble thrown into smooth water. In these cases, more often than in those first described, pus-filled pocks may develop over some portions of the surface, while in others a species of gangrene occurs in consequence of the separation of the derma from the subcutaneous tissues by effused blood. At times pustules of somewhat typical aspect are formed and subsequently filled with blood by a hemorrhage from below. The accompanying symptoms are grave, but less rapidly fatal than in the other types of the disease. Delirium, stupor, an intense fever, and a rapid, feeble pulse are commonly noted. A fatal result is usually reached in from four to five days.

Hemorrhagic lesions, isolated or confluent, are seen also in severe forms of variola, not of the two types described above. Thus, in confluent small-pox, especially when occurring among the unvaccinated, some of the pustules on the face, the back, or possibly the legs, where varicosities of the veins permit a passive engorgement of the tissues with blood, may become the seat of a hemorrhage. For these local causes are often etiologically effective. In other cases the appearance of the hemorrhagic lesions seems to be due to a dyscrasia, such as that recognized in phthisis, chronic alcoholism, and hæmophilia.

Aside from the trivial accidents to which the exanthem may be subject, the hemorrhagic types of variola may be regarded as necessarily grave and in a large proportion of cases inevitably fatal. That they are all truly the results of variolous poisoning is shown, first, by the occurrence of intermediate forms; second, by the occasional transmission of the disease in its typical aspects to the partially protected.

VARIOLOID is that form of variola in which the disease is modified, either in its course, duration, or intensity of symptoms, such modification usually resulting, directly or indirectly, from the protective influence of vaccination or from a previous attack of variola.

The symptoms of the class of patients commonly regarded as suffering from varioloid are all those of variola, modified, however, in the direction of a mitigation of their intensity and dangerous character. It is thus evident that there is no strict line of demarcation between the very mildest physical expression of the variolous poison and that variola vera which presents atypically benign symptoms in any stage of its career. Within this wide range of possibilities cases of varioloid occur which certainly differ from each other by very marked degrees.

The invasion stage of varioloid may be shorter or longer than that occurring in variola vera, and may be insignificant or intensely marked as regards the severity of its symptoms. According to Bartholow[4] the [p. 444] invasion rashes are here of common occurrence; and the more extensive the latter, the less copious the subsequent eruption. It must be admitted that a personal experience has not confirmed us in this view.

[4] *Loc. cit.*

After the high fever and severe cephalic and lumbar pains of this stage there may follow, in the case of varioloid, a complete defervescence and the appearance of a very copious exanthem. With this, however, the apogee of the disease may be reached, and the subsequent symptoms be altogether insufficient in comparison with those which have preceded. Thus, the maculo-papules may never reach a vesicular stage, or, having attained this, the vesicles may not be umbilicated, or may shrivel after their contents have assumed a lactescent color, and be succeeded by light superficial crusts which in a few days fall. Or, again, the pustular stage of the lesions may be fully developed, even with the production of a halo about the pocks, while yet there is no swelling of the skin and but trifling subjective sensations experienced by the patient. The pustules in the course of from four days to a week desiccate and are shed, leaving behind them violaceous pigmentations of the surface without persistent cicatricial sequelæ.

Other cases, again, instead of producing the impression upon an observer of being illustrations of a malady aborted or cut short at some period of its career, seem to exhibit merely a modification in the intensity or distribution of symptoms betrayed in a wellnigh typical career. Thus, there may be a total absence or insignificant reminder of the septic fever usually known as the secondary fever of variola, and the elements of the eruption may be few or appear in scanty number upon the face and more copiously elsewhere. The latter may, however, pursue a perfectly typical career and be followed by characteristic scars.

There is yet another type of varioloid with which many practitioners become familiar who have experience in epidemics of small-pox. The patient exhibits distinct symptoms of malaise in the period of incubation. The fever of invasion, with its characteristic pains and nausea, is equally well marked. Defervescence occurs with a trifling eruption of maculo-papules, which in two days have wellnigh completely disappeared. There is no secondary fever, but the patient is far from well. There is a period of anæmia, mental depression, marked languor, and unmistakable evidences of physical prostration out of all proportion to the precedent symptoms. In these cases it may well be believed that the poison has at last produced a strong impression upon the nervous centres. The most characteristic feature of these cases is the tedious convalescence from an apparently trifling form of the malady.

The identity of varioloid with variola is abundantly shown—first, by the occurrence of intermediate forms of every grade, from the mildest evidence of variolous poisoning to typically developed cases of variola vera; second, by the fact that patients affected with varioloid are capable of transmitting variola to the unprotected; third, by the anatomico-pathological fact that the structure of the pock, when it appears, is the same in all.

A variation as to the form and contents of the lesion of modified variola occasionally occurs as a consequence of individual peculiarities or of the special surroundings of the patient. A number of useless terms have been employed to designate these peculiarities, the most of which [p. 445] are relics of the superstitions of the past. In variola siliquosa the pocks are said to contain air only; in v. pemphicosa, bullous lesions predominate; in v. verrucosa, the papules, after partial evolution and involution, leave minute wart-like papillary masses upon the face; in v. crystallina, there are superficial vesicles only filled with clear serum, which somewhat resemble those recognized as sudamina. The older English writers with as little reason described cases of horn-pox, swine-pox, etc., differing only from those of variola by the anomalous behavior of the exanthem in the course of its evolution.[5]

[5] Besides the terms given above, Hebra gives the following list of Latin adjectives which have been employed to describe special varieties of small-pox, none of which requires special explanation: variola papulosa, conica, acuminata, globosa, globulosa, tuberculosa, cornea, fimbriata, miliaris, lymphatica, vesiculosa, pustularis, rosea, morbillosa, carbunculosa, etc.

COMPLICATIONS AND SEQUELÆ.—The complications and sequelæ of variola are fewer in number and more restricted in range than those of many other maladies. This results from the remarkable unity of the disease as it occurs in its several manifestations among the unprotected, its relatively rapid progress, and its absolute disappearance on the completion of its curriculum. There is no chronic form of variola lingering for weeks and months after the violence of the fever has abated.

Furuncles and abscesses occasionally result during or after the pustular stage of the disease has been reached, sometimes of such extent as to give exit to large quantities of an ill-conditioned pus. The tissues, weakened by the suppurative process which the skin has undergone, may then necrose, and thus lay bare periosteum, cartilage, or bone. Erysipelas, especially about the face, may close the eyes, encroach upon the scalp, or spread extensively over other regions. Muscular paralyses, hemiplegic and paraplegic attacks, albuminuria, diarrhoea, and the inflammations of chronic type affecting the thoracic organs may each supervene, and either greatly prolong convalescence or precipitate a fatal issue. None of them is perhaps more common than a low typhoid and febrile state, in which the patient lies after his variola is practically ended, his skin struggling to regain its normal tone, a fever of remittent type taxing his energies, his bowels in frequent movements discharging a thin and fetid feculent matter, while a low delirium renders him insensible to the gravity of the situation.

Reference has been made above to the implication of the eyes of the variolous, and the possibility of the disorder terminating, after an otherwise favorable convalescence, in total blindness, should not be forgotten. The cornea may be the seat of pustules or a diffuse puriform infiltration resulting in ulceration, and eventually perforation with hernia of the iris. At times it is merely macerated by the pus continually covering it, and in that condition yields to even moderate pressure. At others the deeper portions of the globe fall into inflammation, and there is a resulting cyclitis, irido-cyclitis, or parophthalmia.

In the nose severe destructive effects may follow the pustular involvement of the Schneiderian membrane, including necrosis of the nasal bones and profuse epistaxis.

In a similar way, the external ear may be involved, the tympanum disappear, a severe otitis media supervene, and the mastoid cells become filled with pus and detritus of necrosed tissue.

[p. 446]In the larynx, which may be well lined with pustules, as indicated above, complications may arise in the shape of oedema of the ary-epiglottic folds,[6] laryngo-oesophageal abscess and various diphtheritic deposits lining every portion of the mucous membrane.

[6] J. William White, "Surgical Aspects of Small-Pox," *Medical News*, March 4, 1882, p. 241.

Other disorders noted as complicating variola are hydrocele and orchitis in the male, ovaritis in the female, gangrene of scrotum or labia, hæmaturia, peritonitis, adenopathy and lymphangitis and arthritis, as well as peri-arthritic suppurative inflammation.

PATHOLOGY AND MORBID ANATOMY.—Ours is a day in which bacteria, special to each of a number of infectious diseases (lepra, pemphigus, tuberculosis, etc.), are constantly reported as coming to light under the persuasive influence of modern staining solutions. With respect to variola, it may be said that while Cohn, Klebs, Weigert, and others have, without question, recognized microsphæra, micrococci, and similar organisms in variolous pus, their causative relation to the pathological process has certainly not yet been demonstrated.

The pathological anatomy of the cutaneous lesions of variola has been very carefully studied by Auspitz and Basch,[7] and Heitzmann.[8] The following is a condensed account of the results reached by these observers:

[7] *Virch. Archiv*, Bd. 28.

[8] *Trans. of Amer. Derm. Ass.*, Aug., 1879.

First appear circumscribed patches of hyperæmia, in which the papillary layer of the corium is concerned, and which is followed by some thickening of the rete, the epithelia involved becoming coarsely granular. This granular condition is due to an increase of living matter within the protoplasmic bodies, evident at the points of intersection of the reticulum of which they are composed, the nuclei becoming solid and shining, and the threads traversing this cement-substance between them becoming also increased in thickness. The papillæ beneath increase in size in consequence of their vascular engorgement, and in consequence of the change experienced by the connective-tissue bundles, which are partly transformed into protoplasm, while the protoplasm between them increases also. There is, in brief, a liquefaction of the glue-giving basis-substance, which makes visible the reticulum of living matter formerly hidden within it. In this way the epidermis is raised into the flat solid papules which are the early lesions of the disease.

Then follows an exudation of a serous fluid at one or more points in the papule, the meshes of the reticulum being so stretched and torn that small chambers are formed filled with the liquid exudate containing granules. Between these chambers the separating strata of epithelia are compressed so as to form septa or partition walls. The neighboring epithelia become granular, divested of their cement envelope, and transformed into protoplasmic clusters still connected with the living reticulum by slender threads. An irregular cavity is thus formed in the thickened rete traversed by septa, the contained exudation being filled with granules, coagulated fibrin, and lymph. A few protoplasmic bodies are here also distinguishable, which Heitzmann regards as either débris of destroyed epithelia or colorless blood-corpuscles.

In these changes the connective-tissue beneath participates. The papillæ eventually disappear, the superior portion of the corium being replaced by[p. 447]clusters of medullary or inflammatory elements uninterruptedly connected by threads of living matter.

The pus-corpuscles which eventually appear originate mainly from transformed epithelia. In the process of transformation the increased protoplasm of the epithelia first exhibits shining homogeneous lumps, which, after an intermediate stage of vacuolation, undergo an endogenous metamorphosis into nucleated bodies with a reticulum in each. To the number of these there is possibly an addition by the immigration from below (diapedesis) of leucocytes.

The question of repair with or without the production of cicatrices rests upon the behavior of the connective-tissue elements. If these are not torn asunder, but remain in connection with each other, the re-formation of a glue-giving basis-substance is possible, and new bundles of fibrous connective-tissue take the place of the old. If, on the contrary, the latter are completely destroyed, their place is filled with the cicatricial new growth. The pigmentation, which is such a common transitory sequela of the skin lesions, is due both to the imbibition of the coloring matter of the blood by the epithelia and by direct hemorrhagic exudation into both the rete and derma.

The umbilication of the mature pock is doubtless due to the situation of such lesions at the orifices of the excretory ducts of the skin-glands. The epidermis, in one or more of its strata, dips downward to form a living investment for such glands, and in this situation ties down the centre of the roof-wall of the pustules. Eventually, it too, as a result of the maceration and tension incidental to the complete filling of the pock with pus-elements, is ruptured or stretched, and the umbilication of the pustule disappears.

The anatomy of the exanthematous lesions in hemorrhagic variola is not different from that described above. The pocks in such cases are merely filled with blood instead of with pus or sero-pus. In some forms of hemorrhagic variola, as indeed would be suggested by their clinical observation, there is hemorrhage directly into the tissues of the integument, or, more probably in severe cases, a mere passive leaking of the sanguineous fluid with its coloring matter through the relaxed and weakened vascular walls.

The morbid changes occurring in the viscera are described by Curschmann as follows: The mucous surfaces may be the seat of pustules, diffuse purulent infiltration, and catarrhal, croupous, or diphtheritic inflammation. As regards the extent of diffusion of the pustular lesions, they occur, according to Wagner, in bronchi of the second and even of the third order, rarely in the stomach and intestines, and in the rectum only in its lowest portion. The bladder, urethra, and serous surfaces are always exempt. The lungs, breast, liver, spleen, brain, and spinal medulla are variously involved. Often the tissues of these organs are quite unchanged as regards their macroscopical appearance. At other times the tissues appear swollen, granular, and undergo a fatty degeneration. In purpura variolosa the spleen and walls of the heart, however, are seen to be firm, dark-red, and more or less indurated.

DIAGNOSIS.—The establishment of a correct diagnosis where there is question of variola is one of the most critical and important of the duties of a physician. Upon such decisions have turned, again and again,[p. 448]professional success or disaster. To pronounce that case to be variolous which is not of such a nature is to subject one to the indignation of the few and the ridicule of the many. On the other hand, to be guilty of treating a patient with small-pox, and of remaining ignorant of the nature of the malady, is to subject many ignorant people to the danger of exposure to the disease and to render one's self liable for the redress sought by recourse to the civil authorities and the law. It is difficult to decide which predicament is the graver.

Typical variola vera is readily recognized by its characteristic features. As usual, it is the atypical and modified forms where the difficulty most often arises and where the danger to the physician is proportionately increased.

In the invasion stage of the disease it is often impossible to recognize any symptoms characteristic of variola. High fever with severe lumbar pain, considerable gastric distress, and the appearance of one of the invasion rashes (roseola variolosa) would, however, put the observant practitioner on his guard. I have often noticed in these cases a symptom which, apparently insignificant, has on more than one occasion preceded the eruptive period. It is the occurrence upon the centre of the two cheeks of a vivid damask-red blush, occasionally having a purplish-red hue, and with a very remarkable circumscribed area. This may be recognized in children and adults of both sexes when it occurs in typical aspect, and is undoubtedly a hyperæmia of the character of that producing the rashes in Simon's triangles.

When the variolous exanthem first appears the practitioner should secure as soon as practicable a history of the invasion stage if this has not been subject to his personal observation. He should then make careful inquiry as to the possibility of a neighboring source of contagion, and ascertain by inspection whether the person of the patient exhibits the evidences of successful vaccination. In this connection it is always well to estimate the value of the elements represented by (*a*) the period ascertained as having elapsed since the last successful vaccination; (*b*) the typical or atypical character of the existing cicatrices of vaccinia; (*c*) the unicity or multiplicity of the cicatrices simultaneously resulting from vaccinations performed at one and the same date.

Without question, the first papular lesions of variola resemble those of rubeola or measles to an extent which has often deceived the most expert diagnosticians. The distinguishing points are—(1) In measles, catarrhal symptoms (conjunctival, nasal, laryngeal, bronchial), which are usually absent in the early stages of variola, and later are obviously associated with the irritation set up of the pustules of the maturing period. (2) The difference in the temperature record, that noted in the invasion stage of variola varying from 104° to 105° F., while in rubeola it is rarely registered above 103° F. Moreover, in typical variola the defervescence is marked and characteristic on the appearance of the exanthem, while in rubeola, when the rash appears, the temperature is usually sustained at a maximum, and may even rise. (3) The differences in the rashes of the two disorders. The papules of variola, even in its confluent forms, are, when first observed, remarkably discrete and exhibit not the slightest tendency to grouping, while the maculo-papules of rubeola are (*a*) developed simultaneously on the face and trunk, while those of variola [p. 449]commonly appear first on the face and afterward on the trunk, the older, and larger therefore, in the site of earliest appearance; (*b*) are set in clusters or groups having a distinct tendency to crescentic arrangement, a symptom decidedly best appreciated by the eye when the eruption is viewed in totality or in large areas with the eye of the observer somewhat removed from the surface; (*c*) are often made to disappear or pale beneath the pressure of the finger, while there is greater persistence of color in the variolous papules; (*d*) are surrounded by little or no halo, each elementary lesion of the eruption being abruptly defined upon the sound skin, while the variolous papule is apt to rest upon a circlet of hyperæmic integument.

Even with careful observation of all the specific differences between the two diseases, they may, for a brief time, so resemble each other as to defy the skill of the expert. In all doubtful cases the physician should invariably admit the doubt and defer an exact diagnosis for twenty-four hours. During the delay the variolous exanthem should betray its individuality by the formation of a minute vesicular apex at the summit of several papules.

In scarlatina the uniform diffusion of the exanthematous blush, the absence of papules and vesico-papules, the continuance of the fever after the rash has appeared, the characteristic scarlet or boiled-lobster color of the skin, and the anginose condition of the throat, are all significant symptoms. In hemorrhagic small-pox the color of the integument is a much more purplish and lurid-reddish hue, rapidly reaching that stage where it refuses to pale under the pressure of the finger, and never leaving in the track of the finger-nail quickly drawn over its surface the peculiar transitory yellowish-white line which can be usually obtained in the skin of the patient with scarlatina.

The pustular stage of variola might be confounded with the pustular syphiloderm. But in the latter there should be a history of a chronic rather than of an acute affection, and, as a result, the simultaneous appearance of lesions in very different stages of their career, some distended with pus, others ruptured and crusted, yet others which have recently formed in the immediate vicinity of the oldest lesions, while the latter have been in full involution or have been replaced by superficial losses of tissue.

The resemblance of pustular variola to certain suppurative and other disorders of the sebaceous glands is well attested by the name given by certain French authors to molluscum epitheliale (M. contagiosum, M. sebaceum)—viz. acne varioliformis. But in the case of acneiform disorders the concurrence of comedones, the chronic course of the disease, the absence of fever and systemic disturbance, and the particularly irregular distribution of the lesions upon the face, with failure to appear elsewhere,—all these facts forbid the confusion of the affection with variola. In medicamentous acne, accompanied by the sudden appearance of numerous pustular lesions symmetrically displayed upon the surface, there will indeed be a source of error. In such cases, of course, a history of the ingestion of a medicament capable of producing a rash will afford valuable aid in the diagnosis. In pustular forms of dermatitis medicamentosa there will usually be found a more abundant development of the pus-containing lesions upon the head and both arms and forearms, with [p. 450]no tendency to extension over very large areas of the trunk and lower extremities—a circumstance which a delay of but a few hours will often substantiate.

The absence of marked defervescence is the most characteristic difference between variola in its eruptive stage and typhus, typhoid, and relapsing fevers. Pneumonia, cerebro-spinal meningitis, acute miliary tuberculosis, and gastric fever are all to be differentiated from variola by the occurrence of symptoms characteristic of the involvement of the several organs which in these diseases respectively are more particularly impaired.

PROGNOSIS.—The prognosis of variola is wellnigh inseparably associated with the question of protection by vaccination. Variola vera in the unprotected is an exceedingly fatal malady, the death-rate varying in different epidemics according to the severity of each and the ages and hygienic surroundings of the victims of the disease. Certainly, from 15 to 50 per cent. of unprotected individuals affected with the disease occurring in epidemic form in any given community will perish. This number may, however, be enormously increased, as, for example, among a large number of unprotected negroes crowded together in a filthy prison, or when the malady makes a periodical visitation to an insular community where long isolation has begotten a carelessness with respect to vaccination.

With respect to individual cases it may be asserted, first, that an intense series of prodromic symptoms, followed by the appearance of an unusually large number of cutaneous lesions, is often unfavorable. Confluence of the latter adds to the gravity; hemorrhagic and purpuric symptoms are in the highest degree portentous, and commonly indicate a fatal result. Women pregnant or in the puerperal state, infants at the breast, and persons of both sexes at advanced ages, are little able to resist the ravages of the disease. According to Kaposi, women recently delivered prematurely or who have lately suffered from an abortion succumb more often than others of their sex. Chronic alcoholism among male subjects and the cachexia induced by all chronic visceral and systemic disorders are sources of weakness which largely increase the death-list by adding to the heavy strain upon the vital energies. The prognosis is rendered uncertain or unpromising by extensive involvement of the mucous as well as of the cutaneous surfaces, by marked visceral complications, by evidences of shock or exhaustion before the apogee of the exanthem is reached, by grave sequelæ, and even by simple complications of the malady when, instead of entering promptly upon convalescence, the patient lingers for weeks in a typhoid condition. An unfavorable symptom in any case is the sudden cessation of the processes actively pursued upon the surface of the body. The swelling of the integument then suddenly diminishes and the crusts by which it was covered shrivel. The eruption, in brief, seems to undergo what may be described as a collapse. The pulse at such moments usually flutters feebly, and there are other portents of dissolution which the eye of the physician will hardly fail to interpret correctly. The fluids in such instances mechanically drain away from the surface of the body to seek the deeper parts. This is not peculiar to small-pox. Similar phenomena occur even in the case of other than exudative affections of the skin. In pityriasis rubra the [p. 451]patient dies leaving an integument apparently unaffected, and I have seen a patient dead of even multiple sarcoma of the skin when the tumors were reduced fully one-half in bulk as the result of a similar cause.

On the other hand, the practitioner should never forget that even apparently desperate cases of variola rally and are won back to life. That the exudative process should be in full evolution at the surface of the body is, cæteris paribus, certainly so far a good omen. The most hideous, extensive, and stench-emitting crusts have hidden for a time the forms that have for many subsequent years not only known the enjoyment of life, but have made that life of inestimable value to others. The physician in the presence of this most loathsome and formidable disease should never despair.

PROPHYLAXIS AND TREATMENT.—The loftiest end to be reached by the physician of our day with respect to variola is its complete removal from all civilized countries, and indeed from the face of the earth, by the practice of universal vaccination and revaccination. The evident modifications which the disease has undergone in late years as a consequence of the extraordinary attention given to this subject is an earnest of the future. The day is probably not far distant when the man, woman, and child unprotected by vaccination will properly be regarded as an enemy of the human race, and treated accordingly. Evidences of the most satisfactory character as to successful vaccination should be imperatively required of all applicants for admission to schools, academies, colleges, charitable institutions, public libraries, art-galleries, and places of labor controlled by incorporated institutions; of all members of conventions, legislatures, political, religious, and deliberative bodies; of every purchaser of a ticket for purposes of travel; and of every voter. In addition, there should be in every district a systematic and periodical inspection of all persons registered in the census by persons qualified and competent to perform compulsory vaccination. This is the scientific treatment of variola.

Respecting the therapeutic management of variola, it must be admitted that there are no remedies known to exert the slightest influence in either cutting short the curriculum of the disorder or in checking its progress in any stage. When vaccination is practised after the disease is fully developed, the two disorders, vaccinia and variola, apparently concur, and proceed pari passu to the evolution peculiar to each. Quinia, the sarracenia purpurea, the salicylate of sodium, emetics, diaphoretics, purgatives, and other remedies and methods vaunted as efficacious, have again and again failed to establish the claims which have been put forth respecting the value of each.

The most important of the considerations to be regarded at the outset of the management of the small-pox patient relate to his hygienic surroundings and nursing—considerations which scarcely differ from those recognized as of general importance in the case of all septic, contagious, and filth-producing diseases.

The timid, the fearful, and the unprotected are to be at once dismissed from the bedside, and trustworthy attendants secured who have received protection by either recent vaccination or a prior attack of the malady. The sick chamber should be sufficiently large and capable of the most thorough ventilation by free access of air. Solar light should be excluded[p. 452]as rigidly and completely as possible, since it is reasonably certain that its access to the face has an etiological relation to the pitting of that part, often the most serious sequel of the affection. It is an interesting fact that pitting is much less frequently noted on those parts of the body from which light is excluded by the covering of the clothing. The temperature of the sick room during the febrile stages of the disorder should not rise above 70° F. nor be permitted to fall below 60° F. Between these extremes a variation may be made in accordance with the sensations of the patient.

During the invasion stage of the disease the patient can rarely assimilate food, but if this be possible it should be given throughout the entire course of the disease in the form of animal broths, eggs, nutritious soups, and milk. Iced and acidulated beverages are often grateful to the palate, and small lumps of ice should be permitted to dissolve slowly in the mouth. Lime-water may be required by unusual gastric irritability. As the disease progresses and the palate and buccal membrane become painful and sore by reason of the localization there of pustular and other lesions, various mouth-washes and gargles may be ordered, such as those containing the chlorate of potassium, the tincture of myrrh, the tincture of cinchona, or even the milder demulcent fluids made by the addition of flaxseed, gum acacia, or powdered elm-bark to water. In almost all such cases the skilled nurse will accomplish a grateful result by frequently cleansing the mouth of the sufferer (especially before the deglutition of aliments) by covering the finger with a soft handkerchief, dipping it in pure hot water, and then thoroughly and gently cleansing the entire buccal cavity. The spray of a saturated solution of boracic acid in rose-water may then be directed over the parts.

Applications of cool and iced water to the skin are commonly grateful, and, as a rule, are accompanied by no danger to the patient, though in the early periods of the disease they unquestionably retard the full evolution of the cutaneous symptoms. For the pain in the back, therefore, which is often the most urgent symptom of the invasion stage of the disease, it is usually preferable to make hot applications. The large rubber bags now in common use, filled with hot water and from time to time applied to the lumbar region, may be employed with good effect simultaneously with iced, spirituous, or camphorated applications to the head.

Numerous indeed have been the topical applications made to the surface of the skin in the pustular stage of the malady, both with a view to assuage the soreness and pain and to obviate the tendency to pitting. The opening of the pustules and the evacuation of their contents (practicable only in other than confluent forms of the disease) has been practised from an early date, but is ineffectual from the standpoint of any practical results thus obtainable. The same may be said of the subsequent cauterization of the floor of the pustular chamber, which only adds to the distress experienced by the sufferer in his skin. Medicated unguents, applied to the skin, containing mercury, iodine, and other substances, are not known to be followed by any better results. It may indeed be laid down as a general rule that fatty applications to pus-producing surfaces where the pathological product is virulent are apt to undergo decomposition and otherwise act unfavorably upon the tissues—a fact first pointed out by Ricord in connection with the treatment of the [p. 453]chancroid. Vaseline, as not liable to undergo chemical decomposition, is not open to this objection.

Curschmann, Kaposi, and other authors are in agreement respecting the value of water-compresses over the surfaces invaded by the eruption—a method of topical treatment which I desire to fully endorse after personal observation of its value. Curschmann recommends compresses dipped in iced, Kaposi those moistened with tepid water. The sensation experienced by the patient will prove the best guide to the temperature of this fluid. I prefer a solution containing one drachm of boracic acid to the pint of water as hot as can be discovered to be productive of comfort, a drachm or two of glycerine being added to the solution. The compresses dipped in this (or a carbolated solution, if the latter is preferred by either physician or patient) should be assiduously moistened and changed regularly by the attendants just as long as they can accomplish good. They operate, first, by protecting the part; second, by keeping it moist; third, by maintaining the surface temperature at the point most pleasant to the patient; fourth, by exercising the gentlest degree of equable compression over the surface. When desired, this may be covered with the Lister protective material or a piece of oiled silk to prevent evaporation at the surface.

In Vienna warm baths, administered either by the process of continuous immersion so generally practised there or by immersion for from two to three hours of each day, have been found to furnish the greatest amount of comfort to the patient. The skin is thus speedily relieved of its tension, the exfoliation of the crusts is hastened, and the time required for the evolution of the cutaneous lesions, if not shortened, is at least not retarded by the accidents of exposure to the desiccating influences of the air—ends which for the patient are practically one. In this country, and especially in private practice outside the larger charities with their ampler provision for these emergencies, nearly the same result may be reached by wrapping the patient completely in sheets wrung out of water of the temperature desired.

From first to last in the treatment of variola, all indications should be made subordinate to that most prominently set forth by the general character of the symptoms—viz. the conservation by every possible means of the vigor of the patient. The tax upon all reserves of vital energy is here so enormous and constant that he will gravely err who for a moment loses sight of this fact. Hence it is that anodynes, chloral, opium and its alkaloids, the bromide of potassium, and similar medicaments, introduced either by the stomach or by hypodermic injection, are to be jealously reserved for emergencies when it would seem cruel to withhold the temporary comfort they may impart. Stimulants are of course to be freely employed whenever they are indicated by exhaustion as this may be shown by a weak pulse and other failing functions of the body, but are certainly best reserved for such emergencies. In general, it may be remarked that the fewer the medicaments ingested by the stomach, and the larger the restriction of the labor of this organ to the task of sustaining the nutrition of the body, the better are the chances of a favorable issue.

It is unnecessary to add that all other indications presented in any given case are to be met, subject to the conditions indicated above. Abscesses[p. 454]are to be opened and antiseptically treated; delirious patients are to be sedulously prevented from doing themselves injury; daily movements of the bowels are to be secured; while the diarrhoea of the typhoid state, occasionally resulting from the exhausted condition of the system when the force of the disease is spent, demands proper control.

Cleanliness is to be enforced by every judicious measure. The skin of the patient is to be washed in tepid water and soap as often as practicable in the course of the disease, and under no circumstances are applications of ointments, washes, or lotions to be allowed to collect in strata upon the surface commingled with the pus and crusts of the disease. At the time of such ablution, and occasionally oftener, the linen and other garments of the patient are to be changed. When the crusts are regularly exfoliating from the surface of the body general warm baths may be ordered, after each of which the surface of the body may be anointed with vaseline or covered with a finely-sifted dusting-powder, such as the cornstarch farina sold by grocers.

Inasmuch as hemorrhagic variola is usually hopeless in character, and remedilessly fatal, Kaposi's liberal use of opiates may be recommended when euthanasia is all that can be expected. So long as there is the narrowest chance of recovery resort may be had to ergot, turpentine and the mineral acids internally, combined with the external use of styptics and ice. But little confidence can, however, be placed in these measures, which will prove entirely ineffective in the great majority of all cases.

In all fatal cases of variola the duties of the physician are not ended by the death of the patient. It is for the benefit of the living that he should require destruction or disinfection and long disuse of all domestic articles that were employed upon or about the patient. The lifeless body should be disposed of by cremation, and medical men should exert their influence in favor of legal enforcement of such a wholesome practice.

[p. 455]

VACCINIA.
BY FRANK P. FOSTER, M.D.

SYNONYMS.—Vaccina, Variolæ vaccinæ (Jenner), Cow-pox, Cow-pock, Kine-pox, Kine-pock; *Fr.* Vaccine; *Ger.* Kuhpocken, Schutzpocken, Impfpocken, Schutzblattern; *It.* Vaccina; *Sp.* Vacuna.

DEFINITION.—An eruptive disease characterized by a cutaneous lesion closely resembling that of small-pox, going through the stages of papulation, vesiculation, pustulation, incrustation, and cicatrization; differing from small-pox in the mildness or almost total absence of the constitutional symptoms, by being communicable only by inoculation, and by the fact that the lesions, as a rule, are developed only at the points of inoculation and in their immediate neighborhood.

This definition holds good for the great majority of cases, but in each of its parts we must take account of exceptions. For example, the lesion does not always follow the regular sequence of changes described. It may stop short at the stage of papulation, constituting the so-called raspberry excrescence, which will be further referred to hereafter; it may pass directly from the stage of vesiculation into that of incrustation, without any such change in its liquid contents as can properly be said to form a pustule; desquamation may take the place of incrustation; and, after an evolution otherwise normal, there may be no formation of a scar, simply because the destructive effect of the lesion has not extended deeper than the epidermis. The constitutional symptoms are sometimes severe, but they are always of very short duration. The disease is said to have been communicated otherwise than by inoculation in the case of some of the lower animals. Thus, Chauveau succeeded in producing some of its phenomena in the horse by causing the virus to be inhaled in the form of spray. It is doubtful, however, if it is possible to eliminate all sources of fallacy in such experiments. Finally, a generalized eruption is occasionally observed, although with great rarity. In stating these exceptions no reference is intended to cases in which complications occur.

NATURE OF THE DISEASE.—Many considerations warrant us in classing cow-pox among the varioliform diseases—chiefly its general resemblance to variola, and the fact that individuals who have been affected by it are thereby more or less fully protected against small-pox. It has been thought, indeed, that cow-pox was in reality but a modified form of small-pox; and this idea has been the basis of one of the theories that have been held as to the origin of vaccinia. Before enumerating and discussing those theories it will be well to mention that cow-pox is spoken of as spontaneous, casual, or inoculated, according to its mode of origin, known or assumed, in individual instances.

[p. 456]Spontaneous or original cow-pox is the name commonly applied to the disease as it is met with in the cow in instances in which its mode of origin is unknown. Strictly interpreted, this expression implies a belief that the affection is capable of being developed in a cow independently of contagion or infection—a notion that seems to be held by many physicians, but not, so far as the writer is aware, by those whose study of the subject has been such as to lend any considerable weight to their opinions. Ordinarily, however, the term spontaneous cow-pox is employed simply as a convenient expression to denote the disease as it occurs naturally in cows, without implying any belief or theory as to its mode of origin.

Casual cow-pox is the term applied in cases that have been contracted by accidental inoculation, whether in the cow or in man. It is manifest that the so-called spontaneous cases are really casual, unless we accept the doctrine that infection is not necessary to the development of the disease.

The term inoculated cow-pox implies that the affection has been produced by intentional inoculation. Here, again, we are confronted with an illogical expression, for a disease that is inoculated accidentally is still inoculated, as much as if it had been conveyed purposely. It may be said, indeed, that the casual disease is due to some other form of infection than inoculation, but for such an assertion there is not a particle of proof.

Passing from this unsatisfactory nomenclature to a consideration of the theories that have been held as to the nature of cow-pox, we are first met with that of its being a disease sui generis, like small-pox, measles, scarlet fever, and the like, and, like them, originating only by its own specific contagion, not being capable of development by a modification of any other contagion, however closely it may thus be counterfeited. This seems the most rational theory of the nature of cow-pox, but it cannot be demonstrated except by disproving all opposing theories; and that has not yet been accomplished.

Another theory is, that cow-pox is really small-pox modified, as the phrase runs, "by passing through the system of the cow." It has been thought possible, indeed, to specify in what way the cow's system could impress such decided changes upon the virulent disease small-pox as to convert it into the mild affection that we know as vaccinia; in other words, it has been imagined that the function of lactation accomplished this remarkable result. This notion may have been due to the observation that so-called spontaneous cow-pox is met with only in cows that are in milk. The significance of this fact, however, is really nothing more than that cows in milk are more exposed to accidental inoculation than other bovine animals—namely, at the hands of the milkers. The fact that in such cases the lesions are almost always confined to the teats and the udder, far from affording any ground for the notion that there is some mysterious connection between cow-pox and the function of lactation, is but another proof that the disease is the result of inoculation. The lesions appear at the points of inoculation, the teats and the udder being the parts handled by the milkers. Moreover, there is no difficulty in inoculating young calves or adult bulls, and the lesions so produced do not vary in a single particular from those observed in so-called spontaneous cases.

[p. 457]Men have been so carried away with this milk theory, however, as even to believe that the virus of small-pox might be shorn of its dangerous properties, so that it would produce only the vaccinal lesion when inoculated simply by mechanical mixture with milk. During the late Civil War one of the Confederate Army surgeons actually put this notion to the test of practice on quite a large scale, inoculating large numbers of persons with a mixture of small-pox virus and milk, terming the practice mitigated inoculation. We can scarcely suppose that he did anything else than variolate these persons, just as he would have done had he used variolous lymph without the addition of milk. His experiments show nothing new; they merely furnish a recent confirmation of the well-known fact, familiar to the old inoculators, that inoculated small-pox is sometimes exceedingly mild in a series of cases.

This theory of the variolous origin of cow-pox, and of the practicability of converting small-pox into cow-pox at will by "passing it through the system of the cow," has taken deep root in the minds of men, especially in Great Britain, where the late Mr. Ceely's experiments and Mr. Badcock's experience seemed to give it some color. Some years ago, however, the question was investigated most practically and thoroughly by a commission appointed for the purpose by one of the medical societies of Lyons, Chauveau being the recorder. Their conclusion was—and their reasoning seems to the present writer incontrovertible—that small-pox and cow-pox were wholly distinct from each other under all circumstances, and that it was impossible to convert the one into the other. But the doctrines of the English investigators, reinforced as they were by the ingenious arguments of the late Dr. Seaton, were not easily to be overturned in their own country or in America; consequently, the practice of variolating cows has been resorted to from time to time for the purpose of obtaining a stock of vaccinal virus of unquestionable authenticity—the so-called variola vaccine. This practice is utterly fallacious, and it is also dangerous, since the disease so produced, however mild it may seem to be, is nothing more nor less than small-pox, with its infectiousness by effluvium and its liability to prove serious even when carefully inoculated.

Quite recently the experimental investigation of the question has been undertaken de novo by a well-known English veterinarian, Mr. Fleming; and, since his conclusions coincide with those of the Lyonnese commission, it is to be hoped that we have seen the last of this rough-and-ready method of improvising a case of genuine cow-pox—a method that, in the light of our present knowledge, can only be characterized as downright malpractice.

The third and last theory we have to consider is that which ascribes the origin of cow-pox to infection from the horse. So far back as Jenner's time it was conjectured that cow-pox was due to the accidental conveyance of the virus of the grease (the eaux-aux-jambes of the French) by reason of the cows being milked by persons who were also employed in the care of horses affected with that disease. Grease is an eruptive disease of horses' heels. Doubtless it has often been confounded with a mere eczematous affection by those who have repeatedly failed in their persistent attempts to inoculate cows with it, and, on the other hand, a localized eruption of horse-pox may have been mistaken for it by those who have [p. 458]supposed themselves to have succeeded in producing cow-pox by inoculating cows with the virus of grease, and have consequently given in their adhesion to the grease theory of the origin of cow-pox. At all events, so far as the writer is aware, that theory is not now held by any well-informed writer.

Still regarding the horse as the originator of cow-pox, we must turn our attention to horse-pox (equinia). Several years ago Depaul of Paris took great pains to establish the fact that horse-pox (an affection totally distinct from grease) was an eruptive febrile disease of horses, an exanthem; that the eruption was generalized, and, being for the most part concealed by the hair, generally overlooked; and that it was capable of being conveyed by inoculation, the lesion being indistinguishable from that of cow-pox. He believed himself to have demonstrated also that it was the contagion of horse-pox that gave rise to cow-pox in the cow.

Depaul's investigations were very keen and his conclusions were exceedingly plausible, but they cannot be called convincing, notwithstanding the fact that Constantin Paul succeeded for a time in popularizing a stock of horse-pox virus as material for vaccination. At about the same time the Beaugency case of cow-pox was discovered, and the perfectly satisfactory use that has been made of that stock may have thrown Depaul's theories and Paul's practice undeservedly into the background.

We can only say, in summing up, that the small-pox theory is utterly untenable, that the horse-pox theory has not been disproved, and that the theory that regards cow-pox as derived neither from small-pox nor from horse-pox, but as a disease sui generis, although not proved, is the most rational of all, and the most in keeping with known facts.

ETIOLOGY.—Nearly everything that could be said under this head has already been considered. It may be added that meteorological conditions have been supposed to favor the prevalence of the disease among cows. More precise observations are needed to enable us to determine whether or not there is any truth in this supposition. It has been said that the affection is most apt to prevail during warm and moist seasons. This is contrary to what we might have imagined, as warmth and moisture are quite destructive of the vaccinal virus. Under ordinary circumstances, however, the contagium often proves wonderfully tenacious of life, and the disease, once introduced among a herd of cows, is prone to linger for months, or even years, attacking animals recently added to the stock and young cows during their first lactation. As has already been stated, age, sex, and parturition can be regarded as etiological factors only in so far as they favor the occurrence of accidental inoculation. In the human subject vaccinia occurs generally as the result of intentional inoculation, as will be more fully referred to when we come to the consideration of vaccination. Insusceptibility is occasionally met with, both in the cow and in man, but it is very rare. Perhaps it may be explained in some instances by the subject having really had the disease, or indeed small-pox, either before or after birth, in so mild a form as not to have left the characteristic marks. Certain it is that the lesion does not always leave a permanent scar, especially in the cow.

GENERAL COURSE OF THE DISEASE.—This is best studied in cases that have followed intentional inoculation, for here we know the [p. 459]chronological sequence of events. Depending somewhat upon the method of inoculation, and perhaps also to some extent upon the state of the skin at the site of the inoculation, or even upon a systemic condition (since some vaccinators hail it as a harbinger of success), at the time of the operation a ring-like erythema may be seen surrounding the inoculation. This is exceedingly evanescent, being doubtless due to vaso-motor action, and is not often witnessed.

Ordinarily, no effect whatever is observed until after the lapse of two or three days, when a red papule is formed. This papule increases in superficial area, but not in height, and gradually loses its redness. It assumes a circular form, or, in the case of a compound pock (for that is the proper name for the lesion), a configuration representing segments of several circles, and as it increases in area it becomes more and more raised at the border (the bourrelet of French writers), while the central portion, which also increases in size pari passu with the peripheral annular vesicle, does not become more elevated, but remains depressed, giving the pock as a whole the peculiar shape termed umbilication. Up to the eighth or tenth day, inclusive, the marginal elevation contains a limpid fluid termed lymph, and consequently presents a pearl-like lustre. At this period a rather sudden increase takes place in the corpuscular elements contained in the lymph, causing that liquid to become thick and opaque, so that the elevated margin of the pock, which before had shown the pearl-like lustre alluded to, now comes to look as if made of tallow.

At the same time what is known as the areola forms around the pock, and constitutional symptoms show themselves. The areola is a circumscribed redness of the skin, perfectly circular in form and of five or six times the diameter of the pock itself. It is sharply defined and of a vivid red hue. Usually it is a mere hyperæmia of the skin, but in some instances, especially where the process of pock-formation is decidedly pronounced, a few papillary elevations are to be seen in the immediate neighborhood of the pock, and at that situation there may also be some lividity. After a few hours' persistence in the form of a disc the areola begins to disappear, the redness fading first at the central portion, so that in its declining stage it assumes the shape of a ring which constantly grows narrower and narrower at the expense of its inner portion, and finally disappears altogether. In the cow the areola is only a faint line immediately around the pock.

Constitutional symptoms are invariably present in cases that follow the regular course. The temperature rises one or two degrees Fahrenheit, the appetite becomes impaired, and sleep is somewhat disturbed. In many cases, mostly those of secondary inoculation, the symptoms are more severe; the fever runs higher, and may be accompanied with transient delirium; nausea is experienced, perhaps with actual vomiting; and severe pain is felt in the head and along the spine, the latter being most marked in the cervical region. These symptoms usually last but a few hours, and they are apt to be accompanied by a modification of the areola whereby it loses its disc-like outline and becomes diffused irregularly, especially, if, as is usual, the inoculation has been done on the arm, in a downward direction toward the elbow.

Along with these phenomena intense itching is often felt at the situation of the pock, being an aggravation of the pruritus that in a mild [p. 460]form accompanies the greater part of the whole course of the lesion. Supposing the arm to have been inoculated, the lymphatic glands of the axilla now become swollen and tender, but their suppuration is unusual, and is to be regarded as a complication.

To go back to the pock: some time before the contents of the marginal elevation become opaque the central portion is converted into a crust of a brownish color, and finally, from the tenth to the fifteenth day, the bourrelet itself, having ceased to increase in size, takes part in the process of incrustation, the completed crust representing the form of the pock, having a circular ridge at the border, at which part its color is not so deep as at the centre. The crust usually falls off between the fifteenth and the thirty-fifth day. It is hard, translucent, and of a prune-juice color; thick at the centre and thin at the periphery; smooth on its attached surface and somewhat wrinkled on its outer aspect; surmounted at the centre by the epidermal débris produced by the operation of inoculation, mingled perhaps with more or less dried blood.

After the crust falls off a reddened surface is left of a cicatricial nature, usually somewhat depressed below the level of the surrounding skin, and frequently showing lesser pits, which latter appearance is termed foveolation. Instead of these pits, radiated striæ are frequently left. Gradually the scar loses its red color, and, like other scars, finally becomes paler than the surrounding skin. It is usually permanent.

IRREGULARITIES IN THE COURSE OF THE DISEASE.—Ever since cow-pox first became the subject of medical study deviations from its typical course have been noticed, and have been the theme of a good deal of speculation. The older writers, indeed, bestowed no little attention upon what they considered to be not irregular forms of vaccinia, but distinct affections with which it was liable to be confounded. Their descriptions of these diseases, which they termed spurious cow-pox, are, however, so vague as to possess but little more than an historical interest. In regard to affections met with casually in the cow, we can often determine their nature only by test-inoculations, and even that criterion is not always thoroughly convincing; for, on one account or another, we may fail in the attempt to propagate true cow-pox, and on the other hand, if we admit that there is a radical difference between cow-pox and small-pox, it is manifest, bearing in mind the errors into which experienced investigators have fallen, that we may propagate small-pox through a long series of experiments without once suspecting it to be anything but cow-pox. We may, nevertheless, always determine, provided we succeed at all, whether we are dealing with a disease that protects against vaccinal and variolous inoculation.

In the human subject we seldom meet with affections that counterfeit vaccinia, although, if we take only the lesion into consideration, there are certain contagious forms of herpes that may give rise to doubt, and possibly the same may be true of impetigo contagiosa.

Turning, then, to the irregularities properly so called, we have first to consider the absence of constitutional infection. This must not be confounded with the mere lack of obvious constitutional symptoms; what is meant by the expression is, that in certain instances the local lesion may appear typical, and yet no such impression be made upon the system as to render it proof against subsequent inoculation. Early in the [p. 461]century the possibility of this lack of systemic infection was insisted upon by Mr. Bryce of Edinburgh, who invoked it as an explanation of the occasional failure of vaccinia to protect against small-pox. The practical question was, how to decide, in a given instance, whether general infection had or had not taken place. In the opinion of many observers—and that notion has cropped out every now and then up to the present day—absence of the areola furnished at least presumptive evidence that the constitution had eluded infection. But, whatever may be held theoretically, it must be conceded either that the general system very rarely fails to feel the impress of the disease, or else that the criterion is fallacious. For in an experience of seventeen years the present writer has not known of a single instance in which a vaccinal lesion that pursued a regular course in other respects has failed to be accompanied by the areola. And certainly Mr. Bryce himself must have attached little if any importance to it, for he took great pains to establish a means of determining the presence or absence of constitutional infection—the so-called Bryce's test. This consists in repeating the inoculation at a certain period in the evolution of the disease, the theory being that systemic infection does not take place at once, but only after the lapse of a number of days from the time of the inoculation. Up to that time a repetition of the inoculation is possible, and, if systemic infection results from the first one, both lesions will mature at the same time, the second one following an accelerated course, reaching its acme rapidly, although dwarfed in size. If, on the other hand, the first inoculation failed to infect the constitution, the second one will pursue its course in the usual manner. Moreover, at a certain time, generally about the fifth day, a repetition of the inoculation will fail altogether if the original insertion has really infected the system. The present writer can testify that Mr. Bryce's statements are correct; he has applied the test in many cases, but in no instance has he been led to the conclusion that constitutional infection had failed to take place. He is inclined to think, therefore, that such failure is exceedingly rare.

Passing over the multiplicity of irregularities in the lesion that were described by the older observers, it seems that there are a few that are of practical importance. In the first place, there is a variety of pock to which it is not easy to give a definite name, but which is characterized by a lack of decided elevation above the surrounding skin (a deficiency for which it makes up in superficial area), by the early formation of a thin, flimsy, straw-colored crust, and by the utter failure of the characteristic firm brown crust of the typical variety to become developed. This form of irregular pock has not been seen by the writer of late years, but before animal vaccination came into general use he met with it frequently, mostly in cachectic children. Notwithstanding its sprawly, unsatisfactory appearance, it is undoubtedly genuine, for the typical lesion may be produced by inoculation with its contents.

Another irregularity of the pock is what is familiarly termed the raspberry excrescence. A red elevation forms at the seat of inoculation, and at first promises to follow the typical course, although it may be tardy in making it appearance; but it never advances to full development. It becomes indolent, and may last for several weeks, or even months, in the form of a hard, flat nodule of a bright-red color, not unlike a small [p. 462]nævus. In many instances it has a succulent look, but no lymph can be obtained on puncturing it. No areola appears at any time, and finally the lesion slowly disappears, leaving no trace of its existence. It is probably an abortive form of pock, in which only the papillary layer of the skin takes part, without any exudation into the epidermis. It is seldom, if ever, protective against small-pox, for it constitutes no bar to a subsequent vaccination. This irregular pock has been observed from time to time ever since the early days of vaccination, but for the past six years it has been seen more frequently in New York than for many years before. Now, however, it seems to be growing less common. The writer is not aware of any satisfactory explanation of its occurrence. It is seen in all sorts of subjects, and seems to follow the use of one variety of virus as much as the employment of any other.

What has been termed generalized vaccinia is another form of irregularity. The expression is a vague one, covering as it does not only the very rare cases of true eruptive vaccinia, in which a general eruption of pocks takes place as a consequence of constitutional infection, playing the part of an exanthem, but in addition those instances, not very uncommon, in which pocks are formed here and there on the body, probably as the result of the accidental transfer of the virus from the pock by scratching. Under such favorable conditions—the immediate transfer of lymph from a pock in which the specific evolution is going on vigorously—the slightest penetration of the epidermis with the nails is enough to secure self-inoculation. In view of this facility with which it may be effected, we should be very careful not to jump hastily to the conclusion that in any given case of generalized vaccinia the supplementary pocks are truly eruptive; as a matter of fact, the present writer has never seen an instance in which he was convinced that such was the case. Where the pocks are very numerous, especially in subjects with an irritable skin, much distress may be caused by the itching and by the consequences of scratching, and marked febrile reaction may accompany the process; so that, in view of the great similarity of the lesions to those of the variolous eruption, much doubt is sometimes entertained as to whether the disease is not really small-pox. This question cannot always be definitely settled at first, but the failure of the secondary fever of small-pox, together with the fact that the disease does not spread by infection, will generally suffice to decide it.

Concerning those cases of generalized vaccinia that are manifestly not eruptive, it sometimes happens that the cutaneous receptivity is not exhausted for several weeks, or even months. Such cases set Bryce's test at defiance, in consequence, probably, of an idiosyncrasy. In some of these instances the pocks appear in clusters of successive formation, looking not unlike patches of zoster. Small supplementary pocks in the immediate neighborhood of the original lesion are not at all uncommon.

PATHOLOGICAL ANATOMY.—Avoiding the minute histological details for which the prescribed length of this article gives no scope, but little is to be added to what has already been said in the section on the clinical features of the disease. The lesions of vaccinia are wholly cutaneous. Confining ourselves to cases that follow a regular course, there is, indeed, but one, the pock—a term that seems preferable to vesicle and [p. 463]pustule, since the latter apply only during certain phases in the development of the lesion.

A pock may be regarded as essentially a lesion of the epidermis, for it is in that structure that its most striking features are developed, and in some cases, although doubtless the papillary layer of the derma is congested, there is no permanent alteration of tissue below the Malpighian layer of the epidermis. These are the catarrhal pocks of Rindfleisch, and it is in such cases, if any, that no scar (even of temporary duration) results. The term catarrhal pock, however, is not vitiated by an extension of the morbid process deep enough to produce a permanent cicatrix, and it is probable that in most cases the catarrhal type predominates. By the term diphtheritic pock the same author refers to cases in which the congestion of the papillary layer is so intense as to block the supply of blood to the apices of the papillæ, as a result of which they become exsanguinated and necrosed, forming a white pultaceous layer on the floor of the pock, which is undoubtedly what Ceely referred to when he spoke of a false membrane. In some cases even the subcutaneous tissue undergoes necrosis, a sort of core being included in the substance of the crust that ultimately forms.

Whichever of these forms of pock we take into consideration, always excluding irregularities and complications, we find certain definite changes in the epidermis. The dome of the pock is formed by the unbroken transparent horny layer of the epidermis, unaffected by the morbid process. The cavity of the pock is formed by the squamous cells of the epidermis being forced out of their normal relations by an exudation of lymph between them, some of them being tilted up edgewise while still retaining their connection with the surrounding cells, thus accounting for the multilocular structure of the pock; for it is a fact that the circular bourrelet consists not of one ring-like cavity, but of many separate chambers. The result of this structure is, that the liquid contained within the pock—the lymph—escapes only partly through a puncture made in the wall of the vesicle. In order to evacuate the pock thoroughly it is necessary to make a great number of punctures or a circular incision following the ring-like ridge of the bourrelet.

The lymph contained within the cells of the pock is a liquid which in its gross physical properties differs but little from the lymph which exudes from any traumatic surface shortly after the injury has been inflicted, as in the glazing process that takes place in wounds. Examined microscopically, however, it is found to contain not only the fibrin, the salts, the corpuscular elements, and the débris that ordinary tissue-juice presents, but also certain minute spherical bodies—termed microspheres, microzymes, vaccinads, etc.—that give it its characteristic infective quality and justify the title of virus commonly applied to it. That these minute bodies really constitute the virulent element of the lymph, or at least that they are the vehicle of the contagium, is not a mere matter of conjecture, but has been demonstrated abundantly, notably by Chauveau and Sanderson's diffusion experiments. Inoculation with the supernatant liquid, containing none of these bodies, always fails to convey the disease, but it is not absolutely essential that they should be present in large proportion in the lymph to render the latter virulent, for Chauveau found that lymph diluted with thirty times its bulk of water was not without infective [p. 464]power. It scarcely need be said, however, that the greater the proportion in which they are present, the greater is the probability that the lymph will prove infective on inoculation. These bodies have been supposed to be of a vegetable nature, and Hallier, Kohn, and others have bestowed no little study upon their botanical characteristics. Under favorable circumstances they retain their virulent properties for a long time, especially if kept perfectly dry and not subjected to a high temperature. The present writer has met with success in the use of vaccinal virus seven years old.

The lymph differs somewhat in its gross appearances according as it is produced in man or in the bovine animal. In the former it is clear and limpid, and exudes freely in great drops when the pock is punctured in its peripheral portion; in the latter it is more straw-colored and more viscid, exuding sluggishly, or even refusing to flow without the aid of pressure. Moreover, the vaccinads seem endowed with different properties in the two cases: in man they have a tendency to remain equably diffused through the liquid, while in the cow they tend to separate from it and to be deposited upon any solid surface at hand.

The phenomenon termed umbilication, common to the vaccinal pock and to that of variola, has given rise to some differences of opinion as to the mechanism of its production. The term implies a depression at the centre of the pock. This appearance is not invariable, but it is constant enough to have met with general acceptance as a characteristic feature, notwithstanding the undoubted fact that it is found in lesions that have nothing whatever to do with any of the varioliform diseases. Not to waste space in discussing the various theories that have found supporters, it may be said that they have all been proved to be defective, save only the simple explanation that as the process of evolution advances the centre of the pock undergoes desiccation, whereby that portion of the tissue involved is so glued and drawn together as to become incapable of the swelling that is still going on in the growing peripheral portion of the lesion.

The crust into which the pock ultimately becomes converted is not, as is commonly supposed, mere dried lymph and nothing else; it is dried tissue enclosing concrete lymph. It generally includes also various sorts of débris—broken-down epithelium, blood-corpuscles, pus-corpuscles, and even, in rare cases, a core of sphacelated tissue like that of a furuncle.

As has already been said, the cicatrix is to a certain extent peculiar in that it is usually depressed and foveolated. Too much stress has been laid upon these features, however, and the truth is that some traumatic scars cannot be distinguished readily from that of vaccinia, while, on the other hand, many a genuine pock leaves no permanent trace behind it. Indeed, in the cow it is the exception for a noteworthy scar to form.

SEQUELÆ AND COMPLICATIONS.—The most important sequela of vaccinia is the fact that it protects the subject against small-pox, and on that circumstance hinges the chief practical interest of the disease. This leads us at once to the subject of vaccination, and therefore under that head we shall pursue our consideration of this curious affection.

[p. 465]

Vaccination.

SYNONYMS.—"The new inoculation;" *Fr.* Vaccination; *Ger.*Kuhpockenimpfung, Schutzpockenimpfung; *It.* Vaccinazione; *Sp.*Vacunacion.

HISTORY.—Before giving the history of vaccination itself (meaning by that term the intentional inoculation of vaccinia for the purpose of protecting the subject against small-pox), it may be well to devote a few words to a practice that preceded it—that of the intentional inoculation of small-pox (or simply inoculation, latterly called variolation). In very early times various Oriental peoples became aware of the fact that small-pox might be very decidedly mitigated by inoculation. This was practised in various ways, all of which may be reduced to the process of inserting small-pox virus into a solution of continuity. Lady Montagu, the wife of an English ambassador to Turkey, brought the practice back to England with her, where it soon made its way into popular favor, and whence it spread rapidly over Europe and America. Thus contracted, small-pox was shorn of a great part of its terrors; the eruption was usually trifling in amount, and in every way the disease was mild as a rule. Still, the mortality was something worth considering, and, worse than that, the inoculated disease was communicable by effluvium, so that an inoculated person had to be secluded carefully for fear of spreading the disease in the ordinary way. In all cases, too, careful medical treatment was thought necessary. On the whole, then, while inoculation was undoubtedly a boon, it was fraught with many grave perils. So great, indeed, were these perils, and so thoroughly were they appreciated, that the practice was interdicted by law in most civilized countries so soon as vaccination had become established in popular favor.

In several European countries the common people—at least those of them who had much to do with dairies—gradually became aware of the existence of the disease termed cow-pox, and of the fact that those individuals who had accidentally contracted it were rendered proof against the infection of small-pox. There is even fair testimony to show that some of these people, particularly the English farmer, Benjamin Jesty, relying on their observation to this effect, employed intentional cow-pox inoculation as a protective measure. These facts, however, do not detract in the least from the credit that all Christendom has awarded to a man who subjected the popular impression in question to the test of scientific investigation, proved its truth, and demonstrated its value to the world. That man was Edward Jenner, an English country physician. It was in the last quarter of the eighteenth century that he entered upon his course of inquiry, and on the eve of the present century he published his demonstration to the world. It was not a discovery; it was not an invention: it was more than either, "a matchless piece of induction," to quote the words of Mr. John Simon. Filled as he must have been with the consciousness of his great achievement, Jenner set this good example to all investigators: that he did not make haste to convert the world; he first convinced himself. It may almost be said, indeed, that, like Minerva from the head of Jove, the rational and perfected practice of vaccination sprang complete from Jenner's hands. Doubt and ridicule he had to encounter at first, and afterward envy and detraction; but the force of [p. 466]his facts and the symmetry of his deductions were such that the new inoculation soon spread through the broad world, and has ever since maintained its sway, save with a few fanatical scoffers.

That vaccination really does protect against small-pox observation has taught the whole civilized world, if we leave out of account the few conscientious and intelligent doubters (made such, doubtless, quite as much by the extravagant statements often put forth by those who from time to time think it incumbent on them to defend vaccination, as by their own misinterpretation of facts) who are to be found associated with the noisy little body of actual opponents of the practice. One of the most injurious statements ever made in the advocacy of vaccination is, that it always protects if properly done. When one of these illogical defenders of that proposition is confronted with an instance that disproves his assertion, he falls back on the allegation that in that instance the vaccination was not properly done. The manifest absurdity of such an argument strikes the doubter most forcibly, and inclines him to say to himself, Falsus in uno, falsus in omne. Unbelief founded on this ground would never have arisen if the plain truth had always been adhered to: that the protection afforded by vaccination is not invariable, and that very often it is not permanent. In the infancy of the practice these facts were not known, but it is now many years since they became obvious to every fair-minded observer. The misapprehension of facts lies chiefly in the false deduction from the circumstance that the great majority of cases of small-pox occur in persons who have been vaccinated. But the explanation of this is very simple. Suppose that, of one hundred persons vaccinated, twenty fail to be protected permanently; that all persons not vaccinated are unprotected; and that throughout the civilized world the proportion of vaccinated to unvaccinated persons is as ninety to ten. Making no pretence of arithmetical accuracy, it may certainly be said that all these suppositions are well within the truth. It follows from them that in a community of ten thousand persons there will be nine thousand who have been vaccinated, and one thousand who have not. Of the former, eighteen hundred will have failed to secure lasting protection. Therefore in case of an epidemic there will probably be a proportion of eighteen cases of small-pox in the vaccinated to ten in the unvaccinated; and yet this should not obscure the fact that of the nine thousand vaccinated more than seven thousand were absolutely protected, whereas of the one thousand not vaccinated not one could escape the disease if exposed to it. When we add the further observation that of the eighteen hundred cases of small-pox among the vaccinated not more than thirty or forty would probably prove fatal, while of the one thousand cases in the unvaccinated about two hundred would end in death, we have a striking demonstration of the efficiency of vaccination. As a matter of fact, statistics show that the figures here given err rather in allowing too little than in asserting too much in favor of vaccinal protection.

The question naturally arises, Why it is that vaccination protects some persons and does not protect others?—reference being had, of course, to permanent protection, for it is exceedingly rare for temporary immunity to be attained if we exclude those instances in which the variolous infection has taken place before the operation is resorted to. This [p. 467]question cannot be answered with any certainty, but various theories have been brought forward, some of which call for notice.

In the first place, it has been thought that the revolution of the system termed puberty was fraught with such a radical change as to do away with the mild modification due to vaccination. While this theory has an air of plausibility, it seems to lack proof and not to be upheld by analogy, for we do not find that children who have had scarlet fever, measles, and the like often undergo those diseases a second time on arriving at the age of puberty.

The only remaining theory that our limits will allow a consideration of is that put forward by Marson of London, that the degree and duration of vaccinal protection are proportionate to the perfection of the vaccinal lesion and to the number of insertions made. In a large experience with small-pox Marson found that the disease was more fatal among those whose vaccinal scars were imperfect or few in number than among those who bore evidence that several pocks had been produced and had run a typical course. As to the influence of a perfect evolution of the lesion, but little doubt can be entertained, for we have already seen that in some instances its course is so different from what it should be that no protection whatever seems to result. When we come to consider the number of the pocks as affecting the degree or the duration of protection, however, an obvious source of fallacy arises in the fact that we cannot always be sure that some of the scars on a person having a number of them were not the products of a repetition of the operation several years after the first—that is to say, a revaccination, the efficiency of which in restoring lost immunity is now well established. Nevertheless, as long as the doubt remains the best course to pursue seems to be to act as if Marson's theory were in all respects correct, and vaccinate by multiple insertions.

We have, then, no positive means of ascertaining who those persons are that are likely to fail of lasting protection, or how long a time will elapse before the cessation of their immunity will take place. The only safety lies in revaccination. But after how many years should revaccination be resorted to? It has been thought that this question might be settled by noting at what age, or at what period after primary vaccination, large numbers of people became susceptible of revaccination. This test, however, is not altogether trustworthy, for a renewed susceptibility to vaccinia by inoculation does not necessarily imply that the liability to take small-pox by effluvium has been regained. If it did, modified small-pox (varioloid) would be far more common than it is, for it is certain that revaccination can be made to succeed in a very large proportion of children long before they have reached the age of puberty. The fact is, contrary to the notions of the last generation, that success in revaccination is the rule, not the exception. Formerly it was not expected to succeed, and therefore no special pains were taken to ensure success.

Definite rules cannot be laid down as to the time that should be suffered to elapse before vaccination is repeated, but in the great majority of instances safety may be attained by revaccination every five or six years, and always in the presence of an epidemic, regardless of the lapse of time; also whenever one's mode of life is to undergo a noteworthy change, [p. 468]as in emigrating to a foreign country, on entering the military service, and the like.

To sum up, then, vaccination almost invariably protects against small-pox for the time being; generally for a long term of years; sometimes for a lifetime. Often the protection is absolute; as a rule, it is very nearly so; in rare instances it is trifling. In general terms, it may be said that it is scarcely less protective than variolous infection itself, for death from a second attack of small-pox is by no means rare. Here the question comes up: Is vaccination less protective, either in degree or in duration of effect, than it was at the time of its adoption? Given a typical vaccinia, we may unhesitatingly answer, No; but do we now so invariably produce the disease in all its essential features as was done in Jenner's time? Yes, provided we use proper virus and employ as much care as was taken by the older physicians, who, trained to the practice of variolation (the inoculation par excellence of bygone days), did their work with a gusto now seldom witnessed. But there was a time, now happily at an end, when it was not easy to obtain thoroughly good virus, and when, therefore, the result was apt to vary materially from the standard. This may be conceded without entering upon the vexed question of the general deterioration of the Jennerian stock of vaccine.

Besides immunity from small-pox, there are one or two sequelæ of vaccinia that deserve mention before we proceed to consider what it is better to class as complications. In the first place, vaccination has been supposed to confer temporary protection against whooping cough. The writer is not aware, however, of any precise data going to prove either the truth or the falsity of this supposition.

Secondly, by virtue probably of the inflammation that attends the evolution of the vaccinal pock, vaccination practised in the immediate neighborhood of a small nævus often cures that blemish, and it has been done for that purpose in many cases. It has no advantage over many other measures, however, and there is the disadvantage that the nævus may so mask the pock as to give rise to some doubt as to the satisfactory character of the latter. The practice, therefore, is not to be urged.

COMPLICATIONS.—These are local and systemic. Those of them that are at all serious are rare, and can generally be traced to fortuitous circumstances.

Inflammatory complications are usually due to undue traumatism at the time of the inoculation, to injury of the pock, or to the previous existence of a cutaneous disease or of some dyscrasia. Dermatitis is the most common. It is usually a mere erythema, but in some instances lymphangitis, lymphadenitis, phlegmonous inflammation, with diffuse suppuration, may result. From injury of the pock ulceration and gangrene may take place, and septic absorption may follow in their train. These complications are to be treated as if they had occurred from any other cause. Generally, the mere vaccination is not responsible for them, but in some instances putrescent vaccine may be adduced as their source. In such cases the complications, if they can still be called so, are apt to make their appearance long before the pock matures, even within forty-eight hours of the vaccination. Inflammatory complications supervening on the full development of the pock may invariably be set down as due to some cause not connected with the quality of the virus employed.

[p. 469]An undue amount of dermatitis is best treated with some mildly astringent and anodyne application. The following liniment is excellent for the purpose: Rx. Unguenti

Stramonii oz. j; Liquoris Plumbi Subacetatis fl. drachm ss; Olei Lini fl. oz. iv.—M. fiat linimentum. As a rule, it is best to avoid poultices applied over the pock itself, for they soften the tender structures that make up its dome and render it prone to rupture, with all the consequences that may follow its conversion into an open sore. When the latter accident has occurred, dusting powders will ordinarily suffice to absorb the discharge, and thus prevent putrefaction—either the ordinary toilet powder or salicylized or carbolized powders, the basis of which may be starch with a small proportion of the oxide of zinc. Besides the antiseptics mentioned, iodoform, boric acid, etc. may be used to advantage. Liquid applications are not usually so appropriate, but the writer has known the proprietary preparation termed Listerine to answer admirably.

Circumscribed collections of pus are to be treated as under other circumstances, and burrowing is to be guarded against. It is only in the worst cases that constitutional treatment of any sort is demanded, and in these it should be of a supporting nature.

Passing from the simple inflammatory complications to those of a specific character, we will first mention erysipelas. Genuine erysipelas following vaccination is quite rare, but when it does occur it is prone to prove serious. The writer believes that it always depends on secondary infection—*i.e.* that the vaccinal wound becomes the nidus of an erysipelatous contagium already existing in the patient's surroundings, just as any other traumatic surface might, and that the vaccinal virus has nothing whatever to do with it. Admitting that improper virus is apt to give rise to dangerous inflammatory complications, the latter are not really erysipelatous, whatever guise they may put on. Erysipelas following vaccination calls for no other treatment than what is proper for traumatic erysipelas under ordinary circumstances.

We now come to the subject of vaccinal syphilis. The question of the possibility of conveying constitutional taints along with vaccinia was raised long ago, but, partly relying on certain theoretical tenets, and partly because of the rarity of well-ascertained facts to shake the blind confidence felt in the utter harmlessness of vaccination, the profession fought the suggestion without properly investigating it. In regard to syphilis, the broad assertion was maintained that two infectious diseases could not affect an individual at one and the same time: either syphilis would be communicated alone or vaccinia alone; moreover, it was affirmed that the juices of a syphilitic person were not capable of giving rise to the disease by inoculation unless they happened to proceed from a syphilitic lesion. There was never sufficient basis for the former of these two doctrines, and the latter received a rude shock when it was shown by Pallizzari and the anonymous physician of the Palatinate that the blood of a syphilitic subject was capable of conveying the taint. Meantime, certain horrible outbreaks of syphilis were reported, chiefly in Italy, that could not reasonably be imputed to the ordinary occasions of syphilitic infection. Even these occurrences, however, failed to shake the general incredulity, especially in Great Britain, where until quite recently men's orthodoxy in medical matters was gauged by their obstinacy in refusing to[p. 470]investigate, far less believe, the slightest proposition unfavorable to vaccination, and where, also, observations from beyond the limits of the empire were looked upon as in all probability fallacious.

To a Frenchman, M. Viennois, we are indebted for the first systematic and fair-minded study of the subject of vaccinal syphilis. This writer demonstrated that the Rivalta cases and those of other like outbreaks were certainly due to vaccination, but he concluded that they owed their occurrence not necessarily to the use of lymph from syphilitic subjects, but to the fact that that lymph contained blood. By this time it had come to be recognized that syphilis was inoculable by the blood. But even Viennois's masterly essay, and the facilis descensus it offered to those English authors who found themselves confronted with proof positive of their error, failed to make any noteworthy impression beyond the concession that syphilis might possibly be communicable in vaccination, but that, if it were, the catastrophe might easily be escaped by avoiding the use of lymph contaminated with blood, and that, therefore, the danger was practically no danger at all, for no one in England would think of using bloody lymph! In all this the English were slavishly followed by our own countrymen. It is proper to add, however, that Ballard of London did his best to present the matter in a proper light to the British profession, and that it is largely due to his labors and to those of

Jonathan Hutchinson (the latter of whom supplemented Ricord's discovery that vaccine lymph is never free from blood with abundant clinical evidence of the existence of vaccinal syphilis unavoidable by the mere observance of Viennois's safeguard) that we are now freed from the clog of error in this matter. Nor was it the English alone that so long baffled the recognition of the truth; in the French Académie de Médicine, Jules Guérin and his adherents fought desperately against it.

At the present day we know that syphilis is liable to be communicated in vaccination, and that, too, without regard to visible blood in the lymph employed. There are two ways of avoiding it. One is, to use non-humanized lymph, since the lower animals are insusceptible to syphilis.[1] This is simple. The other is, to select a human vaccinifer that is free from syphilis. This is difficult. Too great reliance, however, should not be placed upon the vaccinifer; it is possible to convey syphilis even in the use of bovine virus. Suppose two persons, A and B, are to be vaccinated at one sitting, A being syphilitic. If A is vaccinated first, and the same lancet, imperfectly cleansed, is used on B, it is plain that B will be inoculated not only with vaccine lymph, but also with A's blood. It is of the first importance, therefore, that this form of vaccinal inoculation of syphilis should be carefully guarded against; and that can be accomplished most certainly by using a fresh instrument for each patient.

[1] Practically, this is certain, although there is some reason to believe that the disease may be conveyed to monkeys.

From a medico-legal point of view it is important to note that constitutional syphilis may follow vaccination, and yet have nothing to do with it. Suppose an infant to be born syphilitic, but with no visible manifestations of the taint. Let that child be vaccinated, and let the syphilitic dyscrasia afterward break forth. The ordinary inference would be that the syphilis was due to the vaccination; and in most instances this view would certainly be urged by the syphilitic parent, since it would [p. 471] free him from suspicion. It is always easy to disprove such an allegation, however, for syphilis communicated in vaccination always shows itself first in the form of a chancre at the site of the vaccination. Therefore in any given case, unless this mode of onset can be proved, the syphilis is manifestly not of vaccinal origin. Some observers, it is true, are of the opinion that vaccination may evoke a pre-existing syphilis, to use Lanoix's term—*i.e.* that it may hasten the appearance of the characteristic manifestations, and even determine their localization at the site of the vaccinal inoculation. But, even allowing the truth of that proposition, in such a case the lesion would be constitutional, not chancrous.

It is well, nevertheless, to take precautions against being placed on the defensive in this way; and it may commonly be avoided by declining to vaccinate infants under three or four months old, since inherited syphilis generally manifests itself by that time. This prudence on our own behalf should not be carried so far, however, as to lead us to deny the benefit of vaccination to very young infants whenever the prevalence of small-pox is such that they are in obvious danger of exposure.

As regards its management, vaccinal syphilis does not differ from the ordinary form of the affection, and hence demands no other treatment than what is proper for the disease contracted in the usual way. It simply originates in an extragenital chancre.

Concerning the conveyance of other constitutional taints in vaccination our knowledge is very limited. The present tendency of pathological investigation is, however, to accord inoculability to many diseases that formerly were not imagined to possess that quality, so that in regard to other affections than syphilis it is prudent to use the utmost care in the choice of lymph. There is one supposed safeguard that does not seem to have the slightest title to be so regarded—namely, the notion that a typical pock cannot be developed on a person affected with a specific cachexia. There is no truth in the doctrine. Over and over again the writer has seen perfect vaccine pocks on persons whom he knew to be syphilitic.

Cutaneous affections of a non-specific character are sometimes observed to result from vaccination; that is to say, they follow close upon its performance, without any other known exciting cause. It may fairly be supposed that in many instances they would have shown themselves even if the vaccination had not been performed, for it is often the case that we are unable to speak positively in regard to the exciting cause of an eruption. Several years ago a striking case in point was related to the writer by a well-known physician of this city, S. S. Purple, in whose practice it occurred. Purple had engaged to vaccinate a child on a certain day, but for some reason the vaccination was not done. In about a week from the appointed day, however, erysipelas made its appearance, beginning on the left arm at the usual site of vaccination, and pursued its course to a fatal termination. To be sure, we are now speaking of non-specific affections, but erysipelas illustrates the proposition perfectly, notwithstanding its specific character.

Children with a tendency to eczema are prone to suffer an outbreak of that disease as the result of vaccination. In Jenner's time, indeed, it was considered not only that there was great risk of causing an aggravation of any slight eczematous eruption by vaccination, but that the mere [p. 472]existence of the eczema, even in the most trivial form, was likely to interfere with the success of the vaccinal inoculation. This has been the general feeling of the profession. Quite recently, however, many observations have been recorded tending to show that the old dread of vaccinating an eczematous child was not altogether warranted. The question needs further study, and, while it is probably best to postpone the operation under ordinary circumstances, nothing should induce us to withhold its protective influence where there is any manifest danger of actual exposure to small-pox.

Although eczema is the most common of the cutaneous affections called forth or aggravated by vaccination, there are various forms of skin disease, some of them difficult to classify, that occasionally result. They are usually vesicular, pustular, or furuncular—that is to say, irritative. In the majority of instances it will be found either that the pock itself has followed an irregular course, being whitish, diffuse, and ending in an exaggerated although superficial incrustation, or that it has been subjected to injury. Still, in some cases neither of these conditions is the precursor of the skin affection. In many instances the latter can only be called nondescript. There seems to be some occult connection between vaccination and the curious skin disease described by the late Tilbury Fox of London under the name of impetigo contagiosa; and, indeed, Piffard of this city has found certain microphytes to be common to the crusting period of vaccinia and that of contagious impetigo. What the relation of the two affections is to each other, however, it is difficult to say.

Apart from impetigo contagiosa, the cutaneous complications that follow in the wake of vaccination possess no distinctive features, and their management differs in no wise from that of the same manifestations due to other causes.

THE TECHNICS OF VACCINATION.—This aspect of our theme involves a number of separate considerations. It will be convenient to give our attention first to the matter of the choice of virus. The question arises at once as to the selection between animal vaccine and the humanized variety. In a broad sense the term animal vaccine includes—1. Virus derived directly from a case of so-called spontaneous cow-pox. 2. Variola vaccine—*i.e.* the virus of an affection of the cow resulting from variolation. 3. The virus of horse-pox (not strictly vaccinal). 4. Retro-vaccine—*i.e.* the virus of an affection produced in the cow by the inoculation of vaccinia from the human subject. 5. The virus of a disease (true vaccinia) propagated through a series of bovine animals from the so-called spontaneous cow-pox, being the virus now commonly understood by the term, and the variety here referred to when it is not stated to the contrary.

By humanized vaccine we understand that which is obtained from the human subject, no matter how short or how long its descent from the cow. As regards animal vaccine, we may practically exclude from consideration all but the last variety mentioned, that being the one to which, in the great majority of instances, the term is now restricted. This narrows the question down to the choice between virus that has been propagated through a number of bovine animals (practically, calves) from the spontaneous disease in the cow, and that which, whatever its original source, has already passed through the human system.

[p. 473]The variety first mentioned, sometimes called primary vaccine, is generally spoken of by authors as not very trustworthy as regards its infective power (that is, not to be counted on to take), and as prone to give rise to undue inflammatory complications when its use does prove successful. These unpleasant qualities might be explained by the supposition that primary vaccine is not apt to be at its best when it is now and then obtained. Practically, however, it may be dismissed without further consideration, for it is seldom to be had.

The second form—variola-vaccine—is manifestly improper to be used whenever genuine vaccine is to be obtained, unless, indeed, we shut our eyes to the accumulating evidence that variola-vaccine, so called, is not vaccine at all. Furthermore, it is a question whether its use, as well as all attempts to produce it, should not be forbidden by law.

The third variety, if such it may be called, it does not seem legitimate to use in the present state of our knowledge, since it is not yet proved satisfactorily that horse-pox possesses the full protective power of cow-pox, or is free from objections that do not arise in connection with the latter.

As to retro-vaccine, while the writer is unable to see any positive reason against its use, neither can he see any reason why it should be superior to humanized vaccine, as such, save that during the period of its bovine propagation it is not liable to become contaminated with the poison of syphilis. The idea that an enfeebled stock of humanized vaccine can have new life infused into it by passing through the system of the cow is not reasonable primâ facie, and there are no particular facts to support it. By ensuring freedom from the danger of communicating syphilis retro-vaccination doubtless served a good purpose at one time, but now, since the remarkable and enduring excellence of the Beaugency stock is so well established, there seems to be no excuse for a further resort to the practice.

The last of our five forms of animal vaccine, that produced by the continued propagation of spontaneous cow-pox through calves, is what is now known as animal vaccine par excellence. Its advantages over the other forms are so obvious that it alone should figure in any comparison between animal and humanized vaccine. That being understood, what are the relative merits of animal and humanized vaccine? It should be stated, in the first place, that bovine virus should be compared with virus that has long been humanized, for lymph of but a few removes from the bovine animal does not show any noteworthy differences from animal vaccine itself.

In behalf of humanized virus it is maintained—1, that it is a more trustworthy preventive of small-pox; 2, that it is superior in its infective property, so that it is surer to take; 3, that it is more prompt in its action, thereby affording more speedy protection to persons who have actually been exposed to small-pox; 4, that its virulent property is easier of preservation, wherefore it is more to be depended on when it is necessary to keep it on hand for a long time or to transmit it to great distances; 5, that its use requires less skill, or, rather, less special knowledge of the peculiarities of the animal virus; 6, that it is less violent in its effects; 7, that it is less apt to give rise to irregular, and therefore more or less abortive and non-protective, forms of pock.

[p. 474]The first of these propositions, which asserts that humanized vaccine confers greater protection against small-pox than the animal virus, was warmly maintained by those who opposed animal vaccination on its first introduction into this country; but now the record of the past thirteen years, during which period bovine virus has more and more borne the brunt of the fight against small-pox, has disproved it in the judgment of all competent and fair-minded observers. So far, indeed, as the facts have been analyzed, they go to show that the reverse is the case—that bovine virus confers a more complete and a more lasting protection. Direct observation on this point is strengthened by the collateral fact that revaccination became at once astonishingly successful when the use of animal vaccine first gained currency, whereas now it is again declining in success; the explanation of which latter circumstance is, that it is now found difficult to revaccinate those whose primary vaccination was done with bovine virus—a striking indication of the permanence of the protection accomplished with the latter.

The second assertion—that humanized virus succeeds more readily than the bovine variety—is still maintained by many, but, it may confidently be said, by few if any whose experience with good animal vaccine has been large. The truth is, that every large public vaccination service in the country is now carried on almost solely with bovine virus, and that results are thus achieved that were not dreamed of in former times. Individual experience cannot weigh against this fact, but may be explained, rather, by what modicum of truth there may be in the fifth proposition, or by the assumption (surely a legitimate one, in view of the number of irresponsible and ignorant purveyors of animal vaccine that have thrust themselves before the profession since the advantages of the practice were established by the labors of others) that those whose observation leads them to a conclusion at variance with that reached by the great majority of trained observers have really been unfortunate in the quality of the virus with which they have been supplied. Whatever the explanation may be, however, there is nothing more certain than that the use of animal vaccine, properly carried out, is daily furnishing results that have never been excelled, if they have been equalled, in the employment of humanized virus on a like scale.

The third suggestion—that the humanized virus acts the more promptly of the two, and is therefore to be preferred for immediate protection—is plausible, since the areola (the alleged sign of systemic infection) forms somewhat later around a pock produced by animal virus than around one that is the result of vaccination with the humanized variety. The difference is one of a few hours only at the most, and it is not by any means a general occurrence; still, we may concede that in this respect the use of humanized virus is to be preferred under certain circumstances.

As to the fourth statement—that humanized virus is more tenacious of its infective property—strictly speaking, there is not a particle of truth in it. In the case of liquid lymph preserved in capillary tubes it has the semblance of truth, but, for reasons that will be more fully set forth hereafter, that is because it is difficult to get the virulent portion of bovine lymph out of the tube. In the form of dried lymph (the only form that ought to be used) animal vaccine may be sent to all parts of the world, and may be kept any reasonable length of time and without [p. 475]special care, without undergoing sensible deterioration, if tested by one who is familiar with its peculiarities and aware of the care that should be taken in using it. Under ordinary circumstances there is no difficulty about preserving animal vaccine with its energy practically unimpaired.

The statement that the use of humanized virus demands less special knowledge than that of bovine virus is conceded at once. That special knowledge is easily mastered, however, and no man fitted to practise medicine will look upon its acquirement as a bugbear or a hardship.

The impression, almost universal thirteen years ago, that humanized vaccine is less severe in its local and constitutional effects than the animal virus has been eradicated from the minds of all but those who still follow the teachings of the older writers rather than yield to what daily experience has been teaching during these thirteen years, or those who reason from exceptional cases rather than from a general drift. The truth seems to be this: with revaccinated adults animal vaccine acts somewhat more severely than the humanized virus; in infants, on the other hand, its action is not so violent as that of the humanized variety.

Concerning the seventh and last claim put forward in behalf of humanized vaccine— that it is less apt to give rise to irregular or spurious pocks—we may say that no form of irregularity has been observed by those who have lately used the bovine virus that was not well known to the older writers, who founded their observations wholly, or almost wholly, on the use of the humanized virus; nor is there any proof that such irregularities are more common now than formerly. The truth seems to be, that these irregular forms of pock seem to prevail at certain times, and not at other times, regardless of the particular stock of virus used, other things being equal. Why this should be so we do not know, but the fact is beyond dispute.

To sum up, then, we can only say that in barely one particular—that of promptness of action—can humanized virus justly be credited with any superiority, while in every other essential respect it is inferior, so far as any difference is to be observed.

What, on the other hand, are the points of superior excellence attaching to bovine virus? Setting aside certain extravagant assertions that have sometimes been made in its behalf, such as that it far exceeds the humanized virus in its protective virtue (which may be true, but is not yet proved), they may be put in general terms in the form of a denial of all the particular claims that we have enumerated as having been put forth for its rival. Such a denial, it has been seen, seems to the writer to be justified, save in the one particular that perhaps we should accord to humanized virus the merit of speedier action, and consequently greater certainty of protection, in cases of actual exposure to small-pox.

Besides these negative points in its favor, the foremost advantage of animal vaccine is the guarantee it gives that, properly used, no syphilitic contamination will result. On this point no argument is needed, for the cow is insusceptible to syphilis.

A second consideration in its favor is, that it can always be had in large quantities at short notice. The young practitioner of the present day can scarcely appreciate the importance of this fact, but whoever remembers the comparative helplessness in which, in past years, he has found himself in the face of a sudden outbreak of small-pox, not knowing which [p. 476]way to turn for an adequate supply of vaccine, will at once concede its force.

On the whole, then, it must be said that bovine virus is entitled to the preference as a rule, but that possibly it is well to resort to humanized lymph of early removes under the special circumstances above referred to. On no account should long-humanized vaccine be used so long as our present stocks of animal virus maintain the excellence they have thus far preserved, nor should humanized virus of any sort be preferred in the general run of cases.

Passing now to a consideration of the various forms of vaccine, disregarding its source, there are practically these three: the crust, liquid lymph preserved in capillary tubes, and dried lymph.

Until recently the crust, or scab, was much used in this country. Its capability of being preserved unimpaired for a long time was a valid excuse for this, especially in regions remote from the great channels of communication, and it was in such districts that the use of the crust was chiefly practised. That excuse scarcely exists now, for there are few physicians who cannot obtain a better form of vaccine within a very short time. The objections to the crust are two: 1. Most crusts are inert. Especially is this true of bovine crusts, which are wellnigh worthless. It must be confessed, however, that when once a crust has proved itself active it may be trusted to retain its infective property for a very long time. The writer has made successful use of crusts seven years old that had made the voyage to Japan and back; and they were bovine crusts too. Still, the rule is, that crusts are untrustworthy. 2. Their use is apt to be followed by undue inflammation, probably of septic origin, for they almost invariably contain putrescent or readily putrescible elements. It has even happened to the writer to cut open a crust that to all appearance was typical and innocent, and to find in its interior a cavity occupied by a pulpy, stinking slough. Manifestly, such material is unfit to be introduced into the system of any human being.

In regard to liquid lymph in tubes, it is not much used in this country, and its employment elsewhere is on the decline. At first thought, it would seem to be the best form of all, but experience does not bear out this view. In this form humanized lymph is vastly superior to animal lymph, but with every possible care in charging and sealing the tubes it is not uncommon to find their contents putrid. There are low vegetable organisms that are supposed to prey on the vaccinad. If there is any truth in this supposition, those organisms are certainly favored in their destructive luxuriance by keeping the lymph liquid, thus furnishing them with the best possible culture-fluid. Be this as it may, the fact is well ascertained that tube-lymph does not keep well. It has been mentioned already that bovine lymph stored in tubes is decidedly inferior to the same form of humanized lymph. This was long ago recognized by propagators of animal vaccine, but the cause remained a mystery until Warlomont of Brussels suggested that it was due to one of the physical peculiarities of animal lymph—that, namely, as already hinted at, by virtue of which its formed elements tend to attach themselves to any surface presented to them, leaving the supernatant liquid a mere inert compound of water, albumen, and salts; so that in the case of tube-lymph the virulent elements remain attached to the glass, and only the inert constituents [p. 477]are really used. This theory is exceedingly ingenious and plausible, but the writer is not aware that it has been proved. He does know, however, that in some South American countries, where calf lymph in tubes is used with success, the custom is to grind the tubes to powder, and inoculate with the resulting magma, glass and all. This practice is certainly not to be commended.

Dried lymph is the most efficient of all forms of vaccine, and, kept as it ought to be, it retains its infective power long enough to answer all ordinary requirements. The writer has used it three years old with success. It may commonly be counted on for six weeks. One fact should be borne in mind, however: the longer dried lymph has been kept the more care is necessary in its use, for by long keeping it becomes very hard, so that it is a work of patience to dissolve it off from the surface on which it was deposited. Failure to accomplish its solution is the most common cause of a lack of success in its employment.

The various forms of stored vaccine are esteemed by the writer in the following order: 1, dried bovine lymph; 2, dried humanized lymph; 3, humanized tube-lymph; 4, humanized crusts; 5, bovine tube-lymph; 6, bovine crusts.

The age and other circumstances under which it is best to vaccinate children constitute a point for practical consideration. It may first be mentioned that pre-natal vaccination has been advocated by some authors; that is to say, the vaccinal infection of the foetus in utero by vaccinating the mother during gestation. There seems to be respectable testimony going to show that the end may thus be accomplished, but a weighty objection arises in the fact that this mediate vaccination of the foetus produces no physical sign of its success, so that doubt must always be felt as to whether or not the procedure has been efficacious. Moreover, it is seldom indeed that a child needs protection before its birth, provided we protect the mother, for it is well known that vaccinia will overtake and destroy the variolous infection, even when the latter has had two or three days' start. The practice has been chiefly urged by Bollinger. It is not likely to come into general use.

There is no special objection to vaccinating an infant at any time after birth, but usually it is well to defer the operation until the child is about three months old, unless there is actual danger of exposure to small-pox. Yet it is not well to postpone vaccination until the period of dentition, for the combined irritation of the two disturbing elements may prove decidedly uncomfortable if not serious.

Something is to be said as to the time of the year to be chosen. In New York the bad custom prevails, especially among the poorer classes, of having children vaccinated only in April, May, or June—just the part of the year in which erysipelas is most rife. The hot months should not generally be chosen, for any source of irritation is apt to be felt more severely by infants during the summer heat. However, no circumstances should be looked upon as a positive bar to vaccination in case of actual danger of exposure to small-pox, and in large towns children should never be taken into public conveyances or carried into any promiscuous assemblage until they have been protected by vaccination.

The next question is as to the part of the body that should be selected for the inoculation. The region of the insertion of the left deltoid muscle [p. 478]is usually chosen—the left rather than the right, because most nurses habitually carry an infant on their own left arm, so that the child's left arm is uppermost, and hence less exposed to injury. The region of the deltoid insertion is comparatively free from the irritation of muscular contraction, and it is easily accessible. If two insertions are made, it is well to make one of them over the deltoid insertion and the other at a point about an inch distant on the line of the posterior border of the same muscle, for there the lymphatic connection with the axillary glands is less free, so that adenitis is not so much to be feared. To avoid a scar in a locality that may be exposed to view on certain occasions some mothers prefer that their daughters should be vaccinated on the lower limb. To this there is no special objection, further than that the lower limb is rather more exposed to rough handling than the arm. If the leg is chosen, the point of junction of the two heads of the gastrocnemius is an eligible situation.

The actual operation is performed in various ways. The old inoculators generally made an incision through the whole thickness of the skin, so that a pellet of subcutaneous fat rolled up into the little wound. This is wholly unnecessary; furthermore, it is objectionable, for it decidedly increases the risk of inflammatory complications. Still more to be avoided are the methods of inserting a seton imbued with the virus and by hypodermic injection or other like procedures. The best way is, simply to remove the horny layer of the cuticle, so as to expose the succulent portion of the epidermis. This surface is somewhat red, and from it a slight exudation of lymph will be observed, but there need not be the least flow of blood. By this procedure it is not uncommon to vaccinate a sleeping child without waking it. It is not only admissible, but preferable, not to wound the derma at all. Such an abrasion is easily made with an ordinary lancet, which, contrary to the advice sometimes given, should be very sharp; but no cutting or scratching should be done with it, only scraping with the convex part of its edge, precisely as in using an ink-eraser. Scratching instruments (such as the rake-like vaccinator often used or a row of needles set in a handle) are not easy to adapt to varying degrees of plumpness of the arm, and are apt to make too deep scratches, one at either side, while the skin between the two is scarcely touched. Whatever instrument is chosen, it should not be used again until it has been thoroughly cleansed—made chemically clean—which can be accomplished only by heating it or by wiping it off and then dipping it into a strong disinfectant solution.

Some individuals are refractory to vaccination, but complete insusceptibility is exceedingly rare. Various expedients have been resorted to in rebellious cases, such as vesication with ammonia-water, maceration of the skin for some hours with glycerine, and the like. The writer has known these devices to succeed, but he has not seen the slightest advantage in the plan recommended by Ceely, that of using a wound some hours old rather than one just made, although he has tried the experiment many times. It is not necessary to make a large abrasion; one as large as the little finger-nail is ample.

The next step is to apply the virus, and it should be so applied as to bring it into contact with every part of the denuded surface. In what is known as arm-to-arm vaccination, or its equivalent, calf-to-arm [p. 479]vaccination (by all means the most successful method, although not often practicable in this country), the liquid lymph, fresh from the vaccinifer's pock, is simply applied, when it will at once become diffused over the abraded surface without any special pains being taken to accomplish that end.

If dried lymph is used, particular care should be taken to see that it is actually dissolved and transferred from the substance on which it was dried to the abraded surface. Failure to accomplish this is the cause of almost all the lack of success that inexperienced vaccinators meet with. The lymph should be moistened with water, or, if it is quite old, with glycerine, before the abrasion is made, so that it may have time to dissolve. It should then be rubbed upon the abraded spot vigorously, and at least for the space of a full minute.

In the use of tube-lymph no other precautions are necessary than in arm-to-arm vaccination, but, simple as this method is, its results are unsatisfactory.

Crusts should be reduced to a powder, and then made into a thin paste with water or glycerine. A convenient way of powdering a crust is to rub it on a file or between two files. The paste is to be well rubbed upon the abrasion. The insertion of a solid piece of crust into a valvular incision is not to be recommended.

When the operation is finished it is well to keep the arm bare for about five minutes, but not necessarily until the spot has become dry. It is not well to apply any sort of plaster, but means should be taken to prevent the underclothing from sticking to the abrasion. For this purpose there is no objection to the shields that are furnished by the surgical instrument-makers. Usually, however, nothing of the sort is necessary.

THE STORAGE AND PRESERVATION OF VACCINE VIRUS.—Lymph should usually be taken on the eighth day, inclusive—never after the areola has formed. On the other hand, the writer's experience does not lead him to coincide with those who state that the earliest lymph that can be obtained is the most energetic. If it is to be dry-stored, the substance to be coated with it (slips of quill, ivory, wood, whalebone, glass, and the like) should be laid gently in the pool of lymph that exudes on puncturing the pock, and allowed to dry, preferably without the aid of artificial warmth. The layer of lymph should be plainly visible after it has dried. A second coating is advisable, as it serves to preserve the first.

Capillary glass tubes are either cylindrical or furnished with a bulbous expansion at the middle, the latter form being most commonly used. To charge a tube make sure that both ends are open, and then submerge one end in the pool of lymph. Capillary attraction will cause the tube to fill, and the process may be facilitated materially by inclining the tube toward a horizontal direction, so that the capillary attraction is not opposed by that of gravitation. Care should be taken to keep the applied end of the tube constantly submerged, or bubbles of air will enter it. The sealing may be done with a blowpipe, by simply holding the ends in a flame, or by means of sealing-wax or some similar substance. The satisfactory charging of tubes demands some practice, but a little patience will enable any intelligent person to succeed.

In regard to crusts, they should never be removed until the surface beneath has become cicatrized and they have been partially detached by the natural process. A crust torn off prematurely should never be used,[p. 480]and the same may be said of secondary crusts—*i.e.* those that form by the desiccation of the discharge from the raw surface left when the primary crust has been removed forcibly.

For the preservation of vaccine in these various forms tubes need only be kept in a cool place. Dried lymph and crusts should be guarded against dampness even more than against warmth. Their preservation may be decidedly favored by over-drying, either in an exhausted receiver or by keeping them in a closed vessel in the presence of sulphuric acid, chloride of calcium, or some other substance having a strong affinity for water. It is needless to say, however, that they should not come into actual contact with any such agent. While this artificial desiccation tends powerfully to preserve dried lymph, it makes it more difficult to use. When dried lymph or a crust is to be sent by mail or other conveyance, it should be wrapped in some impermeably envelope, for which purpose gutta-percha tissue is very convenient. Both these forms of virus should be kept in a cool place. There is no objection to keeping them on ice, provided they are well protected against moisture.

In conclusion, the writer wishes to say that the limited space at his command has compelled the assumption of a dogmatic rather than an inductive form in the construction of this article. To the reader who may wish to pursue the subject further—and it will well repay thorough study—he would recommend the following bibliography:

Ballard: *On Vaccination: its Value and Alleged Dangers*, London, 1868.
Bousquet: *Nouveau traité de la vaccine et des éruptions varioleuses*, Paris, 1848.
Bryce: *Practical Observations on the Inoculation of Cow-pox*, Edinburgh, 1809.
Ceely: *Observations on the Variolæ Vaccinæ*, Worcester, 1840.
Chauveau et al.: *Vaccine et Variole*, Paris, 1865.
Depaul: *Nouvelles recherches sur la véritable origine du virus vaccin*, Paris, 1863; *De l'origine réelle du virus vaccin*, Paris, 1864; et al.: *De la syphilis vaccinale*, Paris, 1865.
Hardaway: *Essentials of Vaccination*, Chicago, 1882.
Hering: *Ueber Kuhpocken an Kühen*, Stuttgart, 1839.
Jenner: *An Inquiry, etc.*, 2d ed., London, 1800.
Sacco: *Trattato di Vaccinazione*, Milano, 1809.
Seaton: *A Handbook of Vaccination*, London, 1868.
Steinbrenner: *Traité sur la vaccine*, Paris, 1846.

[p. 481]

VARICELLA.
BY JAMES NEVINS HYDE, M.D.

Varicella is an acute disorder of infancy and childhood, in the course of which appears a cutaneous exanthem of vesicular type, accompanied at times by systemic symptoms of moderate severity, terminating in the course of from three days to a fortnight, after the formation of relatively few crusts upon the skin, with occasionally persistent cicatrices.

SYNONYMS.—*Eng.*, Chicken-pox; *Ger.*, Windblattern, Schafpocken; *Fr.*, Varicelle; *Lat.*, Variola notha, seu spuria; *Ital.*, Morviglione.

HISTORY.—The literature of the disease which is now best recognized under the title of varicella has been, in the history of medicine, wellnigh inextricably confused with that of variola. In the latter part of the seventeenth and the early part of the eighteenth century the distinction between typical forms of the two disorders became apparent, and was described by Willan and Harvey in England, and other writers in Germany, France, Holland,

and Belgium. Among those who have contributed to its literature may be named Hebra, Kaposi, Trousseau, Simon, Thomas, Güntz, Henoch, Kassowitz, and Boeck.

ETIOLOGY.—Varicella is essentially a disease of early life, occurring almost exclusively in infants and young children. It is a contagious disorder, and at times, especially in hospitals and asylums for children, occurs in apparently epidemic forms. The question relating to the inoculability of the contents of its vesicular lesions is still open, positive and negative results being recorded by different experiments.[1]

[1] The writer has purposely avoided, in the brief space here devoted to the disease under consideration, entering into a discussion of the question respecting the relation sustained by varicella to variola. On one side are the views entertained by the Vienna school of dermatologists, according to which there is but a single virus in these several forms of disease—the variolous poison. On the other are the opinions and the practice, largely based upon the latter, of most English and American physicians, who deny the existence of any relation between the pathological states recognized by them as occurring in two entirely distinct affections.

My personal view may be briefly formulated as follows: Practically and clinically, it is useful to regard these disorders as of a distinct nature. The arguments, however, in favor of such absolute distinction are not irrefutable. There is probably in both forms of disease but a single virus, that of variola; but this, modified by evolution among generations of vaccinated children, has, in this process of natural cultivation or attenuation, produced a malady of tender years whose attacks do not protect from variola and occur irrespective of vaccination.

SYMPTOMATOLOGY.—The period of incubation of the disease cannot be said to be definitely established. At times, without question, an entire fortnight elapses between the dates of exposure and the evolution of the disease, but both longer and shorter intervals have been recorded.

[p. 482]If there be a prodromal stage of the disease, certainly in the vast majority of the little patients it cannot be recognized. During the last month the writer has observed the evolution of the disease in twenty children gathered together in the Chicago Home for the Friendless, no one of whom was recognized as ailing before the eruption appeared. Occasionally the disease is preceded by mild or even severe febrile symptoms, accidents sufficiently common in this class of patients.

The exanthem, commonly the first symptom of the disorder, occurs in the form of reddish puncta, from which rapidly develop rosy-colored maculations, and these become tensely distended, transparent or slightly yellowish vesicles, of the average size of a split pea, though they are occasionally smaller or may enlarge to the dimensions of a bean or small nut. The eruption appears first upon the upper segment of the body, implicating the chest in front and behind, the neck, the scalp, particularly the extremities, and quite sparingly the face also, which may, however, entirely escape. In cases where the eruption is profuse it may be completely generalized, involving largely the trunk and extremities, the lesions, upon the back particularly, being as closely set together as in discrete variola. In many, even the majority, of cases the exanthem is much less profusely developed, not more than a dozen or twenty vesicles springing from the surface.

The vesicles are superficial in situation, the firm papule which precedes the variolous rash being altogether wanting. They are at first transparent, their contents plainly showing through their translucent roof-wall, composed only of the stratum corneum of the epidermis. They are both acuminate and globular, and occasionally rest upon a slightly hyperæmic integument. Umbilication rapidly occurs at the apex, and simultaneously their contents become lactescent and gradually sero-purulent. Occasionally vesicles are transformed into genuine, coffee-bean-sized, pustules. Intermingled with these are often seen illy-developed and abortive vesicles.

By the end of a period lasting from twelve hours to the second or third day involution has usually begun, and the lesions, with and without rupture—more often the latter—desiccate, and are thus transformed into yellowish or yellowish and brown, circular, circumscribed crusts resting upon an apparently unaltered integument. These crusts are often so firmly attached that they do not fall spontaneously before the lapse of from five to eight days. When this exfoliation is ended there are left slightly hyperæmic pigmented patches of corresponding size where the crusts had rested. A destructive process occasionally results upon the surface of the face at the base of such vesiculo-pustular lesions as have formed there, in consequence of which a small depressed and superficial cicatrix is left, which does not differ from that resulting from discrete variola. These scars may be superficially seated and transitory in character, or much deeper and persistent through life.

Throughout the course of the disease systemic symptoms may be altogether wanting, or may occur in a mild, and much more rarely in a severe, type. In some cases the temperature is increased by one or two degrees upon the appearance of the exanthem, and often a febrile movement of moderate grade may persist for forty-eight hours or somewhat longer. Defervescence, however, is always rapid and perfect. In very [p. 483]rare cases there is a subsequent successive new development of scanty vesicles, whose appearance is heralded by mild exacerbations of fever.

Occasionally the vesicles may be recognized upon the mucous surfaces of the lips, inside of the cheeks, tongue, palate, conjunctivæ, and progenital regions of both sexes. Still more rarely the glands of the throat become slightly tumid and painful.

The complexus of symptoms, in the large majority of all these little patients, is that which pertains to a disorder of distinctly mild type. The eruptive lesions are scanty and productive of but trifling subjective sensations. Occasionally they are picked or scratched, and thus become the seat of either pain or pruritus. In the febrile stage the child is noticeably fretful for a period of perhaps twenty-four hours. At the end of that time older children are frequently observed engaged in their customary amusements in the nursery.

Severe types and complications of varicella are in general limited to the little patients who are recognized as suffering from hospitalism. Among these we see erysipelas, severe vaccinal eruptions, lesions of inherited syphilis, and the sequelæ of morbilli and scarlatina, which the disease both precedes and follows.

PATHOLOGY.—The anatomical structure of the lesions in varicella is largely a matter of inference, since there has been but small opportunity of studying the disorder as displayed in sections of the morbid integument. Manifestly, the exanthem is exudative in type, the serum in circumscribed areas lifting the superficial layer of the epidermis from the deeper parts of the derm. Unquestionably, septa occur in typically developed varicella chambers, similar to those seen in variola—a pathological fact which is the corner-stone of the doctrine relating to the unity of the two disorders. The serum contained in these septa possesses an alkaline reaction. The formation of a cicatrix is evidently due to the intensity of the process in certain exceptional lesions, as a result of which the papillæ of the corium are superficially destroyed. These sequelæ are often due to the picking and scratching of the lesions.

DIAGNOSIS.—Varicella is to be distinguished from eczema pustulosum by its mild febrile symptoms, the discreteness of its pustular lesions, the absence of itching, and of infiltration of the skin in patches, and its tendency to symmetrical development.

From impetigo and the impetigo contagiosa of Fox of London it will often be scarcely differentiated. Inasmuch as these disorders are frequently recognized among children suffering from varicella or varicella convalescence, it can scarcely be doubted that these diseases have been in the past often confounded, and that in many cases it is practically impossible to distinguish between them. Decided elevation of bodily temperature, umbilication of symmetrically-disposed lesions, and a rapid involution of the disease point to varicella. The two forms of impetigo occur without fever, are usually scantily developed, and are much more apt to be pustular in type, lacking, moreover, the halo of the varicella lesions. The latter are also, on an average, smaller and more numerous. The two forms of impetigo, finally, never display the generalized eruption of severe varicella. The non-contagious variety of impetigo is much more decidedly pustular in its lesions, and the latter spring from a deeper plane of the epidermis.

[p. 484]As to the eruptions due to vaccinia and vaccination, there can be but little doubt that these also have been frequently confounded with varicella. Efflorescences having origin in this way are very largely impetiginous in type, and the conditions named above are then to be regarded as distinctive differences, so far as any distinction can, under these circumstances, be recognized. Impetigo, impetigo contagiosa, and varicella are all sufficiently common accidents after vaccination. No reliance can be placed upon characteristics described as connected with a certain stuck-on appearance of the crust regarded by Fox as characteristic of the crusts in impetigo contagiosa. In all these vesiculo-pustular disorders of childhood desiccating serum and sero-pus upon the surface result in the formation of crusts which have a similar (so-called) stuck-on appearance.

Variola and varioloid of infants and children are to be distinguished from varicella by the evidence of origin from such contagious maladies; by the occurrence of prodromal symptoms; by the greater rise in temperature during the febrile stage; by the typically papular stage of the exanthem at its outset, and no less typically pustular stage before the occurrence of desiccation; by the confluence of lesions in confluent cases; and by the much longer and evidently graver stadium of the disease. Distinctions between mild varioloid and severe varicella in infancy and childhood will always tax to the utmost the skill of the diagnostician. The sooner it is generally understood that intermediate forms occur which cannot be positively assigned to the one or to the other category, the better it will be for both the profession and the laity. The fact that in the one case there is generation of a variolous poison capable of producing a contagious disease in adults, and in the other a malady which is known to affect children only, renders the decision important. Scattered papulo-vesicular and vesiculo-pustular lesions appearing after a high fever, and pursuing a period of evolution longer than forty-eight hours, should always awaken suspicion. Superficial lesions, on the contrary, distinctly vesicular on the third day, or commingled with minute, very superficial pustules, should be regarded as characteristic of varicella.

The so-called varicella prurigo of Hutchison of London[2] includes several of the disorders considered above under the titles impetigo, impetigo contagiosa, and the vaccine rashes. The irritable condition of the skin resulting from several of the exanthemata leaves it prone to the development of a long list of cutaneous lesions, some of them accompanied by pruritus in various grades, to each of which might be given, according to the caprice of authors, a separate name.

[2] *Lect. on Clin. Surg.*, Lond., 1878, p. 15 *et seq.*

PROGNOSIS.—The prognosis of varicella, per se, is always favorable. Only in the hospital cases, complicated by erysipelas and scarlatina convalescence, may grave results be anticipated. The milder attacks may leave persistent relics of their career in the form of one or more depressed and persistent cicatrices, which become less conspicuous as the patient approaches adult years.

TREATMENT.—Varicella is, in a large proportion of cases, successfully treated by domestic management and the simpler remedies familiar to those in charge of the nursery. Confinement for a brief time to the [p. 485]cradle or bed, and a proper regulation of the temperature of the room and of the diet, are usually all that is required. Special remedies may be indicated in isolated cases, but certainly none such are demanded by the varicella. Efforts should be made to protect the face lesions from the traumatism of picking and scratching, with a view to prevent pitting.

Isolation of patients is not requisite, nor any process of disinfection other than that which is incidental to a fresh supply of pure air. Vaccination should be practised alike in the case of children who have and who have not suffered from the disease.

[p. 486]

SCARLET FEVER.
BY J. LEWIS SMITH, M.D.

HISTORY.—The terms scarlet fever and scarlatina are used synonymously to designate one of the most common and fatal of the eruptive fevers. Whether this malady occurred prior to the Christian era is uncertain. It is believed by some that the plague of Athens, 430 years before Christ, vividly described by Lucretius, and by Thucydides, who was attacked by it, was scarlet fever of a peculiarly malignant type (Richardson); but, as will be seen from the following extracts from Thucydides, the plague differed in important particulars from scarlatina of the present time: "Internally, the throat and the tongue were quickly suffused with blood, and the breath became unnatural and fetid. There followed sneezing and hoarseness; in a short time the disorder, accompanied by a violent cough, reached the chest.... The body externally was not so very hot to the touch, nor yet pale: it was of a livid color, inclining to red, and breaking out in pustules and ulcers." Loss of sight and gangrene of the extremities were common results in those who recovered, and adults appear to have been affected as frequently as children. "The dead lay as they had died, one upon another, while others, hardly alive, wallowed in the streets and crawled about every fountain craving for water. The temples in which they lodged were full of the corpses of those who died in them." Lucretius says of this plague, "If any one for a time escaped death (as was possible, either by reason of the foul ulcers breaking or by means of a black discharge from the intestines), yet consumption and destruction awaited him at last; or, as was often the case, an excessive flux of corrupt blood, attended with violent pains in the head, issued from the obstructed nostrils, and by this outlet the whole strength and substance of the man passed away. He, moreover, who had escaped this violent flux of foul blood was not certain wholly to recover, for still the disease was ready to pass into his nerves and joints, and into the very genital organs of the body. And of those who suffered thus, some, fearing the gates of death, continued to live, though deprived by the steel of the virile part, and some, though without hands and feet, and though they lost their eyes, yet persisted to remain in life, so strong a dread of death had taken possession of them. Upon some, too, came forgetfulness of all things, so that they knew not even themselves."

Gangrene of the extremities, loss of sight, a violent cough, loss of memory, etc. are not symptoms of scarlet fever, so that in my opinion [p. 487]the plague of Athens, if correctly described by the historian, was a different malady.

Caspar Morris, in his essay on scarlet fever, states his belief that Seneca, who lived in the first century of the Christian era, described an epidemic of the malignant form of scarlatina in his portrayal of the pestilence that visited Thebes during the half-mythical age of Oedipus, six centuries before Christ. Seneca's description of the symptoms of this plague is as follows:

> Piger
> ignavos
> Alligat artus languor, et ægro
> Rubor in vultu, maculæque caput
> Sparsere leves; tum vapor ipsam
> Corporis arcem flammeus urit
> Multoque genus sanguine tendit
> Oculique regent, et sacer ignis
> Pascitur artus. Resonant aures,
> Stillatque niger naris aducæ
> Cruor; at venas rumpit hiantes.

Languor, redness of the face, light spots upon the head, distension of the cheeks with blood, distortion of the eyes, a flushed appearance of the limbs, tinnitus aurium, and a discharge of black blood from the nostrils, certainly indicated a very malignant form of disease, but to believe that it was identical with the scarlet fever of the present time requires considerable credulity. From the fact that it devastated Thebes we infer that it occurred largely among adults, differing, therefore, from the modern scarlet fever, whose victims are chiefly children. The same uncertainty hangs over epidemics during the first centuries of the Christian era.

The first clear and undoubted portrayal of scarlet fever is found in the medical literature of the sixteenth century. Sydenham and his contemporaries in the seventeenth century witnessed epidemics of it, studied its nature more thoroughly, and consequently acquired a more accurate knowledge of it than that possessed by their predecessors. It was in this century that measles and scarlet fever were differentiated. During the last two hundred years scarlatina has been the subject of monographs too numerous to mention. It has long been regarded as one of the most important maladies of childhood, on account of its frequency and the great mortality that attends it, so that numerous cases and many epidemics are every year related in the medical journals. By this vast accumulation of observations and the patient and thorough use of the microscope our knowledge of scarlet fever has become full and accurate.

As with most of the infectious maladies, scarlet fever extended to the Western World through European shipping. It was brought to North America about the year 1735. Tardily it spread to South America, where it appeared in 1829, and more recently it has been established in Australia. It entered Iceland in 1827, and Greenland in 1847.

ETIOLOGY.—The evidence is strong that scarlet fever does not originate de novo—that it does not spring from certain atmospheric or telluric conditions, but is produced by a definite specific principle, since countries have been free from it for centuries till it was imported by commerce. That it appears in certain localities without any known exposure is attributed to the fact that the poison is so subtle and transmissible that it is[p. 488]conveyed long distances in articles of merchandise, even in small packages, so that those who chance to open them or come in contact with them are infected. It is believed that reading matter transmitted through the mails has in many instances been the medium of infection.

The theory that the acute infectious maladies are caused by micro-organisms, or, as they are now designated, microbes, commonly discarded at first and believed to be chimerical, is rapidly gaining ground in the profession, and appears to be fully established as regards certain of them. These parasites, barely visible under high powers of the microscope, and ascertained to be vegetable by their behavior under certain chemical agents, exist in immense numbers in the blood, tissues, and secretions of patients suffering from the infectious maladies, especially in the graver cases of them; and the microscope shows that these organisms vary in shape and appearance so as to admit of classification.

The germ theory has now become so important that it cannot be ignored in a monograph relating to so important an infectious malady as scarlet fever. The relation of microbes to the infectious diseases has been made the subject of investigation by Pasteur, Toussaint, and others in France, and by many in Germany, with most interesting results. The belief held by many, and which seemed very plausible, was that the microbes, instead of sustaining a causative relation to the maladies in which they occur, were the result of these maladies—that they sprang into existence in consequence of the vitiated state of the blood and tissues, just as fungi appear on decaying substances or as the Oidium albicans appears in certain morbid conditions of the buccal surface and secretions. Obviously, in order to elucidate this matter and determine the relation of these parasites to the diseases in which they occur, it was necessary to experiment on animals, but, unfortunately, as a bar to successful experimentation many of the most important infectious maladies which afflict the human race, as typhus and typhoid fevers, the marsh fevers, and syphilis, do not occur in animals, or they occur in a changed and mitigated form. Others, however, can be produced in their typical character in animals, as diphtheria, and others still originate in animals and are transmitted from them to man, as anthrax or splenic fever of the herbivora and hydrophobia. Very interesting and important results have been produced by experimental researches with the microbes of certain of these diseases, which, if applicable to the common and fatal infectious maladies of an analogous nature in man, may yet result in immense benefit in mitigating the virulence of those affections which are the scourge of childhood and which sensibly diminish the increase of population. It has been found possible to cultivate the microbes contained in the blood, tissues, and secretions in certain of the infectious diseases, and after a series of cultivations, so that these organisms are far removed from the animal substance which contained them, and with which they were so intimately associated in the individual, they have been employed for inoculation—with this important result, that the primary disease was reproduced. This seems to indicate beyond question the causative relation of these parasites to the diseases in which they occur. Experiments with the result which I have stated have been made with the microbes of splenic fever, chicken cholera, murrain, and certain other maladies.

Pasteur employs as the media for cultivation—(1st) urine neutralized [p. 489]by a few drops of potash solution; (2d) a liquid prepared by boiling for twenty or thirty minutes the yeast of beer in water, neutralizing, and filtering; and (3d) chicken tea, prepared by boiling equal parts of water and the lean of muscles a quarter of an hour, filtering, and neutralizing. A small drop of infected blood is placed in the liquid of cultivation, and the microbes which it contains multiply so abundantly that the liquid becomes turbid in a short time, and they are found in all parts of it. A drop of this liquid is added to another portion of the medium, and this also soon becomes turbid from the immense development of organisms which have the same microscopic appearance and character as those in the drop of blood. The process is repeated many times, until the microbes are far removed from their original source in the blood and tissues, and a drop of the last cultivation, whether it be the fiftieth or the hundredth, is inserted under the skin of a healthy animal selected for the experiment. If it be true, as stated by the experimenters, that the original disease is thus reproduced with the microbes of at least three or four distinct maladies, this age is distinguished by one of the most important discoveries ever made in pathological studies. It remains to determine whether this great discovery is of general applicability to the infectious diseases with which man is afflicted. If so, it is not improbable that we are on the eve of finding a method by which some at least of these maladies may be prevented or mitigated, as small-pox has been since the time of Jenner. The result of experiments made by Pasteur with the microbes of that fatal malady of the herbivora, known under the various names of splenic fever, anthrax, wool-sorter's disease, and charbon, encourages this belief. Originating among the herbivorous animals, it has in many instances been contracted by individuals who have rapidly perished. Many engaged in assorting alpaca and mohair have lost their lives by it, some with all the symptoms of profound blood-poisoning, without external lesions, and others with redness and swelling at some point of infection where a sore or abrasion existed, but with speedy blood-contamination.

The microbe of this malady, the Bacillus anthracis, occurs in the form of straight filaments with little movement or only with oscillation, and producing bright-shining spores. Now comes a very interesting and important result of experimentation: Pasteur states if several days elapse between the cultivations the virulence of the parasite diminishes, so that he has been able to produce by inoculation with it a mild and never fatal form of charbon, which affords immunity in the animal from any subsequent attack. This opinion was sustained by a trial experiment on sixty sheep. Toussaint and Chauveau claim that they produce a similar attenuation of the virus by defibrinating infected blood, heating it to 55° C. (131° F.) and filtering it. These experiments awaken the hope that the time will come when the acute infectious maladies in man, scarlet fever among others, will be rendered less virulent. That one of them—to wit, small-pox—has for nearly a century been under our control certainly encourages the belief that there is some way to mitigate others of the same class which are equally fatal if not so loathsome.

As yet, observers do not agree in regard to the parasite which is supposed to sustain a causative relation to scarlet fever. Klebs states that it is highly probable that both measles and scarlet fever are produced by [p. 490]micrococci, and he has sketched the design and described the development of a microbe which he designates the Monas scarlatinosum.

The *London Medical Times and Gazette* for Jan. 28, 1882, contains an account of the supposed discovery of the scarlatinous microbe by Eklund of Stockholm, an authority in the microscopic examination of parasites. He says that scarlet fever is rarely absent from the Swedish capital and from the barracks and dwellings on the isle of Skeppsholm. In the urine of scarlatinous patients he has constantly found a prodigious number of discoid corpuscles, oval or round, their diameter being less than $1/1000$ millimetre and from $1/30$ to $1/10$ that of a red blood-cell. They are colorless or yellowish white, surrounded by a distinct cell-wall, each containing a well-defined nucleus of a deeper hue. Sometimes one or more microbi may be seen. They exhibit rotatory or oscillatory movements, especially observed when a drop of water is added to the fluid. They multiply, as he has frequently seen, by fission—first in the microbes, next in the nucleus, and lastly in the cell-wall. He cannot say whether they develop into a mycelium. At any rate, the development of fine filaments seems to be exceptional. He has never seen them adhere in moniliform chains nor massed as zooglæa. He considers them to be veritable schizomycetes, and proposes the name Plox scindens.

Eklund asserts that he has found these same organisms in vast numbers in the soil- and ground-water of the isle of Skeppsholm, in the mud of the trenches dug for the water-mains, and in the greenish mould upon the walls of the old barracks, where scarlet fever was most rife. He states that scarlet fever has occurred in children after drinking milk mixed with the ground-water of the island, and he observed a case which followed immersion in one of the trenches of the island and the drying of the clothes in a small room. In another instance scarlet fever broke out in a block immediately after exposure of the ground-water by excavations.

It is evident that the discovery of this microbe under such circumstances does not prove that it is the cause of the disease. This can only be determined by inoculation, or by experiments which furnish the conditions of scientific exactness. Although great progress has been made in parasitology during the last decade, it is evident that several years of observation and experimentation must elapse before it is clearly and definitely ascertained whether or to what extent microbes cause scarlet fever and the other exanthematic fevers with which it is classified.

Whether the specific principle of scarlet fever be a micro-organism or a chemical substance, its mode of action and effects have been ascertained by clinical observations. Without doubt it commonly enters the system by the breath, but it may enter in the ingesta, and it infects the blood. That it resides in the blood has been ascertained by inoculation with this liquid, by which scarlet fever has been reproduced in its typical form. From the blood it enters the tissues and secretions. Hence handkerchiefs or linen containing the saliva or mucus of a patient, the epidermic scales shed abundantly in the desquamative period, and probably also the urinary and fecal evacuations, contain the poison, so as to be highly infectious. Even the discharge of a scarlatinous otorrhoea is thought by some to be contagious for a considerable time.

Scarlatina is communicable not only by direct exposure to a patient, [p. 491]but also by exposure to objects which happen to be in his room during his illness, and to which the poison becomes attached, such as clothing, books, and toys; small packages, even letters, it is believed, from cases which have occurred, sometimes convey and disseminate the contagious principle.

In England observations have been made which show that scarlatina has been communicated by infected milk. The disease occurred in the family of a milkman, and the milk, before it was distributed, remained for a time in a kitchen which had been occupied by the patients. This milk was taken by twelve families, and in six of these the disease occurred almost simultaneously at a time when few cases were occurring in the locality. There had been no direct exposure to the carrier of the milk nor to members of the affected family (Taylor). In another instance a woman and her son had scarlet fever while they were serving milk to several families, and the disease appeared in all these families except one, which consisted of old people (Bell). It is known that milk absorbs volatile substances so as to be flavored by them, as is shown in the experiment of placing it in an open vessel in a box with a pineapple; and it may in a similar manner become infected by the specific principle of scarlet fever, or it may be infected by detached particles of epidermis; which is not improbable when one convalescing from scarlet fever is allowed to milk the cows or prepare the milk for distribution.

The scarlatinous virus surpasses that of any other eruptive fever except small-pox in its tenacious attachment to objects and its portability to distant localities. Hence in the literature of the disease are the records of many cases in which the poison was conveyed long distances, retaining its virulence to the full extent and causing an outbreak of the malady in the localities to which it was carried. In New York, so frequently has scarlet fever as well as measles and diphtheria been contracted from the persons or clothing of well children who come from infected houses, that the Health Board now excludes from the public schools all children who come from such houses, even though they live on separate floors from those occupied by the sick. In one instance that came under my notice a washerwoman whose child had scarlet fever communicated the disease to an infant in the household where she was employed, by placing her shawl over the cradle in which it was lying. A physician of my acquaintance went from a scarlet-fever patient to a family several streets distant, and took one of their children upon his lap. After the usual incubative period this child sickened with a fatal form of the malady, and the remaining children of the household were in time affected. In New York scarlet fever has seemed to me to be not infrequently communicated through school-books, which, profusely illustrated by pictures and rendered attractive to the young, are often allowed to lie upon the bed of a scarlatinous patient and be handled by him during convalescence, or even during the course of the fever if it be mild. The young librarian of the circulating library of a Sunday-school, whose pupils came largely from the tenement-houses, was occupied a considerable part of a day in covering and arranging the books. After about the usual incubative period of scarlet fever he sickened with the disease. His two sisters were immediately removed to a rural township three hundred miles away, and to an isolated house where scarlatina had never occurred. About one[p. 492]month after his recovery, and after his room had been disinfected by burning sulphur and his bed-clothes and linen had been thoroughly washed, and all articles suspected to hold the poison had been either disinfected or destroyed, the brother visited his sisters in the country. Three weeks subsequently to his arrival one of these sisters sickened with scarlet fever, and a week later the other also. It seems that the exposure must have occurred several days after his arrival in the country from some book or other infected article in his possession. About two months elapsed after the last case; the family had returned to the city, the infected room in the country-house had been thoroughly fumigated by burning sulphur from morning till evening, when a little girl from an inland city remained a few days in this house, and probably often entered the room where the young ladies had been sick. In a few days she also sickened with a fatal form of scarlatina. Such histories and experiences are not infrequent. They are common during epidemics of scarlet fever. They indicate an extraordinary attachment of the scarlatinous poison to objects, and show that it is not gaseous nor readily volatilized.

A striking example of this fixity of the poison occurred in the practice of the late Kearney Rogers, formerly a prominent and much esteemed surgeon of New York City. Six children in a family had scarlet fever. Three and a half months subsequently another child, living at a distance, was allowed to return home and occupy the apartment in which the sickness had occurred. One week subsequently to the date of the return this child sickened with the same malady. Elliotson states that a patient with scarlet fever was admitted into one of the wards of St. Thomas's Hospital, and for two years subsequently young persons who were admitted into the ward were apt to take the disease. Richardson of London relates the following experiences of a family whom he attended in a rural district: "At a short distance from one of our villages there was situated on a slight eminence a small clump of laborers' cottages, with the thatch peering down on the beds of the sleepers. A man and his wife lived in one of these cottages with four lovely children. The poison of scarlet fever entered the poor man's door, and at once struck down one of the flock." The remaining children were now removed some miles away, and after several weeks one of them was allowed to return. Within twenty-four hours it also took the disease, and quickly died. The walls of the cottage were now thoroughly cleaned and whitewashed, the floors scoured, and all the wearing apparel either destroyed or washed. Four months elapsed after the last sickness when one of the remaining children returned. "He reached his father's cottage early in the morning; he seemed dull the next day, and at midnight I was sent for, to find him also the subject of scarlet fever. The disease again assumed the malignant type, and this child died." Richardson believes that the contagium was attached to the thatch, which could not be thoroughly disinfected. The fact of this remarkable long-continued attachment of the poison to objects, indicating by this fixity that it is a solid, is consonant with the theory that it is an organism.

INCUBATIVE PERIOD.—The duration of the incubative period varies in different cases. It is sometimes less than twenty-four hours, as in [p. 493]the above case reported by Richardson; in the following well-known case, observed by Trousseau, it was one day. A girl arrived in Paris from Pau, where there was no scarlet fever, and occupied the same apartment with her sister, who was sick with this disease. Twenty-four hours after her arrival she also was attacked with the same malady.

Russeberger attended a child who was exposed at noon to scarlet fever, and took the disease on the following night. B. W. Richardson (*Clinical Essays*, 1861, vol. i. p. 94) gives his own experience: He had applied his ear to the chest of a patient suffering from scarlet fever, and was conscious of a peculiar odor emitted from the patient. He was immediately nauseated and chilly, and from that moment he dated the beginning of an attack of scarlet fever. In the *Transactions* of the Clinical Society of London, vol. xi. 1878, the late Charles Murchison gives the statistics of 75 cases, showing the incubative period, as follows:

In 4 cases it was not more than 24 hours.
In 2 cases it was not more than 30 hours.
In 3 cases it was not more than 36 hours.
In 4 cases it was not more than 40 hours.
In 1 case it was not more than 41 hours.
In 4 cases it was not more than 58 hours.
In 1 case it was not more than 54 hours.
In 1 case it was not more than 2½ days.
In 31 cases it was within (time not accurately ascertained) 4 days.
In 2 cases the incubation did not exceed 4½ days.
In 17 cases the incubation did not exceed 5 days.
In 2 cases the incubation did not exceed 6 days.

In three cases Murchison believes that the incubation was precisely fixed at thirty-six hours, three days, and four and a half days.

Watson says that a man reached Devonshire on mid-day to see his daughter, who had scarlet fever. Two days later he was also attacked. Rehn saw a child who was attacked two days after its grandmother returned from a case of scarlet fever; and Zengerle, a girl of ten years, residing at Wangen, where there was no scarlet fever, who took the disease two days after her mother had returned from visiting a family affected with it. Loochner states that a boy aged four and a half years was attacked one and a half days after admission into the infected wards of a hospital. Armistead, in his annual report on the health of the Newmarket rural district, states that three children, coming from a different part of the district, visited Westley, and stayed next door to a child who had scarlet fever six weeks previously, and who was allowed to play with these children on the evening of Aug. 13th and morning of the 14th. The family then returned home, and on the 18th, four days after the exposure, all three children sickened with scarlet fever (*Brit. Med. Jour.*, Sept. 30, 1882).

Ordinarily, therefore, the incubative period, though varying in different cases, is within six days. Many cases, however, occur in which it seems to be longer. Thus in my practice scarlet fever appeared in a family on April 26, 1882. The patient was immediately removed to the third floor and the other children to the basement. All communication between the infected room and the basement was forbidden, but on May 8th, twelve days after the separation, one of these children sickened with the disease. [p. 494]Many observers—among whom may be mentioned Niemeyer and Copland—believe that the incubative period may be longer than one week, but, on account of the subtlety of the poison and the many modes of transmission, it is possible that in the instances of an apparently long incubative period there were other and unsuspected exposures. When scarlet fever has been communicated by inoculation, as in the experiments of Rostan and others, the incubative period has been about seven days, but Gerhardt states that a man was attacked four days after an abscess was opened by a knife used upon a scarlatinous patient. This variation in the incubative period, which also occurs in some other infectious diseases, as diphtheria, is probably due mostly to individual differences, some being more susceptible than others; but it may be due partly to those obscure meteorological conditions which we designate the epidemic influence. Probably, as a rule, when the disease is quickly developed after exposure, the attack is more severe than when several days elapse.

CONTAGIOUSNESS.—The area of the contagiousness of scarlet fever is small. It apparently embraces only a few feet. Therefore, close proximity is the necessary condition of its propagation. Hence many who are exposed, particularly of those who are remotely exposed, do not contract the disease. There is also an idiosyncrasy in some children, so that they resist infection even when repeatedly and closely exposed. In the *New York Medical Record* for March 23, 1878, C. E. Billington states that of 90 children in 26 families who were exposed to scarlet fever, 43 contracted the disease and 47 escaped; whereas, as is well known, comparatively few unprotected children escape pertussis, variola, varicella, or measles if exposed to either of these diseases. By strict isolation, therefore, the spread of scarlet fever is more easily prevented than that of most other acute infectious maladies. In the New York Foundling Asylum for a number of years children with scarlet fever were isolated in a small room attached to one of the wards. The door between the two rooms was closed, and not opened during the continuance of the sickness. Entrance into the small room was through another door, and a nurse was assigned to the scarlet-fever cases, with strict directions that she should not mingle with the other children. These simple precautions were found sufficient in the various epidemics of scarlet fever which occurred in the city to prevent the spread of the malady through this institution; whereas, similar measures were much less effectual in arresting the spread of measles and pertussis. Consequently, an outbreak of scarlet fever in this institution was usually limited to a few cases, while the extension of measles and pertussis was arrested with difficulty till a more efficient quarantine was established.

VARIATIONS IN TYPE.—The type of scarlet fever varies greatly in different epidemics, and frequently also in cases which occur in the same epidemic, even in the same family. One child may have scarlatina so mildly that little treatment is required and convalescence soon begins, while another has the malignant form, and soon succumbs, notwithstanding the prompt employment of the most efficient and appropriate measures. Ordinarily, however, if the first case in a family be very severe, subsequent cases will present a similar type; but there are notable exceptions. This variation in type in different years and different epidemics is probably not equalled in any other infectious malady. Consecutive [p. 495]epidemics may present this variation, or the same type may continue for a series of years, and then, from some unknown cause, change to one milder or more severe. In England, during Sydenham's life, scarlet fever was so mild that he regarded it as a trivial affection, requiring little attention, like rötheln of the present time, but after the death of Sydenham, Morton and his contemporaries in London found, to their sorrow, that the type of scarlet fever was very different from that described by Sydenham's pen. The late Graves of Dublin and his contemporaries treated a mild type of scarlet fever with a very small percentage of deaths—much less than that during the preceding generation—and they attributed their success to their greater knowledge and more appropriate use of remedies than their ancestors possessed and employed. By and by the type changed, the mortality of former years was restored, and they discovered that their previous success in saving life had been due not to their skill, but to the mild form of the malady. A distinguished physician of New York treated more than fifty cases of scarlet fever in one of the institutions without a single death. A few months afterward the type of the malady changed, and his own son perished from it.

SURGICAL AND OBSTETRICAL SCARLATINA.—After surgical operations, and sometimes in surgical cases not requiring operative measures, a scarlatinous efflorescence occasionally appears upon the whole or nearly the whole body, and remains for several days. The following were cases of the kind alluded to. They occurred in Guy's Hospital, and were published by H. G. Howse in *Guy's Hospital Reports* for 1879: On March 15, 1878, Jacobson performed osteotomy upon a child suffering from extreme rachitis. The operation was followed by a moderate febrile movement (100° to 101°), and after three days by the appearance of an efflorescence, with sore throat and the strawberry tongue. The osteotomy had been performed under carbolic acid spray and with all the details of antiseptic surgery. The rash soon faded, the temperature fell, and the child, temporarily separated from the other patients from the suspicion that the disease was scarlet fever, was brought back to the ward. The subsequent history confirmed the diagnosis of scarlet fever, for the skin desquamated, and on April 1st abundant albumen was found in the urine. The case terminated favorably. Three months previously the same operation had been performed on the other leg, with no unfavorable symptoms. On April 5th, three weeks after the osteotomy, a lipoma was removed from another patient aged twenty-one years. The following day the temperature rose to 101°, and remained at that till April 8th, when it suddenly increased to 103°, and a rose-rash occurred over the body, with sore throat. On April 9th, Howse excised the elbow-joint of a girl of sixteen years having pulpy disease. On the 10th her temperature began to increase, and on the 11th reached 105.8°. Toward evening a roseoloid eruption appeared over her body, and she was isolated. On April 12th, Dr. H. excised a fibroid bursa patellæ from a woman of twenty-nine years. On the following day her temperature was 99°, but on the 14th it rose to 100°, and on the evening of the 15th she had rigors and headache. On the morning of the 16th the temperature was 102.5°, and a roseoloid eruption occurred over the face and chest. The surgeons now perceived that an epidemic of the so-called surgical scarlatina was occurring, so as to justify the postponement of other operations.

[p. 496]In the same volume of *Guy's Hospital Reports*, James F. Goodhart gives the histories of nearly thirty cases of this disease occurring during a series of years in the same hospital. The patients were chiefly children, having the most diverse surgical ailments, among which may be mentioned hip disease and abscess, genu valgum without operation, necrosis of femur, hydrocele with explorative operation, a scald, a sinus over the great trochanter, spinal disease with abscess, tenotomy for club-foot, and vesical calculus with operation. The most common disease was caries or necrosis with abscess. In cases operated on the intervals between the operations and the occurrence of the efflorescence varied from two days to more than two weeks. Goodhart, after a careful examination of these cases, came to the conclusion that they were for the most part examples of true scarlet fever, especially as a considerable proportion of them occurred in groups, and there was a known exposure of some of the patients to children admitted into the hospital with the sequelæ of scarlet fever.

In the *British Med. Jour.* for Jan., 1879, George May, Jr., reported a case of efflorescence in surgical practice which appears to have been scarlatinous. A child was operated on for the radical cure of hernia on Dec. 4th. Toward the close of the same day he became restless, vomited, and his pulse on the following day rose to 136. Forty-eight hours after the operation a rash appeared on the chest and arms, the abdomen became tense and painful, and on the following day he died. The poison, however, in this case may have been septic.

Hillier remarks (*Diseases of Children*): "In the hospital for sick children, of the children who contract scarlatina a very large proportion have been the subjects of a surgical operation within a week before the rash appears." Gee says (Reynolds's *System of Medicine*): "It has been doubted by some whether the scarlatiniform rash which sometimes follows operations is really scarlatinal. The eruption appears from the second to the sixth day after the operation, and in the cases which have caused the doubt is very fugitive and the first and only symptom. Yet that the disease really is scarlet fever would seem to be proved by the following observations: first, that the disease occurs in epidemics; secondly, that in a given epidemic a severe case occasionally relieves the monotonous recurrence of the very mild form; thirdly, that a precisely similar scarlatinilla attacks in the same epidemic patients who have not been subjected to operation and who have no open sore; and lastly, by way of a veritable experimentum crucis, that, however freely these patients are exposed to ordinary scarlet fever contagion afterward, they do not contract that disease." Paget and other distinguished London surgeons who have observed this complication of surgical cases, believe that the patients have been previously exposed to the scarlatinous poison, and that the surgical diseases or operations furnish favorable conditions for the occurrence of scarlet fever, so that the exposure, which probably would have been without result in ordinary health, causes an outbreak of the malady.

Those who have reported cases of this form of efflorescence have for the most part neglected to state whether the patients had had scarlet fever previously, knowledge of which would have aided in the diagnosis; but from an examination of the histories of cases, especially those [p. 497]published in the London journals in the last four or five years, there can, I think, be little doubt that surgical maladies of a certain kind, especially traumatism, do produce a state of system which predisposes to scarlet fever, so that this class of patients are especially liable to contract it. Therefore, in my opinion, a considerable proportion of reported cases of surgical scarlatina are genuine, but in a considerable number, perhaps an equal number of such cases, the histories and symptoms indicated a septic rather than scarlatinous efflorescence, and in not a few instances, when consultations have been held, opinions differed, some diagnosticating scarlet fever, others septicæmia. In some of the cases I find it stated that the fauces presented the normal appearance. Now, faucial redness is so generally present in scarlet fever, antedating that of the skin and coexisting with it, that its absence is strong evidence that the disease is not scarlatinous. Moreover, when, as was true of certain of the reported cases, the rash appeared irregularly upon the surface, and faded away in two or three days with the abatement of the fever, and the conditions for septic absorption were present, the efflorescence was probably septicæmic.

The following were apparently cases of septicæmia efflorescence: A child aged five years (*Brit. Med. Jour.*, Feb. 15, 1879) had inflammation of the lymphatic glands in the groin, which suppurated. At the time when the abscess was fully formed a rash appeared over the entire body. It consisted of numerous red points, but was paler than that of ordinary scarlet fever; temperature never above 99°; no sore throat nor desquamation of cuticle. No child exposed to her took scarlet fever, and her sickness could not be traced to infection. In the *British Med. Jour.*, Jan. 4, 1879, L. Braxton Hicks states that his son, attending school at Reading, was seized with a severe attack of pyrexia, accompanied on the second day by delirium and the occurrence of a rash like scarlet fever over the entire surface. He had no decided redness of the fauces, though it was perhaps slightly flushed. The right buttock was swollen from inflammation, and a large, deep-seated abscess formed near the tuberosity of the ischium. When the delirium abated the boy said that he was standing the day before the fever began with his legs far apart, when a schoolfellow stretched them farther by suddenly pulling on one of them. The rash, which was nearly universal, lasted three days, and was not followed by desquamation. No case of scarlet fever occurred in the school before or afterward. In the same volume of the *British Medical Journal*, Surgeon Frolliott of the East India Service relates the case of a private, aged twenty-three years, and three years in India, who, when on duty in the Punjab, was injured by the explosion of an Afghan powder-magazine. The accident occurred Dec. 21, 1878. On Dec. 25th a bright scarlet rash appeared upon the abdomen and spread over the entire body. The following day the eruption was very vivid, like a boiled lobster, and it lasted five days. The temperature, which in the beginning had been 101°, abated to the normal after the rash appeared. No soreness of throat nor redness of the buccal surface occurred, but the epidermis desquamated even from the palms of the hands and soles of the feet. Now, the febrile movement of scarlet fever does not cease while the efflorescence is distinct. It does not even diminish when the eruption appears, while in the above case it fell to the normal—a common [p. 498]occurrence in septicæmia, even when the blood-poisoning is profound. Moreover, scarlet fever is so rare in India that Frolliott, after twelve years' service, had only heard of one case among Europeans and natives. The surgeons who consulted over the case of this private disagreed in opinion, some regarding the disease as septicæmic, others as scarlatinous. But a better knowledge of the clinical history of scarlet fever on the part of these army surgeons would, I think, have removed all doubt as to the diagnosis.

It is the opinion of some reputable surgeons that the exposure of traumatic patients to the scarlatinous poison sometimes aggravates the inflammation of wounds, causing them to assume an unhealthy appearance even though no scarlatina be produced. The late Solly made the remark, "Whenever a case of surgery in private practice takes on a highly phlegmonous appearance I am always sure to find break out, in the inmates of the house, either erysipelas or scarlet fever" (*British Med. Jour.*, Feb. 15, 1879). We will see that the scarlatinous poison sometimes causes pharyngitis or nephritis without producing the general disease. In a similar manner it seems that it may aggravate open wounds, intensifying the inflammation in them, while there is no efflorescence or other symptom to show that scarlatina itself is present. The poison appears to act entirely locally in such cases.

Paget, in his *Clinical Lectures*, says: "I think it not improbable that in some cases results occurring with obscure symptoms within two or three days after operations have been due to the scarlet-fever poison, hindered in some way from its usual progress." Playfair, in his remarks on the puerperal state, adds: "Mr. Spencer Wells informs me that he has seen cases of surgical pyæmia which he had reason to believe originated in the scarlatinal poison; and his well-known success as an ovariotomist is no doubt, in a great measure, to be attributed to his extreme care in seeing that no one likely to come in contact with his patients has been exposed to any such source of infection." Opinions like these, held by such prominent members of the profession and sustained by many observations, should certainly induce physicians to prevent, so far as possible, any exposure of their surgical patients, especially if they have any sores or wounds, whether by traumatism or the scalpel, to the scarlatinal poison.

OBSTETRICAL SCARLATINA.—Women during convalescence after childbirth are very liable to contract scarlet fever. In the New York Infant Asylum, which has maternity wards, a woman was admitted from a house in which scarlet fever was prevailing, and assigned to a cot next that occupied by one of the waiting women, who was confined soon afterward. Her labor was favorable, but three days afterward she took scarlet fever, and another lying-in-patient contracted it from her. The sore throat and desquamation were characteristic. It has come to my knowledge that a physician of New York, in whose family scarlet fever was occurring, attended three women in succession in their confinement, and all contracted scarlet fever, which presented the characteristic symptoms, and two of them died. Experienced and cautious physicians of New York, aware of the danger, do not go directly from a scarlatinous patient to an obstetrical case, but avoid the risk by intermediate visits to other patients or by remaining for a time in the open air.

[p. 499]Playfair, remarking on this subject, says: "There is good reason to believe that the contagium of zymotic diseases may produce a form of disease indistinguishable from ordinary puerperal septicæmia, and presenting none of the characteristic features of the specific complaint from which the contagium was derived. This is admitted to be a fact by the majority of our most eminent British obstetricians, although it does not seem to be allowed by continental authorities, and it is strongly controverted by some writers in this country. It is certainly difficult to reconcile this with the theory of septicæmia, and we are not in a position to give a satisfactory explanation of it. I believe, however, that the evidence in favor of the possibility of puerperal septicæmia originating in this way is too strong to be assailable. The scarlatinal poison is that regarding which the greatest number of observations has been made. Numerous cases of this kind are to be found scattered through our obstetric literature, but the largest number are to be met with in a paper by Braxton Hicks. Out of 68 cases of puerperal disease seen in consultation, no less than 37 were distinctly traceable to the scarlatinal poison. Of these, 20 had the characteristic rash of the disease, but the remaining 17, although the history clearly proved exposure to the contagium of scarlet fever, showed none of its usual symptoms, and were not to be distinguished from ordinary typical cases of the so-called puerperal fever. On the theory that it is impossible for the specific contagious diseases to be modified by the puerperal state, we have to admit that one physician met with 17 cases of puerperal septicæmia in which, by a mere coincidence, the contagion of scarlet fever had been traced, and that the disease nevertheless originated from some other source—a hypothesis so improbable that its mere mention carries its own refutation."

Parturition, like traumatism, furnishes in an eminent degree the conditions in which septic poisoning occurs, and the efflorescence which often accompanies septicæmia bears, as we have seen, a very close resemblance to that of scarlet fever. Hence in many instances the same difficulty is present in making a differential diagnosis between septic and scarlatinous blood-poisoning in obstetrical cases which occurs in surgical practice. But, according to my observations, an efflorescence occurring during the week following parturition is in most instances septic. It is only in exceptional cases that it is scarlatinous, and there is little danger that the accoucheur, engaged in general practice and visiting scarlatinous patients, will communicate scarlet fever through his person or clothing if he exercise proper precautions. His short stay in the sick room and his out-door exercise in visiting cases prevent infection of his person or dress. But if, as Playfair believes, the scarlatinal poison sometimes produces in parturient women a puerperal fever in which the characteristic scarlatinal symptoms are lacking, and which, in the present state of our knowledge, is not distinguishable from ordinary septic fever, certainly the scarlatinous virus sustains a much more frequent causative relation to childbed fever than has been heretofore supposed.

Infants under the age of six months do not ordinarily contract scarlet fever, although fully exposed, and those under four months nearly possess immunity. Still, this disease has been observed in new-born infants, contracted, apparently, through the placental circulation. [p. 500]Tourtual states that a woman waited upon her own husband and child, both of whom had scarlet fever, during the eighth and ninth months of her pregnancy, till near her confinement. Though she had no symptoms of scarlet fever, her infant had unusual redness of the skin and buccal surface and difficulty of swallowing up to the fifth day. On the ninth day desquamation began, and at a later stage the nails of the fingers and toes separated. A case having a history in some respects similar is related by Megnert, but the symptoms were anomalous for scarlet fever, and the disease may have been ordinary septic fever. On the other hand, in one instance in my practice a mother had scarlet fever, beginning about the third day after her confinement, and although she suckled her infant and it was constantly in bed with her, it had no symptoms of scarlet fever, although it became affected immediately afterward by a severe form of eczema, probably from the altered quality of the milk; and in two instances observed by Murchison new-born infants remained healthy, although their mothers suffered from scarlet fever.

After the age of six months the liability to scarlet fever increases till the close of infancy, children between the ages of six months and one year being less liable to contract the malady than during the second year, and those in the second year being less liable to it than those in the third year. Murchison collected the statistics of deaths from scarlet fever in England and Wales during a series of years ending with 1861. The number of deaths aggregated 148,829, and the percentage of deaths at different ages was as follows:

Deaths under 1 year,	.7	per cent.
Deaths between 1 and 2 years,	4.09	per cent.
Deaths between 2 and 3 years,	6.00	per cent.
Deaths between 3 and 4 years,	5.13	per cent.
Deaths between 4 and 5 years,	1.9	per cent.
Deaths between 5 and 10 years,	5.9	per cent.
Deaths between 10 and 15 years,	.8	per cent.
Deaths between 15 and 25 years,	.6	per cent.
Deaths between 25 and 35 years,	.8	per cent.
Deaths over age of 35 years,	.8	per cent.

Among the deaths were ten cases above the age of eighty-five years, so that scarlet fever, though especially a disease of childhood, may occur in any decade of life; but old age, like early infancy, almost possesses immunity from it.

I have preserved the records of the ages of 145 consecutive cases occurring in private practice. If we add to these 58 cases observed by Prof. Octerlony (*Amer. Jour. of Med. Sci.*, July, 1882) we have the statistics of the ages of 203 cases, which are embraced in the following table:

Age	Cases
Under 1 year,	
From 1 to 2 years,	5
From 2 to 3 years,	3
From 3 to 5 years,	7
From 5 to 10 years,	3
From 10 to 15 years,	3
From 15 to 20 years,	
From 20 to 30 years,	
From 30 to 40 years,	2
Total,	03

[p. 501]CLINICAL FACTS REGARDING SCARLET FEVER.—As a rule, scarlet fever occurs but once, one attack conferring immunity from the disease for life; but there are exceptions. In 1869, I attended a child with fatal scarlet fever who three years previously, it was stated, had passed through a first attack with all the characteristic symptoms. The following case occurred in a family attended by the late Dr. Herzog: R———, a boy of six years, had scarlet fever in a mild form in January and February, 1875, followed by moderate desquamation. In July of the same year he was kicked by a horse in the street, receiving a deep scalp-wound which required three stitches. Three days afterward he had, to appearance, a second attack of scarlet fever, attended by high febrile movement, and followed also by desquamation. It was believed by Dr. H. to be a genuine case, and was so treated. I am not able to state as regards the presence of soreness of the throat, and doubt arises whether this second attack may not have been septicæmic. In April, 1876, a third attack occurred, which I saw from the beginning. It was accompanied by all the characteristic symptoms—injection of the fauces, an efflorescence continuing the usual time, followed by desquamation and albuminuria, the latter continuing several weeks. Richardson states that three distinct attacks occurred in his own person, and a student attending the lecture at which this was mentioned informed the doctor that he also had had scarlet fever three times.

Sometimes a second attack occurs so soon after the first that it has been described as a relapse. The following was a case in point in the practice of Godneff (*Meditz. Vestnik.*, No. iv., *N.Y. Med. Rec.*, April 30, 1881): A youth of seventeen years contracted scarlet fever while taking care of a child. It began with a chill, and he had the usual efflorescence, sore throat, and tumefaction of the cervical glands. An exudation appeared upon his tonsils and uvula, and his temperature reached 104°. The urine contained a trace of albumen, the rash in due time faded, and the epidermis exfoliated. On the fifteenth day, when he was about ready to leave the hospital, he again had a chill, followed by fever. The temperature reached 105.2°, the rash reappeared over the entire surface except the face, diphtheritic exudations occurred upon the fauces, and the urine, the quantity of which was diminished, again became albuminous. This second efflorescence faded on the twenty-fourth day, and on the twenty-seventh exfoliation began. Hillier says: "I have seen a young woman in the fever hospital suffering from a second attack of scarlatina, the first attack having occurred five weeks previously. She had quite recovered from her first illness, and was acting as nurse. In both seizures the rash, the sore throat, and other symptoms were characteristic. The relapse or recurrence was less severe than the primary disease." Cases of a fourth, or even of a greater number of attacks, have been reported. The first seizure is sometimes milder, but in other instances is more severe, than those which follow.

Exposure to the scarlatinous poison not infrequently produces pharyngitis without the occurrence of scarlatina, and the inflammation is apt to be severe, accompanied by pain in swallowing and marked febrile movement. This phlegmasia is distinguished from scarlet fever by its shorter duration and the absence of the efflorescence. It occurs in adults as well as in children, and in those who have had, as well as in those who have not [p. 502]had scarlatina. So far as I have observed, it is very seldom accompanied or followed by any of the complications or sequelæ so common in and after scarlet fever. It cannot be distinguished from ordinary pharyngitis except in the manner in which it occurs, and one attack does not preclude another. The late George B. Wood made the remark that he never attended a case of scarlet fever without suffering from sore throat. The following were examples of this form of pharyngitis: On Jan. 17th, 1882, I was called to a boy of three years with severe scarlet fever, ushered in by convulsions. On the following day his sister, aged seven and three-fourths years, whom I had attended a year previously during a severe attack of scarlatina, and who had been almost constantly with the brother, became very ill, with a temperature of 103.5°. Examination revealed severe inflammation of the fauces, without pseudo-membrane or any other exudation except muco-pus. On Jan. 19th an older brother, nine years, whom I had attended in scarlet fever three years previously, was affected in the same way, his temperature being 104° and his respiration guttural and noisy, especially during sleep, in consequence of the great amount of faucial swelling. At times he was delirious. The inflammation in both cases began to abate about the third day, and had disappeared by the close of the week. That the contagium of scarlet fever may be received into the system and cause pharyngitis, while the patient has immunity from scarlet fever through a previous attack, and that this inflammation may occur any number of times, as in the case of Dr. Wood, are remarkable facts.

Now and then cases occur which appear to show that the scarlatinous poison may affect the kidneys, producing nephritis, while there is no other manifestation of its influence. Thus in my practice a lady of about forty-five years constantly attended her son, sleeping by his side, during an attack of scarlet fever. Her health had previously been good. When the boy was convalescent, as her appetite failed and she was indisposed, a careful examination revealed the fact that she had albuminuria, although she had had no sore throat or other symptom of scarlet fever. After several weeks of treatment her disease was removed, and she has remained well since. In the *British Med. Jour.* for Nov. 29, 1879, it is stated that in a family four girls were found to be suffering from desquamative nephritis. One of them had recently had scarlet fever, but the other three had presented no symptoms whatever of this disease. Such cases, although probably rare, appear to show that, as the scarlatinous poison may produce inflammation of the fauces without the occurrence of scarlet fever, so it may cause nephritis without producing the general disease, or apparently disturbing the functions, or changing the state of other parts, except the kidneys.

SYMPTOMS.—ORDINARY FORM. Scarlet fever usually begins abruptly, so that the exact time of its commencement can be fixed. If any premonitory symptoms occur, they are slight, so as scarcely to attract attention, as languor or the appearance of fatigue. A dusky aspect of the surface may occasionally be observed during the few hours preceding the attack. In some children the first symptom is chilliness, and occasionally a distinct chill occurs. In the adult a chill is ordinarily the first symptom. With or without the initial chilliness, febrile movement occurs, of variable intensity according to the severity of the type, and [p. 503]accompanied by such symptoms as usually arise in a febrile state of system, as cephalalgia, anorexia, and thirst. The pulse rises to 110, 120, or more per minute, the temperature to 102°, 103°, or 104°; the skin is hot, face flushed, and the eyes bright. Even in cases that are not malignant or grave, and that give indications of a favorable result, there is often more or less stupor, with transient delirium and sudden starting or twitching of the extremities, showing that the cerebro-spinal axis is involved.

Vomiting is a common symptom in the beginning of scarlet fever, occurring before the appearance of the efflorescence. It therefore has diagnostic value when the nature of the case is still doubtful. In some patients it is an initial symptom, but in others some hours have elapsed when it occurs. I recorded its presence or absence in 214 patients, with the following result: present in 162 patients, absent in 52. In severe forms of the disease it is rarely absent, and if it do not occur it is probable that the case will be mild, requiring little treatment and having a favorable termination. In epidemics of unusual mildness the number of cases without vomiting may be in excess of those in which this symptom occurs. It appears to be due to functional disturbance of the cerebro-spinal system, and it may therefore be properly regarded as a nervous symptom. In severe cases the vomiting is apt to be repeated, not only on the first but on subsequent days, and we shall see that in cases of great gravity, in which a fatal termination is not improbable, persistent vomiting, by which the food and stimulants so urgently required are rejected, interferes seriously with successful treatment. In a few cases embraced in my statistics nausea without vomiting was recorded. The bowels in ordinary scarlatina act regularly or are slightly constipated. Diarrhoea, which so commonly accompanies the persistent vomiting in malignant cases, if it occur in this form of the malady is slight and transient and due to accidental causes. The food, if it be given in the liquid form and cool, is usually taken readily, on account of the thirst, except when deglutition is rendered painful by the pharyngitis.

The symptoms pertaining to the nervous system vary according to the severity of the disease and the temperament of the patient. Many children during the progress of the common form of scarlet fever present a dull or apathetic appearance. They lie much of the time with their eyes closed; others are more restless, and not a few, if the fever be considerable, have occasional twitching of the limbs and more or less headache. Eclampsia sometimes occurs on the first day, especially in those predisposed to it, even when the subsequent course of the disease is mild and favorable. This complication, very grave and usually fatal when it occurs at a later stage, is in most instances, when it takes place on the first day, readily controlled by proper remedies and with little detriment to the patient. But if it be attended by high elevation of temperature and marked drowsiness, approaching the comatose state, it is very serious upon the first as well as upon subsequent days. Nervous symptoms occurring in the beginning of scarlet fever, when it has the ordinary favorable type, begin to abate in three or four days, but if they supervene at a later date, and especially in the declining stage, they possess more gravity, since they then not infrequently result from and indicate renal complication.

[p. 504]Early in the disease, nearly as soon as the commencement of the fever, the faucial and buccal surfaces become inflamed, as shown by redness, swelling, and tenderness. The physician summoned in the beginning of an attack will already, at his first visit, observe hyperæmia of the fauces, with points of deeper injection than over the general faucial surface, and soon the buccal surface also participates. The inflammation at first produces preternatural dryness, and this is followed by a viscid secretion. The papillæ of the tongue enlarge and become prominent, giving rise to the appearance known as strawberry tongue which is so common in scarlet fever. This state of the buccal and faucial membrane continues throughout the disease. A thin fur appears upon the tongue on the first day, and it increases on the second and third days, after which it is apt to be detached, exposing the surface of the organ, which has a deep red hue, but in not a few patients the fur remains or is reproduced as soon as shed. Except in the mildest cases the Schneiderian membrane also participates in the inflammation as the disease advances, so that a thin, irritating discharge, containing leucocytes or pus-cells, flows from the nostrils. The skin is hot and dry, and cutaneous transpiration nearly checked. The respiratory system is rarely involved in any notable manner unless there be a complication. Many have no cough whatever, while others have a slight cough, due to the fact that the inflammation, of a catarrhal form, has extended from the fauces to the surface of the glottis. Slight acceleration of respiration, corresponding with the degree of fever, may also be observed. The kidneys commonly act regularly and normally during the first days, any serious impairment of their functions being rare before the close of the first week.

When the symptoms described above have continued from six to eighteen hours the efflorescence appears. It is first observed about the ears, neck, and shoulders, in reddish patches fading into the normal hue. These patches extend and unite, and in the course of a few hours the trunk and upper extremities, and finally the legs, are covered. The scarlatinous rash usually, when fully developed, resembles that produced by external heat or the application of a sinapism. It has been likened to the appearance of a boiled lobster, but there are numerous minute points of a deeper or duskier hue than the surface generally. In many patients the rash appears, especially over the abdomen and lower extremities, as minute, thickly-set points, with the skin of normal appearance between them. Henoch of Berlin says of scarlet fever: "In general, the moderate grades of eruption prevail, the skin, when seen from a distance, presenting a diffuse, more or less scarlet redness, while on closer inspection it is found that this redness is composed of innumerable red points closely situated together, and separated from one another by very small paler portions of skin. The dark-red points appear to correspond to the hair-follicles." On passing the finger over the efflorescence no distinct prominences are observed, but a sensation of roughness is sometimes imparted from engorgement of the cutaneous papillæ. The rash disappears on pressure, but it immediately reappears when the pressure is removed. Its slow return is evidence of sluggish circulation, and it indicates a grave and dangerous form of the malady. The color is then usually a dusky instead of a bright red. The efflorescence is most marked in dependent parts, as along the back, over the chest and [p. 505]abdomen, and in the flexures of the joints. Parts pressed upon by the bed-clothes, which confine and intensify the heat, present a deeper coloration than other portions of the surface. Often, especially in mild cases, the rash is absent from portions of the surface where it commonly appears, while it presents a typical character elsewhere. Tardy and incomplete establishment of the rash when the symptoms indicate an attack of ordinary or more than ordinary severity is commonly due to some perturbating cause, especially diarrhoea. In the *London Lancet* for Aug. 16, 1879, cases are related of supposed scarlet fever without the rash, cases in which pharyngitis and stomatitis with the strawberry tongue occurred, without efflorescence upon the skin; but it is to be remembered, as stated above, that the inflammations which commonly attend or follow scarlet fever, particularly the pharyngitis and nephritis, not infrequently occur in those who have already had scarlatina, and occur more than once from fresh exposure to scarlatina patients. These inflammations, occurring under such circumstances, appear to be purely local maladies, produced by the scarlatinous virus; and it seems to me a question whether, in the so-called scarlatina without efflorescence, the inflammations which are present, and which undoubtedly have a scarlatinous origin, are not local in their nature, instead of being local manifestations of the constitutional disease. The burning and itching sensation produced by the rash increases the restlessness of the patient, and is sometimes the most annoying of the symptoms.

The temperature in the common favorable forms of scarlet fever usually varies from 101° in the mildest cases to 103° or 104° in those more severe. If it attain 105° or over, the case is properly designated grave or severe. The febrile movement commonly fluctuates but little from day to day till the fourth or fifth day, when, if the case be favorable and no complication occur, it begins to decline. The temperature is as high in the beginning of the attack as subsequently.

The symptoms pertaining to the digestive system during the initial period of scarlet fever have been sufficiently described. The subsequent symptoms referable to this system do not differ materially from those present in the beginning, except the absence of vomiting. The lips are dry and often cracked. The inflammation of the mouth and throat continues, with anorexia and thirst. With the decline of the disease the appetite gradually returns, but it is not till the close of the second week that it is fully restored. Great and continued disturbance of the digestive apparatus, seriously interfering with the nutrition, pertains to the malignant forms of scarlet fever.

The urine is high-colored, and in robust children during the first days of scarlet fever it frequently deposits urates on cooling. Gee, who has carefully investigated the state of the urine in scarlet fever, says that the quantity of water is diminished and the urea is not necessarily increased during the pyrexia; that the chloride of sodium is diminished till the fourth, fifth, or sixth day, and that the phosphoric acid is diminished during the climax of the pyrexia, though not during the first three or four days. In one case he made a daily estimation of the amount of uric acid, and found it greatly diminished on the second and third days, normal on the fourth, and much increased on the fifth. He believes that similar variations are common in the quantity of the products excreted [p. 506]in the urine. Bile may also appear in the urine, coincident with a yellow tinge of the conjunctiva.[1]

[1] Article on scarlatina in Reynolds's *System of Medicine*.

The duration of scarlet fever varies in different cases. If the attack be very mild, with little efflorescence, the febrile movement may decline by the fourth or fifth day; but if the disease be severe, little or no amelioration of symptoms may occur before the twelfth or fourteenth day, even when no complication has occurred to increase the temperature or cause aggravation of symptoms. Octerlony, who estimated the duration of scarlet fever from the commencement of febrile symptoms to "the disappearance of fever, with marked improvement in leading symptoms," ... "found that the average duration of the disease in forty cases was six and one-sixth days. The minimum duration in a very slightly-marked case was three days: the maximum duration was fourteen days." In general, prolongation of fever beyond the usual time is due to some complication—more frequently to unusually severe pharyngitis, with accompanying cellulitis, than to any other cause.

The malady whose commencement was so abrupt declines gradually. In ordinary cases, by the close of the first week or in the beginning of the second the rash becomes less and less distinct, and finally disappears, as do also the redness and swelling of the buccal and faucial surfaces. The engorgement of the tonsils and of the papillæ of the tongue subsides, the appetite returns, the countenance brightens and becomes natural, and the child, who during the height of the fever scarcely noticed objects or noticed them with indifference or even repugnance, can be amused as before his sickness.

Desquamation succeeds. This begins at about the sixth day, and is not completed till the tenth or twelfth day; often not till the close of the third or in the fourth week. The amount of desquamation corresponds with the intensity and duration of the efflorescence, or rather of the dermatitis which produces the efflorescence. If the efflorescence have been slight and partial, it will be slight, perhaps scarcely appreciable, but if the rash have been general, full, and protracted, exfoliation occurs upon every part. It begins about the face and neck, and within a day or two appears upon other parts. Where the skin is thin the epidermis as it is detached presents a furfuracous appearance; where it is thick, as upon the palms of the hands or soles of the feet, it separates in layers of considerable thickness.

Such is a brief description of scarlet fever when it pursues its normal course without any disturbing element, but there is no other disease in which complications and sequelæ so frequently occur. The liability to them renders the prognosis in every case doubtful. They largely increase the percentage of deaths. They occur both in mild and severe forms of scarlatina.

The difference in type in different cases and epidemics has already been alluded to. Scarlet fever is sometimes so mild, and its symptoms so slight, that the diagnosis is necessarily uncertain. In the spring of 1866 I was called to an infant thirteen months old who had slight pharyngitis and an indistinct rash over a part of the surface. In two days the eruption had disappeared, and the health within a day or two later was apparently fully restored. Diagnosis would have been doubtful except for sequelæ [p. 507]which clearly indicated the scarlatinous nature of the attack. In another instance two children passed through the entire course of scarlet fever playing every day in the street. Although the intelligent grandmother saw the rash upon them, its nature was not suspected, as it was midsummer and cases of prickly heat common, till nearly two weeks afterward, when one of the children had nephritis and anasarca ending fatally. In cases so mild as these the heat of surface is but slightly increased, the pulse but little accelerated, and the rash usually does not occupy so much of the surface as in ordinary cases; the appetite is not lost, though diminished, and the thirst is moderate.

Between scarlet fever so mild that it terminates in four or five days, and that of the grave or malignant type presently to be described, all grades of severity exist. Scarlet fever occurs in all forms from mild to severe, but certain symptoms characterize grave or malignant cases—symptoms which are absent or much less prominent in ordinary scarlet fever. Therefore the grouping of cases according to the type is proper, and facilitates the studying of the disease.

GRAVE FORM (malignant scarlet fever).—This form of the disease is in some epidemics common, while in others it is rare. The symptoms which characterize it are severe from the beginning, those of the nervous system predominating at first, such as intense cephalalgia, restlessness or stupor, sudden twitching of the muscles, and perhaps delirium, or even convulsions. Many pass rapidly into coma and die within two or three days, succumbing to the intensity of the scarlatinous poison while the malady is still in its commencement. The rash is dusky. It disappears by pressure, and returns slowly when the pressure is removed, showing extreme sluggishness of the capillary circulation. Some patients are very drowsy, lying in a semi-comatose state except when aroused, and if aroused are very restless. Others are constantly restless. If placed in one position on the bed, they throw themselves in another in a half-conscious or unconscious state. They do not speak, or they mutter like those affected by the graver forms of typhus, calling the names of playmates or talking incoherently about things which interested them when well. The thermometer placed in the axilla is found to rise above 103°, which is a safe average, to 105° or even 107°, and the heat of the surface is pungent except when the case approaches a fatal termination, when the extremities, ears, and nose may be cool while the trunk and head are extremely hot. The pulse from the first is rapid, ranging from 130 as the minimum in a malignant case to a frequency which can scarcely be counted. A very frequent pulse is nearly always feeble and compressible. Irritability of the stomach is one of the most common symptoms in grave cases, so that many patients immediately reject the nutriment and stimulants which are so urgently required to sustain the vital powers. The vomiting, therefore, if frequent and severe, greatly increases the danger, and in not a few instances this symptom is associated with diarrhoea, which also tends to increase the prostration.

Severe and dangerous nervous symptoms, due to the intensity or activity of the scarlatinous poison, occur chiefly within the first three or four days. Grinding the teeth, sudden muscular twitching, delirium, convulsions, and profound stupor occur for the most part within this time. Afterward the danger is mainly from exhaustion, unless the [p. 508]second week or subsequently, when nervous symptoms may arise from uræmia.

Those who survive the onset of malignant scarlet fever often have in the course of a few days severe pharyngitis, with extension of the inflammation to the lymphatic glands and connective tissue around the angle of the jaw. These inflammations cause more or less external swelling. The faucial turgescence around the entrance of the larynx, with the accompanying secretion of viscid mucus or muco-pus, often causes noisy respiration, and many at this stage of the attack breathe with the mouth constantly open to facilitate the ingress of air.

Ordinarily, no discharge occurs at first from the nasal surface, but as the disease continues, if the type remain severe, defluxion of thin muco-pus takes place from the Schneiderian surface, which frequently excoriates the cheek. The lips also are apt to be sore and swollen.

In malignant cases the disease is more protracted than when the type is mild. Thus in a recent case in my practice the rash was still distinct at the close of the second week, though the temperature had fallen from 105° to 102° and some desquamation had appeared. Long continuance of the febrile movement is, however, oftener attributable to some inflammatory complication than to the primary disease.

In all epidemics of a severe type cases now and then occur in which the poison is so intense, or it acts with such frightful energy, that death occurs even within the first day. The patient is overpowered at the outset of the disease by the virulence of the specific principle, perishing in coma, preceded perhaps by convulsions. The autopsy in such cases reveals hyperæmia of the brain and cranial sinuses, blood of a dark-red color, capillary hemorrhages in various parts, a flabby heart, and perhaps some engorgement of the spleen and kidneys.

Usually, malignant scarlet fever exhibits its severe type from the first, but cases sometimes occur which seem mild and favorable for a few days, when severe symptoms suddenly supervene. This change from a mild to a dangerous disease is, however, most frequently, I think, due to some complication.

IRREGULAR FORMS.—Deviation from the normal type in scarlet fever is usually due to some perturbating cause, which is often a pre-existing or co-existing disease, or a disordered state of system through causes distinct from the scarlatinous disease. Thus, a little girl in my practice had the symptoms of scarlet fever, such as febrile movement and inflammation of the buccal and faucial surfaces, nearly a week before the scarlatinous eruption appeared. During this time the patient had an intestinal catarrh, with diarrhoea, which declined when the rash occurred. This intestinal disease was the apparent cause of the irregularity in the malady. If scarlatina occur during a severe attack of entero-colitis attended by purging, the defluxion from the external surface may be such that no efflorescence appears. Severe scarlet fever itself sometimes appears to cause gastro-intestinal catarrh so as to produce an afflux of blood toward the intestinal tract and away from the skin. Practitioners occasionally meet cases like the following, which I recall to mind: In a family where scarlatina was prevailing a little child early after the commencement of symptoms which seemed to be plainly referable to this exanthem was seized with vomiting and purging, which continued till death [p. 509]occurred on the third day. No efflorescence appeared upon the skin, but the symptoms indicated the presence of severe intestinal catarrh, complicating and masking scarlatina. We are aided in the diagnosis of such cases by observing the faucial redness, and we may discover a faint efflorescence upon parts of the surface, as about the groin or in the flexures of the joints. In another instance an infant in the warm months having protracted entero-colitis, the usual summer epidemic of the cities, had the characteristic symptoms of scarlet fever, which was present in the family, but the diarrhoea continued and no rash appeared.

In one who is much reduced by an antecedent disease, as phthisis, or who has a disease, chronic or acute, which produces a decided afflux of blood away from the surface and toward the interior of the body, the eruption is commonly tardy in its appearance, indistinct, or wholly absent. Thus, severe inflammations of internal organs not infrequently render scarlet fever irregular. On the other hand, some maladies occurring in connection with this exanthem do not change its symptoms, but themselves undergo modification. Pertussis may be cited as an example, the cough of which is sometimes modified by an intercurrent attack of scarlet fever, the symptoms of the latter disease undergoing little change.

Scarlet fever may also be irregular without any apparent perturbating cause. In 1867 I attended a young lady whose previous health had been good, and whose brother was sick at the time with scarlet fever. She had considerable febrile movement, with severe pharyngitis, and, though her surface was repeatedly examined, no efflorescence was seen. Two weeks subsequently she was affected with severe nephritis, anasarca, effusion into at least one of the pleural cavities, oedema of the lungs, and probably hydro-pericardium, the case ending fatally. Rilliet and Barthez state that a second attack of scarlet fever is more apt to be irregular than the first. Probably this opinion is correct, especially if only a short time have elapsed between the two seizures. Still, as we have already stated, both seizures may be typical, and the second more severe than the first.

It would be impossible to make a clear and positive diagnosis of certain cases of irregular scarlet fever, in which cerebral, pulmonary, or gastro-intestinal symptoms predominate, were it not for the fact that they occur in connection with other cases of scarlet fever or are followed by sequelæ which evidently have a scarlatinous origin.

Occasionally, the eruption, if it be intense or if a certain condition of system be present in the patient, is accompanied by more or less extravasation of blood-corpuscles from the capillaries, so that the redness does not entirely disappear on pressure, usually in points. In rare instances certain of the exanthematic fevers present an extreme hemorrhagic character, so as to be beyond the reach of remedies, and of necessity speedily fatal. Hemorrhagic cases of this severe form are probably more common in variola than in the other fevers, but I have met a notable case in what was diagnosticated scarlatina. In June, 1881, a man in his thirty-second year, whose previous health had not been good, though he had no defined ailment and had been able to follow his occupation of harness-maker, suddenly became very ill, with high febrile movement and faucial inflammation, attended by marked prostration. After some hours an intense eruption of a scarlatinous appearance covered nearly the entire surface, and on the following day hemorrhages began to occur. The urine[p. 510]contained a large proportion of blood; each conjunctiva was raised by hemorrhages underneath (ecchymosis), so that its natural color was lost and the eyelids closed with difficulty; and blood flowed from the nostrils, gums, and under the skin, forming hemorrhagic points and blotches. One of the consulting physicians, perceiving the resemblance to hemorrhagic variola as described by Hebra, suspected that we had a case of this formidable malady to deal with, but the time for the appearance of the variolous eruption passed by without its occurrence. Death took place on the fifth day. The temperature during the sickness was high, though the record of it has been mislaid. Fortunately, such severe hemorrhagic cases, which are necessarily fatal, are rare.

COMPLICATIONS AND SEQUELÆ.—Scarlet fever, if its type be severe, is in itself dangerous to life. Many, as we have seen, perish from its direct effects when it produces profound blood-poisoning. But, while the ordinary epidemics of this malady are necessarily attended by a large mortality from the virulence and depressing effect of the specific principle, unfortunately, of all the diseases of modern times, scarlatina ranks first as regards the number and gravity of its complications and sequelæ, so that nearly or quite as many perish from these as from the direct effect of the poison.

Nervous accidents occur chiefly at two periods—to wit, in the first days, when they are due to the severity and malignancy of the malady and to the impressible nervous temperament of the child, and in the declining stage, or after the termination of the fever, when they occur from uræmia. If the type be malignant, delirium, jactitation, profound stupor, and convulsions frequently occur on the first and second days; and they are symptoms which properly excite the utmost alarm and demand all the resources of our art, since they indicate a form of the disease which is apt to end in speedy death. The eyes have a dull or wild expression, the conjunctiva is suffused, the heat of surface pungent, the pulse rapid and compressible or feeble, rising above 150, even to 200, per minute, and the temperature is always elevated to a degree that involves danger, the thermometer not infrequently indicating 105° or 106°. But this severe form of scarlet fever, attended by so great elevation of temperature, is much less dangerous than in former times, even though it be complicated by delirium and convulsions, since we no longer hesitate to reduce bodily heat, when excessive, by the free use of cold baths, and have discovered potent agents in the bromides and chloral for controlling convulsions. Nevertheless, not a few perish in the commencement of scarlet fever with predominating cerebral symptoms, as delirium or eclampsia, followed by coma, under the best possible treatment. Sometimes the symptoms have closely simulated those of acute meningitis, and if the rash have been delayed and the sore throat is as yet slight, the physician may suspect that he is dealing with this disease; but autopsies in such cases show no inflammatory lesions, but only congestion of the cerebral and meningeal vessels.

As is stated in a preceding page, in every case of normal scarlet fever inflammation of the faucial surface is present, as indicated by redness, tenderness, and increased secretion of mucus or muco-pus. It precedes the efflorescence on the skin, and is announced by pain in swallowing and on pressure with the fingers behind and below the angles of the jaw. In that form of scarlet fever which has been designated anginose the [p. 511]pharyngitis is severe, and is a prominent element in the malady, the uvula, the pillars of the fauces, and the faucial surface in general being infiltrated and swollen. Nevertheless, this inflammation, with the accompanying tumefaction, is properly a part of the disease, rather than a complication, if it abates with the subsidence of the scarlet fever or begin to abate soon after, and if it produce but slight destructive change in the tissues of the neck. The secretions from the fauces may be foul and offensive; even superficial ulcerations or gangrene may occur upon the faucial surface, causing it to present a dark brown or jagged appearance, and the tissues of the neck may be infiltrated to a certain extent, and we designate the disease a form of scarlet fever under the title anginose. But when this condition is greatly aggravated, so that there is extensive infiltration and swelling of the tissues of the neck, with an amount of ulceration or gangrene which in itself involves danger, continuing after the primary disease abates, prolonging the fever and reducing the strength, it is proper to regard the state of the throat as a complication. In addition to the pharyngitis, which is severe as described above, the sides of the neck around the angles of the jaw become swollen, hard, and tender. The inflammation has been propagated to the deeper structures of the neck. Poisonous substances, the result of decomposition or vitiated secretions, traverse the lymphatic vessels from the faucial surface, and, being intercepted in the lymphatic glands, cause adenitis, and the inflammation extends from the glands to the adjacent connective tissue, which becomes hard, tender, swollen, and infiltrated with inflammatory products. This tumefaction sometimes begins by the second or third day, but it is usually about the close of the first week or in the beginning of the second week that it becomes so considerable as to constitute a source of danger and anxiety. It is in most cases bilateral, though one side may begin to swell before the other and remain larger throughout.

In severe cases of this complication the tumefaction extends from ear to ear, filling up the space below and around the angles of the jaw and under the chin. Not only is deglutition difficult, but it is difficult to open the mouth sufficiently to inspect the fauces, and attempts to do so cause much pain. The lymphatic glands, which lie in the inflamed area and participate in the inflammation, are greatly enlarged by hyperplasia, the round granular lymph-cells multiplying so abundantly that the glands increase to many times their normal size. Most of the tumefaction is, however, due to extension of the inflammation to the connective tissue of the neck. The cellulitis, which resembles that occurring in other conditions, is attended by distension of the capillaries, the abundant formation of young round cells, and transudation of serum (Billroth). A moderate amount of tumefaction may disappear by resolution, but if it be considerable it seldom abates in this way, but by the tedious and exhausting process of suppuration or gangrene. If the swelling at its most prominent point present a reddish hue, all hope of producing resolution must be abandoned; it cannot be effected by any medicine or appliance within the resources of our art. The abscess which forms is apt to be diffuse, so as to involve danger of pyæmia, unless it be soon opened and properly washed out. With the discharge of the pus the swelling gradually softens and declines. In other cases gangrene results. The vessels in the inflamed part are compressed by the inflammatory products, so that [p. 512]they no longer convey the blood which is required for the purpose of nutrition. It is a law of the economy that whenever the circulation ceases, the tissues which receive their nutritive supply through the obstructed vessels lose their vitality. Hence gangrene occurs in all that portion of the swelling in which the circulation is arrested. The skin over it peels off, the dead tissue underneath is brown or dark, and soon, if life be prolonged, the slough begins to separate. The prognosis as regards this complication depends largely on the size of the slough. If it be large, death will probably result, since the strength of the system is already reduced by the primary disease, and the reparative process will necessarily be slow, while abundant suppuration tends to increase the exhaustion. In some of the worst cases of cervical gangrene which I have seen the slough has laid bare the muscles and vessels of the neck, producing in one case a cavity or excavation sufficiently large to admit a hen's egg. Often the slough extends under the skin, so that the deepest recesses of the cavity are not visible, and occasionally in cases which have ended fatally in my practice severe hemorrhage occurred from the concealed vessels. If the ulcerative or gangrenous process extends so deeply into the tissues of the neck that hemorrhages occur, death is the common result; but if the destructive action be of moderate extent and other conditions favorable, we may expect recovery through cicatrization, with perhaps some deformity by contraction of the cicatrix.

When the inflammation of the connective tissue of the neck is extensive, involving both the lateral and anterior regions of the neck, the patient is in a perilous state. The cellulitis, when extensive and accompanied by much swelling, may produce oedema of the glottis, may obstruct respiration by compressing the air-passages or the laryngeal nerves, may cause compression of the jugular veins, and thus give rise to dangerous cerebral symptoms, or may lay bare and injure important muscles and nerves, as we have seen. If the ulceration or gangrene be extensive, and death do not occur by hemorrhage from arterial or venous twigs, septic poisoning may occur, increasing still more the fatal nature of the malady.

Some cases of this complication are melancholy in the extreme, as one related by Cremen, in which ulceration of the pharynx occurred, allowing the escape of food and preventing deglutition. In severe scarlatinous pharyngitis the inflammation is apt to extend along the Eustachian tube, causing its occlusion. This accident will be considered when we treat of otitis media, another grave complication. It often also extends into the nares, causing catarrh of the Schneiderian mucous membrane, with discharge of muco-pus from this surface. Not infrequently ulceration or gangrene occurs in the faucial surface, producing more or less destruction of tissue and forming excavations which connect with the throat, while the cutaneous surface retains its integrity and is not even reddened. The following case shows how grave the complication which we are now considering sometimes is when the external surface of the neck is not involved, and how the inflammation by extension outward from the fauces may involve the middle ear.

Case 1.—Annie K——, aged two and a half years, an inmate of the New York Foundling Asylum, was well, except an eczema of the scalp, until the night of April 3, 1882, when she was attacked with vomiting and[p. 513]diarrhoea. She was feverish and drowsy, and at 2 P.M. on the 4th the scarlatinous efflorescence appeared upon her neck, body, and lower extremities; tongue coated; pharynx red; temperature (axillary) 103°; pulse 160. The symptoms and aspect indicated a grave form of the malady, and the usual sustaining treatment was ordered. On April 5th the temperature was 102°, pulse 144, tongue less coated, eruption fading, less stupor, no albumen in urine. April 6th, morning temperature 102°, pulse 160; passed a restless night; stools thin and too frequent; has grayish patches in the throat: P.M. temperature 103.2°, pulse 150. April 7th, the diarrhoea continues, and she has a copious muco-purulent discharge from the nostrils; P.M. temperature 103.6°, pulse 160. April 10th, the temperature has continued at about 103°; the patient is very sick, with a constant foul-smelling discharge from the nostrils; breath very offensive; temperature 103.5°, pulse about 180. April 12th, general appearance a little better, but the posterior surface of the fauces is completely covered by a thick pseudo-membrane; had four loose stools last night; temperature and pulse the same as at last record; a dark, offensive, and jagged coating over the fauces, and a dark, foul discharge from the nostrils, as before; examination of the chest negative. April 14th, is much prostrated; temperature 104.5°, pulse rapid and weak; respiration noisy, diminished resonance over lower two-thirds of left side of chest; ulcers upon the mouth and tongue; fauces red and ulcerated. April 17th, pulse 150, temperature 100.5°; general appearance somewhat better, but the diarrhoea continues, and patches of a diphtheritic character have appeared upon the lips; moist râles in left side of chest. The symptoms continued nearly the same until April 23d, when she died. A dull percussion sound and distinct bronchial respiration were observed in the left scapular region during the last days of her life.

Autopsy nine hours after death by the curator, Dr. W. P. Northrup: Body well nourished; the tissues have a jaundiced hue; lips sore; on turning the head to one side pus runs from the left ear and dirty muco-pus from the mouth. Brain normal; on opening the petrous portion of the left temporal bone the middle ear is found full of pus, which communicated freely with the external ear through a perforated membrana tympani; the Eustachian tube cannot be traced in the sloughy tissue, and a passage filled with pus extends from the ear to the fauces; opposite the greater cornua of the hyoid bone are two deep ulcers, each having about the diameter of a ten-cent piece, with sloughy and offensive base and sides; the left ulcer communicates by a ragged and wide sinus with a dark and sloughy cavity of about four drachms capacity; this cavity is located in the neck under the angle of the jaw, apparently occupying the site of a disintegrated gland, and it opens upon the surface of the fauces. The surface of the larynx has a dusky, dirty appearance, sprinkled with little cheesy-looking spots, and covered by a dirty, foul-appearing liquid, as if some of the ichorous pus had escaped into it from the neck; about one and a half inches below the vocal chords there is an unmistakable pseudo-membrane; below this, near the bifurcation, the trachea has a bright-red color, as if a pseudo-membrane had been peeled from it, leaving the surface raw. The detachment of a pseudo-membrane from this part, if it did occur, must have been ante-mortem, for the organ had been carefully handled [p. 514]in making the autopsy. Between the apex of the left lung and the median line the tissues of the neck, dissected upward, are found indurated, yellow, and giving an offensive odor, showing that the cervical cellulitis had extended downward farther than usual. The bronchial glands have undergone hyperplasia, being enlarged and hard. The right lung is normal; about one-half of the left lower lobe is consolidated, and when cut is found to be gangrenous and offensive. The liver is apparently somewhat enlarged; spleen normal in size; gastric mucous membrane has a congested appearance and is covered with mucus; mesenteric glands enlarged, pale, and firm; Peyer's patches swollen and pale; at lower end of ileum some pigmentation of these glands; in large intestine the solitary glands are enlarged, and a few of them pigmented; kidneys pale, cortex thickened, and markings indistinct. Microscopical Examination.—In the pia mater perhaps a little increase of cells; meninges of brain otherwise normal. The trachea shows well-marked diphtheritic inflammation; it contains a film of pseudo-membrane; evidences of inflammation occur also upon the laryngeal surface, though less marked than in the trachea. The solidified portion of the lung exhibits the ordinary lesions of broncho-pneumonia, with some interstitial change. In the kidneys we find parenchymatous nephritis, with some cell-growth in the Malpighian bodies.

The above case has been related at length, not only because it shows how severe and destructive the inflammation of the throat, extending into the tissues of the neck, sometimes is, but because four other complications or sequelæ were also present—to wit, otitis media, diphtheria, nephritis, and pneumonia. We see from the above case how formidable a disease scarlet fever sometimes is when attended by the inflammations to which it so frequently gives rise, for a child older and stronger than this, if thus affected, would necessarily have perished with the best possible treatment.

In localities where diphtheria is endemic, as in New York City and Paris, scarlet fever is often complicated by a pseudo-membranous inflammation of the fauces and air-passages. In severe cases of scarlet fever the Schneiderian as well as the faucial surface is covered with it, so that it can be readily seen on inspecting the anterior nares. Occasionally, the pseudo-membrane appears upon the laryngeal and tracheal surfaces, as in the case which I have related above and in others presently to be related, causing dangerous embarrassment of respiration. This complication sometimes begins almost at the commencement of scarlet fever, but in most instances it does not occur before the third or fourth day, and it sometimes does not appear till in the declining stage of the fever. When it begins, it intensifies the febrile movement and produces general aggravation of symptoms.

The common opinion is, that whenever a pseudo-membrane occurs upon the inflamed mucous surface in scarlatina true diphtheria has supervened; but there are those who hold that scarlet fever itself, when the inflammations which attend it are severe, may give rise to pseudo-membranes, so that what seems to be diphtheritic is but an element in the primary disease. My convictions are strong that when pseudo-membranes occur on any of the inflamed mucous surfaces in scarlet fever, true diphtheria has, with few exceptions, supervened if the patient live in a[p. 515]locality where diphtheria is prevalent. That scarlet fever may occur in an individual along with another acute infectious malady is shown by abundant cases. It often occurs with varicella, and J. Herzog relates the following case, in which measles and scarlet fever coexisted:[2] A boy aged eight years had measles, with the usual catarrhal symptoms, and on the fourth day, as the temperature was returning to the normal, it rose again suddenly, and the scarlatinal rash and sore throat appeared. In due time these subsided, and desquamation occurred. I have seen a similar case in consultation during the current year, so that there is nothing improbable in the theory that scarlet fever may coexist with other infectious maladies; and it is admitted that diphtheria, like erysipelas, may complicate the most diverse constitutional diseases. Moreover, when a child with pertussis, measles, typhoid fever, or tuberculosis suddenly develops a high fever with the occurrence of a pseudo-membranous inflammation upon the fauces or air-passages, all admit that diphtheria has supervened, since such inflammation is not an element in any form or type of either of these diseases; and I see no reason in the nature of the disease why scarlet fever should not be equally liable to this complication.

[2] *Berl. klin. Woch.*, 1882, No. 7.

The elaborate treatise by Sanné of Paris on diphtheria contains a chapter entitled "Secondary Diphtheria." In it the author says, what all who are familiar with diphtheria will agree to, that secondary diphtheria does not differ in nature from the primary form, and that it exhibits a tendency "to occupy the organs which are themselves the seat of the more pronounced local determinations of the primitive malady.... Diphtheria is seen in the course or sequel of numerous diseases. Some appear to have a special proclivity for engendering diphtheria; these are specific maladies: measles, scarlet fever, pertussis." I have tabulated as follows Sanné's statistics of secondary diphtheria:

Diphtheria complicating measles,	100 cases,	83 deaths,	15 cures,	2 doubtful.
Diphtheria complicating scarlet fever,	43 cases,	22 deaths,	17 cures,	4 doubtful.
Diphtheria complicating pertussis,	20 cases,	12 deaths,	6 cures,	2 doubtful.
Diphtheria complicating typhoid fever,	8 cases,	8 deaths.		
Diphtheria complicating tuberculosis,	19 cases,	19 deaths.		

Sanné's statistics relating to the seat of scarlatinous diphtheria are as follows:

Fauces alone	attacked,	15 cases.
Fauces with larynx	attacked,	4 cases.
Fauces with nasal fossa	attacked,	8 cases.
Fauces with larynx and nasal fossa	attacked,	4 cases.
Fauces with larynx and bronchi	attacked,	1 case.
Fauces with nasal fossa and lips	attacked,	1 case.
Fauces with lips and skin	attacked,	1 case.
Fauces unaffected,		3 cases.
Diphtheria generalized,		2 cases.
Larynx only affected,		2 cases.

356

Nasal fossa affected, 1 case.

The opinion of so good an observer as Sanné, that when in scarlet fever, pseudo-membranous exudation appears upon the mucous surfaces which are the seat of scarlatinous inflammation, diphtheria has supervened, and not a croupous form of scarlatinous phlegmasia, carries with it great[p. 516]weight. That it was diphtheria in four instances in my practice I had sufficient proof, for this disease became dissociated from scarlet fever, and extended to other members of these families as idiopathic diphtheria.

Nevertheless, one of the most difficult problems which we have to deal with in certain cases is to distinguish diphtheritic from non-diphtheritic inflammation; and I see no reason why the scarlatinous inflammation when intense may not be sometimes membranous; and those no doubt err who ignore this, and consider every inflammation attended by a pellicular exudation diphtheritic. We know that in some cases of dysentery a fibrinous exudation occurs upon the surface of the colon; that in croupous pneumonia fibrin exudes into the bronchioles and alveoli of the lungs; and that physicians in localities where there is no diphtheria meet, though at long intervals, cases which they designate croupous pharyngitis and laryngitis; and it seems to me that the intense inflammation of anginose scarlatina probably sometimes produces the same exudation. Moreover, it is very difficult to distinguish in the swollen fauces between a membranous exudation and ulceration or superficial gangrene so common in malignant scarlet fever. The grayish-white surface, jagged and foul, may be the one or the other, an exudation or a sphacelus, and in certain instances it is impossible to discriminate between the two conditions at the bedside.

Diphtheria complicating scarlet fever sometimes begins nearly simultaneously with the latter. Henoch states that exceptionally he has observed suspicious patches upon the fauces before the appearance of the scarlatinous eruption upon the skin; and he adds: "I have had repeated opportunities of observing this unusual beginning. In such cases we must ask ourselves whether the first affection was really connected with the second, or whether the former was a true primary diphtheria, rapidly followed by scarlatina. This opinion is favored by the fact that I have only observed such cases in the hospital, in which infection with various forms of contagion can scarcely be avoided."

But usually it is not till the third or fourth day of scarlet fever that this complication begins. The patient has been progressing favorably with the scarlet fever, till on a certain day a marked aggravation of symptoms occurs. A higher temperature, more pungent heat, and the physiognomy of a more serious malady are present. On inspecting the fauces to discover the cause we observe a pellicle forming over the tonsils and perhaps other portions of the faucial surface. Often the entire aspect of the case changes by the occurrence of this complication, a mild case of scarlet fever becoming grave and fatal in consequence. Thus in a case which I saw with Dr. Hardy of New York the membranous inflammation of diphtheria, commencing upon the fauces on the third day of scarlet fever, extended to the Schneiderian membrane, and thence along the left lachrymal sac to the eyelids, producing redness and swelling along the side of the nose and upon the cheek like that of erysipelas. A thick diphtheritic pellicle occurred upon the under surface of each eyelid on the left side, with great tumefaction of both lids, gangrene of the cornea, and destruction of the eye. The case soon ended fatally.

The diphtheritic inflammation sometimes extends to the larynx and trachea, producing hoarseness and more or less obstruction to [p. 517]respiration. A thin film or flakes of fibrinous exudation, rendering the respiration noisy, developed on the laryngeal or tracheal surface, is, I think, not infrequent in diphtheria complicating scarlet fever, but the rapid development of a thick and firm pseudo-membrane, so as to imperil the life of the patient from the stenosis in the air-passages, has been much less frequent in my practice than it is in primary diphtheria and in diphtheria complicating measles or pertussis. The following were cases of this severe complication occurring in a recent epidemic in the New York Foundling Asylum. In these cases the respiration was noisy, but the obstruction to breathing seemed to be due to infiltration and swelling around the aperture of the glottis, rather than to diphtheritic croup, which the autopsies showed to be present.

Case 2.—A child aged three and a half years, who previously had symptoms of mild catarrhal croup, with moderate redness of the fauces, sickened with scarlet fever on Oct. 1, 1882, the rash being profuse and soon covering nearly the entire body. The axillary temperature was 103°, pulse 140; slight stridor in breathing and some cough; fauces very red, but free from membrane. Oct. 2d, restless, sleeping but little; has vomited four times. Oct. 3d, temp. 103.5°, pulse 120; fauces much swollen; still vomiting; rash abundant. 4 P.M., temp. 104.3°, pulse 128; tongue clean; some discharge from nares; urine not albuminous, but its quantity diminished. Oct. 4th, aspect that of very severe sickness; profuse discharge from nostrils; fauces of a deep red color, and a diphtheritic pellicle over tonsils and uvula; tumefaction along the sides of the neck; temp. 104°, pulse 140; breathing moderately stridulous; urine is passed more freely than yesterday; evening temp. 105°. Oct. 6th, croupy symptoms more marked; tonsils and uvula greatly swollen, so that the fauces are almost occluded; temp. 103.5°; breathing difficult, but apparently sufficient oxygen is received; profuse nasal discharge, and other symptoms as before. About 1.30 P.M. he was raised to take some milk, and suddenly became asphyxiated. His face was dusky, his eyes protruded, and he voided urine and feces. Dr. Swift, who attended the child, and to whom I am indebted for this history, immediately performed tracheotomy, which gave temporary relief by the expulsion of a considerable quantity of pseudo-membrane through the opening. On the following day the respiration again became obstructed at some point below the canula, so that it could not be removed; the features grew livid, and death occurred in convulsions twenty-six hours after the tracheotomy.

The autopsy was made by Dr. W. P. Northrup, curator of the asylum, who found the pharynx covered by a membrane which was traced to the posterior nares; larynx, trachea, and bronchial tubes as far as the third divisions also covered with membrane; portions of the tracheal surface denuded, and the mucous membrane underneath of a bright red color and smooth; tonsils sloughy and fetid; mucous membrane of smaller bronchial tubes very red and covered with viscid mucus and pus; a portion of the left lung, extending from the root posteriorly to the surface, gangrenous, discolored, and honeycombed; two or three intensely hyperæmic spots, as large as a bean, in left lung; right lung congested, but not consolidated; slight catarrh of stomach; circumscribed areas of congestion in intestines; solitary glands of intestines swollen, and some [p. 518]of them ulcerated; spleen of normal size, rather pale; liver congested and somewhat enlarged.

Case 3.—Katie, aged six and a third years, was returned to the asylum on Nov. 18th. Three days later (Nov. 21st) she had sore throat, reddened fauces, coated tongue, and a faint rash upon the neck, chest, and arms; eyes injected; temperature 102°. In the afternoon temperature 103°; eruption still faint. Nov. 22d, temperature 103.5°; an eruption on chest, abdomen, arms, and legs in patches. Evening, temperature 104°; voice clear. Nov. 23d, temperature 103.5°; tongue red; fauces deeply reddened, but without any visible pseudo-membrane; eruption of a scarlatinous appearance over the back and abdomen; on the extremities dusky, livid patches. P.M., temperature 104°; is slightly delirious; eruption abundant. Nov. 24th, temperature 103.5°; eruption well out on abdomen; it is the same as yesterday upon the extremities, except perhaps a little more dusky; still no pseudo-membrane to be seen upon the fauces; is restless and delirious. P.M., during the day has been very restless, suffering from dyspnoea; no croupy voice nor croupy cough, though the dyspnoea continues, and a pseudo-membrane is now visible over the tonsils and adjacent faucial surface; eruption dusky; skin cool; pulse very frequent and feeble. From this time she sank steadily, and died at 11.30 P.M.During her sickness her urine seemed to be diminished, but it was not properly examined.

Autopsy Nov. 25th by Dr. W. P. Northrup, curator: Points of redness, apparently a hemorrhagic eruption, over the face, shoulders, and parts of the trunk; a few of the same on the extremities; no pseudo-membrane visible in nostrils or in buccal cavity; brain not examined. Naso-pharynx covered by a thick fibro-purulent membrane. Larynx contains a well-marked pseudo-membrane, but not continuous. Trachea covered by a pseudo-membrane, continuous over most of its surface, but in places broken and flaky. Where it is detached the mucous membrane is seen underneath, dusky and deeply injected. At the root of the lungs the pseudo-membrane can be traced along the tubes about an inch in all directions. Lungs oedematous, with deep congestion in places, but apparently no pneumonia; about two drachms of clear, straw-colored fluid in pericardium; a few stringy decolorized clots in the cavities of the heart; left ventricle contracted. The heart-fibres, carefully examined, microscopically, in the laboratory, are found to be normal, not having undergone granular or fatty degeneration. Liver normal in size; pale-yellow areas upon the superior surface, either from anæmia or fatty deposition. Kidneys of usual size, capsule not adherent; pyramids congested; cortex pale; markings distinct. Spleen enlarged about one-third; consistence normal. Stomach and intestines not examined.

Case 4.—Scarlet fever complicated by diphtheria, nephritis, and broncho-pneumonia. (History by house physician, Dr. Swift.) Phoebe, aged three and a quarter years, was delicate, but in her usual health till Oct. 29, 1882, when she became languid and vomited several times, and her tongue was coated. Oct. 30th, occasional vomiting; fauces reddened; tongue coated. Oct. 31st, remains languid; fauces deeply reddened; a faint scarlatinous eruption over back, wrists, and feet; temperature 100.5°. P.M., eruption of scarlet fever well out over the surface; tongue cleaner. Nov. 1st, [p. 519]rash over entire body; temperature 100.2°. Nov. 2d, fauces deep-red; tonsils and uvula swollen; diarrhoea and vomiting. Nov. 3d, temperature 102.5°; the eruption, which has been bright red, is now more dusky. Nov. 5th, temperature 104.5°; dusky-red color of the eruption; skin beginning to desquamate in places; urine normal; a discharge from nostrils. Nov. 6th, temperature 103.5°; eruption still present, but skin of abdomen and back desquamating; has otorrhoea on both sides; fauces deeply hyperæmic, but no pseudo-membrane visible upon them. Nov. 7th, temperature 103°; respiration and cough have a slight croupy character; other symptoms as yesterday. Nov. 8th, temperature 101°. A careful inspection of the fauces shows that it contains no pseudo-membrane; nostrils discharging a dark-brownish liquid; examination of urine negative. Nov. 11th, eruption, which appears to have been hemorrhagic in points, is fading and the desquamation is less. Nov. 14th, nostrils still discharging; glands of neck swollen. Nov. 16th, temperature 103°; sp. gr. of urine 1010, no casts, nor albumen; the chest seems clear; less discharge from nostrils; fauces clean and but slightly inflamed. Nov. 17th, 18th, temperature 103.5°; vomits; lungs healthy, but breathes with considerable effort, though without stridor; urine diminished; its sp. gr. 1020, albuminous, contains blood-corpuscles and granular casts. Nov. 19th, is very pallid; temperature 104°; very restless; vomits; urine diminished; bowels freely open. Nov. 20th, respiration still embarrassed; subcrepitant râles over the entire chest and percussion resonance not clear; temperature 102.5°. Nov. 21st, physical signs the same; temperature 103.5°; respiration 80. Nov. 22d, urgent dyspnoea; dulness on percussion over top of right lung and over lower part of left lung; is delirious; no perspiration; urine scanty; bowels freely open. From this date the dyspnoea became more urgent, and death occurred at 4 P.M. on the 23d.

Autopsy by Dr. W. P. Northrup, curator: Body well nourished; slight oedema of both legs; swelling at angles of jaws, most marked on left side. Vessels of brain moderately injected; otherwise appearance normal. Cicatrizing ulcers on both sides of fauces; a diphtheritic pseudo-membrane on septum of nose, larynx normal. Trachea, upper half apparently normal; a thin film of pseudo-membrane extends from just above the bifurcation upward to nearly the middle of trachea. About an ounce of fluid in each pleural cavity; on the right side a few loose flakes of fibrin floating in the serum, and consolidation of lung at apex; collapse in one or two places. Left side, recent adhesions over whole of posterior surface and base; surface of lower lobe dark, and when it is detached strings of fibrin adhere to it, and it is consolidated. The cut surface shows marked oedema, injection, increase of mucus in bronchi, and disseminated miliary tubercles in every part; no tubercles in the pleura, and none elsewhere in the body except in the left lung; tubercles in the lower lobe larger and more thickly grouped than in the upper lobe. Decolorized clots in heart, extending from ventricles into auricles of both sides. The capacity of the ventricles seems normal. Liver and spleen, normal. Kidneys rather large; capsules not adherent; superficial veins injected. The cut surface shows congested pyramids and pale cortex; markings indistinct and irregular; about four ounces of clear straw-colored fluid in abdominal cavity, and the solitary follicles of [p. 520]large intestines show pigmentation; two simple intussusceptions, each three-fourths inch in length, in small intestines.

Coryza frequently commences at or about the time of the pharyngitis. The inflammation of the Schneiderian membrane is continuous posteriorly with that of the fauces, and is announced by redness and swelling, inability to breathe freely through the nostrils, and an irritating ichorous discharge. Simple coryza in itself involves little danger, though it is an unpleasant complication, and in the nursing infant it may interfere with sucking. Diphtheritic coryza, on the other hand, which is frequently present when diphtheria complicates scarlet fever, involves danger, since it is apt to cause ulcerations, hemorrhages, and septic poisoning. When the local symptoms are unusually severe and the discharge abundant, it is probable that inflammation has in some cases extended to the antrum of Highmore.

Inflammation of the middle ear is another unpleasant and not infrequent complication. It is attributed to extension of the catarrh from the pharynx along the Eustachian tube to the tympanum. In a considerable proportion of cases of otitis media this tube is occluded by the infiltration and swelling of its mucous membrane, so that the muco-pus escapes with difficulty or is retained. Hence severe earache, an increase of the febrile movement, and outward bulging of the membrana tympani occur. Sometimes headache or other cerebral symptoms arise, probably from the fact that the meningeal artery, which supplies the meninges, is connected by anastomosing branches with the tympanum. In one of the cases related above it will be recollected that the ulceration and abscess extended from the fauces to the middle ear, the entire Eustachian tube having disappeared in the ulcerative process.

Frequently, the otitis escapes detection, its symptoms being masked or obscured by the general disease, until the membrana tympani is perforated and otorrhoea begins; but by careful examination the nature of the complication can usually be ascertained before the ear is injured to this extent, for a patient too young to speak will often press with the fingers against the painful ear or lie with the ear pressed upon the pillow, evidently having an increase of suffering if placed in any other position. One old enough to speak and in proper mental condition makes known the earache as soon as it occurs.

The mucous membrane of the tympanum, red and swollen from inflammation, secretes muco-pus abundantly; and this, pent up in the cavity, must obtain an exit before relief occurs. It is well if this secretion escape, though with difficulty, down the Eustachian tube. The destructive action of the pus upon the delicate structure of the ear is often such that, within a few days, irreparable harm is done and more or less deafness results. Relief can occur, if the Eustachian tube remain closed, only by perforation of the membrane and the discharge of the secretions into the external meatus. When this occurs the inflammation in the most favorable cases gradually abates, the aperture in the drum closes, and the integrity of the auditory apparatus is preserved. In severe cases the mastoid cells participating in the inflammation become filled with muco-pus and tender to the touch, and often the collateral oedema causes tumefaction and narrowing of the external ear, which subside with the discharge of pus from the tympanum.

[p. 521]Unfortunately, there is for many a more melancholy history—a more destructive inflammation, involving permanent impairment or total loss of hearing. This is especially apt to occur in strumous and feeble children. All grades of inflammation and destructive action occur in different cases. The perforation in the drum-membrane may be large or the membrane may be completely destroyed, and the detached ossicles escape one by one into the external meatus, and in a few instances, fortunately rare, this occurs in both ears, producing complete and permanent deafness. In my own practice this has never occurred, but I have met one or two adults who were totally deaf from this cause.

The mucous membrane which lines the bony wall of the middle ear has the function of the periosteum, and therefore, when inflamed and subjected to pressure, is liable to ulcerate. As in other parts of the skeleton under similar conditions, superficial caries or necrosis of the underlying bone is apt to occur. The carious or necrotic process may extend to the mastoid cells. An offensive otorrhoea, continuing for months or years, indicates the persistence of this pathological state of the tympanum, which is rendered so obstinate by the presence of dead bone. A moment's survey of the anatomical relations of the middle ear shows the danger to which these patients are liable. A thin bony septum, perforated with blood-vessels and sometimes containing congenital apertures, separates the tympanum from the cranial cavity above. Posteriorly lie the mastoid cells, connected with the tympanum by one large and several small apertures. Anteriorly is the commencement of the Eustachian tube and in close proximity to the tympanum lies the carotid canal, and at one point also the superior petrosal sinus. Virchow has shown how inflammation extending from the ear in otitis media sometimes produces such compression of the veins or sinuses by the swelling from the infiltration and exudation that the circulation is arrested, and the fibrin contained in the blood of these vessels is precipitated, forming thrombi, with the most disastrous effect upon the individual. Pus may also burrow in the interstices of the bone, causing great pain, or the pent-up secretions, having no outlet for escape, may in time undergo caseous degeneration, producing the conditions in which tuberculosis so often originates.

Death not infrequently occurs in chronic otitis media in another way. The otorrhœa, after months or years, suddenly ceases, the child complains of constant severe headache and is feverish, and the case ends in coma, preceded perhaps by convulsions. Meningitis has occurred, produced by extension of the inflammation through the thin bony septum which divides the tympanum from the cranial cavity, and at the autopsy hyperæmia of the meninges, fibrin, pus, perhaps softening of the brain and an abscess, are formed in the portion of the encephalon adjacent to the tympanum. Therefore, otitis media, though it often ends favorably, is in many patients an obstinate, dangerous, and even fatal sequel of scarlet fever.

The complication known as scarlatinous rheumatism is regarded by some as a synovitis, but its symptoms, especially its shifting from joint to joint, seem to ally it to the rheumatic affections. In some epidemics it is common. It usually begins toward the close of the first week or in the second week, and its common seat is in the ankle, phalangeal, and wrist joints. It is attended by very little swelling in [p. 522]most patients, though the joints are tender and painful on pressure. It does not seem to retard convalescence materially, though it produces suffering and involves danger as regards the heart. It subsides in a few days with the ordinary treatment of acute rheumatism, and even without special treatment, the chief danger being that, as in idiopathic rheumatism, endocarditis may arise, with permanent crippling of the valves. The following was a case of valvular disease having this origin. It occurred in my practice.

Case 5.—Freddy M., aged four years, sickened with scarlet fever March 6, 1879. The usual vomiting occurred on the first day, and the temperature was 104°. The case progressed favorably till March 14th, when he complained of pain in both wrists, both ankles, and both knees. On March 17th the general condition was good, the urine contained no albumen, and apparently few urates, but he still had pain in the joints of the upper and lower extremities and in the back; pulse 140, temp. 103°; breathes with a slight moan; urates in the urine, but no albumen. A distinct mitral regurgitant murmur is now heard for the first time. Under the use of salicylate of sodium the pain in the joints soon ceased, but the mitral murmur is permanent.

The following prescription is for a child of five years:

		Ol.	fl.	
x.	Gaultheriæ		drachm iss;	
	Sodii Salicylat.			drach m iii;
	Syrupi			fl. oz. ii;
	Aquæ			fl. oz. iv. M.

S. Give one teaspoonful every four hours.

Of the serous inflammations occurring in scarlet fever, pericarditis has been, according to Rilliet and Barthez, most frequently observed. In this country it is probably more frequent than is usually supposed, but it is less frequently detected than pleuritis, the symptoms of which are more conspicuous. It is apt to occur in connection with endocarditis.

The following case, showing the liability to pericarditis and other serous inflammation which exists in scarlet fever, occurred in my practice:

Case 6.—C——, girl aged five years and ten months, sickened with severe scarlet fever on April 4th. Was delirious; pulse 158; had vomiting and constipation. April 10th, pulse varies from 124 to 153, no delirium; a considerable quantity of urates in the urine. April 11th, has to-day, for the first time, severe pain in the epigastrium, with tenderness and moderate distension. Otherwise symptoms favorable, but severe; pulse 140; respiration moderately accelerated, and vesicular in every part of the chest. From this date the symptoms continued about the same till April 14th, when the dyspnoea became more marked and the action of the heart rapid and tumultuous. The epigastric pain, distension, and tenderness continued; the percussion sound was dull over the lower part of the chest; the dyspnoea became rapidly worse, although the pulse had considerable volume; and at 5 P.M. death occurred. At the autopsy about one ounce of turbid serum, with a soft deposit of fibrin, was found in the pericardium. Each pleural cavity contained from six to eight ounces of transparent serum, and both lungs were readily inflated, except a little of the posterior portion of each lower lobe, which could not be; no fibrinous exudation over the lungs. The liver extended four inches below the margin of the ribs, and upon its convex [p. 523]surface in the epigastrium, corresponding with the seat of the pain, was a rough patch of fibrin about one and a half inches in diameter. The bronchial mucous membrane was moderately injected, as was also that of the colon, and the kidneys appeared hyperæmic.

Among the serous inflammations which complicate or follow scarlet fever, pleuritis is one of the most important. It usually begins in the desquamative stage, and is apt to be suppurative on account of the feeble state of the patient when it commences. It has always, in my practice, been tedious, as all empyemas are, and it does not differ in its clinical history from the idiopathic disease. I have met cases of scarlatinous empyema in which, from opposition of the family or for other reasons, thoracentesis was not performed, and death occurred; others in which this operation effected a cure, and one at least in which the patient recovered by escape of pus through a bronchial tube. The pleuritis is seldom latent, or so masked by the symptoms of the general disease that it is apt to be overlooked. On the other hand, the cough, embarrassment of respiration, and pain referred to the affected side render diagnosis easy.

Dilatation of the heart is common in grave cases of scarlet fever, such cases as are properly termed malignant. It is indicated by a feeble and quick pulse. Acute infectious maladies, especially those of a malignant type and accompanied by high febrile movement, are very apt to cause parenchymatous degenerations in organs, prominent among which is granulo-fatty degeneration of the muscular fibres of the heart. This weakens very much the contractile power of these fibres. But early in malignant cases, probably before the muscular fibres are damaged, the contractile power of the heart is feeble from impaired innervation, the result of the general weakness. Hence this organ, when weakened by structural change and insufficiently stimulated through diminished innervation, may not fully empty itself during the systole, and consequently it becomes dilated. Dilatation of the heart and imperfect contraction of the auricular and ventricular walls are apt to result in the formation of clots in the cavities of the heart; and this appears to be the immediate cause of death in not a few instances. An ante-mortem clot occurring in any of the cavities of the heart necessarily seriously obstructs the circulation, unless it be of small size. Hence the dyspnoea, which may occur perhaps suddenly, and the change of pulse to one of marked feebleness and frequency. Large, firm white clots are most frequently found in the right cavities. They interlace with the chordæ tendineæ, lie even within the auriculo-ventricular opening, and send prolongations into the pulmonary artery and the cavæ. Associated with the white clots are dark, soft clots and fluid blood. The left cavities may be contracted and empty, or they may contain dark, soft clots or white ante-mortem clots. Clots in the left ventricle are sometimes prolonged into the aorta as far as the brachio-cephalic branches, while those in the left auricle may extend to the pulmonary veins. If dilatation of the heart be so great that clots form in its cavities, speedy death is probable. Sometimes a patient passes through scarlet fever and appears in a fair way to recover, when he succumbs to some exhausting sequel distinct from the heart, and at the autopsy the heart is found dilated and containing whitish clots, which are probably ante-mortem, and which hastened [p. 524]death by obstructing the circulation. Under such circumstances this state of the heart is attributable in great measure to the complication which has weakened its contractile power.

The following was a case in point. It occurred in the New York Foundling Asylum:

Case 7.—R. A., aged three years, had scarlet fever, beginning March 23, 1882. The symptoms were favorable at first, but serious complications and sequelæ occurred, which were fatal. The record of April 18th reads: "Appears well nourished, but is anæmic; has otorrhoea; no oedema; skin desquamating; dulness on percussion over upper third of right side of chest, anteriorly and posteriorly; mucous râles and rude breathing over same area; fine râles posteriorly over lower part of left side of chest; pulse 160, respiration 68, temperature 101.4°." April 20th, is feeble and takes nutriment with difficulty; tongue thickly coated; pulse 160, respiration 68, temperature 101.4°. April 26th, condition about the same as at last record, but he is evidently weaker; the lips are ulcerated and fauces still swollen. May 2d, cannot speak distinctly; a brownish, foul-smelling secretion lodges on the spoon used in depressing the tongue; left side of face swollen. On the following night eight convulsions occurred, attended by orthopnoea, and mucous râles in the chest from pulmonary oedema. Diarrhoea supervened and the patient died about midnight. Autopsy: Body moderately wasted and very white, several dark-blue spots on scalp and face from hemorrhages underneath; lips covered with dry crusts; brain of normal appearance; aperture of the larynx narrowed at the chink by infiltration and swelling of the tissues; surface of the vocal cords covered by a thin white film, apparently a fibrinous exudation; tracheal surface hyperæmic; about a drachm of straw-colored fluid in each pleural cavity; right lung wholly adherent by recent exudation of fibrin; left lung also largely adherent. A careful examination showed the presence of broncho-pneumonia in each lung, with considerable infiltration of the walls of the bronchi, and cylindrical dilatation of many of them; cavities of the heart dilated, so that this organ appears much enlarged, and its shape approaches the globular; its apex is rounded or obtuse; transverse diameter of the right ventricle, when its walls were open and drawn apart, was three and one-quarter inches; that of the left ventricle three and a half inches. Similar measurements of the heart of another child of about the same age, believed to be normal, were about one inch less in each direction. All the cavities contain white firm clots along with soft dark clots. Liver of normal size, pale; the outer surface and all cut surfaces are studded with nodules of the size of a pin's head, of a dull, opaque white color. These white spots, examined microscopically by Professor Delafield, are found to be neither tubercles nor gummy tumors, but to consist of polygonal cells, lying in the meshes of the capillary plexus of veins, which are perfectly preserved. He has not observed a similar case. The walls of the gall-bladder are one line or more in thickness, and the gall-duct is pervious. The microscope shows general hypertrophy of the gall-bladder and hypertrophy of its papillæ. The urine removed from the bladder was found to contain albumen and hyaline casts, and a microscopic examination showed a small amount of parenchymatous inflammation. The spleen was somewhat enlarged. Punctate congestion of small areas of [p. 525]gastric surface, no increase of mucus; mesenteric glands uniformly enlarged; jejunum, ileum, and colon exhibited a slightly increased vascularity. The immediate cause of death appeared to be imperfect contraction of the heart and the formation of clots in its cavities, due, apparently to the pleuro-pneumonia as much as, or more than, to the primary disease, scarlatina.[3]

[3] Dr. Goodhart (*Guy's Hospital Reports*, 1879) reports several interesting cases to confirm his opinion that acute dilatation of the heart is a not infrequent sequel of scarlatinous nephritis, and is the cause of death in some apparently inexplicable cases.

There can be little doubt that nephritis in its milder form is much more common than was formerly supposed. A few years since little attention was given by a large proportion of physicians to the state of the kidneys, and the urine was not examined till dropsy made its appearance, which only occurs in the more severe forms of nephritis and is a late symptom. It is now known that catarrh of the renal tubes frequently occurs in a mild form early in scarlet fever, without causing albuminuria, dropsy, or any notable symptom. It may produce a smoky color of the urine, and the appearance in it of granular epithelial cells, with an increase of mucus, but no albumen. With careful treatment and no exposure to cold, the renal catarrh abates with the decline of the scarlet fever. It is scarcely severe enough to merit the name desquamative, tubal, or parenchymatous nephritis, though it is a mild form of the same pathological state. Steiner states, as the result of many careful examinations of cases, that hyperæmia of the kidneys was always present in those who died early in scarlet fever, and that in a certain proportion of these cases catarrh of the renal tubules was present in addition to the congestion. Even in some who died on the second or third day he found cloudiness of the epithelium in the renal tubes, although the urine had not indicated such a change. The opinion has even been expressed that catarrh of the renal tubes is as common in scarlet fever as that of the bronchial tubes in measles; that is, that it is a uniform element in the disease; but this appears to be an exaggerated statement, for others have failed to find any evidence of renal catarrh in certain cases.

The nephritis which gives rise to symptoms, and therefore interests the practitioner, commonly begins in the declining period of scarlet fever or during the desquamative stage, and is in many instances plainly attributable to exposure to cold or to currents of air. It originates either during this period, or, if it have previously existed as a mild renal catarrh, it now becomes aggravated. Dropsy, which always attracts attention, does not occur till the nephritis has continued for some time.

Why nephritis, with the subsequent dropsy, so frequently occurs after scarlet fever is not fully understood. Rilliet and Barthez attribute to it disturbance of the function of the skin. The fact has long been observed that the kidneys become affected nearly if not quite as frequently after mild as after severe cases. Indeed, the chief danger in mild cases, when the patients are but a short time in bed and are soon allowed to go about, is from the nephritis. Chilling the surface and checking cutaneous transpiration appear to be the immediate cause of this inflammation in a considerable proportion of cases. Therefore, severe attacks of scarlet fever with abundant rash and desquamation, which require the patient to be kept in bed the proper time and in a warm room two or three [p. 526]weeks, appear to be less frequently followed by this renal disease than are milder cases which are more carelessly treated.

The most thorough and minute microscopic examination of the state of the kidneys in scarlet fever which have come to my notice were those by E. Klein, published in the *Lond. Path. Soc. Trans.*, and illustrated by microscopic drawings. It appears from these examinations that the changes in the kidneys are complex, among which we recognize both those of parenchymatous or desquamative nephritis and interstitial nephritis; but we would infer that the interstitial nephritis is mild in degree and quite subordinate, or else confined to portions of the organ, from the fact that so many permanently and fully recover. The following is a resumé of Klein's examinations in twenty-three cases: We conclude from these microscopic researches that the anatomical changes of both parenchymatous and interstitial nephritis are commonly present in greater or less degree in cases of scarlet fever. If they are mild or confined to portions of the kidneys, no symptoms occur; but if they are sufficient in extent or degree to impair the function of these organs, then symptoms, as albuminuria, diminution of urine, etc., appear.

1. Parenchymatous Nephritis, Proliferation of Nuclei, Hyaline Degeneration of Arterioles, the Glomerulo-Nephritis of Klebs.—Klein found increase of nuclei (probably epithelial) upon the glomeruli and hyaline degeneration of the intima of minute arteries, especially marked in the afferent arterioles of the Malpighian bodies. The intima of these vessels was in places so swollen as to resemble cylindrical or spindle-shaped hyaline masses, and cause narrowing of the lumina of the vessels in which this degeneration occurred. Klein observed in some specimens so great hyaline degeneration of the capillaries of the Malpighian bodies that circulation through them was obstructed. In the more advanced or protracted cases this hyaline substance in the glomeruli began to assume a fibrous appearance. Bowman's capsule was considerably thickened. This hyaline degeneration of the Malpighian bodies Klein discovered in the earliest cases which fell under his observation.

Also in the earliest cases the multiplication or germination of the nuclei of the muscular coat of the arterioles was observed, with a corresponding increase in the thickness of the walls of these vessels. This change in the muscular element was observed in the arterioles in different parts of the kidney, but it was most conspicuous in arterioles at their point of entrance into the Malpighian bodies; and it was distinctly observed in other arterioles, both in the cortex and in the base of the pyramids.

In the glandular portion of the kidneys other anatomical alterations were observed, indicating parenchymatous nephritis. There were swelling of the epithelial lining of the convoluted tubes; multiplication of nuclei of epithelial cells, especially in ascending tubules, which lay close to the afferent arterioles of Malpighian corpuscles; granular matter, and even blood, in the cavity of Bowman's capsule and in the convoluted tubes; cloudy swelling and granular disintegration of epithelium in some parts of the convoluted tubes; detachment of epithelium from the membrane of larger ducts of the pyramids in some cases. These parenchymatous changes are already known to the profession through the observations and writings of Dickinson, Fenwick, Johnson, John Simon, and others.

[p. 527]Klein, in commenting on the hyaline degeneration which he observed, states that Neelsen found the walls of the capillaries of the pia mater thickened, highly refractive, and of a lardaceous appearance in certain acute infectious maladies, as variola, typhoid fever, measles, and in one case of scarlet fever.[4] Usually, only a small portion of the capillaries were thus affected, most frequently at the point of division into branchlets. In a few instances Neelsen observed degeneration of arterioles extending a considerable distance, with fusion of the intima, media and adventitia, and chemical examination showed that the substance produced by this degeneration had similar properties to elastic tissue. Although the examinations by Neelsen relate to the pia mater, two of his observations are especially interesting—first, that the hyaline change affects chiefly vessels near their point of branching; and, secondly, that the hyaline substance is of the nature of elastic tissue, for in the kidney in scarlatinous nephritis the arterioles undergo the change in question chiefly near their point of branching into the capillaries of the glomerulus; and the intima being the part which undergoes the hyaline change, it is probable, in the opinion of Klein, that the same substance is produced by the degeneration in walls of the vessels of the kidney which Neelsen observed in the pia mater, and therefore that it is of the nature of elastic tissue.

[4] *Archiv der Heilkunde*, 1876.

This hyaline degeneration of the arterioles is also very marked in the spleen in scarlet fever; and in studying the minute anatomy of the intestines and spleen in typhoid fever Klein has found the same degeneration of the intima of the minute vessels. He believes that this hyaline change and the proliferation of muscle-nuclei which thus occur at an early period in scarlet fever in the renal vessels when the kidneys become affected are due to an irritating cause acting similarly to that in typhoid fever.

Klein calls attention to the interesting examinations of the scarlatinous kidney made by Klebs, who attributed the diminished urination and the uræmic poisoning in certain cases in which the kidneys do not exhibit any marked change to the naked eye, to what he designates glomerulo-nephritis. Klebs says: "In the post-mortem examination the kidneys are found slightly or not at all enlarged, firm, ... the parenchyma very hyperæmic. Only the glomeruli appear, on close inspection, pale like small white dots. The urinary tubes are often not changed at all. Occasionally the convoluted tubes are slightly cloudy. The microscopic examination shows that there are neither interstitial changes nor proliferation of epithelium, the so-called renal catarrh generally supposed to be present in these conditions on account of the absence of other perceptible derangements; and there seems, therefore, leaving out the glomeruli, the congestion of the kidneys alone to remain to account for the symptoms during life." But that mere congestion is insufficient to produce the symptoms appears from the fact that it does not produce them under other circumstances. Klebs finds, "on microscopic examination of the glomerulus, the whole space of the capsule filled with small somewhat angular nuclei, imbedded in a finely granular mass. The vessels of the glomerulus are almost completely covered by nuclear masses."

Klein, commenting on these examinations by Klebs, states that in all [p. 528]early cases which he examined he observed great abundance of nuclei of the glomeruli, but a condition like that described and figured by Klebs[5] he has seen in only a few glomeruli; for a general state of these bodies, as described by this observer, and such an excessive proliferation of the nuclei that the blood-vessels are completely compressed, was not seen in one of the twenty-three cases. Klein therefore questions whether the diminished urination and retention of urea in scarlet fever, when the kidneys do not exhibit any conspicuous catarrhal or other change, is due, unless in exceptional instances, to compression of the vessels of the glomeruli by nuclear germination, but believes, rather, that the obstructed circulation, and consequent diminished urinary excretion, is largely due to the changed state of the arterioles. Klein adds that perhaps undue contraction of the arterioles, through stimulation by the blood-irritant, may also be a factor in causing arrest of circulation in the Malpighian corpuscles. As regards cases that perished early, he found the parenchymatous change slight, so that a careful examination was required in order to detect cloudy swelling and granular degeneration.

[5] *Handbuch der Pathol.*, p. 646, fig. 72.

2. Interstitial Nephritis.—A second set of changes Klein observed in cases that died on about the ninth or tenth day. In such cases he found changes due to interstitial, in addition to those produced by parenchymatous, nephritis. Round cells, lymphoid cells, or whatever else they should be called, were seen in the connective tissue of the kidneys. In the kidneys of those that died at the end of the first week after the commencement of nephritis, infiltration with round cells was observed in the connective tissue around the large vascular trunks. At a later stage this infiltration had extended into the bases of the pyramids and into the cortex. The gradual increase in extent and intensity of this infiltration was so decided in the cases which Klein observed that he has no hesitation in concluding that when interstitial nephritis occurs it begins about the end of the first week, in the manner already stated—to wit, as a slight infiltration of the tissue around the large vascular trunks, and gradually extends, so that portions of the cortex, and rarely portions of the base of the pyramids, are changed into firm, pale, round-cell tissue, in which the original tubes of the cortex become lost.

The infiltration of the cortex with round cells, beginning at the roots of the interlobular vessels, spreads rapidly toward the capsule of the kidney, and laterally among the convoluted tubes around the Malpighian bodies.... In the course of this process considerable parts of the peripheral cortex, occasionally of a more or less distinctly cuneiform shape, with the base nearest the capsule of the kidney, become changed into whitish, firm, bloodless, cellular masses, in which Malpighian corpuscles and urinary tubes are only imperfectly recognized, being more or less degenerated. In some cases attended by this infiltration of the cortex Klein observed a more or less dense reticulation of fibres, especially around the interlobular arteries, containing in its meshes lymph-cells, chiefly uninuclear.

In a child of five years that died after a sickness of thirteen days Klein found evidence of intense interstitial inflammation, and also emboli, consisting of fibrin with a few cells, in the arteries, both in those of large size and in the arterioles, chiefly where they enter the Malpighian corpuscles. [p. 529]He states that in the specimens which he examined the more intense the degree of interstitial change, the greater was the enlargement of the kidneys, and the more distinct also were the evidences of parenchymatous nephritis in the urinary tubes, which either contained casts or were in the process of destruction. By being crowded with inflammatory products, especially cells, the Malpighian corpuscles were obliterated, undergoing fibrous degeneration. A very curious fact observed was the deposit of lime in the urinary tubes, first of the cortex, and then also of the pyramids, at an early stage of scarlet fever, when the kidneys otherwise showed only slight change. Several observers, as Biermer, Coats, and Wagner, have each described a case of scarlet fever with interstitial nephritis, which they consider unusual; but Klein has apparently demonstrated, as we have seen, by a large number of microscopic examinations, that this form of nephritis is common after the ninth or tenth day.

Nephritis, in proportion to its extent and gravity, is accompanied by languor, febrile movement, thirst, loss of appetite and strength. At first the patient experiences but slight pain in the head or elsewhere, and the quantity of urine is not notably diminished; but as the disease continues urination becomes less frequent and the urine more scanty. Albuminuria occurs, while the urea is only partially excreted, and therefore accumulates in the blood. If the nephritis be so severe or protracted that this principle accumulates to a certain extent, grave symptoms occur, as headache, vomiting, apathy or restlessness, and, more dangerous than all, eclampsia, which is not unusual in these cases. Microscopic examination of the urine shows the presence in this liquid of blood-corpuscles, granular epithelial cells, and hyaline or granular casts, or both. The specific gravity of the urine is diminished. But a large quantity of albumen in the urine may render the specific gravity as high or higher than in health.

The altered state of the blood soon gives rise to transudation of serum, first observed in most cases as an anasarca occurring in the feet and ankles. The oedema, if not checked by treatment or through mildness of the disease, extends over the limbs, scrotum, and sometimes upon the trunk. It is well if the dropsy remain limited to the subcutaneous connective tissue, but, unfortunately, it is apt to occur, if the nephritis continue, in and around the internal organs, producing, mentioned in the order of frequency, pulmonary oedema, effusion into the pleural and peritoneal cavities, the pericardium, the encephalon, and lastly into the connective tissue of the larynx, causing that very fatal complication, oedema of the glottis. Although this is the common order in which dropsies occur, exceptions are not infrequent. Even the anasarca may not be the first to appear, although in the vast majority of cases it has the precedence. Thus, Rilliet relates the case of a boy of five years who twenty days after the occurrence of scarlet fever, and six hours after the appearance of bloody and albuminous urine, had double hydrothorax, rapidly developed. As long as the hydrothorax continued no anasarca was observed, but as it declined anasarca appeared. Legendre cites a case in which oedema of the lungs occurred without anasarca or other dropsy. Occasionally, the anasarca and internal dropsies take place nearly simultaneously. The nephritis and consequent serous effusions usually appear within three weeks after scarlet fever ends, but cases occur in which the effusions are first observed as late as the fourth and fifth weeks. The patient may be [p. 530]considered to possess immunity from this sequel if he have reached the close of the fifth week after the abatement of scarlet fever without its occurrence.

The dropsy is usually acute, but it may assume the chronic form, since the nephritis which causes it, happily curable in most instances, may, if neglected, become chronic. Whether the dropsy in itself involve danger depends in great part on its location. Anasarca and ascites may exist a long time with little suffering or danger, but a small amount of serum in certain other localities causes alarming symptoms and speedy death. Oedema of the lungs, hydro-pericardium, oedema of the glottis, and intracranial effusions are always dangerous, and the last two are sometimes fatal within twenty-four to forty-eight hours. Oedema of the lungs has been fatal within twelve hours from the occurrence of the first symptoms of obstructed respiration.

Cerebral symptoms occurring during scarlatinous nephritis are probably sometimes due to the irritating effect of the retained urea on the nervous centre. In other cases the cause appears to be cerebral oedema or compression of the brain by effusion of serum within the ventricles and upon the surface of the brain. Headache, dull or severe, dilatation of the pupils or their oscillation in the same degree of light, vomiting with little apparent nausea, are common symptoms of scarlatinous nephritis when it has continued a few days, and the excretion of urea is so diminished that this substance begins to exert its poisonous effect on the system. Such symptoms are apt to be followed by somnolence, threatening coma, or by eclampsia, unless the patients are promptly and properly treated. In some patients that die of scarlatinous nephritis, death occurring in convulsions or coma, no appreciable lesions are observed within the cranium, unless more or less congestion, the fatal ending being attributable to the uræmia. In other instances we find an effusion of serum within the ventricles or upon the surface of the brain. Although the symptoms in scarlatinous nephritis and uræmia may appear very unfavorable, the prognosis is usually good under prompt and appropriate treatment. Thus severe convulsions and a degree of somnolence that bordered on coma may abate, and convalescence be fully established within a few days, and Rilliet and Barthez announce ten recoveries in thirteen patients affected with convulsions due to this renal affection.

ANATOMICAL CHARACTERS.—Scarlet fever being, as we have seen, a constitutional febrile disease of an ataxic nature, and accompanied by certain inflammations, necessarily affects the composition of the blood; but since this disease varies so greatly in type or severity, the state and appearance of this liquid also vary. At the autopsies of the more malignant cases we find the blood dark and fluid, with small, soft, and dark clots in the heart and large vessels. In other cases the clots are large, firm, and solid, as described in a preceding page. In malignant cases that end fatally Rilliet and Barthez state that both the large and small vessels of the cerebral meninges and the brain are found hyperæmic, but in a variable degree. In those who die in coma, preceded by delirium or convulsions, during the eruptive stage, the intracranial congestion is usually marked, with perhaps some transudation of serum, but without inflammatory lesions. The fibrin in scarlet fever remains in about normal proportion, except as it is increased by inflammatory [p. 531]complications. Andral found an increase in the proportion of blood-corpuscles from 127 to 136 parts in 1000.

The respiratory apparatus, except the Schneiderian membrane, is usually normal when no complications exist. Samuel Fenwick[6] made post-mortem examinations in sixteen cases of scarlet fever, and concludes from them that inflammation of the mucous membrane of the stomach and intestines occurs like that of the skin, followed by desquamation of the epithelial cells, like that of the epidermis. I have had the opportunity of examining the stomach and intestines of those who died of scarlet fever in the eruptive stage, and have not found any unusual hyperæmia of the gastro-intestinal surface, except when gastro-intestinal inflammation, usually indicated by diarrhoea, had occurred as a complication.

[6] *London Lancet*, July 23, 1864.

In some cases the abdominal organs exhibit changes which suggest a resemblance to typhoid fever. The spleen is enlarged and somewhat softened, and Peyer's patches and the solitary glands are thickened and prominent, but less in degree than in typhoid fever. The mesenteric glands also are in a state of hyperplasia. In other patients these parts appear normal.

Klein made microscopic examination of the liver in eight cases, and states that he found granular opaque swelling of liver-cells, and changes in the internal and middle coats of certain arteries similar to those observed in the kidneys, which have been described above. He also found evidences of interstitial inflammation, as an increase of round cells and connective tissue in the liver. He remarks also that he observed hyaline degeneration of the intima of arteries in the spleen. Rilliet and Barthez state that swelling and softening of the spleen are exceptional in scarlet fever, but are sufficiently common to merit attention. In post-mortem examinations which I have witnessed nothing noteworthy has appeared to the naked eye in the state of the liver, nor ordinarily in that of the spleen.

The efflorescence, though one of the anatomical characters, has perhaps been sufficiently described in the foregoing pages. It begins over the neck, chest, and groins as numerous reddish points not larger than a pin's head, closely crowded together, but with skin of normal color between. It is estimated that the aggregate efflorescence and aggregate normal skin over a given area are about equal. If the cutaneous circulation be active and the febrile movement be considerable these spots extend and coalesce, producing an efflorescence like erythema or like the hue of a boiled lobster, to which it has been likened. The efflorescence, less upon the face than upon the trunk, contrasts in this respect with that of measles, in which the rash is full in the face, often causing some swelling of the features. It is also less upon the palmar and plantar surfaces than elsewhere. It scarcely causes any perceptible elevation of the skin, but in certain localities, as upon the backs of the hands and upon the fore-arms, it communicates the sensation of slight roughness. The seat of the efflorescence is mainly in the superficial layers of the skin, but it is said that it sometimes has occurred upon a cicatrix, as that from a burn. In the robust and in favorable cases in which the circulation is active the rash has a scarlet hue, and when the cutaneous capillaries are emptied and the skin rendered pale by pressure with the [p. 532]fingers, the circulation immediately returns when the pressure is removed. In malignant cases the color is not scarlet, but dusky red, and so sluggish is the capillary circulation that the skin when pressed upon recovers the blood very slowly. In grave cases also extravasation of blood in minute points or transudation of its coloring matter is apt to occur in portions of the surface, when of course decolorization is not fully produced by pressure. In cases ending fatally, during the eruptive stage the efflorescence may entirely disappear in the cadaver, or it remains upon parts of the surface, especially depending portions. Desquamation is attributable to the exaggerated proliferation of the epidermis and the loosening of its attachment by the inflammation.

DIAGNOSIS.—In the commencement of scarlet fever, prior to the eruption, no symptoms or appearances exist which enable us to make a positive diagnosis. Positive statement in reference to the nature of the attack should be deferred, for the credit of the physician. Still, if a child with no appreciable local disease sufficient to cause the symptoms a few days after exposure to scarlet fever, or during an epidemic of this malady, be suddenly seized with fever, the pulse rising to 110, 120, or more, and the temperature to 102°, 103°, or 105°, scarlatina should be suspected. The diagnosis is rendered more certain at this early stage if vomiting occur, and especially if the fauces be red, for hyperæmia of the fauces, due to commencing pharyngitis, is one of the earliest and most constant of the local manifestations of scarlatina.

When the eruption has appeared the nature of the malady is in most instances apparent. The punctate character of the eruption before it becomes confluent, its occurrence within twenty-four hours after the fever begins over almost the entire surface, but its absence or scantiness upon the face, and especially around the mouth, serve to distinguish it from other diseases.

Scarlet fever and measles were long considered identical by the profession, and, though the ordinary forms of these maladies can be readily distinguished from each other, cases occur in which the differential diagnosis is attended by some difficulty. But there are differences in the symptoms and course of the two diseases which aid in discriminating one from the other. Measles begins with marked catarrhal symptoms, as if from a severe cold. Mild conjunctivitis, causing weak and watery eyes, coryza, and mild laryngo-bronchitis, with accompanying cough, precede the eruption three or four days and continue during the eruptive stage. The febrile movement in the prodromic stage of measles is remittent, the evening temperature being two or three degrees higher than that in the morning. Contrast this with the invasion of scarlet fever, in which the only catarrh is that of the buccal and faucial surfaces, and there is consequently little or no cough, and the febrile movement, ordinarily high in the beginning, is nearly uniform in the different hours of the day. The scarlatinous eruption appears, as we have seen, within twelve to twenty-four hours about the neck and upper part of the chest, and spreads over the body in a shorter time than that of measles, which appears on the third day. The rash of measles begins to fade at the close of the third or in the fourth day after its appearance, that of scarlet fever not till from the sixth to the eighth day. In nearly all cases of measles, even when the rash is confluent upon the face and a [p. 533]considerable part of the trunk, in consequence of the high febrile movement and vigorous cutaneous circulation, we observe the characteristic rubeolar eruption upon certain parts of the surface, as the extremities, which, in connection with the history, renders diagnosis certain.

Erythema resembles the scarlatinous eruption, but its duration is commonly shorter. It is limited to a part of the surface, and it is accompanied by much less febrile movement. The temperature in erythema does not usually rise above 100°, unless for a few hours, whereas in scarlet fever it continues considerably above 100° for several days. The scarlatinous efflorescence has also a brighter red or more scarlet hue than that of erythema, except in the more malignant cases, in which the severity of the symptoms renders the diagnosis clear. But an important aid in differentiating the one from the other of these diseases is the fact that in erythema there is, with few exceptions, no faucial inflammation, and in the few instances in which it is present it is slight and transient, fading within a day or two.

Scarlet fever is readily diagnosticated from diphtheria, although the affinity is close between these two maladies. The early appearance of the pseudo-membrane upon the fauces in diphtheria, its absence in scarlet fever, and the absence of any appearance resembling it until the fever has continued some days, and the characteristic efflorescence upon the skin in scarlet fever, render diagnosis easy. If scarlet fever have continued some days when first seen by the physician, the diphtheritic pseudo-membrane may be present as a complication, or the fauces may present an appearance like diphtheria from ulceration or sloughing and the presence of foul and offensive secretions, which produce a dark-grayish and fetid mass over the faucial surface. Under such circumstances the character of the disease is ascertained by the history of the case, and especially by the occurrence of the scarlatinous eruption. An erythema transient and limited to a part of the surface sometimes appears in the commencement of diphtheria, and at a later period, as a result of the toxæmia, points of a roseoloid appearance and irregular patches, often located upon the extremities. Both kinds of rash can be readily diagnosticated from that of scarlet fever, for the erythema, as has been stated, is transient and partial, and does not exhibit minute points of deeper injection, while the toxæmic rash differs in form and aspect from that of scarlet fever, and appears at a stage of the case when the scarlatinous efflorescence would have faded or begun to fade.

The efflorescence of rötheln sometimes closely resembles that of scarlet fever, though it is usually more like that of measles; but it is ordinarily accompanied by symptoms which are much milder than those of scarlet fever, and it begins to abate as early as the third, and disappears on the fourth, day. The eyes have a suffused appearance, the temperature may reach 102° or 103°, and the efflorescence may be as general over the body as that of scarlet fever, but there is not the aspect of serious indisposition, and the speedy abatement of the symptoms shows that the disease is not scarlet fever.

PROGNOSIS.—The prognosis depends on the form of scarlet fever, whether mild or severe, the strength of the patient, and the presence or absence of complications or sequelæ. The type of this disease is sometimes so mild throughout an epidemic or during a series of years that[p. 534]death seldom occurs, whatever the mode of treatment; but afterward the type changes, and the percentage of deaths increases and remains high till another mitigation in the type occurs.

Sydenham in the middle of the seventeenth century stated that scarlet fever, as he saw it in London, was so mild that it scarcely deserved the name of disease: "Vix nomen morbi merebatur." Morton some years later, and Huxham in the following century, had abundant reason to regret the change of type, and now throughout Great Britain scarlet fever is one of the most fatal and most dreaded of the diseases of childhood. In Dublin during the present century, prior to 1834, scarlet fever was uniformly mild, so that on one occasion of eighty patients in an institution all recovered. In 1834 the type of the disease totally changed and epidemics of unusual virulence occurred. The type frequently changes from mild to severe or severe to mild, not only in consecutive years, but in consecutive months. A few years since a distinguished physician of New York treated about fifty cases of scarlet fever in one of the institutions without a single death, but a few months later the type of the malady changed, and his own son was among those who perished from it. The prevailing type of the disease should therefore be considered in giving the prognosis when in the commencement of a case we are asked the probability as regards the termination.

Extensive statistics, including those collected by Murchison from various sources, show that in different epidemics the mortality may vary as much as from 3 per cent. (Eulenberg of Coblentz) to 19.3 per cent. (cases seen by myself in New York City in 1881-82, many of which were complicated by diphtheria), or even to 34 per cent. (epidemic in the Palatinate in 1868-69). The hospital statistics of Rilliet and Barthez gave 46 deaths in 87 cases, or about 53 per cent.

Observations have thus far failed to establish any connection in the atmospheric conditions of temperature or moisture and the type of scarlet fever. Grave as well as mild epidemics have occurred in all climates and seasons.

The mortality is nearly equal in the two sexes, but age bears a marked influence on the percentage of deaths. Comparatively few contract scarlet fever under the age of one year, and the period of its greatest mortality, since it is of its greatest frequency, is between the ages of one and six years. The following are statistics bearing on the relation of the age to the percentage of deaths:

		Under 1 year.	From the close of 1st till close of 5th year.	From the 5th to the 12th year.	
Flei	C	8	204	260	

shman,	ases				
	Deaths	6	88	51	
		1st to close of 6th year.	6th to 12th year.	From the 12th to 20th year.	
Kraus,	Cases	13	113	106	40
	Deaths	4	29	10	2
			7th to 16th year.		
Voit,	Cases	5	166	109	
	Deaths	1	24	10	
		1st to close of 5th year.	Over 5 years.		
Röset,	Cases	43	156	88	
	Deaths	16	31	3	
		Under 5 years.	5th to 10th year.	10th to 15th year.	Over 15 years.
Rusigger,	Cases	101	126	47	27
	Deaths	21	20	3	0

[p. 535] These statistics, which I believe correspond with the observations of others, show that although few cases occur in the first year, the percentage of deaths is large, and that a majority of the deaths occur under the age of six years. After the sixth year the greater the age the less the proportionate number of deaths.

Scarlet fever is liable to so many complications and sequelæ that a physician should not predict a certain favorable termination in the beginning, however mild and regular the symptoms may be. But a favorable result may be expected if the attack be mild, the efflorescence appear at the proper time and extend over the entire surface, the angina be moderate and accompanied by little or no cellulitis or adenitis, with pulse under 140, temperature not above 103°, and no marked nervous symptoms.

Whether the complications or sequelæ be dangerous depends upon their character. Rheumatism has never in my practice been dangerous, nor has it materially retarded convalescence, except when it affected the heart, causing pericarditis or endocarditis, when it involves great danger. Nephritis, if it be moderate, attended by little albuminuria and serous effusion, and by the occurrence of few renal casts in the urine, commonly ends favorably under judicious treatment, as we have already stated; but severe nephritis, with abundant albuminuria and casts and serous effusions, soon gives rise to alarming symptoms, and is the cause of death in a considerable number of instances. A similar remark is applicable to the angina, which occurs in all grades of severity. If it be attended by much cellulitis, with considerable ulceration or necrosis, the state is one of danger, in consequence of the difficulty in administering sufficient nutriment, of the diminished assimilation and of the loss of strength from the prolonged inflammatory fever, the septic poisoning, and the occasional hemorrhages. Complication by pharyngeal or nasal diphtheria, now so common where diphtheria is endemic, also greatly increases the danger.

Many cases, even when their course is normal and without complications, involve danger, and some are necessarily fatal, from the direct effect of the scarlatinous blood-poisoning. Such are grave or malignant forms of the disease which the experienced eye recognizes at a glance. Death often occurs rapidly from the toxæmia. Such cases are characterized by high temperature (105° or 106°), rapid pulse, a dusky-red hue of the surface from languid capillary circulation, pungent heat, frequent vomiting, diarrhoeal stools, a dry-brown tongue, and marked nervous symptoms, such as delirium, great restlessness, or stupor. Not a few in this form of scarlet fever take eclampsia, which is apt to be severe and repeated, and to end in fatal coma.

Other inflammatory complications and sequelæ, which have been described in the preceding pages, retard convalescence and jeopardize the life of the patient, such as empyema, endocarditis, pericarditis, and pneumonia. Otitis media is seldom immediately dangerous, although it may be painful and involve serious consequences, even a fatal meningitis, as has been stated above, after months or years of otorrhoea. Anomalous cases are believed to be, as a rule, more dangerous than such as are[p. 536]attended by an early and full efflorescence and have the usual symptoms.

TREATMENT.—PROPHYLAXIS. Since the discovery by Jenner of the prophylactic power of vaccination as regards small-pox, the attention of the profession has been frequently directed to the prevention of scarlet fever. Belladonna has been employed for this purpose by a class of practitioners who believe in the theory that an agent which produces symptoms similar to those of a disease is antagonistic to that disease, and therefore tends to prevent it, or, if it be present, to render it milder; and since this herb causes an efflorescence upon the skin and redness of the fauces, it was selected as the proper preventive and remedial agent for scarlet fever. Its use, however, for this purpose has been fruitless, and it is now nearly or quite discarded.

It is probable, from a considerable number of observations, that scarlet fever occasionally occurs in the domestic animals during epidemics of the disease in children. It is stated that Spinola observed it in the horse; that Heim saw a dog that occupied the same bed with a scarlatinous patient sicken with fever, which was followed by desquamation; that Letheby saw scarlatina in swine, and Kraus in young cattle. Prominent veterinary surgeons, as Williams of Great Britain, admit the occurrence of scarlatina in animals, and the hope has arisen that since small-pox is modified in cattle so as to afford us the vaccine virus, perhaps scarlet fever may also be modified by passing through one of the lower animals, so that a milder and less fatal form of the disease might be produced in man by inoculation from the animal. This theory, though it deserves investigation, is far from being established. It has not yet, so far as I am aware, been shown that scarlet fever is milder in any animal than in man, nor, if we admit that it is modified in the animal, is it certain that the disease could be returned to man in the modified form. In the *N.Y. Medical Record* for March 24, 1883, some experiments are detailed by S. W. Strickler of Orange, New Jersey. He cites the experiments of Caze and Feltz, who injected scarlatinal blood under the skin of sixty-six rabbits, and of these sixty-two died within eighteen hours to fourteen days, which indicated a highly poisonous state of the blood employed, either septic or scarlatinous, and certainly no mitigation of the virulence of the scarlet fever. Strickler obtained from Williams of Edinburgh nasal mucus from a horse supposed to have scarlatina, and with it inoculated twelve children, all of whom had sores at the point of inoculation, with redness of the skin around the sores, and in some instances swelling of the adjacent lymphatic glands. It is stated that the children thus inoculated did not contract scarlet fever subsequently when they were exposed to scarlatina. Obviously, there is a serious objection to such experiments upon children, so that they may not be repeated, but a movement has been made in one of the New York medical societies looking to the appointment of a competent committee to investigate them. Some of the prominent veterinary surgeons of this city do not attach much importance to the experiments thus far made, as they are in doubt whether the virus employed was that of the genuine disease.

It is a matter of great interest and importance, and one not yet elucidated, whether or to what extent disinfectant and antiseptic remedies administered internally prevent the occurrence of the infectious maladies[p. 537]in those who have been exposed, and aid in curing those who are sick with them. Sodium sulpho-carbolate, from which, by decomposition in the system, carbolic acid is supposed to be set free, has been used for this purpose. It is administered to adults in doses of ten to thirty grains, and to children in doses proportionate to their age. Declat has prepared a syrup of phenic (carbolic) acid as a preventive and curative agent in the infectious diseases. It is now employed by several of the New York physicians, but thus far the statistics of its use are not sufficient to determine its efficacy. It is a question whether the so-called antiseptics can, on account of their toxic properties, be used with safety in doses sufficiently large to be antidotal to the specific principle of any of the infectious maladies.

It is not my intention to recommend in this treatise any remedial agent that has not been fully tried and its efficacy determined; but from observations made by myself in nearly twenty families in which scarlet fever was prevailing, I am convinced that boracic acid (acidum boricum), an antiseptic recently introduced into our Pharmacopoeia, deserves trial as a preventive and antidote of scarlet fever as well as diphtheria. The good result in my practice from the use of this agent, which only extends over about six months, may be due to the present type of scarlet fever, but I have been surprised at the favorable progress of the cases which appeared very grave in the beginning, at the small mortality, and at the large proportion of well children exposed to scarlatinous cases that escaped infection, to whom this medicine was regularly administered. Boric (boracic) acid has been recently used by aurists with remarkable success in suppurating and granulating otitis media, and by oculists as an eye-wash. E. R. Squibbs says of it (*Ephemeris*, May, 1883): "A solution saturated at ordinary temperatures contains between 4 and 5 per cent.... It is a very bland and soothing application, whether applied in powder or solution, relieving irritation and reducing suppuration.... It has been administered internally in large doses without any disturbing effects." The preparation which I have employed is one found in the shops, with the name listerine, prepared by a Western pharmaceutical firm. It contains, according to the manufacturers, the "essential antiseptic constituents of thyme, eucalyptus, baptisia, gaultheria, and mentha arvensis," and also two grains of benzo-boracic acid in each drachm. The dose of listerine which I have employed for an adult is one teaspoonful, considerably diluted with cold water. A child of five years can take ten to fifteen drops every two to four hours. I call the attention of the profession to the use of boracic acid as an antidote to the scarlatinous poison, without sufficient experience to enable me to speak positively of its efficacy, but with the hope and expectation, from observing its apparent effects in seventeen families afflicted with scarlet fever, that it will be found a useful addition to our means of controlling this much-dreaded and fatal malady.

In the present state of our knowledge the most reliable and certain prophylaxis is the isolation of patient and nurses, and the thorough and judicious employment of disinfectants upon their persons and in the apartments. All furniture and articles not absolutely required should be removed from the sick room, and no one should be allowed to enter it except the medical attendant and nurses. Constant ventilation should be[p. 538]insisted on by lowering the upper and raising the lower sash of the window two or three inches in mild weather. Even in stormy weather sufficient ventilation can be obtained in this way without exposing the patient to currents of air, which should be avoided.

Since the exhalations from the body, the various excretions, and the epidermic cells shed so abundantly in the desquamative period contain the scarlatinous poison, measures should be employed to disinfect them, in so far as the comfort and well-being of the patient will allow. Vessels which receive the excretions should contain carbolic acid, chloride of lime or other disinfectant, and they should be immediately emptied and cleaned after use. By the frequent application of disinfecting washes to the nostrils and fauces the secretions from these surfaces are to a great extent deprived of their contagiousness. If otorrhoea occur, boracic acid, so serviceable in its treatment, acts as a disinfectant, but in addition the ear should be syringed with warm carbolized water, one drachm of carbolic acid to the pint of water, and this should be continued during convalescence, for cases occur which show that the discharge from the ear is probably the vehicle by which the virus is communicated. Even as late as the fourth week after the disappearance of the rash children in scarlet fever experience relief from inunction of the surface, and if carbolic acid be added to the substance which is employed for this purpose, and the inunction be made twice daily over the entire surface, contamination of the air through the exfoliations and exhalations from the skin is in great part prevented. The late William Budd of Bristol, England, was in the habit of recommending inunction of the surface twice daily with sweet oil, which answered the purpose of preventing dissemination of epidermic particles through the air; and we will presently see how successful were his precautionary measures.

A convalescent child should not be allowed to mingle with other children till three or four weeks have elapsed and desquamation has ceased; and all who are liable to take the malady should be excluded from the room in which a case has occurred for a longer period, and until it has been thoroughly disinfected by burning sulphur or other methods.

The New York Board of Health enforces the following excellent regulations to prevent the spread of scarlet fever as well as other acute infectious maladies:

"Care of Patients.—The patient should be placed in a separate room, and no person except the physician, nurse, or mother allowed to enter the room or to touch the bedding or clothing used in the sick-room until they have been thoroughly disinfected.

"Infected Articles.—All clothing, bedding, or other articles not absolutely necessary for the use of the patient should be removed from the sick room. Articles used about the patients, such as sheets, pillow-cases, blankets, or clothes, must not be removed from the sick room until they have been disinfected by placing them in a tub with the following disinfecting fluid; eight ounces of sulphate of zinc, one ounce of carbolic acid, three gallons of water. They should be soaked in this fluid for at least an hour, and then placed in boiling water for washing.

"A piece of muslin one foot square should be dipped in the same solution and suspended in the sick room constantly, and the same should be done in the hallway adjoining the sick room.

[p. 539]"All vessels used for receiving the discharges of patients should have some of the same disinfecting fluid constantly therein, and immediately after being used by the patient should be emptied and cleansed with boiling water. Water-closets and privies should also be disinfected daily with the same fluid or a solution of chloride of iron, one pound to a gallon of water, adding one or two ounces of carbolic acid.

"All straw beds should be burned.

"It is advised not to use handkerchiefs about the patients, but rather soft rags, for cleansing the nostrils and mouth, which should be immediately thereafter burned.

"The ceilings and side-walls of a sick-room after removal of the patient should be thoroughly cleaned and lime-washed, and the woodwork and floor thoroughly scrubbed with soap and water."

By such measures of prevention there can be no doubt that the number of cases of scarlet fever would be greatly reduced.

Budd for years recommended similar precautions in the families which he attended, and the following is his testimony in regard to the result: "The success of this method in my own hands has been very remarkable. For a period of nearly twenty years, during which I have employed it in a very wide field, I have never known the disease to spread beyond the sick-room in a single instance, and in very few instances within it. Time after time I have treated this fever in houses crowded from attic to basement with children and others, who have nevertheless escaped infection. The two elements in the method are separation on the one hand, and disinfection on the other."[7]

[7] *British Medical Journal,* Jan. 9, 1869.

HYGIENIC TREATMENT.—The room occupied by a scarlatinous patient should be commodious and sufficiently ventilated. Its temperature should be uniform at about 70° during the course of the fever. When the fever begins to abate and desquamation commences, a temperature of 72° to 75° is preferable, so that there is less danger that the surface may be chilled during unguarded moments, as at night, when the body may be accidentally uncovered, since sudden cooling of the surface at this time may cause nephritis or some other dangerous inflammation. Henoch does not believe in the theory that the nephritis is commonly produced by catching cold, but many observations show that those who are carefully protected from vicissitudes of temperature, who remain during convalescence in a warm room, and are protected by abundant clothing, more frequently escape this complication than such as are under no restraint of this kind and are carelessly exposed in times of changeable weather. Nevertheless, it is true that a certain proportion suffer from nephritis however judicious the after-treatment may be. The best hygienic management does not always prevent its occurrence. The patient should not, therefore, leave the house until four weeks after the beginning of the fever, and in inclement weather not till a longer time has elapsed. So long as desquamation is going on and the skin has not regained its normal function the patient should remain indoor, and when finally he is allowed to leave the house he should be warmly clothed.

THERAPEUTIC TREATMENT.—In order to treat scarlet fever successfully it is necessary to bear in mind that it is a self-limited disease, running for a certain time and through certain stages, and that it is not [p. 540]abbreviated by any known treatment. Therapeutic measures can only moderate its symptoms and render it milder. The severity of the disease is indicated by its symptoms, and the symptoms are to a certain extent under our control.

MILD CASES.—A patient with a temperature under 103°, and with only a moderate angina, does not require active treatment, but, however light the disease, he should always be in bed and in a room of uniform temperature, as stated above. Instances have come to my notice in the poor families of New York in which scarlet fever was not diagnosticated, and the patients were allowed to go about the house, and even in the open air, in the eruptive stage, till some severe complication or an aggravation of the type created alarm and medical advice was sought, when it appeared that a grave and dangerous condition had, through carelessness and ignorance, resulted from a mild and favorable form of the malady. The physician, when summoned to a case however mild, should never fail to take the temperature, note the pulse, inspect the fauces, and inquire in reference to the fecal and urinary evacuations, that he may detect early any unfavorable changes which may occur.

Since in all cases angina and more or less blood-deterioration are present, the following prescription will be found useful in mild as well as severe scarlet fever:

x. Potass. Chlorat. drach m ii;

Tr. Ferri Chloridi fl. drachm ii;

Syrupi fl. oz. iv. M.

S. Half a teaspoonful every hour to two hours to a child of three years; a teaspoonful to a child of six years.

Small doses of this medicine frequently administered act beneficially on the surface of the throat and tend to prevent the anæmia which is so common after scarlet fever. If the medicine be given gradually diluted with only a moderate amount of water, the effect is better on the inflamed fauces. Potassium chlorate is known to be an irritant to the kidneys in large doses, causing intense hyperæmia of these organs, with bloody urine or suppression of urine. The melancholy fate of Fountaine, who died from the effects of one ounce of this medicine, is known to the profession. I have seen a similar instance in a child. But doses of one to four grains, according to the age, can be administered with safety to children, so that half a drachm to a drachm and a half are taken in twenty-four hours. A quantity much exceeding this amount involves risk. In mild cases it is not necessary to treat the throat by topical measures, the above prescription producing sufficient local effect, but camphorated oil may be used externally. I ordinarily prescribe quinine in small doses for this form of scarlatina, as in the following formula:

x. Quiniæ Sulphat. gr. xvi;
    Ext. Glycyrrhizæ scrupl e ss;
    Syr. Pruni Virginianæ fl. oz. ii. M.

S. One teaspoonful every fourth hour to a child of three to five years, the potassium chlorate and iron mixture being administered twice between.

The treatment of scarlatina by antiseptic remedies will be considered hereafter.

[p. 541]The itching and dryness of the surface, which increase the discomfort of the patient in mild as well as severe scarlatina, are relieved by frequently anointing the whole body with vaseline, cold cream, or butter of cocoa. Carbolic acid is an efficient remedy for pruritus, while it is also a disinfectant. It may be used in the following formula:

x. Acidi Carbolici drac hm i;
    Vaselin e oz. iv. M.

S. To be applied over the entire surface.

In New York leaf lard has long been employed as an unguent over the entire surface in scarlet fever, and patients experience benefit from it. Alcohol and water or vinegar and water are sometimes employed for the same purpose. The linen should be changed every day and the bed thoroughly aired.

ORDINARY CASES AND CASES OF SEVERE TYPE.—A safe temperature in scarlet fever may be considered at or below 103°. If it rise above this, measures designed to abstract heat are very important—more important even in many cases than the medicinal agents which are commonly used to combat this disease. Since a high temperature retards assimilation, promotes deleterious tissue-change, and causes rapid emaciation and loss of strength, measures designed to reduce it are urgently needed. "The production of heat depends chiefly on oxidation of the constituents of the body" (Billroth). Therefore fever indicates an increase of the oxidation and a molecular disintegration above the healthy standard. Hence the augmentation of urea in the urine and the progressive emaciation and loss of weight which characterize the febrile state. Fever also diminishes the secretions by which food is digested and destroys the appetite, so that repair of the waste is insufficient. Moreover, a high temperature continuing for a time tends to produce degenerative changes, albuminous and fatty, in the tissues, the more rapidly the higher the temperature, so that the functions of organs are seriously impaired. Among the most dangerous of the tissue-changes is granulo-fatty degeneration of the muscular fibres of the heart. In dogs and rabbits that have perished from a high temperature artificially produced by experimenters granular clouding of the elementary tissues has been found after death.[8] A high temperature, therefore, in itself involves danger, and if it occur in an ataxic disease like scarlet fever, and be protracted, it greatly diminishes the chances of a favorable issue.

[8] See experiments by Mr. J. W. Legg, *Lond. Path. Soc. Trans.*, vol. xxiv., and others.

The temperature can be reduced without shock or injury to the child by the judicious use of cold water externally. The cold-water treatment is not necessary if the temperature be under 103°, though useful if judiciously employed by sponging when the temperature is at

102° or 103°; but if it rise above 103° it is required, and the more urgently the higher the temperature. The external use of cold water as an antipyretic in the febrile diseases is now almost universally recommended by physicians, but it still meets with opposition on the part of families, especially in the treatment of the exanthematic fevers, and the directions for its employment are therefore not apt to be fully carried out during the absence of the medical attendant. The old theory that the fevers require warmth and sweating has such a firm hold on the popular mind that some years longer will be required for its removal.

[p. 542]The modes of applying cold water recommended by cautious and experienced physicians are various. Von Ziemssen recommended that the patient be immersed in water at a temperature of 90°, and cool water be gradually added till the temperature fall to 77°. In a few minutes the patient is returned to his bed, his surface dried, and he is covered by the proper bed-clothes, when his temperature will probably be found reduced two or two and a half degrees. If the patient complain of chillness or his pulse be feeble, he should be immediately removed from the bath and stimulants administered, either whiskey or brandy, for if the extremities remain cool and the capillary circulation sluggish, the effect may be injurious, since some internal inflammation may arise to complicate the fever. Under such circumstances increased alcoholic stimulation is required.

The cold pack is also effectual for reducing the temperature. The patient is placed upon a mattrass protected by oil-cloth, and is covered by a sheet wrung out of water at a temperature of 70°. This is covered by one or two blankets. In half an hour he is returned to bed, and will be found to have a temperature two or three degrees less than that before the bath. Another method is to apply the sheet wrung out of water at 90°, and then reduce the temperature by adding water at a lower degree from a sprinkler. In most cases, however, I prefer to reduce the temperature by the constant application to the head of an india-rubber bag containing ice. The bag should be about one-third filled, so that it should fit over the head like a cap. At the same time, as a potent means of abstracting heat, at least when the temperature is at or above 104°, a similar application should be made by an elongated rubber bag lying over the neck and extending from ear to ear. Cold applied over the great vessels of the neck promptly abstracts heat from the blood, while it diminishes the pharyngitis, adenitis, and cellulitis; which is an important gain. At the same time, it is proper to sponge frequently the hands and arms with cool water. If the temperature with this treatment be not sufficiently reduced, one or two thicknesses of muslin frequently wrung out of ice-water should be placed along the arms and upon either side of the face. By such local measures, which are agreeable to the patient and without any shock or perturbing effect on the system, we can reduce the temperature two or three degrees. By adding alcohol or one of the alcoholic compounds to the water the popular objection to the use of cold is overcome.

Trousseau, in the treatment of sthenic cases attended by a high temperature, was in the habit of placing the patient naked in a bath-tub and directing three or four pailsful of water to be thrown over him in a space of time varying from one quarter of a minute to one minute, after which he was returned to bed and covered by the bed-clothes without being dried. Reaction immediately occurred, often with more or less perspiration. This treatment was repeated once or twice daily, according to the gravity of the symptoms. Trousseau, alluding to this treatment, says: "I have never administered it without deriving some benefit." But the application of cold water in a manner that does not excite or frighten the patient seems preferable. Henoch, having a large experience, gives the following advice in reference to the water treatment: "If the fever continue high and the apparently malignant [p. 543]symptoms described above develop, the head should be covered with an ice-bag, ... and the child placed in a lukewarm bath, not under 25° R. (88.25° F.). I decidedly oppose cooler baths, because in scarlatina, which presents a tendency to heart-failure, cold may produce an unexpected rapid collapse more than in any other affection. But I strongly recommend washing the entire body every three hours with a sponge dipped in cool water and vinegar."[9] In grave cases with a high temperature the application of cold should be sufficient to produce a decided reduction of heat, otherwise the full benefit from its use is not obtained. With proper stimulation and proper precautions prostration does not occur from the ice-bags to the head and neck and cool sponging of other parts, so long as the temperature does not fall below 102° or 103°. The danger alluded to by Henoch can only occur from the use of the pack or general bath, and the water treatment can be efficiently carried out and the temperature sufficiently reduced without resorting to these. Even Currie of Edinburgh, who first drew attention to the benefit from the cold-water treatment of scarlet fever in an age when the sweating treatment, and even the exclusion of cool and fresh air from the apartment, were deemed necessary, recommended cold affusion only in sthenic cases with full and strong pulse, and he mentions as a warning two cases with quick and feeble pulse and cool extremities in which death occurred immediately after the use of the water.

[9] *Diseases of Children.*

Sodium salicylate is in some instances a useful remedy for the reduction of heat in the infectious diseases. It seems to be more decidedly antipyretic than quinine in the febrile and inflammatory diseases, though somewhat depressing to the heart's action. James Couldrey writes to the *London Lancet* (Dec., 1882, p. 1064) that he has derived great benefit from its use in seven cases of scarlet fever. He administered it every two hours till ringing in the ears was produced, and afterward every four hours, prescribing one grain for each year in the age of the patient. It is, in my opinion, a proper remedy when the pulse is full and strong and the temperature is not sufficiently reduced by the cold-water treatment.

Aconite and veratrum viride reduce fever, but they are too depressing to be safely employed in grave scarlet fever, and their antipyretic effect is less than that of water. The use of digitalis might be suggested by the quick and feeble pulse in certain cases that are attended by high temperature, but the judgment of the profession is for the most part against its use in such cases. What Stillé and Maisch state of its employment in typhoid fever appears equally applicable to scarlet fever: "Even its advocates have not shown that it abridges the disease or lessens its mortality, while it is abundantly demonstrated to impair the digestion, reduce the strength, and even to occasion sudden death. The use of digitalis in other forms of fever is equally unsatisfactory, and justifies the judgment of Traube, that the true field of action for digitalis is not fever."

Quinine is the medicine which above all others has been heretofore most used, by almost common consent of the profession, to reduce the temperature in malignant scarlet fever, but its use for this purpose is, according to my observations, far from satisfactory. To obtain its[p. 544]antipyretic action it must be administered in large doses, and if any of the quinine salts in ordinary use be administered by the mouth in sufficient quantity, they are apt to be vomited. To a child of five years five grains should be administered twice daily by the mouth, or ten grains of a soluble salt, as the bisulphate, may be given per rectum, dissolved in a little warm water. Administered per rectum, it is frequently not retained unless held for a time by a napkin. A considerable proportion of the malignant cases are attended by not only irritability of the stomach, already alluded to, but by diarrhoea, so that quinine, if administered at all, should be employed hypodermically. The double salt of quinia and urea answers for this purpose, as it is very soluble in water and does not produce inflammation of the connective tissue. When the antipyretic doses of quinine are discontinued, this agent may be prescribed as a tonic in the doses recommended for the treatment of mild scarlet fever.

In severe cases with frequent and rapid pulse, in which ante-mortem heart-clots are apt to occur, the ammonium carbonate is often useful. It should be dissolved in water and given in milk, in as large doses as five grains every hour or second hour to a child of five years. It aids in producing stronger contraction of the cardiac muscular fibres, and thus diminishes the danger of the formation of thrombi. Ten-drop doses of the aromatic spirits of ammonia may be employed instead of the carbonate, given in sweetened water. It is especially useful if the stomach be irritable.

In severe cases attended by considerable angina and foul and offensive secretions upon the faucial surface an antiseptic, as boracic acid in small quantity, should be added to the potash and iron mixture recommended above. If no drink be allowed for a few minutes after the dose, so as not to wash it too soon from the fauces, the antiseptic effect is more certainly produced. Those old enough should be directed to hold the medicine for a moment like a gargle in the throat before swallowing it. I employ boracic acid by preference, as in the following formula:

℞.
Acid. Boracic.	drach m ss;
Potass. Chlorat.	drach m ii;
Tr. Ferri Chloridi	fl. drachm ii;
Glycerinæ Syrupi	aa. fl. oz. i;
Aquæ	fl. oz. ii. M.

S. Give one tablespoonful every two hours to a child of five years.

More minute directions will presently be given for the treatment of the pharyngitis when we speak of the complications.

Alcohol, whether administered in one of the stronger wines, as sherry, or in whisky or brandy, is a most useful remedy in scarlet fever, and is indeed indispensable in all grave cases which are attended by feeble capillary circulation and evidences of prostration. Milk is also the best vehicle for this agent. The wine-whey or milk-punch should be given every hour or second hour. In scarlet fever, as well as diphtheria, comparatively large doses are required, as a teaspoonful of the stimulant every hour or second hour for a child of five years.

During convalescence the hygienic treatment already described is important. Nutritious diet and a moderate amount of alcoholic [p. 545]stimulants are required, while the patient is kept indoors and protected from currents of air as long as desquamation is occurring. More or less anæmia is present in most convalescent patients, so that a mild tonic containing iron will aid in restoring the health. Elixir of calisaya-bark and iron; preparations of beef, iron, and wine, or the following prescription, will be found useful under such circumstances:

℞.
Ferri et Ammon. Citrat., Ammon. Carbonat.	aa. gr. xxiv;
Syrupi	fl. oz. i;
Aquæ	fl. oz. ii. M.

S. Dose, one or two teaspoonfuls, according to the age, every third hour.

ANTISEPTIC TREATMENT.—It is still to be determined whether or to what extent antiseptics, administered internally, antagonize and control the scarlatinous poison, and are therefore curative of scarlet fever. The most important agent of this class, carbolic acid, can only be employed in small doses, for a dose much exceeding a drop for a child, or even exceeding a fractional part of a drop for a young child, might produce poisonous symptoms. Carbolic acid is a cardiac and arterial sedative, and it appears to reduce temperature. Intra-uterine injections of carbolized water in the treatment of puerperal fever are known to reduce temperature, even when there is no septic matter in the uterus to be disinfected and washed away, as in a case related to me in which the fever proved to be due to measles. It is not improbable that the antipyretic action in patients of this class who have no septic substance within the uterus is due largely, if not mainly, to the absorption of carbolic acid from the uterine surface and its sedative action on the vascular system. Whether this agent, so highly extolled by Declat, and to which I have alluded in a preceding page, can be safely employed in doses large enough to be efficient and curative will be determined by future observations. The same remark is applicable to the sulphocarbolate of sodium, whose antiseptic action is supposed to be due, as already stated, to the liberation of carbolic acid in the system. Since boracic acid does not seem to have any deleterious action, this agent has been administered to most of my scarlatinous patients during the last year, in addition to the older and better known remedies, and with a very small percentage of deaths. What may be the result in a more severe type of the disease remains to be seen.

TREATMENT OF COMPLICATIONS AND SEQUELÆ.—Local measures designed to diminish or cure the pharyngitis are important in all but the mildest cases. They are more especially required in the anginose variety and in those not infrequent cases in which diphtheria complicates scarlatina. Formerly it was necessary, in making applications to the fauces, to employ the brush or probang for those too young to use the gargle, but hand-atomizers, as Richardson's or Delano's, which are now in common use, afford a quick and easy method for making such applications. Six or eight compressions of the bulb of a good atomizer are sufficient to cover the fauces with the spray. Those hand-atomizers in the shops which have slender metallic points are apt to prick the buccal surface and cause bleeding if the child resist and toss the head. To prevent this, I am in the habit of directing india-rubber tubing to be drawn over the point in such a way as not to obstruct its action. The following will be found useful mixtures for the atomizer: For ordinary cases,

[p. 546]

x. Acidi Carbolici drachm ss, vel. Acid. Boracic. drachm ii;

Potass. Chlorat. drachm ii;

Glycerinæ fl. oz. ii;

Aquæ fl. oz. vi. M.

If the surface of the throat be covered by foul secretions,

x. Acidi Carbolici drachm ss;

Potass. Chlorat. drachm ii;

Glycerinæ fl. oz. j;

Aquæ Calcis fl. oz. vii. M.

Or else,

x. Tinc. Ferri Chloridi fl. oz. ss;

Acidi Sulphurosi fl. drachm ii;

Potass. Chlorat. drachm ii;

Glycerinæ fl. oz. i;

Aquæ q. s. ad. fl. oz. vi. M.

If diphtheritic exudation complicate the scarlatinous angina, or the surface of the throat in consequence of ulceration or necrosis present an appearance like that in diphtheria when the exudation begins to soften, being foul, jagged, of a dirty brown appearance from dead matter and fetid secretions, the following should be prescribed for use in the atomizer:

℞. Acidi Carbolici drachm i, vel. Acidi Boracici drachm iii;
Liq. Potassæ fl. drachm i;
Potass. Chlorat. drachm ii;
Glycerinæ fl. oz. ii;
Aquæ Calcis fl. oz. viii. M.

Liquor potassæ, although a very efficient solvent of pseudo-membranes, is too irritating for use in the atomizer unless largely diluted. One part to eighty, as in the above mixture, will not be found too concentrated. The following powder, used every third hour through the insufflator, is also useful in cases of diphtheritic exudation:

℞. Acidi Salicylici drachm ii;
Bismuth. Subnitrat. oz. ii. M.

To be used every third hour. It is the favorite remedy of some of the prominent New York physicians in the local treatment of diphtheria.

The following mixture is also beneficial for local treatment when the faucial surface is foul and offensive from the exudations and secretions. It should be applied by a large camel's-hair pencil every three to six hours:

℞. Acidi Carbolici gtt. x;
Liq. Ferri Subsulphatis fl. drachm ii;
Glycerinæ fl. oz. i. M.

In all cases of scarlatinous pharyngitis sufficiently severe to require special treatment, cool applications should be made over the neck from ear to ear, as by two thicknesses of muslin frequently squeezed out of cold water, or by the elongated india-rubber bag already recommended in our remarks relating to methods to reduce temperature.

In the first days of scarlet fever the coryza is slight, and no discharge from the nostrils occurs, so that no local treatment is required; but before the termination of the malady, in cases of ordinary gravity, a nasal discharge usually supervenes, producing more or less redness and [p. 547]excoriating the upper lip. Moreover, in localities where diphtheria occurs, if this malady complicate scarlet fever, it is apt to affect the nostrils at the same time that the fauces are invaded. These conditions require local treatment of the nares. It should be remembered that the Schneiderian membrane is midway in sensitiveness, as it is in location, between the conjunctival and buccal surfaces, and is readily irritated by strong applications. Medicinal applications made to it must be much milder than those which the fauces tolerate. They should always be applied warm, and a teaspoonful of any mixture properly employed is sufficient for each nostril at one sitting. The applications should usually be made every two or four hours, according to the gravity of the case and the amount of discharge. The best instrument for this purpose is a small syringe of glass or brass with curved neck and bulbous tip. The child's head should be thrown back and the piston depressed rapidly, so as to thoroughly wash out the nasal cavity. The application can also be made through an atomizer with a rounded tip or a tip covered by rubber tubing. The following is a useful prescription:

Acidi dra

x.	Carbolici	chm ss;
	Sodii	dra
	Chloridi	chm ii;
	Aquæ	Oj.

The substitution of 2 or 3 drachms of boracic acid in place of the carbolic acid makes a nicer preparation. If the diphtheritic pseudo-membrane appear in the nares, the officinal lime-water, injected every hour or second hour, is beneficial in consequence of its solvent action on pseudo-membranes.

It is evident, from what has been stated above, that the condition of the ear should be closely observed in and after scarlet fever. If the patient have earache, considerable relief may be obtained in the commencement by dropping a few drops of laudanum and sweet oil into the ear and covering it by some hot application, either dry or moist, which will retain the heat. A light bag containing common table-salt, heated, or dry and hot chamomile flowers will also answer the purpose. Water as hot as can be well tolerated dropped into the ear or allowed to trickle from a fountain syringe, so as to fill the ear, is also very beneficial in allaying the pain. If a few drops of laudanum be added it is more useful. If the pain be not quickly relieved, a leech should be applied at the base of the tragus. O. D. Pomeroy, an experienced aurist of New York, says: "Leeching employed at the right time rarely fails to subdue the pain and inflammation. The posterior face of the tragus is ordinarily the best place for applying the leech, but it may be applied in front of the ear or behind, wherever the tenderness on pressure is greatest. In my opinion, paracentesis may frequently be rendered unnecessary by the timely use of one or two leeches applied to the meatus."

If the otitis continue, as shown by pain in the ear, of which children old enough to speak bitterly complain, and which causes those too young to speak to press their fingers into or against their ears, this inflammation should not be neglected, as it may involve serious consequences. Multitudes of children have had permanent impairment or even loss of hearing, with caries or necrosis of the walls of the middle ear and of the mastoid cells, which might have been prevented by prompt and skilful[p. 548]management of the ear in the early stage of the inflammation. If, therefore, the otitis continue without mitigation of pain after the above measures have been employed, paracentesis of the drumhead is probably required. The following directions for performing this operation, which will be useful to country practitioners who may not be able to obtain the assistance of a specialist, are from the pen of Pomeroy: "The forehead mirror should be worn, in order to leave the hands free to operate by either artificial or day light. A good-sized speculum is introduced into the meatus. Then an ordinary broad needle, about one line in diameter, with a shank of about two inches, such as oculists use for puncturing the cornea, should be held between the thumb and fingers, lightly pressed, so as not to dull delicate tactile sensibility. The part being well under light, the most bulging portion of the membrane should be lightly and quickly punctured with a very slight amount of force. The posterior and superior portion of the membrane is most likely to bulge. The chordæ tympani nerve ordinarily lies too high up to be wounded. The ossicles are avoided by selecting a posterior portion of the membrane. After puncture the ear should be inflated by an ear-bag whose nozzle is inserted into a nostril, both nostrils being closed, so as to force the fluid from the tympanum. The puncture may need to be repeated at intervals of a day or two, provided that the pain and bulging return."

Albert H. Buck of New York, in a highly instructive paper read before the International Medical Congress in 1876, writes as follows of paracentesis of the membrana tympani in scarlatinous otitis: "In this one slight operation, which in itself is neither dangerous nor very painful, lies the power to prevent the whole train of disagreeable and dangerous symptoms." Buck relates an instructive example: The age of the patient was three years, and the earache had been complained of only about twenty-four hours. "Toward morning," says he, "I was sent for, as the pain had become constant.... An examination with the speculum and reflected light showed an oedematous and bulging membrana tympani (posterior half), the neighboring parts being very red, though as yet but little swollen. In the most prominent portion of the membrane I made an incision scarcely three millimetres (one-tenth inch) in length, and involving simply the different layers of the membrana tympani. This was almost immediately followed by a watery discharge (without the aid of inflation), which ran down over the child's cheek. At the end of three or four minutes the child had ceased crying, and in less than a quarter of an hour she was fast asleep. At first, the discharge was very abundant and mainly watery in character, but it steadily diminished in quantity and became thicker, till finally, on the fourth day, it ceased altogether. On the tenth day the most careful examination of the ear could not detect any trace of either the inflammation or the artificial opening." The ear had probably been saved from ulceration of the drum membrane, long-continued suppurative otitis, and perhaps from permanent impairment of hearing.

When an opening has been made in the membrana tympani either by incision or ulceration, it is advisable in some instances to inflate the tympanum by Politzer's method, which has been alluded to above. The nozzle of an india-rubber bag, with a flexible tube attached, is introduced into the nostril on the affected side, and both nostrils are compressed[p. 549]against it. The patient fills his mouth with water, which he swallows at a given signal, as after the words one, two, three, spoken by the operator. During the act of swallowing, which opens the Eustachian tube, the rubber bag is forcibly compressed, which forces the air along the tube into the middle ear and facilitates the escape of the pent-up secretions in the tympanic cavity.

If the otitis have continued unchecked by treatment until the secretions within it, after days and nights of suffering, have escaped by ulceration through the drumhead, the opportunity for prompt and certain cure is passed. Still, the patient under these circumstances may quickly recover, or there may be the other alternative described above, in which the ear is badly damaged and chronic inflammation established in the walls of the tympanum, giving rise to an offensive otorrhoea. In this state of the ear internal remedies are indicated, such as surgeons employ in suppurative inflammations of bone occurring in other parts of the system. Cod-liver oil and iodide of iron are required, especially by patients of strumous diathesis, the object being to promote a more healthy state of system, so as to prevent extension of the inflammation and facilitate the healing process. Carbolized solutions, as the following, syringed warm into the ear in which otorrhoea is occurring, are useful in promoting cleanliness and increasing the comfort of the patient:

x. Acidi Carbolici drach m ss;
Glycerinæ fl. oz. ii;
Aquæ fl. oz. iv. M.

But recently a much more effectual curative agent for local treatment has been discovered in boracic acid, by the use of which the discharge more quickly diminishes and the condition of the ear more certainly and rapidly improves than by the use of the carbolized mixtures. When the inflammation is recent and the ear sensitive and painful, the following prescription should be used:

x. Acidi Boracici drach m iiss;
Morphiæ Sulphat. gr. i;
Glycerinæ
Aquæ fl. oz.
aa. i. M.

S. Drop one to three drops into the ear three times daily.

If the acute stage of the otitis have passed, with fever and pain, and no tenderness be present on pressure, the following prescription, which causes too much pain in the acute stage, will be found useful to check the inflammation and otorrhoea and restore a healthy state to the granulating surface:

℞. Acidi Boracici drac hm iiss;
Alcohol.
Aquæ aa. fl. oz. i.

S. Drop one to three drops into the ear three times daily.

The beneficial effects observed from the use of boracic acid in aural surgery have given it nearly the same position as a curative agent to diseases of the ear which atropine holds to diseases of the eye. Recently, aurists are employing finely-triturated powder of boracic acid dusted into the ear. The patient lies upon the side with the affected ear uppermost. The ear is thoroughly cleaned by syringing with tepid water, and by means of a little scoop made of stiff paper or pasteboard or the segment [p. 550]of quill as much of the powder is introduced into the ear as would cover a five-cent silver piece. By working the ear it descends to the drumhead. I can bear witness to its efficacy in the otorrhoea of children when it is used in this manner three times daily.

The following astringent has also been employed with good results for the otorrhoea resulting from scarlet fever as well as from other causes:

℞. Zinci Sulphatis,
Aluminis aa. gr. v;
Aquæ fl. oz. i. M.

A few drops of this should be dropped into the ear, or, if the ear be sensitive and painful, five drops should be added to a teaspoonful of warm water and dropped or syringed into the ear.

But in recent times aurists have discovered a remedy superior to the above in iodoform, the action of which is safe and efficient for protracted otorrhoea with granulations, and it is superseding to a great extent the agents heretofore used in the treatment of this disease. The ear should first be thoroughly cleaned by syringing with warm water and dried, and iodoform, to which a little balsam of Peru is added to cover the disagreeable odor, should be pressed down to the bottom of the auditory canal by any convenient instrument. It is anodyne, astringent, and disinfectant, and should be employed in a dry state in considerable quantity.

The sequelæ of otitis media, such as granulations sprouting out from the drumhead, some of which may be of large size and are known as polypi, may require treatment by the aurist. A polypus may sometimes be removal by the forceps or better by the snare. Polypi not large and favorably located can sometimes be cured by an astringent powder, as iodoform, sulphate of zinc, or alum, or by applying the liquid subsulphate of iron. The otitis externa produced by the irritating discharge which flows from the middle ear soon disappears when the flow ceases.

The renal affection, which, as we have seen, so often commences in the declining period of scarlet fever or during convalescence in mild as well as severe cases, is frequently more dangerous than the primary disease. It largely increases the percentage of deaths. A clear appreciation of its therapeutic requirements is important, since by judicious treatment many recover who would inevitably be sacrificed by improper measures. The family should be informed that the danger from scarlet fever does not cease with the decline of the eruption, and that the kidneys may become seriously affected by too early exposure of the patient to currents of air or sudden changes of temperature, by which cutaneous transpiration is checked. He should therefore be kept indoors in a comfortable and uniform temperature three or four weeks after the termination of the fever, until desquamation has entirely ceased and the new epiderm is sufficiently thick and firm to protect the surface. During the changeable temperature of the autumnal, winter, and spring months even longer confinement at home may be advisable.

The nephritis and consequent albuminuria antedate by some days the occurrence of dropsy, and a physician should never discharge a scarlatinous patient without one or more examinations of his urine. When his visits cease the nurse should be instructed to make the examinations by heat and nitric acid during the ensuing month, and if any evidence, however slight, appear that the kidneys are involved, he should be notified, [p. 551]in order that appropriate treatment may be immediately commenced. Early and correct treatment of the nephritis is attended by much better results than delayed treatment, and many more patients are doubtless now saved than in former times, when little attention was given to the state of the kidneys until dropsy or other prominent symptoms appeared. I have found no mother or nurse so ignorant that she could not properly employ the test of nitric acid and heat, and, if she be solicitous for the welfare of the child, she will not hesitate to carry out the directions and immediately notify the physician if the tests employed produce the least cloudiness or turbidity of the urine.

The patient as soon as nephritis commences, as shown by the state of the urine, should be put to bed in a room of warm and equable temperature (72° to 75° F.). His diet should be liquid, consisting of milk, farinaceous food, and a moderate quantity of animal broths. He may drink liquids freely, especially water not too cool, to which spiritus ætheris nitrosi is added. If he be prostrated by the primary disease, alcoholic stimulants should be allowed.

The indications are to relieve the hyperæmic kidneys by diaphoresis and purgation. To produce the former the patient should be immersed in a warm bath at about the temperature of the body (98° to 100°), in which, if he be quiet and comfortable, he should remain from fifteen to twenty minutes, but if restless and frightened by the water a less time, after which he should be placed in a warm bed and well covered by blankets. If perspiration result, the bath has been useful, and it may be employed in grave cases two or three times daily. If perspiration do not result, it may be produced by surrounding the body either by hot dry or moist air. Hot dry air may be produced by burning alcohol in a thin layer upon a plate under a chair upon which the patient sits while he is surrounded by a blanket, or he may be covered in bed and the hot air introduced under the bed-clothes. In New York a convenient apparatus is used for this purpose, consisting of a small sheet-iron pipe enclosed in a small box of the same material. The box is in the form of a trunk, with a handle for convenience in carrying, and the lower end of the pipe, which extends nearly to the floor, contains an alcohol lamp. Hot moist air may be produced by placing against the patient bottles of hot water surrounded by towels wrung out of water. The steam arising from them and enveloping the body and limbs produces a prompt sudorific effect. There is in use in this city, in the treatment of these and similar cases requiring diaphoresis, a convenient apparatus for generating steam. It consists of a cylinder pierced with holes for the admission of air and containing a spirit lamp, over which is a pan or pail holding a little water. The patient, nearly naked, is placed in a chair with the apparatus underneath, and is covered by a blanket, so that the steam surrounds the body. This gives rise to free perspiration, which continues after the patient is placed in bed. This treatment should be repeated one or more times daily, according to the gravity of the case.

The sudorific effect of the treatment by external warmth described above should be aided by employing diaphoretics. Those which have been most used are the acetates of ammonium and potassium, the bitartrate and citrate of potassium, and spiritus ætheris nitrosi. If employed when the surface is cool, they act rather as diuretics than diaphoretics. [p. 552]These agents, being simple in their action and without deleterious effects, may be given frequently and in large proportionate doses for the age.

But lately a diaphoretic which far surpasses these in efficiency has been discovered in pilocarpine, the active principle of jaborandi. Being soluble in water and tasteless, it is easily administered, and is retained when, on account of the uræmic poisoning present in scarlatinous nephritis, the stomach is irritable and other medicines, as digitalis, are rejected. Ether may be employed with it, or the amount of alcoholic stimulant may be increased at the time of its exhibition in order to guard against any depressing effect. To a child of two years one-fortieth to one-twentieth of a grain may be given every six hours by the mouth. It may also be employed hypodermically, as one-twentieth of a grain to a child of five years. It has both a diaphoretic and diuretic action, while it stimulates both the salivary and mucous secretions. According to one observer, an adult when fully under the influence of pilocarpine secretes from one pint to one quart of saliva within two hours, and Leyden reports a case of diphtheritic nephritis in which the quantity of urine rose from half a pint to five pints daily. But its most prompt and certain action is upon the sweat-glands. Hirschfelder speaks of its beneficial action in relieving various forms of dropsy, and adds: "In one morbid condition of the kidney, however, jaborandi is the remedy par excellence, and that is the acute parenchymatous nephritis which frequently follows scarlatina.... This disease heals spontaneously if the danger that threatens life from reduction of the urine and from the effusions of fluid into the cavities of the body be averted. In this disease jaborandi works wonders." I have also found it an invaluable agent when the older remedies failed and death seemed imminent. The following cases, in which the beneficial action of this agent was apparent, occurred in my practice:

Case 8.—G——, male, aged five years and six months, sickened with scarlet fever on June 2, 1882. It began with vomiting, and was attended by a degree of febrile movement which indicated an attack of rather more than the average gravity. The fauces at one time exhibited a slight exudation like that of diphtheria. In the declining stage of the malady rheumatic pain and tenderness occurred in the wrist and finger-joints, but not in those of the lower extremities. The case, however, progressed favorably, and during the convalescence my attendance ceased. On June 24th my attention was again called to the child, when the urine was found to be scanty and very albuminous. External measures, such as are described in the foregoing pages, were employed, and the infusion of digitalis with potassium acetate ordered to be given every three hours, but this medicine was for the most part vomited. The bowels were kept open by jalap and the potassium bitartrate. The urine, however, continued scanty, and on June 28th severe convulsions occurred. At this time the quantity of urine was only fl. oz. ij in twenty-four hours. The pulse in the convulsions was quick and feeble, the skin very hot, and the axillary temperature 103°. The eclampsia continued one hour, and were controlled by large and repeated doses of bromide of potassium, aided by clysters of five grains of hydrate of chloral in water. Muriate of pilocarpine was now directed to be given in doses of one-thirty-second of a grain every three hours, dissolved in cold water. This agent was not vomited, and it must have been given by the parents in their fright and [p. 553]anxiety in larger or more frequent doses than were directed, for on July 1st the bottle containing one grain was empty. Free diaphoresis resulted from the pilocarpine, and the quantity of urine was increased. The mother stated that the child had taken only two doses, or one-sixteenth of a grain, of pilocarpine when the diuretic effect was apparent and free diaphoresis also occurred. She also stated subsequently that the quantity of urine was larger when the pilocarpine was administered every third hour than when given at a longer interval. A flaxseed poultice on which mustard was dusted was also applied over the kidneys. On June 29th the pulse was 96, temperature 100.5°; occasional convulsive attacks occurred, which were readily controlled by enemata of hydrate of chloral. On June 30th the symptoms were all better; no more attacks of eclampsia had occurred, and the urine was more abundant and less albuminous. The mother remarked that the new medicine (pilocarpine) had settled the stomach and increased the urine. The patient continued to improve, and on July 4th the record states: "Now takes the pilocarpine, gr. 1/32, every six hours; passes urine freely since yesterday; has not vomited since he began to take the pilocarpine; pulse 106, axillary temperature 99°; is playful and takes milk freely, nearly three quarts in twenty-four hours, with some farinaceous food. Digitalis with potassium acetate is also given in occasional doses." July 6th, pulse 92, temperature 99°; perspires much, and urine nearly normal in quantity and character.

Case 9.—Mary S———, aged five years, on Dec. 22, 1882, presented the symptoms of severe nephritis. Her brother had scarlet fever two weeks previously, and she had sore throat at about the same time, but without efflorescence; pulse 98, temperature 98.5°; her urine highly albuminous, and reduced to fl. oz. iv in twenty-four hours; bowels constipated. Ordered a single dose of

	Hydrarg.	
x.	Chlor. Mitis	gr. iii;
	Resin.	gr.
	Podophylli	1/6. M.

The muriate of pilocarpine was also ordered, gr. 1/20, but the patient vomited soon after taking it. Another dose was retained, and was followed by considerable perspiration. Dec. 23d, had one stool from the powder of yesterday. Has taken five doses of pilocarpine, but vomited after three of them. The last dose was administered at 10 P.M., and the mother says she "sweat fearfully" during the night. The patient was kept warm in bed; stimulating poultices of mustard and flaxseed, one to sixteen, were constantly in use over the kidneys, and the pilocarpine was administered three or four times a day. The record for Dec. 26 states: "Took the pilocarpine four times since yesterday morning, and each dose is followed by perspiration lasting from one to one and a half hours; quantity of urine, from fl. oz. vj to fl. oz. viij daily; vomited twice yesterday, not to-day; pulse 104, temperature 97.75°; complains of frontal headache; bowels regular; has considerable salivation. The patient is warm in bed, and the flaxseed and mustard poultice over the kidneys is continued." Dec. 28th, specific gravity of urine 1019; urine still quite albuminous, and containing blood-corpuscles and granular casts, also crystals of oxalate of lime. Dec. 30th, takes gr. 1/20 pilocarpine twice daily, and occasional doses of infusion of digitalis; urine more abundant; its specific gravity 1014, slightly albuminous, and containing [p. 554]very few granular casts and blood-corpuscles; has lost its smoky appearance; reaction alkaline; perspiration slight; patient convalescent.

In another instance, a child of five years, from three to four weeks after scarlet fever was noticed to have anasarca of the face and extremities, with scanty and albuminous urine. One-thirty-second of a grain of muriate of pilocarpine was administered every six hours without the desired sudorific effect. It was then administered every four hours, with an increase of perspiration and urination, so that the nephritic symptoms were relieved and the patient apparently out of danger within three or four days.

In a fourth patient, a girl of three years, having scarlatinous nephritis, with symptoms very similar to those in the last case, the administration of one-twentieth grain doses of pilocarpine in conjunction with the hot-air bath, was followed by increased perspiration and urination, and progressive and rather rapid convalescence. This child had been taking bichloride of mercury in one-fiftieth grain doses, prescribed by a homoeopathic physician, without appreciable benefit. It had been for the most part vomited.

Given, as in the above cases, in moderate doses and with sufficient interval, pilocarpine has never in my practice had any deleterious effect, and I regard it as a very important addition to the remedies for the relief of scarlatinous nephritis. It is apparently the most useful and important diaphoretic for this disease which we possess.

Cathartics, especially those of a hydragogue nature, are also very beneficial. Their action is more certain than that of most diaphoretics and diuretics, and their employment is imperatively required in severe or dangerous cases in which it is necessary to remove as soon as possible the serum or urea which endangers life. Young children or those with delicate stomach, and those much enfeebled by the primary disease, may take magnesia, either the citrate or the calcined. A good cathartic for ordinary cases is a mixture of jalap and potassium bitartrate, the pulvis jalapæ compositus, consisting of one part of jalap and two of cream of tartar. Ten grains of the mixture may be given to a child of five years, and repeated according to circumstances. Its effect is increased by dissolving a teaspoonful of potassium bitartrate in a gobletful of water, and allowing the patient to drink from it. The following is a good cathartic in some instances, especially if the stomach be irritable, so that the more bulky and nauseating cathartics are rejected. Care should be taken to obtain a good article, as some of the podophyllin of the shops is not reliable:

℞. Resinæ Podophylli gr. j;
Sacchari j. scruple M.
Ft. in chart. No. v.—x.

S. Give one powder, and repeat according to circumstances.

In the treatment of one of the cases reported above it will be recollected that the mild chloride of mercury mite was given with the podophyllin, with a good result.

After the use of laxative agents the kidneys, being less congested on account of the diversion that has occurred, often begin to excrete urine more freely. But if the patient be anæmic or enfeebled and the symptoms are not urgent, it is frequently better to avoid active catharsis, which [p. 555]more or less reduces the strength, and employ remedies of a sustaining character, as in the following case, which occurred in my practice: A little boy, pallid and scrofulous, began to have anasarca after scarlet fever, chiefly in the scrotum, accompanied by a moderate degree of ascites. The urine, which was passed in nearly the normal quantity, contained albumen, but not in large amount. This patient gradually and fully recovered, with no treatment except the use of an oil-silk jacket over the kidneys and abdomen to promote diaphoresis, and the use of iron. Such a patient, treated by the powerful eliminatives which we employ for the more urgent and robust cases, would probably have been injured rather than benefited. No treatment can therefore be recommended in a treatise on scarlatinous nephritis which will be strictly applicable for all cases. Variations are demanded according to the state of the patient and the form and gravity of the disease.

Diuretics which do not stimulate the kidneys are proper at an early as well as late period of the renal malady, and digitalis is the one usually prescribed. I do not hesitate to order it from the first day in combination with the acetate of potassium. One teaspoonful of the infusion may be given every third hour to a child of five years. The following formula is for one of this age in good general condition:

℞. Potass. Acetatis oz. ss;
Infus. Digitalis vi. fl. oz. M.

The following formulæ are recommended by Meigs and Pepper:

℞. Potass. Bitart. drach m i;
Spt. Junip. Comp. fl. drachm ii;
Spt. Æther. Nitros. fl. drachm i;
Tr. Digitalis, mini m xv;
Syrupi fl. drachm v;
Aquæ ii. fl oz M.

Dose one teaspoonful every two hours to a child of two to four years.

Potass. drach

x.	Acetat.	m i;
	Tr. Digitalis	fl. drachm ss;
	Syr. Scillæ,	fl. drachm i-ii;
	Syr. Zingib.	fl. drachm v;
	Aquæ q. s. ad	fl. oz. iii. M.

Dose, a teaspoonful every two or three hours to children two or three years old.

Local treatment is important. L. Thomas, Romberg, and others recommend the application of leeches, three or more, over the kidneys. Thomas says: "In many cases the abstraction of blood causes immediate and permanent relief; the fever and the pain in the region of the kidneys cease, the secretion of urine becomes augmented, the albuminuria lessens from day to day, and the moderate degree of dropsy that has been developed disappears." It is only in the more robust children, who have been but little reduced by the primary disease, that leeching is, in my opinion, admissible. In the majority of cases instead of depletion a poultice slightly irritating, so as to cause redness of the skin, should be applied over the kidneys, or for older children, not likely to be frightened by the process, the dry cups may be applied daily. In subacute cases, not attended by any alarming symptoms, sufficient redness may be produced by one of the irritating plasters which the shops contain, constantly worn.

[p. 556]Eclampsia, described in the preceding pages, is produced, as we have seen, during the course of scarlet fever by the irritating effect of the scarlatinous poison upon the nervous centres, but, occurring after the decline of scarlet fever, it is ordinarily produced by the retained urea. The same remedies are required to control the convulsive movements as when they occur under other circumstances. The bromide of potassium should be immediately administered in large and frequent doses whenever eclamptic symptoms arise. During eclampsia a child of three years should take five grains of this agent every five to ten minutes till the attack ceases, and then at longer intervals. The hydrate of chloral is a more powerful agent, and if the eclampsia be not quickly controlled, I commonly employ it per rectum, dissolved in one or two teaspoonfuls of water. For a child of three to five years five grains should be thrown into the rectum by a small glass or gutta-percha syringe, and retained by pressure. Properly administered and retained, it rarely fails to control the eclampsia within ten or fifteen minutes. Subsequently, occasional doses of the bromide should be given to prevent the occurrence of eclampsia while the measures described above are being employed to relieve the uræmic condition.

Rheumatism, endocarditis, and pericarditis, arising as complications or sequelæ, require the treatment which is appropriate when they occur under other circumstances, but the remedies should not be depressing, as the system is already enfeebled by the primary disease. The rheumatism, if mild, usually abates in a few days without medication, and the affected joints require only some soothing lotion and support by a bandage. The following liniment may be applied upon muslin and covered by cotton wadding:

x.	Acid. Carbolici	fl. drachm i;
	Tinc. Belladonna	fl. oz. i;
	Ol. Camphorati	fl. oz. ii;

If the rheumatism be severe and affect several joints, the sodium salicylate should be prescribed, as in the idiopathic disease, with an occasional opiate to procure rest.

Endocarditis and pericarditis require rest in the horizontal position, avoidance of all excitement, the use of the tincture or infusion of digitalis or of the fluid extract of convalaria to procure a slow and steady action of the heart. Three drops of the tincture of digitalis or five minims of the fluid extract of convalaria may be given every four hours to a child of five years. The same external measures should be employed as in acute pleuritis. I prefer the application of a thin poultice of flaxseed containing one-sixteenth part of mustard and covered with oiled silk. The cardiac inflammations, as well as rheumatism, require opiates in sufficient doses to procure rest and sleep.

Pleuritis, which we have stated is apt to be suppurative, demands the same treatment as the idiopathic disease when it occurs in cachectic patients.

[p. 557]

RUBEOLA.[1]
BY W. A. HARDAWAY, M.D.

[1] In the preparation of this article the writer has consulted the following works: Thomas, in *Ziemssen's Cyclop. Pract. Med.*, vol. ii., N.Y., 1875, Am. edit.; Bohn, in *Gerhardt's Handbuch der Kinderkrankh.*, Zweiter Band, Tübingen, 1877; Squire, in Quain's *Dict. Med.*, N.Y., 1883; Ringer, in Reynolds's *System Med.*, vol. i., Phila., 1879; Meigs and Pepper, *Dis. of Children*, Phila., 1882; J. Lewis Smith, *Dis. of Children*, Phila., 1882; Hebra, *Dis. of Skin*, London. 1866; Vogel, *Dis. of Children*, N.Y., 1871; Niemeyer, *Handbook of Pract. Med.*, N.Y., 1869; Trousseau, *Clinical Med.*, Phila., 1871. Other references will be found in the foot-notes to the text.

SYNONYMS.—Rubeola, Morbilli, Measles, Masern, Flecken, Rougeole.

DEFINITION.—Measles is an acute infectious disease involving the skin and mucous membranes, characterized by successive stages and a maculo-papular eruption, which terminates in a fine branny desquamation. In normal cases it runs a definite course, which from the date of invasion to the end of desquamation occupies about fourteen days. It is highly contagious, and occurs, as a rule, but once in the same person.

HISTORY.—The word rubeola is probably of Spanish origin and was formerly written rubiola or rubiolo. The designation morbilli is the diminutive of the Italian il morbo, the plague. Although it is doubtful, as claimed by Willan, that the Greek and Roman physicians were acquainted with measles, there is no question that Rhazes was one of the first to describe the affection correctly. Rubeola is said to have been distinguished from variola by the Arabians in the twelfth century; but, nevertheless, as late as the middle of the seventeenth century we find Sennertus discussing the question "why the disease in some constitutions assumed the form of small-pox, and in others that of measles;" and in a posthumous work of Diemerbroeck, published in 1687, it is asserted that small-pox and measles are only different degrees of the same affection.[2] According to Mayr, the merit of having shown measles to be a distinct malady from scarlatina must be ascribed to Forestus and Sydenham. It is not clear, however, that the two diseases were accurately differentiated till the close of the last century, and notably by Withering in 1792.

[2] *Cyclop. Pract. Med.*, London, 1834, p. 625.

ETIOLOGY.—The exact nature of the measles contagium has never been satisfactorily established, although we are in possession of numerous researches in that direction, which, however, are to a great extent contradictory. A brief examination of these various observations will not prove uninteresting. Hallier found in the blood and sputa numbers of free cocci, which fructified upon various substrata, but was invariably the same fungus—mucor mucedo verus, Fres. In 1862, Salisbury[3] published[p. 558]his observations on the relation of the straw fungus to measles. He recorded instances of inoculation with this organism that resulted, according to him, in the production of a modified form of rubeola, and, moreover, was protective against further attacks of the same disease. In an exhaustive paper bearing on this question H. C. Wood[4] quotes certain experimental inoculations made by William Pepper, which showed conclusively that measles was not propagated in this way, and that where any symptoms were developed they were not those of true measles, nor did they protect the subjects from unquestioned measles. Salisbury also claimed that measles had occurred in camps where damp and mouldy straw had been employed for bedding. J. J. Woodward in his work on *Camp Diseases* points out that camp measles prevailed almost exclusively in regiments from the rural districts, while men enlisted in towns and cities were more or less completely exempt. The explanation was, that those from the country had hitherto escaped the disease, while townspeople had suffered from it at some previous time—a condition of affairs inconsistent with the theory of the straw fungus. Coxe and Felz found numerous bacteria in the blood of measles patients, especially in regions where the eruption was most pronounced. The nasal mucus also contained similar germs. Inoculation of the blood from the subjects of measles upon rabbits did not produce an analogous affection (Thomas). Klebs[5] obtained micrococci from the trachea and from blood taken from the hearts of infant cadavers. "In the latter, collected in flattened capillary tubes, there developed balls of micrococci; in the trachea both micrococci and bacteria were present in large quantities. Under observation, pale, finely-granular micrococcus balls developed and changed very quickly to bacteria, which moved about very actively. These sought the periphery, about ½ mm. distant from the centre of development, and formed a zone, comparable with a hedge or fence that is composed of rods. From this were formed new masses of micrococci, but further no regular process of arrangement or development could be observed."

[3] *Am. Jour. Med. Sci.*, July and Oct., 1862.

[4] *Ibid.*, Oct., 1868, p. 333.

[5] *Würzbr. Verh.*, N. F., v., 1874, quoted by Forchheimer in Supplement to *Ziemssen's Cyclopedia*, W. T., 1881, p. 102.

Braidwood and Vacher,[6] as the result of a number of experiments, believed that they had sufficient evidence for concluding that the most active mode of the transmission of measles was through the breath, and accordingly instituted a series of experiments by carefully examining the breath of children in the acute stage of the disease.[7] With this object in view they coated over with glycerine the inside of several clean glass tubes of a diameter of a half to three-quarters of an inch. As soon as the nature of the eruption was manifest the patient was required to breathe through one or more of the tubes, and so on each day till the eruption had faded. Upon examination of the glycerine with an one-eighth objective every specimen showed numerous sparkling bodies, something like those found in vaccine, but larger. Some were spherical; others were elongated, with sharpened ends. They were most abundant during the first and second days of the eruption. Healthy children and patients suffering from typhoid and scarlet fevers were made to imitate these [p. 559]experiments, but no such bodies were to be seen in their specimens. They conclude from these observations that the small spherical elements discovered in the breath are perhaps the active agents in the propagation of measles. Upon post-mortem of patients who had died of rubeola these germs were found in the lungs and liver, and, particularly, close to the walls of the capillaries. They believe that the "lungs are the favorite breeding-ground of the contagium."

[6] *Brit. Med. Jour.*, Jan. 21, 1882.

[7] Several years ago Ransome of Manchester obtained particles from the breath of two persons suffering from measles (Squire).

That inoculation of morbillous blood may convey the disease was first demonstrated by Home in 1757, which experiments were verified by Speranza in 1822 and by Katona in 1842. The inoculations of the latter are especially noteworthy, as they numbered more than a thousand. No person inoculated by him died, and only 7 per cent. of the inoculations failed. On the other hand, inoculations made by Mayr gave negative results. It is stated that Monro and Locke communicated measles by inoculating with the tears and saliva. Attempts of the same kind were fruitlessly made in Philadelphia in 1801, although the blood, the tears, the nasal and bronchial mucus, and the exfoliated lamellæ of the epidermis were successively employed in the trials.[8]

[8] Rayer, *Diseases of the Skin*, Phila., 1845.

Mayr has shown that the nasal mucus is capable upon inoculation of propagating the disease. He performed the experiment upon two healthy children living at a distance from each other, at a time when the disease had ceased to be epidemic. Some nasal mucus taken from the patient during the stadium flavitionis, and kept fluid in a glass tube, was the same day placed upon the mucous membrane of each of these children. In one of them the first symptom of sneezing occurred after eight days, in the other at the expiration of nine days. Febrile symptoms set in two days later. In each child the rash appeared on the thirteenth day after infection. The inoculated disease was mild and regular in its course.

While it is perhaps true that the contagion of measles is not so tenacious as that of small-pox and scarlatina, it is a matter of observation that susceptible persons are liable to contract the disease, even if not directly exposed to its influence. There is incontestable evidence that it is conveyed by fomites—a fact well worth bearing in mind.

It is but just to say that so excellent an observer as Mayr taught that measles could not be conveyed by clothes, linen, etc. unless transferred immediately from one individual to another. Panum, however, showed that contagion could be carried many miles by an unaffected third person without losing its activity. Aitken[9] has also pointed out the fact that children's clothes sent home in boxes from schools where the disease has raged communicated the disease, and that susceptible children who had slept in the same beds, in the same rooms, after they had been occupied by persons suffering from measles, have taken the malady. Squire observes that the contagium of measles, except in the catarrhal stage, is not far diffusible in the air, but clings to surfaces, and may be thus carried from place to place; on the other hand, children have been brought, while in full eruption, into a house among others, and nursed in a room apart, without any extension of the disease to the most susceptible.

[9] *Science and Pract. of Med.*, Phila., 1868.

[p. 560]Various circumstances render it probable that measles is most readily propagated during the stage of efflorescence; but that it is also highly infectious during the prodromal period is now universally acknowledged.

According to Niemeyer, the probability of infection during the prodromal stage is supported by the wonderful spread of measles through schools; for, while the strictest surveillance is established over children with any suspicious eruptions, and those known to have had the disease are not allowed to return till long past the stage of desquamation, no heed is paid to those exhibiting the premonitory cough and coryza. There is no reason for believing that measles can be propagated during the period of incubation; on the other hand, there is no satisfactory argument for the denial of its infectiousness in the desquamative stage. Although Panum is inclined to doubt its contagiousness at this time—and his observations are worthy of the greatest confidence—other good authorities differ from him materially, and extend the stage of personal infection to a period of from three weeks (Squire) to forty days (Hillairet).

Reasoning from analogy, we would naturally expect that the period of incubation in measles suffered a certain amount of variation; the result of numerous observations confirms this expectation. It is manifestly a difficult matter in densely populated communities to establish with accuracy the date of a given infection, but from a study of more or less carefully noted cases it will be found that the period of incubation may vary from three to thirty days. For the vast majority of cases the average time between the reception of the measles poison and the appearance of the characteristic eruption will be about from thirteen to fourteen days. Panum, under exceptionally favorable surroundings, found it more frequently fourteen than thirteen days. Therefore, deducting the three or four days occupied by the invasion stage, we shall find that the real incubation period is from nine to ten days from the date of exposure. Mayr's two cases of inoculation with nasal mucus showed no departure from this rule, but in the inoculations made by Katona with blood the prodromic symptoms made their appearance in seven days, the cutaneous lesions developing two, and at the most three, days afterward.

Minor epidemics of measles are said to occur every three to five years, more extensive and severe ones every seven or eight years. In the centres of population measles may be said to be endemic; in isolated regions the visitations of the disease may be widely separated. Measles is a less severe disease in warm than in cold climates, and, as a rule, we also find the affection more common and more intense in the fall, winter, and spring than in the summer months.[10] Epidemics of measles are usually short, and it is thought that there is a definite relation between the severity of their onset and their duration, this being in general short in proportion as the given epidemic was at first severe (Mayr). Intestinal complications are more frequent in summer, and involvements of the respiratory organs more common in winter. The varying aspects of different epidemics—[p. 561]sthenic, asthenic, etc.—depend on changes in the weather, season of the year, the presence of complications, and other agencies not very clearly understood. Epidemics of whooping cough may precede, accompany, or follow in the wake of measles, and it has therefore been suggested that it stands in some peculiarly close connection with the latter; but, aside from this often-observed coincidence, we are not justified in our present state of knowledge in assuming any definite relation of cause and effect between the two diseases.

[10] Aitken (*op. cit.*, p. 295) declares that the mortality returns from England and Wales show that the influence of season is most trifling. Occasionally it has been found that the deaths in summer exceeded those in winter, but we believe that the statement made above is, in the main, correct. For instance, Parson's figures for Berlin for the years 1863-67, inclusive, are: spring, 11.9 per cent.; summer, 13.3; autumn, 33.4; winter, 41.4. Voit's statistics in an average of thirty years at the Children's Clinic at Würzburg establish the same general principles (Thomas).

There would seem to be neither geographical nor racial bar to the propagation of measles, for it has been observed in all countries and among all peoples. As in the case of other zymotic diseases, a tolerance is established for measles in countries where the disease is more or less constantly prevalent; but where the affection becomes epidemic for the first time, or reappears after many years, it rages with terrific violence. This fact was particularly exemplified in the epidemic in the Faroe Islands, and more especially in the recent (1877) visitation of the Fiji Islands, where one-fourth of the population succumbed in a comparatively short time.

It is quite probable, as asserted by Mayr, that children affected with scrofulous complaints, as well as those who are the subjects of diseases of the respiratory organs—pertussis, bronchitis, or tuberculosis—are eminently susceptible of measles; but his statement that sufferers from epilepsy, chorea, and paralysis exhibit an unusual power of resistance cannot be accepted without reservation. Acute diseases often appear to delay the outbreak of measles, so that the latter does not appear till convalescence from the former (Thomas). The development of vaccinia is occasionally interfered with by an attack of rubeola; on the other hand, the two diseases may be seen running their courses together.[11] The emphatic statement made by Hebra, that measles is never seen to occupy a patient simultaneously with another acute exanthem, has not been confirmed by other observers. My own experience furnishes several examples. Measles may also occur during the course of other acute or chronic maladies. From a study of the literature of measles complicating pregnancy and parturition Underhill[12] finds it to be quite uncommon, due probably to the fact that most adults are insusceptible of further attacks; but when it does occur in pregnancy he regards it as a very serious and frequently fatal complication. Underhill believes measles to be most fatal when it supervenes soon after delivery, while those who are confined during the course of the malady stand a better chance of recovering from it. That puerperal women are not always unfavorably affected by measles is well shown in two remarkable cases reported by Nelson[13] of St. Louis and Chantier[14] of Geneva, in which the mothers were safely delivered, though suffering from measles contracted at the end of their pregnancies.

[11] Hardaway, *Essentials of Vaccination*, p. 60.
[12] *Obstet. Jour. Great Britain and Ireland*, July, 1880.
[13] *St. Louis Courier of Med.*, Sept., 1879.
[14] *Annales de Gynécologie*, May, 1879.

All ages are susceptible to the measles poison, and the apparent exemption enjoyed by adults is due to the fact that most grown-up people have already suffered the disease in childhood; but in Panum's epidemic, mentioned above, it was discovered that nearly all who had not had measles [p. 562]elsewhere, or were not old enough to have been exposed at the last visitation, sixty-five years before, acquired the affection regardless of age. It is quite probable, however, that the law of decrease of susceptibility with age holds good for measles as well as for variola, etc., but to a less degree. It will therefore be seen that measles is not essentially a disease of childhood. Although there is no special limit to the susceptibility of rubeola at one extreme of life, it would seem to be quite well established that it is much modified at the other—namely, that infants under six months are rarely attacked. This latter fact is conceded by individual experience, by the records of epidemics, and by the testimony of most observers.[15]

[15] On the other hand, as quoted by Forchheimer (*loc. cit.*), H. C. Fox publishes some tables which show that for England and London a much larger number of young children are attacked by measles than other statistics would lead us to believe.

	England.		London.	
	Males.	Females.	Males.	Females.
Under one year	2022	2530	2571	2987
One and under two years	5086	5825	8630	8050
Two and under three years	3178	3255	4683	4757
Three and under four years	1730	1851	2594	2620
Four and under five years	80	1028	1358	1466
Five and under ten years	55	278	301	316
Ten and under fifteen years	9	38	4	32
Fifteen and under twenty years		13		11
Twenty and under twenty-five years		9		7
Twenty-five and under thirty-five years		8		7
Thirty-five and under forty-five years		5		3

Even sucklings do not enjoy a complete immunity from measles. Steiner[16] states that he has met with it in children only four or five weeks old. Monti has recorded ten cases of rubeola in children under two months of age. A case is reported by Kunze where a mother in the stage of efflorescence gave birth to a child, which contracted the disease five days afterward. Quite a number of cases of congenital measles have been put on record from time to time; but Thomas, after a careful investigation, says that he has been able to discover but six authentic accounts of such occurrences.[17] That children born to mothers suffering at the time of parturition from measles may yet escape it themselves is proven by the cases of Nelson and Gautier mentioned above. Whether a pregnant woman attacked by measles transmits the disease to the foetus in utero, thereby securing immunity from it in after life, is a question difficult of decision, especially as we have not yet been able to decide this same inquiry, with infinitely better opportunities, for vaccinia.[18]

[16] *Compendium of Children's Diseases*, N.Y., 1875, p. 396.

[17] I believe that, under certain circumstances, the erythema papulatum of the newborn is often mistaken for measles.

[18] See experiments of Burckhardt, Rickett, Gart, and others, quoted in Hardaway's *Essentials of Vaccination*, p. 38.

There is no good reason to believe that sex is of much importance in establishing a predisposition to measles, although the statement has been repeatedly made that males are more frequently attacked than females.[p. 563]Fox's statistics show a slight preponderance in favor of the male sex; but a careful examination of accessible statistics proves, as would be expected, that this degree of susceptibility varies at different times in obedience to circumstances not readily understood.

By the older writers (Willan, Rosenstein, Fuchs) it was very dogmatically asserted that one attack of measles completely extinguished all future susceptibility to the disease. Of late years this dogma has met with much opposition, and numerous observations have been recorded which, if entirely trustworthy, would lead us to believe that rubeola may occur not only twice, but several times, in the same individual. While from analogy and actual experience we are quite sure that the recurrence of measles is not so uncommon an event as it was once held to be, a closer examination of the question in all its bearings clearly confirms us in the belief that subsequent attacks are much more infrequent than is now thought to be the case by many, and that other diseases, more or less resembling true measles, are largely responsible for errors of diagnosis in this regard. Panum found that all the old people who had measles during the epidemic on the Faroe Islands in 1781 escaped it in 1846. Both Rosenstein and Willan declared that they had never witnessed an instance of the true recurrence of measles. Among other facts, it may be stated in this connection that Woodward (*loc. cit.*) has shown that during our late war, while members of regiments recruited from the rural districts, who had never before had measles, largely took it when exposed to its influence, regiments from the cities, who had presumably acquired the disease in childhood, remained almost entirely exempt.[19] Other arguments of a similar sort could be readily adduced. There is no question that mistakes in diagnosis have occurred from confounding rötheln, roseola, etc., which closely simulate measles, with that disease. Those particularly engaged in the treatment of cutaneous affections could multiply instances of such errors. It is quite significant that for certain analogous infectious diseases—*e.g.* variola and scarlatina—the same frequency of recurrence is not claimed, although as a matter of fact they do occur. The explanation would seem to lie in the fact that neither small-pox nor scarlet fever is so closely counterfeited by other skin affections, notably by rötheln, as is measles. But it would be entirely contrary to analogy and indubitable experience to go to the extreme of the older writers and absolutely deny the possibility of second, and even third, attacks of rubeola. The frequency of such cases is, however, as Henoch[20] truly states, much overestimated.

[19] These observations of Woodward were made without any reference to the question at issue.

[20] *Lectures on Diseases of Children*, N.Y., 1882, p. 282.

Occupying quite a different position from the measles induced by reinfection from without are the so-called relapses of rubeola. These relapses, which may occur in from two to four weeks after the original invasion, are analogous to the similar occurrences in scarlatina and typhoid fever. I am cognizant of but a single case of this sort, but Steiner and other accurate observers record a number of such instances.

SYMPTOMS AND COURSE.—It is generally stated that the stage of incubation exhibits no symptoms whatever; but it is undoubtedly true that the patient will sometimes appear dull and listless, and, on occasion, even give evidence of some slight and ephemeral elevations of temperature. [p. 564]As a rule, however, this period is devoid of any marked indication of the presence of the measles poison in the system.[21]

[21] Some writers describe a much more marked train of symptoms as prevailing at this time than seems warranted by general experience, and Rehn has gone so far as to declare that the prodromal period, as usually understood, properly commences in the stage of incubation. Bohn is inclined to a similar view. The prodromic stage of authors is, then, to be looked upon as the "period of the mucous membrane exanthem."

The prodromal stage is usually ushered in by symptoms of general malaise, fretfulness, more or less frontal headache, shiverings, nausea, loss of appetite, excited sleep, and sometimes delirium. Vomiting is not so common in measles as in scarlatina, and may occur at any time previous to the appearance of the rash. The tongue is apt to be coated, although it may remain clean; the taste is bad, and pressure over the stomach and bowels occasionally elicits considerable pain; an aching pain over the sternum is also noted. As a general thing, at this time patients are drowsy and inclined to sleep much. Meigs and Pepper found this a very constant symptom, which they state is in no way alarming unless associated with other more serious symptoms of local or general disturbance. Constipation is present in some cases, or the bowels may be relaxed or remain in their natural state.

The prodromal fever of measles follows a peculiar course. It is remarkably remittent in character, and is rarely of such intensity as to threaten life, as is often the case in scarlet fever. The temperature will rise on the first day to 102°-104° F., and the height of the fever at this time will measurably foreshadow the character of the subsequent course. On the second day of the prodromal stage the fever suffers a marked remission, or may even entirely disappear, to again rise in the evening. Smith has observed two exacerbations in the day. Again, in some instances, after the high initiatory fever, the temperature may remain normal till just before the rash comes out (Bohn). It is this peculiar behavior of the fever, together with the fact that the child may regain its usual vivacity in the fever-free intervals, which so often misleads the physician into the diagnosis of malarial poisoning.

The most pronounced feature of this stage of the disease is, beyond all others, the catarrhal affection of the mucous membranes. The mucous membranes of the eyes, nose, mouth, and air-passages are all more or less involved, and the patient suffers in varying degrees from photophobia, coryza, hoarseness, cough, and pain in swallowing. Sneezing is frequent and annoying, and slight epistaxis is not uncommon. The cough usually appears on the first day, simultaneously with the fever. It is not very troublesome at first, but by the fourth day it becomes more frequent, assuming a hoarse, barking, paroxysmal character. Expectoration is scanty, and auscultation reveals a harsh vesicular murmur or else sibilant râles. Alarming but not dangerous attacks of false croup may come on during the night. Many observers have called attention to the red spots (papules) in the oral cavity, which make their appearance during the period of invasion. According to Bohn, usually on the second or third day from the beginning of the fever there appear upon the slightly hyperæmic mucous membrane of the soft palate, palatal arch, and uvula small or large, dark, red spots that spread to the mucous membrane of the cheeks, and sometimes to the hard palate, lips, and gums. Soon they become more defined, and are to be distinguished by shape and coloring [p. 565]from the membrane upon which they are situated. According to the same authority, they also afford an index to the intensity and extent of the coming cutaneous eruption. It is also stated that if the latter partakes of a hemorrhagic character, the spots on the mucous membrane may also become livid. This same punctate reddening has been demonstrated in the epiglottis, larynx, and trachea (Gerhardt), and upon the bronchi and small intestines of children who had died during this stage of the eruption. It is also to be noted on the conjunctivæ. It has been assumed that this period of this disease is not to be looked upon as the stadium prodromorum, but as the period of the "exanthem of the mucous membrane." This view of the pathology of measles seems to me most reasonable; but in whatever way we may look upon the question, the practical importance of this precutaneous eruptive stage is to be insisted upon for diagnostic purposes, just as is the analogous eruption upon the mucous membrane in small-pox.

In ordinary cases of measles we do not find such profound reaction of the nervous system as in scarlatina. I believe that convulsions in the prodromal stage are much more common than available statistics would have us believe; at least, this is my own experience. Meigs and Pepper met with convulsions but five times in 314 cases at the beginning of the eruption, while Rilliet and Barthez observed but one convulsion in 167 cases. Thomas says that convulsions are almost always absent. On the other hand, Trousseau and Bohn expressly declare that they are very common, the former stating that they occur with greater frequency than in scarlatina. I consider that convulsive seizures occurring in connection with marked catarrhal affection of the mucous membranes are very important aids in forecasting a probable attack of rubeola. Fortunately, convulsions at this stage are not very serious unless repeated or injudiciously treated.

The duration of the period of invasion in regular cases is from three to five days, with an average of about four, but in perfectly uncomplicated attacks this period may be extended to six or eight days, or even longer. But that the duration of this stage may be much shorter than the average is not sufficiently insisted upon by writers. Ringer,[22] for instance, says that he had an opportunity of testing the earliest appearance of the rash in an epidemic of measles in a large public school for boys under twelve. In every case during the epidemic the rash appeared on the first day, the cases being severe, though of short duration, the temperature rising to 103° and to 104° F. In some instances the rash preceded (?) the fever. Thus, several of the boys feeling poorly, their temperature was carefully taken night and morning under the tongue, and in several cases the rash appeared in the morning about the face and collar-bone, while the temperature remained normal, and did not rise till the evening, when it ran up to 101°-103° F., and even higher. These cases certainly resemble rötheln more than measles. In two cases, which I observed under very favorable conditions, the eruption commenced to appear on the morning of the second day, and more or less similar experiences are recorded by others.

[22] *Handbook of Therapeutics*, 6th ed., London, 1868—note to p. 26.

The skin eruption, which appears, as a rule, on the third, fourth, or fifth day of the attack, is ushered in with an increase in the general and [p. 566]local symptoms of the disease. It is particularly to be remarked that the fever does not subside at this time, as is the case in variola. The eruption appears first upon the face, about the cheeks and forehead, then on the chin and neck, and thence gradually overspreads the trunk, and finally reaches the extremities. When the eruption is intense no part of the body is free from it, the rash being found upon the palms and soles and upon the hairy scalp. The cutaneous lesions proper consist at first of hyperæmic spots of about a line in diameter, which gradually increase in size, until at their full development they may attain a diameter of from one-twentieth to a quarter of an inch. In the beginning they bear a very close resemblance to the sub-papular lesions of small-pox. The maculo-papules, when fully developed, are slightly elevated above the level of the skin, the elevation, however, being more appreciable to touch than sight, have a smooth velvety feel, and are so arranged as to enclose areas of healthy skin. In the individual spots we may frequently observe one or several minute, darker-colored papules, due to follicular congestion, which when more intense constitutes the morbilli papulari presently to be described. The maculæ are, as a rule, roundish, or they may be moon-shaped, or their borders may present an indented or notched appearance. Where the capillary circulation is active—on the cheeks, for example—or upon parts subjected to pressure, the eruption may become confluent; that is to say, the usually pale intervening skin becomes injected or the papules coalesce, and in this way produce a uniform redness over large single tracts of skin. This scarlatinoid rash, however, never occupies the whole surface of the body, but only limited regions, and in other situations may be detected the characteristic discrete papules of rubeola; the color is not uniform, but is broken here and there by the darker streaks and spots of the measly eruption. The rash, which disappears upon pressure to return when the pressure is removed, is of a more or less rosy red, with a tendency in some to deep red, and has occasionally a purplish hue. According to Mayr and Hebra, it is of the precise color which is obtained by adding a little yellow or brown to a red pigment.

According to the researches of Thomas, Squire, and Wunderlich, as abstracted by Seguin, the fever of the eruptive period is divided into a moderately febrile stage and the fastigium or acme. The moderately febrile stage averages thirty-six to thirty-eight hours, and is made up of one or two exacerbations of 100.4° to 102.2° F., but not quite so high as the initial fever. If there are two exacerbations, the second one is the higher; the intervening remissions are not so low as those of the prodromal stage, yet even now the norm may be noted on a single occasion. The fastigium commences early in the day or in the evening; if the rise should occur in the morning, the evening temperature rises still higher, with or without a slight remission the following morning, and the next evening attains the maximum. If the acme begins in the evening, the remission on the next morning is either absent or very slight. The greatest height of the fever in normal cases corresponds to the greatest intensity and development of the eruption. This rule is not invariable, however, for sometimes the fever is higher soon after the eruption appears, and has fallen when the exanthem has reached its highest point. The whole fastigium lasts from one and a half to two [p. 567]and a half days, so that the complete eruptive fever occupies from three to four and one-half days.[23] The pulse in general preserves a proportionate correspondence to the temperature, and never attains the great frequency to be observed in scarlatina.

[23] According to Ringer, the highest temperature reached in normal cases is 103° F. Thomas places it as high as 104° F., but states that it may go up to 105° F. without the intervention of any complication.

The general symptoms, with the exception of the fever, do not greatly differ from those common to the prodromal stage. The skin is hot and more or less swollen, particularly about the face; there are anorexia, photophobia, lachrymation, and sometimes epistaxis; the cough continues, and is generally frequent and harassing, and attended with little or no expectoration; the voice is hoarse. The tongue is coated, principally in the middle, through which the swollen papillæ protrude, while the tip and sides are red. The blotchy redness of the oral cavity is visible for some days, and finally becomes indistinguishable from the surrounding congestion. The tonsils sometimes become considerably enlarged, though suppuration must be rare. Enlargement of the glands behind the jaw and in the neck and groin are to be observed. At the outset of the eruption a profuse diarrhoea supervenes in most cases—a symptom which Trousseau rightly insists to be an essential feature of measles. This occurrence is interpreted by some writers as an evidence of the implication of the mucous membranes in the specific exanthem of the disease. This flux, which is sometimes accompanied by a little blood and tenesmus, rarely continues long, and may be succeeded by a degree of constipation. The respiration is generally somewhat accelerated, mostly in correspondence to the amount of fever present. Some degree of deafness is not uncommon, owing to the extension of inflammation along the Eustachian tubes. The urine is scanty and high colored; there is sometimes scalding in urination and vesical tenesmus, and at the acme of the fever traces of albumen may be detected.

The eruption, in fact, generally occupies the skin an average of four days, and, although this period may be shortened materially, it is less apt to be lengthened. The duration of the eruption at its maximum of development over the whole surface is about half a day, more or less, and, as a rule, corresponds with the greatest elevation of the temperature. The retrocession of the rash takes place in the order of its appearance—viz. first from the face, then from the trunk and upper parts of the extremities, and last from about the feet and hands, where, indeed, it may remain vivid, or even progress for a short time longer, after the eruption has begun to subside in other situations. Sometimes the almost faded spots will be temporarily renewed by an abnormal rise in the temperature.

With the decline of the eruption the other symptoms begin to subside. The cough loses its hacking, paroxysmal character, and becomes less and less frequent, and gradually disappears. The voice regains its normal tone, the tongue loses its fur, cleaning up in patches, and expectoration, which was absent or scanty and viscid in the beginning, increases and is free, the masses coughed up being coin-shaped and floating in a clear watery mucus—a symptom much dwelt upon by the older writers. The behavior of the temperature at this period—the stage of decline—is quite[p. 568]characteristic. The fall usually begins at night, and generally the next morning it has reached the norm or else fallen below it. On the other hand, the descent may be less precipitate, and the fall continues less rapidly all through the day; or there may be a slight rise again in the evening, the norm being reached the following morning. The termination by lysis—that is, slight elevations in the evening for several days—is much rarer, and while it may occur in perfectly regular cases, it should put the medical attendant on his guard against complications.

The comparatively normal course of measles portrayed in the preceding paragraphs does not always occur, but, on the contrary, the disease may depart from the more usual type in one or more particulars, either in especial stages of its progress or in the greater or less intensity of the malady as a whole.

In addition to those cases of measles where the eruptive and catarrhal symptoms are so slight as to almost escape observation, except for the existence of other cases in the same house or family, there are to be recognized two other trivial varieties of the disease—namely, measles without the catarrh, and measles without the rash.

That the eruption of measles should occur upon the skin without implication of the mucous membranes seems to be much more doubtful than that the catarrh should appear without the eruption. It is quite probable, at any rate, that many so-called cases of rubeola sine catarrho are merely instances of rötheln, which we know may occur without any reference to an existing epidemic of measles. But that this form of measles does exist is admitted by trustworthy observers, although its diagnosis under any circumstances must be a matter of great difficulty. Measles without the eruption (rubeola sine eruptione) is more readily recognized, especially and only, however, when a susceptible person is exposed, and as a result acquires the characteristic catarrhal symptoms. Since in recent years more attention has been paid to the eruption on the mucous membranes, it may be that its discovery in these situations may lend positive assistance to the diagnosis in such cases. It is hard to understand how this variety of measles, which presents no inflammatory changes in the skin, should be followed by desquamation; yet this observation has been made. The assertion that these anomalous forms of the affection afford no protection against subsequent attacks seems to be founded in error, and is undoubtedly due to the confusion existing between measles and rötheln or other exanthems.

Continental writers, especially, describe a form of measles called by them inflammatory or synochal. It is simply an exaggeration of the symptoms, particularly those appertaining to the mucous membranes, found in ordinary measles (morbilli vulgaris). The prodromal stage is much more violent, the nervous symptoms more threatening, the implication of the mucous membranes more pronounced and persistent, the febrile movement is of a higher inflammatory character, and the eruption, which instantly covers the whole body (Vogel), is made up of dark-red or purplish spots which fade slowly. It is this form of measles, according to Niemeyer, which is chiefly attended by croupous instead of catarrhal laryngitis, in which the inflammation of the air-passages often extends to the alveoli of the lungs, and in which the gastric and intestinal coats are often affected with catarrh.

[p. 569]Let the contagion of measles be a grade more virulent, or perhaps the resisting power of the patient more feeble, and the case will assume the features of the septic, typhous, or hemorrhagic variety (rubeola nigra). It is said that the hemorrhagic measles is most apt to occur in epidemics; certain it is that the dreaded black measles of former times is very infrequent now-a-days, due, no doubt, to a more rational treatment and a better hygiene. Isolated cases, however, are occasionally encountered. As a rule, from the beginning all the symptoms evidence an overwhelming of the system by the virulence of the poison—a condition of things much more common in scarlatina. The pulse becomes weak, thready, and frequent; the temperature lacks the typical remittent character of normal measles; there is unusual prostration; and the nervous centres are profoundly concerned, as shown by delirium, convulsions, and coma. The eruption lags, and finally makes its appearance in an imperfect or irregular manner. The spots are of a livid hue, interspersed with larger or smaller ecchymoses. Hemorrhages from the mucous cavities take place, and the patient dies in convulsions or sinks into fatal coma. It has been said that the grave constitutional symptoms do not generally make their appearance till the eruptive stage, but I know from experience that the patient may be overwhelmed quite early, as in purpura variolosa.

Too much stress should not be laid on these different types of the disease, whether mild or grave, since they depend upon a common cause, however much modified in one way or another; but they may be allowed to stand for the sake of clinical convenience.

Measles may also present certain irregularities in its various stages without necessarily departing from the otherwise benign character of the disease.

As stated elsewhere, it is believed by some writers that a greater part of the period of incubation is occupied by symptoms which already indicate the activity of the measles poison in the system, and that, therefore, this stadium in reality lasts but a few days. This opinion does not seem to be generally accepted; at any rate, I think we are quite safe in saying that in the majority of cases no departure from the usual latency is observed. The deviations in the stage of invasion have been considered above, and mostly concern its duration and the character of the temperature. Evanescent rashes, which have nothing in common with the specific exanthem, are sometimes observed at this period. The eruption of measles may present certain peculiarities. First, as to localization. Instead of coming out on the face first, it may primarily develop on other parts of the body, provoked into existence, as it were, by local exciting causes; thus, where ointments or plasters have been applied or upon a part subjected to constant pressure. It may affect only one-half of the body, or entirely spare paralyzed extremities (Mayr). In some instances the papules are so sparse, indistinct, and short-lived as to be scarcely appreciable.

Second, as to the physical characters of the eruption. Hebra and Mayr recognize the following modifications:

Morbilli lævis. The efflorescence is smooth and flat, and the individual lesions are separated from each other by normal integument. This is the common form of measles.

[p. 570]Morbilli papulosi. The papules are dark red and more elevated, are about the size of hempseeds, and situated at the mouths of the hair-follicles.

Morbilli vesiculosi. In this variety the mouths of the hair-follicles are filled with fluid and produce delicate transparent vesicles.

Morbilli confluentes. The maculæ are here so crowded together that no healthy skin intervenes.

Morbilli hæmorrhagici. The efflorescence consists of maculæ or papulæ of a dark-red color, due to extravasations of blood, and do not fade on pressure. It is well to mention in this connection the fact, particularly noted by Meigs and Pepper in this country, that hemorrhages into the skin may occur in cases which otherwise run a benign course. They are best seen after the eruption has faded. In some cases the efflorescence of measles may remain visible for a week or ten days.

As heretofore observed, there may be a relapse of the measles eruption after some weeks, accompanied by fever. It is said that the spots appear on parts of the skin hitherto normal (Thomas). So far as I know, Hebra was one of the first to point out the fact that the so-called striking-in of the eruption was the result, and not the cause, of some complication in the disease; for, as this author states, before the rash fades or disappears the internal disease is always present. It is well known, for instance, that syphilitic eruptions will sometimes disappear upon the supervention of some acute intercurrent affection, such as pneumonia, acute rheumatism, etc.; but no one will suppose for a moment that the retrocession of the syphilides was the cause of these affections.[24] The pathological explanation seems obvious.

[24] See Bumstead and Taylor on *Venereal Diseases*, 4th edit., p. 513.

COMPLICATIONS.—The complications of measles consist, as a rule, in the exaggerated morbid action of organs or parts that are essentially implicated in the disease; therefore we are most apt to encounter such affections as laryngitis, bronchitis, pneumonia, etc. Inflammation of serous membranes, on the other hand, are rare; thus, pleurisy is infrequent unless in connection with a lobar pneumonia.

The exact causes of the complications are not always obvious, but in many instances can be traced to the previous bad health of the patient, to the influence of insanitation, or, finally, to certain ill-understood features attendant upon some epidemics.

Simple bleeding from the nose, not associated with the hemorrhagic diathesis, is not an uncommon accompaniment of the prodromal stage, and is rarely a dangerous symptom—rather the contrary. It may also arise after the development of the rash, and occasionally proves a complication of serious import.

The aural complications, unlike those in scarlatina, are generally not sufficiently prominent at first to attract attention. The symptoms, particularly pain and deafness, are apt to be masked. Purulent processes and consequent perforation may occur during the eruption, but are more frequent at the stage of desquamation (Spencer).[25]

[25] Oral communication.

Various disorders of the skin have been observed during the course of measles—viz. miliary vesicles, and even pustules, as already described; herpes facialis, zoster femoralis (Thomas), and erythematous rashes, which [p. 571]may precede, accompany, or, it is said, follow the eruption. Of considerably more importance is the pemphigoid eruption mentioned by several observers. In Henoch's[26] case, a girl of four years, the usual remission of the fever on the evening of the second day was absent, and from the third day there appeared over nearly the whole surface blebs filled with a limpid fluid, which varied in size from a hazel-nut to a thaler, and even larger. The cheeks and the backs of the hands were each covered with a single bleb. The exanthem was of a hemorrhagic character, and the intervening skin was red and the face swollen. The bullæ appeared not only where the eruption existed, but also on parts of the body free from it. The fever remained at the same height till the fifth day, when, upon the cessation of the bullous eruption, it fell to 100° F. A.M., and 101° F. P.M.The child died on the eighth day of a pneumonia which developed between the sixth and seventh days. Other cases have been reported by Steiner, Klüppel, and Löschner. Henoch rejects the theory that the bullæ are the result of the morbillous dermatitis, but thinks that they are merely instances of the coincidence of a contagious pemphigus.

[26] *Berl. klin. Woch.*, No. 13, 1882.

The severe affections of the eye described by continental writers—blennorrhoea, keratitis, iritis, etc.—are certainly very rare in this country as complications of measles. Various so-called strumous disorders of this organ, as will be seen hereafter, not uncommonly, however, come under the care of the ophthalmologist as sequelæ of the disease.

The tonsils and the mucous membrane of the pharynx may become severely inflamed. The tonsils are sometimes very much enlarged, but suppuration, if it occur, is certainly rare. Slight ulceration of the gums close to the teeth is occasionally noted, also aphthous ulcerations on the lips, tongue, and gums (Ringer).

Some degree of laryngitis is an accompaniment of all cases of measles. It has already been stated that catarrhal or false croup is frequently observed during the stage of invasion. Inflammation of the larynx may be present in all grades of severity. Rilliet and Barthez found ulcerations and erosions, especially of the vocal cords, upon post-mortem examination of a large proportion of measles subjects; and Gerhardt, both during life and by autopsy, has verified these observations. Loeri[27] states that inflammatory changes are more marked in the larynx and trachea than in the pharynx. According to his examinations, hemorrhages or ecchymoses seldom occur, but more frequently superficial or even deep catarrhal ulcers, especially on the anterior aspect of the posterior wall of the larynx at the apices of the cartilages of Santorini, or on the posterior portion of the vocal cords. The physical condition of these parts readily accounts for the frequent and harassing cough and attacks of spasmodic laryngitis which are such frequent complications of the invasion and eruptive stages of measles.

[27] *Jahrb. f. Kinderheilk.*, xix. B., 1 H.

There may be an extension of the tracheo-bronchitis to the finer bronchial tubes, thus producing capillary bronchitis (suffocative catarrh). It is apt to prove fatal to very young children. It occurs more generally during or after the eruption.

Pneumonia is one of the most frequent and, directly and indirectly, most dangerous complications of measles. Catarrhal pneumonia (broncho-pneumonia) is, for obvious reasons, more common than the lobar or[p. 572]croupous variety. Pneumonia may develop at almost any stage of measles, but experience does not confirm the statement occasionally made that it is most frequent in the initial stage. Most observers will agree as to its greater frequency just at the end of the eruption or during the desquamative period. The occurrence of epileptoid convulsions, or an untoward increase of the fever, or an unexplained continuance of the same, should direct the attention of the attendant to the chest, if his anxiety have not already been aroused by a change in the character of the respiration or other symptoms. It may be mistaken for meningitis (Squire). In estimating the prognosis it should be remembered that croupous and catarrhal pneumonias run quite different courses. The influence of inflammation of the lungs upon the rash is quite decided. If an intense pneumonia should develop in the initial stage, the eruption will be pale and sparse, or else absent; if the eruption is already out at the time of the attack, it may become temporarily more vivid, to rapidly fade later.[28]

[28] A scanty rash by no means indicates an unfavorable course of the disease; this symptom is only serious when evidently due to some complication.

Chadbourne[29] has the merit of calling attention to the occurrence of heart-clot and subsequent pulmonary oedema as a fatal complication of measles. In a number of autopsies he found that in each case the heart contained clear gelatinous clots of a very firm consistence, which in most instances extended to the pulmonary arteries, and in some to the extent of one and one-fourth inches. In the series of cases observed by him pneumonic consolidation was mostly absent, and there was very little evidence of collapse, but the lungs were exceedingly oedematous. But Keating has also found heart-clot to be the cause of death in some cases, and believes, as the result of his investigations, that the presence of large numbers of micrococci in the blood and in the white blood-corpuscles is responsible for this condition.[30]

[29] *Am. Jour. Obstet.*, Oct., 1880.
[30] *Phila. Med. Times*, Aug. 12, 1882.

There is a strong tendency in measles to intestinal catarrh. As already stated, a quite sharp diarrhoea is not uncommon at the beginning of the eruptive stage; but, unless it should prove very profuse and long-continued, it is not to be looked upon as of very serious import, especially if the other general symptoms of the disease are following a normal course. In other instances the bowel affection may be much more severe, giving rise to tenesmus, bloody stools, and the other phenomena of colitis. In weakly children the early diarrhoea may persist in spite of treatment for many days; indeed, under the influence of high temperatures it may take on a true choleraic character. Diarrhoea is a very frequent and grave complication of the broncho-pneumonia of measles.

Acute miliary tuberculosis as an immediate concomitant of measles is rare. According to Thomas, the disease at times immediately follows the exanthem, and reaches a fatal issue in a few days or weeks. The tubercles are more particularly to be found in the lungs and in the membranes of the brain.

Among the more common disturbances of the nervous system convulsions play an important rôle. The epileptoid seizures of the prodromal stage generally terminate favorably, but in some cases of a malignant character the onset of the disease may be ushered in with fatal [p. 573]convulsions. Convulsions in the later stages are apt to have a lethal termination, as they usually occur in connection with some grave complication, particularly of the thoracic organs.

Diphtheria is an exceedingly grave complication of measles, although not necessarily a fatal one. It is of less frequent occurrence than in scarlatina. It may attack any of the usual oral, nasal, or laryngeal regions, sometimes extending into the bronchi, but suffers no modifications in its symptoms and course from the primary disease. It may also rarely involve other parts—*e.g.* genitals, eyelids, etc. There is reason to believe that it is most prone to attack those cases in which the mucous membranes have undergone the greatest inflammatory alterations.[31]

[31] Loeri (*loc. cit.*) says that diphtheria may appear at any stage of measles, and commences generally in the larynx, and sometimes in the trachea simultaneously; seldom in the pharynx, as in primary diphtheria or in that complicating other diseases than measles.

Many other complications of measles have been recorded in literature (see Thomas, *op. cit.*); but it is no doubt true, as observed by Bohn, that very few of them have a real essential connection with that affection, and might as readily be associated with any other malady, especially in already vitiated constitutions. In the above sketch the endeavor has been made to indicate those disorders which from the nature of measles would seem to have a more or less close and definite relationship to it. It is certain that the more serious complications and sequelæ of measles are comparatively infrequent in private practice in America, although common enough in continental Europe, and to a certain extent in the children's asylums and foundling hospitals in this country.

SEQUELÆ.—It is a difficult matter to dissociate the complications and sequelæ of measles. Properly speaking, the sequelæ are to be looked upon as the complications which have continued in existence after the subsidence of the exanthem; but it is also customary to include under this head certain affections that are the result of the derangement of the system by the morbillous process.

As would be expected, among the most frequent sequelæ of measles are those diseases which have their seat in the mucous membranes. Thus, we may observe various grades of inflammation and ulceration of the larynx, trachea, and bronchial tubes. According to Loeri, follicular ulcers of the larynx always give a bad prognosis, for these cases usually succumb to tuberculosis. It is not uncommon to observe a bronchial catarrh, apparently simple in nature, which persists with frequent exacerbations for many months. The very frequent broncho-pneumonia, which occurs as a complication, always remains as a sequel, or it may develop after the morbillous process has come to an end. In favorable cases recovery may take place in two or three weeks, or, preceded by hectic and progressive emaciation, the disease may prove fatal after a number of months. But even here it is not impossible for affected persons to recover.

Chronic pulmonary tuberculosis is one of the most formidable and frequent sequelæ of measles. It is a not uncommon occurrence that, with the exception of some trivial bronchitis, a patient may apparently recover his health completely, and only after a lapse of time slight daily elevations of temperature, accompanied by loss of appetite and emaciation, [p. 574]first give warning of the impending danger. This form of phthisis may follow either croupous or catarrhal pneumonia. Granular meningitis or general miliary tuberculosis also frequently follows in the wake of measles, connected in many cases with foci of caseous degeneration in the involved lymphatic glands or unabsorbed pneumonic exudation.

Various gangrenous affections, particularly of the oral cavity (noma) and genitals, but also of the skin, subcutaneous connective tissue, cartilages of the nose, ear, etc., are often to be observed after an attack of measles. Cancrum oris is to be especially noted.

Albuminuria is not an essential sequel of measles, although it may occasionally occur as the result of great exposure and neglect.

A large group of chronic affections may follow in the track of measles, either in the form of sequelæ to the complications which arise during the course of the disease or in the nature of secondary accidents. Some few, perhaps, are more common after measles than after any other complaint, but the majority are such as might arise in weakly children subsequent to any specific disturbance of the health. In addition to those already mentioned we may especially designate chronic intestinal disease, together with ulcerations and strictures of the bowel; chronic coryza, in varying degrees of obstinacy and severity; chronic ophthalmia, under which title may be included ciliary blepharitis, granulations, trachoma, phlyctenular conjunctivitis, ulcers of the cornea, etc. (Michel[32]); aural affections in the form of chronic suppurative inflammation, and, more rarely, chronic catarrh of the middle ear (Spencer); certain cutaneous diseases, more especially in my experience furunculosis and pustular eczema; chronic bone and joint disorders (strumous), which, according to Gibney,[33] may not only be evoked in the already hereditarily predisposed, but also induced when the diathesis has not heretofore existed; and, lastly, various derangements of the nervous system.

[32] Oral communication.

[33] See valuable statistical article in *N.Y. Med. Record,* June 3, 1882.

In Thomas's valuable and freely-quoted monograph on measles (*op. cit.*) it is stated that secondary measles can exert various influences upon the primary disturbance. In most instances when measles attacks a person already the subject of some other disease, particularly when the latter belongs to the common complications of the former, it usually is aggravated. This is a matter of common experience; but this author further declares—and supports his assertion with numerous references—that, on the other hand, should measles appear during the existence of a disease to which it does not usually give rise, it may favorably influence the course of the latter. In spite of the cases quoted in support of this view, such results would appear to be contrary to pathological laws.[34]

[34] Thus, while Thomas seems to be without personal experience in the matter, he quotes without dissent a number of observations in support of his assertion—viz.: Behrend saw a chronic eczema of the scalp permanently disappear after measles; Rilliet found that a chronic coxitis improved noticeably after measles; various chronic skin symptoms, and also chorea, epilepsy, incontinence of urine, mania, worms, dropsy, joint diseases, ophthalmia, gonorrhoea, etc., have been known to recover under the same influence. Gibney (*loc. cit.*) in his valuable paper states that he can readily believe that, occasionally, any acute disease, occurring in the course of a chronic one, will prove beneficial to the other, but that he is far from considering this to be anything more than an exception to a very general rule to the contrary. Chronic joint disease, he continues, is especially a disease of exacerbations, and any one not familiar with their natural history may interpret the post hoc as a propter hoc. Gibney has collected 24 cases of chronic bone disease in children, 21 of whom were under ten years of age and all under thirteen. On analysis he found that 12 of these came out of the intercurrent disease in a worse condition, 11 were unaffected, and 1 only seemed a little better. In my personal experience I have invariably seen the eczemas of children made worse by measles. I have no wish to dispute the trustworthiness of the statistics quoted by Thomas; indeed, I regard them as mostly thoroughly reliable instances of exceptions to a general pathological law; but I wish it to be clearly understood that they are such, and that measles is not a disease to be slightly regarded as to its effects upon the system.

[p. 575]MORBID ANATOMY.—The normal rash of measles is not to be observed on the dead body, and the only lesions of the skin to be noted are those resulting from extravasation of blood into that tissue. Examination of the skin removed during life from a patient with measles reveals the following anatomical changes, according to Morris.[35] In the earliest stages are found usually slight hyperæmia around the orifice of a sebaceous follicle, with slight swelling from effusion of plasma. Occasionally swelling alone is present, and more rarely hyperæmia only. Round the small hyperæmic papule thus developed—often pierced by a hair—a roseolar patch, due to congestion of the papillary body, soon makes its appearance. Slight exudation of plasma, with a few corpuscles, usually follows, and produces elevation of the papule itself. As most of the deaths in measles are due to the presence of some complication, the post-mortem changes will be found to correspond to the lesions produced by these diseases, principally affections of the respiratory organs and intestinal tract.

[35] *Skin Diseases*, Phila., 1880, p. 57.

DIAGNOSIS.—As a rule, the diagnosis of measles offers no great difficulties, especially if a correct clinical picture of the disease has been thoroughly impressed upon the mind. The salient points may be thus summarized: A period of incubation of about fourteen days—*i.e.* from the date of infection to the commencement of the eruption; a prodromic stage of about four days, ushered in with fever and marked implication of the mucous tract, notably cough, coryza, epistaxis, and photophobia; in this stage may also be noted the punctated redness of the conjunctivæ and of the palatal mucous membrane, which is to be regarded as a diagnostic sign of great value and importance; finally, there appears at the conclusion of the stage of invasion, simultaneously with increase of the febrile movement, a characteristic eruption upon the cutaneous surface, this eruption coming out first upon the face, and composed of large maculo-papules of brownish-red color, arranged in a crescentic form with tracts of normal integument intervening. Of all the symptoms of measles, the catarrh of the mucous membranes is undoubtedly the most pathognomonic. In the colored races, where the recognition of the skin lesion is often a matter of difficulty, this combination of symptoms should be borne in mind.[36]

[36] Corre (*La Mère et l'Enfant dans les races humaines*, Paris, 1882) states that measles and scarlatina exist in all climates and among all races; however, they are less frequent in warm than in cold climates. This relative rarity may be only apparent, and has only been established by reason of the difficulty of recognizing exanthems among dark-skinned peoples. In the

negro the eruption (of measles) often escapes observation, but the general symptoms, the angina, coryza, and bronchitis, and the special coloration of the bucco-pharyngeal membranes, permit the establishment of the diagnosis. The skin appears more tense, and the face especially is puffed and glossy; in passing the hand over the different regions of the body slight elevations are felt—a difference in the level of the skin exists in the affected and unaffected portions. On examining the surface of the body obliquely at a well-pronounced angle of incidence, these elevations can be perceived by the eye. Desquamation, which is very manifest in the negro, also confirms the diagnosis; this desquamation is formed of epidermic débris; it gives rise to a white dust, which is well defined against the black skin. The skin itself seems to have lost its gloss; it is completely dry, and no longer gives the abundant and odoriferous secretion characteristic of the subjects of that race.

[p. 576]In the way of conjectural diagnosis, the presence of an epidemic of measles in the community should be taken into account. Although measles possesses features so characteristic and pronounced, there are a number of other diseases with which it may be confounded, especially in its earlier stages.

There is no other disease which presents so close a resemblance to measles as does rötheln, and it must be confessed that under certain circumstances the question of diagnosis is a perplexing one. In rötheln the appearance of the eruption is often the first symptom of the affection, whereas in measles there is a prodromic period, having a peculiar remittent type of fever, which continues for three or four days. According to Liveing, the short duration of the febrile attack before the eruption appears is one of the most constant and distinctive features wherein rötheln differs from ordinary measles. In some instances, in rötheln the premonitory fever is not at all appreciable. The catarrhal involvement of the mucous membranes is not nearly so marked as in measles, while the very frequent sore throat bears more resemblance to the angina of scarlet fever. In many instances, although by no means constantly, the eruption of rötheln first appears on the chest, and not on the face, as is the rule in measles. It is quite evident that the eruptive spots of rötheln have presented different physical features in different epidemics; but, as a general thing, it may be said that they are smaller than those in measles, of a paler color, and, according to Thomas, not so angular, less indented, and not so often provided with processes, therefore less apt to assume the crescentic arrangement so often seen in measles.[37] The incubation period is longer in rötheln than in measles.

[37] According to Curtman (*St. Louis Courier Med.*, June, 1882), the eruption of rötheln consists, when not confluent, of single papules, each separated by a distinct small red areola. Not infrequently the papules are large, and sometimes a few pass into vesicles or pustules. In measles the papules are very small, mostly confluent, from four to six landing on a single areola, which is larger than that of rötheln.

In scarlet fever the incubation stage is shorter than in measles, and the constitutional symptoms are apt to be more pronounced; the temperature is higher, the pulse more rapid, and vomiting more frequent. The stage of invasion in scarlatina is but twenty-four hours; in measles, seventy-two. There is absence of the characteristic catarrh of measles, and the presence of severe sore throat, strawberry tongue, and swelling of the lymphatics at the angle of the jaws. In measles the rash begins on the face; in scarlatina, on the neck and chest. In measles the eruption consists of large papules arranged somewhat crescentically, with intervening normal skin, followed by bran-like desquamation; in scarlatina the rash is made up of large patches formed of minute red spots on a bright red, hyperæmic base, and is followed by desquamation in large lamellæ. In measles the rash is brightest on exposed parts; in scarlatina, most vivid on covered regions. The sequelæ of the two diseases are quite different.

There is no great difference in the duration of the invasion stages of variola and rubeola; but in the former disease we have the marked lumbar and sacral pains and vomiting, while in the latter the catarrhal symptoms and photophobia are pathognomonic. When the eruption of [p. 577]small-pox appears there is subsidence of fever; in measles, an exacerbation. A point of great importance in the diagnosis of variola is found in an examination of the mouth and pharynx, for in these situations on the fourth day we will often find the vesicles fully developed, while on the skin they are still in the stage of papulation. When measles assumes the papular form (morbilli papulosi, rougeole bouttoneuse), it is often confounded with the papular stage of small-pox. I have seen a number of such mistakes made. Attention to the general symptoms of the two diseases, however, and particularly an examination of the mucous membranes, will generally clear up any doubt. At any rate, the question will generally settle itself in the next twenty-four hours, for if it be variola the papules will have undergone their specific development and the rubeolous elevations will have become more decidedly macular.

Typhus sometimes offers a certain resemblance to measles. According to Buchanan,[38] the eruption of typhus is occasionally, though not commonly, a good deal like that of measles, and appears about the same time after invasion. Coryza, when present and distinct, points to measles. The eruption of typhus is of a smaller pattern, discrete, and not raised; that of measles, often coalescent, crescentic, and elevated. Subcuticular mottling is present in typhus, and absent in measles. The palatal mucous membrane should always be examined in suspected measles.

[38] Art. "Typhus" in *Reynolds's System Med.*, Am. ed., p. 262.

As I have never been able to convince myself of the existence of an independent disease called roseola, I am at a loss to give the points of differential diagnosis; on the other hand, the various forms of symptomatic erythema, occurring either as the result of numerous slight derangements of the system, or in connection with grave constitutional disease, should be carefully considered. In the first group of cases the absence of premonitory symptoms, catarrh, etc., and the presence of the smooth, rose-colored macules, mostly on the trunk, and in the latter the existence of symptoms belonging to the primary disease, should prove of assistance. The erythema papulatum of new-born children I have seen mistaken for measles, but the fact that rubeola is exceedingly rare in sucklings, and the absence of fever and catarrhal disturbances, are sufficient grounds for a differential diagnosis.

The erythematous syphilide (roseola syphilitica), particularly when accompanied by fever, may bear some resemblance to the rash of measles; but the history of the case, the circumscribed, indolent character of the syphilide, in many instances sparing the face, the absence of pathognomonic catarrhal symptoms of measles, and the coexistence of other features of syphilis, are quite distinctive.

PROGNOSIS.—The prognosis of normal uncomplicated measles is very favorable. Thus, of 257 cases observed by Meigs and Pepper (*op. cit.*), all terminated favorably. But in coming to any conclusion in regard to prognosis a number of different factors must be taken into consideration. Among the more important are—the hygienic surroundings of the patient, the age, the nature of the complications, whether the measles be primary or secondary, and the character of the epidemic. In the first place, rubeola in foundling hospitals and among the poorer classes in large cities gives a larger ratio of deaths than among the well-to-do members of the community. For instance, Bartels has shown that catarrhal pneumonia, one [p. 578]of the most frequent causes of mortality in this disease, is particularly prone to occur among those dwelling in crowded, poorly-ventilated houses. Then, again, the asylums and hospitals for children are peopled in many instances with the victims of depraved constitutions, who readily succumb to intercurrent maladies.

Leaving out of consideration sucklings under six months of age, in whom measles is rare and said to be slight, most deaths from the disease occur among very young children, from their greater liability to complications. According to Beddoes,[39] the mortality from measles is, beyond all comparison, greatest in the second year of life, and by the tenth has become quite trifling. An examination of the statistics bearing on this question coincides with this general statement; but Fox's tables, already quoted, would show that more infants under one year of age die of measles than has hitherto been supposed. The susceptibility to measles decreases with years, perhaps on account of the fact that most adults have already contracted the disease; but when it does attack the unprotected adult it may prove fatal. This statement is borne out by the large death-rate in the so-called camp measles of our late war.[40] The ravages of measles in virgin communities have been referred to in preceding pages. The general temper of the epidemic must also be considered, since it is well recognized that the essential character of epidemics differs much as to severity.

[39] Art. "Mortality" in *Quain's Dictionary Med.*, p. 1002.

[40] In the general field hospital at Chattanooga the death-rate was 22.4 in 100 cases. In General Hospital No. 1, at Nashville, it was 19.6 in 100, or nearly 1 in 5. Many died or became permanently disabled from the sequelæ (Bartholow).

Such complications as diphtheria, catarrhal pneumonia, diarrhoea, convulsions, etc. necessarily affect the prognosis of measles most seriously. More patients die of measles in the second than in the first week of the disease. The careful studies of temperature made by Thomas, Bohn, and others show that an unusually high and increasing fever in the prodromal stage is of ill omen, particularly on the second and third days, and a fever heat measuring over 105° F. at any stage should be considered as very unfavorable.[41] Particularly to be feared is continuation of the fever after the subsidence of the eruption, or a sudden elevation after the normal curve has been reached. In fact, it is a safe rule to look upon all anomalies of the curve with suspicion. Secondary measles, or measles grafted upon some serious existing affection, is particularly fatal.

[41] In adolescence a body heat of 107° F. has been safely passed during the decline of measles with no marked complication (Squire).

TREATMENT.—There is no remedy which will destroy the susceptibility to measles. The future may develop some form of vaccination against rubeola, for, certainly, the hopes held out by the inoculation of measles upon the healthy subject have not been realized, as this procedure merely reproduces the original complaint, without any diminution in its intensity, and does not lessen the probability of complications (Mayr). The matter of carrying out a practical and efficient quarantine in measles is one of unusual difficulty, for the reason that the disease is capable of active propagation at a time—the prodromal stage—when it is not yet sufficiently characteristic for positive diagnosis. But, as measles is by no means as trivial a disease as would seem to be the common impression, I hold it as a well-established principle of preventive medicine that a [p. 579]strict isolation should be enforced whenever, from the nature of the case, it is at all possible; certainly, very young children and those suffering from or showing a tendency to other diseases should be jealously shielded from exposure.

The usual precautions as to disinfection and purification of the room, bedding, and utensils used by patients should be observed, as in other infectious diseases. Squire is of opinion that there is danger of personal infection for perhaps a month, and Hillairet that isolation for forty days should be enjoined. It is quite certain that inunction lessens the danger of infection, and Kaposi[42] is authority for the statement that a warm bath administered after the completion of desquamation, or about fourteen days from the beginning of the attack, will effectually prevent contagiousness.

[42] *Pathologie u. Therapie der Hautkrankh.*, Wien, 1880.

The apartment occupied by a patient suffering from measles should be kept at a uniform temperature of from 66° to 70° F., and free ventilation, at the same time avoiding draughts, should be enforced. The room should be kept moderately dark. The bed-clothing should be light, yet sufficiently warm, and the old notion of keeping the patient in a profuse sweat the better to bring out the eruption should be discouraged. The diet should be bland and nutritious, and may preferably consist of milk, gruel, tapioca, and such like substances. As convalescence progresses there may be a gradual return to more substantial food. The patient may be allowed cool water in moderation, as it is cruel and useless, and even harmful, to restrict one suffering with fever to warm or sweetened drink. The patient should be confined to his room until convalescence has been fully established, and should not be allowed to leave the house, both on his own account and that of others, until the usual health has been regained. Any of the lingering results of the disease, such as bronchitis, otorrhoea, conjunctivitis, etc., should receive prompt attention; iron and cod-liver oil should be prescribed for the weakly and strumous, and regular hours of sleep, careful diet, and appropriate bathing and exercise should be advised. It may be said, without exaggeration, that neglect of the after-care of measles patients is, in some instances, more to be deprecated than a similar neglect in the actual treatment of the disease itself.

Since we are powerless to cut short an attack of measles by any remedial agents at present known to therapeutics, the intervention of the physician is limited to assisting the cases through to a safe termination. Quite a number of cases, as seen in private practice, require no special medicinal treatment, or at most one that is merely symptomatic. The value of the so-called specific treatment, such as by carbonate of ammonium, etc., has not been verified by experience.

In ordinary uncomplicated attacks, if the temperature should run high, in addition to the general rules as to diet and hygiene referred to before it will usually be found advisable to put the patient on some diaphoretic mixture, to which may be added a mild opiate. I know of nothing better than the formula found in the work of Meigs and Pepper on the *Diseases of Children:*

[p. 580]

x.	Potass. Citrat.		drachm i;
	Spt. Ætheris Nit.	ii;	fl. drachm
	Tr. Opii Deodorat.	vel xxiv;	minim xii
	Syrupi	ii;	fl. drachm
	Aquæ	ii. M.	fl. oz.

S. A teaspoonful every two or three hours for a child of five years of age.

Aconite in small doses has been well spoken of in this connection, but I have no personal experience in its use. Bromide of potassium, together with a few drops of syrup of ipecac., dissolved in syrup of wild cherry, acts pleasantly both on the cough and the nervous system.

The inunction of fatty substances, as originally proposed by Schonemann, and recently urged by Milton,[43] is an excellent routine practice, and in addition to adding very much to the patient's comfort, has, perhaps, the merit of lessening somewhat the danger of infection to others. For this purpose one may use leaf lard, cold cream, or vaseline, to each ounce of which it is well to add a few minims of carbolic acid.

[43] *Archives of Dermatology.*

Stimulants are rarely needed in uncomplicated measles, but Squire very wisely calls attention to the great value of wine in the depression following upon the crisis.

In spite of some excellent authority to the contrary, I cannot see that any benefit is to be derived from using severe measures to bring out an eruption that has undergone retrocession. As stated in another part of this article, the so-called striking-in of the rash is the result of the supervention of some complication, and not the cause of it; therefore, a rational course of action would be to ascertain the nature of the complicating trouble, and to endeavor to correct it, which, at the same time, would be the very best means of restoring the normal course of the disease.

Quinia is of great value in controlling the excessively high temperature which is sometimes observed either in connection with, or independent of, complications. If the quinia should prove ineffectual or else be rejected by the patient, the physician should not hesitate to abstract heat by cold water in the shape of the wet pack or the general bath. I think the latter method is to be preferred. It is but to employ the gradually cooled bath of Ziemssen, perhaps, commencing at 90° F. and going to 80° or 70° F. The condition of the patient, as ascertained by the thermometer and also the state of the pulse, must be the guide as to the duration and repetition of the baths. In Germany excellent results are claimed for the treatment of hyperpyrexia in measles by the cold pack, even when the excessive temperature is due to such a complication as broncho-pneumonia.

There is little hope from therapeutical interference in malignant forms of measles, but the medical attendant should endeavor to reduce temperature and support the strength by free stimulation and nourishing food.

It will now be advisable, at the risk of some repetition, to call attention to the treatment of some of the more prominent disturbances and complications of measles.

Epistaxis, if severe, should be checked by cold applications and astringents. Plugging will rarely be found necessary. Trousseau recommends the injection of water as hot as can be borne. Ergotine by the mouth or hypodermically will sometimes prove highly valuable.

The lids should be anointed with vaseline or cold cream to prevent their sticking together, and it is well to occasionally evert them to see that no[p. 581]serious mischief has happened to the eye. If the conjunctivitis is intense, the discharges should be removed and cold compresses applied.

Since aural complications are due to extension of inflammation from the oral and nasal cavities, Spencer urges the importance of early and systematic treatment of these parts. He advises astringent applications (Monsell's solution 1 to 4 of glycerine) to the pharyngeal mucous membrane. Ointments of boracic acid, zinc, or iodoform are likewise useful when introduced through the nostril. Earache will require warm opiated poultices and inflation. Otorrhoea is best treated after the dry method.

For sickness of the stomach a spice poultice may be applied and small bits of ice given to suck. If constipation exist, a little oil or syrup of rhubarb or some stewed prunes, or an enema, may be ordered. Active purgation should be withheld.

The early diarrhoea need give little concern, as it usually soon ceases; but if it should persist, recourse must be had to more energetic measures, such as the use of opium by mouth or enema, given cautiously in the case of children, vegetable and metallic astringents, and the application of hot poultices to the abdomen. The diet should be carefully guarded.

The cough, even in mild cases, generally requires some slight palliative, such as syrup of ipecac., and an occasional small dose of Dover's powder. Loeri very properly advises against the use of irritating expectorants. I think it advisable to keep the chest well smeared with camphorated oil, over which should be worn an oil-silk jacket. These simple measures, perhaps, diminish the tendency to thoracic complications. The sometimes violent paroxysms of false croup are very satisfactorily managed, after the manner of Graves, by gently pressing a sponge, soaked in very hot water, under the chin and over the front of the neck. When the dyspnoea is alarming, emetics, and the general warm bath should be brought into requisition.

Convulsions in the early stage require little treatment other than the warm bath and appropriate doses of the bromide of potassium; occurring later, they are very fatal under any treatment, as they generally supervene in connection with some of the grave complications of the disease. Chloral, preferably by enema, and chloroform may be tried. The management of the severe bronchitis and pneumonia of measles requires great care and circumspection on the part of the physician. The application of a well-made flaxseed poultice, which should be neither too heavy nor too hot, is to be regarded as invaluable. To the flaxseed may be added a small quantity of mustard. Over the whole is to be placed an oil-silk jacket. Alcoholic stimulants, nourishing, easily-digested food, and expectorants containing carbonate of ammonium are to be recommended.

For the treatment of the other complications and sequelæ of measles the reader is referred to the appropriate sections of this work.

[p. 582]

RÖTHELN.[1]
BY W. A. HARDAWAY, M.D.

[1] In the preparation of this article the author has consulted the following authorities: Emminghaus, in *Gerhardt's Handb. der Kinderkrankh.*, Zweiter Band, 1877; Thomas, in *Ziemssen's Cyclop. Pract. Med.*, vol. iii., Am. ed., 1875; Squire, in *Quain's Dict. Med.*, 1883. References to current literature will be found in foot-notes to the text.

SYNONYMS.—Rubeola, Rubella, Roseola, Epidemic Roseola, German Measles, French Measles, Hybrid Measles, False Measles, Rubeola Morbillosæ et Scarlatinosæ.

DEFINITION.—Rötheln is an acute infectious disease, presenting an eruption of reddish macules upon the skin, accompanied by mild catarrhal symptoms, and usually producing but slight disturbance of the general system. It is self-protective, and occurs but once in the same individual. It has no relationship to measles or scarlatina.

HISTORY.—A rapid glance at the interesting historical evolution of rötheln to a specific position among the acute infectious diseases is all that our space will allow. Some writers have attempted to show that this affection was known to the Arabian physicians; but since it is only in comparatively recent times that the contagious epidemic exanthemata in general have been thoroughly differentiated, it is quite likely that the modern conception of it was not held by them nor by other medical men till many centuries later. Indeed, in our day, physicians are yet to be found, though the number is rapidly diminishing, who refuse to recognize in rötheln a distinctive specific malady. Certain German observers in the middle of the last century (De Bergen, 1752; Orlow, 1758) favored the idea of specificity, but these views were soon disputed. In the years following a number of other physicians announced their belief in the specific nature of rötheln, while, on the other hand, various noted authorities still insisted upon its connection with scarlet fever or measles. In 1815, Maton, an English physician, most unequivocally declared that he had observed cases of an eruptive disorder which resembled neither measles, scarlatina, nor roseola, and which was worthy of a new designation.[2] In the second and third decades of this century Hildebrand, and afterward the celebrated Schönlein, taught that rötheln was a hybrid of measles and scarlatina, although at this time Wagner (1834) advocated the essential independence of rötheln. There is no doubt that under the name of rubeola sine catarrho Willan, Bateman, and later writers described what we now call rötheln, for they stated that this variety of measles was not self-protective. Space will not allow of a detailed mention of the various writers who, during the first half of this century,[p. 583]have contended for or against the autonomy of rötheln. It will be well to state, however, that Hebra, from the standpoint of the dermatologist, very properly regards the manifold roseolæ of Willan as in many instances merely symptomatic erythemata, or else as irregular forms of measles or scarlatina; but he also fails to recognize the distinctive features of rötheln. Even so recent a writer as Niemeyer declares that roseola arising from infection consists in a modification of measles or scarlet fever. It is only in the last twenty years that our present exact ideas of rötheln have obtained. For example, while Trousseau[3] asserts that rubeola (rötheln) is a perfectly distinct nosological species, he speaks of the rash as appearing and disappearing alternately for some days, of its frequent recurrence in the same individual, etc. American physicians were almost entirely ignorant of rötheln till within the last ten years, when they were made acquainted with it through the medium of a careful paper on the subject from the pen of J. Lewis Smith of New York.[4] Before this time, however, cases had been described by Homans, Sr., of Boston (1845), and in 1853 and 1871 by Cotting. Very few authorities now dispute the distinctive specific nature of rötheln; which statement is borne out by the fact that at the last meeting of the International Medical Congress, held at London in 1881, there were but two dissentients to this view in the section before which it was discussed.[5]

[2] Squire, *Trans. Internat. Med. Congress*, London, 1881.

[3] *Clinical Medicine*, vol. ii.

[4] *Archives of Dermatology*, Oct., 1874.

[5] See especially Kassowitz's paper, "Die Wirkliche Stellung der sogenannten Rubeola," etc., *Trans. Internat. Med. Cong.*, 1881.

ETIOLOGY.—The contagium of rötheln is unknown, but that the disease is contagious has been fully demonstrated by numerous observations of epidemics and sporadic cases. From my own experience I should judge that unprotected persons are not so susceptible of it as is known to be the case under similar conditions in measles;[6] yet cases are recorded which would prove that the contagion may be conveyed through a third person and for some distance. It is probable that the vehicles of contagion are the same as in measles. At what period of its course the disease is most capable of transmission has not been satisfactorily determined. Squire is of the opinion, however, that the disease is contagious before the appearance of the rash, and may continue so for some days or for two or three weeks. Rötheln may be called a disease of childhood for the same reason that the other contagious exanthemata are—namely, that the majority of adults have already been attacked. From an examination of available statistics I am inclined to regard the ages between five and fifteen—the years of school attendance—as the period of life most susceptible of the influence of rötheln, although, of course, no time of life is entirely exempt. The non-susceptibility of sucklings, as in measles, holds true as a rule, although I am in a position to supply exceptions to this from my own experience, as well as from that of others. Sex seems to be without influence in determining liability to the disease.

[6] In this regard it resembles scarlatina more than measles, for I have a number of times seen the disease introduced into families, where it would attack one or two of a number equally exposed. J. L. Smith regards it as feebly contagious, and quotes Chadbourne's experience to the same effect. Liveing declares that rötheln is more distinctly epidemic in Great Britain than either measles or scarlet fever, although probably less contagious.

The period of incubation is not very definitely settled, and, indeed, [p. 584]owing to the generally trivial character of the affection, evidence on this point is difficult to obtain. Taken as a whole, it is probably longer than is observed in measles. According to J. Lewis Smith, in the epidemic observed by him the incubation period varied from seven, or less than seven, to twenty-one days; Emminghaus places it at from two to three weeks; Thomas, from two and a half to three weeks; Squire, mostly a fortnight, the extreme being twenty-one days; Cheadle, from eleven to twelve days.

There is nowhere recorded a trustworthy instance of a second attack of rötheln, although from analogy such an event is to be expected. As in measles, true recurrences of rötheln—that is, the result of a fresh infection—are not to be confounded with relapses. I have never witnessed a relapse, but cases of such a nature have been recorded by other observers (Lindwurm, Emminghaus, Körtlin, Kingsley).

Rötheln is a disease sui generis, and is in no way related to either measles or scarlatina; that is to say, it is not an irregular form of either of these nor a hybrid of them, nor has it ever been observed to propagate anything but itself. That it is not connected with any of the symptomatic skin eruptions—the so-called roseolæ—is proved by its contagiousness and epidemic character. I quite agree with other observers in declaring that rötheln has very little clinical resemblance to scarlatina, and that, on the other hand, in the greatest number of cases the points of likeness are with measles. In the section on diagnosis the differential points between rötheln, measles, and scarlatina will be considered; therefore in this place it will only be necessary to call attention to certain general facts. Thus, aside from the marked divergence in clinical symptoms—incubation, invasion, fever, eruption, complications, and sequelæ—we are at once met by the positive fact that epidemics of rötheln, while always presenting identical features, prevail without regard to the existence of similar epidemics of measles and scarlatina—following or preceding them—and that attacks of rötheln offer no bar to the reception of their contagions, or vice versâ. Literature is so full of examples of this statement that it need scarcely be dwelt upon. By way of illustration, however, the accurate observations of J. Lewis Smith may be quoted in this connection. Of 48 cases recorded by him prior to May 1st in the New York epidemic of 1874, 19 had had measles. Rötheln in the N.Y. Foundling Hospital in 1873-74 followed an epidemic of measles. During the epidemic of 1880-81 the same fact was observed—namely, that a previous attack of measles, as well as scarlatina, afforded no protection from rötheln. I could multiply such examples from my own experience. A single interesting instance may be noted here. A physician asked the writer to examine his child, suffering, as he thought, from measles. A careful investigation revealed a typical rötheln. A number of weeks later an older child got measles, from which the rötheln patient acquired a characteristic attack of the same. In the following year both children were taken with scarlet fever.

The only escape for those who would deny the autonomy of rötheln is in the bold assertion that both measles and scarlatina more frequently recur in the same individual than universal experience and observation will allow; and this leaves them in the dilemma of determining to which group rötheln must be relegated. The hypothesis of the hybrid nature [p. 585]of rötheln cannot be accepted by the pathologist nor the clinician, if for no other reason than that no one has ever seen rötheln generate anything but rötheln, and in no case give rise to either scarlatina or measles.

SYMPTOMS AND COURSE.—As already stated, the probable average duration of the incubation period in rötheln is about fourteen days, varying, however, within the limits of from six to twenty-one days. In this respect rötheln resembles scarlatina more than measles, the period of latency in the latter observing considerable uniformity. No deviations from the general health are to be noted in the incubation stage.

In most cases prodromal symptoms are entirely absent, the presence of the eruption being the first thing to show the existence of rötheln in the system. On the other hand, in a certain proportion of cases there will be present for a half day, or even longer, the general symptoms of malaise, such as slight nausea, some sore throat, pain in the limbs, stiffness of the neck, etc. Vomiting is generally absent. J. L. Smith records one case of convulsions in the stage of invasion, and I have notes of a single case in which the prodromal stage was initiated by mild delirium and fever, the latter anticipating the eruption for two days and a half, and disappearing when the rash came out. As Thomas well observes, however, such cases are anomalous, and indicate either abnormal sensibility on the part of the patient or are due to a secondary rötheln.

Most observers (Emminghaus, Thomas, Smith, Squire) describe the rash as coming out in the order usual in measles—namely, first upon the face, scalp, and neck, then the trunk and arms, and finally the legs. Others (Liveing, Morris) have stated that the rash first appears upon the back and chest. In many cases in my own experience this has seemed to be true. It is quite probable that the situation of the exanthem in rötheln, as in measles and scarlatina, may present various irregularities; but I am inclined to believe that a careful investigation will in most instances show that the normal course of the eruption is as first stated. Now, a marked characteristic of the rash of rötheln is that, unlike that of measles, there is no period, however short, in which its maximum is simultaneous over the whole body; on the contrary, the eruption will have reached its full development upon the face, and will be almost or quite faded again, before the exanthem, for example, will have blossomed upon the trunk, and especially upon the lower extremities. The duration of the eruption upon individual parts of the body is probably from a few hours to half a day at most (Thomas). A consideration of these facts explains, according to Emminghaus, how different observers have described the eruption as having its seat upon this or that region of the body; in other words, it is probable that in a certain proportion of the cases in which the rash was supposed to have begun on the chest it had already run its course upon the face. The eruption usually continues altogether about four days, sometimes disappearing sooner, and sometimes being visible, especially as a fine mottling, for some days longer. So far as the individual lesions of the eruption are concerned, there is no question that they present, within a certain range, varying aspects; and this clinical fact has been taken advantage of by the opponents of the idea of specificity in order to make it appear that the disease is not sui generis, inasmuch as it lacks uniformity of expression. Such an argument wants force when we consider that in making up a given diagnosis we lay stress [p. 586]not upon special, but upon the ensemble of, symptoms. For example, no one would deny to measles an independent position because the eruption, as is well known, may assume this or that form (morbilli lævis, m. papulosi, etc.); on the contrary, we recognize a particular case or series of cases to be measles from a due appreciation of all the symptoms present. So it is to be expected that while the cutaneous lesions will present a certain similarity of feature, as they do, there will also exist minor differences in detail.

In the greatest number of cases in my own experience the exanthem is composed of ill-defined, roundish, punctate macules, without special grouping. These are usually discrete, but in certain situations they may coalesce. The color is of a pale rosy red, quite difficult to describe, but less purplish than in measles, and not so livid a red as in scarlatina. I have occasionally observed large irregular spots not unlike those of measles.[7]

---

[7] According to Emminghaus (*op. cit.*, p. 345), the eruption generally forms roseolæ of pin-head, lentil, or small bean size. They are mostly round, sometimes oval, and bordered by well-defined or by blurred edges. The intervening skin is not always unchanged, for here and

there we find upon it small dilated blood-vessels, and from the spots processes extend with a certain regularity to other spots in such a way as to give the skin a marbled appearance.

Thomas distinguishes three types of eruption—one with large spots, which is rare; one with medium-sized spots; and one with small spots. Emminghaus describes a discrete and a more confluent variety. I have observed one case where the maculæ on the back had undergone a vesicular transformation. Others have mentioned this occurrence. Itching of the skin is marked in some cases, and a fine desquamation is observed after the rash, but by no means invariably.

The mucous membranes are implicated to a slight degree in rötheln, but the amount of involvement varies considerably. In some cases that I have observed the catarrh of the mucous membranes has been barely appreciable. As a rule, however, the eyes are somewhat suffused, and there is slight lachrymation and photophobia. Sneezing may be noted, but there is little discharge from the nose. Sore throat is not uncommon, perhaps the most constant feature, and, according to Liveing, is apt to persist after the subsidence of the rash. The fauces are injected, and the tonsils are red and swollen, but with no evidence of ulceration. J. Lewis Smith and others state that the buccal mucous membrane shows a more or less diffuse patchy and spotted redness. The tongue may be, and usually is, covered by a white fur, through which protrude a few enlarged red papillæ. There may be slight cough. Loeri[8] describes the mucous membranes of the pharynx, larynx, and trachea as presenting a spotted or uniform hyperæmia. There is no marked participation of the intestines in the catarrh. Some few writers have noted a transient albuminuria, but it is safe to say that such cases are entirely anomalous, if not, indeed, in some instances, examples of mistaken diagnosis.

[8] *Jahrb. f. Kinderk.*, xix. Bd., 1 Heft.

A very constant feature is the swelling of the lymphatic glands of the neck, especially those back of the sterno-mastoid; the swellings may come on before the rash appears. In all the cases that have fallen under my notice this symptom has not been absent in a single instance. Less constantly, and it would seem in proportion to the development of the rash, engorgement of the glands may be noted elsewhere.

[p. 587]There is but slight disturbance of the temperature in rötheln, and when it does occur it is usually limited to the first few hours of the eruption. This has been the rule in my observation, and certainly holds good for the majority of cases. In a minority, varying degrees of fever may be present; thus, the temperature may reach 102° F. or 103° F., and then rapidly sink by the second day of the disease, or, having fallen a degree, it may continue at this point till the subsidence of the rash, or, it is said, may retain its initial height till the end of the disease. During the following week Squire states that the temperature may be readily disturbed—either elevated by exertion or depressed by fatigue or chill. A relapse or recrudescence of the rash may be looked for at this time.[9]

[9] Cheadle (*Trans. Internat. Med. Congress*, London, 1881) has reported an epidemic of rötheln of a very severe type, all the symptoms of the disease as ordinarily recognized being very much exaggerated.

COMPLICATIONS AND SEQUELÆ.—In the vast majority of cases neither complications nor sequelæ have been observed in connection with rötheln. J. Lewis Smith has recorded instances of diphtheritic inflammation as a complication, which, however, as he justly remarks, may, when prevalent, attack any inflamed surface. Pneumonia and bronchitis have been occasionally reported as complicating or following rötheln. Liveing and Duckworth mention albuminuria, but, so far as I know, they are alone in this experience. I have known otorrhoea and ciliary blepharitis to occur as sequelæ. It would not be a matter of surprise that in weakly children various chronic ailments should be set up by rötheln, as by any other disturbance of the general health.

DIAGNOSIS.—There is no other disease which so much resembles rötheln as measles. Especially is this true of atypical cases occurring sporadically. In rötheln the whole course of the disease is much milder than in measles, the incubation is longer as a rule, and the fact of a previous attack of rubeola is of much importance, since we know that recurrences are very rare. In measles there is a prodromic period, having a characteristic temperature curve, and presenting pathognomonic catarrhal symptoms, which precedes the eruption for three or four days; in rötheln the appearance of the rash is often the first sign of the affection. The sore throat of rötheln resembles that seen in scarlatina more than the angina of measles, and the general catarrhal implication of the mucous membranes, so marked a feature of measles, is either absent in rötheln or exists to a very trivial extent. Measles is essentially a febrile disease, having a peculiar type of fever; rötheln may run its whole course without appreciable rise of temperature. As will be seen in the preceding pages, the development and progress of the exanthem of measles differs materially from that witnessed in rötheln. In measles the lesions are larger, more vivid, more angular and indented, more frequently provided with processes, and therefore more apt to assume the crescentic arrangement, than in rötheln. Finally, it must be urged that the tout ensemble of the case should be taken into consideration, and not some special feature of the skin eruption.

The incubation period of scarlet fever is much shorter than in rötheln, and all of the constitutional symptoms are, as a rule, infinitely graver. In scarlatina there is a febrile invasion stage of twenty-four hours; in rötheln, if fever is present at all, it is most generally simultaneous with [p. 588]the rash, and rapidly disappears, while in the former it persists for a number of days longer. Vomiting is common in scarlet fever, rare in rötheln. In scarlet fever the lymphatic glands are notably involved at the angles of the jaw, in rötheln at the sides and back of the neck. Sore throat is a feature common to both scarlet fever and rötheln, but it is very much less marked in the latter. Thomas[10] says that in scarlatina only the posterior parts, the uvula, the arches of the palate and their vicinity are affected, while in rötheln the anterior parts are also affected, and both in much the same degree. In scarlet fever the rash, which mostly begins on the neck and chest, is made up of large patches formed of minute red spots on a bright-red hyperæmic base; in rötheln the eruption is composed of roundish pea-sized macules, with normal integument intervening. In cases of doubt—for example, when the rash of rötheln consists of very small spots which have become confluent—the further development and persistence of the scarlatinal efflorescence, the temperature, the pulse, the angina, and the character of the desquamation must be taken into consideration. The complications and sequelæ are very different in the two diseases.

[10] Article "Scarlatina," *op. cit.*

The symptomatic eruptions of the skin which pass under the name of roseola bear no resemblance to rötheln. They usually occur as the result of some trivial derangement of the system or in the course of some primary affection. They are not contagious, the lymphatic glands and the mucous membranes are not involved, and the rash is quite different in character.

PROGNOSIS.—The prognosis of simple uncomplicated rötheln is invariably good. Complications arising in delicate children necessarily affect the prognosis, as would any other disturbance of the general health.

TREATMENT.—Simple cases of rötheln require no treatment, as the patients are rarely sick enough to be confined to bed. Graver forms of the disease must be met by such measures as are indicated by the symptoms present. The after-management must be conducted on general principles having reference to the previous and present condition of the person attacked.

[p. 589]

MALARIAL FEVERS.
BY SAMUEL M. BEMISS, M.D.

In the medical nomenclature of this country the term malaria is synonymous with swamp or ague poison.

Malarial affections, therefore, comprise all those diseases or morbid manifestations which the swamp poison produces in the human organism.

This article is not designed to notice in a systematic manner any of these disorders which are not properly classifiable under the head of malarial fevers. It will, however, be necessary to make such references to the pathology of chronic malarial toxæmia as may serve to explain the influence this condition exerts in occasioning departures from type in the febrile attacks.

When a poison generated outside the human system obtains admission to it, and produces deleterious effects, three questions naturally arise: What is the essential character and natural history of this noxious agent? How does it obtain access to the human system? What is its mode of action when received?

In reference to the first of these questions, it must be admitted that the substantive essentiality of the malarial poison remains as yet undemonstrated. It is true, however, that the attempts at an objective study of this poison by means of the microscope and the cultivating retort point to the conclusion that it is an organism.

Its subjective or analogical study affords quite incontestable evidence in support of this conclusion. The leading features in the natural history of malaria are closely coincident with those of certain known organisms. It requires for its production suitable conditions of moisture, temperature, and a properly circumstanced breeding-place. Within certain bounds these conditions are requisite to the life and perpetuity of all organisms.

Again, when all the above-enumerated conditions correspond apparently in the most favorable degree, their continuous concurrence for a lapse of time is necessary before the poison manifests its presence. It is not improbable that this period of development may differ in different climates, but in this country we assume it to be about thirty days. If these facts related to some noxious organism visible to the eye, no doubt would be entertained that the presence of its germs in the places where it appeared was the indispensable condition. It would then follow that the concurrence of suitable meteorologic and telluric conditions with sufficient time for its growth and maturity were merely accessories to its perfect development. According to this theory, the coincidence of five circumstances is necessary before malaria can be fully matured—viz.: Its own [p. 590]specific germ; suitable soil or pabulum; suitable moisture; suitable temperature; sufficient time for its growth and development.

Certain physical qualities which pertain to the malarial poison can also be profitably made points of subjective study. These are very closely connected with the answer to the second question, or "How the malarial poison obtains access to the human system." They will therefore be briefly noticed in relation to the instrumentality of each in conveying malaria into the system.

The first to be mentioned is ponderability, which the following facts prove that malaria possesses:

Those different atmospheric states which affect the range of diffusion of known airborne yet ponderable substances exert similar influences upon the malarial poison.

Altitude illustrates the ponderability of malaria by powerfully retarding its diffusion.

High readings of the barometer favor its aërial dissemination.

Fogs, smoke, dust, or floating particles presumably more buoyant than this poison may exert greater or less influence in overcoming the obstacle which ponderability attaches to malaria as an air-borne agent.

Currents of air passing continuously and steadily in one direction over the breeding-places of malaria increase the limits and intensity of toxic range.

The atmosphere is undoubtedly the medium by means of which malarial poison is most frequently brought into the human system. Liability to intoxication is increased in direct ratio to the proximity of points of exposure to places of development; to similarity of level; to situation in the line of prevailing winds which have traversed the breeding-ground; and, lastly, to the extent and fertility of the locality of production.

Whether malaria passes through the respiratory apparatus directly into the circulation, or is lodged upon the fauces and absorbed through some other surface, is not clearly ascertainable. It is certainly not deprived of its noxious qualities by stomach digestion, and therefore, sometimes at least, may reach the blood through the alimentary canal.

Malaria is miscible with water. It is capable of being carried by currents of water through distances and periods of time altogether undetermined, without losing either its toxic effects or, perhaps, the faculty of reproduction. It is more than likely that this means of conveyance has effected its distribution to continents and islands too widely separated to justify a belief that it was wind-wafted. No observations need be adduced to establish the water-borne habit of the malarial poison, or the positive liability to its toxic effects when received into the stomach through this medium. These facts have been well understood from the time of Hippocrates.

The matter of communicability of malaria by means of drinking water should not be dismissed without some allusion to the great probability that other fluids or solids are open to a similar charge. There is a widespread popular prejudice, especially notable in the southern part of the United States, that drinking milk occasions attacks of the endemic fevers. It is the usual custom to pour the evening supply of milk into broad uncovered pans, and allow it to remain exposed in the open air for [p. 591]consumption at the morning meal. This viscid fluid, so tenacious of ordinary air-borne particles, may well be suspected of entangling sufficient quantities of swamp poison to produce sickness if exposed where it is rife during a whole night.

A similar popular prejudice exists in regard to the muscadine grape, which flourishes best in swampy localities. The rough skin of this fruit, frequently covered with its own juice, offers favorable conditions for the adhesion of air-borne particles.

The malarial poison is not reproduced within the human system. This proposition is undeniable, since no intensification of the poison is produced by any degree of crowding of the sick which can be practised; neither do any conditions of contact with the sick ever impart malarial affections.

Malarial poison is specific. This allegation is sufficiently established by its specific effects on the human economy. There is no other agent known which is capable of originating morbid phenomena characterized by such marked diurnal periodicity.

It is not interchangeable with other specific poisons. This statement may be rested upon all fairly collected clinical observations.

There are no facts which justify the belief that malaria is capable of becoming mixed in the atmosphere, or outside the system, with any other specific morbific germ, so as to produce a third something which may give rise to compound forms of disease.

The answer to the second question which is best supported is, that the malarial poison is brought into the system principally by breathing an atmosphere impregnated with this miasm.

It is also ingested by being held in suspension in fluids used as drink or food; perhaps also by eating certain fruits or vegetables in their natural state whose external surfaces afford favorable conditions for its lodgment.

MORBID EFFECTS AND PHENOMENA WHICH FOLLOW ITS INTRODUCTION INTO THE HUMAN SYSTEM.—The discussion of the morbid process established by the malarial poison involves some difficult problems. A period of incubation must be admitted to follow the inception of the ague germs. But this period has no definitely marked limits. Perhaps it is a shifting one, according to the quantity or quality of the poison received, or the sudden or gradual manner in which it is received, or the state of receptivity of the system.

Certain facts seem to indicate very clearly that malarial poison is very slowly removed from a system which has been brought under its influence. These evidences of long systemic residence of the poison are principally displayed in those attacks which occur after long periods of removal from any surrounding where intoxication was possible. Vernal attacks may be classed in the same connection. In many instances the subjects of these long-delayed attacks have never suffered a paroxysmal seizure, and yet when some accidental derangement of health occurs, as from a fit of indigestion or a sudden wetting, they fall sick with one or another form of malarial fever.

It does not appear to me that we are justified in assuming that such attacks as I refer to are to be ascribed to secondary changes produced in either the fluids or solids of the system by the malarial poison. In so [p. 592]far as the clinical phenomena are worth anything in demonstrating the presence and agency of the specific malarial poison in these deferred attacks, they are precisely similar to those observed in paroxysms arising after a few hours' or a few days' exposure to marsh miasm.

But we find further proofs of the long-continued and silent manner in which malaria exerts its pathological influences in those enlargements of the spleen which occur without specific attacks of sickness. The alterations of nutrition in this organ are so characteristic of malaria that they can scarcely be supposed to depend upon those chances which determine the nature of secondary blood-impurities.

Intermittent Fever—Simple Forms.

The clinical phenomena of intermittent fevers afford strong support to the opinion that this type of malarial attacks illustrates more strongly than any other the primary influence of the poison upon the human system. Fits of ague often occur very shortly after exposure in infected localities, and the persons thus suddenly attacked may present little or no evidence of cachexia before or after the paroxysm. Indeed, they frequently resume their ordinary avocations after the paroxysms, apparently as well as if they had not occurred.

It is therefore my opinion that the pathology of an intermittent fever does not necessarily involve an hypothesis that the attacks are the results of certain changes which the poison undergoes after its inception, nor, on the other hand, that certain perversions of systemic chemistry are required to inaugurate the paroxysms.

In accordance with these conclusions, it seems likely that the phenomena of intermittent malarial fever result from the primary effects of its specific poison exerted directly upon the fluids and solids of the system, and disturbing their functions, and especially the nerve-function.

Those malarial attacks which ensue almost immediately after exposure are principally manifested in persons exposed at points of unusually abundant evolution. The rule of malarial attacks in temperate latitudes is, that they require repeated exposure to infection for their production. The long residence of the poison in the system may render additional doses possible, until a point of saturation is reached which occasions paroxysmal explosions. In these cases the period of incubation is reckoned from the first date of exposure, thus forming the most striking contrast with the incubative periods of the cases occurring almost immediately after exposure.

Whether the quiescent period after exposure to malaria be long or short, attacks are seldom abrupt in their announcement. The symptoms which usually precede pronounced attacks consist, for the most part, in some derangement of the functions presided over by the organic nervous system. Derangement of digestion, vitiated taste, coating of the tongue, loaded urine, and sallow skin are ordinarily found among the prodromic symptoms. Next in succession come feelings of malaise, hot and cold flushes, and those neuralgias which precede and attend malarial paroxysms.

The symptoms of an ordinary or typical malarial paroxysm are so characteristic, as to be generally readily interpreted. Creeping, chilly,[p. 593]sensations over the surface, especially along the spine, yawning, livid coloration beneath the finger-nails, retreat of blood from superficial capillaries, and that consequent papillary elevation which is commonly called goose-skin, comprise the earliest symptoms. Then decided shiverings with chattering of the teeth come on, and the patient asks for blankets to be heaped upon him and hot applications to be made, even though the atmospheric temperature may be decidedly elevated.

Nausea and vomiting are frequent symptoms, no doubt due to the fact that the portal system of blood-vessels is so often the seat of congestion during a chill. No intelligent practitioner can watch a patient during the cold stage of a malarial paroxysm without realizing how important the attendant congestion is as a pathological state. It should first be considered that every chill necessarily implies a condition of congestion in some part of the system. The blood driven from the surface and extremities must be accounted for elsewhere;

and the amount of blood which is lost from one part of the circulatory tree must correspond with that accumulated elsewhere. But in treating of the pernicious forms of malarial fevers this question will again receive notice.

In our present state of knowledge we are no more able to explain those perversions of the normal action of the physical forces of the system which occasion the phenomena of a chill than we are to explain how the altered circulation in the first steps of an inflammation is brought about. The theory which Cullen adopted is quite as explanatory and consistent as any which has been promulgated since his time. According to this, a state of spasm of the arterioles and capillaries causes the chill, while the fever is merely the rebound of functions held in abeyance during the chill.

After a variable length of time there occurs a change in these symptoms: the patient begins to remove the blankets which covered him; the face shows signs of returning circulation; the veins of the whole surface gradually fill again, apparently beyond their normal state. But the reaction goes far beyond any normal physiological state. The face becomes flushed and the eyes injected, and the patient complains of headache, thirst, dryness and heat of the surface; he will not permit any covering, and constantly shifts his place in the bed in the hope that some new position may afford him more comfort. Nausea and vomiting are commonly present. If the fever runs high, delirium is apt to occur. The thermometer seldom shows a temperature above 105°, but I have seen 106.5° recorded in the axilla in the hot stage of a paroxysm of simple intermittent fever.

The duration of the hot stage is different in different cases. According to Aitken, the mean duration is three to eight hours.

There is a very old and quite well-supported opinion, that the cold stage is shorter in the quotidian than in the tertian type, and also that the hot stage is longer in the former than in the latter. It may certainly be affirmed that in individual cases of either type there is no fixed relation between the duration of the chill and that of the hot stage.

The decline of the hot stage begins by the appearance of a gentle perspiration, limited at first to the forehead, face, and neck. This gradually extends itself over the surface and increases in quantity until the whole body is bathed in a profuse sweat. During this period the [p. 594]patient's symptoms, both subjective and objective, undergo wonderful mitigation, and, although this stage is usually short, it often happens that by the time it is concluded a restoration to ordinary health seems to have occurred.

The sweating stage terminates a malarial paroxysm. The intermission now begins, and lasts until the inauguration of another paroxysm. The intermission is longer or shorter accordingly, first, as the paroxysm occupies less or more time; and, second, as the interval may affect it. The interval is that period of time which reaches from the beginning of one paroxysm to the beginning of another. It therefore furnishes the basis of classification of simple intermittents into the following forms: quotidian, tertian, and quartan.

Statistics gathered from a great many sources and relating to many countries and climates indicate that quotidian intermittents are more common than tertian. It may then be assumed that the natural type of intermittents is that form characterized by diurnal paroxysms. It must be remarked, however, that if any natural law does exist establishing the quotidian as the typical form of intermittent fevers, it is very often set aside by unknown influences. In certain epidemics the tertian cases preponderate, and under all circumstances convertibility may be witnessed between the various forms.

It is probable that the statistics gathered by the medical staff of the United States Army during the late Civil War afford the most valuable data which we possess touching these points, in so far as they relate to this country. During three years of the war 724,284 cases of intermittent fever were recorded, tabulated as follows:

Quotidian, 370,401 cases, 388 deaths—equivalent to 1047 + deaths per 1,000,000 cases.

Tertian, 318,704 cases, 324 deaths—equivalent to 1007 + deaths per 1,000,000 cases.

Quartan, 35,179 cases, 79 deaths—equivalent to 2245 + deaths per 1,000,000 cases.

It has been remarked by several writers that quartan attacks have a smaller ratio in the Southern States than in other parts of the Union. My observations on this point have not been sufficiently well recorded to make them especially authoritative, but they support such a conclusion.

The morbid anatomy of malarial fevers is more properly discussed in treating of the graver forms, since the paroxysms of simple intermittent do not often occasion death.

TREATMENT.—This must necessarily vary with the stage of the paroxysm and condition of the patient at the time of the first visit.

Let us suppose this to be the incipiency of the paroxysm, or the early part of the cold stage. However little the danger to life from the paroxysm of a simple intermittent attack, the practitioner should not forget that whatever danger does exist is to be ascribed to damages suffered during or in consequence of the chill. There are few exceptions to this rule, and those will be noticed presently. With this fact in view the practitioner's duties are much simplified. He should first endeavor to remove any complications present which tend to aggravate the cold stage. If the chill has come on after a full meal or after eating indigestible food, the stomach should be promptly emptied; otherwise the cold stage will [p. 595]be prolonged and rendered more violent. Large draughts of warm water will frequently produce sufficient emesis. If this should fail, ipecacuanha may be added. The warm infusion of eupatorium perfoliatum answers well as an emetic, producing also a laxative effect. But it is disgusting to the palate, and sometimes prolongs its action beyond desired results. The effect of an emetic in abridging a chill by revulsive action are uncertain, and I avoid resorting to them for this purpose alone in simple intermittents.

The patient's subjective complaints of suffering should receive a due degree of attention. Additional blankets and warm applications should be allowed when solicited. I always discourage hot or heating drinks, except for the purpose just mentioned. I especially oppose alcoholic stimulants, because they seldom do any good in mitigating the chill, oftener aggravating the patient's symptoms during the hot stage, particularly the headache and vomiting, and sometimes directly occasioning perplexing perturbations. For example, I have seen convulsions speedily follow a strong brandy toddy given to shorten a chill.

While the removal of complications is imperatively indicated, it is also important to use promptly those means which are designed to modify and shorten the chill. It is a remarkable fact that all the agents found to be useful for this purpose are such as directly influence nervous function. Opium in some form enters into all prescriptions which I have found efficient in modifying a chill. It is quite efficacious when given alone, but I think its therapeutic energy and certainty are increased by the addition of other agents of the same class. I have often exhibited twenty to thirty drops of chloroform with an equal quantity of laudanum with excellent results. The tincture of opium may be combined with aromatic spirit of ammonia, or with bromide of potassium, or with chloral hydrate. In combination with either of the latter medicines it may be given by rectal injection. If the stomach is intolerant, or by preference because of facility of dosage and quickness of effect, the opiate may be given hypodermically. For this purpose one-sixth to one-quarter of a grain of morphia may be given, together with one-sixtieth to one-fortieth of a grain of atropia. It is rarely necessary to repeat the dose whichever form may be adopted.

After much experience in these methods of mitigating and abridging the chills of intermittent fever, I feel entitled to say that, whether the objects be achieved or not, no injurious consequences ensue.

The conditions of the circulatory and digestive organs are not favorable for the introduction of quinia or of any preliminary purgative which may be supposed to be necessary, and I therefore delay their exhibition. It may be excepted, however, that sometimes a very obstinately irritable stomach or exceedingly vitiated state of the fluids can be appropriately met by gr. x to xx of calomel.

The hot stage of a simple intermittent seldom calls for medical interference on account of excessive temperature. If the headache is very violent or the vomiting troublesome, a subcutaneous dose of morphia will bring speedy relief. The existence of high temperature does not contra-indicate its use.

I am in the habit of giving opium in the following combinations:

        Morphiæ   gr. ss;

x.	Acet.	
	Liq. Ammon. Acet.	fl. oz. iv. M.

S. Two tablespoonfuls every second hour.
[p. 596]Or, occasionally, the following:

x.	Sodii Bicarb.	gr. xx.
	Morphiæ Sulph.	gr. i;
	Aquæ Lauro-Cerasi,	
	Aquæ Menth. Pip. *aa*.	fl. drachm iv. M.

S. Teaspoonful pro re nata.

I do not limit the use of opiates in the hot stage to old and infirm subjects, as Dickson suggests, but give them in all cases where vomiting, headache, or other neuralgias are excessive, or where unusual restlessness and jactitation are present.

The propriety of giving purgatives as a preliminary measure of treatment during the hot stage must be determined by symptoms connected with individual cases. In the majority of cases falling under my care purgatives are avoided. When regarded necessary, gentle purgation is solicited by administering bitartrate of potassium in lemonade or by combining mild mercurial doses with antiperiodics when these latter are resorted to during the fever. In some cases a very furred tongue, sallow skin, and costive bowels indicate more active purgatives, which may be exhibited during the febrile stage.

The most important question which relates to medication during the hot stage is in respect to the administration of antiperiodics. It may be safely stated that practitioners of this country were the first to adopt this method of procedure in malarial fevers. Here it has been well demonstrated that a competent dose of quinia, given during any part of the hot stage, is so often followed by the defervescence of the fever that it would be illogical to attribute the change to any other cause. Sometimes the remedy fails in producing this result; then excessive physiological disturbances may follow, and perhaps some general aggravation of the patient's symptoms.

There are four different circumstances, each of which, in my opinion, calls for the exhibition of quinia during the hot stage, whether the fever has reached its maximum point or not:

First. If the period which has elapsed since the beginning of the paroxysm is so considerable that further delay might prevent sufficient cinchonism to intercept the next accession.

Second. When the fever is so excessive that quinia should be given as an antipyretic.

Third. When apprehensions exist that the fever will occasion some complication or accident.

Fourth. When the tongue is clean and the state of the system is favorable to absorption.

The hot stage is not usually favorable to absorption, and consequently the economical use of quinia must not be attempted. It should be given in doses varying from ten to twenty grains, preferably in solution. I may remark that I have seldom failed in getting good results from the powder or pills if lemonade or some fluid facile of absorption be given at the same time. The mixtures previously formulated answer this purpose very well, and at the same time mitigate the disagreeable physiological effects of the quinia.

Allusion has been made to certain symptoms occasionally connected [p. 597]with the hot stage which involve danger. Convulsions are among the most important of these. They occur most often among children, but occasionally with adults. They should be met by chloroform, cold to the head, hypodermic injection of morphia, and cupping or leeching if the face is flushed, the eyes injected, and the carotids pulsating forcibly.

The sweating stage may be classed with the intermission in respect to medication. No time should be lost in securing cinchonism. From the moment the sweating stage announces itself the fluids of the system begin to resume their normal physiological functions. Absorption from the intestinal surfaces is again restored, and remedies may be administered with confidence in their effects.

The question is now no longer whether antiperiodics should be administered, but how they shall be given. Many practitioners prefer exhibiting them in one large dose; others think it better to give them in repeated small doses. I have usually adopted the latter method. Beginning with the sweating stage, I give three grains of quinia every hour or two hours, until eighteen grains have been taken. This would occupy periods of five to ten hours to complete the doses, ordinarily quite a sufficient length of time to obtain cinchonism before the advent of another paroxysm. If the physician elects to give his antiperiodic in one or two large doses, he should not trust to so small an amount as eighteen grains. Allowance must be made for the loss incident to the probable over-taxation of the power to dissolve and receive a large amount into the circulation.

Purgation should not be induced to a sufficient degree to hurry the quinia off before absorption takes place. Some practitioners favor the employment of adjuvants to the quinia. Very few of these have appeared to me to be of service except opium. A very convenient formula is a solution of quinia in peppermint-water by addition of dilute sulphuric acid, in such proportions that fl. drachm j of the solution shall represent five grains of quinia and seven and a half drops of laudanum.

But, however we may boast of the efficacy of cinchona as the anceps remedium for malarial diseases, we are forced to admit that it is not certainly an immediate cure, and very commonly fails in producing a permanent curative effect. If we could in all cases discern and remove the impediments to its immediate or temporarily curative action, its claims to be regarded as a practical specific would be undeniable. It is probable that these impediments generally rest upon the fact that either the remedy does not gain admission to the circulation or that some complication exists not within the range of its therapeutic action.

The failure of cinchona to cure a malarial attack in such a permanent manner that it shall not be liable to return is probably owing to the incompetent action of the drug because of its transitory stay in the system as compared with that of the malarial poison. Some objections apply to this theory, because when the succession of intermittent attacks is broken by quinia and it is continuously administered afterward, the paroxysms occasionally recur in spite of its presence in the system. These objections may be answered by pleading that under these circumstances secondary blood-poisons precipitate the attacks, and cinchona should not be expected to cure these conditions.

The best methods of practice I know of to prevent a recurrence of[p. 598]intermittent fever after having interrupted the succession of attacks are, first, to continue the cinchona for at least forty-eight hours, giving at least three three-grain doses a day. After this no medicine need be given except such as may be required to correct chronic toxæmic states of the system or to act as blood-restoratives until such time as prodromes of another paroxysm may exhibit themselves. At the instant when these manifest themselves ten to fifteen grains of quinia in solution should be taken. In order that no loss of time should occur in applying this method, I always advise patients to keep a solution of quinia within immediate reach. The following prescription has sometimes appeared to effect a permanent exemption from recurrence of paroxysms:

x. Ferri Redacti xl; gr.
    Acid. Arseniosi j; gr.
    Quiniæ Sulph. xl; gr.

Ol. Pip.   gtt.
Nigr.   x. M.
Ft. pil.
No. xx.

S. One pill three times daily.

It seems sometimes to occur that intermittent attacks so impress the nervous system that they become, like epilepsy, more liable to recur because of an established habit. I have known chills to occur when the ears were ringing with quinia. Strychnia fails to arrest them; arsenic has more value, but frequently fails. Pure nitric acid, properly diluted, in doses of six to ten drops, given every four to six hours without regard to the stage of the paroxysm, succeeds more often than any medication I have ever resorted to.

Before dismissing the subject of the treatment of simple intermittent fever it may be proper to mention that I have made trials of cure by carbolic acid, administered by mouth and subcutaneously, and also of the sulphites, with no results worthy of recommendation.

Remittent Fever.

The difference in definition between the words remittent and intermittent expresses the clinical distinction between these two forms of fever in a very satisfactory manner.

Remittent fever exhibits oscillations of temperature regulated as to hours of recurrence by laws similar to those which govern the periodic returns of intermittent fever; but there is no complete defervescence of the fever. While the lowest angles of the fever curve approximate the normal body heat more or less closely, they never decline to a standard of apyrexia.

That remittent fever is a malarial disease, produced by a cause identical with that which produces intermittent fever, is well proven by the following facts:

First. Cases occur in close relation with cases of intermittent fever in populations similarly exposed to malaria, and at the same periods of the year.

Second. The two forms of disease are readily convertible, the one with the other.

In non-tropical countries remittent fever cannot be regarded as the [p. 599]natural type of malarial fevers. At least, it may be affirmed that the proportion of cases which begin as remittent attacks is so small that we are warranted in looking upon them as departures from type. In the United States army during the years 1861-66, inclusive, there occurred 286,490 cases of remittent fever. The fatal cases were 3853, being a mortality-rate of 13,450 per 1,000,000 cases. By comparing these statistics with those of intermittent fever recorded in a previous section it will be found that remittent fever is more than twelve times as fatal to life as the simple intermittent forms.

If we accept this view of the pathology of remittent fever, it is of interest to the sanitarian or practitioner to endeavor to arrive at the causes which occasion these departures from type. Some of these are undoubtedly extraneous to the system, and relate wholly to circumstances affecting the malarial poison as a disease-producing agent. Increased quantity of malaria is well understood to enlarge the ratio of remittent cases. There is also strong presumptive evidence supporting the hypothesis that different annual crops of malaria vary in respect to the noxious qualities of this agent. The same presumption relates to all crops produced in certain localities as contrasted with others. Other causes which determine remittent rather than intermittent attacks are personal to patients. They may be classed as follows:

First. Unusual personal receptivity or impressibility to malaria may exist, either because of some constitutional idiosyncrasy or of some state the system at the time of exposure.

Second. Want of timely medical treatment or of proper medical treatment may convert intermittents into remittents.

Third. The rapid occurrence of secondary blood infections, extraordinary in character or amount, may cause the fever to be continuous.

Fourth. The existence of complications, inflammatory in their nature, may change intermittent into remittent attacks.

However various or complex the causes may be which operate to convert intermittent attacks into remittent forms of fever, each one must be supposed to act by disturbing the functions of those centres which preside over the normal physiological and chemical changes of the system.

SYMPTOMS AND DIAGNOSIS.—Attacks of remittent fever are, as a rule, more abrupt in their advent than intermittents. When prodromic symptoms exist, they are similar to those which precede ordinary cases of ague.

The chill is seldom attended by such violent symptoms as the cold stage of intermittents. The duration of the cold stage is also more brief. In a small proportion of cases severe vomiting with large bilious ejections complicate the cold stage. The chill is quickly followed by the hot stage.

The mildest cases of remittent fever are not readily distinguishable from the intermittent forms. In these cases the temperature curves are marked by sharp angles and long tracings between the lowest and highest records. As cases become more decided in diagnosis, and consequently represent higher degrees of departure from the intermittent type, the angles of temperature curves become more obtuse and exhibit a more or less high average range. The accompanying temperature diagram (Fig. 23) shows the thermometric record of an unusually protracted and grave case. The patient was a near relative of my colleague, Prof. Logan, a leading practitioner of New Orleans, and the clinical records may be [p. 601]accepted as altogether accurate. It is somewhat to be regretted that the records of temperature were not begun at an earlier period, but the gravity of the case was not manifest until the continued type of fever was found to exist. The latter part of the diagram illustrates the lapse of the remittent fever into an intermittent. This is so commonly a mode of cure that the practitioner watches with solicitude for increasing oscillations of temperature to announce mitigations of severity in his gravest cases.

[p. 600]

FIG. 23.

Temperature chart showing the lapse of a remittent fever into an intermittent.

NOTE.—From the third to the fifteenth day after attack a half drachm of quinia was given daily. Observing no good result, it was omitted until the twenty-ninth day, on which date two doses of eight grains each were administered. On the morning of the thirty-fourth day eight grains were again given; on the thirty-fifth day one scruple was given.

The differential diagnosis of intermittent and remittent fevers may be looked upon as practically unimportant. All cases so near the borderline as to make differential diagnosis a question should receive identical treatment.

There are, however, two other very grave forms of fever which are liable to give trouble in differentiation from remittent fever. These are typhoid and yellow fevers. The sanitary protection of communities exposed to cases of the latter, and also the practical treatment of the sick, call for early and correct differentiation.

But it is only in the early stages of the pathological processes of these affections that difficulties of diagnosis are liable to obtain. The facial expression of patients suffering with remittent is sufficiently characteristic to afford some diagnostic inferences. During the pyrexia the face is flushed and the eyes injected, but the redness is more vivid and the countenance more animated than in either typhoid or yellow fever. It would not be inaccurate to say that, however great may be the flushing or other alterations of the countenance in remittent fever, the natural facial expression is better preserved than in either of the fevers under comparison with it. Sallowness of the skin is an early and almost constant event in remittent fever. It comes on as a secondary manifestation, and appears in a large ratio of cases to bear some relation to the high temperature preceding its occurrence. The icteric hue is seldom intense, indeed very infrequently equalling the orange-yellow of jaundice resulting from obstruction. There is an exception to this statement in those cases in which remittent fever attacks a person already jaundiced. I have seen many cases in which the jaundice preceded the remittent fever, and became more strongly marked after its incursion, particularly in those persons who had remained for some time in a malarial region and suffered repeated attacks. In all cases of remittent fever it seems reasonable to ascribe the more or less jaundiced state to one or both of two factors, viz.—the accumulation of excrementitious material and bile constituents in the blood from primary derangement of its chemistry; and that excessive activity of the liver which the malarial poison appears to induce. Whether the latter mentioned factor results from some action of malaria directly affecting the nutritive processes of the liver, as it does those of the spleen, or whether the altered blood-currents during the paroxysms cause this supposed hypersecretion of bile, we certainly know that to malaria only can we ascribe those fevers which are marked by such peculiar symptoms of biliousness or superabundance of bile as to justify the prefix bilious fever or bilious remittent fever.

The state of the alimentary tract may properly receive notice after these remarks. In the early stages of remittent fever the tongue may be moist and large, and covered with a white or lead-colored or yellowish coat. The edges may be indented with imprints of the teeth. This is [p. 602]Osborne's malarial tongue, and its appearance is worth something in diagnosis.

Later in the progress of remittent fever the tongue may become dry, brown, cracked, and difficult of protrusion, but seldom showing the tremulousness of a typhoid-fever tongue, and differing also from the yellow-fever tongue in the fact that in this disease the appearance of the tongue is usually indifferent as a symptom, except that in advanced stages it is liable to be smeared with blood.

The stomach is irritable from the very beginning of an attack, and the acts of emesis are generally in striking contrast with those of typhoid or yellow fever, both in respect to their violence and to the relative amount of bile they eject.

The bowels are ordinarily costive, and when moved by purgatives the stools contrast strongly with those of typhoid or yellow fever by presenting evidences of the bile-coloring principles which attend all excretions in malarial fever, and are found in the urine, the perspiration, and occasionally the sputa.

Some unusually violent cases of malarial fever, which may become remittent, are inaugurated with convulsions, profuse diarrhoea, and coma.

Before closing the remarks concerning the digestive organs in remittent fever I should mention that in the long array of cases I have treated I cannot recall one solitary instance of black vomit. It is, however, true that I have observed hemorrhage from the bowels in quite a number of cases. These occurred late in protracted cases, and were sometimes the cause of death. Whether it be merely a coincidence I am unable to say, but it is true that the majority of these cases have been in young females just after the establishment of the catamenia.

Hemorrhage from the nose is frequent in remittent fever, but I have never seen a case with general tendency to hemorrhage.

The pulse in remittent fever differs from that of the typhoid or yellow fevers by being more synochal in character, firmer, and more resisting to pressure. The longer the duration of the case the less is this characteristic discernible.

The nervous system shows less ataxia. Delirium may occur in any stage of the disease, but differs from the delirium of typhoid and yellow fevers in showing a lessened degree of perversion of the reasoning faculties. The neuralgias have nothing special.

The urine is acid, high-colored, and scanty. I have never found much albumen in the urine of a case of remittent fever, unless there was some other cause to account for its presence. A small amount may be detected during excessive fever. Blood is a rare constituent.

Mild cases of remittent fever should terminate in recovery in from five to seven days. Fatal attacks usually end from the fifth to the tenth day. Many cases pursue a course which lasts from twenty to forty days. Under proper treatment the usual termination is in recovery, either directly or by conversion into the intermittent type.

POST-MORTEM APPEARANCES.—When death occurs in remittent fever the post-mortem changes generally consist of those which are principally due to chronic malarial toxæmia and those ascribable to the acute attack.

Under the former division are permanent enlargements of the spleen and liver, and pigmentary matter in the blood and deposited in various [p. 603]organs. Under the latter are to be classed hyperæmic or even inflammatory states of the stomach and intestines, and those degenerative changes which are the consequence of continuous hyperpyrexia. The post-mortem changes which are so uniformly found as to be most often appealed to in the establishment of diagnoses are enlargements of the liver and spleen. These may be due in part to hyperplasia and in part to blood-engorgement. The brown or slate color of an enlarged liver is strongly diagnostic of malarial affections. It contrasts strongly with the yellow and natural-sized liver of yellow fever and with the negative liver of typhoid fever.

The skin is generally yellow, sometimes quite intensely icteric, but seldom showing the ecchymotic extravasations of yellow fever. In remittent fever we never find the cadaver oozing blood from the nose and the mouth, nor are the stomach or intestines ever found to contain black vomit.

TREATMENT.—The indications of treatment in remittent fevers differ from those of intermittents in two leading essentials.

First. It is a far graver form of fever, and calls for more promptitude and energy in treatment for its successful management.

Second. The important pathological condition to be combated is the hyperpyrexia, and not the cold stage, as in intermittents.

But even with a clear realization of the practical importance of these facts in governing the treatment of remittents, the practitioner must still exercise care and self-control, lest he shall unconsciously adopt the doctrine that inflammatory lesions must be present to occasion such violent pyrexia as often exists. The physician who comes directly from a case of pneumonia or rheumatic fever and finds a patient suffering from remittent fever, with temperature higher and pulse more bounding than those of the patient he has just left, is pardonable for finding it difficult to realize that these furious symptoms are not also associated with inflammation.

Attempts to cure remittent fevers by an exclusively antiphlogistic treatment either result fatally or induce long periods of confinement and suffering before recovery is reached. The great indication is to secure cinchonism as promptly and completely as possible. Nothing should divert our attention from this object. The condition of the patient as it respects fever, delirium, or state of the tongue, should form no bar to the administration of quinia. There are no practitioners who have had much experience in treating these grave forms of malarial fever after this method who are not able to recall the numerous instances of most astonishing and gratifying amelioration of symptoms as soon as saturation with quinia was brought about. The dry tongue becomes moist, the skin is bathed in gentle perspiration, the delirium ceases, and the patient sinks into a quiet sleep.

The amount of quinia necessary to produce cinchonism must be estimated for each particular case according to the measure of its severity or to states of the system more or less favorable to its absorption. It must be borne in mind, however, that questions concerning the patient's safety are paramount to those of economy. In the mildest cases I never trust to a smaller amount than from twenty to thirty grains. In violent attacks I have administered scruple doses every fourth hour until a [p. 604]sufficient test had been made of its capability to arrest or modify the febrile paroxysm. I have never met with any of those exaggerated physiological effects which some observers teach us to fear from the exhibition of cinchona preparations during fever. Certainly, I can declare that no permanent deafness or other lasting lesion of nerve-function has ever occurred under my observation. I must also add that I know of no reasons why remissions afford more favorable conditions for the administration of quinia, beyond the fact that the system is in a better state for its absorption and assimilation. The quinia is preferably given in solution, but may be exhibited in the form of pills, or in powder suspended in black coffee, or in the thick mucilage of the slippery elm.

The considerations of treatment which are naturally connected with those just advocated relate to measures which it may be proper to associate with the quinia. The answers to the two following questions comprise all that is necessary to be said on this point—viz.:

Are conditions of the system present which may interfere with the specific treatment by quinia, and which are not, in themselves, curable by it?

Are any medicines to be given as succedanea to the specific remedy for the purpose of rendering its action more sure or prompt?

In regard to the first inquiry, it must be admitted that in quite a large proportion of cases of remittent fever specific treatment fails to cure. I suppose that may be a reasonable proposition which holds that in the majority of these cases the presence of secondary blood-impurities annuls the ordinary specific effects of cinchona. These must be gotten rid of by depurative medicines. The intestinal canal, the skin, and the kidneys are the emunctories through which elimination must be effected. It is therefore proper for the physician to endeavor to recognize cases where such impurities exist, and to so modify his treatment as to remove them. The indications for depurative treatment are jaundiced skin and eyes, furred tongue, costive bowels, and scanty, loaded urine. These are more or less positively expressed symptoms in a large majority of cases. It is therefore proper that in this large majority of cases of remittent fever depurative treatment should be conjoined with the specific treatment. In my opinion, no drugs meet this indication so well as mercurials and saline purges and diuretics. Calomel or blue mass may be given either simultaneously with the quinia or in alternate doses.

There are three very important rules to be observed in regard to cathartics: They should never be carried to such an extent that absorption of the quinine is interrupted. They should not be given in such large or repeated doses as to produce prolonged irritation, or it may be even inflammation, of the alimentary canal. Purgatives should be used for their depurative effects, and never as antiphologistics.

Opium exercises excellent effects in preventing local irritation or hypercatharsis, and in relieving derangements of nerve-function and insomnia. It is preferably given in small doses, combined either with purgatives or with the quinia.

I have found bitartrate of potassium the most grateful and efficient saline for depurative action. I have generally given it in lemonade in such amounts as to secure a gentle aperient and diuretic effect. I hold strongly to a conviction that all drugs as soluble as this facilitate the absorption of those less soluble—as, for example, of quinia.

[p. 605]If the first efforts to break the febrile paroxysms fail, it is better to discontinue the quinia and place the patient under symptomatic treatment, and await conditions of the system more favorable for its repetition. Of course the high temperature is generally the symptom requiring most care and attention.

Vomiting is one of the troublesome symptoms of remittent fever. As internal medication minute doses of morphia, dry upon the tongue or in solution in cherry-laurel water, or in combination with eight or ten drops of chloroform, are generally efficacious. Swallowing pellets of ice or frequently taking iced effervescing mixtures are good measures of treatment. Occasionally, a mild emetic, such as warm chamomile infusion, or warm water alone, will arrest the vomiting temporarily. It is doubtful, however, whether this relief is secured by the ejection of any offending matter from the stomach. It is more than probable that the forced dilatation of the stomach has arrested the spasms, for filling this viscus with cold drinks to repletion will often effect the same result.

Of all applications to the epigastrium, a cold wet towel occasionally sprinkled with chloroform is the best.

A tympanitic or tender abdomen requires stupes wrung from warm water. They may be dashed with turpentine at first, and afterward consist of warm water with whiskey. I have occasionally given two or three doses of turpentine emulsion with benefit, but from much observation I am forced to protest against the turpentine treatment, as it is called, which is to give twenty drops of turpentine every two to four hours as a curative agent.

Hemorrhage from the bowels must be met by hæmostatic treatment—preferably, in my experience, by the use of five grains of gallic acid in half an ounce of camphor-water every two hours, of morphia subcutaneously, and of cold cloths over the bowels. As in all diseases liable to cause death from exhaustion, careful attention must be paid to the nutriment, and stimulants must be administered as required.

Pernicious Malarial Fever.

Certain departures from the ordinary types of malarial fever are termed pernicious, because of their great tendency to inflict more than usual systemic damage and danger to life upon those who suffer such attacks. The word pernicious is used in its common English sense of being hurtful or injurious.

It is entirely unnecessary to enter upon a discussion respecting the propriety of employing this adjective to designate a class of cases of disease which are primarily due to the same poison which produces simple intermittent attacks. The extreme hurtfulness and danger of the attacks to be described in this section, and the awful suddenness with which they often occasion death, form striking contrasts with the more typical forms of malarial fever, and appear fully to justify the use of the qualifying adjective pernicious.

While all these various departures from type to be grouped under the term pernicious possess the quality ascribed to them, they nevertheless differ so widely in their modes of inflicting injury that it seems desirable to arrange them under distinct sub-classifications.

[p. 606]Some cases of pernicious malarial fever preserve the periodicity of simple attacks sufficiently well to enable one to classify them as intermittent or remittent in form. But more commonly it is impossible to determine this classification, and for practical purposes it is unimportant to attempt to make any such distinction.

The classification which appears to me most true to nature is the following:
First. The algid or congestive form;
Second. The comatose form;
Third. The hemorrhagic form.

The algid or congestive form occurs more frequently than either of the others. Its perniciousness is due to an aggravation or sheer exaggeration of the cold stage of an intermittent attack.

The following brief clinical histories of two cases will serve to illustrate the symptomatic phenomena of this form of pernicious malarial fever:

M. S., aged fourteen, had accompanied his father to a malarious locality in the country, and had remained with him during September and a portion of October. Shortly after his return I was asked to visit him because of some unusual symptoms attending a chill. I found him in a stupor, from which he was with difficulty aroused sufficiently to be able to swallow a dose of quinia combined with laudanum. His face was pallid and inexpressive; the skin cool and moist; extremities shrunken and cold; pulse small, easily obliterated by pressure, and irregular; tongue large and moist; and pupils rather dilated.

My second visit was at 12 M., one hour and a half later than the first. Patient was found in a deep stupor; surface cold; extremities and face shrunken and blue; pulse barely perceptible; large liquid and offensive stools occasionally escaped from the bowels without the consciousness of the patient. Death at 3 o'clock P.M.

Miss H., living in a malarious situation, complained about noon of September 19th of great cerebral fulness and unaccountable sleepiness and debility. She retired to her room, and after a few hours' sleep resumed her household occupations. On the 20th similar symptoms manifested themselves, but earlier in the day. She again slept for some hours, but complained of great prostration after the sleep. On the 21st, about 10 A.M., she complained of a return of the stupor, and while retiring to her room requested that I should be called if she did not awake in a better condition. At 1 P.M. she was found profoundly comatose, with cold extremities and surface and bathed in perspiration. When I reached her residence at 3 P.M. she had expired.

There is a common belief among non-professional people that the third congestive chill is necessarily fatal. There is no foundation for this opinion, except in the fact that when congestive chills are waxing in their perniciousness the subject is seldom able to survive the third recurrence if the second or first should not prove fatal.

It is difficult to account for the pathological dissimilarity between the simple and congestive types of malarial fevers. If we say that congestive chills are produced by an intensification of those causes which produce and govern an ordinary chill, we make an explanation which, however unsatisfactory, represents very nearly the full extent of our knowledge on this point.

[p. 607]It cannot be admitted that alterations of quantity or quality of the malarial poison exercise the sole influence in determining the occurrence of congestive cases. All experienced practitioners understand that certain constitutional conditions may pervert simple chills into congestive forms by producing prolongation or aggravation of the states of congestion always present in ordinary chills. Weakened cardiac function, from whatever cause, may be reckoned among these conditions. In these cases the feeble vis a tergo yields readily to those perturbations of vaso-motor influence which occasion passive blood-accumulations in the small veins and capillaries. I may say further, in speaking of the influence of the vaso-motor nerves in governing the phenomena of a chill, that we know that in congestive chills the cerebro-spinal system is much less the seat of symptomatic phenomena than in simple attacks. On the other hand, the organic system is far more profoundly affected.

However we may account for the perversions of normal circulation underlying and producing congestive chills, the great degree of injury they are liable to inflict is so well understood as to awaken the most serious apprehensions whenever we are called upon to treat them. Congestion, however occasioned, may destroy life through abolishment of function by the sheer physical change of infarction, or, again, through those inevitable consequences which arrested circulation entails upon the blood. Blood-stasis is followed by separation of its constituents, and its disqualification as a circulatory fluid in a degree proportionate to the duration of the stoppage, and probably also to the actual extent of the passive engorgement. Thence result the formation of coagula in the congested vessels and deposits of pigmentary matter. If partial reaction should occur, portions of this blood-débris may be floated to various parts of the circulatory system, and give rise to greater or less important alterations of function.

Among the white soldiers of the United States army from May 1, 1861, to June 20, 1866, 13,673 cases were diagnosed as congestive intermittent fever. Of this number, 3370 died, being a mortality-rate of 23.91 per cent. The aggregate number of malarial cases returned was 1,255,623. It would therefore appear that 1 case in not quite 372 was congestive in its type, or 1.08 per cent. The late Dr. Cook of Washington, La., estimated 2 per cent. of his malarial cases to be of the congestive type. It can scarcely be doubted that the ratio of congestive attacks is greater in the more southern belts of latitude than in the middle or northern parts of the United States. Chronic malarial toxæmia and the enervating effects of long-continued heat upon the circulation must occasion an increased proportion of such attacks, but my own observations show slightly more than 1 per cent. of the cases treated in the Charity Hospital to have been of the congestive form.

The cure of a congestive chill is one of the most difficult problems the physician can possibly encounter. It is nothing less than the proposition to remove a perverted state of the blood-vessels which is dependent upon some influence exerted through a nervous apparatus whose therapeutics and experimental physiology are imperfectly understood. While a satisfactory solution of this problem will probably be a remote achievement in medicine, it was long ago empirically ascertained that certain [p. 608]agents exercised some degree of control over the cold stage of febrile attacks. For the most part, these agents are addressed to those perversions of nerve-function which constitute so important a part of the pathology of a chill. They are identically the same remedies whose aid we invoke to allay many other forms of perturbed nervous action. Opium, chloroform, belladonna, chloral hydrate, and bromide of potassium have proved more or less valuable, according to the idiosyncrasy of the patient or the circumstances under which they have been used. I consider opium the most valuable of these remedies. It should be given in moderate doses, and preferably combined with chloroform or ammonia, or, if more expedient to administer per rectum, combined with solutions of chloral hydrate or bromide of potassium. One-sixth of a grain of morphia, combined with one-fortieth or one-fiftieth of a grain of atropia, is an available and useful prescription when given hypodermically. Rubbing the extremities or the spine, or indeed the whole surface, with ice, is a mode of practice well worthy of attention. In the event of inability to procure ice, douches of cold water, followed by frictions with coarse towels, may be substituted. I have used nitrite of amyl by inhalation, but its effects are too transitory to prove serviceable.

Some practitioners speak highly of alcoholic stimulants. My own experience has not been favorable to their use. Perhaps their benefits are altogether restricted to those cases in which previously weakened heart-function existed. But it is important that alcohol be added in all those cases of pernicious malarial fever, whatever the type may be, where cardiac stimulation and improvement of nutrition are leading indications.

I am sure I have often derived benefit from enemas consisting of four ounces of well-prepared beef essence with a half ounce of whiskey or brandy and a half ounce of strong infusion of coffee.

The value of the hypodermic syringe in treating congestive chills must never be lost sight of. The suspension, or even reversal, of normal systemic currents is made evident by the serous vomiting and purging attending congestion of the abdominal cavity. Medicine placed in the stomach under these circumstances is virtually thrown away.

The term comatose is applied to certain cases of pernicious malarial fever because they present coma as a marked symptom. To appreciate the propriety of this classification, it must be well understood that the coma present is not due to cerebral congestion. Further than this one restriction upon the application of the word there is in its employment no declaration of any pathological views respecting the cases it is intended to define. While, therefore, the term is unquestionably liable to criticism, I suppose its use may still be admitted, provided it is accompanied by a satisfactorily explicit account of the symptoms and probable pathological conditions of the cases included under its caption.

There is a sharp line of distinction between the symptoms and conjectural pathology of comatose cases and of those of the congestive form of pernicious fever. The following notes of cases will sufficiently establish this statement:

C. L., fisherman, aged forty-four, brought into Ward 20, Charity Hospital, in an insensible condition, November 18, 1875. Temperature at time of admission 104.8°, pulse 120, respiration 40; able to swallow liquids placed far back in his mouth. Ordered scruple ij of quinia in [p. 609]solution, ten grains to be given every fourth hour. Nov. 19th, patient has taken and retained all the quinia ordered; is perspiring profusely; temperature 97.8°, pulse 88; more conscious; takes food and water when offered him. Ordered blue mass, comp. extr. colocynth., *aa* gr. v, to be taken at once. To drink through the day bitartrate potass. oz. j, dissolved in lemonade, until bowels are moved. Evening temperature 99.3°. Nov. 20th, temperature 98°; patient placed under convalescent treatment; discharged from hospital Nov. 29th.

Another comatose patient was admitted to Ward 19 on the 29th of October, entirely insensible. He was treated by large doses of quinia in solution per rectum, and by calomel gr. xx, sodii bicarb. gr. v, placed upon base of tongue, and caused to be swallowed by a tablespoonful of water trickled over the powder. As the patient began to recover it was noticed that his right arm was paralyzed. A history subsequently obtained showed that the patient was an engineer, and had been engaged in making some land surveys in a swampy portion of the State of Louisiana, and had been often obliged to wade or swim across the bayous and to sleep at night in the open air, sometimes without any protection from the weather. He had previously enjoyed good health, and was altogether unable to account for the paralysis of his arm. During convalescence he was treated with iron, strychnia, and preparations of cinchona, and by cold douches and frictions to the paralyzed arm. Convalescence was slow, but he was discharged, completely recovered, on November 20th.

In typical cases the differential diagnosis between the congestive form and the comatose is made without difficulty. In a congestive chill the surface is cold, blue, or livid, the pupils dilated, and the pulse generally slower than natural and irregular. In the comatose form the surface is preternaturally warm, of a muddy, semi-jaundiced hue, and the pulse and temperature both indicate the feverish rather than the algid state.

The subjects of attacks of the comatose form of malarial fever are for the most part persons who, having contracted attacks of fever in malarial regions, continue to reside in the same localities and yet use no proper medication, either for cure or for prophylaxis. We have in these cases accumulations of secondary blood-poisons quite sufficient to greatly impede brain-function, and the additional doses of the primary toxic agent must exercise more or less influence in determining the phenomena of the attacks.

Very little need be said of treatment, beyond a recommendation of the courses pursued in the cases cited. Hypodermic medication must be resorted to when necessary. Efforts to nourish the patient must never be relaxed. One must see many of these cases before he can realize how often they recover, from conditions apparently utterly hopeless, when promptly treated and properly nourished.

The hemorrhagic form of pernicious malarial fever can scarcely be regarded as an original type. Malaria is not a hemorrhage-inducing poison. Indeed, it may be positively stated that malaria never establishes the hemorrhagic diathesis as a primary effect; and it is only by changes effected in the human economy by its prolonged influence that it appears to become capable of doing so. The most experienced and accurate observers of malarial affections concur in the opinion that this rule is almost without exception.

[p. 610]The morbid conditions whose concurrence entails upon malarial fevers a tendency to hemorrhages may be classed together as follows: First. The blood-changes of chronic malarial toxæmia so alter the consistency of that fluid as to favor the occurrence of hemorrhage. Second. The long persistent states of malnutrition in chronic malarial cachexias produce textural weakening of the vascular walls and increased liability to their rupture. Third. There should be added to these one other factor, which is mainly operative during a malarial paroxysm—namely, the increased blood-pressure put upon the vascular walls by passive congestions.

Two of these factors, as above enumerated, are more or less general to the system, being the consequence of general cachectic states. The third factor acts in a purely dynamical manner in causing hemorrhages, and must necessarily have its area of influence confined to some certain portion or portions of the vascular tree, since the congestions of malarial paroxysms cannot by any possibility be general. It is an interesting fact that the influence of this last-mentioned factor is so frequently paramount in producing malarial hemorrhages. These hemorrhages occur in such immediate relation to chills that we are forced to the conclusion that while altered blood and weakened blood-vessels were previously present, yet some increase of pressure beyond the normal was required to precipitate the hemorrhage.

More than once in the presence of medical classes I have illustrated the influence of these various factors, respectively, by showing the arm of a patient suffering with chronic malarial cachexia, with no extravasation of blood, but upon which the slightest suction with the lips would produce exaggerated ecchymoses. This explains the fact that hemorrhages in malarial fevers are never general, but only manifest themselves upon those surfaces or into those structures which are the seats of congestion during the cold stage of an intermittent.

I do most earnestly assert that during a practice of almost half a century, nearly all of which has been passed in malarious localities, I have never once seen a malarial-fever patient with a general hemorrhagic tendency, if yellow fever and other hemorrhage-inducing diseases could be authoritatively excluded. The medical profession cannot be too watchful in guarding itself against erroneous entries upon mortuary records to account for deaths from fevers accompanied by hemorrhages from multiple surfaces of the body. Such aliases as hemorrhagic malarial fever, climatic fever, rice fever, hæmatemesic paludal fever, and many more of the same character, should receive the severest examination before approval and adoption.

When hemorrhage does attend malarial fevers, it may occur from one or another of a variety of surfaces or into shut cavities or in parenchymatous structures. Some years ago I visited a gentleman who was suffering from an attack of malarial fever, with hæmaturia. He made a rapid and, apparently, a complete recovery. Disobeying my injunctions, he returned to the intensely malarious locality where he had formerly resided. After a few weeks he was seized with a chill, followed by apoplectic symptoms, hemorrhage, and death on third day. It is hardly to be doubted that his death was caused by cerebral hemorrhage. But, however much in consonance with ascertained facts the foregoing remarks may appear to be, there are certain points of pathology connected with [p. 611]malarial hemorrhagic fevers not easy of explanation. Within the last score of years hæmaturia has been a far more common form of hemorrhage in malarial fevers than formerly. In many localities and during certain seasons it has been very prevalent.

In the present state of our knowledge it is not at all possible to explain why it is that different epidemics of malarial diseases should give rise to such a diversity of phenomena, so that one epidemic will be characterized by a peculiar train of symptoms which shall be absent in another, being there replaced by different symptoms equally distinctive of the second epidemic. Whatever may be the cause of these epidemical peculiarities, it must rest in a something which is capable of acting as a force upon the human system. We must think of that unknown agency which exercises this force and gives it some peculiar direction as possessing at least a conventional essentiality. It is not satisfactory to say that the renal blood-vessels are the first to give way, because they are accidentally more weakened than other parts of the vascular system, or accidentally more often the seat of congestion. When accidents become as numerous as these cases sometimes are, they acquire the authority of laws.

The following notes of two cases of malarial hemorrhagic fever may be found of interest:

C. E., aged twenty-six years, was admitted to Ward 19, Charity Hospital, Nov. 18, 1872. Had been in America more than a year, and for several months had been working in an intensely malarial district preparing the bed of a railroad; has had malarial diseases for several months, and suffered a severe chill the day before admission. A few hours after admission temp. 103°, pulse 120, respiration 29; effusion in both thoracic cavities, and very marked in abdominal cavity; lower lobe of right lung oedematous, legs anasarcous, pitting greatly on pressure, with several ulcers of long standing. Urine loaded with albumen and showing under the microscope abundant blood-corpuscles; considerable jaundice present, which the patient states to have occurred suddenly. Ordered five grains each of calomel and bicarbonate of sodium, to be followed after catharsis with ten grains of quinia in solution every two hours. Nov. 22d, patient has taken and retained one hundred and eight grains of quinia; secretion of urine abundant; no blood present, and only a trace of albumen; ordered twenty drops of tincture of chloride of iron three times daily. Discharged cured December 12th. The above comprises the whole treatment in this case, except one important measure, which consisted in determined and persistent efforts at forced nutrition. Meat essences, milk, eggs, and milk-punch were given as methodically as drugs.

H. K., fifteen years of age, was admitted to Charity Hospital Sept. 15, 1872; has a history of malarial poisoning for several months; was considerably jaundiced at time of admission, with anasarcous legs. Under the administration of a mercurial, followed by quinia and iron, he improved so greatly that he was discharged from my wards and placed upon some duty in the hospital. Dec. 19th, at 11 A.M., had a chill which lasted several hours; this was followed by violent fever, with rapid but compressible pulse; much jactitation; incessant vomiting of a greenish-black fluid; urine loaded with blood; and sudden supervention of intense jaundice. Ordered quinia gr. xij by hypodermic injection; [p. 612]small doses of calomel and soda to be placed upon the base of the tongue and washed down with ice-water. Secretion of urine ceased on the morning of the 20th, followed by death at 11 P.M. Autopsy showed both kidneys dark-colored and swollen from complete blood-engorgement.

The treatment of hemorrhagic malarial fevers may be included under the following indications:

First, to secure cinchonism as early as possible;

Second, to arrest the extravasation of blood;

Third, to sustain the patient's strength, and to preserve the systemic fluids at as near a healthy standard as may be possible.

The first-mentioned indication is certainly the first in importance. If the hemorrhage originates during a chill, or exhibits degrees of aggravation in such close relation to the cold stage of malarial paroxysms as to point to a relation of cause and effect, then that course of treatment which breaks the recurrence of paroxysms will at the same time mitigate the hemorrhage, if, in truth, it should fail to stop it entirely. Quinia should be given in large doses by the mouth or rectum, or both, or subcutaneously if demanded by the urgency of the symptoms. I have generally used carefully prepared solutions of the sulphate for hypodermic injections, but many practitioners prefer solutions of the hydrobromate for this mode of exhibition. I have never witnessed any symptoms following the administration of cinchona salts which justified a belief that they increased the hemorrhage. My rule of practice has invariably been to endeavor to prevent the occurrence of another paroxysm, without regard to this very questionable charge.

In regard to the second indication, it may be stated that patients are not likely to die from actual loss of blood in any form of hemorrhagic malarial fever. The blood which is poured out on free surfaces and escapes by some outlet is seldom so much as to endanger life, but the hemorrhagic process is likely to involve deeper-seated vessels. This is especially true in malarial hæmaturia. Hemorrhages into the stroma of the kidneys, the Malpighian tufts, and the uriniferous tubules arrest urinary secretion, and thus entail death. In order to prevent these results hæmostatics should be resorted to as often as attendant circumstances will permit. Generally these are such as to admit of the use of hæmostatics without prejudicing the effects of other remedies. In my experience ergot in combination with gallic acid and dilute sulphuric acid has been very efficient. The following prescription has been usually given:

x. Ext. Ergot. Fluid. fl. drachm iv;
Acid. Gallic. gr. xl;
Acid. Sulphuric. dil. fl. drachm j;
Syr. Zingiber. fl. drachm iij;
Aquæ q. s ad ij. fl. oz. M.

S. Dessertspoonful every four hours, diluted with water.

Some practitioners place a very high estimate upon the hæmostatic effects of turpentine. This is undoubtedly a most valuable and accessible remedy. Dr. Schnell of Plaquemine Parish, La., has found the tincture of chloride of iron the best hæmostatic. He places fl. drachm ij in fl. oz. iv of water, and directs a dessertspoonful every hour as long as the hemorrhage continues. In a great majority of cases of malarial hæmaturia occurring under my observation solutions of bitartrate of potassium have [p. 613]been given with great apparent benefit. Its action is certainly not that of a direct hæmostatic, but by setting up currents through the kidneys, and perhaps by some solvent power over exudations in the uriniferous tubules, it has acted as a renal deobstructive.

In the arrest of renal secretion diuretics, cupping over the lumbar region, and large injections of warm water into the bowels may be resorted to. Some practitioners state that they have found buchu beneficial.

The third indication involves a twofold duty. One relates to judicious and vigilant attention to the patient's nutrition; the other relates to such measures for depuration as may be called for in each particular case.

It must be admitted that there is a degree of antagonism in the measures of practice proper to effect these two purposes, which renders their coincident exercise a difficult practical question. In many cases of hemorrhagic malarial fever a competent supply of properly prepared foods is sufficient. In other cases—and this is especially true of malarial hæmaturia—depurative medication becomes paramount. A person suffering under the effects of chronic malarial poisoning is seized with a chill; this is followed by bloody urine, and in the course of four or five hours intense jaundice appears. Incessant vomiting, delirium, and jactitation also occur. The experienced physician is at once brought to the conclusion that he has to deal with a case of blood-poisoning bearing a close resemblance in symptoms to uræmia. To render this conclusion still more absolute, he has only to recall the suddenness of the occurrence of the jaundice and to inquire what has occasioned it. Its appearance is too rapid to permit us to ascribe it to obstruction. It is altogether improbable that it is due to sudden hypersecretion in such pathological states of the system as are present. If, however, we account for it by saying that the addition of a new toxic constituent, urea and its congeners, to an already profoundly poisoned fluid suddenly arrests those processes which dispose of bile in physiological conditions of the system, it seems to me that we adopt the most rational theory. It is then jaundice from lack of consumption. The mere probability of truth in this theory will impress the practitioner with the great importance of eliminant practice in these conditions.

Calomel has been the medicine to which I have principally trusted. I give it merely as a depurative, and not as an alterative. Doses of from two to ten grains may be repeated at suitable intervals until catharsis has been produced. Bitartrate of potassium, Seidlitz powders, or solutions of citrate of magnesia may be also administered if indicated. After purgation the vomiting is mitigated, if not altogether relieved. On this account, and because of bettered states of the system for absorption and assimilation, the way is now clear to the physician. He can ply his antiperiodics, his properly prepared sustenance, and his alcoholic stimulants according to the exigencies of each particular case.

The following propositions may seem not inappropriate in closing this section:

1st. Attacks of pernicious malarial fever are attended by more danger to life or subsequent health than simple attacks; therefore more prompt and energetic efforts should be made to cut them short by cinchonism.

2d. The blood depravations of pernicious malarial fevers far exceed those of simple cases; and therefore it becomes a leading indication of treatment to correct faulty conditions of this fluid as early as possible. [p. 614]In endeavoring to secure this end assimilable foods, stimulants, and depurants must have a shifting scale of value according to the exigencies of each particular case.

3d. The complications of attacks of pernicious fever are far more important than those of simple forms; and therefore symptomatic treatment is often urgently required.

4th. Attacks of pernicious fever may be greatly diminished in number by properly directed treatment of chronic malarial toxæmia, and especially also by the removal of persons suffering under this cachexia to non-malarious localities.

Typho-Malarial Fever.

The prefix typho- is properly applicable to a class of malarial fevers which are complicated by the specific poison which produces typhoid fever.

This term was introduced into medical nomenclature by Surgeon J. J. Woodward of the United States Army. His classical paper on this subject has been published in the *Transactions* of the International Medical Congress at Philadelphia in 1876. The following extract from the proceedings of this congress will show the interpretation of this term by Woodward:

"On motion of Dr. Woodward, seconded by Dr. Pepper, the following was adopted as expressing the opinion of the section: Typho-malarial fever is not a specific or distinct type of disease, but the term may be conveniently applied to the compound forms of fever which result from the combined influence of the causes of the malarious fevers and of typhoid fever."

It follows, therefore, that the term should be so restricted as to define a disease compounded of the two pathological factors which when acting separately produce either typhoid or malarial fever.

When understood in this sense, and carefully employed, the term appears to me unobjectionable. Perhaps, indeed, it may be a convenient addition to medical nomenclature. If such a name had not been introduced, we would be forced to speak of these cases of compound disease as complications. As it is customary to regard the minor or less important affection as the complicating disorder, we would often have confusion in determining whether the case should be typhoid fever complicated by malaria or malarial fever complicated by typhoid. This term leaves all questions of precedence or predominance in abeyance.

There are no facts, however, which support a conclusion that the malarial poison is capable of forming combinations with the particular poisons of other specific fevers and give birth to a new special poison, which may be perpetuated by successive generations, and thus produce epidemics of a new but compound disease.

The importance of a proper use of the term typho-malarial implies co-ordinate care in diagnosing the true nature of the malady it should define.

It may be said, in brief, that the diagnosis of typho-malarial fever must rest upon the blending of the symptomatic phenomena peculiar [p. 615]to each one of the two fevers which enter into combination. In other words, if the differential diagnosis between the two diseases when they are distinct is made by contrasting the symptoms peculiar to each, the compound disease is to be recognized by more or less positive combinations of these symptoms.

These blended symptoms should not be expected to exhibit the results of a copartnership in which each member exerts equal influence. It is well understood that when two diseases coincide, that one which is more violent or excessive in its morbid process holds so much sway as in some cases almost to extinguish the symptoms of the weaker member of the combination. Consequently, in typho-malarial fever, the typhoid, being the graver of the two forms of disease, ordinarily rules the pathology.

The following notes, accompanied by a temperature chart, will illustrate the clinical course of a case of typho-malarial fever:

J. L., aged thirty years, of French nativity, but a resident of New Orleans for three years, was admitted to Ward 21, Bed 311, Charity Hospital, on the night of December 10, 1881. Had been ill some days with ague. The house-surgeon administered gr. x. of quinia in solution and gtt. xv. of tincture of opium.

The records and temperature date from the 12th of December. During the 11th he took drachm ij sulph. cinch. in solution.

[p. 617]

FIG. 24.

PART I., showing the temperature curve from December 12th to 31st, inclusive, during which time the more characteristic typhoid symptoms predominated.

PART II., showing the temperature curve in same case from January 1st to 20th, inclusive, during which the influence of the associated malarial poison was prominent.

Dec. 13th, tenderness and gurgling in ileo-cæcal region; epistaxis; rose spots on abdomen; deafness and ataxia; no stools since 11th. Ordered

                    Acid.
x.   Sulphuric. dil.,
            Syr. Aurantii   fl.
        Cort. *aa.*   drachm ij;
            Tinct.   fl. oz.
        Cinchonæ Co.   j.   M.

S. Teaspoonful in water every four hours.
Also ordered beef-essence, milk-punch, and milk.

Dec. 13th, two very offensive liquid stools; ataxia greater; skin yellow and countenance dull and listless. Dec. 14th, fresh rose spots; tongue brown and dry; three stools; much jactitation. Dec. 15th, more ataxia; some delirium; pulse 100, weak. Gave gr. iiss quinia in solution, with tincture opium gtt. iii, every two hours. Dec. 16th, pulse 128, weak; delirious. Dec. 17, new rose spots; belly tympanitic; tongue brown, dry; sordes on teeth and lips; eyes injected; very delirious. Treatment continued; nutrition and stimulants given methodically. From 17th to 22d but little change in condition or treatment. Diet and stimulants administered regularly. Dec. 22d, coma vigil; completely delirious. Ordered

	Liq. Morphiæ	
x.	Sulph.,	
	Tinct. Digitalis *aa.*	fl. drachm iij;
	Spts. Æther. Nitrosi	fl. drachm ij;
	Liq. Potass. Citrat.	fl. oz. iij. M.

S. Tablespoonful every three hours.

As the oscillations of temperature became more marked, quinia was resorted to, apparently with good effect. The patient was discharged from the hospital Feb. 8, 1882.

It should be observed that after the 14th of December the patient's bowels were rather costive, and the stools occasionally moulded and very [p. 616]dark in color. On the forty-fifth day after admission the patient had a severe chill, followed by a rise of temperature to 104°. This yielded to competent doses of sulphate of cinchonidia.

This was a typical case of typho-malarial fever. The blended symptoms, as well as those special to each disease, are sufficiently exhibited in the clinical account. The presence of typhoid fever was established by the rose spots and the marked nervous symptoms. The typhoid process seems to have been unusually mild in so far as evidence of bowel lesions were made manifest.

The history of the patient before admission, the color of his skin and stools, and the temperature curves gave abundant proofs of the malarial element in the pathology of the case.

Perhaps nothing need be added on the subject of diagnosis. I may, however, remark that I am very cautious in asserting the diagnosis of typho-malarial cases unless the nervous symptoms, positively-marked bowel symptoms, or rose spots are present to vindicate such a decision. The presence of malarial poison may be determined with less difficulty from the previous history of the case and its special symptoms in the early stages of an attack. But if the morbid processes of the typhoid poison are violent, there are likely to be stages of the disease when it is not possible to detect symptoms which indicate the presence of malaria. On the other hand, it is unquestionably true that the typhoid condition, as it is termed, which so often complicates malarial fevers, can very generally be differentiated from true typhoid fever. While certain cases, or even epidemics, of malarial fevers are attended by remarkable adynamia, often manifesting itself from the very incipiency of attacks, it differs widely from that utter nervous ataxia which characterizes typhoid fever. Again, the adynamia of malarial attacks is generally ascribable to some cause not essential to those affections. Imperfect reaction from a chill, long persistent hyperpyrexia, diarrhoea or vomiting, or chronic paludal cachexia, or, it may be, some epidemic influence, may produce it. The ataxia of typhoid fever is part of its morbid process.

Woodward's statistics show that 49,871 cases of fever diagnosed as typho-malarial occurred among the white forces of the United States during the late Civil War. Of this number, 4059 proved fatal, a mortality-rate of 8.13 + per cent. Among the colored troops 7529 cases occurred, with 1301 deaths, a mortality-rate of 17.27. Statistics borrowed from the same excellent authority give the number of cases of unmixed typhoid fever (or fever classed as typhoid without reference to any complication) as 75,368 among the white troops, with 27,056 deaths, a mortality-rate of 35.89. Among the colored troops 4094 cases occurred, and 2280 died, a mortality-rate of 55.68. These figures show very singular comparative results. They prove that typhoid fever as an uncomplicated malady, was four and a half times as fatal among the whites as the same disease when in combination with malarial poison. Among the colored troops typhoid fever was three and a half times more fatal than typho-malarial fever.

It is highly probable that inaccuracies exist in statistics gathered in the confusion of a great civil war, but I am not prepared to say that the conclusions they point to are incorrect. When an acute inflammation is complicated by malaria, its prognosis is rendered more grave. This, no doubt, [p. 618]is due in part to degradations of the fluids of the system by the malarial poison, and in part to the revulsions of circulation during paroxysms. But it does not follow from this fact that the presence of malaria in the blood, or its effects upon that fluid, exercise an unhappy influence upon diseases due to other specific poisons. It may, on the contrary, be ascertained in the future that it modifies the typhoid process, so as to deprive it of some of its most dangerous features.

Further investigations are required to determine the facts in regard to these questions. But it may be premised that if such a conclusion shall ever be reached, it will influence our expectations of cure rather than our practice. If the malarial poison is capable of modifying the toxic effects of the typhoid poison, it must do so in the very formative stages of that affection, if not in its incubative period, so that, having accomplished all the good it is capable of effecting, we may proceed at once to rid ourselves of its presence.

In entering upon the treatment of two diseases compounded in the same patient, if one should ordinarily be amenable to specific treatment, it must certainly be wise practice to endeavor to simplify the case by subtracting that one from its composition. This is more especially true if the treatment does not affect the course of the other disease in any injurious manner. It is therefore proper to begin the treatment of a case of typho-malarial fever by administering large doses of quinia. A scruple may be given every fourth hour, until its effects in eliminating symptoms ascribable to malaria, and also as an antipyretic, have been sufficiently tested. In the early stages of typho-malarial attacks the febrile exacerbations conform to those laws of periodicity which govern uncomplicated malarial fevers. After the first week, or when the typhoid process has become well established, periodic returns of the fever are less plainly observable. It is possible that in some cases in which the typhoid process manifests itself with great severity the temperature curves may be very characteristic of that disease. I am satisfied that the indications for giving quinia to eliminate the malarial element must be based upon the fever curves which mark the case. Perhaps a more frequent application of the thermometer would often exhibit malarial periodicity where it may otherwise remain unsuspected. I know this to be very often the case in pneumonia complicated by a malarial fever.

Whether thorough cinchonism in the early progress of the attack rids the case of symptoms due to malaria or not, only a very few days are likely to elapse before oscillations of temperature call for its repetition.

The typhoid processes require very much the same measures which are applicable in uncomplicated cases of that disease. The stools of the early stages of attacks should not be checked unless excessive, and mercurials and laxatives should be more freely used than in simple typhoid fever. The effects of the malarial fever and of the hyperpyrexia of typhoid fever, when combined, must almost necessarily entail more accumulation of excrementitious material in the blood than would occur either disease existing separately. On this account eliminating treatment is an important indication. When it becomes necessary to check the diarrhoea because excessive or on account of failing strength, diuretics subsequently prove serviceable. Effervescing solutions of potassium or ammonium, lemonade, Apollinaris water, iced tea, strawberry, mulberry, or raspberry juice, are [p. 619]grateful beverages and increase renal activity. The mineral acids may be given during the ulcerative periods of the disease. Insomnia must be relieved by opiates, chloral hydrate, or other hypnotics.

Tympanites should be met by warm stupes, large enemas of warm water with fl. drachm j tincture of asafoetida or fl. oz. j of whiskey. Small doses of turpentine in emulsion are often beneficial.

In the early progress of cases the diet should consist of farinaceous foods, with milk and the pulps or juices of fresh fruits, given either cooked or in their natural state as the physician may determine for each patient. Methodical and forced nutrition becomes necessary at more or less early periods in different cases.

The stools and all ejecta of the sick should be disinfected and disposed of with the same care and for the same purpose as those of unmixed typhoid fever.

[p. 620]

PAROTITIS.
BY JOHN M. KEATING, M.D.

The term parotitis is applied to a condition of painful enlargement of one or both parotid glands, inflammatory in nature, acute in its course, and usually subsiding by resolution, but sometimes ending in suppuration. The different methods of termination, together with certain etiological distinctions, form the basis of a division of the affection into two sub-classes—namely, 1, idiopathic parotitis; and 2, symptomatic or metastatic parotitis. These demand separate consideration.

I. Idiopathic Parotitis.

Idiopathic parotitis, parotitis epidemica, or mumps, as it is variously named, is an acute contagious inflammation of one or both parotid glands, which usually appears but once in a lifetime, and which, although by no means limited to children, is commonly met with between the second year and the age of puberty. In certain exceptional cases the disease affects the submaxillary glands alone.

NATURE.—The undoubted contagiousness of mumps, with the fact of its frequently occurring in extended epidemics, entitles it to a place among the zymotic diseases, from which it differs, however, in the marked disproportion between the local and constitutional symptoms, the former being well developed, the latter but slight or altogether absent.

ETIOLOGY.—While it is more than probable that, like the other diseases of the zymotic class, mumps is due to a contagium that finds its way into the body in the inspired air or with the food or drink, nothing is known of the nature of this infecting principle.

The predisposing agencies are better understood. Age is one of these, the greater number of cases occurring, as already stated, between the second and the fifteenth year. Infants at the breast are almost entirely exempt, and so, too, are individuals advanced in years. In extended epidemics it is not unusual to meet with cases in adults, but it will generally be found on careful examination that these patients have escaped the disease during childhood. Sex exerts some influence, a much larger percentage of males being attacked than females. Epidemics appear more frequently in the spring and fall than at the other seasons of the year, so that cold and dampness of the atmosphere must be looked upon as predisposing causes. Mumps bears a peculiar relation to measles, scarlet fever, and diphtheria, epidemics being apt to occur directly before, during, or immediately after the prevalence of either of these affections, especially [p. 621]the first. The popular idea of mutual protection is entirely without foundation.

Certain peculiarities are presented by the disease in its mode of occurrence and in the duration and intensity of its epidemics. Thus, some localities are visited annually, others only at intervals of thirty years or more; again, one epidemic may last but a few weeks and affect a small number of individuals, while another extends over months and attacks all the children and many of the adults in the affected region.

ANATOMICAL APPEARANCES.—The exact pathological lesion in mumps is obscure, since the trifling nature of the disease and the almost invariable termination in recovery afford no opportunity for post-mortem investigation. According to Foerster, who seems to have made examinations in cases where mumps occurred as one of the accidental complications of other and fatal diseases, the affected gland at first becomes hyperæmic, and is then the seat of serous exudation. It is reddened, swollen, and on section presents a uniform flesh-like, moist appearance, in place of the ordinary granular aspect. The tumor is often greatly increased in size by a simultaneous serous infiltration of the periglandular connective tissue, and occasionally this tissue alone is involved, the gland itself being entirely free from lesion. The great point in favor of this view of the pathology is the rapid and complete subsidence of the parotid swelling by resolution—a termination to be expected only when the inflammatory process stops short of suppuration or fibrinous exudation.

Virchow regards all cases of parotitis as the result of an extension of a more or less malignant catarrh originally affecting the gland-ducts. This is undoubtedly true in some cases, but that it is far from being the rule is proved by the infrequency of parotitis as a secondary complication of catarrhal affections of the mucous membrane of the mouth.

COURSE AND SYMPTOMS.—The course of the disease is susceptible of a division into three stages—a period of incubation, of invasion, and of actual attack.

The stage of incubation extends over a period variously estimated as from seven to fourteen days. It is marked by no symptoms, though sometimes a history of impaired appetite and digestion, irregular bowels, and languor during the last two or three days may be obtained.

The period of invasion is short, lasting only twelve, or at the most twenty-four, hours. The patient is pale and languid, has slight rigors, pains in the breast and head, and loss of appetite; later, local pain in the parotid region on moving the jaws or on taking acid liquids into the mouth. The surface temperature increases from hour to hour, and just before the glandular swelling appears it reaches 100° or 101° F. In some cases the invasion is characterized by the same train of symptoms that ushers in the acute exanthemata, such as repeated vomiting, diarrhoea, restlessness and anxiety, a disposition to syncope, and, in very irritable children, convulsions. Contrasted with this violent invasion other cases are met with, in which there are no prodromes whatever except a gradual rise in temperature, imperceptible without the use of the thermometer.

The first symptom of actual attack is a peculiar slight stitch-like pain in one parotid region, usually the left. This radiates toward the ear of the affected side, and is increased by movements of the jaw, as in [p. 622]chewing or talking, and by external pressure. The pain rapidly grows more intense, and soon becomes associated with swelling. The tumor first appears in the depression between the mastoid process and the ramus of the jaw, which it fills up, and at the same time thrusts outward the lobe of the ear. As the gland alone is swollen at first, the tumor has the outline of a triangle, with the apex directed downward and forward; soon, however, the connective tissue becomes oedematous and the swelling is greatly extended, involving the cheeks and neck, in the latter region, in severe cases, running forward as far as the median line, downward nearly to the shoulder and backward toward the spine. The most prominent point is directly in front of the ear. The oedema also extends internally, involving the pharynx, the tonsils, and sometimes even the larynx. The skin covering the tumor is either perfectly natural in color or slightly reddened. The central portion is firm and elastic to the touch, the periphery doughy, and pressure here often produces pitting. There is but moderate tenderness. The swelling reaches its height in three days, remains stationary for two days longer, and then rapidly declines, the oedema first disappearing and afterward the glandular swelling, the process of resolution occupying four or five days and being attended with a slight desquamation of the cuticle.

While mumps almost uniformly begins on one side, both glands are, as a rule, affected during the attack. The second tumor begins to develop twenty-four to forty-eight hours after the first, though its appearance may be delayed much longer, even until resolution has begun on the side primarily affected. As the course of the inflammation is similar in both parotids, the whole duration of the attack will depend on the time of involvement of the second gland.

Among the other symptoms an alteration of expression is prominent. At first, the head is inclined toward the affected side; later, when both glands are involved, it is held perfectly erect, and, as the slightest movement increases the pain, it is maintained stiffly in this position. The swelling of the cheeks prevents all play of the features, and this, combined with widely-open, staring eyes and increased thickness of the neck, gives the patient a stupid, almost idiotic, expression. The swelling of the neck is sometimes so great that its diameter exceeds that of the head, and the shoulders, neck, and head, viewed together, have the outline of a truncated pyramid.

As any movement of the lower jaw greatly augments the suffering, the mouth is kept closed, often so tightly that it is impossible to see more than the tip of the tongue. All efforts at mastication are suspended, and deglutition is so painful, especially when the tonsils become enlarged, that the sufferer bears the pangs of hunger and thirst rather than endure the agony entailed in satisfying his wants. The act of speaking even augments the pain; the voice, when heard, has a nasal tone. The acuteness of hearing is impaired, there are singing noises and shooting pains in the ears, headache, and sometimes, in extreme cases, symptoms of cerebral hyperæmia due to pressure upon the cervical veins.

The tongue is heavily coated, the mouth is either dry or there is an increased flow of saliva, and the fluid dribbling from the mouth adds another element to the idiotic expression already referred to. There is loss of appetite, increased thirst, occasionally vomiting, and commonly[p. 623]constipation. The temperature is elevated and the pulse increased in frequency, both to a moderate degree. The respiration is unaffected, except when the oedema has invaded the submucous connective tissue of the larynx; then the movements are increased in frequency and difficult.

Throughout the attack the pain, unless intensified by some extraneous influence, as pressure or the act of speaking or swallowing, is only moderately severe. In ordinary cases the patient rests quietly and sleep is undisturbed, unless the tonsils are enlarged, when it is liable to interruption from loud snoring. When the attack is severe and in nervous, excitable children there is restlessness, sleeplessness, and slight delirium at night.

The general symptoms keep pace with the local in their increase, but they commence to subside before, beginning to disappear while the swelling remains stationary. As soon as resolution sets in the general and local improvement are both rapid, and by the end of the week nothing is left but a trifling weakness and pallor, which disappear in a few days more, leaving the patient perfectly well.

Besides the ordinary symptoms, mumps in certain instances shows a peculiar tendency to metastasis, or secondary involvement, of the testicle and scrotum in males, and the mammæ, vulva, and ovaries in females. This metastasis occurs much more frequently in males than in females, and is usually met with in pubescents and adults, being very rare either in childhood or old age. It generally begins six or eight days after the appearance of the parotid tumor. The latter, as a rule, subsides on the occurrence of any of these metastatic affections, though occasionally the two run a simultaneous course. This occurrence, together with the fact of the secondary inflammation appearing at the date on which the parotitis naturally begins to disappear, tends to support Niemeyer's view, that the two affections are in reality due to the same cause, and that no true transference of inflammation takes place from one point to the other. Occasionally, the parotitis disappears a variable time before the onset of the metastatic affection; then the interval is marked by grave symptoms of depression and cerebral disturbance, but there are no proofs of actual meningeal involvement. In these cases there is, at times, an excessive elevation of temperature, which may account for the brain symptoms.

The most constant secondary manifestation is swelling of the testicle proper, or true orchitis; less frequently there is epididymitis, and with it acute hydrocele and oedema of the scrotum. The orchitis in most cases is unilateral, the right testicle being affected, just the opposite to the parotids, of which the left is the one first involved. When the orchitis is double, both testicles do not become swollen at once, the one preceding the other by an interval of several days.

The course of the orchitis is very similar to that of the mumps, the inflammation increasing gradually for from three to six days, then undergoing rapid resolution, the gland returning to its normal condition by the end of two weeks.

The local symptoms are swelling, the testicle being enlarged to two or three times its natural size, dull pain, and moderate tenderness, while in very severe cases there is burning on micturition and a purulent discharge from the urethra. The spermatic cord does not sympathize in the[p. 624]inflammation, and neither the swelling, pain, nor tenderness is so great as in specific orchitis.

The general symptoms are confined to a moderate elevation of temperature and increase in the frequency of the pulse, thirst, and loss of appetite. This fever is separated from that of the parotitis by an interval of two or three days.

The course of bilateral orchitis is longer by forty-eight hours than that of the unilateral form, and the attending fever is more intense.

The rapid return of the testicle to its natural size and shape shows that, as in the parotid glands, the inflammation does not extend beyond the stage of serous exudation.

THE DIAGNOSIS of mumps is easy after the disease is sufficiently developed to produce the characteristic alterations in the facial expression. In the earlier stages the position of the swelling, immediately beneath and in front of the ear, its triangular shape, and the elevation and outward displacement of the lobe of the ear of the affected side, distinguish it from the enlargement of the cervical lymph-glands so liable to occur in strumous subjects. The acute onset and course of mumps are the points of distinction between it and morbid growths, or the very rare condition of chronic hypertrophy of the parotid gland. The metastatic orchitis cannot be mistaken for gonorrhoeal orchitis if the least care is taken to investigate the history in either case.

THE PROGNOSIS is extremely favorable, there being no record of a fatal case of uncomplicated mumps. Suppuration may occur, but it is an exceedingly rare event. In scrofulous children the course may be protracted for several weeks, and in them resolution is occasionally imperfect, a degree of enlargement and induration of one or both parotids remaining for some time.

Metastatic orchitis, as a rule, leaves the testicle in a normal condition, but, according to Vogel, in some epidemics complete atrophy results.

Dogmy reports an epidemic which raged in a garrison of Mount Louis in January, 1828. Of sixty-nine bilateral and eighteen unilateral cases of parotitis, metastasis to both testicles occurred in four cases, all of which resulted in atrophy of the affected testicle.

THE TREATMENT is simple. The patient should be kept in a uniform temperature, confined to one room, or, better still, to bed, until resolution is well established. While the difficulty in swallowing and fever continue the food should consist of milk and beef-tea; later, other nutritious articles of diet may be added as the appetite demands. Water, iced carbonic acid water, or lemonade may be allowed as freely as the patient will take them, to allay the thirst. A daily evacuation of the bowels must be secured by the use of saline laxatives. During the early stage, if the fever be high, tincture of aconite-root should be cautiously administered; afterward liquor potassii citratis will sufficiently fill the indications for a febrifuge. Tonics are required during the decline of the disease; of this class of remedies, syrup of the iodide of iron, bitter wine of iron, and ferrated elixir of cinchona are most useful.

Special symptoms may demand attention. For example, headache and delirium should be relieved by hot mustard foot-baths and moist cold to the forehead; difficult deglutition from enlargement of the tonsils, by the frequent swallowing of bits of ice, or, if possible, by the application of[p. 625]astringent lotions, as tannic acid and glycerine (one drachm to the ounce); sleeplessness, by the administration of bromide of potassium, with or without small doses of hydrate of chloral in children and of some preparation of opium in adults.

In the way of local treatment the best results and greatest relief to suffering will be obtained by gently rubbing the swollen glands with a mixture of tincture of opium and sweet oil (one drachm to the ounce), three times daily, and in the mean while keeping the parts enveloped with a moderately thick layer of cotton wadding covered by oiled silk. Water dressings or light poultices may be used with advantage. When resolution begins a more stimulating lotion will hasten the disappearance of the swelling.

In the exceptional instances in which the skin covering the tumor becomes tense and red, and suppuration is threatened, two or three leeches may be applied behind the ear of the affected side. When suppuration has actually taken place the abscess should be immediately opened to prevent further destruction of the gland-tissue and perforation into the external auditory meatus.

If, particularly in strumous subjects, resolution be incomplete and glandular enlargement and induration remain after the cessation of the acute symptoms, cod-liver oil and iodide of iron are demanded for internal administration and the compound ointment of iodine for external application. It is well to dilute the latter sufficiently to prevent its causing irritation of the skin, and to apply it twice daily.

When metastasis occurs, the return of fever calls for the same general treatment as in the early stage of parotitis. In addition, an emetic should be given, as this often cuts short the fever or causes it to disappear more rapidly. The patient must be kept at perfect rest in bed, with the scrotum elevated by a cushion and covered with warm anodyne lotions. Salines must be administered sufficiently often to secure regular and free action of the bowels.

When the mammæ or ovaries are secondarily attacked, the seat for local treatment is of course different, but in all other respects the management must be the same.

For the uncommon cases in which the transference of the inflammation is attended with depression stimulants are required, and for those in which meningitis is threatened cutting off the hair and the application of cold to the head, hot mustard foot-baths, local and general venesection, drastics, and irritants to the cutaneous surface, are necessary.

II. Symptomatic or Metastatic Parotitis.

Symptomatic, metastatic, malignant, or suppurative parotitis, as the condition is variously designated, is an inflammation of the parotid gland which occurs during the course of different grave acute diseases, is usually unilateral, and terminates in suppuration, or much more rarely in gangrene, of the gland involved.

ETIOLOGY.—It may occur in association with typhus, typhoid, relapsing, puerperal, and scarlet fevers, or with the plague, measles, dysentery, cholera, and pyæmia, springing into notice at different periods of the[p. 626]course of these affections, which may be regarded as predisposing causes. The exciting cause is perhaps mechanical in nature—namely, the excessive dryness of the mucous membrane of the mouth so common in the severe fevers. This dryness may lead to an occlusion of the orifice of the parotid duct, with retention of the saliva, which fluid, undergoing decomposition, may act as an irritant, producing inflammation, and finally suppuration, of the glandular tissue. This is a likely enough explanation of the causation in some cases, but dryness of the mouth is such a uniform symptom in fever, and suppurative parotitis such a comparatively rare complication, that it cannot be a very active or common cause. Nevertheless, it is impossible to fix upon any other direct cause, though the altered condition of the blood in the conditions mentioned must not be lost sight of as an important etiological factor.

ANATOMICAL APPEARANCES.—The character of the pathological lesions have been well established, owing to the frequent opportunities that arise of examining the diseased gland at different stages of the inflammatory process. When the inflammation has lasted a short time, a day or two, the tubes and acini of the gland are seen on section to be swollen and reddened, and the connective tissue infiltrated with serum and yellowish-red in color; a fluid, either viscid, ropy, grayish in color, or more purulent in character, fills the duct, and may be forced out into the mouth by stroking it in the direction of the orifice. If of several days' longer duration, purulent softening will be noticed in the centre of the acini; this gradually extends until each acinus is converted into a little sac of pus. Then the interacinous connective tissue breaks down, and the multiple, minute, purulent collections become converted into a single large abscess or into two or more smaller ones. Next, the pus seeks an outlet. The position of pointing may be on the cheek or in the external auditory meatus—a very common location; again, the abscess may break into the mouth, the pharynx, the oesophagus, or into the anterior mediastinum, the pus burrowing its way along the sheath of the sterno-cleido-mastoid muscle.

While the parotid abscess is forming, suppurative inflammation is apt to be set up in the masseter, pterygoid, and temporal muscles, and from these positions the pus forces its way upward to the temporal or zygomatic fossæ. The periosteum of the neighboring bones, and even the bones themselves, may become involved, and sometimes the cranial bones are partially destroyed, and there is an extension of the inflammation to the brain or its membranes. The middle ear may participate in the general destruction, and the patient is left permanently deaf, if indeed he escape with his life.

The lymphatics, veins, and nerves traversing the parotid are affected by the suppuration in the gland. Irritation of the lymph-vessels results in swelling, tenderness, and suppuration of the lymph-glands. Thrombi form in the jugular vein and its branches, and by breaking down lead to septicæmia and ichorization of the sinuses of the dura mater. The nerves resist for a long time, but seem to act as paths of conduction of the inflammation, the facial nerve leading it to the ear, and the branches of the trifacial to the brain. When gangrene of the gland takes place, the traversing nerves as well as the gland elements are rapidly destroyed.

SYMPTOMS.—Symptomatic parotitis, occurring during the course of [p. 627]any of the diseases already named, produces no change in the general symptoms; if, on the other hand, it occurs during convalescence, the onset is marked by a moderate elevation of temperature and increase in the frequency of the pulse, by thirst, loss of appetite, and sluggish bowels. The tumor, which occupies the same position and thrusts outward the ear-lobe as in mumps, is hard, dense, well defined, and the seat of considerable pain until suppuration takes place, when the latter subsides greatly. The skin over it is red, hot, and tense, and there is much tenderness and little or no pitting on pressure. After the abscess has formed there is well-defined fluctuation on palpation, and at the position of pointing the skin becomes very thin and assumes a bluish-red hue. Gangrene of the gland is manifested by the cadaverous odor, blackening of the skin, the formation of a cavity, and the discharge of ichor and shreds of tissue. The alteration in the expression, the pain in the ear, the difficulty in moving the jaw and in swallowing, are as constantly present here as in idiopathic mumps. It must not be forgotten, though, that when the disease arises during the course of any of the severe infectious diseases, the brain may be so overcome that the subjective symptoms are frequently not complained of.

The course is usually rapid, the abscess pointing on the fourth or fifth day after the appearance of the parotid tumor; occasionally, however, the inflammatory process is much slower, extending over a period of several weeks. The course is also much protracted when secondary abscesses form in other parts of the gland or in the surrounding tissues, when the abscess is transformed into an ichorous cavity, and when gangrene sets in. Ordinarily, where the pus is evacuated by spontaneous rupture or by incision the abscess heals quickly by granulation, leaving the gland enlarged and indurated for some time.

THE PROGNOSIS depends upon the gravity of the original disease, the period of the disease at which the complication occurs, and whether or no mortification sets in. When the vital processes are greatly impaired by the primary disease, the onset of the parotitis, trifling in itself, may prove sufficient to determine a fatal result. The danger of such a result is much increased, too, if the inflammation begins in the earlier stages or during the height of the disease which it complicates, while if it commences during convalescence by far the most frequent result is recovery. Gangrene of the gland involves great risk of life—a risk which increases in proportion to the early date of its onset in the course of the original disease. Even when the gangrenous process ends in recovery, the face is much distorted, the hearing is lost in the ear, and the facial muscles are paralyzed on the affected side. Bilateral symptomatic parotitis has naturally a graver prognosis than the unilateral form.

DIAGNOSIS.—The disease is readily distinguished from idiopathic mumps by the history, the less marked degree of the enlargement and surrounding oedema, the greater degree of pain and tenderness, the hardness of the tumor, the red discoloration of the skin covering it, and the termination in suppuration. Further, it never displays an epidemic tendency.

TREATMENT.—The general treatment of this form does not differ from that of the disease it complicates, though the employment of stimulants in increased quantities may be indicated.

[p. 628]Before the first appearance of tumefaction of the parotid the introduction of a probe or canula into the duct of Steno, associated with pressure on the gland from the outside, may, by forcing from the duct a collection of mucus or muco-pus, abort the inflammation. If this is unsuccessful, a poultice should be applied over the gland to encourage suppuration and pointing externally. As soon as the abscess points the pus must be evacuated by an incision, and, as this has a tendency to close again, a piece of lint must be kept between the lips of the wound.

The enlargement and induration left after the healing of the abscess require the application of tincture of iodine or of compound iodine ointment to the surface.

When gangrene occurs it demands the same treatment, both local and general, as when it is seated elsewhere.

[p. 629]

ERYSIPELAS.
BY JAMES NEVINS HYDE, M.D.

DEFINITION.—Erysipelas is an acute disorder, characterized by the systemic symptoms common to the febrile state, and by an involvement of the integument and deeper parts, the affected surface being tumid, hot, reddened, painful, and often the seat of well-defined bullæ, the process terminating either in complete resolution after cutaneous desquamation or in a fatal result commonly due to complications of the malady.

SYNONYMS.—*Eng.* St. Anthony's Fire; *Fr.* Érysipèle; *Germ.* Rothlauf;*Ital.* Risipolo.

CLASSIFICATION.—Erysipelas is properly recognized as one of the acute infectious diseases. Though by its symptoms and career it would seem to be properly assigned to the category of the exanthemata, it is yet by most authors set apart from the latter—first, because its career is less specifically defined; second, because its contagiousness is less demonstrable in every case; third, because one attack is not known to confer upon its victims immunity against a second; fourth, because the occasional prevalence of the disease in apparently epidemic form is evidently due to extrinsic causes, and does not depend exclusively upon its sudden appearance among the unprotected; fifth, because no definite period of incubation precedes its earliest manifestations; and, sixth, because at times it appears in local manifestations apparently unaccompanied by systemic phenomena.

HISTORY.—The earliest writers on medicine bear witness to the fact that the disease was recognized at the date when men first made record of human ailments. It has occurred in all parts of the world and at all seasons of the year, sparing neither age nor sex in its development. Zuelzer[1] refers to epidemic occurrences of the disorder, described by Rayer, as visiting the Paris hospitals in 1828; by Schönlein, as existing in Zürich in 1836; by Gintrac, as spreading in Bordeaux in 1844-45; and by Trousseau, as prevailing in the Maternité in Paris in 1858.

[1] *Cyclop, of the Prac. of Med., Ziemssen*, vol. iv. p. 424.

ETIOLOGY.—Authors have in general assigned different causes to the forms of erysipelas hitherto regarded as either idiopathic (or medical) or traumatic (or surgical). The modern view, however, is that which regards all cases as alike produced by the absorption of the toxic agent capable of exciting this peculiar inflammation of the skin. The peculiarly well-characterized symptoms of the disease—for example, when it affects the head and face—were long regarded as etiologically distinct from the affection which complicates surgical injuries and wounds. But [p. 630]a closer study of many of the cases first named has again and again disclosed the fact that they originated in such traumatism, for example, as the piercing of the lobule of the ear for the insertion of an ear-ring, a carious tooth, an alveolar abscess, or a pathological product in the antrum of Highmore.

The disease is equally common—apart from the puerperal state—in both sexes and at all ages, and occurs under favorable circumstances in all seasons of the year. It is unquestionably at times spread by direct contagion, either from the living or dead body affected with the disease. Such contagion may occur mediately or immediately. It is, however, not readily shown to be producible by the media of clothing and other articles which have been in contact with a diseased surface. The contents of the bullous lesions which appear upon the erysipelatous surface are inoculable; and the disease has in this way been transferred not only to men, but also, by Orth and others, to the lower animals, and even from one of the latter to another of the same species.

Certain it is, however, that the disease does occur, characterized by symptoms indistinguishable from those to be recognized in the contagious type of the malady, where the most careful investigation wholly fails to reveal the cause, and where the disorder rapidly spreads if the conditions for its extension are favorable. Under these circumstances it is wisest at present to admit that the exact etiology of erysipelas is unknown. Its relative frequency in the puerperal state is unquestionably to be explained by the favorable local conditions which at such times exist in the female for the development of all septic disorders.

As regards the circumstances which might be supposed to specially favor its development, these the capriciousness of the disease, which is its striking characteristic, often quite disregards. Thus, on the one hand, it may and often does prevail, year after year, in certain hospitals, and even in certain wards of a single hospital, especially where these are crowded with patients. But it may also repeatedly spare masses of men affected with disease of a different type when the latter are gathered together in prisons or camps, and indeed even may appear among such individuals and fail to spread to others who are in close proximity to them.

With respect to the propagation of erysipelas from infected to sound individuals, a contrast is exhibited when the transmission of variola, for example, is compared with it. Thus, it is well known that the mildest cases of varioloid may be sources of malignant forms of variola to the unprotected, while those who are partially protected and exposed to the virus of confluent forms of the disease may exhibit the mildest symptoms of varioloid. In erysipelas, however, it is tolerably certain that there are different degrees of virulence to be recognized in different cases, and that the disease at times is transmitted in its different types. Thus, traumatic erysipelas is much more closely related to childbed fever than the varieties of the disease appearing upon the head and face, which cannot be attributed to traumatism, surgical accidents, dental abscesses, or local injuries of the antrum of Highmore. Parturient women frequently escape infection when the erysipelatous disorder is of the so-called medical type. Per contra, it is to be noted that women who are prone to the relapsing and so-called chronic forms of erysipelas are [p. 631]particularly apt to suffer from that involvement of the genital organs, peritoneum, spleen, and febrile movement whose sudden occurrence after confinement is so portentous.

SYMPTOMATOLOGY.—The disease is usually announced by the occurrence of a chill, which may precede by a day or but a few hours the appearance of the cutaneous disorder. The rigor may be severe or mild in grade, so that it may even be forgotten by the patient till his attention reverts to it in connection with the resulting symptoms. There may be simultaneously some gastric distress, rarely of severe character. These symptoms are commonly followed by a febrile reaction. In other cases the first recognized symptoms of the malady occur in the skin, the patient scarcely recalling the fact of a slight preceding malaise.

The cutaneous lesions appear in the form of a circumscribed oedema and redness of the surface, often preceded and usually accompanied by a sensation of tension, heat, and burning pain. This macule, plaque, or patch of diseased integument is in its typical features characteristic. It is distinctly or irregularly circumscribed; its oedematous condition elevates its level decidedly above that of the adjacent integument, so that there is a somewhat sudden descent from the former to the latter for a space of from one to two or more lines. The redness is also of a bright crimson hue, and the reddened surface has a sheen or glossy appearance uniformly displayed over its area. It disappears under the pressure of the finger, leaving a yellowish-white color in the region of impact, the erysipelatous blush rapidly returning when the circulation at the surface is restored. This smooth and shining condition of the reddened patch is so characteristic of erysipelas that it arrests the attention of the diagnostician as soon as he observes it. According to Zuelzer, it is caused simply by the tension of the epidermis. When first observed it may occur in the form of circular, small or large coin-sized patches, or in streaks, striæ, and radiations, or as very irregularly disposed, rosy, and shining marblings or mottlings of an oedematous surface.

The skin thus affected is hot to the touch, tender, firm, and smooth. It is occasionally the seat of pruritic sensations, more commonly of a peculiar sensation of heat and burning.

In the course of two or three days the involved area spreads uniformly or irregularly and centrifugally from the point first involved, after which time, in mild cases, the disease persists without apparent change for a few days more, prior to its decadence by resolution. This final stage of the malady is characterized by a progressively diminishing fever, moderate desquamation, gradual disappearance of the oedema, and a color-change to the darker shades of bluish-red or to a light brown. In this form of the disease the erysipelatous patch, after being fully developed, does not tend to spread from the affected to the unaffected surfaces; and, as a consequence, the affection may complete its entire career in less than a fortnight.

In other cases, however, a remarkable tendency is developed to the progressive spreading of the inflammation from one point or surface of the body to another, the parts first affected paling as the disease passes on to involve those in the vicinity, or being yet deeply involved while the process of peripheral extension is in progress. In yet other cases the red blush sweeps away from its first position in tongue-like projections over a[p. 632]tumid and painful skin, while the region first invaded becomes paler, though still preserving its oedematous features. In still another class of cases the advancing ribbon or band of elevated and reddened integument passes over to a new area, leaving the regions it has traversed tumid, painful, and here and there streaked with rosy lines, patches, or irregular gyrations.

In yet severer types of the malady the intensity of the inflammatory process is such that the epidermis is raised from the tissues below by the free exudation of the serum of the blood. In this way vesicles, or, more commonly, bullæ, develop upon the surface. Bullæ thus formed may be typically perfect, but are often exceedingly irregular in contour, having an appearance which is suggestive of the blistering of a surface by boiling water. The bullæ may be well distended and filled with a perfectly limpid serum. This fluid may, however, in the course of a few days become purulent, the contents in such case drying into crusts. In the severest types of the disease gangrene results from the intensity of the dermatitis, and the loss of tissue which thus occurs is repaired by the processes of granulation and cicatrization.

The migration of erysipelas from one part to another of the surface is sometimes so extensive as to invade from time to time the larger part of the superficies of the body. Erysipelas of this ambulant character may also, after invading the entire surface of the body, be relighted at the point where it first appeared. In other cases this phenomenon of recurrence or reawakening on patches of skin traversed by the disease may be noticed only after moderate extension from a given point. Reddish or rosy-colored islets then appear as new centres of a fresh extension-process upon an integument whose swollen tissues still exhibit the evidences of the prior invasion. In still other cases similar islands of fresh disease are recognized in advance of the elevated edge and tongue-like prolongations which mark the onward progress of the erysipelatous inflammation over areas previously unaffected.

The swelling of the involved tissues is one of the most characteristic features of erysipelas. By this is meant not the tumefaction simply of the superficial portions of the integument, nor the tumefaction which may be measured by the height of the affected above the level of the unaffected skin at the edge of the involved area, but a swelling much more than this, involving the entire skin, and often indeed the subcutaneous tissues, differing, of course, in the extent to which it advances in different cases. In those of severe grade the swelling is enormous, an affected limb assuming the elephantiasic aspect, while the deformity thus induced in the head is fully as great as that seen in the height of confluent variola. In such cases the neighboring ganglia are, as a rule, enlarged and often painful.

It is indeed this swelling which gives to erysipelas of the head and face its peculiar physiognomy. The disorder is apt to find its starting-point in the ear, the side or point of the nose, or one cheek. At this moment it may be possible to recognize the fact that the adjacent mucous membrane is also involved. Thence the disease progresses over the face, and possibly over the scalp also, the resulting tumefaction being occasionally, as already stated, enormous. Thus the eyes are usually closed and sealed by the swollen lids and the orbital depressions are effaced. The lips, enormously pouting and reddened, project from the swollen visage to as [p. 633]great an extent as the tumid ears, which, for similar reasons, depart from the usual plane. The mouth, nares, and eyes alike are covered with mucous secretions, possibly commingled with the contents of bullæ which have formed and broken. Crusts may thus collect near the mucous outlets. The tongue is dry, parched, and cracked, and exhibits a reddish-brown hue. In less severe cases it may be seen to be covered uniformly with a thick yellowish or yellowish-white paste. The fauces and buccal membrane are reddish in color, glazed, and dry.

The patient having this serious form of the malady is indeed in a critical condition. There is usually a coincident coma or delirium. The pulse is either greatly accelerated and full, or thready, fluttering, and destitute of rhythm. The temperature rises to 105° F., and even higher. In this condition a fatal issue may be heralded by collapse, with decadence of the external evidences of the disease, or by the occurrence of blood-filled blebs, or indeed by larger or smaller areas of the surface falling into gangrene. This latter accident may also involve the mucous surfaces, large patches of the buccal membrane, the gums, and even the palate, losing their vitality and showing as greenish-black, insensitive tracts, quite firmly attached to the healthy tissue. These accidents may be of very rapid occurrence, more particularly in the case of individuals prone to exhibit the severest forms of the malady, such as very young infants and those enfeebled by advanced age, by alcoholism, or by any of the cachexiæ.

Other types of erysipelas, chiefly noticeable by reason of their location, are those spreading from the umbilicus, the genital region, the sites of vaccination, of varices of the lower extremities, and the surfaces near the seat of surgical accidents and operations.

The various names which have been, especially by older writers, given to the several expressions of this disorder relate almost exclusively to their external characteristics. Among these may be mentioned—E. ambulans, e. erythematosum, e. bullosum, e. glabrum, e. levigatum, e. miliare, e. oedematosum, e. pemphigoides, e. phlyctenulosum, e. puerperale, e. vaccinale, e. variegatum, e. verrucosum, and e. vesiculosum.

The resolution of erysipelas in favorably terminating cases is accomplished by very gradual amelioration of symptoms. The swelling begins to subside, usually between the third and sixth days. The blebs that have formed then disappear by absorption, bursting, desiccation, or crusting, and subsequent exfoliation. Desquamation of the involved surface may be a prominent or a very insignificant feature. When the patient with erysipelas capitis enjoys a favorable crisis in his disease, there is occasionally noted a very rapid amelioration of the symptoms. The tumefaction speedily subsides, the features become recognizable, and defervescence is complete. Throughout the course of all attacks the febrile process and the erysipelatous blush proceed pari passu with but little deviation of the severity of the one from the intensity of the other.

The complications and sequelæ of the disease are less numerous than they are grave. In erysipelas of the head there is usually a rapid shedding of the hair, though in convalescence the growth of the hair may be restored. An obstinate seborrhoea sicca may, as after variola, linger long afterward upon the scalp; here also, as in other [p. 634]portions of the body, one or many abscesses may form in the subcutaneous tissue after the resolution of the dermatitis; while in phlegmonous erysipelas these abscesses may accompany the disease at its height.

Lymphangitis and adenopathy are common complications of erysipelas, the former betrayed in thickened and often knotted cords, which may be felt radiating from involved areas to neighboring glands. A singular modification is often undergone by the integument affected with erysipelas which has also been the seat of other cutaneous disorders. In this way lupus, psoriasis, chronic eczema, and some of the syphilodermata have been relieved.

Besides the surfaces of the nasal, pharyngeal, and buccal mucous membranes which have been indicated as at times involved by the disease, the inflammatory redness and swelling may extend to the epiglottis, the larynx, and the trachea. Croupous and other forms of pneumonia, pulmonary oedema, and pleuritis have been not rarely noted. In erysipelas of the head the membranes of the brain may inflame and serous effusions distend the ventricles.

The joints may be inflamed either by sympathy or by direct extension of the erysipelatous inflammation to the periarticular tissues, or yet by the occurrence, in or about them, of metastatic abscesses in septicæmic conditions.

The peritoneum may be also acutely or subacutely inflamed in erysipelas, though it is doubtful whether the accident occurs in consequence of the extension of the disease to this membrane from the skin of the abdominal wall. The same may be said of the endocarditis and pericarditis noted by several authors. Of all other complications, it may be said that they can usually be assigned to the occurrence of either septicæmia, or pyæmia, or to the development of metastatic abscesses.

With respect to the eyes, a distinction should be drawn between those attacks originating in deep or superficial affections of the globes and those in which the visual organs are merely involved as by accident in the extension of the disease. In the former case deep orbital abscesses or inflammatory affections of the iris and retina may be followed by erysipelas of the lids or neighboring parts, while in the latter event the issue is more commonly a transitory conjunctivitis, lachrymation, and photophobia, which soon disappear when the disease has declined. The cornea, being unmacerated with pus as in severe variola, commonly escapes perforation.

Erysipelas is a disorder which, without question, produces in a certain proportion of patients a susceptibility to recurrent attacks. This susceptibility, however, is less a systemic tendency to the development of the disease than a peculiar liability to recrudescence originated by chronic local ailments. Thus catarrhal, ulcerative, and other affections of the nasal mucous membrane are particularly apt to originate repeated erysipelatous attacks in the integument covering the nose, and the same is true of the skin in the vicinity of the orifices of fistulous sinuses and varicose veins.

The forms of disease which are often described as instances of chronic erysipelas belong to several classes. There are, first, those in which are observed recurrent attacks of true erysipelas. Second, those in which a chronic eczema or dermatitis produces a circumscribed patch of infiltration [p. 635]in a skin having a lurid reddish hue, which is also the seat of marked subjective sensations, chiefly itching. The well-known forms of chronic eczema erythematosum of the face in middle years or advanced life are commonly, and erroneously, regarded as erysipelatous in character. Third, there is a peculiar dermatitis, of the cheeks chiefly, with regard to whose identity as an erysipelatous affection there is much doubt. The skin is infiltrated in a circumscribed patch, and has a peculiarly glossy red hue. It is essentially a chronic disorder, the affected patch remaining unchanged for months at a time, and then exhibiting aggravation in consequence of accidental exposure to heat or traumatism. These patches may be relics of relapsing forms of erysipelas; and in my experience are more commonly encountered in the subjects of chronic alcoholism.

PATHOLOGY AND MORBID ANATOMY.—The pathological changes exhibited in the erysipelatous skin are those of an exudative process involving the cutaneous and subcutaneous tissues. Nothing specially different from the phenomena observed in a simple dermatitis can be recognized by the microscope alone. Biesiadecki's careful investigations[2]certainly do not disclose any such specificity. The epithelia are swollen with serous fluid, and the exudate, though largely serous, contains also the corpuscles recognized in plastic lymph. It is this serum, rapidly invited to the surface by the acuity of the exudative process, which raises the epidermis into the bullæ described above. The nuclei of the bodies recognized in the exudate are evidently in a state of division and consequent multiplication. The epithelia of the rete mucosum are swollen and stretched. The connective-tissue elements in the derma are also swollen, and exhibit reversion to the embryonal state. There is within each a relative increase of protoplasm, as a consequence of which they undergo a species of liquefaction. The blood- and lymph-vessels enlarge and are crowded with corpuscles. The subcutaneous tissue participates in this process, its elements being filled with finely granular cells disseminated or in aggregated masses. The chief peculiarity of this exudation, and of these changes in the tissue-elements where it recurs, is the rapidity with which, when involution is in progress, the fluid is absorbed and the inflammatory elements disappear. When abscess or gangrene complicates the erysipelatous inflammation the changes are not different from those recognized in dermatitis calorica.

[2] *Sitzungsber. d. k. Acad. der Wissen.*, Wien, ii., 1867.

The changes noted in the viscera are also of a congestive and inflammatory type. According to Ponfick,[3] there is at times a parenchymatous degeneration of the muscular tissues of the large vessels, and of the extremities, as well as of the kidneys, liver, and spleen, the latter organ occasionally undergoing softening. The mucous surfaces of the mouth, larynx, lungs, and alimentary canal have also been found affected with oedema, congestion, and infiltration, rarely terminating in ulcerative changes.

[3] *Deutsch. klin.*, No. 20, 1868.

DIAGNOSIS.—The diagnosis of a typical case of erysipelas is so simple that the nature of the malady is often recognized by those unskilled in such matters. It is difficult to mistake for any other affection the circumscribed, swollen, shining, and rosy-reddish patch of skin, accompanied by fever or marked malaise, with adenopathy of near glands, and often with a history of traumatism to which the origin of the disorder may be readily referred.

[p. 636]It is to be distinguished from dermatitis in its various forms (venenata, medicamentosa, phlegmonosa, suppurativa) by its characteristic features, and by the frequent absence in these inflammations of a febrile reaction and of a shining, rosy-red hue of the skin, and by the peculiarities described above of the elevated margin of the erysipelatous area.

Eczema, especially in its chronic erythematous forms, exhibited in the face of adults in middle and later life, is of much slower development, is productive of itching, is ill-defined in contour, and is not accompanied by fever.

Erythema in all its varieties is a purely hyperæmic affection and unaccompanied by fever. In erythema multiforme there is an exudative process by reason of which various papules, nodosities, and at times even bullæ, appear upon the surface. None of them, however, are accompanied by a diffused area of redness spreading at the periphery. All of its lesions are circumscribed, and rarely affect the face.

Pemphigus could only be mistaken for the form of erysipelas bullæ, but its lesions do not rise from a broadly inflamed area; they rather have attended with each a distinct individual halo when the integument from which they spring is at all congested. They are also rarely accompanied by a febrile process.

Scarlatina, though a febrile affection, is readily distinguished from erysipelas by the appearance of its exanthem, symmetrically and generally developed over the entire surface of the body, or progressively and symmetrically from the upper to the lower segment of it. The exanthem has also a dull scarlet color or the boiled lobster hue, differing thus from the rosy-red and shining patch of erysipelas.

Urticaria also is often of symmetrical development, is rarely accompanied by fever, and is characterized by typical wheals, which, however closely packed together, never have the smoothness of the surface affected with erysipelas.

PROGNOSIS.—The prognosis of a simple case of uncomplicated erysipelas occurring in an individual in fair health and possessed of a reasonable degree of vigor may be regarded as favorable. Even in the weakness of infancy a large area may be involved in the disease and a high degree of fever be aroused without alarming results.

Erysipelas should, however, always be regarded as a serious disease or a serious complication of any existing malady. It is often a grave feature in surgical injuries. Erysipelas involving the entire surface of the face and head is always a formidable affection. In the puerperal state it is dreaded by every accoucheur.

All these circumstances are rendered more portentous by the existence of the disorder as a complication of any other grave malady, or by its occurrence among the subjects of alcoholism, struma, phthisis, or various other cachexias, and among the aged. Occurring in epidemic form among the inmates of prisons, camps, and hospitals, the mortality of the disease may be increased tenfold.

TREATMENT.—The prophylaxis of erysipelas is that of all contagious diseases. It involves isolation of the affected individual, disinfection of body- and bed-clothing before the latter are again employed upon the persons of others, and destruction by fire of all dressings which have been in contact with the integument.

[p. 637]The hygienic management of the patient is not to be neglected. The complete ventilation of the sick chamber is to be secured, and its temperature uniformly sustained at a point between 65° and 70° F.

The general treatment of the sufferer need not greatly differ from that commonly pursued in the febrile state by modern therapeutists. There is but little confidence to-day in the methods by venesection and purgation, upon which at one time reliance was placed. Cool or cold water may be freely employed when there is hyperpyrexia, either by general bathing or by wrapping the patient in sheets dipped in and wrung out of the same fluid. The results are favorable as regards the bodily temperature, and are not productive of danger, though water thus applied has no effect upon the local disorder of the skin. Iced or cool water, by the ice-bag or compresses, is specially indicated as a topical application for the head when there is delirium or other indication of disturbance of the cephalic centres, irrespective of the invasion of the scalp and face by the erysipelatous inflammation. The sulphate of quinia in full doses is indicated especially when there is any tendency to remittence in the febrile accessions, but is not known to possess any power to cut short the disease. In many cases of erysipelas the febrile condition is readily managed by the administration of the simpler remedies found grateful to the palate of the sufferer, such as iced, acidulated, and effervescing draughts, with perhaps the employment of the spiritus Mindereri or the spirit of nitrous ether. In other cases the mineral acids can be substituted with advantage for the latter. With many American physicians it is customary to add to these remedies the tincture of the root of aconite, with a view to its effect upon the pulse.

Few internal remedies, however, have in this country enjoyed as much popularity with the profession in the treatment of erysipelas as the muriated tincture of iron in full doses. Its use, first suggested for this purpose by Bell in 1851, has here steadily gained in favor since its general adoption. It is well to give it in doses of not less than 20 or 30 drops, repeated every two or three hours, diluted with water. When there is high fever, and especially if the secretion of urine is scanty, the following formula will be found valuable:

               Tr. Ferri
x.   Chloridi;

               Sp. Ætheris
Nitrosi;

            Glycerinæ   fl. drachm
       aa.   i.   M.

S. A teaspoonful in water every three hours.

This preparation of iron certainly seems, in many cases, to shorten the disease, but, per contra, it is to be remembered—first, that in many other cases it has been found to exercise no control whatever over the severest manifestations of the disease; second, that in other countries, especially in Germany, where it is rarely employed, the mortality from the disease is no greater than elsewhere.

The widest difference in practice has obtained relative to the local treatment of the affection. They who have had the fortitude to content themselves with watching the evolution of the specific dermatitis, merely protecting the skin by dusting over it a simple powder or leaving it covered with a cold compress, have certainly no worse results to tabulate than those who entertain a belief in the efficacy of the abortive treatment of the local disorder.

[p. 638]No remedies, locally applied, can be recognized as certainly possessing the power to cut short the inflammation. Those which enjoy the highest reputation for topical employment are saturated solutions, hot and cold, of the hyposulphite of sodium, of boracic acid, and of the bicarbonate of sodium; salicylic acid; iodoform in powder; and, quite lately, resorcin. Hot fomentations of the erysipelatous patch are in general most grateful to the patient, and with these an opiate and astringent effect can be obtained, as by a hot lead and opium wash or by solutions of the sulphate of iron or of alum and tannin. Useful methods of applying these are by the medium of borated cotton, oakum, tow, or spongiopiline, covered with oiled silk or the Lister protective material.

Other medicaments which have enjoyed favor in the topical treatment of the disease are lime-water and linseed oil (carron oil), sulphur in powder, carbolic acid, camphor, the oil of turpentine, collodium, cataplasms and ointments containing mercury, lead, zinc, tar, and tannin.

Respecting the measures adopted with a view to checking the extension of the disease at the periphery of the patch, the belief in such a possibility has been wellnigh abandoned. For this purpose the nitrate of silver, caustic potash, tincture of iodine, and similar substances have been boldly and broadly applied, alike over the sound and affected integument, with the production of an artificial dermatitis intended to supplant that which was previously in progress. Again and again has the local inflammation transgressed these artificial limits; and when they have been by it apparently respected there has been little ground for believing that the result was due to the treatment pursued. Inasmuch as the disease is often self-limited and distinctly limited in its progression over the surface, it is manifestly difficult to determine that its limitation in any given case is the result of topical agencies. These agencies have, moreover, the marked disadvantage of adding their irritative effects to those incidental to the dermatitis.

The surgical treatment of erysipelas invading special regions of the body or the deeper tissues is a matter of importance. Free incisions are requisite for the liberation of pus, and all abscess cavities should be treated antiseptically and stuffed with iodoform or resorcin. Great tension of the lids demands free incisions in the long diameter of either, and the same surgical procedures are often demanded in erysipelas of the scrotum or of the labia in the female. Gangrene and sloughing are to be treated in accordance with the principles recognized as important in the management of these accidents in general.

The mouth when involved may be benefited by gargles containing the chlorate of potassium, alum, tannin, the compound tincture of cinchona, or by the use of the spray with a saturated solution of boracic acid in rosewater. Kaposi lays stress, in all cases of erysipelas of the face, upon the importance of searching for and evacuating all dental abscesses and pustules seated upon the Schneiderian membrane. Crusts in the nasal cavity are to be soaked with vaseline and removed by washing, their re-formation being prevented by the insertion of small tampons smeared with a bland ointment or oily fluid. Abscesses in other portions of the body, not suspected as being etiologically significant, are to be carefully searched for and emptied, whether occurring about the anus, the genitals, or the legs.

[p. 639]Subcutaneous injections of carbolic acid and other antiseptic solutions have not been rewarded by such results as to establish in any degree their special efficacy.

In all ordinary cases the expectant treatment recommended by Zuelzer is abundantly to be commended. The inflamed tissue is to be dusted with finely-powdered starch, and protected by a layer of soft cotton-wool which exercises a moderate degree of pressure upon it. Antiseptically, the highest ends are thus reached.

The diet of the patient should consist of animal broths, soups, milk, and eggs, with a view to the reparation of the waste incidental to the febrile process. Stimulants are to be freely used in all asthenic conditions. In convalescence the warm water and soap bath is to be employed, followed by dusting of the surface with starch powder or by inunction with vaseline.

[p. 640]

YELLOW FEVER.
BY S. M. BEMISS, M.D.

Yellow fever is a specific, infectious, and communicable disease of one febrile paroxysm.

This definition includes some of the most prominent characteristics of the disease. The malady, however, derives its name from a symptom not mentioned in the definition. The yellow color of the skin and scleroticæ which appears in advanced stages of grave cases of yellow fever, and which becomes especially marked in the cadaver, has ruled its nomenclature. Whatever objections may be urged against the term "yellow fever" as being founded upon a symptom of the disease not always present, it is too strongly fixed in both medical literature and popular usage to justify efforts to change it.

Neither is it liable to beget confusion as long as it is understood that it is to be restricted in its application to a specific fever induced by a specific poison, and that as an incident of its morbid process it produces yellow coloration of the surface so frequently as to suggest the prefix yellow to its title.

ETIOLOGY AND SYMPTOMATOLOGY.—In this day of almost general belief in the theory which holds that each specific disease has its own specific poison or morbific germ, it is scarcely expedient to occupy much space in discussing the propriety of classing yellow fever among the specific maladies.

Whether we rest the decision of this question upon the uniformity of those circumstances and conditions which originate and develop epidemics of yellow fever, or upon the sameness of its symptomatic phenomena wherever observed, we find very nearly as substantial claims to a specific individualization of the disease as any one of the eruptive fevers possesses. Not only are its morbid phenomena so characteristic that even non-professional observers designate it by such epithets as Bronze John, Yellow Jack, Vomito Prieto, etc., but it is inconvertible with other specific affections. This inconvertibility of yellow fever with other diseases is absolute, and affords irrefrangible evidence of the specificity of that germ or poisonous principle which produces it.

The study of yellow-fever poison after the objective method has hitherto been unproductive of definite results. When such experienced and truthful observers as Sternberg, Woodward, and Schmidt, working with the most approved microscopes, have failed to identify any organism or object peculiar to the products from the bodies of yellow-fever subjects or to the circumfusa of the sick, this declaration is sufficiently supported.

[p. 641]But when we turn to a subjective method of investigating that toxic agent which causes yellow fever, it is found to possess sufficiently well-marked characteristics to justify practically valuable conclusions. Some of these characteristics or modes of behavior merit notice.

1st. The human system is a field of reproduction and multiplication of yellow-fever poison. This is sufficiently established by two facts:

(a) A person in the incubative stage of yellow-fever intoxication may be divested of all fomites and yet originate other cases after a developed attack.

(b) The infection is intensified by aggregation of the sick.

These propositions are indisputably true.

2d. The poison or infection undergoes some change after leaving the human system. This appears to be susceptible of proof, because communication of the disease from person to person is not a common event. When this does apparently occur, there is often very strong reason for a belief that the contagion was resident in some fomites connected with the patient's bed or clothing.

3d. There are no sustained observations which prove that yellow-fever poison is ever created de novo.

The autochthonous birthplace of the poison is unknown. The suggestion of Niebuhr, that yellow fever may have been one of the causes of death during the plagues of Athens, can not be authoritatively denied. It may have been called into existence at the moment when all things else were created which were to perpetuate each its kind.

4th. Some of those conditions and circumstances which favor or retard the development or maturation of yellow-fever poison outside the human body are quite well understood. Warm, damp weather is most prominent among those climatic conditions which are favorable to the growth of yellow-fever epidemics.

5th. A freezing temperature ordinarily destroys the contagium of yellow fever. A high degree of artificial heat produces a similar result. It is highly probable that certain chemical agents would also effect its destruction if brought in contact with it.

6th. If yellow-fever fomites are hermetically enclosed in situations protected from cold or other agents which are destructive to their infection, its vitality may be preserved for an undetermined length of time, and its toxic qualities again made manifest when unacclimated persons are exposed to it.

7th. Yellow-fever poison possesses ponderability. This characteristic is so distinctly marked that it has been frequently termed a "low-lying poison."

8th. It is incapable of being air-borne through any great distance, at least without being deprived of its toxic effects.

9th. It is transportable in fomites through great distances, either on sea or land, and as often as its toxic effects are manifested after these portations they are so uniform as to be promptly recognizable.

A great number of different materials in common use may act as fomites, such as loose wool, cotton, or hair, or textile fabrics of various descriptions.

The following facts, which illustrate how yellow-fever infection may be conveyed in the most unsuspecting and innocent manner, are well[p. 642]authenticated. There can be no ground for accusation of error except in the hypothesis that the infection was encountered simultaneously in some unexplained manner. The facts are furnished by Dr. Shannon of Ocean Springs, Mississippi: "On the 14th of October, 1883, Maj. J. B. B. died of yellow fever in Ocean Springs, Miss. I moved the family at once to the healthy locality where you saw Miss B., not allowing them to take any article from the room where the husband and father had died. The children applied to me for a lock of their father's hair, which I refused, but the oldest daughter, now dead, prevailed upon the nurse to give it her. She placed it in an old envelope that had been torn open at the end and carefully folded the torn end down, thus practically sealing it, and laid it away among other old letters. On Sunday, the 4th of November, at 12.30P.M., she brought this envelope out upon the open gallery, and opened it for the first time to examine the lock of hair and show it to her aunt, Miss S., who was visiting her, and upon inhaling the concentrated poison confined in the envelope and emanating from the hair, exclaimed, 'Oh, what a peculiar smell!' She then handed the envelope to her aunt, Miss S., who, unconscious of danger, also inhaled the 'messenger of death' with a similar exclamation, when Mrs. B., who was standing near, reached out her hand for the envelope, but was prevented from getting it by the entreaties of a fretful child to be taken up in her arms. This gave time for sufficient reflection, and she admonished the young ladies of the possible danger. The envelope was then carefully folded, and with its fatal contents replaced in the drawer where it had been since the 14th of October. This drawer had been almost daily opened. On the following Saturday night, Nov. 10th, at 9 P.M., Miss S. was taken sick with a chill, and Miss B. at about 2 A.M., some five hours later, the period of incubation being less than seven days in both cases. No other person handled the fatal envelope or in any way came in contact with it, and there is, after the most careful inquiry, no suspicion of any other source of infection in these two cases. Miss S. died on Oct. 14th, Miss B. on Oct. 16th."

10th. These qualities of yellow-fever infection, and especially its faculty of reproduction (which only organisms possess), furnish almost conclusive evidence that yellow fever is a germ disease produced by a specific contagium vivum.

Many facts are patent which sustain the generally accepted opinion that yellow-fever poison gains admission to the system through the medium of atmospheric air. On the other hand, I know of no observations which prove that the disease is ever communicated by food or drinks, or through any other vehicle than atmospheric air.

In respect to atmospheric infection by yellow fever, localizations of aërial impregnation are often observable, not common in other air-infecting diseases. A certain district of a large and populous city may become the seat of a sweeping and fatal epidemic, and yet no case occur outside of this area of prevalence. It is customary to speak of these points of epidemic prevalence as infected localities. If unprotected persons visit such infected places, even for a short period of time, they are liable to attacks of yellow fever, although they may take neither food nor drink within the limits of infection and bring no fomites away with them. Under these circumstances atmospheric impregnation is conclusive.

[p. 643]But it is difficult to determine how this infection of a locality has been produced in the first place, and how, in the second place, it is maintained sometimes for periods of from one to three months, with so little apparent diminution or change in the liability to communicate yellow fever to unprotected visitors within the limits of infection.

It seems highly probable that yellow-fever poison, after its exit from the human body, attaches itself to various solid surfaces in proximity to the sick, where, under suitable climatic conditions, it undergoes more or less speedy processes of maturation in toxic qualities. The poison thus matured is capable of being preserved with but little change for the periods indicated above, and is communicable through the atmosphere for short distances. It is also capable, by virtue of some unexplained process or quality, of spontaneously extending its area of infection. But this is at all times slow, and is readily interrupted by streams of water, high walls, or even by much-travelled thoroughfares.

There are no instances in which the water-supply of cities has been shown to have distributed yellow fever.

The periods of time which may intervene between exposure to yellow-fever poison and attacks of the disease are extremely variable. The shortest period of incubation which has come under my observation was about twenty hours. In three cases in which I was able to fix the hours of first exposure with precision attacks followed in 72 hours, 83 hours, and 101 hours, respectively. Of 55 unacclimated physicians who exposed themselves at Memphis during the epidemic of 1878, 54 suffered attacks of yellow fever. In these cases the periods of incubation varied from one to twenty-five days, the average duration being ten days. These physicians all remained steadfastly at their posts of duty; consequently, the attack which occurred on the twenty-fifth day was postponed for that length of time during constant exposure in a locality most intensely infected.

It must be true that many cases of individual resistance to the effects of yellow-fever infection depend upon states of the system or idiosyncrasies which diminish liability to the action of the poison. In other words, their personal receptivity to it is lessened by certain constitutional states.

That this position is correctly taken is proved by the fact that many circumstances which violently disturb the system determine attacks in persons who may have for a long time enjoyed immunity from them. Anxiety, grief, fright, fatigue, or exposure to sudden wettings or cold may precipitate attacks, either by disturbing vital processes by which the system is ridding itself of the poison—so far, at least, as to prevent an accumulation great enough to occasion attacks—or by lowering powers of resistance through enfeeblement of nerve-force.

But it can be affirmed in regard to yellow-fever poison that it is not more capricious or eccentric in its behavior as an infection than that of scarlet fever. Each of these diseases may appear in a large family of unprotected persons with a degree of violence which results in death in every instance, and suddenly cease, leaving a greater or less number of the household without attacks, though equally exposed with those who have died.

One attack of yellow fever confers immunity from the disease during after life. A person who has suffered an attack is said to be acclimated [p. 644]or protected. Neither of these terms should be applied to those who have not suffered attacks, however long they may have withstood exposure during epidemics. It often occurs that persons who have escaped attacks through many years of renewed exposure at last succumb to the disease. On the other hand, I know of three well-authenticated instances of immunity in a sweeping epidemic of persons whose mothers had suffered attacks during the gestations which respectively resulted in their births.

While negroes are susceptible to yellow-fever infection, attacks are far less fatal than among whites.

SYMPTOMS IN MILD OR SIMPLE CASES.—Yellow fever is usually sudden in its onset. Persons are liable to be seized while pursuing their ordinary avocations, or, as often occurs, the attack may begin during the night. The initial symptoms are chilliness or cold sensations, seldom amounting to a decided rigor. Reaction is usually prompt and decided, the temperature reaching within a few hours 102° to 105° F. Yellow fever is not a disease in which it is very common to observe excessive body heat.

As the fever is established, the countenance becomes flushed and the eyes injected and glistening. Frontal headache and lumbar pain are experienced very early in the attack, and are liable to become more intense during the progress of the fever. Muscular neuralgias, especially in the lower extremities, are not uncommon.

During the early period of the attack the tongue is indifferent as a symptom. It is generally moist and free from any coating. In cases attended by much furring of the tongue careful investigation is pretty sure to disclose the fact that it has been brought about by some pre-existing state of disease.

The bowels are generally inactive, though naturally impressible to cathartic drugs. The stomach is querulous from the inception of the attack to its conclusion. Vomiting may not occur spontaneously, but it is easily provoked by repletion of the stomach with any description of ingesta or by harsh or disgusting medicines. The acts of emesis are sudden and short in duration. Bile is a very uncommon constituent of the matters ejected. Whether vomiting has occurred or not, patients nearly always express repugnance to the weight of the physician's hand over the epigastrium. In the very mildest cases it seems to excite gastric distress and a tendency to emesis. The stomach and bowels are liable to distension by flatus, sometimes to the extent of producing colicky pains. Gaseous eructations are common.

During and shortly succeeding the cold stage the urine may be somewhat increased in amount, but after the fever is established both the quantity and the specific gravity are notably lessened. Albumen seldom appears in the urine during the first twenty-four hours of an attack. In very mild cases it is altogether absent throughout.

Delirium is not unusual during the fever. Among children attacks are often ushered in by convulsions. In such cases delirium may be persistent and alarming in violence.

The pulse in the early stage of yellow fever is slower in proportion to the temperature than in most other acute diseases. This is more especially true in respect to mild cases. Another characteristic feature of the pulse in[p. 645]yellow fever is that it declines in frequency before the fever has reached its maximum. In the mildest forms of the disease the temperature will attain its highest record within twelve hours. It then rapidly defervesces, never to return again. But in some cases of a moderately mild form the body heat does not reach its acme of intensity until the second day, occasionally not until the third or fourth day. In these cases also the pulse is apt to decline in frequency before the fever has culminated. There are therefore no fixed laws which govern the duration of the hot stage of yellow fever. Those which relate to the pulse are more uniform.

The following clinical reports of two cases support this statement. The detailed account of the symptoms establishing their diagnosis as mild cases of yellow fever is omitted.

Susie W——, white, aged seventeen years, was admitted to Charity Hospital on August 28, 1878. First observation, nine hours after the beginning of the attack, pulse 100, temperature 104.6°. Morning of 29th, pulse 94, temperature 102.8°; evening, pulse 80, temperature 101.5°. Sanguineous discharge from vagina began on 29th; patient supposed it to be her proper period. Aug. 30th, pulse 80, temperature 99.2°; convalescent and dismissed from further observations. In this case the urine presented a trace of albumen early on the second day, but as the menses appeared shortly after the urine was obtained, the presence of albumen may be in that manner accounted for.

Bessie L——, white, age twenty-seven years, admitted to Charity Hospital on August 28, 1878. First observation, twelve hours after beginning of attack, pulse 100, temperature 100.6°. 29th, pulse 76, temperature 102.3°. 30th, pulse 64, temperature 101.5°. Sanguineous discharge from vagina began on 30th and continued until Sept. 4th; this was two weeks before the patient's regular period. The urine showed traces of albumen at date of admission. Discharged, cured, Aug. 31st.

It may also be stated of the pulse of yellow fever that it is easily compressible and often gaseous in character.

Perspiration is probably an incident in the natural clinical history of a case of yellow fever. It occurs spontaneously if the patient's surface is protected from those influences which conflict with its appearance. It is not critical in any sense of the word, and may coexist with high temperature.

Yellow fever is considered to have two clinical stages. The first is the paroxysm. This is made to include the cold stage and succeeding fever. The cold stage is often almost or quite inappreciable, and when this is not the fact it is in simple cases a very unimportant event. It is therefore quite convenient to include it with the fever under the term paroxysm. The paroxysm of a simple case is terminated by a subsidence of the fever to nearly or quite a normal temperature. Sometimes the temperature falls below the normal standard.

The neuralgias and subjective sufferings are greatly mitigated or cease altogether. Thirst and restlessness are relieved, and the patient sees before him a delicious, but too often treacherous, mirage of restoration to perfect health. This is termed the stage of calm, perhaps because it often precedes a tempest of fatal symptoms.

In mild cases convalescence begins at the termination of the paroxysm, and may proceed without interruption until complete re-establishment of[p. 646]health has been accomplished. But in the very mildest cases the process of recovery is easily interrupted.

In these simple forms the tendency to hemorrhage first manifests itself in the calm stage. The gums become red, tumid, and spongy, the tongue pointed and red at the tip. Epistaxis is liable to occur. The eyes and skin may be slightly yellow, and the urine may show traces of albumen. However mild the other symptoms may appear, the tendency to hemorrhage, to albuminous urine, and to jaundice in the calm stage bears a direct relation in frequency of occurrence and in degree to the blood-stasis, or sluggish capillary circulation, of the first stage.

The foregoing is a recital of the clinical phenomena of typical and simple forms of yellow fever. The departures from type have been divided by different writers into a variety of forms. The most important of these will be referred to in connection with suggestions as to treatment.

PROGNOSIS.—Prognosis is variable in different epidemics, this observation being understood to apply to the same localities. Some of those circumstances which affect epidemic force, so as to increase the mortality-rate, are appreciable. If an epidemic invades a population after an interval of exemption sufficiently long to allow a large number of unprotected persons to have accumulated in its midst, the crowding of the sick will increase the death-rate. We may naturally assume that this is attributable, first, to sheer multiplication of the infection; second, to lack of proper attention to the sick, and to fright, grief, exhaustion, etc.

Tabulated Abstract of Practice in Yellow-Fever Epidemic of 1878, New Orleans Charity Hospital.

AGES.	July.		August.		September.		October.		Total.		per cent.
	No. treated	No. fatal	No. treated	No. fatal	No. treated	No. fatal	No. treated	No. fatal	No. treated	No. fatal	
White Under 5	..	..	7	3	..	..	1	0			0.0
5 to 10	..	..	2	1	..	..	3				6.66

10 to 20	8		26		25		7	..	66	6	4.2
20 to 40	8	1	246	41	175	1	61	4	500	65	3.0
40 to 60	9		75	5	83	5	18	0	185	106	7.3
60 to 80	2		7		5		1		15	10	6.66
Total.	37	0	363	303	292	45	87	5	779	703	1.7
Black.											
10 to 20	1	..	..	2	..	5	..	1	..	8	..
20 to 40	2	..	..	11		8		5		24		0.8
40 to 60	2	..	..	2		1		3		6		0.0
Total.	5	..	..	15		14		9		38		1.0
Grand total.										817	11	0.3

[p. 647]Prognosis is especially bad in hospital practice. The foregoing statistics of cases admitted to the Charity Hospital of New Orleans during the greater part of the epidemic of 1878 illustrate the usual results of hospital practice.

Many of these patients were conveyed to the hospital in extreme conditions; occasionally they were moribund on admission. It is hazardous to the life of a yellow-fever patient to transfer him over the rough streets of a city, often for two or three miles, unless this is done in the very earliest hours of the attack.

Prognosis is seriously influenced by the condition of the patient at the moment of attack. If pregnancy exists or delivery has just occurred, it is, under most circumstances, extremely unfavorable. Fatigue, anxiety, despair, or grief, all render prognosis more gloomy.

The march of temperature is also important in determining fatal results.

The following statistics show the influence of temperature in relation to mortality from yellow fever:

	First day.	Died.	Second day.	Died.	Third day.	Died.	Fourth day.	Died.	Fifth day.	Died.
106°	..	..	3				2		..	..
105°			5				2			
104°	8	0	23	3			2			

03°	4	1	1			3		..

It will be seen from this table that the danger line of temperature in yellow fever descends as the case progresses.

It may again be stated that yellow fever, like scarlet fever, exhibits such striking contrasts in its mortality-rate that it is hardly possible to assert any average standard. It is true that in this disease, as in all others, statistical accumulations tend to correct their own errors in exact proportion to the magnitude of the collections.

In 1878 some 36,000 cases occurred in Louisiana, of which number not less than 6000 were fatal, a percentage of 16.66. The results of private practice in New Orleans are exhibited in the following statistics: Four of the principal practitioners in the city treated in private practice 975 patients—909 white and 66 colored. Of the former, 92, or 10.11 per cent., died; of the colored only 2 died. The cases and deaths among the whites, classified by age, were as follows:

AGE.	Cases.	Deaths.	Per cent.
Under 5 years of age	206	26	12.67
From 5 to 10 years of age	233	20	8.61
From 10 to 20 years of age	183	9	4.9
From 20 to 40 years of age	232	39	16.7
From 40 to 60 years of age	47	6	12.7
From 60 to 80 years of age	4	2	50

The physicians above quoted lived in different parts of the city. All of them extended their visits and professional services to the sick to the [p. 648]very limits of physical endurance, and consequently included in the above lists some patients who were not able to procure the comforts and attention necessary to the sick. Some cases also were included to which the physician was only brought that he might sign the death-certificate and so avoid the coroner's inquest. After making allowance for increase of mortality on these scores, I think it safe to assert that the best results obtained in private practice varied from 7 to 10 per cent. of mortality-rate.

DIAGNOSIS.—While there is no one symptom pathognomonic of yellow fever in every stage of the disease, its differential diagnosis is nearly always possible. The morbid action of its special poison produces phenomena sufficiently characteristic to prove its presence. The sudden attack, the slight cold stage, the frontal and lumbar pain, and the capillary congestion are important diagnostic symptoms.

Even in mild attacks this capillary blood-stasis is usually sufficient to alter the patient's countenance to such a degree as to attract attention. A great many different adjectives are used in description of the countenances of yellow-fever patients. While no one among them is constantly applicable, the presence of a changed facial expression should enlist the physician's attention and incite investigation. If this altered countenance be associated with watery or glistening injected eyes, the probability of yellow fever is increased.

The slow pulse which coexists with elevated temperature is a point of much diagnostic value. But it must be remembered that this symptom is not peculiar to yellow fever. I have noted this lack of correlation of pulse and temperature in several cases of dengue. It is also not infrequently found in ordinary cases of jaundice. The slow pulse of yellow fever must be attributable to the special action of the poison upon the nervous system. The heart's action may be slowed by influences exerted directly or through the retrograde effects of the delay of blood-currents in the capillary distribution.

Albuminous urine is a symptom of much diagnostic importance.

A tendency to hemorrhage may be safely stated to exist in all cases of yellow fever. In the mildest cases hemorrhage may not actually take place unless the patients be non-gravid females within the ovulating limits of life. These patients seldom pass through yellow-fever attacks without sanguineous vaginal discharges. But even in the mildest cases yellow fever establishes the hemorrhagic diathesis to an extent sufficient to render the occurrence of hemorrhage an imminent event. This fact is shown first, by the congested and tumid gums, from which blood can be readily pressed, and also by the still more important circumstance that medical or hygienic mismanagement is so quickly and certainly followed by black vomit or by hemorrhages from other parts of the system. Capillary congestion is undoubtedly an important factor in the production of hemorrhages in yellow fever, since we cannot otherwise account for the liability to hemorrhage which is so general in this disease.

The yellow color of the skin and eyes during life, and of the tissues and serum of the cadaver, is probably due to the coincident influence of two causes: first, to the coloring matter of the red corpuscles diffused in the serum of the blood; second, to an accumulation of secondary blood-poisons. The occurrence of the yellow color and its intensity bear a [p. 649]direct relation to the sluggishness of capillary circulation during the paroxysm. It appears likely, therefore, that the yellowness is principally ascribable to coloring principles derived from dissolution of the blood, to which capillary obstruction would so strongly predispose this fluid.

Schmidt has made a very careful résumé of the pathological changes found after death from yellow fever. The most important and uniform of these affected the nervous system, liver, and kidneys. They consisted for the most part of hyperæmic conditions, not infrequently attended by points of extravasation and of degenerative changes. The latter are principally found in the liver, and bear some relation to the duration of the case, and it may be also to the degree and persistence of the pyrexia. When the liver is the seat of fatty degeneration, it is yellowish in color in whole or in parts. It is then sometimes spoken of as the café au lait or the box-wood liver.

In cases which run a very rapid course these changes are not observed, but only those which indicate congestion are found, and often hemorrhagic puncta. In these instances the depending portions of the body have dark or livid ecchymoses.

TREATMENT.—There are two propositions to which due attention should be given before formulating rules for the treatment of yellow fever. The first of these is, that yellow fever is strictly a self-limited disease, and therefore is insusceptible of jugulation. Both clauses of this proposition are indisputably true. Cases have been observed in which mitigation of symptoms and abridgment in duration appeared to follow spontaneous diarrhoea. Such events must be extremely uncommon, since in my large experience I know of but one such instance supported by good testimony.

Efforts to abort the disease by purgatives, bleedings, cold baths, quinia, etc. have all signally failed. Among the possibilities of the future is the discovery that some drug or combination of drugs is capable of meeting yellow-fever poison in the field of the circulation and antagonizing it sufficiently to rescue the victim from its fatal toxic effects.

The second proposition is, that the formative stages of the disease—that is, the early hours of the paroxysm—afford the most precious moments for instituting such medication as may be considered proper. This proposition applies no doubt to a number of other acute affections, but in no one among them all is it so important to be regarded as in yellow fever. The primary effects of the poison are so boldly outlined that it appears highly probable that the damage it exerts upon the economy is chiefly inflicted during the paroxysm. This affords an additional reason why efforts at medication should be principally restricted to the paroxysm and to the earliest periods of that stage.

It is probable that during an attack of yellow fever the patient's hold upon life is more or less secure in direct ratio to the number of functions which retain their physiological integrity fairly well. The suggestion of such a fact should exclude all scholastic or routine rules of treatment.

In simple forms of yellow fever the first desideratum of the practitioner is to become acquainted with the patient's condition at the moment of attack. If this has occurred after eating indigestible food or after a hearty meal of any description, the stomach should be emptied. Ipecacuanha may be given in warm water or chamomile infusion until this result [p. 650]has been accomplished. After emesis, provided this should have been considered necessary or as a first step of treatment under other circumstances, a purgative is usually given. The benefits of purgation are, in my opinion, limited to the act of ridding the bowels of any fecal accumulations present. For this purpose those purgatives which combine a due degree of efficiency with inoffensiveness in operation have appeared to me to be the best. Castor oil is at the head of this class. An ounce may be given to an adult in some acceptable vehicle. This may be followed by an enema of tepid water when required. Salines are more agreeable to the palate, but far too unmanageable in their cathartic effects to be adopted generally.

Some very good practitioners believe that a mercurial purge at the onset of the attack impresses the subsequent career of the case in some favorable manner. I do not share in this opinion, but I do select calomel as the preliminary purgative in cases where much gastric irritability attends the early periods of the attack. I exhibit it also in those cases in which previous indisposition had occasioned coating of the tongue, or in which other conditions of systemic derangement existed for which calomel is usually prescribed.

In many cases it is desirable to avoid the disgust at taking a purgative or the perturbation it may occasion by its action. Enemas of tepid infusion of linseed or of milk and water may be substituted, with the addition of castor oil when necessary.

In the early hours of the attack warm pediluvia are always grateful and proper. They are to be given by placing a basin of warm water near the foot of the bed, beneath the covering of a light blanket or sheet, and allowing the patient's feet to remain immersed for ten or fifteen minutes. If the feet are cold, mustard should be added. During the foot-bath the patient usually falls into a perspiration which is sometimes profuse and general.

Perspiration is a desirable event during the paroxysm, although it is not, like the sweatings of the malarial fevers, critical, in the sense of being accompanied by a marked decline in temperature. The idea that sweating is beneficial is so strongly and generally prevalent as to give countenance to the erroneous practice of resting the cure of the disease upon its production and maintenance. I have seen valuable lives sacrificed by obstinate persistence in measures to promote diaphoresis, more especially in the later hours of the paroxysm or in the succeeding or calm stage. It is quite sufficient to encourage the perspiration by the pediluvia and by a moderate allowance of cool, palatable drinks. Much value is attached by non-professional persons to a warm infusion of orange-leaves or some other warm and grateful beverage. When agreeable to patients I permit them in moderate amounts, but do not regard them as especially valuable.

Jaborandi has been used in yellow fever. Strong hopes were quite naturally based upon the action of this drug in exciting excretory functions, especially diaphoresis, but the observations of my friend Dr. Thomas Layton and of others show that it possesses no special value, while it frequently increases the vomiting and has to be discontinued.

After the bowels have been relieved of fecal accumulations it is good practice to exhibit a scruple of quinia in solution with ten to thirty [p. 651]drops of tincture of opium, by rectal injection. Infusion of linseed or mucilage of elm-bark or gum-arabic are the best vehicles.

The combined action of the quinia and opium mitigates the patient's headache and lumbar pains. But the influence of these drugs is not limited to their effect on the nerves of sensation. In quite a proportion of cases reaction is not so prompt or complete as usual; or reaction may be quite pronounced, and still the surface may alternate between a dry and a perspiring state. These oscillations of function of the organic nerves are also often corrected by this prescription. In the great majority of simple cases no other medication than this is requisite or proper, for no medication is proper in yellow fever unless it is requisite.

When the neuralgias are excessively violent, opium may be again administered, preferably by enema, and in combination with bromide of potassium or chloral hydrate. But the effects of opium in limiting excretory function must always be borne in mind and carefully avoided.

External applications are very efficacious in relieving the neuralgias. In the southern part of this country the "eau sedative" of Raspail is greatly used. This is a mixture of ammonia, camphor, and common salt in solution, and may be prepared extemporaneously. The applications may be made hot or cold, but if used cold they must be continuously kept up. It is therefore better to use them warm if sufficiently effective. Stimulating embrocations of turpentine or mustard, or dry or wet cups, are sometimes resorted to for relief of pain.

Excessive temperature demands attention and antagonistic treatment in direct measure with its persistence, its degree, and its occurrence in advanced periods of an attack.

In the epidemic of 1867, I used gelsemium as an antipyretic in fifty cases or more, but the results were so unsatisfactory that I have quite abandoned its exhibition. I have given quinia as an antipyretic, but never in doses of more than a scruple. In these doses it has failed to accomplish the desired result in the great majority of the cases. Perhaps its antipyretic effects are limited to those cases in which malaria is a known or an unknown complication.

I have exhibited small doses of digitalis with apparent benefit, but aconite and veratrum viride I have long since discarded. The physician cannot afford to sacrifice gastric quietude and competency of function to the use of remedies whose value as antipyretics is, to say the most, quite doubtful.

Cold has for a long period of time been brought into use as an antipyretic in yellow fever. Its positive value and instantaneous action should be constantly borne in mind, and in the hyperpyrexia of yellow fever it constitutes by far the most reliable remedy, though its mode of application must be carefully adapted to the degree of fever present and to the susceptibilities of the patient. Cold drinks in limited quantities, but frequently repeated; cold spongings of the surface, or the use of the cold pack, especially in very high degrees of body heat; large injections of cold water per rectum, which may be passed off and repeated once in two to four hours,—form safe and effective modes of treatment.

Hemorrhages are a constant source of anxiety in yellow fever. It is very true that persons do not often die from actual loss of blood. I do not know that I have ever witnessed such an event except when the [p. 652]blood was poured out from a recently-emptied uterus. But the chances of recovery are lessened, because the hemorrhagic state indicates a degree of spoliation of both the fluids and solids of the system incompatible with maintenance of life. When this condition of constitution is once established, the stomach rarely escapes, and in a majority of instances it is the first, and sometimes the only, bleeding surface. The treatment should be directed, first, to the great indication of correcting the hemorrhagic diathesis; secondly, to quiet gastric irritability, in order that vomiting shall not cause rupture of capillaries. To meet the first indication I regard nutrition and stimulants as the most important measures of treatment. The mode of administration will be specially referred to under the head of alimentation.

Hæmostatic remedies, given as specific treatment, generally fail in accomplishing the purpose for which they are administered. It has always appeared to me that those therapeutic agents which are capable of controlling hemorrhage where yellow fever is not present are completely neutralized by the effects of its toxic agent upon the vaso-motor nerves. Consequently, while ergot, turpentine, gallic acid, and other like remedies may be resorted to, too much hope should not be entertained as to their good effects.

Some excellent practitioners rely greatly on preparations of iron. The tincture of the chloride is undoubtedly the best. This may be given in water or upon shaved ice in doses of five or ten drops every half hour. To allay the gastric irritability pellets of ice should be swallowed. Effervescing drinks may be given with benefit.

I have often used with good results the following prescription:

℞.
    Sodii Bicarb.   gr. xx;
    Morphiæ Sulph.   gr. ss.
    Aquæ Lauro-Cerasi,
    Aquæ Menth. Pip. aa. fl. drachm iv. M.

S. Teaspoonful after every act of emesis.

Occasionally I have given the following prescription:

℞.
    Creasoti   gtt. viij;
    Tinct. Opii Deodorat. gtt. xl.
    Aquæ Menth. Pip.,
    Muc. Acaciæ aa.   fl. drachm iv. M.

S. Teaspoonful after every act of emesis in iced Seltzer or Apollinaris water, or in champagne.

Sometimes a few drops of chloroform in a spoonful of iced mucilage of acacia act favorably.

In cases which appear utterly hopeless the physician, acting desperately, is sometimes able to save life by treatment which could scarcely be safely recommended. I once administered a fourth of a grain of morphia to a child of seven years, who, after a sleep of ten hours, ceased to throw up black vomit and recovered.

External applications to the epigastrium usually afford some relief to nausea at any stage of yellow fever. Mustard or aromatic cataplasms may at all times be used with hopes of favorable effects. Towels wrung from cold water are very efficacious. Sometimes a drachm or two of chloroform dashed over them increases their anti-emetic action.

Suppression of urine is generally a symptom of fatal import. [p. 653]Attempts may be made to establish the secretion by dry or wet cups in the lumbar region, by warm applications around the loins, or by mustard cataplasms or blisters. If the condition of the patient's stomach is such as to permit this practice, copious diluent drinks and diuretics should be given. Lemonade holding bitartrate of potassium in solution is generally the most acceptable, and probably the most efficient. Some physicians think they oftener obtain good results from small and frequently repeated doses of turpentine. I can bear testimony to the good results which sometimes follow large rectal injections of warm or cold water, the latter being preferable when there is high fever.

In certain cases of yellow fever reaction from the cold stage is feeble and imperfect, or perhaps may not occur at all. This departure from type is very fatal. The patients are stupid, sometimes semi-comatose and incoherent, from the earliest hours of the attack. The face is listless, drunken, or idiotic in expression. The color of the skin is dark olive and almost livid. The print of a hand on the chest is very slowly effaced. Sometimes the surface is covered with a peculiarly unctuous perspiration. The pulse is feeble and compressible; the temperature seldom more than one or two degrees above the normal standard. Albuminous urine is found during the first day. Death, attended by convulsive rigors, generally closes the scene within seventy-two hours from the moment of seizure.

Hot mustard-baths should be resorted to. Blood may be drawn by cups or leeches from the back of the neck or temples, and this may be followed by the application of a blister. Morphia and atropia may be exhibited subcutaneously in small doses, to be repeated as often as proper. Quinia may be administered per rectum or by the hypodermic method.

Lastly, pilocarpine may be thrown into the tissues in sufficient doses to procure its vigorous physiological action.

Almost in precise symptomatic contrast with these cases of failure in reaction is another form of attack, in which violent disturbances of nerve-function occurs; such cases often being characterized as congestive in type. The most typical of these attacks are among children or adolescents. If attended by noticeable chill, it is ordinarily slight. Reaction is quick and excessively violent. The face is flushed, the eyes injected, and convulsions with delirium are liable to occur as early symptoms. I have watched with much interest the alternate flushings and pallor of the countenance occurring in these cases, such as are often observed in basilar meningitis.

The treatment in this type of attacks should include chloroform by inhalation in sufficient amount to control convulsions. Chloral hydrate may be administered by enema, or morphia hypodermically. Cathartic doses of calomel often exert a beneficial effect. Leeches or cups, to be followed by cold applications or by blisters, may be applied about the head or neck. But cupping and leeching should only be resorted to in the treatment of grave symptoms, since obstinate hemorrhage is liable to occur from any and every point from which the cuticle has been removed.

Yellow fever is often masked during the paroxysm by some pre-existing disease. Malarial fevers, the febrile states of pulmonary consumption or of the recently-delivered female, may all mask the early clinical [p. 654]phenomena to such a degree that the most experienced and vigilant practitioners are sometimes astonished to find black vomit, suppression of urine, and all those symptoms which mark the last stages of the disease, suddenly developed.

Walking cases should be classed in the same category as masked forms. In these instances the early symptoms are so slight as to be overlooked or neglected by their subjects. They continue to prosecute their usual pursuits until, by sheer exhaustion, they are driven to beds from which they seldom arise.

The hygienic and dietetic management of yellow-fever patients is extremely important, and the strictest attention must be paid to the condition and discipline of the sick chamber. In this disease those occurrences and circumstances which in other affections would be reckoned as unimportant and trivial become matters of serious magnitude.

The physician, by a composed and cheerful demeanor, often decides which end of the balance shall go down. But an intelligent, experienced, and faithful nurse is equally as important as the excellent physician.

The patient should be confined in strictly recumbent positions, and all drinks and foods must be given through tubes or from pap-cups. It frequently occurs that patients are unable to void the bladder in such positions. In these cases the catheter should be used, rather than suffer any violation of the rule which demands a maintenance of unbroken decubitus.

The sick room should be kept freely ventilated, and the patient's bedding should be changed, when requisite, by removing him to one side of the bed while the other is renovated. If the patient's night-shirt becomes soiled and disagreeable, it may be cut so as to remove it, and another, cut in the same manner, may be substituted and stitched together. The room must be kept quiet, and useless visiting entirely forbidden.

Cool and grateful drinks may be given in any stage or state of yellow fever if demanded by patients. The quantity allowed at one time should be small, since over-distension of the stomach almost certainly causes vomiting. Effervescing drinks are nearly always grateful, and are better tolerated than others. Seltzer-water and lemonade, or Seltzer or Apollinaris on shaved ice, are to be recommended. Sometimes patients call for sparkling wines or beers. I never refuse them or any other alcoholic drink asked for in any stage of the disease. Wine surely possesses valuable therapeutic effects in yellow fever.

Alimentation must be severely controlled by the physician, and the tolerance and effects constantly watched. Even to the most experienced physician the kind of food to be selected, and the time and manner of administration, constitute difficult problems. In simple forms of the disease food had better be strictly withheld during the continuance of the paroxysm. Even after the stage of calm has been reached, sufficient time should be allowed to elapse to enable the physician to form some estimate of the degree of damage his patient has suffered and his competency to retain foods and be nourished by them. This question can seldom be answered in a decided manner, except through a cautious trial of some bland and inoffensive food.

[p. 655]On the third or fourth day of sickness a single tablespoonful of iced milk may be given, and the immediate consequences closely watched. If no retching or gastric uneasiness should ensue, it may be repeated at the end of thirty minutes. Some physicians prefer to begin with spoonful doses of equal parts of sweet milk and thin barley-water. In my own experience chicken-water has proved to be the most universally acceptable, as well as the most beneficial, of all the various forms of nutriment to be chosen as a first venture. I have frequently combined this with barley-water when first given. In this cautious and tentative manner even the most experienced physician prefers to proceed, rather than to attempt to prescribe rules of diet in an abstract and arbitrary manner.

If these light articles of diet are well borne, they are to be gradually and watchfully exchanged for beef-essences, the blood of a rare beefsteak, and the more substantial broths. Solid articles of food should not be allowed during the first ten days after an attack, and for still longer periods patients should be admonished against excesses in eating, and especially in respect to indigestible articles. Those lesions of the blood and of the stomach, and those grave disorders of nerve-function which occasion hæmatemesis in yellow fever, are slowly repaired. Instances are reported in which black vomit and death have followed excessive eating and drinking ten or twenty days after dismissal from treatment.

There are, however, certain conditions which are liable to complicate yellow fever which demand a course of dietetic procedure different from that which I have recommended. Thus, children cannot bear privation of food until the paroxysm is over if its duration is long. In like manner, a more supporting course is required in most of those cases in which yellow fever occurs as an intercurrent affection, in all those cases which are termed typhoid or adynamic per se, and, more emphatically still, in every case in which hemorrhages are occurring. A failing pulse should in all instances admonish us to resort to nourishment and stimulants.

It is a fortunate circumstance that in yellow fever the lower bowel is generally in a state favorable for the retention of nutritious enemas. In the most trying and critical hours of desperate cases I have seen patients tided through by the use of skilfully prepared and skilfully administered injections of some suitable meat-essence. When insomnia exists, chloral hydrate or bromide of potassium may be conveniently given in these vehicles.

It is evident that the discussion of the vastly important sanitary questions pertaining to the prevention of yellow fever cannot be appropriately discussed in the present article.

[p. 656]

DIPHTHERIA.
BY A. JACOBI, M.D.

DEFINITION; SYNONYMS; HISTORY.—Diphtheria is a specific, infectious, and contagious disease, characterized principally by epithelial changes in, and the exudation of fibrin on and into mucous membranes, the surface of wounds, and the rete Malpighii, thereby constituting the so-called pseudo-membrane. Under the names ulcus syriacum, ulcus ægyptiacum, garotillo, morbus suffocans, morbus suffocatorius, affectus suffocatorius, pestilentis gutturis affectio, pedancho maligna, angina maligna, angina passio, mal de gorge gangréneux, ulcère gangréneux, angina polyposa, angine couenneuse, cynanche, croup, diphtheritis, and diphtheria, the disease has been known and described at different periods by the writers of different nations. The Hippocratic writings and some remarks in the

Talmud allow of some doubt in regard to their explanation. Whether their authors observed or recognized diphtheria cannot be proven. There is less doubt in regard to Archigenes, quoted by Oribasius. Aretæus of Cappadocia is notably the first, if we except Asclepiades only, who is said to have performed laryngotomy. The description of the pharyngeal and laryngeal manifestations furnished by the former, however, can leave no doubt in our minds that he knew diphtheria and recognized it. Galen, in his remarks on the Chironian ulcer, tells us that the pseudo-membrane was gotten rid of by coughing when the respiratory passages were affected by the disease, and by hawking when the disease was in the pharynx. Cælius Aurelianus recognized diphtheria of the pharynx and larynx, as well as the diphtheritic paralysis of the soft palate; it is to him we are indebted for the information that Asclepiades resorted to scarification of the tonsils, and even to laryngotomy. Aëtius in the fifth century distinguished white and grayish patches and gangrenous degeneration, observed paralysis of the soft palate, and advised against energetic local treatment and the forcible removal of the deposits before they were in a condition to fall off spontaneously. The Arabs and Arabists contain no allusions to the subject, but early chronicles tell of an epidemic raging in St. Denis in 580, subsequent to a great inundation. There appear to have been memorable epidemics in Rome in 856 and 1005, in Byzantium in 1004. The former are mentioned by Baronius, the latter by Cedrenus.[1]

[1] Haeser, *Lehrb. a. Gesch. du Med. u. d. Epidem. Krankh.*, 3d ed., vol. iii., p. 434.

According to Morejon, Gutierrez wrote his *Tradado del enfermedad del garrotillo* in the second half of the fifteenth century. A malignant form of angina raged in 1517 in Switzerland, along the Rhine, and in the Netherlands; in 1544 and 1545 in Northern Germany and on the Rhine; [p. 657]in 1557 in France, Germany, and Holland; to the latter refer the reports of Tetrus Fosterus. Antonio Soglia, quoted by Chomel, describes an epidemic in Naples and Sicily (1563), which spread in the following year as far as Constantinople; Joannes Wierus, epidemics in Dantzic, Cologne, and Augsburg (1565); Ballonius (Baillon), in Paris (1576). At the same time this disease was frequent in Denmark. From Spain there are reports on severe epidemics between the years 1583 and 1618; the year 1613 was long known as the year of diphtheria (anno de los garrotillos).

Mercado (1608) speaks of a child that had communicated the disease to his father by biting his finger. Casealez advised gargles containing alum and sulphate of copper. Herrera described diphtheria of the skin and of wounds, and looked upon the pseudo-membrane as the essential characteristic of the disease. Heredia, in 1690, recognized the suffocative and asthenic forms, as well as the paralysis of the soft palate, the pharynx, and the limbs; he also called attention to the occurrence of relapses, which he attributed to the absorption of the morbid products, and endeavored to prevent by cauterization.

Naples had diphtheria 1610-45, in its worse form 1618-20, together with erysipelas, and diphtheritic affection amongst cattle. About those times tracheotomy was often performed by Severino, the same who found pseudo-membrane in the larynx at a post-mortem examination made in 1642. In 1620 the disease was in Portugal, Sicily, and Malta; in 1630 in Spain, according to Fontechu, Villa Real, and Herrera. It was remarked that in some instances no membranes were perceived in the throat, but the cases were liable to terminate fatally with large glandular swellings round the neck and general symptoms of adynamia. Sicily was again invaded in 1632, Rome in 1634, Italy from 1642 to 1650, Spain in 1666. The Italian reports emphasize the marked contagiousness of the disease and its tendency to depress the vital powers, also the weakness of the mental faculties left behind. In Germany the disease was described by Wedel in 1718. The epidemics observed by him were not very instructive, yet they sufficed to teach the importance of isolating the sick.

In the New England States diphtheria appeared in the seventeenth century. Samuel Danforth lost the four youngest of his twelve children by the "malady of bladders in the windpipe" within a fortnight in December, 1659, in Roxbury, Mass. John Josselyn mentions an epidemic in New England, mainly in Maine, which lasted at least until the year 1671. Mr. Douglass reports another, which commenced on the 20th of March, 1735, in Kingston township, about fifty miles east of Boston, and extended all over, and also to Boston, where it was mild at first. But in 1738 it was very severe, and remained so for some time. Indeed, it did not abate for a long time, to judge from a letter of Cadwalader Colden written in 1753 to

Dr. Fothergill, and the two letters of Dr. Jacob Ogden, written in 1769 and 1774 to Mr. Hugh Gaine of New York; as also from John Archer's "Inaugural Dissertation on Cynanche Trachealis, commonly called Croup or Hives," published in 1798.[2] In 1809 there was a severe epidemic in Philadelphia;[3] in 1816 in Crete.

[2] For extensive quotations from these and other writers on diphtheria at a very interesting period of our medical literature, see A. Jacobi, *A Treatise on Diphtheria*, New York, 1880.

[3] Caldwell, in ed. of Cullen's *First Lines of the Practice of Physic*, Philadelphia, 1816, 1, p. 260.

[p. 658]The reports of Le Cât concerning epidemics in Rouen in 1736 and 1737 being doubtful, the first great epidemic must be set down, in France, for 1745. It commenced in Paris, and invaded the provinces afterward. Chomel gave an accurate description of the diphtheritic paralysis of the soft palate, and reports a case of strabismus. Epidemics are reported from the Netherlands in 1745, 1746, 1769, 1770, 1778-86; from Spain in 1764-71; from England in 1744-48 (by Starr), from Plymouth, England, in 1751-53 (Thurham) and 1776. Dropsy and glandular swellings were frequent; emetics and pure air were the sheet-anchors of treatment. The Netherlands, France, and the West Indies were invaded from 1770-80 by the disease, which was found often complicated with scarlatina; Portugal in 1786 and 1787; France again in 1787 and 1788; Northern Germany in 1790. At that time, particularly in France, the main reliance was had on the internal administration of cinchona and the insufflation into the throat of alum.

Epidemics have been described since from different localities in different years: in Glasgow, 1812 and 1819; Switzerland, 1823-26; Norway and St. Helena, 1824; New York and Kentucky, 1826 and 1828; French provinces, 1834; Paris, 1841; several parts of Europe and North America, 1845-56; Paris, 1853-55; England, 1854 and 1859, when 95 per cent. of all the cases of nasal diphtheria proved fatal; Netherlands and Sweden, 1855; all Western Europe, 1855-65, up to the present time, and all Europe since; California, 1856 and 1857; Portugal and France, 1856; Eastern Prussia, 1850, 1852, 1856, 1857; and all the countries with a cold or moderate climate to this very day.

During the second half of the eighteenth century but two writers are worthy of especial notice—Home, a Scotchman, 1765, and Samuel Bard, an American, 1771.

Home deserves credit for having distinctly drawn the line between the pseudo-membranous and the gangrenous affections. He also endeavored to prove that croup and angina maligna were two distinct diseases, notwithstanding all that had been said since the time of Aretæus in favor of their identity. The false membrane of croup he looked upon as an aggregation of mucus. He sought for it exclusively in the respiratory tract, and disregarded any connection between it and the false membrane found in the pharynx.

Bard's experience was very extensive; he saw membranous pharyngitis, laryngitis, and pharyngo-laryngitis; he speaks of the membrane as met upon the skin, of paralysis of the muscles of deglutition and of the larynx, and likewise of paralysis of the lower extremities, as sequelæ. He looked upon the morbific process as the same whichever were the mucous membranes attacked, and made a distinction only according to the localization of the disease. The influence which he might have exercised in shaping the professional opinion on the nature of the disease did not make itself felt, partly because of his classical modesty, and partly because of his remoteness from the centres of European learning. Not before 1810 was his book translated into French (by Ruette). While his style is classical in its simplicity, his observation is astonishingly correct, and his conclusions as to the actual identity of all the diphtheritic processes in the most various clinical symptoms unimpeachable this very day. His description of the various forms of pharyngeal diphtheria is painfully [p. 659]good, his observations on cutaneous diphtheria very accurate, his few dissections well recorded, particularly when he speaks of tracheal and tracheo-laryngeal diphtheria, and his historical reviews very judicious indeed. "Upon the whole, I am led to conclude that the morbus strangulatorius of the Italians, the croup of Home, the malignant ulcerous sore throat of Huxham and Fothergill, and the disease I have described and that first described by Douglas of Boston, however they may differ in symptoms, do all bear an essential affinity and relation to each other, or are apt to run into each other, and, in fact, arise from the same leaven. The disease I have described appeared evidently to be of an infectious nature, and, being drawn in by the breath of a healthy child, irritated the glands of the throat and windpipe. The infection did not seem to depend so much on any prevailing disposition of the air as upon effluvia received from the breath of infected persons. This will account why the disorder sometimes went through a whole family, and yet did not affect the next-door neighbors. Here we learn a useful lesson—viz. to remove young children as soon as any one of them is taken with the disease, by which many lives have been saved and may again be preserved."

Jurine, in his prize essay of 1807, denies the gangrenous nature of angina maligna and emphasizes the frequent complication of membranous croup with membranous pharyngitis. It was reserved for Bretonneau to enforce attention to the ideas of Bard by asserting (though he did not mention either his monograph or its French translation of 1810) the identity of angina maligna, or by whatever other title it may be known, with membranous laryngitis, and by inaugurating his theory with a new name for the disease to perpetuate the views expressed therein. First and foremost, he called attention to the continuity of the membrane (according to him, composed of coagulated mucus and fibrin) of the nose, pharynx, and respiratory tract, its identity with certain morbid conditions of the skin, and promulgated the theory that "diphtherite"—the name dates from that time—is a specific disease, an affection sui generis, and differs both from a catarrhal and a scarlatinous inflammation.

The modern history of diphtheria may be dated from June 26, 1821, when Bretonneau read his first essay on that subject before the French Academy of Medicine, and gave to the disease the name it now bears. His second and third (Nov. 25th) papers belong to the same year; his fourth was read in March, 1826; his fifth appeared in the *Archives gén.* of January and September, 1855. It was only in 1826 that the material, previously gathered, was summed up in his celebrated monograph.[4] Before this time, however, the separate essays had received prominence from the reports and commentaries of Guersant, who laid particular stress on the statement that diphtheria was a non-gangrenous affection, identical, and even synchronous, with croup in the majority of epidemics. Since that epoch the literature on the subject has assumed enormous proportions. It is a matter of regret that the limited space allotted to this subject should exclude much historical detail of the etiology, pathology, and therapeutics of diphtheria. If the history of any disease is interesting, and the neglect of its study has ever punished itself, it is diphtheria. [p. 660]Particularly would the treatment have been more successful if the knowledge of former times had been available and more heeded. As long ago as in the seventeenth century depletion in diphtheria was condemned, and in the seventeenth and eighteenth centuries the local treatment with muriatic acid and the internal administration of cinchona, camphor, and roborant diet were held to be the only admissible ones. Bretonneau urged the same principles, and still in our own times, for want of historical knowledge, we had to learn the old lesson over again.[5]

[4] P. Bretonneau, *Des Inflammations spéciales du tissu muqueux, et en particulier de la Diphthérite, etc.*, Paris, 1826.

[5] See history and bibliography of diphtheria in Chatto; Sanné, *Traité de la Diphthérie*, Paris, 1874; Jacobi, in *Gerhardt's Handb. d. Kinderk.*, vol. ii., 1877; Seitz, *Diphtheric und Croup gesch. u. Klin. dargest*, Berlin, 1879; *Index-Catalogue of the Library of the Surgeon-General's Office*, U.S.A., vol. iii., Washington, 1882.

The following is a brief review of the main points of discussion upon subjects connected with the symptomatology and pathology of diphtheria since Bretonneau's first paper:

Bourquoise and Brunet express their belief (1823) in the contagious character of this disease. Desruelles (1824) sees a diagnostic difference between the sporadic and the epidemic forms in the participation of the brain in the latter. Louis referred a number of cases of croup in adults to pharyngeal diphtheria as their source. Mackenzie considers that croup has its origin in the fauces, and urges the employment of lunar caustic. Billard (1826) denies the specific character of diphtheritic inflammation. Hamilton describes cases that terminated in suppuration, and which he therefore distinguishes from Bretonneau's cases. He describes two modes of termination of the disease—one in croup, the other in a state of debility arising from the effect of the absorbed secretion on the respiratory nerves. Pretty looks upon those cases of croup that have their original seat in the tonsils as contagious.

Bland (1827) explains the difference between croup and diphtheria. Deslandes declares them to be identical. Bretonneau publishes a work in which he compares diphtheria with scarlatina anginosa, and recommends the use of alum. Emmangard is the first one of the physiological school who, likening diphtheria to typhoid and claiming its origin in a malarial infection, calls it angina gastro-enterica. Abercrombie is in favor of distinguishing diphtheria from croup, but reports a number of cases of diphtheria of the pharynx that terminated fatally by stenosis of the larynx. Ribes, who encountered the disease in nine members of a single family, asserts that croup rarely occurred without a preceding diphtheria in his experience; he advises an examination of the throats of apparently healthy individuals. Fuchs relates the history of epidemics of angina maligna, and declares croup to be a genuine angina maligna trachealis, which only does not run through all the stages. Broussais opposes the identity of croup and diphtheria (1829), and gives a report of cures by means of antiphlogistic regimen and laryngotomy. Diphtheria and gangrenous angina are synonymous with him. Gendron expresses a belief in the identity of diphtheria and gangrenous angina. Roche considers the membrane rather of hemorrhagic than of inflammatory origin, and consisting of discolored fibrin. About the same time Trousseau is endeavoring to clearly establish the diagnosis between diphtheria and scarlatinous angina. Shortly after (1830), he reports cases of diphtheria which originated in blistering wounds, and of diphtheria of the skin giving rise to throat affections, and [p. 661]diphtheria of the throat followed by skin disease. T. F. Hoffmann cites a severe case, that ultimately recovered, with consecutive paralysis of certain cranial nerves. Cheyne (1833) makes a stand against the "confounding of croup and cynanche maligna under the name of diphtheritis." Bourgeois witnessed an epidemic succeeding mumps.

Fricout and Burley (1836) declare their belief in the contagiousness of the disease. Bouillaud attacks the theory of its specific character on the ground that abstraction of blood produced favorable results. Stokes makes a distinction between primary and secondary croup according to the original seat of the affection (1837). Kessler advocates (1841) the view of its contagious nature, and Rilliet and Barthez adduce evidence of the occurrence of ulceration and gangrene in the course of the disease. Taupin, like Ribes, enjoins a methodical examination of the throat of every patient during the prevalence of an epidemic of diphtheria, whatsoever be the disease from which the child suffers. Boudet (1842) opposes Bretonneau's hypothesis that croup is a descending diphtheria, and holds to the identity of diphtheria and gangrenous angina. In this contest Durand (1843) also takes sides against Bretonneau, and lays particular stress on the point that the diphtheritic patient succumbs rather from the severity of the constitutional symptoms than from suffocation. Rilliet and Barthez, on the other hand, rally to the support of the attacked master, asserting that the usual form of croup and that resulting from a descending diphtheritis are one and the same, while they claim that diphtheritis and gangrenous angina are distinct affections.

Meanwhile, the strife regarding the nature of the disease continued. Guersant and Blache (1844) describe the stomatite couenneuse (noma, stomacace, according to them, the rarest kind of gangrenous angina) as a form of Bretonneau's diphtheritis, and Landsberg raises the question whether a nerve-inflammation, present in a certain case, was to be looked upon as an accidental or an essential feature of the disease, and finally comes to the conclusion, with Schönlein, that it was a neurophlogosis dependent on the disease. Bouisson (1847) reports a case of diphtheritic conjunctivitis resulting in loss of the eye. Robert publishes his observations on diphtheria of the skin and of wounds, which he attributes to an atmospheric contamination in crowded wards of hospitals, and looks upon it, with Delpech and Eisenmann, as a form of hospital gangrene. Virchow, in the same year, distinguished the catarrhal, croupous, and diphtheritic varieties of the disease. Meanwhile, reports of paralysis of the soft palate after diphtheria came from Morisseau, from Trousseau and Lasegue, and lastly (1854-59) from Maingault. The subject of diphtheritic conjunctivitis was studied by A. v. Graefe (1854), who encountered the disease as a complication of diphtheria of the pharynx, nose, and skin, and hence considered it a part of the general disease rather than an independent local affection. Diphtheria, in its effects on the system, had at the same time been investigated by Trousseau, who sums up with the statement that the principal source of danger lies in the invasion of the larynx, and that the large majority of cases of croup began as a diphtheria of the pharynx, but that, even without the occurrence of a laryngeal localization, many cases terminate fatally owing to adynamia.

Outside of France, too, the subject had attracted attention. West, who had never seen the disease occur primarily, describes diphtheria as a [p. 662]complication of measles. Bamberger (1855) divides the inflammations of the mouth and pharynx into the catarrhal and croupous forms, and considers croup and diphtheria to be subdivisions of the latter form, differing only in degree. The paralysis of the muscles of deglutition is discussed by Dehænne (1857) who had contracted the disease, and the paralysis of other muscles by Faure. A case of diphtheria of the tonsils, nipples, and vagina in a woman recently confined, followed by infection of the new-born and the death of both, is reported by Mathieux; and cases of diphtheritic conjunctivitis by Grichard, Warlomont, and Testelin. The same year Isambert published a work in which he divided the diphtheritic affections into three forms— viz. angine couenneuse, scarlatinous angina, and diphtheritic angina. The last-mentioned is further subdivided into a croupous-diphtheritic angina, in which croup of the larynx plays an important part, and into that form in which death results from adynamia; in the latter form there is a marked swelling of the lymphatic glands. Apparently, at this time the epidemic in Paris underwent a considerable change, for the croupous form does not occur by far so frequently as Bretonneau had asserted, and croup of the larynx without a preceding diphtheria of the pharynx was observed more frequently than he would lead us to believe.

The various changes in the symptoms of the epidemics of diphtheria which were observed in different places and countries, and at different times, explain many of the differences of opinions in regard to the nature of the disease. The literature of that subject is in the last twenty-five years simply stupendous, and a few more notes must suffice for the elucidation of the drift of theories and observations. Beale was the first to look for organic beings as the cause of the disease, without finding any. Laycock sees it in the bacilli and spores of oidium albicans; Wilks, however, found the same parasite in other affections. Cammack declares the diphtheritic membrane to be herpetic. Feron also calls Bretonneau's mild form of the disease a herpetic angina with pseudo-membrane; so does Gubler. Bouchut writes against the identity of diphtheria, croup, and gangrene. Condie describes the disease as occurring with scarlatina. Litchfield claims that it is a concealed scarlatina, and Hillier that it has some connection with it. Millard cites one case in the course of which gangrene occurred, and another in which skin, mouth, pharynx, respiratory passages, oesophagus, and vulva were affected at the same time. Harley vainly endeavored to inoculate the disease in animals. Stephens declares the disease to be infectious. Sanderson looks upon it as identical with the angina maligna of the aged. Farr considered the exhalations from sewers an important etiological factor. Sellerier, Kingsford, and Harley (1859) report paralyses as sequelæ. Maugin speaks of a specific eruption; Ward, of an accompanying purpura. Bouchut and Empis remarked the frequent presence of and danger from albuminuria; so did Wade. Maugin calls attention to the fact that, when present in diphtheria, it occurs early, whereas in scarlatina it is seen during the period of desquamation, and is not of frequent occurrence even then. Gull gives an account of cases in which death resulted from asthenia, and speaks of a nerve-lesion which he attributes to the severity of the local inflammation. Hildige describes diphtheritic conjunctivitis as seen in Graefe's practice, and looks upon it as contagious. Magne denies its contagious or [p. 663]infectious character. Mackenzie, while probably having seen false membrane appear on the conjunctiva when in a state of inflammation, yet refuses to recognize diphtheritic conjunctivitis as a distinct disease.

In the same degree that observations of cases and epidemics increased in number, the nature of the disease and its cause commenced to be studied. The assumption that the latter was a chemical poison was soon doubted, and the parasitic nature of diphtheria considered by many as proven.

After Henle had (1840) expressed his belief in the existence of a contagium animatum, and morbid processes had for some time been compared with the phenomena of fermentation, Schwann demonstrated the presence of lower organisms in fermentation and putrefaction. The discovery of the cause of the silk-worm disease by Bassis, of the achorion by Schönlein, of the acarus by Simon, of bacteria in malignant pustule by Pollender, Brauell, and, above all, by Davaine, in relapsing fever by Obermeier, the teachings of Pasteur concerning the conditions under which putrefaction occurs,—all tended to explain the various infectious and contagious diseases by analogy also, and to stimulate the search for a vegetable organism in diphtheria. Buhl was the first to discover schizomycetæ in diphtheritic membrane, but expressed no opinion as to the part they played in the process. Hüter found them in the gray diphtheritic covering of wounds, in the surrounding apparently healthy tissues, and in the blood. Hüter and Tomasi found them in the diphtheritic membranes of the pharynx and larynx, inoculated them on the mucous membranes of animals, and described them as small, round or oval, dark-colored, active little bodies. The latter observers look upon these organisms as a part of the infectious element. Oertel found them in diphtheritic membrane and in inflamed mucous membranes in the lymphatic vessels, lymphatic glands, kidneys, and other organs; he considers them as the contagious element of diphtheria. Nassiloff, too, after inoculations in the cornea resulted in an enormous multiplication of the microscopic organisms and their appearance with pus-cells in the lacteals and in the lymphatics of the palate, and even in the bones and cartilages, asserts that the development of organisms is the primary step in the diphtheritic process. Eberth made successful inoculations in living tissues; the micro-organisms, introduced into the cornea, proliferated actively and caused an inflammation of irritative character in the surrounding tissue. He asserts, with the positiveness of an evangelist, that diphtheria cannot occur without bacteria. Klebs inoculated the micrococci in pigeons and dogs, and found them in the blood of the animals after death. Orth found them in the pleura, lungs, kidneys, and urinary bladder. But what their action is, whether they are directly pernicious, or deprive the body of certain elements (as of oxygen in malignant pustule, according to Bollinger), or injure mechanically by acting on the coats of the blood-vessels (either directly or by means of altering the blood), thus depriving whole territories of their blood-vessels, is a question upon which the principal advocates of the parasitic theory have not yet agreed. Even Oertel acknowledges the impossibility of explaining the manner in which bacteria act (Ziemssen, *Handbuch*, ii., 1, p. 581, 2d ed.). This much is positive, at any rate: that no one has yet proven that the vegetable organisms alone, and not other, free or fixed, parts of the [p. 664]diphtheritic membrane, are the vehicles of the infecting elements (Steudener); and even now the question has not been decided whether the bacteria met with in diphtheria constitute the cause of the disease, or are a part of the process, or co-effects of the poisonous action—whether they are the carriers of the poison or entirely indifferent entities.

The most important observations made by those who deny a direct etiological connection between micro-organisms and septic diseases in general, and diphtheria in particular, are those of Hiller and Billroth. The latter has proven the morphological identity of the various kinds of bacteria, although it cannot be denied that the apparent similarity may mask a yet unknown difference. Hiller calls attention to the fact that large numbers of micrococci have been found in the cadaver where death has not been the result of septic disease, and also that septic infection is not always severest where the bacteria most abound, but where an extensive chemical decomposition or a mass of putrefying tissue is found. This would indicate that the septic process is rather dependent on chemical decomposition than on the presence of bacteria.

Panum, Bergmann, and Schmiedeberg have isolated poisons that contained no bacteria. Rawitsch and many others prove that septic infection is not dependent on the existence of bacteria. Davaine has shown that an infinitely small amount of a chemical poison, free from bacteria, can kill quickly.

The presence of cocco-bacteria (Billroth) in the blood during life has not once been proven, not even in pyæmia or septicæmia. Yet their being swept into the lungs with the atmospheric air is indisputable. It would therefore seem as though living blood had a greater tendency to destroy bacteria than to allow itself to be decomposed by them. Not only, however, would it seem so, but P. Grawitz (*Virch. Arch.*, vol. lxx., p. 546) proves that sporules do not grow in the (tissue and) blood, but that they are in part dissolved, in part eliminated through the kidneys, and that this result is accomplished through the combination of the following four factors—viz. the elasticity of the blood, its constant motion, the absence of oxygen in sufficient quantity in the circulating blood, and the presence of living animal cells. All of these factors appear to be of great importance. Thus it is that, where the constant motion of the blood and the animal living cells are not present (as in the anterior chamber of the eye or in the humor vitreous) a rapid proliferation and accumulation of bacteria can take place. They are also known to increase rapidly and emigrate into the liver when deposited in the abdominal cavity.

The destruction of bacteria in the circulating blood, into which they may have penetrated, accounts for some microscopical facts in connection with (actually or apparently morbid) blood. Their remnants are probably the pale and dark particles which are discovered in the blood alongside the red and white blood-corpuscles. They could not be identified as micrococci, while in the tissue they are more recognizable. In autopsies they have been found in the urinary tubules, pressing forward and piercing the walls, not occupying a nidus of inflammation, however, and probably are even here a post-mortem phenomenon. A direct necrosis or inflammation by the inoculation of diphtheritic elements can only be produced in the cornea, as was shown by Recklinghausen, and particularly Eberth. Besides, there is nothing characteristic in the cocco-bacteria of[p. 665]diphtheria, with the exception, perhaps, of their browner color, to justify their being looked upon as a distinct variety, certainly not as another species. It is more likely that a difference of action is not so much to be sought for in a different parasite as in the peculiarity of the corneal tissue. When fluid containing cocco-bacteria was injected into the eye of a rabbit, in twenty-four hours the eye was destroyed. If injected into the eye of a dog or guinea-pig, only a slight inflammation resulted (Billroth and Ehrlich). If these experiments were continued on a larger scale, we might eventually, by analogy, infer, and even prove, that the immunity against certain diseases enjoyed by some animals is owing to peculiarities in the very structure of their own tissues. In a similar manner I shall prove hereafter that even peculiarities and variations in the tissue and epithelium of the human body give rise to different shades and variable clinical symptoms in the diphtheritic processes.

The views of Curtis, Satterthwaite, and Charlton Bastian fully agree with those of the above observers. The latter is rather inclined to look upon bacteria as an effect of the disease than as a cause. Similar views were expressed by Burdon Sanderson.

Nor are the researches of Weissgerber and Terls, Lukomsky, Weigert, Lücke, any more conclusive; and, finally, Fürbringer, in his most recent and careful studies of diphtheritic nephritis, insists upon this, that it is not caused by immigration of fungi into the kidneys, that the very best methods employed for the finding of parasites result in the absence of micrococci from the inflamed organ, and that the renal inflammation following diphtheria is the result of a chemical process.

H. C. Wood and Henry F. Formad, in Supplement 7 of the *National Board of Health Bulletin* (1880), declare it altogether improbable that bacteria have any direct function in diphtheria—*i.e.* that they enter the system as bacteria and develop as such in the system, and cause the symptoms. It is, however, possible that they may act upon the exudations of the trachea as the yeast-plant acts upon sugar, and cause the production of a septic poison which differs from that of ordinary putrefaction, and bears such relations to the system as to, when absorbed, cause the systemic symptoms of diphtheria. Now, these bacteria may be always in the air, but not in sufficient quantities to cause tracheitis, but enough when lodged in the membrane to set up the peculiar fermentation; whilst during an epidemic they may be sufficiently numerous to incite an inflammation in a previously healthy throat.

The same authors publish a number of other experiments and conclusions in Suppl. 17 (Jan., 1882): "There is no proof as yet that the micrococci are the cause of the disease. Their presence in the exposed dead tissue is no evidence, for the membrane represents but the necrotic mucous lining.... Indeed, when the healthy mucous membrane of the mouth or trachea is destroyed by caustics—for instance, ammonia—the eschar into which it is converted—really a pseudo-membrane—contains the same micrococci as are found in true diphtheria, as Wood and Formad have learned. Moreover, in the scrapings of the healthy tongue the same micrococci can be seen. Of more significance is the detection of the same or similar micrococci in the blood of the living patients during severe attacks. But since these parasites were found only in the more severe cases, and not in all instances of the disease, were seen also [p. 666]in the blood of other septic disorders, and since no cultures have been made with the fresh blood, there is not yet enough evidence for any decision. In the internal organs bacteria are not found with any regularity in diphtheria."[6]

[6] H. Gradle, *Bacteria and the Germ Theory of Disease*, Chicago, 1883, p. 186.

O. Heubner, while studying both the local affection and the general infection of diphtheria, availed himself of the methods of Cohnheim and Litten, who produced diphtheritic deposits by cutting off the circulation of the blood. He ligated the neck of the bladder in rabbits for two hours. On the first day he noticed a hemorrhagic oedema of the mucous membrane, with loosened and tumefied epithelium; on the second a firm and coagulated exudation took the place of the normal tissue; on the third there were genuine diphtheritic spots in the mucous membrane. The newly-formed pseudo-membrane exhibited all the morphological elements of human diphtheria (genuine or scarlatinous) and epidemic dysentery.[7] Thus Heubner's results agree with the definition of diphtheria as the compound of severe inflammation and necrosis. The inoculation of his diphtheritic artefacts he found sterile. Animals, however, which were inoculated with diphtheritic masses taken from the diseased human patient fell sick with tumor of the spleen, hemorrhages, and general sepsis, besides a local diphtheritic affection. Scarlatinal diphtheria used for the same purpose had the same effect. Bacilli were developed, but they were not found in the blood-vessels (differing in that respect from the bacilli of anthrax), in spite of continued examination. Thus, Heubner refuses to accept the bacilli as the diphtheritic poison; they are, in his opinion, the result of the morbid process, and not its cause. Thus, though he believes the diphtheria poison to be organic, he concludes that its nature is not yet explained; contrary to the assertions of many prolific prophets of the bacteria literature, who now and then claim for this year's microscopic revelations the same infallibility which was claimed for last year's opposite views.[8]

[7] *Die Experimentelle Diphtherie*, Leipzig, 1883.

[8] L. Letzerich recognized in former years the specific parasites of diphtheria, whooping cough, and typhoid fever as if they were labelled. Then, again (*Arch. f. Experim. Pathol. u. Pharmacol.*), he admitted the great difficulty in discriminating the specific schizomycetæ of diphtheria, croupous pneumonia, epidemic influenza, and typhoid fever.

E. Rindfleisch[9] expresses himself as follows: "The microphytes of diphtheria, septicæmia, and pyæmia have not been isolated and cultivated as yet. But experimenters are convinced that there are a great many species of microphytes underlying genuine putrefaction. In producing septicæmic conditions in animals their efficacy differs. Not every animal is influenced by the same microphyte. Thus it becomes probable that the human organism is endangered by a certain number of the putrefaction microphytes. Some one may have a particular predilection for granulating wounds and mucous membranes, and thereby produce a diphtheritic inflammation. Another may enter the blood from a recent wound and give rise to a septicæmic fever with rapidly fatal termination. The third may invade the body by means of a phlegmonous inflammation, purulent infiltration, thrombosis, embolism, and metastatic abscesses, accompanied with a pyæmic fever of a remittent type."

[9] *Die Elemente der Pathologie*, Leipzig, 1883, p. 301.

After all, it does not appear to me that the bacteria question has come [p. 667]any nearer its solution in the last few years, in spite of the most eager researches and the fact that some of the best medical names in the world of medicine take the parasitic nature of diphtheria for granted. For instance, in the second Congress for Internal Medicine (Wiesbaden, 1883) C. Gerhardt rises in its favor. He makes the statement, or rather admits, that several parasites have been found by different men, that every one considers his the genuine one, that several writers assume that there are several diphtheria parasites, and suggests that, in his opinion, the disease may be produced by different varieties of bacteria. At the same time, he contends that the essence of the disease consists in the erosion (and change) of the epithelium and the emigration of leucocytes. If that be the case, I understand less than ever why diphtheria is, or is to be called, a parasitic disease.

Panum's words seem still to be the soundest expression of all our knowledge on the subject when he says: "It is a matter of rejoicing that physicians have come to the conclusion that certain microscopic organisms, be they considered vegetable or animal, and designated as bacteria, fungi, monads, micrococci, or vibriones, do not exist merely in the minds of theorists as causes of disease, but are in reality enemies that must be combated with all the known efficient weapons in our possession. But, while thus rejoicing, it must be borne in mind that we have but a feeble insight into the relation between these organisms and diseases, and in order to effect that much-desired advance in scientific knowledge—a matter of considerable importance in the practice of medicine—it is necessary not only to grasp at isolated data, but carefully and deliberately to observe and study all the facts before us, and even to devote some attention to those which would tend to prove that there are bacteria and fungi which, under certain circumstances, are perfectly harmless, and that even some of the malignant ones among them do not commit all those outrages with which they are charged, directly and personally."

SYMPTOMS.—In the majority of cases the disease has a prodromal stage, which usually lasts a day or two, and may run a similar course to that of a catarrhal pharyngitis. The patient feels somewhat indisposed, has slight fever, is dejected, complains of painful deglutition, more marked when swallowing fluids than solids or semi-solids, has headache and occasionally vomiting. The occurrence of the latter, however, is very much less frequent than in the outbreak of scarlatina. In very severe cases convulsions have been observed, chills very rarely; elevations of temperature of from 102.5° to 104° F. are frequent; higher ones, from 105° to 107°, rare. At this time it is often difficult or impossible to distinguish a catarrhal angina from a diphtheritic by the subjective symptoms. Slight glandular swellings under the jaw may occur in either. The characteristic objective symptom of the latter disease is the presence of membrane on the reddened mucous membrane of the fauces, which, usually, is markedly injected over all or part of the surface. The arches of the palate and the tonsils, less frequently the posterior wall of the pharynx, are so affected. A distinctly localized redness cannot be but either traumatic or diphtheritic. Larger or smaller deposits are found thereon, lying loose on the surface or deeply imbedded according to the locality. At times the first examination reveals their presence in large numbers; at other times but a single one can be [p. 668]detected, which is soon followed by others, however. Within a certain period of time, as a rule twenty to twenty-four hours, the single deposits coalesce and form a membrane of greater or less extent. Mostly in the same proportion to its increase in size it increases in thickness. On the uvula, soft palate, and the posterior wall of the pharynx the membrane is located superficially, and at times can be easily removed; on the tonsils it has a firmer hold, and is usually amalgamated with their uppermost tissues. On the other hand, there are cases in which no actual membranous formation is observed; in such cases the tissues are more or less swollen, the surrounding portions more or less reddened, and the grayish-white discoloration is the result of an infiltration of the tissues themselves, and cannot be removed.

There are still other cases in which deposits of membrane and tissue infiltration are found at the same time, and where both history and evidence indicate that these two phenomena are the result of one and the same process. When the uvula takes part in the process the swelling is, as a rule, more marked than when the remaining parts of the fauces only are implicated. Its circumference is very considerable, and amounts sometimes to the treble or quadruple of the normal, in consequence of the oedematous condition of the entire tissue.

We have to deal, then, with three different manifestations of the diphtheritic process: first, with a membrane lying on the mucous membrane, and removable without causing much injury to the epithelium or any to the basement membrane; such membranes were given by some the name of croupous deposits; secondly, with a membrane implicating the epithelium and upper layers of the mucous membrane; to this the title of diphtheritic membrane has been given by preference; thirdly, with a whitish or grayish infiltration of the surface and the deeper tissue, which, if abundant, may give rise to a necrotic destruction of the tissue.

The severity of the disease does not always depend on the predominance of one of these three forms, for any of them may accompany a mild or a severe attack. By a severe attack we understand one attended with chills, temperatures as high as 105° and 107° F., and marked nervous symptoms, such as vomiting and convulsions. It is characteristic of such cases that when the membrane is accidentally or forcibly removed it is speedily reproduced;

the lymphatic system, in addition, takes an active part in the process. The neighboring glands become swollen; the periglandular tissue does likewise, so that the circumference of the neck becomes enormous, and the space between the lower jaw and the clavicle appears one immense tumefaction. These are the cases in which, as a rule, loss of strength and general debility speedily ensue, and death occurs from exhaustion. The membrane in cases of this description frequently undergoes changes in appearance; under the influence of the atmosphere and of foreign substances, and by admixture of blood, its color becomes yellowish or brownish. The odor of the membrane and surrounding parts becomes sweetish and musty, and occasionally so fetid that it contaminates the atmosphere of the room, and the air in its transit through the nose and over the pharynx becomes by inhalation dangerous to the patient. His throat becomes more swollen, his respiration loud; he keeps his mouth open constantly, has an indifferent expression; the saliva dribbles continually, the color of the skin is sallow and livid, the [p. 669]appetite very poor, and pulse both frequent and small. When the symptoms are of long duration, and a deep infiltration of the affected parts occurs, hemorrhages not infrequently make their appearance. These may be slight although frequent; occasionally, however, larger blood-vessels are encroached upon in the process of destruction, and dangerous, nay even fatal, hemorrhages may be the result. The septic forms which I have here described are more dangerous than the mild ones previously mentioned. Still, even in the latter bad results may ensue from a direct absorption into the blood of putrid substances and by the penetration of fetid gases to the lungs.

Occasionally, where the infiltration has been extensive, we meet with a condition that can only be considered as gangrene. In such cases we see collections of a grayish pulpy mass, which on falling off leaves a considerable loss of tissue, the further course of the disease being either favorable, or dangerous through absorption of septic material, or accompanied by local hemorrhages. When, after a time, health is completely restored, marked cicatrices are left behind. Such loss of tissue is generally seen in the tonsils only, but it may also be encountered in the soft palate. Its cicatrices on the soft palate are always a source of inconvenience, partly in swallowing, partly in speaking. Actual local perforation of the soft palate I have seen but five times in twenty-five years, sloughing without perforation very often.

The diphtheritic membrane not infrequently spreads from the pharynx to the neighboring organs. From the posterior aspect of the soft palate or pharynx the disease gradually ascends to the nasal cavities; this is particularly apt to occur when the uvula is the seat of extensive deposits, and by forced inspiration and deglutition its posterior surface becomes affected. In such cases the membrane which extends thence to the nasal cavities is very dense, and capable of narrowing the capacity of the nasal cavities anteriorly, and occasionally even to close them entirely; as a rule, however, several days elapse before the membrane assumes such a condition. Usually, when this form of nasal diphtheria is in its incipient stage, it is impossible to diagnosticate it; the most important sign thereof, besides a more nasal articulation and sometimes greater difficulty in deglutition, and the result of close ocular examination while the uvula is turned sideways or drawn forward, is a swelling of the deep facial glands at the angle of the lower jaw; when these swell rapidly it can be asserted positively that the nasal cavities have been invaded. There is little or no discharge from the nostrils under these circumstances.

The picture is a very different one, however, when the nose becomes primarily affected. This usually occurs only where an acute catarrh with but little secretion, not so often where a chronic catarrh, has preceded infection. When the secretion is thin and serous, the diphtheritic infection renders it no thicker, but makes it slightly flocculent, and it may become very profuse. This form is frequently attended with a disagreeable odor, equally unpleasant to the patient and to those around him. During the prevalence of an epidemic one must always be prepared to see an acute nasal catarrh or an influenza, or even a chronic nasal catarrh, become complicated with diphtheria or pass into it. Schuller reports the case of a five-weeks-old male child who, having had a nasal catarrh since birth, became affected with diphtheria of the nose. The glandular [p. 670]swelling of which I spoke above is a very important diagnostic, and likewise a decidedly unpleasant symptom, which becomes very marked inside of twenty-four hours; frequently a partial swelling remains long after the disappearance of the diphtheritic membrane. Such glands rarely suppurate or undergo a necrotic degeneration; sometimes they become permanently indurated. This induration and a chronic pharyngeal and nasal catarrh are very serious matters in many instances. Both of these conditions are starting-points for a number of acute or subacute attacks of diphtheria in the same person. It is they which constitute the liability of persons once affected to be taken sick again. Not only are they liable to be affected themselves, but they are a constant danger to all around them. Diphtheria, in a large family of children living in one of the best houses of the city, after having returned half a dozen times in the course of a year, disappeared instantaneously, not to return, when a seamstress living in an infected neighborhood and suffering from occasional sore throats was relieved of her daily work in the house. Oedematous swelling of the mucous membrane and submucous tissue is often observed for a long period to come; elongated uvulæ, enlarged tonsils, often date back to such an acute attack. Thus it is with the upper portion of the larynx about the posterior insertion of the vocal cords (see below); its large amount of loose submucous tissue is liable to swell considerably in acute attacks. Frequent spells of croupy cough and a certain degree of dyspnoea are often observed for years afterward. Though the cases of genuine cicatrization between the arytenoid cartilages, as described by Michael,[10] be rare, with their result of permanent paresis of the thyroarytenoid interni muscles, when they do occur they are either obstinate or altogether incurable.

[10] *Deutsch. Arch. f. klin. Med.*, 1879, xxiv. p. 618.

Diphtheritic conjunctivitis occurs either primarily or as a complication of pharyngeal or nasal diphtheria. Fortunately, it is not of frequent occurrence; the cornea may become destroyed either by pressure through the considerable swelling of the eyelid or by diphtheritic keratitis. Usually the upper eyelid is the first to suffer; it is red, rigid, swollen. In the beginning the conjunctiva palpebræ is smooth, dry and pale, while that of the eye is chemosed; afterward diphtheritic deposits take place either in floccules or in solid masses. Knapp distinguishes between croup and diphtheria of the eyelid according to the facility or impossibility of removing the deposit. In favorable cases the membranes begin to macerate and the eyelids to soften after a few days. In those less favorable perforation of the cornea, prolapse of the iris, or total destruction of the eye take place.

The ear is but rarely the primary seat of diphtheria. A girl of three years died of laryngeal diphtheria on Sept. 6, 1882, after an illness of four days. A girl of seven years was removed from the house on Sept. 6th and returned on Sept. 8th. On the afternoon of the 10th an earring taken from the corpse was attached to the left ear of the sister, after having been washed with soap and water only. About noon on the 11th the lobe of the left ear reddened, on the 12th it exhibited a membrane and became swollen, and some glands enlarged in the neighborhood. On the right mastoid process the skin was not quite healthy, a vesicatory having been applied three weeks previously. This surface became [p. 671]diphtheritic on the 12th, without consecutive glandular swelling. On the 13th the membranes grew thicker; on the 14th the pharynx was also affected, and the physician called in.

Most diphtheritic affections of the ear, however, are secondary. In pharyngeal and nasal diphtheria the narrow orifice of the Eustachian tube is easily obstructed by either catarrhal swelling or diphtheritic deposit. The disease may invade the middle ear and the drum membrane with perforation, caries, and deafness following.

The descent of the diphtheritic process into the respiratory organs may give rise to various conditions. The membrane is not always found to pass uninterruptedly from the mucous membrane of the fauces into the larynx; not infrequently isolated diphtheritic spots are found in the pouches on either side of the attached extremity of the epiglottis, or on the epiglottis, or in the larynx. At such times the epiglottis is moderately swollen, its margins hard and reddened. Occasionally the redness is interrupted by small diphtheritic deposits, which may remain isolated for a considerable time, but generally coalesce so as to coat the edges of the epiglottis with a continuous membrane. As a rule, the upper surface of the epiglottis is not completely covered by membrane, while only now and then diphtheritic deposits are found on its under surface.

The subjective symptoms accompanying the affection of the epiglottis are not always in direct proportion to the extent of the membranes. Dyspnoea and hoarseness occasionally occur where the only abnormal condition is a marked oedema at the entrance of the larynx, particularly of the posterior wall near the arytenoid cartilages and the attachment of the vocal cords. The oedematous condition causes a functional paralysis of the vocal cords, together with marked dyspnoea on inspiration. The difficulty of breathing may become so excessive that the clinical diagnosis of croup is unquestionable, and tracheotomy resorted to, while expiration is comparatively free and the voice not markedly affected. Furthermore, cases occur in which there is no marked oedema, but merely a general catarrh of the epiglottis and larynx; here, too, the subjective symptoms of hoarseness and dyspnoea may become severe and necessitate the performance of tracheotomy. Still, bearing this in mind, I have on several occasions refrained from performing this operation where I judged that, aside from the diphtheria of the pharynx, I had to deal with a moderate oedema of the glottis or a laryngeal catarrh.

Frequently, however, membranes form in the larynx in the same way as in the pharynx or nose; then inspiration and expiration are equally interfered with, and hoarseness is a more constant symptom than in the above-mentioned cases. Fever and pain are not necessarily prominent symptoms; in fact, they are frequently unimportant, but in proportion as the degree of narrowing of the larynx increases the respiration becomes more difficult, long-drawn, and loud.

It may happen that the trachea and bronchi may become affected, although diphtheria of the fauces does not exist. This does not occur as rarely as Henoch and Oertel seem to believe. They think that diphtheritic tracheo-bronchitis is mistaken for the primary condition, because the throat is not examined early enough.

Oertel is of the opinion that the membrane in the fauces is [p. 672]overlooked in such cases. Steiner,[11] too, asserts that "the tendency of the times is to question, nay, rather to deny, the existence of croup extending from below upward." Now, on the contrary, repeated experience enables me to assert with positiveness that diphtheritic tracheo-bronchitis may occur without an affection of the pharynx at the same time. I do not deny that it may last for days without giving rise to dangerous symptoms. I know it does. But when the process reaches the larynx, the symptoms of suffocation become so urgent that tracheotomy may be absolutely required at once, and, in spite of the operation, death soon after occurs.

[11] *Ziemssen's Handb.*, iv., 1, 126.

Of course these cases are exceptions; as a rule, laryngeal and tracheal diphtheria result from a descent of the disease from the fauces. More or less uncomplicated cases of primary laryngeal diphtheria, or so-called sporadic membranous croup, were, however, observed before the end of the sixth decade of this century. They were then almost the only cases of diphtheria, and linked former epidemics and the present one together.

Inflammatory affections of the lungs may occur at various times and in various forms during an attack of diphtheria. That which appears after tracheotomy is usually a broncho-pneumonia, and results from rarefaction of the air in the respiratory passages during the period of impeded respiration, with consequent collapse of pulmonary tissue and dilatation of the blood-vessels, and hence a disturbance of the circulation. It may not fully develop until after tracheotomy, and is a frequent cause of death on the second or third day after the operation. Now and then a case of lobular pneumonia will result from the aspiration of pieces of membranes into the smallest bronchi. It can be easily recognized when the trachea is opened, but previous to the operation the auscultatory signs are of little or no value, being masked by the laryngeal râles. Percussion is equally useless, for a dulness may just as well indicate collapse of the lung as infiltration. The second form of pneumonia associated with diphtheria is from the beginning fibrinous in character. Here, too, auscultation and percussion are of little assistance in establishing a diagnosis when there is a laryngeal diphtheria at the same time, for the above reasons. Where, however, the dulness on percussion is accompanied by high fever, and the long-drawn inspiration is replaced by rapid respiratory movements, the diagnosis of pneumonic complication is justified.

Diphtheria of the mouth, as a primary affection, is not of very frequent occurrence; not rarely, however, is it associated with diphtheria of the fauces and nose, mainly when they have assumed a septic or gangrenous character; it appears on cheeks, tongue, angles of the mouth and gums, and, after the fetid discharges have excoriated the skin, on the lips also. In all of these localities it appears less in the form of an extensive, thick membrane than an infiltration of the tissues. It is most apt to occur where, from the start, the mucous membrane of the mouth was eroded or ulcerated. The ulcerated base of a follicular stomatitis is very frequently the starting-point of a general diphtheria of the mouth. It is always a disagreeable symptom, points to a long duration of the whole process, and threatens septic absorption.

The oesophagus and the cardiac portion of the stomach are the seat[p. 673]sometimes of very massive and extensive, mostly fibrinous exudations, in typhoid fever, dysentery, cholera, measles, and scarlatina, or after injuries following contact with mineral acids, alkalies, corrosive sublimate, or antimony. When the normal tissue was not injured I never saw any that were not superjacent and could not easily be peeled off (croupous). In cases of extensive pharyngeal and laryngeal diphtheria the upper part of the oesophagus is often covered to a distance of half an inch or an inch with membrane, the lower part of which is thinning out into a mere film. A case of local diphtheritic deposit near the cardiac portions of the oesophagus, upon the seat of a stricture, I have described in my *Treatise*, p. 83. Actual diphtheria of the stomach is rare. So is that of the intestine, which is much more liable to be affected in animals than in man. In the cow intestinal diphtheria is frequent (Bollinger). In the gall-bladder, resulting from the irritation produced by calculus, it was seen by Weisserfels. The diphtheritic form of inflammation of the human colon and rectum—dysentery—is frequent enough, but will be the subject of discussion in another place. But, besides this, in the lower portion of the small intestines and in the colon long, tough, coherent membranes are sometimes found in the male and female (not in the hysterical female only). As a rule they are not diphtheritic, but consist mostly of nothing but mucus hardened and flattened down by protracted compression. The few cases of intestinal diphtheria I have met with gave rise to the usual symptoms of enteritis, and were diagnosticated as such.

Wounds of all kinds are easily and rapidly infected by diphtheria; for instance, vaginal abrasions and erosions of the external ear, tongue, and corners of the mouth. Scarification or removal of part of the tonsils is followed in half a day or a day by a deposit of diphtheritic membrane on the wound. The wound caused by tracheotomy becomes liable to be infected with diphtheria within twenty-four hours. Leech-bites, skin denuded by vesicatories, removal of the cuticle by scratching during cutaneous eruptions, all furnish a resting-place for diphtheria in a short time. What Billroth has described under the name of muco-salivary diphtheritis, as it occurs after the extirpation of a large portion of the tongue and resection of the lower jaw, belongs to this class.

At times immediately at the beginning of an invasion of diphtheria, at other times only on the second or third day, an erythematous eruption, more or less general, appears on the skin. Now and then it appears on the chest, shoulders, and back; at other times it covers the body, and has not infrequently led to its being confounded with scarlatina. It is not always accompanied by much fever, and cannot therefore be mistaken for that form of erythema which frequently appears in children with delicate skins during high fever from any source. I cannot say that I have found this complication to give a more malignant character to the disease, but true erysipelas does. I am not prepared to prove that the two processes, erysipelas and diphtheria, are identical under some circumstances, but the complication of the two, and the ferocity with which they combine, renders a close relationship probable. I have seen an infant dying from an erysipelas added to a post-auricular diphtheria, this being due to a slight abrasion of the surface. Erysipelas originating in the tracheotomy wound, though ever so carefully disinfected and secured, is [p. 674]frequently observed after two or three days, and is a very ominous symptom. Erysipelatous surfaces, denuded of their epidermis by spontaneous vesication or injured by ever so slight a trauma, are very liable to be covered with diphtheritic membranes.

An eruption resembling urticaria in the beginning is as innocent as erythema, but purpura in the latter stage is a symptom of mostly ominous nature.

On the vulva and vagina of little girls diphtheria is sometimes met with; probably in every case it is due, under the epidemic influence, to a local catarrh or erosion. In but few cases, comparatively, the inguinal glands are swollen. There are not many cases of vaginal diphtheria which are followed by the pharyngeal affection. Diphtheria of the vagina in puerperal women is liable to become the cause of general sepsis, and is a dangerous disease; it is seldom complicated, but uterus, Fallopian tubes, and peritoneum may become the seat of inflammatory and septic disturbances. In the bladder it may occur when the urine is alkaline, in chronic cystitis, after lithotomy, urethotomy, the operation for vesico-vaginal fistula, and in ectopia vesicæ. This form has a marked tendency toward localization, but by extension of the phlegmon, when of putrid character, to the retro-peritoneal cellular tissue, peritonitis may ensue and terminate fatally. Sepsis from absorption is also frequent. Vesical diphtheria is sometimes quite unsuspected. A man of sixty had urinary trouble a long time; his urine was frequently very offensive, containing blood and pus. About five days before his death he suddenly collapsed. I found the bladder well filled, and introduced a catheter, but succeeded in removing but a few drops of fetid liquid. Assuming the presence of a malignant tumor at the neck of the bladder, I attempted to draw off the urine by puncturing above the symphisis pubis; again without success. At the post-mortem examination a thick membranous lining of the bladder was found detached in the form of a sac containing about a quart of urine. During life the beak of the catheter evidently passed into the space between the bladder and the membranous sac, which accounts for the unsuccessful attempts at catheterization.

Diphtheria of the placenta was observed by Schüller. The membrane was between uterus and placenta, and attached to the latter. It resulted from puerperal sepsis. Balanoposthitis is liable to result in local and general diphtheria; so are circumcision wounds. They are apt to become affected either primarily, without apparent cause, or when other members of the family are suffering from the disease.

The kidneys may become affected in various ways. Albuminuria is not always of significance, as it occurs in severe and mild cases alike, both before and after tracheotomy, and therefore is not connected always either with the height of the fever or the degree of dyspnoea; at times it disappears in a few days, in other cases it is of longer duration. It is not invariably complicated with changes in the kidney, neither do we always discover casts or degenerated epithelial cells in the urine. In other respects also it does not behave like albuminuria in scarlatina. In the latter it appears seldom before the second week of the process, and frequently later, while in diphtheria it is often seen early. It sometimes lasts but a few days, particularly in many cases which set in with a high fever, which rapidly diminishes, and terminates in speedy recovery. In [p. 675]these occurrences the presence of albumen appears to attend the rapid elimination of the poison.

Albuminuria seldom lasts longer than a week, and is not often complicated with oedema, but sometimes it is but a symptom of a local or general nephritis, and then hyaline, epithelial, and fibrin casts and granular cells are found in the urine. Nephritis then assumes as serious a character as it possesses in scarlatina. Cases of nephritis, fortunately rare in a very early period of diphtheria, are liable to run a rapid and often fatal course.

The heart and blood are affected in various ways by the diphtheritic process. Where the disease runs a slow course, accompanied by high fever, a granular degeneration occurs, similar to that appearing in other acute infectious disorders—typhoid, for example. In diphtheria, however, it would seem that this condition may arise even without marked elevation of temperature. The pathological changes in the heart produced by diphtheria are not always the same. Ecchymoses, cellular hypertrophy, and granular degeneration have frequently been noticed after death where the symptoms had been severe. The result, of course, is considerable weakness of its muscular tissue, evidenced by the formation of local (Beverly Robinson) thrombi, general sluggishness of the circulation, dyspnoea, muffled heart-sounds, a cool and pale skin, and sudden death, preceded by a very feeble and frequent, sometimes, however, by a very slow, pulse. Aside from this, there is actual endocarditis during the course of diphtheria or convalescence therefrom. It affects especially the valves, and among them particularly the mitral. It is characterized by high fever, precordial pain, attacks of syncope, and a systolic murmur.

The rapid decrease of red blood-cells and a moderate increase of leucocytes were demonstrated by Bouchut and Dubrisay, but the disproportion was not such as to necessitate the diagnosis of leucocythæmia. Wunderlich reports two cases of Hodgkin's disease, the pseudo-leukæmia developing during diphtheria. And the slowness of final recovery in many cases, even of but short duration and not complicated with nervous disorders, appears to point to a serious disintegration of the elements of the blood. The dark color and defective coagulation of the blood in autopsies of diphtheria cases have often been remarked.

The direct and rapid introduction into the blood of a foreign substance has amongst its earliest symptoms fever. This reaction of a nervous system depends both on the quantity and quality of the substance or poison introduced, and on the susceptibility of the patient. High temperatures are, however, not the only, nor are they the most dangerous, nervous symptoms. To the latter belong the different shades of paralysis met with during or subsequent to diphtheria.

Sudden and unexpected collapse is sometimes observed, not infrequently in the earlier part of the disease. The changes found in autopsies, such as a dark color of the blood, deficient coagulability, extravasations into and friability and granular degenerations of the tissues, accumulations of degenerated cells, and granules between the fibres, degeneration mainly of the heart-muscle, the presence of heart-clots, thrombi in remote veins,—they all show to what extent the disease can destroy life in the shortest time possible. In the heart either the pneumogastric or the ganglionic[p. 676]nerves may be affected, and the symptoms will vary accordingly. Paralysis of the former will accelerate the pulse, degeneration of the sympathetic will diminish its frequency, yet death may ensue in either.

The usual form of diphtheritic paralysis makes its appearance during the period of convalescence, at a time when all danger seems to have passed by. As a rule, the soft palate and the muscles of deglutition are the first to be attacked, while the condition of these organs is apparently normal (and no longer oedematous, and thereby inactive, as in the first period of the disease). While they are recovering, or before, the accommodation muscles of the eyes become paralyzed. Sometimes, however, these are the first to be affected. This paralysis does not, as a rule, follow severe cases; on the contrary, it is not uncommon to observe it after apparently mild attacks of the disease. In consequence of the former paralysis, deglutition becomes difficult; fluids are expelled through the nose or enter the larynx and bronchi, thereby giving rise to pneumonia; in the latter there is strabismus. The upper and lower extremities become paralyzed afterward. As a rule, a number of muscles are affected at the same time, and improvement will take place in about the same order in which the individual muscles became affected. After paralysis has become affected, circulation begins to suffer. The extremities now and then become bluish, cool, emaciated; rarely atrophy and fatty degeneration have been observed. The muscles of the neck also become paralyzed; the head cannot be carried, or with difficulty only. The fingers are but seldom affected. The same holds good of the bladder and intestines. The respiratory muscles are not frequently attacked. Their paralysis is very ominous, and may prove fatal in a short time from apnoea.

Not only motory but sensory paralyses may occur. Anaesthesia, amaurosis, deafness have been observed; a number of cases of locomotor ataxia are on record, and but lately Hadthagen[12] publishes a case which he claims as disseminated sclerosis.

[12] *Arch. f. Kinderheilk.*, vol. v., 1883.

Sometimes the nervous affection in diphtheria is localized in a peculiar manner; it seems as if there is a predisposition on the part of a certain nerve to become diseased. The case of a boy, active and healthy, in the practice of H. Guleke, is very interesting. In the course of three years he had three attacks of diphtheria. In the very beginning of the disease he always became soporous with an almost normal temperature and a slow but regular pulse. Probably the heart's ganglia are the first to submit to the influence of the poison and exhibit symptoms of flagging function. In most of the cases of diphtheritic paralysis the prognosis is good; the large majority will run a favorable course in from six to ten weeks.

INVASION.—Is diphtheria, primarily, a local or a constitutional disease? Mercado's well-known case of diphtheria, engendered by the biting of a finger, has been alluded to. I know of one case in which the vagina became first affected, and later the pharynx. Bayles saw denuded portions of skin assume a membranous character, and general diphtheria develop afterward. Fresh wounds become diphtheritic, and the general disease arises from this source. Even paralysis will follow. I had a death from diphtheria when a long incision into a phlegmon of the thigh had become diphtheritic. A little girl, who had a considerable amount [p. 677]of discharge from a catarrhal vagina, and sore thighs in consequence, exhibited first, during the epidemic of 1877, membranes on the denuded cutis, and afterward general diphtheria. Brehm reports the case of a woman on whom he performed colotomy. The wound became thoroughly diphtheritic and gangrenous, but the pharynx and respiratory organs remained intact. A few days after, her daughter, who attended her in her sickness, was infected. In her the pharynx was the seat of disorder. Besides, the tonsils are very frequently coated with a membrane without any general symptoms in the beginning, fever and general illness occurring only later on. Now, all of these facts tend to show that there are cases in which the origin of the disease is purely local.

It must, however, not be forgotten that during the prevalence of an epidemic every one is more or less under its influence, and but little is wanting to call forth the disease. Some years ago a well-known physician, with whom I was intimately acquainted, died from facial erysipelas and meningitis which had originated in a slight abrasion of the upper lip. During an epidemic of typhoid we daily see persons with fever, headache, and lassitude. Diarrhoeas are frequent during an epidemic of cholera. An epidemic of diphtheria is accompanied by a great number of cases of pharyngitis. When, in the year 1860,[13] I reported two hundred cases of bonâ fide diphtheria, I at the same time observed one hundred and eighty-five cases of non-membranous inflammations of the throat. Such occurrences may be considered as possible or incipient cases of pharyngeal diphtheria. Therefore, contrary to the view of a local origin of diphtheria, it may be claimed that the individual taking the disease was already saturated with the poison, and the local membrane represented perhaps nothing but a symptom, or at the utmost the causa proxima. Accordingly, then, there are undoubtedly cases in which the pharyngeal membrane is the first cause and symptom of the final affection, and others in which the poisoning of the blood through inhalation is the first step in the development of the disease, amongst the symptoms of which the pharyngeal or nasal membrane counts as one.

[13] *Amer. Med. Times.*, Aug.

In these cases the first complaints of the patients relate to their general condition. Sometimes they are ignorant of any local trouble when they consult a physician. When it is perceptible, however, it is usually found on the visible pharyngeal and respiratory mucous membranes. This would seem to indicate that the infectious elements while being inhaled are there deposited. Thus there is a possibility of simultaneous affections of both the throat and the blood in the lungs, in either equal or variable proportions. We are easily led to defend at least a partial admission of the poison by the respiratory act, when we reflect that the membranes which are swallowed are rendered innocuous by the action of the gastric fluids, and, therefore, the alimentary canal, from the oesophagus downward, cannot be made responsible for the admission of the poison into the system. Thus it is that the general symptoms—as fever, lassitude, etc.—precede the local phenomena in very many cases, while there are exceptional cases in which the membrane appears first and the fever later. This is especially the case when the tonsils are very large and occupy a prominent position in the throat.

Those cases which begin with high fever and moderate or no local[p. 678]symptoms must be looked upon as constitutional diseases. If a person, in the course of several hours or a day, be taken with high fever and a moderate membrane-formation, these symptoms subsiding in one or two days, leaving the patient weak and exhausted, but fully restored to health at the end of a week, we would be justified in assuming (cæteris paribus) that there was a rapid absorption of a large amount of poison, and an equally rapid elimination thereof. They are, moreover, the same cases in which the second or third day of the disease furnishes albuminuria, with rapid elimination and speedy recovery. When, however, the process is slow in developing, accompanied by moderate fever, and the course is indolent, we have reason to infer that moderate amounts of the poison are being continually taken into the system and making their influence felt to a moderate degree, but for a longer period. Such are the cases which, without any violent symptoms, are accompanied by frequent local relapses, or run, when the absorption is constant as well as copious, a septic course, or terminate in paralysis.

Thus there are cases in which a local infection of the skin or of a wound may be one of the causes, or the only cause, of the disease, and there are cases in which the poison, in passing through and caught in the pharynx, gives rise to local phenomena before the system at large gives evidence of infection. But, as a general thing, diphtheria must be looked upon as a constitutional disease, giving rise to local phenomena, in the same way as scarlatina does on the skin, on the mucous membrane of the alimentary canal, and in the uriniferous tubules; measles on the skin and respiratory mucous membrane; or typhoid in the lymph-follicles and on the mucous membrane of the intestine; or, in other words, the diphtheritic poison may enter the system locally through a defective, or sore, or wounded integument or through the lungs.

Is diphtheria contagious? Undoubtedly it is. The contagious element is liable to be directly communicated by the patient; it also clings to solid and semi-solid bodies, and in this way is transmitted even after a long time. There is hardly any disease which can cling so tenaciously to dwellings and furniture; it can be transported by the air, though probably not to a great distance, and hence in houses artificially heated, while the windows and doors are mostly closed, rises from the lower to the upper stories; and it is for this reason advisable to keep the sick on the top floor. It is certainly transmitted by spoons, glasses, handkerchiefs, and towels used by the patient. The contagious character increases directly in proportion to the neglect of proper ventilation. That it is spread by the feces is not clearly established in my mind. I can give personally no examples of its being carried by visitors or by the attending physician; this is said to have occurred, however. The character of the disease communicated, and the local manifestation, do not depend on that of the original sufferer; thus mild cases may produce severe ones, and vice versâ, and convalescents can convey the disease in its full force. Naturally, the softer character of the tissues in children renders them more susceptible to infection, and the activity of their lymphatic system more liable to severe forms of the disease.

Many tragic cases are recorded in literature of infection by direct contact from pharynx to pharynx, or from the opening in the trachea to the mouth of the surgeon; and one of the saddest cases, perhaps, is that of [p. 679]the much-lamented Carl Otto Weber. Myself and others have contracted diphtheria from sucking tracheotomy wounds.

In regard to the length of the incubation periods, there can be no better authenticated facts than those contained in a report of Elisha Harris to the National Board of Health, an abstract of which is found in No. 1, *National Board of Health Bulletin*, June 28, 1879. The report says that in the fourth school district of the township of Newark (Northern Vermont), amidst the steep hills where reside a quiet people in comfortable dwellings, the summer term of school opened on the 12th of May. Among the twenty-two little children who assembled in the school-room in the glen were two who had suffered from a mild attack of diphtheria in April, and one of them was, at the time school opened, suffering badly from what appeared to have been a relapse in the form of diphtheritic ophthalmia. Besides, it is proved that these recently sick pupils had not been well cleansed, one of them having on an unwashed garment that she had worn in all her sickness three weeks previously. At the end of the third day of school several of the children were complaining of sore throat, headache, and dizziness, and on the fourth day and evening so many were sick in the same way that the teacher and officers announced the school temporarily closed. By the end of the sixth day from school opening, sixteen of the twenty-two previously healthy children became seriously sick with symptoms of malignant diphtheria, and some were already dying. The teacher and six of the pupils were not attacked, nor have they since suffered from the disease.

A case[14] is reported of a surgeon who, while attending a diphtheritic child, had some secretion thrown into his face. Twelve hours after his right eye was inflamed and painful. The affection proved diphtheritic, and recovery was completed after several weeks only. In a case seen by me, with Dr. L. Bopp, a child removed from a house infected with diphtheria was attacked after fourteen days and eight hours.

[14] *Würt. Med. Corresp. Bl.*, 1878, No. 2.

It would then appear that, in the direct communication of the disease to healthy or nearly healthy mucous membranes—as healthy as the prevailing epidemic will allow—the period of incubation is from one or two to fourteen days. In only a small number of cases the disease has an even shorter period of incubation than this, as when tonsillotomy or a similar operation is undertaken during the prevalence of an epidemic. One may rest assured that any operation on the tonsils while an epidemic of diphtheria is at its height will be followed within twenty-four hours by diphtheritic deposits on the wounded part. To what extent we are justified in considering this a bonâ-fide incubation of the disease in a previously healthy body is, of course, another question. It seems to me that these cases positively prove that the operation is only the causâ proxima of a diphtheritic affection, and that we may take it for granted that during an epidemic every individual is more or less under its influence and affected by it, so that it needs but a wound or an accidental abrasion of the surface of the mucous membrane to call the disease into action. In a similar way, fresh wounds or morbid conditions of the mouth may call forth the disease. The ruptured vesicles of a follicular stomatitis are liable to serve as resting-places for diphtheritic membranes, and thus I have seen the complication of a follicular stomatitis with oral diphtheria; and any[p. 680]lacerations of the vagina during labor may become diphtheritic within twenty-four hours. If now, on the one hand, incubation depends on the condition of the affected surface, it is probable, on the other hand, that the intensity of the poison at the time plays an important part in determining the period that is to elapse between infection and the invasion of the disease.

ETIOLOGY.—Diphtheria is pre-eminently a disease of early life; in this respect it is said to differ from the genuine fibrinous bronchitis, which by some is held an absolutely different disease, and stated to occur but rarely in children. But even this statement is probably incorrect. In the spring of 1879 I met with four cases of fibrinous bronchitis in children under three years of age. The number of cases of diphtheria in adult life is not very large, while in old age it is very small. Of 501 deaths in Vienna in 1868, only 1 had reached the age of sixty-two; of more than 300 cases in which I performed tracheotomy but 2 were over thirteen years old.

I do not know that sex exerts any predisposing influence over diphtheria, yet of the six hundred cases or thereabouts of laryngeal diphtheria in which I either personally performed tracheotomy or observed the progress of the disease in the practice of others, I found the majority in males, and the recoveries in inverse proportion to the number thereof, the mortality being greater among boys. As far as age is concerned, nearly all the zymotic diseases are seen most frequently in children. They exhibit a greater disposition to submit to diphtheria than adults, if we except those under ten months. Where, however, the disease has occurred previous to the seventh or eighth month, the greater number of cases has been found under three months. Tigri reports the disease in a child of fourteen days. A child of fifteen days was seen with diphtheritic laryngitis and oesophagitis by Bretonneau, one of seventeen days by Bednar, one of eight by Bouchut, one of seven days by Weikert; Parrot mentions several cases, and Sirédey[15] reports eighteen cases of diphtheria in the newly-born. They occurred in the Hospital Lariboisière in the spring of 1877, and were probably infected by the nurses of a neighboring children's asylum. Membranes were found on the soft palate, tonsils, or larynx, and also on both pharynx and larynx. One case occurred where the posterior nares alone were affected. I have met with four cases of diphtheria of the pharynx and larynx in the newly-born myself. One of these became sick on the ninth day after birth, and died on the thirteenth day; the other died on the sixteenth day after birth; the third was taken when seven days old, and died on the ninth day. The predisposition to diphtheria during childhood[16] seems to be explainable by several circumstances. The mucous membrane of the mouth and pharynx in the child is more succulent and softer, and frequently the seat of a congestive and inflammatory process. The nasal cavities are small and frequently affected by catarrhs, the buccal cavity often the seat of catarrh and of stomatitis, and insufficient cleanliness leads here to irritation of the mucous membrane. Any abnormal state of the mucous membrane, with [p. 681]the exception of an atrophic condition and cicatricial changes, affords an excellent abode for diphtheria. The tonsils are proportionally large; in fact, we rarely see the tonsils in children completely sheltered by the arches of the palate. On the other hand, the pharynx is anything but spacious, and while the protuberant condition of the tonsils affords a resting-place for the invading disease, the remaining space is so small that it becomes a source of uneasiness to the well in many instances, and very much more than that to the child during diphtheritic tumefaction. Furthermore, we must take into consideration the large number and size of the lymphatics, which can be more easily injected in the child than in the adult, according to Sappey, and the fact of greater intercommunication amongst the lymphatics and between them and the system; for S. L. Schenck has found that the network of lymphatics in the skin of the newly-born, at least, are endowed with stomata, loopholes through which the lymph-ducts can communicate with the neighborhood, and vice versâ.[17] These circumstances, although they may have no influence in calling the disease into existence, yet assist in its development and in adding to the severity of the symptoms.

[15] Thèse, Paris, 1877.

[16] W. N. Thursfield (*London Lancet*, Aug. 3d, 10th, 17th, 1878) collects 10,000 cases of diphtheria in England between the years 1855 and 1877. Of these 90 per 1000 were under a year, 450 per 1000 from 1-5 years, 260 from 6-10, 90 from 11-15, 50 from 16-25, 35 from 26-45; 25 per 1000 were 45 years and over.

[17] *Mittheil. aus d. Embryol. Instit.*, i., 1877.

On the other hand, while the above reasons go to prove that diphtheria attacks children by preference, there is again an anatomical and physiological condition—to wit, the free slightly acid secretion of the mouth, beginning with the third month—that acts as a hindrance to the frequent occurrence of diphtheria after the third month. A poison or poisonous product of whatever nature can less readily find a hiding-place so long as it can be readily—we might always say must surely be—washed away. During these months of eruptive secretion from the mouth diphtheria, therefore, is not very frequent; thus teething, in the case of diphtheria, cannot be held responsible by mothers fond of diagnosticating dental diseases. In this connection the remark of Krieger ought not to be overlooked, who explains the relative scarcity of the disease in the first year of life by the fact that cumulative influences will produce a great number of cases, and cumulation requires time. Undoubtedly, however, an important etiological consideration is the fact of having had the disease previously. We can cite a host of zymotic diseases the occurrence of which once serves as a protection against future attacks. Not only can no such security be expected after one attack of diphtheria, but, cæteris paribus, the disease shows a preference for those who have survived a previous attack. The statement that only the mild cases, with but slight elevation of temperature and freedom from severe constitutional symptoms, are likely to suffer a relapse is founded on error. True, I have more frequently seen relapses after mild cases—which, fortunately, are in the majority—but the disease has also recurred where originally high fever and an extensive lymphadenitis proved it to be a severe case. Besides, second attacks of membranous croup are also recorded (Guersant, N. F. Gill, Quincke).

As there are individuals, so there are families, which have a predisposition to diseases, as there are others in whom, notwithstanding ample exposure, infection does not easily take place. Yet in the families in which diphtheria is of frequent occurrence it cannot always be attributed to enlarged tonsils and a tendency to pharyngeal or nasal catarrh.

[p. 682]Still, catarrh and the vulnerability of mucous membranes must be considered as a frequent source of diphtheria; children will get numerous relapses often after a nasal or pharyngeal catarrh. Sudden changes in the temperature of the atmosphere or of the surface of the body are therefore dangerous in predisposed persons. And thus it is that while severe epidemics have spared no climate or land known to us, the majority of cases have occurred in winter and spring; in other words, at a time when catarrhal disorders are of most frequent occurrence. In my experience at New York, the first quarter of the year yielded more cases than any other. Still, they are frequent enough in warm seasons. Krieger insists upon the injurious influence of hot summers and dry hot rooms. I do not doubt the correctness of his views, which cannot but be strengthened by the damaging results of our furnace-heating. But the influence of season on the invasion and course of diphtheria is but indirect and conditional, and may be, perhaps, after all, compared with that exerted by filth—a term which is lately used to express all sorts and forms of nastiness, from filthy bodies of men to their clothes, their habits, their food, and the air they breathe, whether polluted by carbonic acid, by excrementitious gases, or by exhalations of sewers.

Cases of diphtheria which are traced to exhalations from sewers (or even to filthy habits of life) are very frequent. Yet typhoid is attributed to the same causes. So is dysentery. Can, then, foul exhalations produce alike diphtheria, typhoid, and dysentery? Do these diseases arise from a common poison? Or is the poison of a treble character, so that a part may give origin to diphtheria, another part to typhoid, a third to dysentery?[18]Have we to deal, in such occurrences, with specific influences, or only with a lowering of the standard of health, thereby affording other morbid influences an opportunity to exercise their power? These questions are still involved in darkness, and constitute problems the solution of which still engages the minds of both individual writers and authorities. A report of the Board of Health of Massachusetts, closely adhering to the results of exact observations,[19] leaves them doubtful, and the affirmative reports of some modern writers do not bear scrutiny.[20]

[18] In regard to the causal connection of the two latter diseases with sewer exhalations we can be more positive than in regard to the former.

[19] Author's *Treatise on Diphth.*, p. 35.

[20] M. A. Avery, *Med. Jour. and Obst. Rev.*, Feb., 1882.

Air polluted by bad drainage or leaky sewers has been considered responsible for diphtheria as well as for typhoid fever and dysentery. Not only the impairment of general health, but the direct and unmistakable disease, has been attributed to it. Thus Bayley refers, in the endemic of Bromley,[21] the first cases to unventilated sewers and cesspools. Schoolchildren multiplied the disease. Thursfield attributes the diphtheria at Ellesmere[22] to the accumulation of excrements under the school-room, and to deficient supply of water, which, moreover, was of bad quality. Tripe (like Railton, Bailey, Russell, Bell) accuses sewer gas;[23] others polluted waters or bad drainage.[24] I have not been convinced, however, that diphtheria can be considered a sewer-gas disease, in the same way as typhoid fever. The deterioration of the general health resulting from the inhalation of foul air is sufficient to explain the outbreak of the individual attack during a prevailing epidemic.

[21] *Sanit. Record*, Aug. 10, 1877.

[22] *San. Rec.*, 158, 1877.

[23] *Ibid.*, June 14, 1878.

[24] *Ibid.*, April 18, May 2, 1879.

[p. 683]In regard to polluted water, I do not think that pathologists who attribute infectious diseases to bacteria only are justified in condemning it. It may not be so guilty, after all, for the admixtures, inorganic and organic, minerals, admixtures of wood and plants, also lower fungi and their products—algæ, infusoria—would render water rather disagreeable, but not exactly unhealthy. The latter effect can be accomplished—always assuming the bacteria theory correct, for the sake of argument—by bacteria only. But when they arrive in the stomach, their doom is sealed; they are decomposed. The only places where, possibly, they could take root would be diseased or ulcerated places in either the oral cavity or the upper portion of the oesophagus.

Not only water, but the milk of animals also, has been accused of being the direct cause of diphtheria. Powers concludes, though a connection between diphtheria and the consumption of milk have not been proven as yet, that it is very probable indeed. His careful investigations into the causes of some local epidemics in North London exclude any other source from which the people could have been affected. Perhaps one of the forms of garget, cow mammitis, is of an infectious character. His reasoning, however, is not accepted by A. Dowrus,[25] who still believes that the milk which gave rise to diphtheria at a distance may have been soiled and infected. For though the connection between milk and scarlatina and typhoid fever had been known for years and variously studied, no observation of the kind had yet been made in regard to diphtheria. Besides, where the young, in England, drink much milk—viz. in the cities—diphtheria was very much less frequent than where little or no milk was taken—viz. in the country. Even in the country the well-to-do classes, who drink milk, had but little diphtheria, while the children of the poor, who obtained none, suffered a great deal from it.

[25] "Diphtheria and Milk-Supply," *Brit. Med. Journ.*, Feb. 1, 1879.

In regard to this transmission of diphtheria by means of milk O. Bollinger[26] hesitates to express any opinion, except that the matter is very doubtful indeed. Probably the possibility of contracting diphtheria directly from animals is very much greater than the danger from water or milk. On a Pomeranian farm, during the winter 1875-76, every newly-born calf died of diphtheria. The superintendent of the farm and the woman who attended to the calves were taken with diphtheritic angina.[27] Similar occurrences have been recorded. Bollinger reports a mycotic disease of the trachea and lungs in birds.

[26] *D. Z. f. Thiermed. u. vergleich. Pathol.*, vi., 1879, p. 7.

[27] Damman, in *D. Zeitsch. f. Thiermed.*, 1876, p. 1.

Friedberger's report,[28] presented to the Veterinary Society of Munich, on croup and diphtheria of domestic fowls, leaves no doubt as to its frequency, particularly amongst the nobler varieties.

[28] *D. Zeitsch. f. Thiermed.*, v., 1879, p. 16.

Nicati[29] studied an epidemic diphtheria amongst hens which had similar symptoms and a course very much like that in man; it could be inoculated into other animals, and was contemporaneous with the outbreak of the epidemic amongst the human population of Marseilles. Trasbot[30] succeeded in inoculating a healthy hen from a diphtheritic one, but the[p. 684]attempts at transmission to dog, pig, and man were unsuccessful. The*Med. and Surg. Journal*[31] contains the following: In a house at Ogdensburg, N. Y., five children were ill with diphtheria. Three kittens who had been playing with them from time to time took the disease and died. Post-mortem examination showed diphtheritic membranes in their throats.[32]

[29] *Revue d'Hygiène et de Police sanitaire*, 1879, p. 3.

[30] "De la transmission de la Diphth. des Animaux à l'Homme," *Gaz. hebdom.*, 1879 Avril 25.

[31] *Med. Rec.*, Nov. 8, 1879.

[32] An elaborate description of the croupo-diphtheritic inflammations of mucous membranes in hens, turkeys, pheasants, and pigeons may be found in *Zürn. Krankh. d. Hausgeflügels*, 1882, p. 104.

Gerhardt[33] reports the following: 2600 hens were imported from Verona, Italy, into a village, Messelhausen, in Baden. Some of these hens were affected with diphtheria when they arrived. Within six weeks 600 of their number died of diphtheria, and 800 more soon after. In the following summer 1000 chickens were raised by artificial breeding, all of which died of diphtheria within six weeks. Five cats kept in the place also died of diphtheria; a parrot fell sick with it, but recovered. An Italian cook, suffering from diphtheria, in the month of November, 1881, while being subjected to local treatment with carbolic acid, bit the head-nurse's left foot and hand. Both these wounds became diphtheritic, the man falling sick with high fever, and requiring three weeks for his gradual recovery. Besides, four of the six workingmen employed in taking care of the hens of the establishment were taken with diphtheria. Not a single case, however, occurred in the neighboring village. Thus, it is safe to assume that the diphtheritic disease of hens can be transmitted to man.

[33] *Verhandlungen des* (ii.) *Congresses für Innere Medicin*, Wiesbaden, 1883, p. 129.

Diphtheria may be also produced by outside influences. In this regard the attempts at generating pseudo-membranes by artificial means are very interesting indeed. As early as 1826, Bretonneau, by the introduction of tincture of cantharides and olive oil into the trachea, succeeded in producing a "dense, elastic, reed-like membranous concretion." Delafond called croup into existence by the use of ammonia, oxygen, chlorine, corrosive sublimate, arsenic, and sulphuric acid. On the other hand, H. Mayer asserts that it is impossible, by means of ammonia, to produce a croup in the windpipes of animals which in the slightest degree resembles that occurring in human beings. Trendelenburg, however, after producing membranes in the trachea by the use of a solution of corrosive sublimate (1:120), succeeded in hardening the entire mass with bichromate of potassium, which it was impossible to do with the most tenacious mucus.

Rey observed croup in horses that inhaled smoke in a burning stable.[34] In the collection of the veterinary school of Zurich there is a croup membrane from a heifer which had been exposed to a fire; at Munich, one from the trachea of a horse, produced by forcibly injecting medicines into the nose. Hahn made an observation on cows, W. Ammon on horses, of long croup membranes after the animals had been exposed to smoke and fire; and Oertel constantly insists on there being "no actual difference between croup as it ordinarily occurs and that excited in the windpipe of a rabbit by means of ammonia. The color and texture, the physical, chemical, and histological characteristics, are identical."

[34] *Journ. de méd. vét. de Lyon*, 1850, p. 249.

[p. 685]MORBID ANATOMY.—Either the membrane or the granular infiltration is characteristic of diphtheria. The statement that the former occurs only when atmospheric air can gain access thereto, as A. d'Espine and C. Picot still hold,[35] is plainly contradicted by its appearance on the mucous membrane of the lower intestines. The condition of the membrane is not unalterable, any more than the clinical symptoms of the disease, for, according to different circumstances, epithelium, mucus, blood, and vegetable parasites are added thereto. The membrane can either be lifted from the mucous membrane on which it lies or is imbedded into and underneath it. In the first instance, it consists to a great extent of fibrin, the result either of epithelial changes or derived directly from the exuded blood-serum. E. Wagner, who makes no anatomical distinction between croup and diphtheria, considers epithelial changes the principal source. The pavement epithelium becomes altered in a peculiar manner. It becomes turbid, larger, dentated, and dissolves into a network; it is at first uninhabited, but serves later as the vehicle of newly-formed cells; there also occurs a considerable infiltration of the mucous membrane pus-cells and granules; besides, the cellular tissue is studded with granules, the granular degeneration resulting sometimes in necrotic destruction, which is looked upon by Virchow as the most important element in severe forms of diphtheria. The several conditions or degrees may occur independent of each other, associated or in succession. Classen shares Wagner's views, but, according to Boldygrew, the pseudo-membrane consists of successive coagulations of a fibrinous fluid which exudes from the diseased surface. Steudener also opposes the views of Wagner. He does not believe in the probability of an exclusively endogenous origin of the cellular elements of croup membrane; in fact, he doubts the occurrence of an endogenous formation of pus-globules in epithelium. Croupous membrane, according to him, is formed by the migration of numerous white blood-globules through the walls of the vessels in the mucous membrane, and by a direct formation of fibrin from the transuded plasma. In addition to this, the mucous membrane is stripped of its epithelium (except at the mouths of the acinous glands) and infiltrated with migrating cells. Fresh croupous membrane consists of a delicate network of homogeneous structure and shining appearance, in which numerous cells and the epithelium of the various layers of the trachea are imbedded. In old membranes the cells are destroyed by granular degeneration and general maceration. Tenacious mucus with pus-cells and detritus are then found. C. Weigert looks upon the deposits as analogous to those on serous membranes. Every inflammation yields an exudation which may coagulate when the coagulating ferment is added. This latter is probably produced by the white blood-cells when in disintegration. But he does not say why it is that there is no such coagulation in suppurative processes, where the leucocytes are more numerous. He believes himself justified in establishing pathological differences of croup, pseudo-diphtheria, and diphtheria. A croupous inflammation means destruction of epithelium, which gives rise to a fibrinous exudation upon the surface, while the cellular tissue remains intact. The only difference between it and the pseudo-diphtheritic inflammation is looked for in the larger number of emigrated white [p. 686]blood-cells. The superficial deposit consists, to a great part, of them and the fibrinous exudation. When there are but few leucocytes the deposit is a network of fibrillæ (croup). When there are many, the masses are more solid and voluminous (pseudo-diphtheritis). When, however, the tissue is changed into a hard substance resembling coagulated fibrin, when the exudation does not exist on the surface, but takes place into the mucous membrane, the process is diphtheria. Zahn also establishes three varieties—viz. 1st, such as result from a peculiar degeneration of pavement epithelium; 2d, such as originate in the solidification of a muco-fibrinous, and, 3d, of a fibrino-purulent, exudation. Each of these varieties may contain colonies of micrococci, but these organisms are neither essential nor are they constantly found.

[35] *Man. prat. des mal. de l'enfance*, 1877, p. 81.

The diphtheritic process does not merely consist of the membranous changes in the pharynx and air-passages. Its fatal cases have afforded marked evidence of the implication of most of the organs. Reimer's 17 cases give the following post-mortem results: the lungs were hyperæmic in 8 cases, twice the seat of pneumonia, and three times of embolic infarctions; in addition, emphysema in 12, oedema in 6, atelectasis in 7, subpleural ecchymoses in 7, pericardial ones in 4. The heart-muscle had undergone fatty degeneration in 6, and was the seat of ecchymoses of the size of a pin's head in 3. In addition to frequent hyperæmic conditions of the abdominal viscera, emboli of the liver in 3 (with capillary hemorrhages of the peritoneal covering in 1), emboli of the spleen in 5, desquamative nephritis in 7 (in 6 of which there were colonies of micrococci in the uriniferous tubules), cellular hyperplasia of the cervical and mediastinal glands in 14 (complicated in 6 with capillary hemorrhages in the glandular tissue). The blood was frequently normal, very often watery and dark, at times leucocythæmic. Thus the disease exerts its influence everywhere.

Rindfleisch defines diphtheritic inflammation as that form of inflammation which produces a coagulating necrosis in the tissues by the immigration of schizomycetæ. The coagulating necrosis differs from the usual form of necrosis in this, that the change from life to death is accompanied with the coagulation of fluid albuminoids. This process takes place mainly in the interior of cells and other parts of tissues, and therein differs from the coagulation of fibrin. In the cells there is taking place a peculiar homogenization of protoplasm; at the same time the nuclei disappear, and are changed into irregular masses liable to cohere and form membranous conglomerates, which owe their peculiar wax color to the invasion of a solid albuminoid endowed with a strong tendency to refract the light. Coagulating necrosis is found in circumscribed localities, and gives rise, in the neighborhood, to a marked amount of inflammation and suppuration, which leads to the expulsion of the necrotic part, with more or less loss of substance—either mild or phagedenic ulceration.

Leyden describes a gray degeneration of the muscular tissue which he believes to be truly inflammatory, and Unruh has lately published an account of some cases in which myocarditis occurred. In Leyden's cases, the muscular nuclei were increased, became atrophied, and underwent fatty degeneration, giving rise thereby to extravasations, softening, dilatation and debility of the heart, with general debility, collapse, and—[p. 687]probably by reflex action on other branches of the pneumogastric—vomiting. Micrococci he found neither in the heart nor in the kidneys.

In the heart, particularly on the right side, numerous thrombi are frequently found in various stages of development; its muscular tissue is often in a state of fatty degeneration or the seat of parenchymatous inflammation and hemorrhages. Bridges first called attention to the occurrence of endocarditis in diphtheria.[36] This complication, which, however, occurs more frequently with rheumatism, puerperal fever, diphtheria of wounds, pyæmia, and old valvular affections than in the course of an acute diphtheria, does not, as found in the latter affection, consist simply of a fatty degeneration and subsequent ulceration, but is considered a genuine diphtheritic process (Virchow), affecting the mitral valve more frequently than the tricuspid or pulmonary valves. It begins with hyperæmia and the exudation of plasma in the cellular elements, so that they appear larger and darker. The granulations which form are frail and easily destroyed, so that ulcers form on which fibrin is deposited, and whence it is conveyed as emboli into the terminal arteries (Cohnheim) of the spleen, nerves, brain, and eye. Infarctions may also occur in the valveless veins of these organs, giving rise rather to small multiple abscesses than to large purulent collections. Suppuration but rarely takes place in the heart; the granular mass found there resists the action of æther and alcohol, and spreads throughout the cardiac parenchyma, so that perforation of the septum and of the right auricle and aorta has been observed.

[36] *Med. Times and Gaz.*, ii. p. 204.

Bouchut and Labadie-Lagrave, out of 15 cases of diphtheria, met in 14 with a plastic endocarditis, which became the source of emboli. Thus, there were infarctions of the lungs, at times in their centre colorless, at other times in a state of purulent degeneration; superficial thrombi of the small veins of the heart, subcutaneous connective tissue, pia mater, brain, and liver; and in addition, moderate leucocytosis.

The lungs exhibit (post-mortem) all sorts of inflammatory and congestive conditions, with their consequences, as oedema, catarrh, broncho-pneumonia, atelectasis, emphysema, ecchymoses, and large infarctions.

The spleen (and occasionally the liver) is frequently large, congested, and friable, and studded with infarctions to a greater or less extent.

The kidneys are either simply congested or the seat of nephritis or infarctions. The same forms of inflammation which accompany scarlatina—to wit, the desquamative and the diffuse—are here observed. The diffuse form is not of so frequent occurrence as in scarlatina, but is sometimes extensive and dangerous.

The muscles occasionally exhibit ecchymoses, and are at times the seat of parenchymatous inflammation, gray degeneration, and atrophy.

The lymphatic glands are frequently inflamed and swollen, either hard or doughy, oedematous or congested. Large abscesses are rare. It is more especially the gland tissue, and less the connective tissue of the glands, which takes part in the pathological process. The periglandular tissue very soon becomes involved, however. Necrotic foci have been described by Bizzozero. When the entire surface of the mucous membrane of the mouth and of the air-passages, from the nose to the trachea, is the seat of the disease, there is an impregnation of the mucous membrane, from the epithelial surface to the submucous tissue, of the entire [p. 688]tongue, borders of the lips, and frequently of the lips and cheeks, as well as of the tonsils, the lower portion of the nasal cavities and the upper, and especially the anterior, portion of the larynx. The fossæ Morgagni and the posterior aspect of the soft palate are more frequently affected in the same way than the anterior aspect. Small isolated spots are found on the tonsils and occasionally on the posterior wall of the pharynx. The so-called croupous form—that is to say, the one in which the membranes deposited may either be removed in large patches or lie macerated in the profuse secretion of subjacent mucous glands—is found partly in the nasal cavities, on the posterior surface of the soft palate, and also in the trachea and its subdivisions.

The character of the mucous membrane varies with the locality. Its different elements, as the epithelium, the basement membrane, the connective tissue mingled with elastic fibres, the blood-vessels, the nerves from the cerebro-spinal and sympathetic systems, and the papillæ and ducts of numberless glands, all influence the pathological process going on upon the surface. Their distribution in the oral cavity and the respiratory organs is a very interesting study, and in a table already published,[37] I have exhibited it in a condensed tabular form.

[37] *Treatise on Diphtheria*, p. 126.

Where elastic tissue predominates, diphtheritic impregnation is slow to take place, and recovery is also slow when the tissue has finally submitted. Pavement epithelium yields the easiest foothold to diphtheritic membrane. Thus it is that the tonsils, not from their prominent situation alone, favor the reception and development of the infection. But the elastic and connective fibres when once affected are apt to harbor the disease a long time. Still, there is another reason why the diphtheritic process should favor the tonsils. For Th. Höhr has demonstrated that their epithelium exhibits interruptions in its continuity. Through them round cells may emigrate. Wherever the epithelial covering of the integuments (skin or mucous membrane) is intact and unbroken, diphtheria takes hold with difficulty. But where a defect is established, large or small, diphtheritic formations will be apt to take place according to the size of the abrasion. This is one of the modes of the formation of small diphtheritic deposits on the tonsils, which it has been the tendency of many, both practitioners and authors, to honor with special names.

Ciliated epithelium is not so liable to be affected. It occupies a higher rank in the scale of animal formations, has a more complex function and a greater power of resistance. The presence of a large number of mucous glands impedes, as a rule, by the presence of the normal secretion, an extensive destructive action upon the tissues. The secreted mucus assists in removing epithelial masses, and even fibrinous exudations, from the surface. Thus it is that the deposits in the respiratory portion of the nasal cavities are frequently cast off through the nostrils, and in a similar manner the membranes that have formed in the trachea are ejected in a semi-solid condition through the opening made by tracheotomy. The large number of mucous glands in the larynx and trachea is unquestionably the reason why the lymphatic vessels of the mucous membrane are not influenced by the overlying loosened masses, and will not absorb; hence laryngeal and tracheal diphtheria, when not complicated, have decidedly a local character, and are usually devoid of constitutional symptoms. For the [p. 689]same reason the usual form of tonsillar diphtheria is a mild disease. On the other hand, the large number and size of the lymphatic ducts of the Schneiderian mucous membrane, as well as their direct communication with the lymphatic glands of the neck, accounts for the dangerous character of nasal diphtheria.

Diphtheria of the intestinal canal is characterized by fibrinous deposits on the surface and in the tissues of the intestine, with subsequent granular degeneration. It is mostly preceded by a catarrhal process. The same condition is found in the urinary organs.

There are but few autopsies of cases which have died of, or during, diphtheritic paralysis. In some instances there was considerable thickening of the spinal nerves at the junction of the posterior and anterior roots, with hemorrhages. The superficial connective tissue in these places exhibited a diphtheritic exudation (Buhl). There was in the sheath of the nerves of the cerebral and spinal meninges and in the gray substance of the cord voluminous nuclear infiltration; in one case there were extensive hemorrhages in the spinal meninges, with nuclear proliferation in the gray substance of the cord (Oertel). Disseminated meningitis with perineuritis of the neighboring roots, characterized by infiltration of nuclei between the nerve-fibrillæ was found by Pierret; and degeneration of the palatine nerves and fatty degeneration of the palatine muscles by Charcot and Vulpian. Dejerine, in five autopsies, records an atrophy of the anterior roots secondary to a myelitic degeneration of the ganglia of the anterior horns. E. Gaucher found the same in the case of a boy who died with paralysis of the muscles of deglutition, of the extremities, and of the trunk. In a child of two years with paralysis of the palate and extremities the autopsy was negative. In two cases Dejerine reports finding changes in the intramuscular nerves, such as liquefaction of myelin and loss of axis cylinders.

Thus, Buhl, Charcot, Vulpian, and Dejerine are unanimous about an affection of the peripheric nerves and muscles. Oertel, Dejerine, and Gaucher believe in a disease of the spinal cord. It is true that a disease of the gray substance would fully explain the symptoms of the bad cases, but what we know of poliomyelitis anterior, with which this affection would be identical, precludes the idea of the rapid and almost certain complete recovery. Therefore, in most cases, diphtheritic paralysis consists of a trophic affection of the motor system, almost always seated peripherally in the nerves and muscles, seldom, if ever, in the centres. This affection must be compared, in most of its relations, with the degenerative processes taking place in the muscular tissue after typhoid fever, or in the renal epithelium after infectious diseases, both of which give rise to serious results, with usually a favorable termination.

DIAGNOSIS.—The characteristic sign of diphtheria is either the membrane or the gray infiltration, with more or less injection of the surrounding parts. In regard to this greater or less injection, I will say that pharyngeal congestion, when it is uniform, may or may not point to imminent diphtheria. When it is local, confined to one side mainly, it is either traumatic or diphtheritic. White spots which are easily washed away, or which can be removed with a brush, or squeezed out of the follicles of the tonsils, into which a probe can be introduced sometimes to the depth of one-half inch, soon announce their true character—viz. either a [p. 690]simple catarrhal secretion or suppuration. Even though the superficial deposit contain oidium or leptothrix in considerable numbers, it can easily be removed; I have only known the totally inexperienced to mistake muguet (thrush) for diphtheria. In the larynx muguet is, moreover, very rare indeed, and always circumscribed. It is sometimes seen on the true vocal cords. The gray discoloration of superficial follicular ulcerations, as observed in the ordinary form of stomatitis follicularis, can hardly fail to be recognized. Such patches are very numerous in the fauces and on the lips and cheeks—never on the gums, except in ulcerous stomatitis (which is not follicular). They are accompanied, too, by vesicles containing more or less serum which have not yet ruptured. It must be remembered, however, that the mucous membrane, when deprived of its superficial covering, is liable during an epidemic of diphtheria to become infected, like every other wound. I have seen cases in which stomatitis and diphtheria existed side by side, the latter having invaded the surfaces exposed by the former. The examination of the entire throat is not always easy. Very young children vomit frequently and persistently before the whole surface is exposed to view, and not infrequently repeated examination with the spatula is absolutely necessary. In general, however, the slight attempts at vomiting suffice to cause a great part of the swollen posterior portion of the tonsils to become visible. I have heard that the pale surface of old hyperplastic tonsils has been mistaken for diphtheria; I merely mention the fact. When a discoloration happens to be the result of a deposited flake of mucus, a drink of water will remove it.

Fever is not always a prominent symptom; as a rule, simple diphtheria of the tonsils is accompanied by very little fever. Still, there are plenty of exceptions. But the differences of temperature are not more striking than in most other infectious diseases, whose either mild or severe invasion may offer an obstacle to immediate diagnosis. As the height of the fever does not absolutely determine, or even indicate, the character of the subsequent course of the disease, but little importance is to be attached to the temperature unless there be a very marked elevation. A sudden rise frequently occurs with lymphadenitis. High fever in the beginning may render the diagnosis difficult or may postpone it.

The absence of glandular swelling does not exclude the diagnosis of diphtheria, for when the tonsils are affected by the disease there is usually little or no swelling of the neighboring glands. Swelling of the glands enables us to locate the affection in a mucous membrane richly endowed with lymphatic vessels. It is very marked when the nose is affected. A few hours' duration of nasal diphtheria suffices for the development of a severe lymphadenitis, especially at the angles of the jaw. When the latter condition is found to exist, the throat should be examined with the idea of finding a membrane extending upward; nasal diphtheria is very liable to complicate an affection of the uvula and arches of the palate. The membrane cannot well be seen by looking through the nostrils; highly serviceable for this purpose is a very short, broad rhinoscope reaching upward to the bony structure of the nose. However, nasal diphtheria may frequently be diagnosticated some days before the membrane becomes visible, by the rapid development of lymphadenitis; this may be done even where the sweetish, musty odor of certain forms [p. 691]of diphtheria is absent. Still, nasal diphtheria may occur without much lymphadenitis; as, for instance, when the blood-vessels are very numerous and superficial, and thereby give rise to slight hemorrhages at the very beginning of the sickness. In such cases the lymphatic vessels are little, if at all, required to transmit the poison, the open blood-vessels replacing them in the function of absorbing. Naturally, there are cases in which an ocular examination cannot be satisfactorily made. In the journals we read of brilliant results of rhinoscopic and laryngoscopic examination; in practice we see but few. This holds good especially for the cases of dyspnoea accompanying laryngeal diphtheria, where the diagnosis may be doubtful when no membrane can be detected in the fauces; even if membrane be observed there, symptoms of suffocation may still arise from a laryngeal stenosis independent of membranous deposits in the larynx. If aphonia and difficulty of both inspiration and expiration be present at the same time, there is certainly membranous occlusion. If aphonia appear late, or even toward the very last, and only inspiration be impeded while expiration is comparatively free, there is an oedematous saturation of the ary-epiglottidean folds and of their copious submucous tissue, and consequently of the posterior attachment of the vocal cords. Although a general oedema glottidis in connection with diphtheria is of exceedingly rare occurrence, the above condition is not at all uncommon, and has forced me to tracheotomize many times; but, again, a comprehension of the true condition, where it occurred in not very severe cases, has on several occasions enabled me to avoid an operation. This local oedema may sometimes be detected by palpation in the region of the swollen posterior wall of the pharynx.

One of the diagnostic symptoms of membranous laryngitis, believed in and referred to by Krönlein, does not exist—viz. the swelling of the lymphatic glands, which in his opinion is pathognomonic. Not only is that not the case, but the absence or scarcity of lymphatics on the vocal cords and in their neighborhood renders the absence of glandular swellings a necessity, provided the latter do not depend on complicating diphtheria in other localities. In uncomplicated diphtheritic laryngitis I expect no lymphadenitis. The character of the laryngeal pseudo-membrane does not depend at all on the condition of the pharynx. The latter may have membranes of any description or consistency without permitting the diagnosis of the condition of the larynx. I lay stress on this fact because no less a writer than Krönlein believes that where there is but little or no membrane in the pharynx, that in the larynx is rather loose and movable.

One of the diagnostic symptoms of diphtheritic laryngitis, or membranous croup, is the relative absence of fever. Catarrhal laryngitis, or pseudo-croup, is a feverish disease. A sudden attack of croup with high temperature, provided there is no pharyngeal or other diphtheria present, yields a good prognosis; without much fever, a very doubtful one.

The diagnosis of diphtheritic paralysis offers very little difficulty in most cases. Its occurrence after an attack of diphtheria, its beginning in the fauces or in the muscles controlled by the ciliary nerves, the immunity of the sphincters, the gradual development, the irregularity of its progress, are good diagnostic points. Examination by the interrupted or continuous current is not conclusive. Very frequently in the [p. 692]beginning the response to the interrupted current is normal, sometimes deficient; to the continuous current, exaggerated. After some time the power of both to excite contraction is diminished. When we reflect on the numerous causes which may underlie diphtheritic paralysis, and that we have not to deal with one and the same anatomical change in all cases, it becomes apparent that no reliable conclusions can be based upon electrical examination.

PROGNOSIS.—In general, the prognosis in diphtheria is favorable when the affected surface is of small extent and where such parts are the seat of disease as have little communication with the lymphatic system. To the latter class belongs simple diphtheria of the tonsils. Marked glandular swelling, particularly if arising suddenly, is always an unfavorable sign, and calls for the utmost caution in prognosis, especially if the region of the angles of the jaw be speedily and markedly infiltrated. This, as we have seen, is particularly apt to occur with nasal diphtheria, whether developed primarily, (and then accompanied by a thin fetid discharge), or, as is more commonly the case, secondarily from an affection of the pharynx and palate which ascends into the posterior nares. With the appropriate local disinfection this form of the disease is neither so alarmingly dangerous as Oertel depicts it, nor so assuredly fatal as Roger but a few years ago taught in his clinique, or as Kohts appears to believe,[38]yet it is ever grave. With energetic treatment many cases will, however, get well. Diphtheria of wounds, complicating diphtheria of the pharynx, is always an unfavorable sign; that of the mouth and angles of the mouth, associating itself with a previously existing diphtheria, having an indolent course, and producing more frequently a deep impregnation of the tissues than a thick deposit, causes a painful and serious condition. Diphtheria of the larynx, whether it be of primary origin or the result of extension from the fauces, is nearly always fatal. In severe epidemics the mortality is 95 per cent. Tracheotomy, too, saves but few of those who take the disease at such a time. In fifty consecutive tracheotomies from 1872 to 1874 I did not see one recovery. In the last few years I have seen few good results. In average epidemics tracheotomy will save 20 per cent. A pulse of 140 to 160, and high fever immediately after the operation, render the prognosis bad; so does absence of complete relief after the operation. An almost normal temperature the day after the operation is an agreeable symptom, but does not exclude a downward extension of the diphtheritic process, and hence cannot be looked upon as assuring a favorable prognosis. A marked elevation of temperature is apt to indicate a renewed attack of diphtheria or a rapidly-appearing pneumonia, and is an unfavorable symptom. A dry character of the respiratory murmur some time after tracheotomy indicates the approach of death within from twelve to twenty-four hours from descent of the membrane; so does cyanosis, whatever be its degree of intensity. Diphtheria of the trachea, which ascends to the larynx, is positively fatal. It has a rapid course, and tracheotomy only postpones the end for a little while, if at all. The general health and strength of the little sufferer have no influence whatever.

[38] Gerhardt, *Handb. d. Kinderkr.*, iii., 2, p. 20, 1878.

Thick, solid deposits need not of themselves render the prognosis so unfavorable as do septic and gangrenous forms. Even in the nose they [p. 693]are not of as serious import as the thin, putrid discharge. I have seen recovery ensue in cases where I was obliged to bore through the occluded nasal cavities with probes and scoops. Fetid, putrid discharges are unfavorable, but in no wise fatal; conscientious disinfection accomplishes a great deal. Slight epistaxis indicates the possibility of rapid absorption through the blood-vessels; but here, too, the final result depends on whether the disinfection be equally rapid and thorough. The same holds true for the sweetish, fetid odor of the breath, whether of the nose or mouth, which, on the one hand, demonstrates the significance of the disease, while, on the other hand, it indicates the possibility of infection by inhalation.

The height of the fever is not in proportion to the danger in any individual case; some have a favorable, some an unfavorable termination, without fever of any account. Simple catarrh of the pharynx and larynx frequently begins with a sudden and marked rise of temperature; diphtheria in the same parts but rarely. There are cases, however, in which the height of the fever and the deposited membranes are in inverse proportion to each other. In these cases the fever may subside rapidly, owing to a speedy elimination of the poison. Young children only are in danger of death from convulsions or a rapid tissue-degeneration due to hyperpyrexia. If the temperature rise suddenly after some days of sickness, either a complication or a fatal termination is to be apprehended. Yet, there are as many deaths in cases with comparatively low as with very high temperatures. Whether collapse has resulted rapidly or slowly, the patient dies often with low temperature. Thus, a rapid elevation is hardly a more unfavorable sign than a rapid fall. The pulse, too, may be very variable. True, a small, rapid, and irregular pulse is always unfavorable, because it indicates a weakening of the cardiac function; yet as long as it retains an approximately normal relation to the frequency of respiration a rapid pulse gives no cause for alarm. Moreover, the pulse is not always rapid when the strength gives way. It occasionally becomes slower, and sometimes very slow, and may then become a dangerous symptom.

Every complication adds to the danger. Bronchitis and pneumonia are not infrequent, yet I have seen cases of laryngeal diphtheria recover in which I had suspected pneumonia before performing tracheotomy, and was enabled to diagnosticate it after operating. Albuminuria in the early part of a diphtheritic attack with high fever is of little significance; nephritis, later in the course of the disease, partakes of the character of scarlatinous nephritis; cases of acute diffuse renal disease are fortunately infrequent, and the remainder are very submissive to treatment. The cases of diphtheria complicated with endocarditis in my practice have ended fatally. An early affection of the sensorium, not dependent on pressure upon the jugulars by greatly swollen glands, is an unfavorable symptom. Purpura, with profuse hemorrhages and a livid hue of the skin, is ominous; icteric discoloration, together with marked glandular and periglandular tumefaction, is absolutely fatal.

Most cases of diphtheria of the pharynx and of the tonsils have a favorable termination, yet a positive prognosis can in no case be given with certainty. Still, even in malignant epidemics the mortality is not very great, for even though there be a large number of severe cases in [p. 694]any one epidemic, yet it is greatly overbalanced by the number of moderately severe and mild ones. True, not a few cases end fatally in several days, owing to the high fever, or to septic absorption, or nephritis, or croup, but the majority of cases end in recovery in one or two weeks. Yet diphtheria does not always take so regular a course; not infrequently, after the pulse has become stronger, the appetite improved, and the pharynx cleared, and the patient is apparently on the high road to recovery, another attack occurs accompanied by fever, as before, and a rapid formation of membrane. Occasionally two or three such relapses may occur in the course of three, four, or five weeks; not to speak of the fact that those who have once suffered from diphtheria are more susceptible to the action of the poison than those who never suffered before.

TREATMENT.—Every case should be treated on general principles; thus, it is not possible to lay down a routine treatment for every individual case. High fever should be reduced by sponging and bathing, quinia, and sodium salicylate; collapse speedily treated, and severe reflex symptoms, as vomiting, etc., checked at once. Whether to employ for this purpose ether, wine, cognac, champagne, or coffee must be decided by the physician in individual cases. The administration of the remedy, whether by mouth, by injection into the bowels, or subcutaneously, as I have employed cognac, ether, alcohol, and camphor dissolved in ether or alcohol, in some cases with decided and rapid success, must depend on the condition of the organs and on the urgency of the case. However, all the above remedies are frequently of no service, because administered too late and in too small doses. If I have ever had cause to feel contented with the results of treatment in diphtheria, it is owing to the fact that I lost no time. No medicines, however, must be resorted to which are apt to derange the digestion of the patient; alcoholic stimulants must be given in fair dilution only, for that reason. The nourishment of the patient is a matter of very great importance. On general principles it is true that care must be taken in regard to food administered to febrile patients, but we must bear in mind that, when the lymphatic vessels are kept empty and no new and proper material is introduced into them, the absorption of locally-existing poisonous substances is proportionately increased. Hungry lymph-vessels are the organism's fiercest enemies.

I dwell particularly on the foregoing remarks for the reason that in diphtheria, unlike certain diseases having a typical course and those of a simple inflammatory character, expectant treatment should not be indulged in. Oertel's advice, that when neither high fever nor complications are present we should quietly wait, and "act only when new and most alarming symptoms present themselves," is decidedly perilous. A mild invasion does not assure a mild course. Never has a "possibly superfluous" tonic or stimulant done harm in diphtheria, but many a case has a sad termination because of a sudden change in the character of the disease, putting the bright hopes of the physician to shame. Only the philosopher may be a passive spectator; the physician must be a guardian. When I again read, in the work of the same meritorious author, "that when in exceptional cases, in children and young people, death is imminent, not from suffocating symptoms in the larynx and trachea, but from septic disease and blood-poisoning, it is necessary to resort to [p. 695]powerful stimulants," it strikes me that he is frequently too dilatory with his remedies, and, furthermore, that his experience concerning the terrible septic form of diphtheria which is so frequently met with in some epidemics must have been very limited at the time he was writing. In New York, during the past twenty-five years, for every death from diphtheritic laryngeal stenosis (membranous croup) there have been three from diphtheritic sepsis or from exhaustion.[39]

[39] We have to improve somewhat on the plan of Thomas Wilson, though his general instructions be good (as laid down in his *Tentamen medicum inaugurale de cynanche maliqna*, Edinb., 1790, p. 24): "Cum hactenus nullum inventum est remedium quod contagionem in corpus receptam suffocare possit; cum medicamenta pleraque quæ putredinem corrigere dicuntur, corpus ejusque functiones manifesto roborant; et denique cum hunc morbum comitantur virium prostratio, et, etiam ab initio, summa functionum debilitas, qualis evacuantia omnigena prohibet, indicationem curandi unicam, scil. debilitatis effectibus obviam ire, proponam. Hinc corporis conditioni obviam itur præcipue tonica et stimulantia administrando." (As no remedy has yet been found which can extinguish the contagion after it has been received into the body; as most medicines which have the reputation of correcting putrefaction are roborants for the body and its functions; and, lastly, as this disease is attended with great prostration and such debility of functions as to preclude the use of all sorts of evacuants,—I propose but this one indication for treatment—viz. to meet the effects of debility. This is fulfilled by the administration mainly of tonics and stimulants.)

In regard to the dose of stimulants, it is a fact that there is more danger in diphtheria from giving too little than too much. When the pulse barely begins to be small and frequent they must be administered at once. A three-year-old child can comfortably take thirty to one hundred and fifty grammes (fl. oz. j-v) of cognac, or one to five grammes of carbonate of ammonium, or a gramme of musk or camphor (gr. xv) and more, in twenty-four hours. In the septic form especially the intoxicating action of alcohol is out of the question; the pulse becomes stronger and slower, and the patient enjoys rest. In those cases in which the pulse is slow, together with a weak heart's action, the dose can hardly be too large. The fear of a bold administration of stimulants will vanish, as does that of the use of large doses of opium in peritonitis, of quinia in pneumonia, or of iodide of potassium in meningitis or syphilis. I know that cases of young children with general sepsis commenced immediately to improve when their one hundred grammes (fl. oz. iij) of brandy were increased to four times that amount in a day.

The remarks I have made in reference to the general treatment of diphtheria naturally render superfluous a discussion of the value of abstraction of blood. To be sure, it could only be a question of local bleeding. For nobody would dare to resort to jugular venesection, as our predecessors did in the last century. It may be safely asserted of the latter that it has no influence on the process, but frequently increases the local swelling and makes the patient more anæmic. There is no case in which a resort to it would not be criminal. I can distinctly recall the time when bleeding and calomel formed the groundwork of the treatment. Until the year 1862 the death-rate in Rupert, Vermont, from diphtheria was 90 per cent., according to the reports of the local physicians, and particularly of my pupil, Dr. Guild, who at that time finished his studies in New York and commenced practising. When, in the same epidemic, bleeding and calomel were replaced by stimulants and iron, with the chlorate of potassium, 90 per cent. recovered.

That attention must be paid to the general condition mainly during a[p. 696]retarded convalescence from previous sickness is self-evident. Any complications, too, must be subjected to early treatment. Diarrhoea must be mentioned among these; it reduces the patient's strength very quickly; likewise, the early appearing nephritis, which may suddenly end life.

In this connection I must allude to the great danger of self-infection, which may occur in every variety of cases, severe or mild. The poison is diffused by expiration and expectoration. Though care may have been taken to disinfect the linen, towels, handkerchiefs, the bedstead and bedding, chairs and wall-papers, and carpets and curtains, even the clothing of the attendants will be infected. While the patient is getting well he will be infected again, and have a more serious relapse; and a third one, and succumb. I have met with such cases often, and with some which went from one attack into another, and would certainly have perished but for their removal to a distant part of the town. Where there are vacant rooms the indication is to change rooms every few days and to thoroughly disinfect (with sulphurous acid) that which has been used and infected.

One important axiom must be borne in mind—namely, that prevention is easier than cure. I do not refer simply to the removal of the healthy members of the family beyond the danger of infection or to the isolation of the patient. If the latter becomes necessary, the first indication is his removal to the top floor of the house. There are, in addition, however, certain prophylactic measures which will prove valuable in the hands of every good physician. It is necessary under all circumstances that the mouth and pharynx of every child be constantly kept in a healthy condition. Eruptions of the scalp must be treated at once, and glandular swellings of the neck caused to disappear. Some cases of laryngeal diphtheria have been traced directly to the presence of suppurating bronchial glands, with or without perforation.[40] The same rule applies to nasal and pharyngeal catarrhs, the treatment of which should be commenced in warm seasons, when general or local remedies yield better results. Enlarged tonsils should be resected, or, where that can not be done, scraped out with Simon's spoon, at a time when no diphtheritic epidemic is raging. It is important that this take place at a time when, even though sporadic cases of diphtheria occur, the danger of infection is not great; for during the height of an epidemic every wound will give rise to general or local infection. This holds good for any part of the body as well as of the mouth. I avoid, therefore, an operation at such a time, provided it can be postponed.

[40] Weigert, in *Virch. Arch.*, vol. lxxvii., p. 294, 1879.

Prevention, after all, is not the business of the physician only, but just as much that of the individual or the complex of individuals—viz. the town, the state, and the nation. Those sick with diphtheria must be isolated, though the case appear ever so mild, and, if possible, the other children must be sent out of the house altogether. If that be impossible, let them remain outside the house, in the open air, as long as feasible, with open bedroom windows during the night, in the most distant part of the house, and let their throats, and those of their nurses, be examined every day. The watching eye of a father or mother will discover deviations from the norm, so that the physician can be notified. Let the temperatures [p. 697]of the well children be taken once a day, toward evening. Ten minutes of a mother's time are well paid by the discovery of a slight anomaly which may require the attention of the physician. Happily, there are now many mothers who keep and value a self-registering thermometer as an important addition to their household articles. The attendant upon a case of diphtheria must not get in contact with the rest of the family, particularly the children, after his visiting and handling the patient, for the poison may be carried, though the carrier remain well or apparently well. Unnecessary petting of the patient on the part of the well ought to be avoided, and kissing must be forbidden; the bed-clothing and linen should be changed often and disinfected, the air of the sick-chamber should be cool and often changed, and if possible the chamber itself should be changed every few days.

The well or apparently well children of a family that has diphtheria at home must not go to school nor to church. The former necessity is beginning to be recognized by the authorities and teachers, and also, in consequence of partially enforced habit, by parents; the latter will be resisted longer. Schools ought to be closed entirely when a number of cases have occurred. Even when the school-children have not been affected to a great extent, but an epidemic of diphtheria has commenced in earnest, it will be better to close the schools for a time. If that be not advisable, the teacher ought to be taught to examine throats, and directed to examine every child's throat each morning, and to send home every one with even suspicious appearances.

In times of an epidemic every public place, theatre, ball-room, dining-hall, or tavern ought to be subjected to supervision. Where there is a large conflux of people there are certainly many who carry the disease with them. Disinfection must be enforced by the authorities at regular intervals. Public vehicles must be treated in the same manner. That it should be so when a case of small-pox has happened to be carried in them appears quite natural. Hardly a livery-stable keeper would be found who would not be anxious to destroy the possibility of infection in any of his coaches. He must learn that diphtheria is, or may be, as dangerous a passenger as variola. And what is valid in the case of a poor hack is more so in that of railroad-cars, whether emigrant or Pullman. They ought to be thoroughly disinfected in times of an epidemic, at regular intervals, for the highroads of travel have always been those of epidemic diseases, and railroad officers and their families have often been the first victims of the imported scourge. Can that be accomplished? Will not railroad companies resist a plan of regular disinfection because of its expensiveness? Will there not be an outcry against this as despotic and as a violation of the rights of the citizen? Certainly there will be. But so there was also when municipal authorities began to compel parents to keep their children at home when they had contagious diseases in the family, and when a small-pox patient was arrested because of endangering the passengers in a public vehicle. In such cases it is not society that tyrannizes the individual; it is the individual that endangers society. And society begins at last, even in America, to believe in the rights of the commonwealth, and not in the rights of the democratic person only. The establishment of State and National Boards of Health proves that the narrow-hearted theories of the strict constructionists [p. 698]have not only disappeared from our politics, but also from the conscience and intellect of society.

The sick room must be kept cool, the windows kept open—more or less—by night as well as by day, the floor frequently washed, the linen soaked at once, the excrements removed. Dead bodies ought to be kept moist, for infectious material, chemical or otherwise, will spread more easily when dry. Attendants must not talk unnecessarily over the mouth or diphtheritic wounds of the patient, and will do well to carry a little dry loose cotton—to be changed often—in each of the nostrils, for it aids in protecting those who are necessarily exposed to infection.[41]

[41] Wernich, in *F. Cohn's Beitr.*, iii., 1859, p. 115.

A very important mode of prevention consists in disinfection. The experiments of Schotte and Gaertner, and of Sternberg, prove the inefficiency of small doses of most of the disinfectants in common use. The popular idea, sometimes even shared by physicians, that the faint odor of chloride of lime or of carbolic acid in a sick room or in a foul privy is evidence that the place is disinfected, is entirely erroneous. Particularly in regard to the latter agent, it may be stated at once that its employment for disinfecting purposes on a large scale is impracticable, both on account of the expensiveness of the pure acid and the enormous quantities required to produce the desired effect. For in regard to its efficiency it does not rank very high in comparison with a great many other articles, as may be seen from a table of the disinfectant properties of different chemicals published by Miquel in the *Semaine Médicale*.

For practical purposes I know of no better or simpler rules for disinfection than those published by the National Board of Health. In its *Bulletin* No. 10, of September 6, 1879, the following instructions for disinfection were published: Deodorizers, or substances which destroy smells, are not necessarily disinfectants, and disinfectants do not necessarily have an odor.

"Disinfection cannot compensate for want of cleanliness nor of ventilation.

"I. Disinfectants to be employed:

"1. Roll-sulphur (brimstone) for fumigation.

"2. Sulphate of iron (copperas) dissolved in water in the proportion of one and a half pounds to the gallon; for soil, sewers, etc.

"3. Sulphate of zinc and common salt, dissolved together in water in the proportion of four ounces sulphate and two ounces salt to the gallon; for clothing, bed-linen, etc."

Carbolic acid is not included in the above list, for the following reasons: It is very difficult to determine the quality of the commercial article, and the purchaser can never be certain of securing it of proper strength; it is expensive when of good quality, and experience has shown that it must be employed in comparatively large quantities to be of any use; it is liable by its strong odor to give a false sense of security.

"II. How to use disinfectants:

"1. In the sick-room.—The most available agents are fresh air and cleanliness. The clothing, towels, bed-linen, etc. should, on removal from the patient and before they are taken from the room, be placed in a pail or tub of the zinc solution, boiling hot if possible.

"All discharges should either be received in vessels containing copperas[p. 699]solution, or, when this is impracticable, should be immediately covered with copperas solution. All vessels used about the patient should be cleansed with the same solution.

"Unnecessary furniture—especially that which is stuffed—carpets and hangings, should, when possible, be removed from the room at the outset; otherwise they should remain for subsequent fumigation and treatment.

"2. Fumigation with sulphur is the only practical method for disinfecting the house. For this purpose the rooms to be disinfected must be vacated. Heavy clothing, blankets, bedding, and other articles which cannot be treated with zinc solution should be opened and exposed during fumigation, as directed below. Close the rooms as tightly as possible, place the sulphur in iron pans supported upon bricks placed in wash-tubs containing a little water, set it on fire by hot coals or with the aid of a spoonful of alcohol, and allow the room to remain closed for twenty-four hours. For a room about ten feet square at least two pounds of sulphur should be used; for larger rooms proportionately increased quantities.

"3. Premises.—Cellars, yards, stables, gutters, privies, cesspools, water-closets, drains, sewers, etc. should be frequently and liberally treated with copperas solution. The copperas solution is easily prepared by hanging a basket containing about sixty pounds of copperas in a barrel of water.

"4. Body- and bed-clothing, etc.—It is best to burn all articles which have been in contact with persons sick with contagious or infectious diseases. Articles too valuable to be destroyed should be treated as follows:

"A. Cotton, linen, flannel, blankets, etc. should be treated with the boiling-hot zinc solution; introduce piece by piece; secure thorough wetting, and boil for at least half an hour.

"B. Heavy woollen clothing, silks, furs, stuffed bed-covers, beds, and other articles which cannot be treated with the zinc solution, should be hung in the room during fumigation, their surfaces thoroughly exposed and pockets turned inside out. Afterward, they should be hung in the open air, beaten, and shaken. Pillows, beds, stuffed mattresses, upholstered furniture, etc. should be cut open, the contents spread out, and thoroughly fumigated. Carpets are best fumigated on the floor, but should afterward be removed to the open air and thoroughly beaten.

"5. Corpses should be thoroughly washed with a zinc solution of double strength; should then be wrapped in a sheet wet with the zinc solution, and buried at once. Metallic, metal-lined, or air-tight coffins should be used when possible; certainly when the body is to be transported for any considerable distance.

"It might have been added here that no public funeral must be permitted."

In this connection I have to speak of a remedy which I class among the prophylactic agents—namely, the chlorate of potassium or the chlorate of sodium. I cannot say that I rely on either of these remedies as curative agents in diphtheria, and yet I employ them in almost every case. The reason lies in the fact that the chlorate is useful in most cases of stomatitis, and thereby acts as a preventive.

There are very few cases of diphtheria which do not exhibit larger surfaces of either pharyngitis or stomatitis than of diphtheritic membrane. There are also a number of cases of stomatitis and pharyngitis, [p. 700]during every epidemic of diphtheria, which must be referred to the epidemic, sometimes as kindred diseases, and sometimes as introductory stages only, which, however, do not, or do not in the beginning, show the characteristic symptoms of the disease.

When, in 1860,[42] I wrote my first paper on diphtheria, I based it upon two hundred genuine cases, and at the same time enumerated one hundred and eighty-five cases of pharyngitis, which I considered to be brought on by epidemic influences, but which, the membrane being absent, could not be classified as bonâ fide cases of diphtheria.

[42] *Amer. Med. Times*, Aug. 11th and 18th.

Such cases of pharyngitis and stomatitis, no matter whether influenced by an epidemic or not, furnish the indication for the use of chlorate of potassium. They will usually get well with this treatment alone. The cases of genuine diphtheria, complicated with a great deal of stomatitis and pharyngitis, also indicate the use of chlorate of potassium; not, however, as a remedy for the diphtheria, but as a remedy for the accompanying catarrhal condition in the neighborhood of the diphtheritic exudation. For it is a fact that, as long as the parts in the neighborhood of the diphtheritic exudation are in a healthy condition, there is but little danger of the disease spreading over the surface. Whenever the neighboring surface is affected with catarrh or inflammation, or injured so that the epithelium gets loose or thrown off, the diphtheritic exudation will spread within a very short time. Thus chlorate of potassium or sodium, the latter of which is more soluble and more easily digested than the former, will act as a preventive rather than as a curative remedy. Therefore it is that common cases of pharyngeal diphtheria will recover under this treatment alone; and these are the cases which have given its reputation to chlorate of potassium as a remedy for diphtheria.

The dose of chlorate of potassium for a child two or three years old should not be larger than half a drachm (2 grammes) in twenty-four hours. A baby of one year or less should not take more than one scruple (1.25 grammes) a day. The dose for an adult should not be more than a drachm and a half, or at most two drachms (6 or 8 grammes), in the course of twenty-four hours.

The effect of the chlorate of potassium is partly a general and partly a local one. The general effect may be obtained by the use of occasional larger doses, but it is better not to strain the eliminating powers of the system. The local effect, however, cannot be obtained with occasional doses, but only by doses so frequently repeated that the remedy is in almost constant contact with the diseased surface. Thus, the doses, to produce the local effect, should be very small, but frequently administered. It is better that the daily quantity of twenty grains should be given in fifty or sixty doses than in eight or ten; that is, the solution should be weak, and a drachm or half a drachm of such solution can be given every hour or every half hour or every fifteen or twenty minutes, care being taken that no water or other drink is given soon after the remedy has been administered, for obvious reasons.

I have referred to these facts with so much emphasis because of late an attempt has been made to introduce chlorate of potassium as the main remedy in bad cases of diphtheria, and, what is worse, in large doses (Seeligmüller, Sachse, L. Weigert, C. Küster, Edlefsen.)

[p. 701]Large doses of chlorate of potassium (2 drachms daily to an adult I claim to be a large dose, particularly when its use is persisted in for many days in succession) are dangerous. In several of my writings I have given instances of its fatal effects.[43] I have seen fatal cases since, and scores have been published in different journals. The first effects of a moderately large dose are gastric and, more especially, renal irritation; the latter it was which I experienced when I took half an ounce twenty-five years ago. Fountain of Davenport, Iowa, experienced the same before more serious symptoms developed, of which he died.[44] The symptoms are those of acute diffuse nephritis, with suppression of urine, or scanty secretion of a little black blood, and uræmia deepening toward death in fatal cases. My earlier cases I considered as primary diffuse nephritis, and I have even been inclined to attribute the frequent appearance of chronic nephritis, amongst all classes and ages, in part to the influence of the chlorates, which have become a popular domestic remedy and are found in every household. But the experimental researches of Marchand[45] and others prove that, at least in many instances, the extensive destruction of blood-cells is the first and immediate result of the introduction into the circulation of the chlorate, and that the visceral changes are due to embolic processes.

[43] *C. Gerhardt's Handbuch der Kinderkrankheiten*, vol. ii., 1876; *Med. Record*, March, 1879; *Treatise on Diphtheria*, 1880.

[44] Stillé, *Therap. and Mat. Med.*, 2d ed., 1874, p. 922.

[45] *Sitzungsber. d. Naturforsch. Ges. h. u. Halle*, Feb. 8, 1879, and *Virch. Arch.*, vol. lxxvii.

Special Treatment.—The first axiom in the treatment of diphtheria is that there is no specific; the second, that in no other disease the individualizing powers of the physician are tested more severely.

The treatment is both internal and external. The local remedies are either such as dissolve the mucous membrane, or such as thoroughly modify the mucous membrane from which the pseudo-membrane has been removed, or real antiseptics, with the power of destroying either chemical or parasitic poisons.

The number of remedies recommended in diphtheria is immense. No other proof of its dangerous nature is needed. In the following I shall review those which I consider it worth while either to reject or to recommend.

Steam is used partly to soften the membranes, but principally to increase the secretion from the mucous membrane, and thereby throw off the superjacent membrane. This can be done to advantage only where there is a natural tendency to it; that is, where there are a great many muciparous follicles under a cylindrical or fimbriated epithelium. This is the condition on part of the pharynx, but not on the tonsils; and in a small portion of the larynx, in the trachea and bronchi, but not on the vocal cords. Wherever there is pavement epithelium on the normal surface, and where the membrane is imbedded into the tissue, steam can hardly be expected to do good. In the other cases it will. Thus, the locality of the diphtheritic process determines to a great extent whether steam is indicated or not. If it be used, the necessity of a full supply of atmospheric air must not be disregarded. Steam, with an overheated room and without pure air, is liable to be as injurious as steam in pure air is beneficial in a number of cases.

[p. 702]There can be no better proof for the necessity of individualizing, and the impossibility of treating all cases alike, than the fact that many will do well under steam treatment, and others are certainly injured by it. I have repeatedly had the joy of seeing children with croup become less cyanotic after their removal from an atmosphere of vapor, and I can readily see that pure atmospheric air would be more agreeable and wholesome to a child with stenosis of the larynx than an atmosphere laden with steam. Of course this remark does not apply to cases of pseudo-croup and bronchitis, which are generally benefited by a warm, moist atmosphere. Those, however, who deem it judicious to employ steam as a vehicle for carbolic acid, salicylic acid, chloride of sodium, chlorate of potassium, or lime, had best resort to the atomizer for applying these remedies. It can be used without trouble; most children are sufficiently intelligent to allow the spray to be directed upon the fauces and larynx every ten or fifteen minutes in case of necessity. When it is deemed advisable to administer steam, I warn against the use of gas stoves. They require a great deal more oxygen than an alcohol lamp, which ought to be preferred when a stove or slaking lime or hot iron or bricks immersed in water are not available.

Water may be made serviceable in different ways. Its effect on the skin, when taken in large quantities, under normal or abnormal circumstances, is a matter of daily experience. Copious perspiration is its immediate result. The very same effect is produced on the mucous membranes. In diphtheria, besides professional hydropathists, I know of but one[46] who favors the plentiful use of water, 100-200 grammes (3-6 ounces) every hour or oftener, either by itself or mixed with an alcoholic beverage.

[46] C. Rauchfuss, in *C. Gerhardt's Handb. d. Kinderkr.*, iii. 2, 1878.

Severe inflammatory symptoms, such as redness of the throat, great pain, swelling of the glands, require cold applications, either an ice-bag or ice-cold cloths well pressed out and frequently changed. They must, however, be placed where they can do most good—in laryngeal diphtheria around the neck, in pharyngeal diphtheria with glandular swelling over the affected part. In the latter, therefore, the flannel cloth which covers the whole of the application must be tied over the head, and not behind. When ice-bags are used, care is to be taken lest they should be too large; if so, they will not affect the desired spot at all. Small pieces of ice frequently swallowed are greatly relished by the patient; water-ices in small quantities will render the same service; ice-cream, in half-teaspoon or teaspoon doses every five or ten minutes, adds to the necessary nutriment. When the fever is high and the surface hot, sponging with tepid or cold water, or water and alcohol, will mitigate both. For the cold bath or the cold partial pack (trunk and upper part of the thighs) the general indications hold good. As a rule, I favor the latter, for many cases have such a tendency to debility and collapse that sometimes the circulation of the surface of the body is badly interfered with by cold bathing. Therefore, a contraindication to cold bathing must be found at once in cold feet, either before or after a bath. When, unfortunately, the feet do not recover their normal temperature in a very short time, they ought to be warmed artificially, and the cold bath not repeated. In such cases the cold pack, however, is still indicated. A linen or cotton cloth, [p. 703]large enough to cover the trunk and half of the thighs, is dipped in cold water, well pressed out, and the body of the patient wrapped tightly in it. The arms remain outside; the whole body is then wrapped up in a blanket; the feet may be warmed meanwhile when necessary, and the cold pack repeated as often as required to reduce the temperature—viz. once every five minutes, every half hour, every hour.

The contraindications to the use of cold have in part been alluded to. Very young infants bear it but to a limited extent. The beginning of recovery contraindicates it, unless for some local cause; for instance, an inflamed gland. The extensive use of cold water or ice is also forbidden when there is no fever, where there is perhaps an abnormally low temperature, where we have to deal with the septic or gangrenous form of diphtheria, where the vitality is low and the mucous membranes pale or even cyanotic. In such cases, on the contrary, while unlimited internal stimulation is required, the hot bath, or hot pack and hot injections into the bowel, will be found beneficial.

Lime-water, glycerine, lactic acid, pepsin, neurin, papayotin, chinolin, and pilocarpine are all solvents of pseudo-membrane, but whether there is sufficient time and opportunity to produce a curative effect by every one of them is a question open for discussion. Of lime-water and glycerine I have employed a mixture of equal parts in considerably more than a hundred cases after the completion of tracheotomy, directing the remedy through an atomizer into and below the canula, but cannot say that the descent of the membrane into the trachea or bronchi was prevented by it. Lime-water may be used in the nose and throat as an injection, spray, or gargle, but its solvent effect is greatly diminished by the action of the carbonic acid of the breath on the lime. I have no doubt that if water alone was used with the same persistence as lime-water, its effects would be nearly the same. Still, what little effect the minute dose of lime (1:800) in the lime-water may have may just as well be utilized. What I object to is the omission of more powerful agents. If lime is to be used, slaking lime frequently in the presence of the patient is attended with vastly more benefit, inasmuch as by that proceeding a large amount of powdered lime is projected into the air of the room and the mouth and respiratory organs.

Lactic acid also, in from ten to twenty-five parts of water, has yielded no better results in my hands. Those cases of tracheotomy which I afterward treated with lactic acid spray terminated no better than such as were treated with lime-water and glycerine. Of the solvent effect of pepsin I have not been able to convince myself so as to recommend it. The accounts of neurin have not encouraged me to try it at all. Chinolin (tartrate) has been used locally by O. Seifert,[47] Müller, and others. It is said to remove the membranes and relieve the fever. For a gargle it is dissolved in five hundred parts of water, or it is mixed with ten parts of water and alcohol each, and applied by means of a sponge. To relieve the burning sensation ice is swallowed afterward. The local applications of alcohol have the same drawback. There are but few patients who do not suffer intensely from its local contact.

[47] *Berl. klin. Woch.*, Nos. 36, 37, 1883.

Papayotin has been recommended by Rossbach for the purpose of dissolving membranes in a one-half per cent. solution. It peptonizes[p. 704]albuminoids, and macerates meat, intestinal worms, and croup membranes in both neutral and feebly alkaline solution. In concentrated solutions it has a caustic effect. It is recommended, not as an anti-diphtheritic, but merely as a solvent remedy.[48] Whatever reliance may have been placed upon it has, however, been jeopardized by Rossbach's remarks[49] on the variability of the preparations in the market. Not only are the specimens very unequal, but each of them is variable, easily spoiled, and particularly affected by moisture.

[48] *Berl. klin. Woch.*, March 10, 1881.

[49] *Transactions of the Congress for Int. Medicine*, 1883, p. 162.

Muriate of pilocarpine was recommended for this purpose three years ago. It was praised by Juttmann as a specific, and has failed. The quackish recommendations of the drug have, indeed, earned for it a certain amount of distrust which it does not deserve in all cases. It is expected to increase the secretion of the mucous membranes to such an extent as to float the pseudo-membranes. It sometimes succeeds in so doing, but only in those cases in which the membrane is deposited upon the mucous membranes. When the tissue is impregnated the drug fails. It also fails in septic cases, and mostly for the reason that it diminishes and paralyzes the heart's action. It ought, therefore, never to be given unaccompanied with large amounts of stimulants. Where the patient is strong, and the heart healthy, it may be tried; I know that a few cases of moderate laryngeal diphtheria improved with pilocarpine, steam, and turpentine inhalations. The dose is 1/30 grain, dissolved in water, every hour.

Turpentine inhalations were recommended by C. Edel.[50] Fifteen drops of oil of turpentine are inhaled from a common inhalation apparatus, which is placed at a distance of three inches from the mouth of the patient, for a period of ten minutes every hour. He claims recoveries in from twelve to forty-eight hours. I allow the patient to remain in his bed, and keep water boiling constantly on an alcohol lamp, on the stove, or over the gas. A tablespoonful of turpentine, more or less, is poured on the water, care being taken that nothing is spilled in the fire. Thus the room is constantly filled with a penetrating odor of turpentine, which is not at all disagreeable, even when in great concentration. The effects are very satisfactory indeed. Where circumstances allowed or required it I have raised a tent over the bed, large enough not to give inconvenience to the patient and to admit either the whole apparatus or the tube containing the mixed vapor of water and turpentine.

[50] *Med. Rev.*, Jan. 19, 1878.

Ammonium chloride may sometimes be used to advantage for its softening and liquefying effects. Its internal administration in bronchial and tracheo-laryngeal catarrh is so old that it has several times been obsolete. Of late, more stimulant effects have been attributed to it than it actually possesses. But its liquefying action, in cases where the secretion of mucus is defective and expectoration scanty and viscid, is undoubted. Thus it proves valuable in many cases of simple catarrh, both when administered internally and inhaled. The latter mode I have often resorted to, and believe that its macerating influence has been of service to me in cases of laryngeal diphtheria. Half a teaspoonful of the pure salt is spread on the stove or burned over alcohol [p. 705]or gas. It evaporates immediately, and fills the room or the tent with a white cloud, which, when dense, excites coughing. But it does not irritate to any uncomfortable degree, and the process may be repeated in an interval of an hour or more.

Not all cases of diphtheria are septic or gangrenous, nor are all the cases occurring during an epidemic of the same type. Some have the well-pronounced character of a local disease, either on the tonsils or in the larynx. The cases of sporadic croup met with in the intervals between epidemics present few constitutional symptoms, and assume more the nature of an active inflammatory disease—very much like the sporadic cases of fibrinous tracheo-bronchitis. These are the cases in which mercury deserves to have friends, apologists, and even eulogists. Calomel, 0.5-0.75 gramme (gr. viij-xij), divided into thirty or forty doses, of which one is taken every half hour, is apt to produce a constitutional effect very soon. Such doses, with minute doses, a milligramme or more (gr. 1/60), of tartar emetic, or ten or twenty times that amount of oxysulphuret of antimony, have served me well in fibrinous tracheo-bronchitis. But the mucous membrane of the trachea and bronchi is more apt to submit to such liquefying and macerating treatment than the vocal cords. The latter have no muciparous glands like the former, in which they are very copious. And while the tracheal membrane, even though recent, is apt to be thrown out of a tracheal incision at once, the pseudo-membrane of the vocal cords takes from six days to sixteen or more for complete removal. Still, a certain effect may even here be accomplished, for maceration does not depend only on the local secretion of the muciparous glands, but on the total secretion of the surface, which will be in constant contact with the whole respiratory tract. Thus, either on theoretical principles or on the ground of actual experience, men of learning and judgment have used mercury in such cases as I detailed above, with a certain confidence.

If ever mercury is expected to do any good in cases of suffocation by membrane, it must be made to act promptly. That is what the blue ointment does not. In its place I recommend the oleate, of which ten or twelve drops may be rubbed into the skin along the inside of the forearms or thighs (or anywhere when their surface becomes irritated) every hour or two hours. Or broken doses will be useful, such as given above, or hypodermic injections of corrosive sublimate in ½ or 1 per cent. solution in distilled water, four or five drops from four to six times a day, or more, either by itself or in combination with the extensive use of the oleate, or with calomel internally. Lately, the cyanide of mercury has been recommended very strongly. I hardly believe that it will work more wonders than any other equally soluble preparation. Within the past few years the internal administration of bichloride of mercury has been resorted to more frequently and with greater success than ever before. My own recent experience with it has been encouraging, and so has that of some of my friends. Wm. Pepper[51] gave 1/32 grain of corrosive sublimate every two hours in a bad form of diphtheritic croup, with favorable result. But in this very bad case, desperate though it was—child of five years, resp. 70, pulse 160—large membranes, "evidently from the larynx," had been expelled before the treatment was commenced on the [p. 706]seventh day of the disease. The remedy ought to be given in solution of 1:5000, and in good doses. A baby a year old may take one-half grain every day for many days in succession, with very little if any intestinal disorder and with no stomatitis.[52] A solution of the corrosive chloride of mercury in water is frequently employed of late as a disinfectant. It acts as such in a dilution of 1:20,000. As healthy mucous membranes bear quite well a proportion of 1:2000-3000, any strength between these extremes maybe utilized. A grain of the sublimate in a pint or more of water, with a drachm of table-salt, will be found both mild and efficient. As a gargle or nasal injection it will be found equally good. But it has appeared to me that frequent applications give rise to a copious mucous discharge; hourly injections into a diphtheritic vagina became quite obnoxious by such over-secretion, which ceased at once when the injections were discontinued. Thus, when it is desirable not only to disinfect but also to cleanse the diseased surface, the injections with corrosive sublimate appear to yield a result inferior to less irritating applications.

[51] *Trans. Am. Med. Ass.*, 1881.
[52] *Med. Record*, May 24, 1884.

Chloride of iron is undoubtedly a valuable remedy in diphtheria, but in its administration it must by no means be forgotten that small doses at long intervals are out of the question. I have not the least doubt but that the failure of the remedy may be attributed in most cases to the fact that the doses were too small and administered too seldom. A dose of from five to fifteen drops, properly diluted, every fifteen minutes, half hour, or hour is indispensable for a proper estimation of its effects. Gargles are not of much service, for the simple reason that they do not come into sufficient contact with the affected parts, and reach at the utmost to the anterior pillars of the soft palate. A direct application of the remedy to the mucous membrane of the pharynx may also be desisted from, thereby avoiding any irritation, the internal administration at short intervals causing the pharynx to be sufficiently influenced by local contact with the remedy. It must, of course, not be expected that the chloride will remove the membrane, but it can frequently be seen to reduce the hyperæmia and swelling and prevent the reproduction of exuded material. The chloride of iron exerts a decided influence on the vital contractility of the blood-vessels. This increased contractility certainly assists in diminishing the rapidity of absorption of putrid fluids through the blood-vessels, which constitutes the principal source of danger from the disease.

It cannot yet be positively asserted that the chloride of iron exerts a direct effect on the lymphatic vessels. Naturally, this was claimed when the remedy was recommended, in the treatment of diphtheria, on account of its therapeutic effects in erysipelas, with the accompanying inflammation of the lymphatic vessels of the skin. Although we know of no direct compression of the lymphatic vessels due to the action of the chloride, yet it may be assumed that perhaps the compression of the blood-vessels exerts a similar influence upon the neighboring lymphatics. In consequence of this there would be an impediment to the absorption and further development of poisonous substances in the lymph. The chloride, like the sulphate of iron, is a tolerably powerful disinfecting agent. If this observation be correct, it may go very far toward explaining the action [p. 707]of the chloride of iron in septic diseases, which are accompanied by an exalted activity of the lymphatic vessels and an increase of the white blood-corpuscles. Furthermore, Saase has endeavored to show that the ferrous salts possess the power of converting oxygen into ozone. They share this power with the blood-globules exclusively, and could hence, to a certain degree, supply a deficiency of the latter. Pokrowsky, too, has shown that iron increases the process of oxidation in the body by demonstrating that in health there is an elevation of temperature and an increase of the percentage of urea in the urine during its administration. In anæmic persons, to whom iron has been given for the purpose of increasing the amount of blood, the above phenomena may be observed before this object is accomplished. Thus iron appears to replace the blood-corpuscles to a certain extent. Now, in infectious disorders of the blood, where the red globules are perpetually menaced with destruction, it seems plausible that the preparations of iron should exert an antiseptic action.

Finally, it has been found that of all the preparations of iron the chloride possesses the greatest power of stimulating the nervous system. Possibly this effect may be traced to an increase of the arterial pressure in the nerve-centres. It has been said that this effect has been vividly illustrated in certain forms of chlorosis. If this be true, iron would be all the more indicated in diphtheria, since it would act as a prophylactic against a series of nervous phenomena that so frequently present themselves, both during and subsequently to the diphtheritic process. Thus it is that for many years the muriate of iron has constituted the main element, with me, of internal medication in most cases of diphtheria, both of the mild and the most dangerous septic type. A common formula is, for a child of two years,

x. Tinct. Ferri Chloridi m ij; drach

Potass. Chlorat. xx; gr.

Aquæ v; fl. oz.

Glycerin. Pur. j. fl. oz. M.

S. A teaspoonful every fifteen, twenty, or thirty minutes.

Carbolic acid exerts a powerful influence on the vitality of all living elements, and hence also on rapidly proliferating epithelium, which constitutes a part of the diphtheritic membrane. It is of great advantage for local use. Its local effect, undiluted or diluted with equal or larger parts of glycerine or alcohol, in shrinking and removing membranes, is sometimes very useful; in mild solutions in water (½, 1, or 2 per cent.) it is very efficient in nasal injections or for external applications or mouth-washes. Rothe's prescription for external use is carbolic acid and alcohol each 2 parts, water 10, tincture of iodine 1. Its internal administration to the extent of five to twenty grains daily, given largely diluted, in small and frequent doses, is of less positive value.

Salicylic acid, in a solution of 1:30-50, is caustic. A milder solution, 1:200-300 relieves or removes foul odor from the nose or throat, but it does not detach membranes or shorten the duration of the disease, apparently. Internally, it acts no longer as a disinfectant, but is changed into a salicylate and is an antipyretic. It is then better to replace it by the sodium salicylate. With its administration (for a child of 2 years 3 grains every hour until 20 or 25 grains are taken) it ought not to be [p. 708]forgotten that serious brain troubles, collapse, and irregular and paralytic breathing, as well as gastric and intestinal disturbances, may follow its use. It ought not to be given without careful watching and the simultaneous free use of alcoholic stimulants.

Binz found, as the result of experiments with solutions of pure quinia varying from one part in a hundred to one in a thousand, that the latter sufficed to prevent the development of bacteria in fluids capable of undergoing putrefaction; but even estimated thus, a patient with eighteen pounds of blood would require one hundred and thirty-eight grains of quinia circulating therein in order to satisfy the conditions of Binz's experiment. If Binz considers two grammes (half a drachm) of quinia per day sufficient for an individual weighing one hundred and twenty pounds, his calculation is founded on experiments with dogs, in which septicæmia was avoided by the injection of quinia. It is also necessary to bear in mind that Binz makes a distinction with regard to the preparations of quinia employed. He warns against the use of the bisulphate as being the most inactive. No matter which preparations are used—I prefer the muriate—I have come to look upon quinia as of no great service in reducing the temperature in infectious fevers. The main indication for its use can only be found in inflammatory fevers. When it is given, however, salicylate of sodium may be added for a short time to obtain a speedier effect.

On the part of bromine Wm. H. Thompson claims the following advantages: 1. When applied locally, it promptly arrests fetor by arresting directly the gangrenous process, and thus lessens risk from absorption. 2. It acts as an anti-putrefactive likewise in the fluids of the body generally—*i.e.* blood, interstitial circulation, and secretions—owing to its high rate of diffusibility, equal to that of sodium chloride itself. 3. It locally destroys the communicable property of the discharges, shown by the immunity of attendants from any sore throat when it is used, and from its checking the spread of the disease in the locality. He orders two solutions to be used: the first of equal parts of Lawrence Smith's solutio bromini and of glycerine, applied with a hair pencil to the membrane, as gently as possible. Sometimes he uses the solution full strength. The brush should be washed at once in water, and does not last more than one day, owing to the action of the bromine on the hair. If, however, the membrane be very extensive and the parts much swollen or difficult to reach, he resorts instead to douching with a Davidson syringe, using half a drachm to one drachm of the solution to a pint of warm water. By beginning gently with the stream directed against the buccal mucous membrane, the child soon becomes accustomed to the current and allows it then to play against the deeper parts.

Internally he orders from six to twelve drops of the solution in a half ounce of sweetened water, every hour, two, or three hours, according to the urgency of the case, and continuously.

The most convenient way of making Smith's solution is: Take two ounces of a saturated solution of potassium bromide in water; add to this, very slowly, in a bottle and with constant shaking, one ounce of bromine. It is better to add a part, and then let it stand a while before adding the rest; then fill up gradually, and with constant shaking with water, until it measures four ounces.

[p. 709]Ozone has been used as an anti-fermentative in inhalation during three or five minutes every hour or two, by Jochheim.

Boric (boracic) acid, in saturated (1:25) or milder solutions, has some antiseptic effect. It is mild, and not very injurious when swallowed by necessity or mistake. In diphtheritic conjunctivitis it is valued highly, and in nasal injections I have found it very useful. It is less repugnant than most other substances administered in that way.

Sodium benzoate cannot be relied on either as an anti-diphtheritic nor as an antifebrile. The doses which were recommended were two scruples or a drachm daily for a child a year old.

Sulphur has been used locally. It gives rise to coughing and vomiting.

Cubebs have been given in incredible doses, two drachms of the powder to a child a year old. The drug disorders the stomach and kidneys.

Local Treatment.—The mechanical removal of the membranes is not permissible unless they are almost detached. It is best to avoid their being cast off, unless partly loosened membranes in the larynx or trachea afford an indication for an emetic. Scratching and eroding the mucous membrane of the neighborhood give rise to new deposits. Even after spontaneous elimination of a membrane a new one may be formed within a few hours.

To cauterize a diphtheritic membrane or infiltration I consider wrong, unless I shall be able to do so thoroughly and to limit the action of the caustic to the diseased surface. Therefore potassa or chromic acid cannot be utilized, because of the impossibility of limiting their effect. Nitrate of silver and mineral acids can be restricted in their effects, but these are not sufficiently thorough, particularly as but few patients will consent to have the remedy applied properly. When I do cauterize, I prefer a mixture of equal parts of carbolic acid and glycerine or the undiluted acid. The membrane crumbles and falls off in pieces. Force must never be used. Where it would be required in the case of obstinate children mild washes must be employed instead of the caustic. Besides, the internal medication detailed above meets every indication. When there is a slight swelling of the lymphatic glands, cold water or ice applications are usually all that is needed. The latter should be made according to general indications. The glandular and peri-glandular swellings are less the result of an actual filling up with foreign matter than of secondary irritation. Ice has a happy effect in such cases, both on internal administration, in the form of frequent small quantities of ice-water, ice-pills, ice cream, and iced medicaments, and also externally by ice-cold cloths or india-rubber bags filled with ice.

In general, the treatment of the swelled glands must be both based on its causes and adapted to the present condition. The adenitis and peri-adenitis is of secondary nature, the irritation being in the mouth, pharynx, and nares. In these localities is where the main treatment is required. The sooner the primary affection is removed or relieved or rendered innocuous, the better it is for the secondary complaint. Frequent doses of chlorate of potassium or sodium, or biborate of sodium in mild doses frequently repeated, according to the principles laid down in another part of this article, mouth-washes, gargles, nasal injections with water, salt water, or solutions of disinfecting substances, are not only [p. 710]indicated, but highly successful. When the case is recent, cold applications are required, but no washes. When it is of older date, stimulant embrocations are in order. Iodine ointments are absorbed but slowly; mercurial plasters do good in some cases; iodide of potassium dissolved in glycerine (1:3-4), frequently applied, iodine in oleic acid (1:8-12), iodoform in collodion or flexible collodion (1:12-15) applied twice daily, the latter frequently with very good result, are beneficial. Copious suppuration is very rare. Cases in which a free incision meets with an abscess ready to heal are very uncommon. But numerous small abscesses with gangrenous walls and pus mixed with a sero-sanguinolent or sero-purulent liquid, are more frequently found. In such cases a probe introduced into the lancet wound enters easily into the broken-down tissue in every direction, to a distance even of three to six centimetres, (several inches), according to the size of the tumefaction. I have seen fatal hemorrhages from such gangrenous destructions; therefore the treatment must be both timely and energetic. The incision must not be delayed too long. When the skin assumes a purplish hue or is simply discolored, it is time to incise and to apply concentrated or nearly concentrated carbolic acid to the interior, unless the neighborhood of very important blood-vessels or nerves yields a contraindication to concentrated applications. In that case a milder preparation is advisable, but the application should be repeated often, until the suppuration becomes more normal. Then mild disinfectant injections into what has now become a cavity will be found satisfactory, particularly when meanwhile the general condition of the patient has been improved.

Treatment of Nasal Diphtheria.—Especially during the prevalence of an epidemic of diphtheria must we be careful not to allow a nasal catarrh to have its own way; we must likewise guard against considering the thin and flocculent discharge in infected cases as a mucous secretion. Whatever be the origin of nasal diphtheria, whether primary or the result of a similar affection in the throat, local treatment should at once be instituted, and if this be done the great majority of cases will terminate favorably. The danger in this form of disease consists in an excessive absorption of putrid substances and in the breathing of contaminated air. The interior of the nasal cavities must be thoroughly cleaned and disinfected. If this be commenced early, the original seat of the affection may be reached, and the disinfectant process will, as a rule, have good results. It is not necessary to select very energetic disinfectants; a solution of twelve to twenty-five centigrammes (two to four grains) of carbolic acid in thirty grammes (an ounce) of water is at once mild and effective, and hardly gives rise to more discomfort than lukewarm water. Nasal injections must be made very frequently, until each time the stream of fluid has a free exit through the other nostril or through the mouth. They must be made at least every hour, and even oftener if necessary; at the same time it is advisable to be careful that the fluid does not enter the Eustachian tube. This can be prevented, to a certain extent, by compelling the patient to keep the mouth open during the procedure. I have seldom seen evil or even disagreeable results from the administration of nasal injections in diphtheria. It is likely that the mucous membrane of the pharynx is swollen as far as the openings of the Eustachian tubes to such a degree as to render the entrance of fluids into the latter improbable. [p. 711]The hardness of hearing, which is of so frequent occurrence in the course of a severe catarrh or of a diphtheritic attack, seems to indicate that the mucous membrane of that part is in a state of swelling. An ordinary syringe will suffice. However, when administered by parents or nurses the blunt nozzle of an ear syringe is preferable. Occasionally here, as in local applications to the mouth and pharynx, the atomizer may be used to advantage, but the tube must be properly introduced into the nostrils. There are cases of nasal diphtheria, however, which are far more troublesome to manage than the foregoing would seem to indicate. I have seen cases in which the nasal cavities, from the anterior to the posterior nares, were filled and completely occluded by a dense, solid membranous mass. I was then compelled to bore a passage with a silver probe, to gradually introduce a larger-sized one, and then to apply the pure carbolic acid, in order to remove the densest and thickest masses, and finally was able to make injections; even in such cases I have had the gratification of being able to give a favorable prognosis. The dangerous secondary swelling of the glands will often subside after a steady employment of disinfectant injections for from twelve to twenty-four hours. It will be found that children frequently do not object to this method of treatment; I have even met with some who, after convincing themselves of the relief afforded thereby, asked for an injection. When we are about to bring each injection to a close it is well to press together the nasal cavities for an instant with the fingers. By this procedure the fluid is forced backward to the pharynx, and is swallowed or ejected through the mouth, and thus washes the pharynx and mouth at the same time. Frequently, however, this latter object is obtained with every injection; for, the palate being swelled, oedematous, and paretic, the fluid is not prevented from reaching the pharynx, even in the average case. In regard to the choice of a disinfecting agent, I have but a few words to say. I believe that no one of them has important qualifications above the others. I avoid those which stain or which produce firm coagula. For the latter reason I do not use the subsulphate and perchloride of iron; for the former, the permanganate of potassium. I employ, as a rule, carbolic acid in solution, of the strength above mentioned. Where there is but a slightly fetid odor I have frequently employed lime-water or water with glycerine, or a solution (1:100, 1:50) of chloride of sodium, or of bicarbonate of soda or of borax, or a saturated solution of boric acid. Disinfecting agents and antiseptics, whether carbolic acid, salicylic acid, or iron, are of no service when administered internally only, unless the seat and cause of the septic infection be attended to previously. Under the local employment of antiseptics, as described, or by simply washing out with water or salt water, most cases recover; without them, death will result. Of late, in many cases, the local applications, injections, etc. of the corrosive chloride of mercury in water (1:5000-10,000) has proved very effective. It has this advantage over carbolic acid, that the swallowing of the former is not so dangerous. This much, after all, my experience has assured me of, that there is a certain number of cases which terminate fatally; but it is likewise true that the mortality need not be excessively great. I cannot grant that it is hard to carry out the exact and apparently barbarous treatment necessary for a favorable result, for it is certainly more barbarous to sacrifice than to save life.

[p. 712]It is a positive fact that when children suffering from nasal diphtheria, with its peculiarly septic character, are permitted to sleep much—and they are apt to be drowsy under the influence of the poison—they will certainly die. To allow them to sleep is to allow them to die.

The first symptom of improvement is often a rapid diminution of the glandular swelling wherever it exists. It is not present in all cases, but chiefly in those in which a bloody serum was discharged in an early period of the disease. In these the blood-vessels appear to be very vulnerable, superficial, and apt to absorb; these are also the most dangerous cases, and require the greatest attention and care, and also prompt disinfection.

Treatment of Laryngeal Diphtheria.—The severest form of diphtheria is that located in the larynx, constituting membranous croup. Its general treatment, whether the disease has originated primarily in the larynx or trachea or has been communicated from the pharynx, does not differ from that laid down for diphtheria in general. Naturally the larynx calls for special treatment on account of the symptoms of suffocation which result from its stenosis. The main indication of removing viscid mucus or partly-detached membranes is best met by the administration of an emetic. Such is their only indication in my experience. The selection of the emetic, when indicated, is of great importance. Antimonials ought to be avoided because of their depressing and purgative effect. Ipecacuanha is but rarely effective. The sulphates of zinc and copper, and particularly the latter, deserve preference. Turpeth mineral acts promptly and satisfactorily. When no emesis can be obtained the prognosis is decidedly bad. Recourse must then be had to tracheotomy, the good results of which are however only too often delusive and transient.

When, after the operation, there is scarcely any relief, and particularly when the case takes a very rapid course, it is probably one of ascending croup which commenced in the trachea. Mechanical relief by pushing down a hen's feather or a bundle of them, and turning it about and twisting, must be tried. It is a much better instrument than pincers of all sorts and shapes. But what relief will be accomplished is but of very short duration. When fever sets in within a few hours it means very much more frequently pneumonia than diphtheritic fever. It is apt to be soon complicated by that disproportion between pulse and respiration so characteristic of inflammatory diseases. Then quinia in larger doses, 0.25 or 0.5 (grs. iv-viij) every two, four, eight hours, at the same time doses of sodium salicylate 0.25-0.40 (grs. iv-vj) every hour or two hours until the temperature goes down, and small doses of digitalis where the heart requires it, must be given at once. Procrastination is dangerous; the patients want careful watching; many of them die within two days after the operation.

Diphtheritic conjunctivitis requires great attention and permits of no loss of time. Cold applications to the affected eye must be made constantly. Pieces of linen or lint kept on ice (better than in ice-water) of little more than the size of the eye, must be changed every minute or two day and night. The danger to the cornea is so imminent that constant watchfulness is required. Boric acid in concentrated solution should be dropped into the eye once every hour. Care must be taken that the well eye shall not get infected; for that purpose it is best to cover it [p. 713]with lint and collodion, or with lint or cotton held in place by adhesive plaster.

Cutaneous diphtheria requires the destruction of the membrane or of the infected surface by carbolic acid, either concentrated or somewhat diluted with glycerine, or the application of the actual cautery. After that the use of ice or iced cloths, or diluted carbolic acid, is indicated. As soon as the surface is no longer diphtheritic the local and general treatment is to be continued on general principles.

Diphtheritic paralysis is invariably complicated by anæmia and debility, and the diet and medical treatment must be regulated accordingly. However, neither overfeeding nor a sameness of diet are to be permitted, for not rarely the muscular coat of the stomach suffers with the rest of the muscular tissue, and the secretion of gastric juice is very deficient in anæmic individuals. While, therefore, iron is indicated, we must not neglect to pay particular attention to nutrition and digestion, and to aid the latter with pepsin and moderate amounts of muriatic acid, well diluted. Quinia in small doses and stimulants are appropriate whenever there is no contraindication to their employment. The treatment of the paralysis itself will naturally depend on the diagnosis of the condition present in each individual case, which we have seen to differ considerably. This alone can explain why various modes of treatment, the electric current among others, after being recommended by some authors, are branded by others. Where we have to deal with those rare changes in the brain and spinal cord, the utmost care is necessary in order not to make the condition still worse; and in such cases there would be a contraindication to the use of the faradic current, though this would not hold true with regard to the use of the galvanic current in short sittings. Besides, central paralyses are by no means so frequent as peripheral ones. In most cases there is not the slightest elevation of temperature during the course of the paralytic phenomena. I lay great stress upon this point, for I am aware that many cases of central congestion and even of inflammation exhibit but very insignificant elevations of temperature. But, as the diagnosis will depend on a positive knowledge of whether there have been changes of temperature, I rely on the rectal temperature only, for many a myelitis runs its course with no greater elevation above the normal than one-half or one degree. In all cases in which the temperature is normal or subnormal, I do not hesitate for a moment to employ the faradic or the galvanic current. In addition to the internal administration of iron I advise by all means the employment of strychnia. When there is no necessity for haste, we may give moderate doses, gradually increasing them, and using iron in combination. When there is danger in delay, recourse ought to be had to subcutaneous injections of the sulphate of strychnia, once or twice daily. They are mainly indicated in paralysis of the muscles of deglutition and of respiration. Of course, where the former are affected it is necessary to nourish the patient artificially, partly perhaps by nutrient enemata, but principally by means of the stomach-tube. In using the latter it is unnecessary to introduce it into the stomach, as it only requires to be passed a few inches below the affected parts, when the oesophagus will usually be found able to undertake the further disposal of the food. In these cases strychnia should be injected subcutaneously in the neck, [p. 714]once or twice daily. In a similar manner it should be injected in the region of the chest, diaphragm, or neck in paralysis of the respiratory muscles or of the glottis. In paralysis of the muscles of accommodation (in which Scheby-Buch claims to have seen the process cut short by the use of the Calabar bean, considered as inert by Hassner) they may be given in the forehead or temples.

Frictions dry and alcoholic, hot bathing, friction with hot water, kneading of the affected parts, will be found beneficial and pleasant.

[p. 715]

CHOLERA.
BY ALFRED STILLÉ, M.D., LL.D.

DEFINITION.—Cholera is an epidemic disease, characterized by the transudation of serum into the stomach and bowels, and usually by the profuse discharge by vomiting and purging of a liquid resembling rice-water, followed by a tendency to collapse. It is endemic in India, but has been conveyed thence to almost every part of the world.

SYNONYMS.—Cholera algida, C. asiatica, C. asphyxia, C. maligna, C. spasmodica. In English it is generally spoken of as Asiatic cholera.

HISTORY.—It is sometimes stated that Hippocrates, Galen, Celsus, and the Greek, Roman, and Arabian medical writers generally record "the fact of the presence of cholera in the various countries in which they lived" (Macnamara). Nothing could be more contrary to the truth. All of these writers describe "cholera morbus" in nearly identical terms; they all include bilious discharges among its symptoms, and no one of them speaks of it as a mortal or even as an epidemic disease. (Compare, especially, Celsus, Aretæus, Cælius Aurelianus, and Paulus Ægineta.) Their description of sporadic cholera morbus is very precise. For example, Cælius Aurelianus says: "Cholericam passionem aiunt aliqui nominatam a fluore fellis, per os et ventrem effecto."[1]

[1] *Acut. Morb.*, lib. iii. cap. xix.

Asiatic epidemic cholera is a very different disease. It seems to have been known in India from a very remote period, but no detailed account of it was published until the beginning of the sixteenth century. During that century many successive descriptions of the disease exhibited its extreme violence and mortality. It is believed to have occurred repeatedly, if not annually, in the same localities down to the present time. The invasion of India by the Portuguese, and afterward by the English, contributed to spread the disease throughout the Peninsula, partly by military occupation and partly through commercial channels, by which it was also carried to the islands in the Indian Ocean. It prevailed in Batavia in 1629. Between 1768 and 1790 numerous epidemics of cholera occurred. About the former date no less than 60,000 persons are said to have perished near Pondicherry, and in 1783 it is reckoned that 20,000 victims to the disease fell in a single week during the religious gathering at the sacred city of Hurdwâr, where, as will be seen hereafter, it became in later years more fatal still. The English armies extended their conquests in Hindostan, and established commerce between that country and Western Asia and Europe, and by the year 1817 opened new channels of [p. 716]communication in every direction, both within and beyond the Peninsula. Along them the disease was carried; it invaded Ceylon and the Burmese empire, and extended to Batavia, Java, and China on the east, and advanced westward to Persia in 1821. In that year also it was carried from Arabia into Africa, and at various later periods penetrated more and more deeply into the Dark Continent, always following the track of pilgrims returning from Mecca, the routes of armies engaged in war, or those of trading caravans.[2]

[2] Christie, *Cholera Epidemics in Africa*, 1876.

In these cases, as in others elsewhere, the spontaneous origin of the disease has been assumed by certain writers, but at every stage of its progress careful investigation led uniformly to the conclusion that it was propagated directly or indirectly from pre-existent cases of cholera. From Persia it moved northward as far as the shores of the Caspian Sea, and westward to the Levant in 1823, and there for a time its ravages were stayed. Meanwhile, it prevailed at various places throughout Hindostan, and, assuming a greater degree of violence in 1826, it advanced steadily in a north-western direction across Afghanistan and Persia in the following year. In 1829 it reached Orenburg, to the north of the Caspian Sea, and was speedily conveyed into the interior of the Russian empire, where it raged with great violence in 1830. In 1831 it prevailed at Mecca among the pilgrims, who had brought it from India, and so virulently that one-half of them are computed to have perished. Hence it speedily passed with returning pilgrims to Alexandria and Constantinople, and was carried to St. Petersburg, to Sweden, to Hamburg, and other places in Northern continental Europe. From Hamburg and other seaports it was conveyed to commercial towns on the eastern coast of England, whence it extended to Edinburgh in the north and London in the south.

In 1832 cholera prevailed in France, and within the year caused 120,000 deaths, 7000 of which occurred in Paris in the space of eighteen days. In the spring and summer of that year it was reproduced in England, and extended to Ireland. From Liverpool, Cork, Limerick, and Dublin five vessels filled with emigrants sailed for Quebec, Canada, and they, together, lost 179 passengers by cholera during the voyage.

The immediate results of this importation and first appearance of cholera on the American continent are described by Dr. Peters as follows: "All these ships and their passengers were quarantined at Grosse Isle, a few miles below Quebec. On June 7th the St. Lawrence steamer Voyageur conveyed a load of these emigrants and their baggage, some to Quebec, but the majority to Montreal on the 10th. The first cases of cholera occurred in emigrant boarding-houses in Quebec on the 8th, and the same pest-steamboat, the Voyageur, landed persons dead and dying of cholera at Montreal, a distance of two hundred miles, in less than thirty hours. Over this long distance, thickly inhabited on both shores of the St. Lawrence, cholera made a single leap, without infecting a single village or a single house between the two cities, with the following exceptions. A man picked up a mattress thrown from the Voyageur, and he and his wife died of cholera; another man, fishing on the St. Lawrence, was requested to bury a dead man from the Voyageur, and he and his wife and nephew died. The captain of a passing boat requested an Indian to bury a man from on board; this man and five other Indians were attacked [p. 717]and died. The town of Three Rivers, halfway between Quebec and Montreal, forbade steamers to land, and escaped for a long time. From Montreal the great influx of emigrants were forwarded away, by the Emigrant Society, as fast as they arrived, and by them the pestilence was sown at each stopping-place. Kingston, Toronto, and Niagara soon became affected. In the end, over 4000 persons died of cholera in Montreal, and more than an equal number in Quebec. The epidemic reached Detroit in the same way, ... and continued west along the Great Lakes, until in September it reached our military posts on the Upper Mississippi.... Fort Dearborn, near Chicago, was temporarily reoccupied in 1832, and it was here that epidemic cholera displayed its most fatal effects among our troops. Out of 1000 men, over 200 cases were admitted into hospitals in the course of seven or eight days.... When these troops again marched for the Mississippi, they appeared in perfect health, yet the cholera broke out again on the way, and when the command reached the Mississippi it had been as fatal as it had been at Fort Dearborn."

Meanwhile, an emigrant ship with cholera on board reached New York, whence the disease spread up the Hudson River, and was also carried southwardly to Philadelphia and the West. The mortality in New York City from this epidemic is stated at 3500. In 1833 the disease broke out in the cities of Havana and Matanzas in Cuba, and is said to have destroyed one-tenth of the entire population. Hence it was carried to Mexican and American towns on the Gulf of Mexico, and up the Mississippi and Ohio as far as the western border of Pennsylvania. In the following year it was again introduced at the port of Quebec by a vessel filled with emigrants, of whom many had died during the passage. It prevailed in Canada and the State of New York and spread over the whole country in 1835 and 1836. In the former of these two years it was confined to several Southern cities, whither it was brought, as on a former occasion, directly from Cuba. It then gradually subsided, and at last disappeared for the space of nearly ten years.

But in 1845 it was known to be advancing on its former path, which it steadily pursued, and entered England in October, 1848, at Sunderland, the very town at which it first appeared in 1831. "During the second epidemic in Europe, in 1848, two vessels sailed from Havre, where cholera prevailed—one, the New York, for New York, and the other, the Swanton, for New Orleans. Both contained large numbers of German emigrants. On one vessel the cholera appeared when it was sixteen days out, with fourteen deaths; on the other, in twenty-six days, with thirteen deaths. The New York arrived at Staten Island Dec. 2, 1848, and a severe epidemic broke out, but was confined to the quarantine grounds. The Swanton arrived at New Orleans Dec. 11th; no quarantine was instituted, and in two days its sick were taken into the Charity Hospital. This was the beginning of a severe epidemic, which increased in power all winter, till, in June, 1849, 2500 died of it in New Orleans. December 20, 1848, it reached Memphis by steamboat from New Orleans, and for twenty-five days was confined to the landing-place of the former city, whence it afterward spread. In the spring it was carried to St. Louis and Cincinnati and the whole Mississippi Valley. In October it reached Sacramento, Cal., by means of overland emigrants, and, almost at the same time, San Francisco, by the U.S. steamer Northerner from [p. 718]Panama. The Chinese of California suffered most severely" (Peters). In April, 1849, cholera reappeared in the public stores at the quarantine station, Staten Island, N.Y., and in the city of New York, where it was fatal to 5000 persons.

A pause now took place in the ravages of the disease which lasted until 1853. In that year it destroyed no less than 11,000 persons in the Persian city of Teheran. At Messina its victims numbered 12,000, in France 114,000, and in England about 16,000. In 1854 it was introduced by emigrant ships into New York, causing a mortality of 2000 persons, and was carried to Philadelphia, where its victims numbered 500. It extended to many towns in New

England and westward along the great channels of emigration. In Montreal the deaths were 1300, and in the then small town of Detroit, 1000.

After an interval of quiescence longer than any previous one the cholera again broke out among the pilgrims to Mecca in December, 1864. It appeared in Alexandria during May, 1865, and thence was carried to many parts of Europe, and from them to North America and the West Indies. This period of exemption included that of the Civil War in the United States, when, if ever, the local causes which have been erroneously assigned to the disease existed in all their forms and in the most intense degree. It was only when its specific germs were once more imported that cholera began to prevail again. Official records show that in 1866 it was introduced from Europe into Halifax, N.S., the city of New York, and the military posts of New York harbor. Thence it was carried in troop-ships to various Southern ports, from which its progress could be traced to Texas and other Gulf States, and to the towns on the Mississippi and Missouri Rivers. From New York, also, the disease travelled westward to Cincinnati and the U.S. barracks at Newport, on the opposite side of the Ohio River, whence it advanced in a south-westerly direction to meet the trail that, coming from the South, followed the great rivers of the Mississippi Valley. During the summer of 1867 cholera again prevailed, although less fatally, at most of the points, especially of the Mississippi Valley, which had been invaded the previous year, and some cases occurred at the military posts around New York in recruits who had shortly before arrived from places in the West where cholera prevailed. Thus did the disease complete the circuit of the United States.

Meanwhile, cholera prevailed to a greater or less extent in the east of Europe between 1865 and 1874. After the latter date it seems to have been confined to Syria, Arabia, and the African shore of the Mediterranean. In 1877-78 it existed to a limited extent among the pilgrims at Mecca, and since then it has not been known in Europe. The latest appearance of cholera in the United States was in 1873, when it occurred at three points far distant from one another. It was introduced in the effects of immigrants. The vessels that brought them were in a perfect sanitary condition. The passengers themselves were healthy, and remained so after landing and until they reached the distant points of Carthage, Ohio, Crow River, Minn., and Yankton, Dak., where their goods were unpacked. At each place, "within twenty-four hours after the poison particles were liberated, the first cases of the disease appeared, and the unfortunates were almost literally swept from the face of the earth" (E. McClellan).

[p. 719]In 1881 cholera was brought from Hindostan to Arabia by pilgrims on their way to Mecca, where it soon afterward broke out and caused the death of about 8000 persons. In the following year several vessels from Bombay evaded the quarantine and reached Djeddah, the port of Mecca, and the pilgrims on reaching the latter city disseminated the disease. The unusually small number of persons who were there at the time, and their prompt dispersion before the danger, limited the mortality, and gradually cases of cholera ceased to appear. In 1882, the English at that time carrying on war in Egypt, very rigid sanitary precautions against the importation of cholera were enacted and successfully enforced, but in the following year, the same urgent necessity no longer commanding, they were considerably relaxed. At the end of June, 1883, the cholera made its appearance at Damietta (at one of the mouths of the Nile), and soon afterward at Rosetta, Port Said, and Mansourah. During July it spread to various places in direct communication with those named. At Cairo it was peculiarly fatal, and on July 20th it was reported to have caused 600 deaths. For several days the daily mortality varied between 500 and 600. The disease prevailed somewhat in Alexandria during the height of the epidemic, and near the end of October it was fatal to numerous European residents of that city, and some deaths occurred in the British army of occupation. In all Egypt, during the week ending Aug. 13th, the total mortality is said to have been 5000, but in the following week it fell to 2000. It is estimated that the epidemic destroyed at least 20,000 lives. The germ of this epidemic has not been accurately determined. Some regard it as a survival of the cholera of the previous year—a supposition which is at least plausible and sufficient; but certain "sanitarians" have attributed the outbreak to the ordinary causes of disease intensified by the civil war which had recently devastated Egypt. It is sufficient here to say that while such causes have in all ages generated typhus and typhoid fevers and dysentery, they never produced cholera. Some, more unwise than judicious, declared that the Egyptian disease of 1883 was not cholera. It is alleged, on the one hand, that several East Indian merchants from Bombay arrived at Damietta on June 18th, or three days before the disease was recognized in that city. It is also said that a stoker from on board an English steamer from Bombay introduced the cholera into Damietta. But the judgment of Surgeon-General Murray carries with it greater weight.[3] He is of the opinion that the Egyptian epidemic of 1883 was simply a revival of the Arabian epidemic of 1882. He shows that cholera existed in several villages on the Damietta branch of the Nile in the latter part of May and during June, and that it broke out in the capital itself, during a fair which had lasted for eight days, on the 22d of June, and was spread by the people on their return from Damietta to their villages. This, adds Mr. Murray, "is a literal transcript of the accounts of many of the severe epidemics that have raged over India." It also appears from M. Proust's narrative[4] that the Ottoman government had already, as early as April, notified the government of Egypt that certain Indo-Javanese pilgrims were on their way to Mecca, and that ought not to be allowed to land without quarantine. The French delegate to the sanitary council also begged that those of the pilgrims who reached Suez without previous quarantine should be isolated and kept under [p. 720]surveillance for three days. But owing to the opposition of the English delegates these measures were not duly enforced, the council did not meet again, and no protective system was adopted.

[3] *Times and Gazette*, Feb., 1884, p. 209.

[4] *Le Cholera*, 1883.

ETIOLOGY.—The essential cause of cholera is unknown, unless the investigations of Koch, described below, may have revealed it. Its secondary causes, or the conditions of its dissemination, are better understood. Some general propositions concerning them will here be laid down, and illustrated so far as the argument requires and the available space will allow.

Cholera is endemic in no other country than India, and more particularly in Bengal. When it has occurred elsewhere it has invariably been carried from India. The cholera poison has been imagined to be of an aërial nature, but its diffusion has no relation whatever to the velocity or the direction of the wind. In no instance whatever has its rate of progress exceeded that of man on land or water, nor has it ever taken a direction different from that of commercial or military movements. On land it has usually crept from place to place, and if sometimes it has seemed to leap across wide spaces, and even seas and oceans, it has never invaded any inland town or seaport without having been brought thither from a point already affected with the disease. Nor, having once entered an inland or seaboard town, does it spread equally therein in all directions, but prevails chiefly in the quarter immediately surrounding the place of its entrance. If appropriate sanitary measures are enforced, it is sometimes confined to that quarter, and, in the case of quarantine stations, it has repeatedly been prevented from extending beyond them. This statement may be illustrated by the fact that of fourteen epidemics of cholera at Staten Island, the quarantine station of New York, all but four were prevented from reaching that city.[5] When the disease does overleap the barrier opposed to it, its origin and subsequent course can usually be traced.

[5] Peters's *Notes, etc.*, 2d ed., p. 94.

A high atmospheric temperature is everywhere associated with the prevalence of cholera. Its origin in the hot climate of Hindostan and its general progress prove this conclusively. In nearly all of the places where a great difference exists between the summer and the winter temperature the disease has disappeared during the cold season, and attained its greatest intensity during the hot months of the year. The only apparent exception to this rule is, that cholera has prevailed in several Russian, Swedish, and Norwegian cities during the winter. But these very exceptions confirm the rule; for in the countries mentioned the intense cold of the winter compels the inhabitants to seal their houses by every possible means, while the atmosphere within them is kept at a high temperature by huge stoves, which hinder ventilation, and indeed render it almost impossible. Difference of temperature likewise explains the fact that of two cholera-ships arriving from Havre, the one at New York and the other at New Orleans, in December, 1848, the former did not disseminate the disease, but the latter formed the starting-point of an epidemic which lasted all the winter.

A good deal has been written of the predisposing causes of cholera, and poverty, crowding, filth, intemperance, and depression of spirits have been given prominent places in the catalogue. But to any one familiar[p. 721]with the history of epidemic diseases it will at once be apparent that every one of these conditions favors the spread of all communicable infectious diseases. There is not the slightest evidence that these agencies, singly or combined, can generate cholera or favor its spread apart from the presence of the specific poison of the disease and the facility with which it is transmitted from the sick to the well whenever the population is crowded, poor, of filthy habits, and weakened by dissipation. Because among such people intemperance prevails, this vice has been regarded as predisposing to cholera. Apart from the brutish mode of living of drunkards, there is nothing to show that they are more liable to cholera than the most abstemious of water-drinkers. On the contrary, it is notorious that during cholera epidemics drunkards in the better classes of society enjoy a certain degree of immunity from the disease; which it is easy to explain on the ground that they imbibe but little water, which is the main channel through which the infectious principle of the disease is spread.

The specific cause of cholera is taken into the alimentary canal, and acts through it to produce the characteristic symptoms of the disease. It is conveyed from the sick to the well by means of the gastro-intestinal discharges, either moist or dry; in the former state, by means of drinking-water, and in the latter through the air, whose suspended noxious particles are received into the fauces and swallowed. There is reason to believe that the poison does not enter the system through the lungs, or through any other channel than the gastro-intestinal canal. W. B. Carpenter[6] appears to hold, however, that the poison may be absorbed through the lungs. To this view there are two objections: 1, That whatever is taken into the mouth or throat by inspiration may very well be swallowed; and, 2, that all the primary lesions of cholera affect the digestive and not the respiratory apparatus. It is not at all necessary to the propagation of cholera that its excreta should be furnished by persons laboring under the fully-formed disease. A specific choleraic diarrhoea is as infectious as the evacuations which occur in completely developed cholera. But neither will propagate the disease through the air to a distance. The tendency to its propagation in this manner depends chiefly upon the concentration of the poison; thus, it much more frequently occurs in close than in well-ventilated rooms or than in the open air. It has been argued that cholera is not contagious, because so few, comparatively, of the attendants upon cholera patients contract the disease. On the other hand, as some of them are attacked, this positive fact outweighs an indefinite number of negative instances. It should also be noted that different diseases enter the system and infect it through different channels—some through the lungs, others through the alimentary canal, etc. Small-pox, the most contagious of all diseases, is introduced through the air-passages, and is probably harmless when its virus is taken into the stomach. That the converse of this proposition applies to cholera is sustained by the whole history of the disease. Cholera poison may be taken to considerable distances in either a moist or a dry condition. In the former state it is mainly conveyed by water, as in rivers, water-pipes, etc.; in the latter, by fomites and especially by clothing saturated or merely soiled with cholera discharges, and which may retain their infectious quality for an indefinite time.

[6] *The Nineteenth Century*, Feb., 1884.

[p. 722]Great stress has been laid upon the humidity and foulness of the soil, a damp atmosphere, filth, crowding, etc., as elements in the production of cholera, but in reality they have no more essential relation to it than to any other disease that occurs epidemically. Cholera may prevail whether they are present or absent. It is evident that from the earliest historical periods all of these causes of disease have existed, and in Europe much more generally and excessively than during the present century, and that they have never been removed in Asia Minor, Egypt, Arabia, and Africa. Yet cholera never was known in any of these countries until it was brought into them about the end of the first third of the present century.

According to Pettenkoffer, cholera is most prevalent when the subsoil water is lowest, and least so when the subsoil water is highest. It would be more descriptive of the fact to say that, so far as cholera has anything to do with the condition of the soil, it is most apt to be severe and prevalent when very dry weather follows a very wet period. Such circumstances are the most favorable to putrefactive fermentation and the dissemination of its products, which thus reach wells of drinking-water, and even rivers, especially when sewers empty into the latter. The identity of this explanation with that which is generally accepted for the dissemination of typhoid fever is too evident to be insisted upon. We might go farther, and say that, in typhoid fever as in cholera, the disease is communicated, although exceptionally, by the air of the sick room and by the exhalations of the soiled fomites of the patient. Now, if typhoid fever resembled cholera not only in being transmitted by means of the dejections, but also in its poison being derived from one primary source only, the analogy between the causes of the two diseases would be very striking indeed. But, in point of fact, the typhoid-fever poison may probably be generated de novo by fecal fermentation and other forms of putrefaction, and the disease is only exceptionally communicable; whereas, the poison of cholera, once received, is conveyed from man to man and far and wide through various channels; but, so far as is known, it has but one primary source, and that is in India. Lebert states that he did not find the localities that are the ordinary seats of typhoid fever peculiarly liable to invasions of cholera. But it must be noted that typhoid fever is very far from being exclusively a disease of the poor, squalid, and vicious. Like death itself, "regum turres pauperumque tabernas æquo pede pulsat;" while cholera much more commonly plants itself and disseminates its seeds in the rank soil of moral and physical degradation.

All morbid causes whatever, derived from race, climate, religion, dwellings, food, clothing, habits of living, etc., have no more to do with the development of cholera than with that of the eruptive fevers, and even less than with the causation of typhus and typhoid fevers and dysentery. The eruptive fevers are caused, as cholera probably is, by specific germs which no known combination of natural causes has ever developed, while the poisons of the other diseases named appear to be generated anew whenever certain more or less definite physicial conditions coexist. It would seem that cholera differs radically from all of these affections by the fact that its cause does not enter the circulation, but confines its direct operation to the gastro-intestinal mucous membrane. In this way it becomes intelligible that while, on the one hand, physicians and nurses of[p. 723]cholera patients, although often, in fact, yet in relation to their numbers, are comparatively seldom infected, provided they duly observe proper sanitary rules, the disease, on the other hand, spreads like wildfire among those who drink water polluted by cholera excretions, and only a little less rapidly among people crowded into ill-ventilated apartments along with cholera patients.

The special fomites of the cholera poison are articles of clothing and furniture soiled with the discharges of the sick, and the emanations from privies, sewers, etc. into which these discharges have been cast. Many considerations render it probable that a very small quantity of cholera matter may suffice to render infectious a very large quantity of liquid, and especially of matters in process of putrefactive fermentation, and that the gaseous or vaporous emanations from them become diffused in the atmosphere and infect all who imbibe them. But water contaminated by cholera discharges is the most rapid and efficient agent in disseminating the disease. Innumerable instances of this mode of action are furnished by its history in Asia and Africa, where water is often scarce, and naturally so impure that its additional defilement by cholera dejections is apt to pass unnoticed. From the illustrations of this proposition which might be adduced only a few of the more striking will here be selected.

Hurdwâr is a town in Northern India at the base of the Himalayas, where the Ganges begins its course in the plains. It is the seat of a great Hindoo pilgrimage, which takes place annually in April, when sometimes from 2,000,000 to 3,000,000 of people occupy an encampment of about twenty-two square miles, comprising a low flat island in the Ganges and the opposite banks of the river. Bathing in the sacred stream on a certain day is the main object of the devotees; which day, in the year 1867, fell on the 12th of April. The bath was taken early in the morning. From noon on that day the pilgrims began to disperse so rapidly that on the morning of the 15th the encampment was quite deserted. It appears that up to the former date the health of the encampment was excellent, and it was the opinion of the reporter (Dr. Cunningham) that cholera was introduced into the camp by pilgrims from the neighboring districts going late to the fair. He believed that the cholera excreta may have been buried in the trenches and carried by a heavy rain into the river, and there swallowed by the pilgrims; for to drink of the water of the Ganges as well as to bathe in it is a religious obligation.

Immediately after the breaking up of the camp cases occurred in the surrounding districts, the epidemic widening in all directions. The pilgrims were almost always the first persons attacked in any locality, and the cholera attended them on their route wherever they went. In all the districts where the disease prevailed no cases occurred until ample time had been given for the pilgrims to reach them. In a word, "the cholera first showed itself among them; it followed their lines of route only, and did not outrun them; their progress was its progress, and their limits its limits." The mortality caused by this epidemic among the whole civil population of the North-western Provinces of the Punjâb has been estimated at about 117,181.[7] The history of the religious festival of 1879[p. 724]was identical with that just sketched, except that the number of the pilgrims was smaller and the deaths proportionally less.[8]

[7] *Brit. and For. Med. Chir. Rev.*, Jan., 1870, p. 137.
[8] Murray, *Practitioner*, xxvi. 309.

Out of the numberless illustrations of the manner in which cholera is disseminated by water the following may be cited: In 1865 about 100,000 pilgrims were assembled at Mecca, of whom from 10,000 to 15,000 fell victims to the disease, two-thirds of them within a period of six days. Some cause acting simultaneously upon the whole number of persons must be admitted to account for so extraordinary a fact, and such a cause is not far to seek. At a certain sacred well "one hundred thousand people had skinfuls of water poured over them at the side of the well, and every one of them then drank largely of water drawn from the well. Much of the water poured over the pilgrims must have found its way by soakage back into the well, and if any of the pilgrims were at the time suffering from cholera, or had cholera-tainted garments about them, the well would be exposed to pollution."[9]

[9] Christie, *Cholera Epidemics in East Africa*, p. 488.

In the cholera epidemics of Zanzibar the disease produced the greatest havoc among the negroes, the Persians, and the East Indians; very few Europeans were attacked, and quite as few of the sect of the Banyans, who drank only water drawn from their own wells. The persons among whom the disease prevailed so fatally used chiefly the water of a certain well which was highly prized, but which on this occasion had become polluted by soakage from an adjacent cesspool into which the dejections of cholera patients had been thrown. It appears, also, that in Zanzibar the streams are very rarely bridged, and hundreds of negroes, in passing backward and forward, wade through them and pollute them. In these streams, also, the negroes wash their clothes and all the foul clothing of the contiguous town. While this business is going on "a gang of negroes may be at work at not many hundred yards' distance filling water-casks for the shipping." Subsequently to the watering of the ships in this manner sailors were attacked with cholera, and others who used water drawn from the stream below the place where it became polluted were attacked, and many of them died; while Europeans living on shore, and who drank the water of the same stream, but drawn from a much higher point in its course and after having been filtered, escaped the disease.[10]

[10] *Ibid.*, pp. 320, 492.

The history of the disease in Europe furnishes a multiplicity of similar cases, and even more distinctly exhibits the dissemination of cholera by contaminated water.[11] In Holland not less than five epidemics of the disease occurred between 1832 and 1869, all of them causing a great mortality, to which the epidemic of 1866 alone contributed not less than 20,000 deaths. This was about 55 deaths for every 10,000 inhabitants. Such exceptional mortality over so wide a territory has been ascribed to the extreme porosity and humidity of the soil, which is nearly all below the level of the sea. Such a soil must necessarily retain longer than other soils whatever it absorbs, and thus tend to render the well-water habitually impure. If, then, to the ordinary impurities a specific [p. 725]poison is added, its characteristic effects may assuredly be looked for. The conditions now stated explain the conclusions of Ballot of Rotterdam, drawn from a study of the several epidemics referred to. They are as follows: "1. Holland is highly affected by the cholera at every epidemic, chiefly in those parts where they drink water directly from the rivers and canals or from ground saturated with sewage. 2. In places where rain-water is generally drunk the disease is far less violent. 3. Places where there is no other drinkable water but rain-water are not affected by the epidemic; the single cases occurring there are imported. 4. When places affected by the cholera were supplied with pure water instead of the vitiated water the disease disappeared."[12] In like manner, we find that the cholera epidemic of 1873 in Germany seemed specially to select those situations where the subsoil was impregnated with decomposing organic matter; and it is evident that, in cities especially, such situations would include the most poverty-stricken districts, while the higher, drier, and at all times more salubrious localities are inhabited by the classes enjoying the greatest material prosperity.[13]

[11] It is of interest to note that on the first appearance of cholera in England, at Sunderland, in 1831, a surgeon of that place, Mr. Ainsworth, collected and published conclusive proofs of the importation of the disease, of its communication from the sick to the well, "and of its propagation by clothes, and even by emanations, from the dead" (*Observations on the Pestilential Cholera*, London, 1832).

[12] *Med. Times and Gaz.*, May, 1869, p. 459; June, 1869, p. 626.

[13] "Report of the German Imperial Commission," *Practitioner*, xxvi. 153.

This mode of infection has been traced in numberless individual cases of cholera. In London there was a certain well into which the liquid contents of a sewer had been percolating for months. Of the water of this well hundreds of persons had been drinking without obvious injury. At last a case of cholera occurred hard by; the discharges were thrown into a privy which communicated with the sewer and indirectly with the well, whereupon more than 500 persons who drank water drawn from that particular well were attacked with cholera within three days. So in 1856 cholera prevailed in the county jail of Oxford, Eng., the drain from which emptied into a pool from which the water was drawn to supply the city prison. In the latter institution cholera began to prevail, but declined as soon as the pipes conveying the water were cut off, and soon afterward ceased entirely.[14] Again, in Constantinople in 1865 the clothes, mattrasses, etc. of cholera patients were washed at a fountain the basin of which was divided into two parts by a wall; one part was used for washing clothes and the other for drinking purposes. Unfortunately, the waste-pipe of the former being obstructed, the foul water of one side communicated with the clean water of the other, and in one day 60 people died of cholera in the small portion of the city which was supplied from the infected source. The striking case has often been cited which occurred at Epping, Eng., where a woman brought the disease from a distance into a perfectly healthy house and neighborhood, and of ten persons affected with it seven died, including a physician in attendance upon one of them. An examination of the premises "discovered, below the pipes leading from the water-closet and from the eye-hole of the sink through which the choleraic dejections had been passed, a leakage which extended under the foundations of the building and entered the well. The sewage was distinctly traceable on the side of the well corresponding with the leakage in the drain." After this discovery and the disuse of the foul water not another case occurred.[15] In 1868, Dr. [p. 726]Farr, in his *History of the London Cholera Epidemic of 1866*, showed that water into which cholera dejections find their way produces cases of cholera all over the district in which it is distributed for a certain period of time, and that if the distribution is in any way cut short the deaths from cholera begin to decline within about three days of the date at which the distribution is stopped.[16]

[14] *Edinb. Med. Jour.*, i. 1122.

[15] *Trans. of the Epidemiological Soc.*, ii. 428.

[16] *Lancet*, April, 1868, p. 217.

Analogous instances are furnished by every cholera epidemic of which the history has been accurately observed, including that which extended so widely over the United States in 1873. Most of the following are cited from the official reports prepared, under the direction of the Surgeon-General of the army, by Surgeon Ely McClellan and Dr. John C. Peters. Several of the first cases, however, are foreign.

In 1861, at a station in India, some fresh cholera dejecta found their way into a vessel of drinking-water. Early on the following morning a small quantity of this water was swallowed by nineteen persons, five of whom were attacked with cholera between the first and the third day afterward.[17] In 1876 an outbreak of cholera took place in a village in Hindostan, which followed the arrival of wedding-guests, one of whom was attacked, and

514

from whom it rapidly spread. The soiled clothes of one or more of the patients were washed in a pool from which all the villagers obtained their drinking-water, and on the discontinuance of this source of water-supply cholera speedily diminished in frequency and fatality.[18] In the German epidemic of 1873 many cases occurred where persons deriving their drinking-water from special sources were attacked with cholera, while their neighbors, supplied from a different source, remained free. Again, it has frequently happened that outbreaks of cholera have been checked by the prohibition of the suspected water and the substitution of a pure supply.[19] It seems probable that a very small portion of cholera discharges suffices to infect a very large body of water and maintain its infectiousness for a considerable time.

[17] Macnamara, *op. cit.*, p. 196.
[18] Surg.-Major Cornish, *Practitioner*, xxiv. 215.
[19] *Practitioner*, xxvi. 159.

In December, 1871, an outburst of cholera occurred which was confined to the inmates of three excellent houses in a fine block of buildings in Calcutta. There had been no cholera in that neighborhood for four years. Within forty-eight hours a majority of the lodgers were sick, and on investigation it was found that the disease was carried in the drinking-water and in the milk diluted with it.[20] The particular locality in which Dr. Koch made the discovery of the microscopic representative of cholera furnishes an example of the same nature: "At Saheb Ragau, a locality which has repeatedly been visited by cholera during the last hundred years, numerous cases of the disease were reported, and these, on inquiry, were found exclusively in the huts situated round a certain tank. Of the few hundred people who dwelt in these huts, as many as seventeen died of cholera, though the disease was not at that time prevalent in the neighborhood, or indeed in the whole police district of Calcutta. It was proved that, as usual in such cases, the dwellers around the tank used it for bathing, and drew thence their drinking-water; it was also elicited that the linen of the first fatal case, befouled with cholera dejections, had been washed in the tank."[21] In June, 1873, a new [p. 727]hotel was opened at Vienna, and many of the guests became affected with diarrhoea that was attributed to the drinking-water, which was offensive to the taste and smell. After a fortnight a gentleman died of cholera in the hotel, and two days later several of the guests were attacked with the disease, of whom fourteen died. The gentleman who first died was believed to have brought the poison with him into the hotel, so that the drinking-water, which previously had been polluted with ordinary fecal discharges, became specifically affected through him.[22] The discharges of one ill of cholera were thrown into, and the vessels used by him were washed near, a well from which all the residents of a farm-house drank. The wooden curbing of the well had rotted, and the ground immediately around had sunken; a heavy rain burst the curb, overflowed the well, and washed into it the entire surface-drainage of the surrounding ground. No attention was paid to this, and the water was used as before. It became so offensive that its use was forbidden, but too late to save the family, nine of whom died of cholera.[23]

[20] *U.S. Report*, p. 85.
[21] *Times and Gaz.*, April, 1884, p. 527.
[22] *Times and Gaz.*, p. 86.
[23] *Ibid.*, p. 140.

At Farmington, Tenn., a man arrived who had contracted the cholera at Nashville; his illness ran its course at a point just forty paces from a well. Families that obtained their water from this well suffered in nearly all their members; where only certain members drank of it, they alone were affected.[24] At Huntsville, Ala., during an epidemic of cholera, the city authorities forbade the use of well-water, and supplied pure water from another source, but only for one week. During this time no new cases of the disease occurred, and the negroes, thinking themselves secure, resumed the use of the well-water, and within four days six fatal cases of cholera occurred in the vicinity. The use of the well-water was again prohibited, and again the progress of the disease was arrested.[25]

[24] *Ibid.*, p. 172.
[25] *Ibid.*, p. 408. For other examples of the spread of cholera by means of drinking-water see Macnamara, p. 149 and seq.

It has already been intimated that the cholera poison may be diffused through the air from either moist or dry sources, and especially from contaminated clothing, and then be taken into the throat and swallowed. Dr. Richardson refers to a local epidemic in England in which "the persons most constantly and fatally attacked were the women who washed the clothes of the sick;" and this circumstance has been largely confirmed by other observers.[26] In a village not far from Marseilles, and in an isolated place, a peasant and his wife who had not left the country sickened and died of the disease. The woman, who was a laundress, had received a bundle of linen belonging to a person recently arrived from Egypt, and the husband opened the bundle and unfolded the pieces. During the Crimean War many of the washermen attending to the washing of the French hospitals were attacked by cholera. In the post-office at Marseilles none of the clerks who handled the outgoing mails were attacked, but of those who sorted the mails coming from the East, where the disease prevailed, one after another suffered from cholera.[27]

[26] *Trans. Epidem. Soc.*, ii. 429.
[27] Read, Boston, 1866.

The cholera was introduced into Guadaloupe by clothing contained in a trunk belonging to a person who died on the voyage thither from Marseilles, where the cholera then prevailed. The woman who washed the clothing died, with all her family. Attracted by the circumstances of [p. 728]the case, many came to her house, and of these several died. From this point the disease spread over the island.[28] A sailor died at some port in Europe of Asiatic cholera in 1832. A chest containing his personal effects, clothing, etc. was sent home to his family, who lived in a small straggling village on the Atlantic coast of the State of Maine. It reached them about Christmas, and was opened on its arrival. The inmates of the house were all immediately and suddenly seized with a disease resembling Asiatic cholera in all its malignity, and died. There had been no cholera in the State. The last case of cholera that occurred in the garrison at Malta in the epidemic of 1865 was that of a woman who had stolen a chemise the property of one who had died of the disease. She put on this fatal garment, probably soiled with cholera discharges, and certainly unwashed, many days after the death of its former possessor; she took the disease and died.[29]

[28] *Med. Times and Gaz.*, April, 1874, p. 387.
[29] *Lancet*, Feb. 17, 1866.

It is sometimes said, and oftentimes repeated, that cholera is not directly contagious—is not communicated by the sick to the well. No statement could be more unfounded. The whole history of cholera proves that the physicians and nurses of cholera patients are often affected by the disease. "In Constantinople no less than twenty-seven physicians and medical assistants were attacked and died during their attendance on cholera patients; and in Paris and Toulon similar results followed. At Halifax, N.S., two of the physicians who volunteered in aid of the steamer England, which put in there disabled by the ravages of cholera among the officers and crew, as well as among the steerage passengers, took the disease, and one died" (Read). In 1832 the cases of cholera in Edinburgh were in the proportion of 1 to every 1200 of the population of the city, while among those in attendance upon the sick the proportion was 1 to 5. In 1848-49 one-fourth of the nurses employed in the cholera hospital took the disease, while in the general hospital, only a few paces distant, where no cholera patients were received, not a single attendant was attacked. In the London Hospital, in 1866, none of the medical officers, volunteer nurses, or sisters were attacked. Of the (regular) nurses five contracted the disease, and of these four died.[30] In 1849 a severe and fatal epidemic broke out in the Philadelphia Almshouse. The resident physicians of the hospital were abundantly occupied with the care of the sick of other diseases, and it was thought prudent not to allow any, even an indirect, communication between them and the cholera patients. The latter were therefore removed to an isolated building in the middle of the quadrangle, and attended by physicians from the city who had volunteered their aid. Three or four of these physicians had attacks of cholera, and two of them died.[31] At this time there was no cholera at all in the city, and the young physicians could not have become infected outside of the almshouse. They were attacked while attending the sick of cholera, but the regular house-physicians, who seldom visited the cholera patients, escaped altogether.

[30] *London Hosp. Rep.*, iii. 439.
[31] *Philada. Med. Examiner*, Nov., 1849.

The importance of recognizing the communicability of cholera is so great that no apology need be made for introducing the following additional illustrations of it furnished by Griesinger in his article on the dangers of cholera to medical men. They are the more important because [p. 729]in many other instances cholera physicians have suffered little for their devotion to duty: "At Moscow, in 1840, hospital attendants contracted the disease to the extent of 30 or 40 per cent., while in the general population only 3 per cent. were attacked; at Berlin, in 1831, in Romberg's hospital, 54 out of 115 persons were attacked: in 1837 one-fifth of the attendants took the disease, and on one occasion no less than seven of them fell ill on a single day. In La Charité Hospital in Paris, in 1849, one-sixth of the attendants had the disease, while only one-twenty-fifth of the general population of the city suffered from it; at Mittau, in 1848, one-half of the physicians took the disease; in 1842, at Toulon, ten health officers out of thirty-five were ill with cholera, and five of them died, while of thirty workmen who were employed to carry the dead bodies one-third succumbed; at Stockholm, in 1853, of 536 attendants one-eighth took the disease, and half of that number died; at Vienna, in 1854, out of thirty-six nurses, seven caught the disease, and seven men employed in removing the dead became affected with a prolonged and exhausting diarrhoea; in 1849, at Strasburg, five nurses out of ten were attacked, etc." ... "Physicians, nurses, students, etc. are less frequently affected, however, than patients ill with other diseases who are lying in the wards where cholera patients are treated, and are therefore more constantly exposed to the emanations from the discharges; and physicians usually suffer less than the attendants who are constantly waiting on the cholera patients."[32]

[32] *Traité des Maladies infectieuses*, 1868, p. 409.

It may be added that Surgeon-General John Murray, who served continuously for thirty-eight years in British India, caused upward of five hundred circulars to be addressed to the local governments and filled up by the local medical officers. From these returns it appeared that the belief in the communicability of cholera, in one way or another, was practically unanimous; for of the whole number, those who believed that it is conveyed from person to person were 75 per cent.; from place to place, 85 per cent.; through the atmosphere, 80 per cent.; with the drinking-water, 85 per cent.; by the evacuations, 92 per cent.; and by clothing, 98 per cent.[33] This gentleman has more recently furnished additional facts supporting the same conclusion. For example: Out of fourteen cases that occurred at Ramleh during the Egyptian epidemic, eleven occurred in patients already in the hospital for other diseases. In 1856, after visiting the dead-house where the bodies of fourteen cholera patients lay, as he entered the cholera ward he felt a sudden shock in the epigastrium, followed by a deadening sensation that rapidly spread over the whole body. On another occasion he saw a clergyman who was talking to a cholera patient suddenly seized with vomiting of a watery liquid. Several analogous instances are related by him.[34]

[33] *Practitioner*, xix. 470.
[34] *Med. Times and Gaz.*, March, 1884, p. 281.

It has been objected to the communicability of cholera that its dissemination does not always follow the deposit of cholera discharges in privies, wells, etc., and also that when infection does take place, it may occur between remote extremes as to time, and therefore cannot be attributed to infectious germs. Such objections are frivolous, because we know nothing of the nature or vitality of cholera-germs, and they are, moreover, drawn from exceptional cases. The power of infected fomites to develop [p. 730]the disease has been preserved, in a journey from Arabia into Africa, for at least twelve days, and for even a longer period in passing from Germany to Chicago, as already related. It is true of every infectious and contagious disease that it may possess one or both of these qualities in various degrees—that at one time it is only exceptionally communicated, and that at another time it appears to propagate itself virulently. So the phenomena of cholera may consist of little more than a watery diarrhoea, which may be so mild as hardly to disable the patient from working, while at other times the attack may include all those terrible and fatal symptoms which have won for the disease the name of malignant. That a certain quantity, or "dose," of the cholera poison is required to develop the disease, but one that varies considerably in different cases, may be inferred from these facts: 1. Out of a certain number of persons equally exposed to receive the disease, only a portion may be attacked at all, and these in very unequal degrees. 2. Persons so slightly affected as to be ignorant of the nature of their sickness, and believing it to be an ordinary diarrhoea, may nevertheless become the innocent, because ignorant, disseminators of cholera. The explanation of such facts may be manifold: they may depend upon the dose or upon the energy of the morbid poison, on various possible conditions of its recipient, and so on; but, however explained, their reality is none the less certain. The receptivity of persons exposed to the contagion of cholera is very different. It is well known that some persons appear to be proof against other contagious diseases, while others seem never to acquire an immunity from them. On this very important point the conclusions of Fauvel directly bear.[35] They include the following propositions: The East Indian ports where cholera exists as an endemic disease are never the seat of an extensive epidemic among the native population. But strangers to these localities are liable to the disease, and such are the Mussulman pilgrims who come to Bombay to take ship for Mecca. A severe epidemic of cholera confers upon the locality in which it has taken place an immunity which in India appears to be of several years' duration. Such an epidemic in any country is a proof that the cholera is not endemic there.

[35] *Mémoire lu à l'Académie des Sciences*, 1883.

If a contagious disease preserved its virulence undiminished, it might continue to prevail indefinitely. But we know that all other contagious epidemics do come to an end sooner or later, and hence we must conclude that their specific cause progressively loses its virulent qualities. There is every reason, therefore, to believe that the same is true of cholera. Its communicability, and therefore its diffusion, may vary with climatic, seasonal, local, personal, and other conditions; but of what nature those conditions are, and especially of the last and most important, the personal, hardly anything is known. Nor need we too curiously investigate them, so long as the fact remains that outside of, and independent of them all, there is but one essential cause of cholera—a morbid poison as specific in its nature as that of any of the eruptive fevers—a poison which no determinable conjunction of circumstances has ever engendered, and which was unknown in Europe and America before it was carried to them from India. In just such a way did small-pox first arise in the Western World. It had never appeared in Europe until the latter part of the [p. 731]sixth century, when for a short time it prevailed in Marseilles and the neighboring country. Afterward it was not heard of until it was reintroduced by the Crusaders on their return from Palestine in the twelfth century, since which period it has hardly ever ceased. The history of the diffusion of cholera is closely analogous to this in several particulars, and we may reasonably expect that what was in the last generation a new disease will henceforth be liable to prevail again and again as the intercourse increases between the nations of the West and the immemorial source of cholera in Hindostan.[36]

[36] Additional illustrations of the communicability of cholera are contained in the *Brit. and For. Med. Chir. Rev.*, July, 1872, p. 56.

In the preceding discussion of the origin and dissemination of cholera the broad facts of its specific nature and its contagion by means of excreta have been chiefly insisted upon. Little has been said either of the nature of the contagium or of the conditions that modify its activity. These points will be considered hereafter. But it is proper in this place to state that, in the opinion of most investigators, the contagious element has the power of multiplying itself, not only within the body, but wherever it is in contact with decomposing organic matter, provided that the degree of heat and amount of moisture present are adapted to promote such a change, which is certainly analogous to fermentation, if not identical with it. And the facts already mentioned may be recalled, which show that the contagium cannot be a light and subtle substance, since, as has been stated, the immediate attendants upon cholera patients are not as apt as might be expected, on that hypothesis, to contract the disease, while washerwomen inhaling, and probably swallowing, the moist fumes from cholera fomites much more frequently do so; that fomites saturated with the dried discharges are very infectious; and that water is the principal vehicle by which cholera-germs are carried into the stomach.

SYMPTOMATOLOGY.—Like other diseases, cholera occurs under very dissimilar aspects and with various degrees of gravity. Like those especially which are caused by specific morbid poisons, it may be so insignificant as to escape recognition, or, on the other hand, it may give rise to violent and distressing symptoms which come on without warning and hurry the patient to inevitable death. Whenever epidemic diseases present such opposite extremes of severity in their symptoms, it may reasonably be inferred that the differences depend mainly upon the quantity of the poison that has been received into the system, precisely as the dose which has been taken of a narcotic or acrid poison may be estimated by the gravity of its effects. Individual peculiarities, constitutional or acquired, may modify the characteristic phenomena, and sometimes a careful inquiry may be necessary even to detect their existence; but a study of cholera in all its grades shows that its symptoms are all the effects of one and the same cause, and that the cholera poison acts primarily upon the gastro-intestinal mucous membrane. It follows, as a matter of course, that, being thus applied, it will occasion symptoms differing in degree and in kind according to the energy of its action, and that this, again, will depend partly upon the inherent virulence of the agent and partly upon its quantity. In fact, this feature in the clinical history of the disease can be explained only by the operation of a special irritant acting with different degrees of power upon the gastro-intestinal [p. 732]mucous membrane. In other words, the different forms under which it is convenient clinically to recognize and describe cholera are nothing more than different degrees of the operation of one and the same poison, modified more or less by the peculiarities of individual patients. In the most typical of the fully-formed cases of cholera there is a stage of diarrhoea, a stage of cholera morbus—*i.e.* of vomiting and purging—with more or less evidence of stagnation of the blood, which is followed either by reaction and recovery or collapse and death. The phenomena of those several stages will now be described, after which certain symptoms will be more particularly considered.

It has more than once been pointed out that, however mild an attack of cholera may be, the dejections accompanying it are infectious, and may produce in other persons the gravest types of the disease. Hence the importance, not only to the patients, but also to others, of recognizing it in the earliest stage; for while this knowledge may suggest measures for preventing an extension of the disease, it leads to the prompt use of remedies at the only period in which their success can at all be counted upon. The characteristic of this stage, which has generally been called either choleraic diarrhoea or cholerine, is a diarrhoea remarkable for its profuseness and the frequency and serous quality of the stools, which are, however, of a more or less yellow color. They are preceded by rumbling and gurgling noises in the abdomen, are voided without colic or tenesmus, and are followed by a remarkable sense of exhaustion or faintness, which is sometimes also accompanied with nausea, and, if they are very frequent and copious, cramps are apt to be felt in the calves of the legs. In this variety or stage of the attack, as a rule, there is not any vomiting; there is complete anorexia, but urgent thirst, a white and clammy tongue, and a peculiar alteration of tone, a huskiness, faintness, or hoarseness of the voice. The stools vary from six to twelve a day, and, as above stated, are slightly yellow; they are also alkaline, and on standing deposit a granular sediment which consists largely of the débris of intestinal epithelium. Unless the attack is very severe the temperature is not lowered by much more than 1° F. The symptoms now described, especially in their milder grades, may last for a week or even longer, and then, according to circumstances, end either in cure or in fully-developed cholera; but under appropriate treatment they usually subside in a day or two, and more or less rapidly according to the degree of damage done to the digestive mucous membrane.

Between the above, which is the mildest type of epidemic cholera, and the fully-developed disease must be placed that grade of the disease which is more appropriately called cholerine, comprising cases in which vomiting occurs as well as purging, with increased debility and a tendency, more or less decided, to collapse. The matters vomited, after the rejection of undigested food, are at first bilious, but they gradually become less and less so the longer the attack lasts, and, together with the stools, assume the appearance of rice-water—*i.e.* they consist of a pale grayish, semi-transparent liquid in which white flocculi are suspended. Its reaction is alkaline, and it has a faint albuminous or spermatic smell. Along with these symptoms the other effects of serous depletion arise—debility with pallor, duskiness, coldness, profuse perspiration, and a sodden condition of the skin, while the secretion of urine is diminished, [p. 733]and all the symptoms that belong to the first stage of cholera are present in an aggravated degree.

A curious feature of this disease is that sometimes the onset even of its graver forms is not attended by any evacuations, although the stomach and intestine may be filled with liquid. It is perhaps chiefly in such cases that the patient experiences a rapid depression of all the mental and physical faculties. The senses are irritable, the head aches and is confused, there is a disinclination to sleep, the limbs totter under the weight of the body, the pulse is frequent and feeble, occasionally fainting takes place; the skin is cool and bedewed with perspiration. In other cases, again, the attack is sudden; the patient is smitten with an unaccountable feebleness, speedily followed by profuse vomiting and purging and general spasms, and dies without any suspension of the symptoms or any tendency to reaction.

But more usually the attack begins with the diarrhoea and vomiting described above, which then assume, more or less rapidly, a high degree of violence, expressed by their frequency and excess. The stools with proportionate rapidity lose all their fecal qualities and acquire the rice-water appearance before mentioned, and the liquid rejected by vomiting in all respects resembles them. It is poured forth less by an ordinary act of vomiting than by gushes, as if it overflowed from the throat and mouth; and it often escapes from the stomach and the bowels at the same instant. Such profuse evacuations necessarily occasion an urgent thirst which cannot be satisfied, for liquids are thrown up immediately on being swallowed. Sometimes a distressing hiccough accompanies these symptoms. It is indeed only one of the many spasms which may affect the muscular system. They generally begin in the fingers and toes, which become bent and stiff; they seize upon the muscles of the calves of the legs, and render the muscular wall of the abdomen as hard as a board. The pain they produce is extremely severe, and unless the patient is exceedingly prostrated he endeavors to assuage it by a constant change of position.

At this period the debility is very great, and progressively increases, and the patient is unable to rise, or even to move at all except under the stimulus of the painful spasms. The features are shrunken; the nose is sharp and pallid, and bent to one side; the dusky, lack-lustre, and sunken eyes, the thin lips, the hollow cheeks, and the contracted muscles that stand out like cords under the tense and clammy skin, present a physiognomy that belongs to no other disease in the same degree. The hands and feet grow cold, and steadily the coldness creeps upward toward the trunk; the temperature falls to 94° or 95° F.; the feeble and even flickering pulse ranges from 100 to 120. The integuments of the limbs are shrivelled and damp, and look as if they had been macerated in water; and if a fold of the skin is pinched up it subsides very slowly indeed. The eyes grow dull and dry, the tongue has a pasty or sticky feel, and the urine is almost suppressed. If any of this excretion can be obtained for examination, it is found to contain both albumen and sugar. As the attack advances the patient falls into a dull, listless, and motionless state, which may be mistaken for insensibility or even unconsciousness but is really due to exhaustion of all the faculties of mind and body. He may express no interest in anything, and hardly notice the [p. 734]attention or the distress of his friends, yet he will generally give clear, although languid, answers to questions, and fall again into an inert and unobservant state.

As these symptoms continue and the fluids of the body decrease, the blood accumulates and stagnates in the veins, giving to the hands and feet, the nose and lips and other features, to the neck, and even to the entire surface of the body, a bluish, leaden, or violet tint, precisely like that of cyanotic children. The pulse, that was already weak and thready, is no longer perceptible; the carotids even and the impulse of the heart cease to be felt, and the second sound of the latter becomes inaudible. The skin is everywhere cold; the hands, feet, and face are sometimes of an icy coldness, and yet the patients seldom perceive that they are so; indeed, complaint is more apt to be made of suffering from internal heat. Even the breath as it issues from the nostrils feels cold. The blood no longer circulates, and the heart seems still. If a vein is opened a few drops of black and viscid blood will trickle from the wound, which if it coagulates, yields but little serum, and in place of a firm clot only a diffluent jelly. The voice has sunk to a mere whisper or is quite extinct. The features assume a distorted and frightful expression; the temples and cheeks are hollowed; the nose is twisted and pointed, and the nostrils are obstructed with dry and powdery crusts; the eyes are also dry, dull, and sunken behind the half-closed and purple lids; the conjunctiva is no longer moistened by its secretion and becomes bloodshot; the temperature in the mouth may fall to 79° or 80° F.; a viscid exhalation bedews the icy and marbled skin; and the whole body is so shrunken from its natural proportions as to lose all the marks by which its identity has been recognized. From this pulseless, exhausted, cold, and cyanotic condition there can be but one step to death. It generally comes on gradually, the patient sinking into the state of apparent insensibility before mentioned; on the other hand, he may expire suddenly on attempting to make some unusual effort.

At any period in the progress of cholera, except that of complete asphyxia, the contest between the system and the disease may be decided in favor of the former. If this occurs before profuse evacuations have taken place or blueness of the skin appeared, the recovery may be gradual and present no special phenomena. The pulse regains by degrees its natural force; the skin grows warm again, first upon the trunk and afterward upon the extremities; the breathing becomes easy, and, the diarrhoea having already ceased, convalescence is established. But in proportion to the severity of the symptoms, the intensity and duration of the cold stage, the cramps, and the evacuations, will there be a tendency to febrile reaction, with more or less passive congestion of the internal organs, and therefore a slower return to health. If the attack has been very severe, and particularly if the algid stage has been prolonged, fever of a low type is apt to occur, and indeed may terminate fatally. This fever presents all the characters of the typhoid state, and is marked by dryness of the tongue, a brown crust upon the teeth and gums, jerking of the tendons, delirium, and coma. These symptoms are partly evidences of exhaustion, of inability of the system to resume its normal action, and perhaps also they denote the retention of the effete products of nutrition in the blood; but sometimes they appear to be associated [p. 735]with, and caused by, a local and latent inflammation of low grade, established usually in the lungs. Again, the nervous system seems to bear the brunt of the reactionary effort, and the patient is attacked by convulsions or perishes in an apoplectic fit. These phenomena appear to be due in most instances, if not in all, to renal obstruction, and, as it is supposed that their immediate cause is the retention of urea in the blood, they have received the title of uræmic. In other cases a wasting diarrhoea, due probably to the damaged state of the intestinal mucous membrane, is superadded to the already existing typhoid state. Occasionally the parotid glands become enlarged and painful, and sometimes a measly or roseolous eruption appears upon the skin.

It frequently happens that the convalescence from cholera is slow and irregular. The system seems to be shattered by the trial it has passed through; the nervous susceptibility is for a long time morbidly increased, or, what is still more usual, the digestive function is greatly impaired. The appetite is capricious and the digestion feeble. The mouth is pasty, the abdomen tympanitic, the bowels are irregular and alternately confined and relaxed. Finally, patients who leave the bed too soon or indulge prematurely in their ordinary diet are liable to a relapse, perhaps fatally, into the original disease. It has sometimes happened that such a relapse has taken place several days after an apparent restoration to perfect health.

COMPLICATIONS AND SEQUELÆ.—In a small proportion of cases, as above stated, cutaneous eruptions have been observed during the attack of cholera, or rather during its decline, for they coincide with the reaction or follow it, and may be regarded as indications of increasing vitality. They belong to the exanthematous class, and comprise roseola, erythema, urticaria, and rarely vesicular eruptions.[37] But, instead of them, there may occur destructive tissue-lesions in the form of abscesses or ulcers. These affections are more usual on the limbs than on the trunk or face, but some of them may appear even in the mouth or fauces. Profuse sweats have been noticed elsewhere, and the important fact that they carry off large quantities of urea, which they deposit upon the skin. Diphtherial exudation has also been met with upon tender parts of the skin and in the fauces, as well as in the stomach and intestine. In some epidemics of cholera suppuration of the parotid gland is occasionally observed, while in others it may be entirely absent. Instances have been reported of double parotitis, and in several of them the termination of the attack was fatal. Still more rarely suppuration of the submaxillary or the cervical glands has been met with. Another sequela of cholera is a tetanic contraction of the flexor muscles of the limbs.

Between the tenth and fifteenth days of convalescence the patient is attacked with a tearing, rending pain in the hands and forearms, the legs and feet, followed by tonic contraction of the flexor muscles of these parts. The sensibility is not impaired. The attack lasts for one or several days, and seems always to end in recovery (Guterbock).

[37] Compare *London Hosp. Reports*, iii. 457.

Some of the individual symptoms of cholera call for a more detailed notice than they have received in the foregoing epitome, in which the continuity of the narrative could not be interrupted by a description of variations depending upon the stage and grade of the disease.
[p. 736]The first to be considered is the temperature. The animal temperature in cholera varies according to the part of the body at which it is taken more than in any other disease. In cases of average severity it rarely falls below 95° F. in the axilla. The temperature under the tongue does not furnish trustworthy indications. In the stage of asphyxia it seldom exceeds 87.8° F., and even in cases that recover it may fall to about 78.8° F. (Wunderlich). In the cold stage it is not uncommon for a difference of temperature to be noted of nearly ten degrees between the axilla and the rectum. In a female aged thirty-two the temperature in the axilla was 93° F., and that in the vagina 102.8° F. (Mackenzie). In other cases a vaginal temperature of 104° F., and even of 108.32° F., has been reached (Guterbock). Such high temperatures furnish an unfavorable prognosis. As Wunderlich has pointed out, during the algid stage temperatures taken in the mouth do not give an accurate idea of the general temperature; the rectal and vaginal temperatures are more nearly correct. The following are some results of thermometry in 74 cases of cholera: Lorain found the minimum rectal temperature in 1 case 93.2° F., in 2 cases 95°, and in 10 cases 96.8°. In 47 cases the normal temperature was preserved; in 27 it rose to 100.4°; in 15 cases to 102.2°; and in 1 to 104° F. Leubuscher gives the average temperature in the armpit 92.7° F.; under the tongue, 90.5°; upon the tongue, 81.5°, in the nostrils, 79.2°; and on the palm of the hand, 84° F. These numbers, however, only represent averages. It should be noted that the low temperature of the mouth and nostrils is caused not only by the evaporation from the surface of those cavities, but also by the relative coldness of the expired air, due to the partial suspension of the passage of blood through the lungs, and therefore to the heating of the air contained in them. According to Leubuscher also, the lowest temperature is found in the nostrils, and next under the tongue, and at the latter point it may vary from 79° F. to 90.5° F. In death by asphyxia the vaginal and rectal temperatures may rise to 104°-108° F. The axillary fluctuates less than the internal temperature. It is remarkable that during the algid stage the patients, at least before the temperature has reached its minimum, are not conscious of their coldness, but, on the contrary, complain of internal heat, precisely as happens in the congestive forms of periodical fever. When the febrile reaction assumes a typhoid type the temperature in many cases is normal or only slightly elevated, and it is of serious import if the temperature then sinks again below the normal grade (Wunderlich). On the whole, the maintenance of a uniform temperature, neither much above or below 90° F. in the axilla or under the tongue, may be regarded as favorable, yet recoveries have taken place even when the temperature at these points has fallen to 79° F. If the temperature of the parts just mentioned should rise rapidly to 104° F., it may be regarded as a very unfavorable sign.

The skin, as has elsewhere been described, is pallid, bluish, shrunken, and cold, and quite destitute of its natural firmness and elasticity, so that when it is pinched into folds they subside very slowly, as if they had been made on the skin of a corpse. It is curious that, although the drain of liquids through the bowels is so great, the skin not only remains moist, but generally is bathed in a profuse cold sweat. Although the secretion of urine is reduced or quite suspended, that of milk is said to be not [p. 737]always so. Large quantities of urea have been found in the urine, and in some cases it has been visible upon the skin in the form of white scales. During convalescence the skin may be the seat of the various eruptions already enumerated. Of a graver nature, but, fortunately, of rarer occurrence, are erysipelas, boils, abscesses, ulcers, and gangrene. These several affections seem to result from the alternate obstruction and freedom of the cutaneous circulation. They commonly appear first upon the limbs, and afterward upon the face or trunk; they may affect even the cavity of the mouth. Some observers have noted a relatively frequent occurrence of diphtherial exudations in this disease, while others do not allude to their existence. The former describe the false membrane as affecting not only the mouth and fauces, but also the stomach, the intestine, and the female organs of generation. A case is reported by Joseph of a young man who, after an attack of cholera, was affected with a blenorrhoea, due to a diphtherial inflammation of the urethra.

The character of the heart- and pulse-beats in this disease is quite peculiar. Their rate does not increase indefinitely, as it does after hemorrhage; the pulse usually varies from 90 to 110, and indeed seldom exceeds 120, but its volume, tension, and force progressively decline until the beats become imperceptible at the wrist, and even in the brachial and femoral arteries. At the same time, the rhythm of the heart is interrupted, the energy of its impulse declines until it can no longer be felt, and its sounds grow weaker and weaker until they become quite inaudible. Sometimes, it is said, a pericardial friction sound may be heard, which is attributed to the dryness of the pericardium. That the decline and suspension of the heart's sounds and impulse are due not only to the weakness of the cardiac muscle, but also to the lessened volume of the circulating blood, is proved by the fact that they persist, sometimes for many hours, after reaction has commenced, and only become audible again when the arteries have been replenished with blood.

In the description of the symptoms of cholera it has been mentioned that the cyanotic color of the skin is produced by an accumulation of blood in the veins. Many years ago Magendie, and after him Dieffenbach, on examining the arteries of persons in the advanced stage of cholera, found those vessels empty of blood. It might be supposed that, under the circumstances, not only the right side of the heart, but also the lungs, would be gorged with blood, and that extreme dyspnoea would result. But, in point of fact, the respiration in cholera is hurried and shallow rather than oppressed and labored, while after death the lungs are not engorged with blood, but rather in a bloodless condition. The pulmonary artery and its branches are also empty, although the right side of the heart may be filled with dark and soft coagula. These singular conditions seem to be due, on the one hand, to the greatly diminished mass of the blood in the vessels, and to its accumulating and stagnating in various parts of the venous system, and, on the other hand, to the weakness of the heart, which is shown by its suppressed impulse and sounds, and which lessens its power to propel the venous blood into the lungs. The infarction of the systemic veins and the threatening suspension of the circulation necessarily impair the activity of all the functions, including those of nutrition and disintegration, so that the effete detritus of the economy tends to accumulate in the blood. This tendency is [p. 738]doubtless counterbalanced not only by the diarrhoea, but also, more or less, by the almost total suspension of nutrition, due to the inability of the cholera patient to digest or even to retain food, as well as by the diminished oxidation of the blood in the lungs. It has already been observed that, to a certain extent, the impediment to the passage of the blood from the right side of the heart into the ramifications of the pulmonary artery tends to prevent congestion and infarction of the lungs. But this obstruction is precisely what occurs during the stage of reaction in many cases, which then terminate fatally by asphyxia, as in the previous stage still more perish by apnoea.

In the milder attacks of cholera vomiting may not occur, and in the most severe it not unusually is suspended for some time before death, although the diarrhoea may continue. In the most malignant cases, indeed, there may be no vomiting at all, in consequence of the extreme muscular exhaustion, although the stomach may be distended with liquid. When rejected, the liquid has the general aspect of rice-water, which the stools also present. Its reaction is alkaline or neutral, and it is said to contain a less proportion than the stools of solid matter, but a larger proportion of urea. The act of vomiting is strictly one of regurgitation, which is performed without effort or pain. Sometimes, indeed, it seems to relieve the sense of weight caused by the accumulated contents of the stomach. It is readily excited by attempts to drink, and even by slight changes of posture. The vomited liquid at first contains the various articles of food the patient may have eaten. Their half-digested remains have sometimes suggested the announcement of strange specific forms of cholera germs. The liquid, after ceasing to be colored brownish or greenish, becomes gray, and subsequently, in favorable cases, more or less green again; while during the stage of reaction in grave and ultimately fatal cases it is more or less reddened by an admixture of blood. Its most usual and characteristic appearance is that of a grayish liquid containing whitish flocculi. The nature of this liquid, whether discharged by vomiting or by purging, has been variously estimated. Formerly, some persons held the white granules to be leucocytes, but the greater number agree that they are mainly epithelial fragments. When the vomited liquid is allowed to stand, a sediment forms in it which is composed almost entirely of epithelial scales, more or less modified in their appearance by the accidental contents of the stomach, and a film covers its surface in which globules of fat and phosphatic crystals may be detected. They are frequently associated with sarcinæ, produced by fermentation in the contents of the stomach, and after standing for some time the liquid becomes crowded with vibrios (Lindsay).

Although the propensity of the sick to discover a cause for every symptom often leads cholera patients to attribute their diarrhoea to some particular exposure to cold, error of diet, etc., yet, in fact, this symptom, so far as it belongs to cholera, is primarily an effect of the cholera poison alone, although it may be aggravated by causes like those mentioned. It is of great practical importance to bear in mind that a specific choleraic diarrhoea—that is to say, a diarrhoea produced by the cholera poison alone—may continue to be very slight as long as it lasts, which may be for several weeks; and hence, as elsewhere insisted upon, a person who is not suspected of being affected with cholera may, quite ignorantly, sow[p. 739]the seeds of a deadly epidemic of the disease. The danger in cholera is proportioned to the volume of the discharges rather than to their frequency, just as a single profuse hemorrhage is more serious than the loss of an equal amount of blood divided among several successive days. The special danger, however, is not, as in hemorrhage, from syncope, but from the progressive loss by drainage of the water of the blood, rendering it unfit to circulate, and therefore causing it to stagnate in the veins. The spoliative operation of the diarrhoea has occasionally been productive of benefit instead of injury, as in the following case of Barlow: A man suffering from dropsy was attacked with cholera, "and passed gallons of liquid by stool, had cramps, and became livid and clammy, but his pulse did not disappear, as in profound collapse, and he eventually rallied, and left the hospital apparently well. When he began to recover from cholera his appearance was almost ludicrous, from the manner in which the integument hung loosely about him."

The stools pass through a series of changes corresponding to those of the matters vomited, being fecal at first, and then becoming colorless and watery. During reaction, if that occurs, they regain more or less of their proper color, but if typhoid febrile symptoms prevail they are usually bloody. Decomposed blood sometimes renders them dark, tarry, and fetid; this condition has caused them sometimes to be described as being composed of vitiated bile, which is, however, a product not of the liver, but of the imagination.

In the intestine after death considerable quantities of epithelium are found floating in the contained liquid or else loosely adherent to the mucous membrane. It is usually in flocculi, but sometimes in fragments large enough to form a continuous membrane. A microscopic examination of cholera stools shows that their turbidness depends chiefly upon desquamated epithelium, with which is mixed white corpuscles and bacteria. It is remarkable that although the stools are drained directly and so rapidly from the blood-vessels, they nevertheless contain but little albumen, indeed hardly more than a trace of it. If, however, blood is mixed with the stools, as happens in rare instances, more albumen is present. Oil-globules are most abundant in cases that have passed beyond the stage of collapse into that of reaction with fever. In these it is said that oily matter may be found either in concrete masses or as a scum of liquid oil. Of inorganic constituents they contain crystals of the triple phosphate of ammonium and magnesium and chloride of sodium in greatest abundance, but the proportion of ammonium and potassium salts is small. Indeed, the total amount of solids does not exceed 2 per cent. As the quantity of water in the blood and solids is limited, and as in this disease the stomach will not receive nor retain any liquid, it follows that the more profuse the evacuations are, the shorter must be the duration of the attack, for the sooner then does the blood become too thick to circulate.

It has several times been stated that in cholera the urine is diminished, and that, therefore, the blood retains a larger proportion of effete products than in health. But it has also been remarked that the amount of these products is abnormally small, on account of the interference with nutrition of the abnormal state of the circulation. Doubtless, as in other cases of renal obstruction, an increased proportion of effete matter is eliminated by the skin, if not by the bowels. When the amount of [p. 740]urine excreted is only diminished, its specific gravity may vary between remote extremes, as 1.012 and 1.030. Usually, however, when its quantity is very greatly reduced, symptoms which are described as uræmic are apt to arise, and the urine is found to contain the usual products of renal congestion—viz. albumen, sometimes traces of blood, hyaline and granular casts, and epithelial scales, with less chloride of sodium and more urea than normal. It is remarkable that at the beginning of convalescence the urine, which had been suppressed or greatly diminished, may become for a time abnormally abundant. Rarely, if ever, does the derangement of the kidneys now described denote or produce an organic lesion in those organs. Like the disorders elsewhere, these are due to the loss of balance between the arterial and the venous sides of the circulation; both, indeed, have lost their functions more or less, the one by lack of blood, the other by an excess of blood unfit for circulation.

The occurrence of cramps in cholera, which has bestowed upon the disease one of its titles, spasmodic, has, however, no distinctive relation to the Asiatic disease. Spasmodic phenomena occur in many cases of poisoning by corrosive and irritant agents and in ordinary cholera morbus, and in cholera infantum they are among the most alarming symptoms, assuming, as they often do, the character of general convulsions. In most of these cases they are clonic and general, and therefore probably of central origin, primary or reflected; but the spasms of cholera are tonic, and affect the muscles of the upper and lower limbs, and most frequently the flexor muscles of these parts, and especially those of the fingers and toes, which become rigidly bent. The larger muscles contract into hard lumps, and even those of the chest and abdomen do not escape the terrible spasms. When they are severe they extort cries from patients who at other times seem quite apathetic. It is stated by Macnamara that the natives of Southern Bengal and other people of relatively loose fibre are much less apt to be attacked by them than the natives of the upper country or than Europeans. It may be debated whether their immediate cause is a reflex irritation emanating from the gastro-intestinal mucous membrane; or whether it is due to the rapid diminution of the supply of blood to the nervous centres, or to the infarction of those centres with thick and imperfectly oxygenated blood; or, finally, whether it is occasioned by a diminished supply of blood, and that blood of bad quality, to the muscles themselves. Probably all of these factors are associated causes in producing the spasmodic phenomena of cholera. It is well worthy of notice, however, that spasms, which are so frequent in all infantile diseases, and especially in those affecting the stomach and bowels, rarely attack children suffering from cholera. This would seem to prove that the spasms in question are not reflex, but either central and spinal, or else muscular—an inference which is strengthened by their being tonic and not clonic. As stated, the spasms, or cramps, frequently affect the limbs, but comparatively seldom involve the muscles of the chest or abdomen, and those of the face hardly ever. They are almost the only causes of pain in the disease, which in not a few instances runs its whole course, even to a fatal termination, without their occurrence.

As a rule, the abdomen is not so much retracted as might be expected from the profuse discharges. Probably in some degree its form is maintained by the constantly recurring accumulation of liquid in the[p. 741]gastro-intestinal cavity. In protracted cases, however, the abdomen becomes sunken and hollowed. At all stages of the disease it is somewhat sore under pressure, especially at the epigastrium, and it generally has a doughy feel. As to the functions of the digestive organs, they are completely suspended during a typical attack of the disease. Not only are these organs incompetent to digest food, but they cannot even retain it.

Throughout such an attack not only is sleep apt to be prevented by the pain of the cramps and the frequent evacuations, but, as a rule, the patient is wakeful, and yet, apart from the restlessness which accompanies the paroxysms of pain, there is, on the whole, a tendency to a placid quietness. Mental excitement and delirium are probably unknown during the primary attack, but sometimes a degree of somnolence or of apathetic tranquillity exists, which, however, is quite distinct from coma. When the attack is prolonged, and especially when it merges into a typhoid state, the eyes become inflamed by their exposure to the air. The conjunctiva then grows blood-shot, and occasionally the cornea is ulcerated.

MORBID ANATOMY AND PATHOLOGY.—The appearance after death of a person who has died in the collapse of cholera is very characteristic. It comprises a shrunken aspect of the whole body, its prevalent grayish or leaden pallor contrasting with the livid hue of the abdomen and back, the fingers and toes, the lips and eyelids, and ears; the eyes are sunken deeply in their orbits; the nose is sharp and bent, the temples are hollow, and the skin seems to cling tightly to the bones beneath it. The connective tissue is very dry, and the muscles are hard as well as dry, and, owing to the wasting of the softer parts, stand prominently out. In consequence of the absence of moisture decomposition takes place very slowly. Cadaveric rigidity is very marked and persistent. A very notable phenomenon is the occurrence of muscular contraction after death. It may be excited mechanically or may occur spontaneously. A case is related (Eichhorst) in which three hours after death the fibres of the biceps were observed to move tremulously, and then the entire muscle contracted, causing flexion of the forearm. Even the fingers performed movements like those made in piano-playing. The lower jaw has also been observed to move, causing the mouth to open and shut repeatedly. The late Sir Thomas Watson long ago described this singular phenomenon as follows: "A quarter or half an hour, or even longer, after the breathing had ceased, and all other signs of animation had departed, slight, tremulous, spasmodic twitchings and quiverings and vermicular motions of the muscles would take place, and even distinct movements of the limbs, in consequence of these spasms."[38] It was carefully studied by Barlow, from whose narrative the following is taken: The patient was a strong man; the course of his attack was rapid, and he suffered most cruelly from cramps. "Within two minutes of his ceasing to breathe muscular contractions began, becoming more and more numerous. The lower extremities were first affected. Not only were the sartorius, rectus, vasti, and other muscles thrown into violent spasmodic movements, but the limbs were rotated forcibly and the toes were frequently bent. The motions ceased and returned; they varied also: now one muscle moved, now many. Quite [p. 742]as remarkable were the movements of the arm: the deltoid and biceps muscles were peculiarly influenced; occasionally the forearm was flexed upon the arm—flexed completely, and when I straightened it, which I did several times, its position was recovered instantly. The fingers and thumbs were now and then contracted, and at times the thumbs were separately moved. The fibres of the pectoral muscles were often in full action; distinct bundles of them were seen at intervals beneath the skin.... After I had taken leave of the body the nurse was horrified by a movement of the lower jaw, which was followed by others; and I thought for a moment that the man was alive. The facial muscles became generally affected, and at length all was still."[39] These muscular contractions succeed one another in a regular order, beginning in one lower extremity and extending to the other, then to the upper limbs, and finally to the face. Their degree varies from a slight quivering to a powerful contraction, and their duration from a minute or less to an hour and a quarter. Cases have occurred in which the legs were so forcibly retracted that they could with difficulty be straightened again. In one case, six hours after death movements took place in one leg, and the hand was drawn across the chest; in another, "the forearms were powerfully flexed, and the hands, approximating, gave the attitude of praying to the body."[40] Again, Mr. Ward reports: "I saw the eyes of my dead patient open and move slowly in a downward direction. This was followed, a minute or two subsequently, by the movement of the right arm (previously lying by the side) across the chest." In the same paper Barlow says: "Mr. Lawrence mentioned to me that a gentleman who died in 1832 of rapid cholera was turned after death completely on the side by a strange and forcible combination of muscular contractions."[41] These muscular phenomena after death form an interesting feature in the history of cholera, but they are by no means peculiar to that disease. They have been observed in other diseases, and especially in yellow fever—an affection in which the pathological condition is quite unlike that of cholera. In both diseases they have been manifested in robust persons and when the course of the fatal attack was both rapid and severe. Thus, Dr. Dowler of New Orleans not only found that they could be developed in such cases of yellow fever by striking the muscles, but he observed their spontaneous occurrence in several, of which the following is a remarkable example: "Not long after the cessation of the respiration the left hand was carried by a regular motion to the throat, and then to the crown of the head; the right arm followed the same route on the right side; the left arm was then carried back to the throat, and thence to the breast, reversing all its original motions, and finally the right hand and arm did exactly the same."[42] In 1860, Drasche alleged that not unusually the skin covering the contracting muscles became reddish, while the local temperature rose $\frac{1}{2}°$, and that as soon as the contractions ceased the temperature fell below the normal and cadaveric rigidity set in. According to the same observer, analogous contractions affect the unstriped muscular fibres, in those of the skin producing a projection of the papillæ, and in the genital organs a discharge of semen. This phenomenon is said to have occurred an hour and a half after death.

[38] *Lectures*, Am. ed. of 1872.
[39] *London Med. Gaz.*, Nov., 1849, p. 798.
[40] *Ibid.*, Jan., 1850, p. 185.
[41] *Ibid.*, pp. 185, 186.
[42] *Experimental Researches*, 1846.

[p. 743]On opening the abdominal cavity of persons who have died in the collapse of cholera one is struck by the general pink or rose tint of the peritoneal coat of the intestines. It is produced by a repletion of the minute branches of the portal venous system. Sometimes the color is rendered very dark by the pitchy blood contained in the veins. The surface of the peritoneum, like all the tissues, is singularly dry, and often has a soapy or sticky feel, caused by a layer of albuminous matter, which forms a lather when rubbed between the fingers, and causes the intestinal folds to adhere to one another. If death takes place during the stage of reaction, these appearances are less distinct, and the intestines, which in collapse are usually retracted, are then somewhat distended.

The stomach generally contains a thin, partially transparent liquid of a greenish or grayish color, and occasionally reddish, holding in suspension portions of coagulated mucus and an unctuous substance of an albuminous nature, which adheres to the walls of the cavity. Fatty globules may be observed floating in the liquid, which under the microscope reveals epithelial débris, granular corpuscles, and fragments of gastric glands. Under heat and nitric acid coagulation of the liquid occurs, and on chemical examination it is found to contain urea. The gastric mucous membrane is of a dark violet or pale pink color, according to the stage of the disease; its follicles are enlarged, and patches of superficial abrasion may be observed on it.

The intestinal canal of those who die during the collapse of cholera is, in the majority of cases, partially filled with liquid which has the aspect of turbid serum, more or less mixed with the previous contents of the bowel if death has taken place very rapidly, but otherwise it is almost colorless. On the whole, however, it is less pale and watery than the stools. It contains, like these discharges, more or less epithelial flocculi, and generally more than were observed during life in the dejections. The mucus scraped from the lining membrane of the intestine and mixed with water renders it turbid with epithelial débris. The same mucus examined microscopically contains fragments, larger or smaller, of epithelium. These conditions are said to predominate in the large intestine. Indeed, the proportion of liquid increases from above downward. Hence in the more prolonged cases the contents of the bowel at its upper part are less liquid and are darker in color. There is, indeed, a striking contrast between the appearance of the intestine in cases which have terminated in collapse and its aspect in persons who have died during the stage of reaction. It has been clearly presented by Dr. Sutton.[43] When death took place in "the cold stage the mucous membrane was unusually pale in three cases; in two it was healthy-looking; in other two it was pale throughout, excepting that one or two of Peyer's patches were congested; and in the remaining three there was more or less congestion of the mucous membrane. When the mucous membrane was pale throughout the entire intestine, the valvulæ conniventes looked swollen and oedematous, and the color of the membrane was dead white. The solitary glands were very distinct and prominent. Those of the duodenum were remarkably so. In cases of imperfect reaction the mucous membrane of the intestine was usually found very much congested and ecchymosed. The congested portions were sometimes [p. 744]granular, and apparently denuded of epithelium. The mucous surface had often a dark port-wine color, due to the extravasated blood and the hyperæmia, and here and there the surface was covered with a dirty gray membranous substance, likened to a diphtheritic deposit. I have, however, seen no decided false membrane, such as could be peeled off, as in diphtheria. The surface was also occasionally bile-stained, and the greenish-yellow color of the bile and the deep red color of the congested surface presented a very striking appearance. The solitary glands were very prominent, and in some cases apparently enlarged." The general paleness of the intestinal mucous membrane in the stage of collapse, and its congestive redness whenever the signs of reaction have existed before death, have a very important bearing upon the pathology of this disease, for they demonstrate conclusively that the gastro-intestinal evacuations in cholera have no relation whatever to inflammation. On the other hand, they render it altogether probable that the serous flux is in the nature of a sweat, an intestinal ephidrosis.

[43] *London Hosp. Clin. Lect. and Reports,* iv. 497.

The nature of the exfoliation found in the intestinal canal has been the subject of much discussion. As long ago as the first American epidemic of cholera (1832-35) Dr. W. E. Horner, Professor of Anatomy in the University of Pennsylvania, described an exfoliation of the epithelial lining of the alimentary canal, whereby the extremities of the venous system of the part are denuded, as being characteristic of cholera alone. In 1849, Dr. Samuel Jackson, Professor of the Institutes of Medicine, and Dr. John Neill, Demonstrator of Anatomy in the University, in conjunction with Dr. William Pepper and Dr. Paul B. Goddard, presented a report to the College of Physicians of Philadelphia, in which they, too, showed that the "epithelial layer of the intestinal mucous membrane was either entirely removed or was detached, adhering loosely." This important fact—the most important, perhaps, in the mechanism of cholera—was confirmed seventeen years later by the eminent pathologist Dr. Lionel S. Beale,[44] who, when referring to "the remarkable characters of the matter discharged from the intestinal tube, and to the fact that the small intestines almost always contain a considerable quantity of pale almost colorless gruel-, rice-, or cream-like matter," added: "This has been proved to consist almost entirely of columnar epithelium, and in very many cases large flakes can be found, consisting of several uninjured epithelial sheaths of the villi.... In bad cases it is probable that almost every villus, from the pylorus to the ilio-cæcal valve, has been stripped of its epithelial coating during life.... These important organs, the villi, are, in a very bad case, all or nearly all left bare, and a very essential part of what constitutes the absorbing apparatus is completely destroyed.... It is probable that the extent of this process of denudation determines the severity or mildness of the attack.... It seems probable also that the epithelium may become detached in consequence of the almost complete cessation of the circulation in the capillaries beneath, but the death of the cells may occur in consequence of their being exposed to the influence of certain matters in the intestine or in the blood, in which case they would simply fall off."

[44] *Med. Times and Gazette,* Aug., 1866, p. 109.

In this connection, and as complementary of the statements now made, should be considered the further description by the same author—viz.:[p. 745]"Remarkable changes have occurred in the smaller vessels, especially in the capillaries and small veins of the villi and submucous tissue. The blood-corpuscles appear to have in a great measure been destroyed in the smaller vessels, and in their place are seen clots containing blood-coloring matter, minute granules, and small masses of germinal matter evidently undergoing active multiplication. Some of the arteries are contracted, but here and there small clots destitute of blood-corpuscles may be seen at intervals." Hence, the gastro-intestinal lesions in cholera, according to their extent and degree, they remove the natural obstacles to exhalation in the mucous membrane, and also, and in the same degree, prevent the absorption of the contents of the alimentary canal. It must not, however, be forgotten that this lesion is not altogether peculiar to the intestinal mucous membrane. Dr. Beale long ago called attention to the fact that in this disease there seems to be a tendency to the removal of epithelium from the surface of all soft, moist mucous membranes, but not from the follicles of the glands. The first statement appears to be explicable by the shrinkage of all the mucous membranes during cholera collapse, for by this merely mechanical agency the inelastic epithelium must necessarily become detached. As to the second statement, the remark may be made that the whole follicular structure furnished with columnar epithelium is an absorbing and not an eliminating apparatus, and that, since its functional activity is from the beginning of the disease diminished by an inadequate blood-supply, it can have but a small and indirect share in generating the phenomena of the disease.

In 1884, Dr. Koch, during his investigations of cholera in India, found bacilli in the bowel which he believed to be peculiar to the disease, and which presented the following characters: they were not straight, like other bacilli, but curved or comma-shaped; they proliferated rapidly and displayed very active movements. Bodies of persons who died of various other diseases did not present them, although abounding in different bacteria. The bacilli were not found, or only exceptionally, in the stomach, but abundantly in the intestine, and most so in the diarrhoeal discharges that occurred at the height of the disease. As soon as the stools began to be fecal the specific bacilli disappeared from them. After death at the height of the disease they were most abundant in the intestinal contents, and especially in the lower part of the small intestine. When death took place at a later period none of them might be detected in the liquids in the bowel, but they would still be present, in considerable numbers, in the tubular glands. They were not found at all in cases fatal from some sequela of the disease.[45]

[45] *Times and Gaz.*, Mar., 1884, p. 398.

Other abdominal lesions in cholera possess a very subordinate importance. The isolated and the agminated glands are both prominent, chiefly because they are swollen by the liquid imbibed from the bowel. A whitish substance which they sometimes contain may perhaps be the albumen or fat which they have taken from the intestinal liquid. A very similar condition of the mesenteric glands is probably due to a like cause. The liver is pale and flaccid when death takes place in collapse, and it is also described as presenting a "dirty grayish-red, homogeneous appearance, and indistinctness of the lobular structure, as if some glutinous matter had been poured throughout the tissues of the organ"[p. 746](Sutton). This appearance would seem to be due to the total suspension of the blood-supply through the portal vein.

At all stages of the disease the gall-bladder is usually found full of bile, which is apt to be dark during the collapse and more watery after reaction has commenced.

The spleen is small, pale, and, as a rule, firm, but occasionally it is soft.

The kidneys present no marked changes when death has taken place early in the attack, or at most only exhibit a lighter color than usual of the cortical substance and a darker one of the pyramids. They show that the arteries are comparatively empty and that the veins are congested. Similarly contrasted appearances are met after death from obstructive disease of the heart and other causes that produce obstruction of the venæ cavæ. In the tubules, later on, fatty degeneration of the epithelium has been observed, and some cylindrical casts. These alterations, especially of the tubules, are most marked when death occurs in the stage of reaction, and are then apt to be accompanied by more or less hemorrhagic transudation. The urinary bladder is always contracted after death in collapse; after febrile reaction its mucous membrane may be more or less coated with false membrane.

The brain and the spinal marrow offer nothing peculiar; their venous systems are everywhere more or less engorged, and sometimes effused blood has been found in the spinal canal.

In the state of the respiratory organs the most important facts are that in algid cholera the lungs are always more or less collapsed, "shrunk and small, and lying back in the chest, toward the spine," and that, so far from being congested, they are (with the exception of a small portion of their posterior part rendered dense by hypostasis) singularly bloodless, dry, and tough. As might be inferred from these conditions, they are also lighter in weight than natural. To Dr. Parkes belongs the credit of having first described this very important fact in the morbid anatomy of cholera, as follows: "In fourteen cases the lungs were completely collapsed, appearing in some cases like the lungs of a foetus. In three cases they were considerably, in eight slightly, collapsed, and in the remaining fourteen cases the collapse was in some altogether, and in some partially, prevented by old adhesions."[46] So Dr. Sutton found that the average weight of the two lungs during collapse was about twenty ounces, and after reaction—that is, after the passage of the blood into the pulmonary artery had become completely re-established—about forty-five ounces. In the latter condition also the lungs presented the usual signs of congestion of those organs, being dark-red throughout or in portions only. Sometimes also they contained masses or nodules of apparent hepatization, and of these some may have undergone partial softening.

[46] *Med. Times*, 1848, p. 378.

In absolute conformity with the condition of the lungs that has been described is that of the heart. If the lungs are bloodless, it follows necessarily that the left side of the heart must be empty, and almost as necessarily that the right side of the heart must be distended with blood. All careful investigators of the subject agree that such is the condition of the heart when death takes place in cholera during the stage of [p. 747]asphyxia. All report that the pulmonary artery is either empty or that it contains a small quantity of dark and usually of thick blood; that the right side of the heart and the coronary veins are distended with blood of the same description, while numerous ecchymoses exist along the course of the coronary veins; that the venæ cavæ are filled with half-coagulated blood of a tarry aspect; and that even the femoral and splenic veins contain similar blood. On the other hand, the left ventricle of the heart is usually contracted, and contains a very little semi-fluid blood, with perhaps a small and pale clot. This engorged condition of the right cavities and emptiness of the left cavities of the heart diminish very slowly during the passage from collapse to reaction, during which time the pulmonary blood-vessels are being gradually replenished. Besides the thick and tarry aspect of the blood above described, it has been observed that when the blood is withdrawn by means of a pipette, its globules rapidly subside and are surmounted by a transparent serum, and that such blood may remain for a long time uncoagulated. The red corpuscles are said to be pale and viscous, but not adhesive, and the white corpuscles abnormally numerous and easily crushed. In the free intervals are observed "very pale little objects, slightly elongated and constricted in their middle," which multiplied in blood kept for one or two days at a temperature of 38° C. (100.4° F.).[47] If death does not take place until reaction is far advanced or has merged into a febrile condition, the left ventricle is usually found not contracted, and it contains a quantity of blood. The term "usually" is employed to show that even to this rule there are some exceptions, and that, as in all other diseases, the issue does not depend absolutely and exclusively upon a definite degree of any anatomical lesion, but upon the aggregate condition of all the functions upon which life depends. The pericardium, like the pleura and the peritoneum, may be covered with a saponaceous film which is albuminous.

[47] *Rapport sur le Cholera d'Égypte en 1883*, par M. le Dr. Strauss, etc.

In looking now over the field that has been traversed in the foregoing pages, and searching for some link that will unite in a consistent whole the causes, symptoms, and lesions of cholera, it is evident that only one factor can possibly be so described. That factor is the gastro-intestinal flux. This it is that produces the vomiting and the purging; that prostrates the patient and wastes away in a few hours the fullest and the firmest form; that chills the limbs and afterward the trunk; that thickens the blood so that the capillary vessels can no longer convey it, and that spreads a cyanotic shadow over the whole surface of the body; that cuts off the supply of blood from the lungs and heart; that paralyzes the nervous system, ganglionic as well as cerebro-spinal; that obstructs the kidneys and arrests their secretion; and that, acting through the several links of this pathological chain, becomes the cause of death. But the question still recurs, What is the cause of the gastro-intestinal flux? To this also, in the light of observation, it is possible to give only one answer. It is a specific poison which originates in Hindostan, and, being taken into the stomach and bowels, not only produces in the individual the symptoms and lesions of cholera, but is capable of multiplying itself and rendering infectious the discharges from the stomach and bowels of the subjects of the disease, so that it may be transmitted from [p. 748]one person to another round the whole circumference of the globe. Regarding the form and nature of that poison little or nothing is definitely established, beyond what has already been stated as the result of Koch's observations. As far as they go, they harmonize with a long-prevalent opinion that the cholera poison consists of certain microscopic germs, which, on being received into the bowels, propagate their kind and destroy the epithelium. It is believed by some that these bodies are products of the rice-plant on the banks of the Ganges, and that, having once originated the disease, the germs contained in the discharges become mixed with water or are borne upon the wind, and enter the system of new victims, who, in their turn, disseminate the plague. This theory will be further considered below.

Another view, that of B. W. Richardson, is that, "as pus undergoes changes which convert it into a septic poison, so the excreted matter from the alimentary canal is equally capable, under peculiar conditions of oxidation, of producing an alkaloidal organic poison, which, soluble in water, but admitting of deposit on desiccation," becomes the agent for disseminating the disease. In these theories a false datum and a hypothesis are offered us in place of the fact which we seek. The cryptogamous nature of the essential cause of the disease has no positive proof, but only the probability of coincidence in its favor. There is no proof, because one after another organic form has been alleged to be the essential generator of the disease, and each has been proved to be either not peculiar to cholera or has been shown to be present in other diseases than cholera.

At the present time (1884) it is the fashion to trace every disease to specific bacteria or analogous organisms. But it may be that the occurrence of cholera only furnishes the occasion for the development of these organisms, just as a certain temperature, hygrometric condition, and deficient light and air will cause mould to form on bread and other organic substances. The judgment pronounced by Dr. Beale in this question as long ago as 1866 appears now, as it did then, to approach the truth upon this point: "There is no good reason for supposing that the bacteria in such numbers in the alimentary canal in cholera have anything to do with this disease or with the falling off of epithelium from the intestinal and other mucous membranes. Bacteria are developed in organic matter which is not traversed and protected by the normal fluids of the body, and they invade the cells and textures in cholera after those cells and textures have undergone serious prior changes, just as they would invade textures removed from the body altogether. Nor would it be in accordance with known facts to infer that cholera was due to the invasion of some peculiar form or species of bacterium."[48]

[48] *Times and Gazette*, Aug., 1866, p. 167.

We repeat, then, that while nothing can be simpler than the mechanism of cholera viewed as a gastro-intestinal hyperidrosis, nothing is more mysterious than the mechanism of the primary cause which gives rise to it. That its real nature has been correctly described is rendered all the more probable by the fact, presently to be insisted upon, that sporadic cholera morbus, which is always the consequence of a direct irritation of the gastro-intestinal mucous membrane, is often with difficulty distinguishable from Asiatic cholera, which, indeed, differs from the former [p. 749]disease chiefly by the intensity of its cause as measured by the gravity of its symptoms and by the nature of the special agent that produces it.

The above views regarding the essential cause of cholera were substantially indited before the Egyptian epidemic of 1883, but they are in accord with the more definite conclusions arrived at by the German and French commissions on the subject. Before their reports appeared, however, a communication was made by Dr. Kartulis of the Greek hospital in Alexandria, setting forth that the drinking-water and the stools and blood of the cholera patients contained, the first a mass of micro-organisms, and the others bacteria and micrococci, which, however, presented no distinctive characters.[49] The German report was prepared by Dr. Koch, the French by Dr. Strauss.[50] The former, alluding to the enormous quantity of micro-organisms found in the contents of the bowels and in the stools, did not perceive any connection between them and the phenomena of the disease. On the other hand, he did assign this relation to a species of bacterium found in the walls of the intestine, and which he compared to the bacilli of glanders. They were lodged in great quantities within the intestinal glands and behind their epithelium, as well as upon the surface of the villi and within them, and sometimes even in the muscular coat. They were most numerous at the lower end of the small intestine. Dr. Koch concluded that although these bacilli, beyond doubt, are in some manner associated with the development of cholera, they are by no means shown to be its cause, and may indeed be themselves the product of the morbid conditions belonging to cholera. All his attempts at that time to develop cholera in animals by inoculating them with the organisms gave only negative results. The conclusions of Dr. Strauss were in entire conformity with those of Dr. Koch, but involved an additional and very important statement—viz. that the shorter and the more violent were the fatal attacks of cholera the fewer were the bacteria found in the intestine. It is evident that this fact is the very opposite of what should have been found had bacteria been essential in the causation of cholera. The more recent investigations conducted in Calcutta by Dr. Koch, which have already been cited, led him, however, to attribute to bacilli of a specific form the absolute origination of the disease. He poses the question in the following manner: Either these "comma bacilli" are a product of the cholera process, or "the disease only arises when these specific organisms have found their way into the bowel." The former alternative he rejects, because, in his judgment, it assumes that the bodies in question must be pre-existent in every person who becomes affected with the disease—a hypothesis which he rejects, because they have never been found except in cholera. He therefore concludes that they are the cause of cholera. He points out that their first appearance coincides with the commencement of the disease, that they increase with it, and that they disappear with its decline.[51] The statement of Strauss quoted above does not, however, appear to harmonize with this conclusion, since the bacteria are said by him to have been fewest in the more violent and fatal attacks of the disease. Another of Dr. Koch's remarks is also open to criticism. After showing how rapidly the cholera bacteria multiply when kept moist, he states that they die after drying more quickly than almost any other form of bacteria. "As [p. 750]a rule, even after three hours' drying every vestige of life has disappeared." It is evident that this statement is not in harmony with the numerous facts, several of which have been cited, that cholera fomites have preserved their infectious qualities after several weeks. Dr. Koch endeavored to produce in animals, artificially, with these bacteria, a disease analogous to cholera, but without success; and he adds, "If any species of animal whatever could take the cholera, it would surely have been observed in Bengal, but all inquiries directed to this point met with a negative result." Dr. Vincent Edwards, who, however, is of opinion that the cholera poison is "not an organism, but of the nature of a chemical compound of comparatively unstable nature," reports that he produced fatal cholera in pigs by giving them the dejections of cholera patients.[52] But the *Times and Gazette* inclines to question that the pigs employed in Dr. Edwards' experiments were affected with true cholera.

[49] *Medical News*, xliii. 377.
[50] *Archives gén.*, Dec., 1883, pp. 713, 722.
[51] *Times and Gaz.*, Mar., 1884, p. 398.
[52] *Notes on the Poison contained in Choleraic Atomic Discharges.*

DIAGNOSIS.—The most characteristic symptoms of Asiatic cholera have repeatedly been mentioned in the foregoing pages. They are rice-water evacuations by vomiting and purging, rapid emaciation of the whole body, a cadaverous hollowness of the cheeks and eyes, a livid color of the face, hands, and feet, a feeble, thready, and at last absent pulse, an icy coldness of the extremities, face, and even the breath, a loss of the elasticity of the skin, a thin and feeble voice, and intense thirst. But every one of these symptoms may occur in cholera morbus produced by a direct irritation of the stomach and bowels. It is rather their nature, we repeat, than their phenomena that distinguishes these two affections from each other. In attempting to separate Asiatic cholera from other forms of cholera we must endeavor to dismiss from the mind the erroneous notion that the term cholera denotes a definite disease identical in its cause, phenomena, and results. It is no more a disease than dropsy or fever is a disease. It is a complex group of symptoms which have in common the fact that they proceed directly from gastro-intestinal irritation, whose degree of severity— *i.e.* the presence or absence of certain grave symptoms—and, above all, its issue, depend chiefly upon the nature and intensity of the cause of the attack, and also, necessarily, upon the degree of resistance opposed to it by the subjects of the disease. Nothing has led to more error in regard to epidemic cholera than the ignorance of this pathological fact by some and the disregard of it by others.

In the first portion of this article it was shown that the Greek, Roman, and Arabian conceptions of cholera morbus included a discharge of bile, the very symptom for the absence of which Asiatic cholera is notorious; and also that the classical cholera, or cholera morbus, ended in recovery even more frequently than Asiatic cholera terminates in death. But local epidemics of cholera morbus sometimes take place which are of a severe and even of a grave type, and which also appear to originate in some peculiar atmospheric influence, for they prevail to a limited extent and in connection with vicissitudes of weather. Still more circumscribed epidemics have been traced to unwholesome food and drink, and innumerable instances of individual attacks have been caused by irritants that are ranked as poisons and others which are reckoned as food or medicines. Now, under these various circumstances, which have in common gastro-intestinal irritation, there may be produced, if the irritation is excessive, [p. 751]a series of symptoms closely resembling, if not identical with, those of Asiatic cholera.

In illustration may be cited the comparatively familiar description of Sydenham.[53] These are his words: "There is vomiting to a great degree, and there are also *foul, difficult,* and *straining motions* from the bowels. There is *intense pain* in the belly, there is *wind,* and there are *distension,* heartburn, and thirst. The pulse is quick and frequent, at times small and unequal. The feeling of sickness is most distressing, and is accompanied with heat and disquiet. The perspiration sometimes amounts to absolute sweating. The legs and arms are cramped and the extremities cold. To these symptoms, and to others of a like stamp, we may add faintness." ... "As the summer came to a close the cholera morbus raged epidemically, and, being promoted by the unusual heat of the weather, it brought with it worse symptoms, in the way of cramps and spasms, than I had ever seen. Not only, as is generally the case, was the abdomen afflicted with horrible cramps, but the arms and legs, indeed the muscles in general, were afflicted also." ... At the risk of repetition an additional passage may be quoted from Sydenham's later definition of cholera morbus: "This is *limited* to the *month of August* or the first week or two of *September.* Violent vomiting, accompanied by the dejection of *depraved humors, difficulty on passing them, vehement pain, inflation and distension of the bowels,* heartburn, thirst, quick, frequent, small, and unequal pulse, heat and anxiety, nausea, sweat, cramps of the legs and arms, faintings, and coldness of the extremities, constitute the true cholera—and it kills within twenty-four hours."

[53] *Works,* Sydenham Soc. ed., i. 163; ii. 8, 266.

In spite of the general likeness between this description and the symptoms of Asiatic cholera, there are differences of considerable importance which have been italicized in the quotations. These differences are such as may be attributed to the action of a harsh irritant in the case of cholera morbus, while in the epidemic (Asiatic) disease the distinctive phenomena are the result of a sudden and profuse intestinal flux. Macpherson, who had a long and extensive experience of epidemic cholera in India, after contrasting in detail its phenomena with those of cholera nostras, sums up the discussion in these words: "Cholera indica is essentially a very fatal disease, while cholera nostras is usually a mild affection and is seldom fatal, although it was called *atrocissimus et peracutus,* and has undoubtedly killed in from eight to twenty-four hours."[54] In regard to the individual symptoms this very competent reporter does not recognize a single one as being absolutely peculiar to either disease. Even the ancients, already referred to, after describing bilious evacuations as being characteristic of cholera nostras, add that sometimes also they are whitish; and modern writers, both before and since the advent of Asiatic cholera in Europe, have made a similar observation. Thus, Quinquaud, in his description of cholera nostras, of which a slight epidemic occurred in 1869 at the Hospital St. Antoine in Paris, says: "The principal symptoms were vomiting and purging, sometimes of a bilious and sometimes of a rice-water liquid; a shrivelled and cyanotic skin, the latter appearance being sometimes strongly marked; anxiety, coldness, cramps, altered voice, and suppression of urine."[55] In 1875 thirty-three cases of this[p. 752]disease occurred at Valenciennes, near Paris, and its symptoms were thus summarized by Manouvriez:[56] "Repeated vomiting, first of food, and then of a dark-green liquid; diarrhoea, which was at first fecal and then bilious, but afterward serous and like rice-water;

533

painful tension of the epigastrium and tenderness of this part; headache, cramps in the legs, suppression of urine; pallor, coldness, and dryness of the skin, especially of the limbs; pinched features, a blue circle around the eyes, a small and scarcely perceptible pulse, and a faltering and whispering voice." Yet of the thirty-three cases only two were fatal—the one a child of four years and the other an infant of as many months. The substantial identity of nature of these two local epidemics, and the almost equally close relation of their symptoms to those of epidemic cholera, must be quite apparent.

[54] *Times and Gaz.*, Dec., 1870, p. 725.
[55] *Archives gén.*, Mars, 1870, p. 308.
[56] *Archives gén.*, Sept., 1877, p. 298.

Yet the contrasts are neither slight nor unimportant; and the most striking and significant is the trifling mortality of the European as compared with the Asiatic disease, notwithstanding the grave symptoms present in the former. It may be regarded as certain, we think, that the reason of this difference of danger lies in a corresponding difference in the nature of the causes of the two forms of disease. The rapid recovery from cholera morbus produced by changes of weather, acid fruits, and indigestion renders it certain that no material lesion of the gastro-intestinal mucous membrane has been produced; while, on the other hand, inspection after death from epidemic cholera or by corrosive poisoning renders it equally certain that the damage to that membrane is substantial and widespread, as well as often irreparable, and that, therefore, "the powers of life that resist death" must be engaged in a very unequal and often fruitless struggle. The cramps in cholera nostras are, as a rule, less severe than in epidemic cholera, while the colicky, and in general the abdominal, pains are greater in the former than in the latter disease. The reason of this difference appears to be that muscular spasm is the natural result of depletion, whether sanguine or serous, while colic is an effect of irritation of the surface of the mucous coat of the bowel, and not of its destruction, such as occurs in epidemic cholera.

It is true only in a limited degree, and indeed only upon a superficial survey of the symptoms, that the effects of irritant poisoning are like those produced by Asiatic cholera. The analogy between the two was pointed out, among others, by Sedgwick in 1867.[57] The resemblance appeared so striking to the vulgar eye that in Paris, and perhaps elsewhere, a popular tumult followed the first violent outbreak of epidemic cholera, and it was charged that the wells had been poisoned. The cases that most resemble cholera are the following: "Acute poisoning by corrosive sublimate, by arsenic, and by mineral acids, especially nitric acid; the effects which follow the eating or drinking of poisonous animal matters, such as tainted or simply unwholesome meat or fish, and milk which has undergone some injurious but yet unknown change, decomposing vegetables and some of the poisonous fungi, and the excessive action of certain drugs, for the most part belonging to the class of drastic purgatives," as elaterium and croton oil. The effects produced by these agents constitute a cholera morbus, and therefore resemble cholera, and have been occasionally, and almost unavoidably, mistaken for it. It [p. 753]is remarkable that suppression of urine may occur among them, as well as vomiting, purging, and collapse. As Griesinger and others have pointed out, the order in which the symptoms occur is a valuable, and generally an available, ground of diagnosis. In cholera, diarrhoea always occurs before vomiting, while in the various irritant poisonings mentioned vomiting precedes diarrhoea. In irritant poisoning also there is generally severe abdominal pain—not so much colicky and paroxysmal as constant and burning; the stools are not so copious as in cholera, and they do not possess the rice-water aspect, but are rather dark, bloody, and fetid, and are voided with tenesmus or with heat in the anus; and even when the urine is suppressed it is less persistently and completely so than in cholera, and attempts to void it are attended with vesical tenesmus and strangury. In a doubtful case it is important to ascertain whether a metallic or other unpleasant taste is perceived in the mouth, whether this cavity or the throat bears marks of corrosion, whether any unusual article of food has been used, etc. Moreover, it is of extreme importance to learn whether Asiatic cholera prevails, not merely in the immediate neighborhood, but at any place from which diseased persons or infected goods may have arrived. The instances should not be forgotten in which cholera-infected clothing from Europe has developed the disease in the valley of the Mississippi. Nor should those still more numerous cases be overlooked in which travellers affected with choleraic diarrhoea have disseminated the disease at great distances from their starting-point, although unconscious of the nature of their own ailment, whose seed they were sowing along their route.

[57] *Med.-Chir. Trans.*, li. 1.

PROGNOSIS.—Like the diseases called septic, of which the eruptive fevers may be taken as examples, and also like the effects of irritant poisons, the gravity of cholera must mainly depend upon the amount and the activity of the specific poison that is received into the system. It is most probable that the cholera poison is organic, and that it has a limited power of reproduction and term of existence, a period also of intense activity and a period of exhaustion; in a word, that either by progressive dilution as an inorganic substance or by organic senescence it finally ceases to exist. By no other theory is it possible to explain the numerous degrees of severity which cholera exhibits, from a mild indisposition to a malignant and rapidly fatal disease. On the one hand, the patients, if they may so be called, are hardly prevented from attending to their customary occupations. They may even be able to travel and carry the disease to distant places, and so appear to justify the erroneous and irrational doctrine of the atmospheric or spontaneous origin of cholera. On the other hand, the entire apparent duration of an attack may not exceed two or three hours, during which all the distinctive symptoms of the disease may be crowded together in the most appalling forms. Such grave cases are always most numerous at the commencement of an epidemic. These statements are true not only in regard to individual cases in the greater number of epidemics, but they represent the distinctive character of particular epidemics, some of which are as remarkable for their benignity as others are for their extreme malignity. For such contrasts no plausible reason can be suggested, unless it be a difference either in the essential virulence of the morbid poison or in the dose of it imbibed. That they are due to the activity rather than to the quantity of the poison seems to [p. 754]be proved by the progressive weakening in the gravity of the cases; for if the quantity of the poison remained the same some malignant cases might be expected to occur even during the decline of an epidemic.

These considerations help to explain the extreme diversities of mortality in different epidemics. The extremes may be stated at 10 and 90 per cent., and they would perhaps be still wider apart if all the mild cases, which are never reported—many of which, indeed, do not even fall under medical observation—were included in the reckoning. The general or average mortality of cholera is about 50 per cent. According to Allbu, the epidemics in Berlin from 1831 to 1873 gave a total of 28,753 cases and 18,916 deaths; that is, a mortality of 65.8 per cent. (Eichhorst). It should be noted that, as in other epidemic diseases, there is no uniform proportion between the extent and the mortality of cholera epidemics. Some of very limited extent have been proportionally the most destructive. It should also be remembered that the disease is far more fatal in infancy and old age than at any other period of life, and for a similar reason it is very dangerous to all who are weakened by any cause, such as an inherited morbid diathesis, a chronic debilitating disease, etc. There seems to be a doubt whether its male or female victims are the more numerous. In this connection it may be suggested that while males are more likely to contract the disease by drinking contaminated water, etc., more women are exposed to its contagion by their intimate relations with the sick, by their handling and washing infected fomites, by carrying away the cholera discharges, etc.

Undoubtedly, the class of society to which cholera patients belong is not without influence on its prognosis. Not only is the total mortality greater among the laboring classes, but the individual belonging to those classes has a less chance of recovery, because he is not apt to resort to treatment on the appearance of the premonitory signs of the disease, and because the treatment he receives is less intelligently and sedulously pursued by his physicians and friends.

In regard to the particular symptoms which are favorable or unfavorable, nothing need be added to what has already been stated in detail, unless it be that during the height of the attack the danger is to be measured by the degree of prostration and of the stasis of the blood, and, during reaction, by the grade of the typhoid state. Gradual reaction, as denoted by the state of the skin and the pulse and a more natural aspect of the stools, is generally indicative of improvement.

Finally, a word of caution may be given to those who are apt to attribute all the favorable changes in the conditions of an epidemic to the sanitary or medicinal measures they have instituted. Cholera epidemics are remarkable for the comparatively short period of their duration, which may be stated at less than a month in the same place. Doubtless, judicious sanitation and timely treatment save a great many lives, but the qualifying fact, already insisted upon, must not be overlooked, that the mortality occasioned by the disease in a given place is greatest during the first period of its prevalence, and that thenceforth it gradually declines. Yet it is of essential significance that the disease rarely attacks a large number of persons simultaneously; the epidemic proper is usually preceded by a few scattering cases which are apt to become foci of ignition that presently unite to form a widespread conflagration. The recognition [p. 755]of these cases, their isolation, and the proper treatment of the localities where they occurred have frequently stamped out what might have been the commencement of a deadly epidemic.

PREVENTION.—The history of cholera demonstrates conclusively that since the disease, outside of India, never arises spontaneously, it must be more or less preventible, partly by excluding its seeds and partly by rendering the soil in which they are planted more or less unfit for their development; in other words, by quarantines and sanitary cordons and by various measures of local sanitation.

In regard to the former there would be comparatively little difference of opinion, at least theoretically, if both measures were alike efficacious. But there would seem to have prevailed a tendency in official quarters to undervalue the efficiency of both. Those who made and administered the sanitary laws relating to cholera seem to have forgotten the emphatic question, "What will not a man give for his life?" or at least to have considered that whatever value some men may set upon their own lives, the lives of other men become of no account when balanced against the needs, or even the conveniences, of commerce. The ethics which justified the introduction of opium into China by the English and the American gift of alcohol to the Indian to gratify a lust for lucre or for land is only paralleled by those contained in the official protests against cholera quarantines. At the International Medical Congress held in 1873 at Constantinople, it was almost unanimously resolved that "the practice of (land) quarantine as now carried out ought not to be maintained, because, on the one hand, it does not constitute a real protection, and, on the other hand, *it is directly opposed to the interests of commerce and industry.*" A leading critic, in commenting upon this, remarks that if a quarantine were possible it would give no real security, because it would be evaded, just as customs laws are evaded by smuggling.[58] A logical deduction from this curious argument would be that customs laws should be abrogated. In 1880 was published the report of the German Imperial Commission on the cholera epidemic of 1873 in Germany, edited by Hirsch, from which we learn that "all the German medical experts agree in condemning the employment of quarantine, for, while largely detrimental to the *interests, welfare, convenience,* and *happiness* of a community, it is *quite inert* and *inefficient* as a safeguard against the further diffusion of cholera."[59]Whether this opinion refers only to land quarantine or not is left in doubt, but the spirit of subordinating the lives of the people to the commercial interests of a country is just the same as, and is not less worthy of condemnation than, the spirit which has more than once blinded customs officials to the disease on board of vessels from which it has afterward issued to destroy thousands of lives.

[58] *Practitioner*, xii. 226.

[59] *Ibid.*, xxvi. 159.

It seems to be overlooked that in national as well as in personal affairs "honesty is the best policy," and that if, instead of concealment or false statements regarding the sanitary state of ships, their passengers, and cargoes, and equally false assertions respecting the contagiousness of cholera, and a contemptuous neglect of well-tried preventive measures,— if, instead of this delusive and disastrous policy, all nations had honestly carried out the rules prescribed by experience for the exclusion of the disease, and for its management after it had passed the frontiers of a country, [p. 756]there can be little doubt that its ravages would ere this have been confined to the region in which it originated. As we have seen, there is urged against the enforcement of a rigid quarantine by land or sea the singular argument that it has not always excluded the disease. A more logical inference would seem to be that since it succeeded, not completely, but yet partially, its inefficiency should be charged to its imperfect execution; or, even granting that the absolute exclusion of cholera is impracticable in every instance, including cases of choleraic diarrhoea, contaminated clothing and merchandise, does it therefore follow that the transit of men and things should be unimpeded? As well might it be maintained that because one or more houses cannot escape destruction by fire, therefore no effort should be made to save the remainder of a threatened city; as well might it be argued that because some men must be killed in battle, no precautions should therefore be used to preserve the rest of the army; as well abstain from all local sanitation intended to mitigate the ravages of the disease, because, do what we may, some victims it will surely have. This is taking counsel from despair; is a stupid fatalism which one might imagine to have been imported with the disease from the East; or it may be a sign of the unconscious blindness of Mammon-worshippers, who, neither fearing God nor regarding man, have as little pity for the victims of cholera, permitted, if not invited, by them to scourge the nations, as devout Christians once felt for the negroes who were bought or kidnapped in Africa to toil and die under the lash of the slave-driver.

Probably no sanitary cordon nor any quarantine will invariably and completely exclude cholera, since it is transmissible by living men and by water and by fomites of various descriptions, and, worst of all, by men who neither exhibit its characteristic symptoms nor are conscious of the poison which they conceal and disseminate. But, as has already been urged, it is no argument against preventive measures that they are not absolutely perfect in their efficiency. If they sometimes succeed in arresting the progress of cholera, and if they always, when honestly executed, lessen the number of channels through which the infection can be conveyed, and thereby reduce to a minimum its fatal effects, they ought to be maintained and perfected, and not decried or abolished. It is difficult to characterize that state of mind which concludes against the use of a salutary measure because its efficiency is not absolute, the more so when it is admitted that its inefficiency is not intrinsic, but due to negligent, and even fraudulent, administration. The preponderance of official and personal authority is altogether on the side of the necessity of a quarantine, not in its literal, but in its technical, sense. The International Medical Congress of 1874 declared as follows: "Quarantine ought to be limited to the time requisite for the examination and disinfection of the ship, the crew, and the passengers; and if there be no disease on board the latter should be released immediately after disinfection. But if there be cholera or sickness of a doubtful nature on board, it will be necessary to isolate and disinfect the ship also." The same congress, however, wholly condemned land quarantines, apparently upon the sole ground of the extreme difficulty of rendering them efficient—an argument, as before remarked, that touches not the principle of the measure, but only the manner of its execution. In this respect the congress occupied a lower position than its predecessor of 1866, which held that the futility of[p. 757]quarantine in "arresting the march of cholera" arose "rather from the unintelligent application of the measure than from any fallacy in its principle."[60]

[60] *Practitioner*, xxviii. 393.

It would burden this narrative even to enumerate the instances in which a strict quarantine has protected places to which cholera has been carried by sea. In the United States numerous examples might be given of seaports into which cholera was brought from foreign countries, and within whose quarantine stations it was confined by rigid sanitary regulations; but it is sufficient to cite the case of New York, through whose quarantine at Staten Island nine-tenths of all emigrants to America have passed. Writing in 1867, Dr. Peters said: "There have been fourteen epidemics of cholera at Staten Island, and only four have reached New York." A large number of illustrations has been collected by Dr. Smart, Inspector-General, R. N.,[61] who sums up the matter as follows: "Believing that cholera has frequently been excluded from islands by quarantine, and as often introduced by its non-observance, I regard it as a truly preventive measure; but, recognizing the impracticability of exacting it under many circumstances, I would insist on the most strict isolation of all the first cases or units of disease, whether introduced from without or originating from relationship to introduced cases, or persons or goods imported from infected countries."

[61] *Lancet,* April, 1873, pp. 555, 659; *Times and Gazette,* April, 1874, p. 387. Compare also Colin, *Brit. and For. Med.-Chir. Rev.,* July, 1874, pp. 42-44.

While experience demonstrates the efficacy, and therefore the necessity, of quarantine against cholera in seaports, it has also shown that the same agent of prevention need not be invariably and rigidly applied. When quarantine meant literally a detention, and almost an incarceration, for forty days, it often failed through its very rigor at a time when proper methods of disinfecting ships, cargoes, crews, and passengers were either unknown or inefficiently applied. It is now certain that quarantine may be reduced to a fraction of its original duration, and yet possess a much greater degree of efficiency, its length depending upon the number and the sanitary condition of the crew, etc., the nature of the cargo, etc. It is evident that a ship carrying only cabin passengers is less open to suspicion than one crowded with filthy emigrants, although both may have sailed from the same cholera-infected port. A more liberal rule may govern the one than the other; and in the second case a rigid inspection and cleansing of luggage may be imperative which would be superfluous as well as vexatious in the first case. The importance of such a treatment of emigrants' effects has already been illustrated by cases in which they caused an outbreak of cholera after having been carried from a seaport into an interior town many hundreds of miles distant.

In regard to the time during which a vessel that has had cholera on board within a week or ten days should be detained under sanitary inspection and treatment, including a thorough cleansing of the passengers and their effects, no absolute rule can be laid down; but it would appear that if no suspicious cases arise within a week, there need be little apprehension that any will occur.

The sanitary measures which should be undertaken wherever there is reason to fear an invasion of cholera are, in the first place, such as are[p. 758]equally appropriate in anticipation of any infectious and contagious epidemic disease, and relate especially to the removal of all sources of putrid emanations, whether in stagnant ponds, in streets, markets, shambles, sewers, privies, cellars, or inhabited rooms; for these influences, although they do not cause cholera, yet, by lowering the vitality of persons exposed to them, create an abnormal susceptibility to disease. Many instances in Europe might be cited to prove that whole cities, which in the earlier epidemics were devastated by cholera, were either spared entirely in the later ones or suffered in a far less degree. The measures which proved most efficient were an improved water-supply and a better system of sewerage; and this fact strongly corroborates the belief that contaminated water and fecal emanations are the principal agents in propagating this disease. Cleanliness is the best disinfectant, but during epidemics of cholera, as of other diseases, the popular faith is very strong in numerous articles called by that name. The real value of these preparations is commercial rather than sanitary, but, indirectly, they are useful by prompting those who use them to be more diligent in searching out and removing many sources of air-contamination that perhaps invite and intensify attacks of cholera.

The disinfectants in common use comprise chlorine gas, chlorinated soda, chloride of zinc, sulphate of iron, permanganate of potassium, carbolic acid, and the fumes of burning sulphur. Some of them—and especially the chloride of zinc, sulphate of iron, the permanganate of potassium, and carbolic acid—are supposed to be capable of destroying the infectious principle of the vomit and stools. Another method is to receive such matters in vessels containing saw-dust, which, after being dried, is consumed by fire; and still another is to mix them with dry earth and bury them. If they are thrown into water-closets or privies, they should have added to them a portion of sulphate of iron. Whatever has been used by cholera patients should be destroyed, unless of value, and in that case it should be thoroughly purified by hot air or boiling water and long exposure to the sun. The importance of having large and well-ventilated rooms for cholera patients is very great, but less, perhaps, for the patients themselves than for their medical attendants and nurses. All persons should be excluded from them who are not required by the duties of the sick chamber, and in case of death funeral assemblages ought not to be allowed; nor, during a cholera epidemic, ought crowded assemblies for any purpose to be permitted.

During epidemics of cholera, as of some other diseases, the liability to be attacked is greatest when the vital powers are depressed by mental or by physical causes. Hence it is desirable that one's courage and confidence should repose upon a consciousness of having done whatever is recognized as proper to ward off the disease—not by a minute, watchful, and anxious attention to rules at every step, but by such a general care of the health as good sense and experience enjoin. Undoubtedly, other things being equal, the weak, sickly, careless, and imprudent are more liable to suffer than the strong and cautious, and therefore it is incumbent upon all to maintain as high a degree of health as possible, avoiding not only all probable sources of contagion, direct or indirect, but excessive fatigue, catching cold, depressing emotions, sexual excesses, etc. During the first cholera epidemics in this country it was considered so [p. 759]dangerous to eat fruit and fresh vegetables that many persons lived entirely upon meat, rice, and bread. Such a regimen intensified choleraphobia, and was also an unsuitable midsummer diet. There is no reason to believe that any intrinsically wholesome food need be prohibited during the prevalence of cholera.

The one article of diet about which the greatest and most peculiar care should be taken is water. It is the first duty of towns supplied with water from a common source to be sure that it is, and continues to be, uncontaminated. Well-water should be used as little as possible after the disease has made its appearance, and, as an additional precaution, no water should be drunken that has not previously been boiled. Where ice can be procured it may be used to restore the boiled water to an agreeable temperature for drinking. Filtered water, provided that it be properly filtered, may likewise be regarded as innocuous.

TREATMENT.—If regard be had to the various methods and particular medicines which have been used in the treatment of cholera, it will appear that in hardly any other acute disease has a greater number or variety been employed. If, on the other hand, we endeavor to learn what measures have been really and generally curative in cholera, and what are they to which, on the occurrence of an epidemic of the disease, we may turn with confidence in their power to cure, the result of the investigation is disheartening, and adds to the accumulated proofs that the power of medical art is exceedingly restricted. To this conclusion we must assent at whatever cost to a faith which is strong in proportion to the ignorance out of which it grows. Nor, if we consider the matter rationally, ought we to be surprised or humiliated on account of the comparative helplessness of medicine in this disease, since, if we reflect upon it, the case is by no means peculiar or exceptional. Every disease that may become mortal occurs more or less frequently with phenomena which place it beyond the resources of therapeutics as completely as cholera is in its most malignant forms; and yet no one lays it to the charge of medicine that the various fevers, for example, are at times utterly uninfluenced by the most rational and judicious treatment. Nor does any one bring a railing accusation against medicine when accident fatally damages a part essential to life.

One accident of frequent occurrence presents a certain analogy to cholera in its effects, and that is a burn or scald involving a very large portion of the skin. In cases of this sort experience assures us that death is almost inevitable, and that the duty of the physician is to avoid officious and meddlesome treatment, and address himself to soothe the patient's suffering and maintain his strength, if haply the powers of nature may triumph over the effects of the injury. This, too, is the lesson, substantially, which experience has taught respecting cholera. It is certain that in this disease the function of the whole gastro-intestinal mucous membrane is reversed, and that it is no longer a secreting and absorbing organ, but one almost exclusively exhaling, and that through it the liquid which is essential to carrying on the functions is rapidly running away. If the lesion on which this symptom depends is complete, if the gastro-intestinal mucous membrane has entirely lost its natural function, evidently it is quite futile to address any treatment to this organ. But if, as probably happens in a great majority of the cases, the [p. 760]disorganization takes place gradually, it is evident that there is more to hope from remedies when the disease is gradually developed than when it reaches its acme at a single bound and leaves no time for medical intervention. The one unmistakable lesson that experience teaches respecting the treatment of cholera is, that its success depends upon its prompt and early application. Almost as distinctly does observation teach that subsequently to the first (or diarrhoeal) stage the comparative value of different methods and individual medicines is very uncertain. And, finally, it would seem that in this, as in other acute diseases, intelligent and careful nursing and regimen are quite as important as any medicinal treatment whatever. However a false notion of the power of medicine may blind us to the fact, it is none the less a fact, that if different methods of treatment are compared, that method gives the best results which is least perturbative. For example, in England, on board of a hospital ship, were 85 cases, of which 19 treated by quinine gave 12 deaths, 12 by calomel gave 2 deaths, 12 by carbolic acid gave 3 deaths, and 37 by "Nil" gave 1 death.[62] Or, again, in 1865, at the London Hospital, 159 patients were treated—48 with a mixture containing logwood, ether, aromatic sulphuric acid, camphor, and capsicum, of whom 31 died; 56 with sweetened water, of whom 28 died; 21 with castor oil, of whom 14 died; and 20 with "saline lemonade," of whom 6 died.[63] In the last example the deaths during the use of the astringent mixture were twice as great as under sugar and water, and under castor oil twice as great as under "saline lemonade."

[62] *Times and Gaz.*, Dec., 1866, p. 590.
[63] *London Hosp. Reports*, iii. 444.

We shall first give an account of the management of cholera in general, and then consider some of the particular medicines used in its treatment.

The essential elements of all plans of treatment for this disease, as for so many others, are rest and abstinence. Whatever else may be done, nothing avails without them. This remark applies emphatically to the premonitory diarrhoea; if it is neglected it may readily be converted into the full-formed disease. It is therefore essential, during the prevalence of cholera, that whoever is attacked with diarrhoea should at once give up all active occupation, and confine himself to a recumbent posture and to the use of food of the blandest quality, such as mucilages and similar preparations, especially of rice, which, less than any other vegetable food, is liable to fermentation during digestion. It is prudent to drink no water that has not been boiled. If there is reason to believe that the bowels retain feces from before the attack, it is generally thought advisable to administer a laxative dose of castor oil, to procure the discharge of matters which would act as irritants. Except for this purpose purgatives are neither indicated nor expedient. In a large number of cases nothing more is necessary than the use of means to check the action of the bowels, and which should consist of absorbents or antacids, astringents, and opiates as they are contained in the officinal chalk mixture, with the addition of tincture of kino or catechu and a small proportion of laudanum. This medicine should be given in dessertspoonful doses at intervals of not more than an hour.

If, instead of a diarrhoea which differs from ordinary dyspeptic diarrhoea chiefly by its watery character, there should also be colic and profuse discharges, it is proper to add to the medicines just suggested some which are of a decidedly stimulant character, such as the essential oils of [p. 761]cajeput, cloves, cinnamon, peppermint, etc., with which chloroform, ether, or Hoffman's anodyne may be associated. At the same time rubefacient embrocations may be applied to the abdomen, which should also be compressed slightly with a broad flannel bandage. Instead of these stimulants, and perhaps more efficiently, may be used a simple epithem made by dipping a large towel several times folded in cold or cool water, applying it so as to cover the whole abdomen, and then enveloping it and the body with a dry towel. This application is more soothing than any liniment and its action is more constant. Instead of any of these agents dry heat may be used, obtained from bags of hot salt or sand, or moist heat from thick poultices of flaxseed meal or Indian corn meal or similar substances enclosed in flannel bags and applied to the abdomen while they are as hot as can be borne. It is difficult to determine which of these applications is the most useful. But, on the whole, heat is preferable to rubefacients, and moist to dry heat. The cold-water dressing is probably best suited to young and robust persons.

It must be remembered that between choleraic diarrhoea and cholera in its complete form there are several grades, in one of the most common of which a tendency to vomit, and even a certain amount of vomiting, accompanies the diarrhoea. Anti-emetic remedies are then indicated. They may consist externally of rubefacient and aromatic applications to the epigastrium (especially the spice poultice); and it is claimed that a hypodermic injection of morphia in this part is very efficient. Internally, the best remedies are ice swallowed in small pieces and small but frequent draughts of iced carbonated water or iced champagne. Where these liquids cannot be procured, effervescing powders used in the same way form a very good substitute for them. If, notwithstanding such remedies, the diarrhoea continues or if it tends to increase, astringent and absorbent medicines may be substituted for them; for example, bismuth may be given instead of chalk, and if this also fails acetate of lead may be prescribed. The last may be used by the rectum as well as by the mouth, but with very questionable advantage. Meanwhile, especial care should be taken to avoid giving so much of any opiate as will induce sopor or excite nausea.

Whoever has had the care of cholera patients has probably, at first, felt sanguine of success in their treatment, even after the characteristic discharges and the symptoms of collapse had set in; but a little more experience has proved their hope to be deceptive, and revealed the reason of it in the absolute suspension of the sensibility and absorbent function of the digestive canal. Hence the dismal unanimity of all medical authors, who from actual observation of cholera have declared that no treatment avails to arrest the fully-developed disease. And yet there is some encouragement in the fact that recoveries sometimes occur from even the most desperate state of collapse and under the most dissimilar methods of treatment; so that the physician is warranted in not yielding to discouragement and in cheering his patients with hope even to the end of life. The popular dread of this, and indeed of all epidemics, is sure to be exaggerated, and it therefore behooves the physician to combat the fears of his patients, and by a cheerful manner as well as encouraging words administer the cordial of hope, which often proves stronger than pharmaceutic elixirs.

[p. 762]It may be well to enumerate, as many do, the indications of treatment in the active stage of cholera, but they really need no such specification. It is evident that they consist in combating the symptoms—the vomiting, the purging, the debility, the cyanosis, the cramps, etc.; and the only means by which the carrying out of such indications can even be attempted are neither more nor less than would be used to relieve the same symptoms in other affections. If the evacuations could be controlled, evidently the cramps and the collapse would not occur; but this essential and preliminary step cannot be secured. The medicines introduced into the stomach or rectum are not absorbed, but are speedily rejected; those which are administered subcutaneously are not taken up by the stagnant blood as freely as in other diseases; the nervous system gives little or no response to the mechanical and physiological stimulants applied to the skin. Yet, in spite of these obstacles, the physician must persist in the use of rational methods, in the hope, however faint it may be, that he may succeed in restraining, and possibly in arresting, the fatal course of the attack. For this end he has hardly any means at command except those, or such as those, which were recommended in the first stage of the disease—the anti-emetic and anti-diarrhoeal medicines, which he is only too likely to see rejected as soon as administered. Yet he must not cease to allay the thirst by the repeated administration of small quantities of carbonated and cold liquids, water, or champagne wine, or morsels of ice swallowed whole. The application of pounded ice in a bladder to the epigastrium is a measure of an analogous sort, and is sometimes as efficient as generally it is soothing. In other cases the aromatic poultice seems to answer better. Of irritants little can be said that is favorable, but the combined irritant and anæsthetic action of chloroform is useful, and morphia should be applied to the epigastrium as well as given hypodermically.

If the vomiting tends to become less frequent, acetate of lead may be prescribed, in the hope that it will exert some constringing action upon the gastro-intestinal mucous membrane. The distressing symptom, hiccough, cannot with any certainty be controlled by medicine, but perhaps the inhalation of chloroform is more efficient than any other remedy, as it also is for the cramps in the limbs. For the latter purpose it is preferable to the frictions with flannel or with stimulating liniments which are generally employed. If such liniments are used, care should be taken that they do not contain ingredients that may disorganize the skin either immediately or subsequently. A dangerous compound of the latter sort introduced during the first epidemic of cholera in this country became officinal under the name of liniment of cantharides.

The loss of the water and of the salts it holds in solution in the blood is, as has now been frequently repeated, the chief pathological element of the disease, next after the conjectural cause which injures the mucous membrane of the stomach and bowels. It was rationally indicated, and therefore a method was early practised, to supply this loss by injecting into the veins a solution of sodium salts. The method was seductive as well as rational, for its primary effects were extremely encouraging; it nevertheless failed, and probably for the very reason that suggested its use. Indeed, there is no more reason, if there is as much, to suppose that a liquid artificially introduced into the blood-vessels will be retained when[p. 763]the natural liquor sanguinis cannot be so. Necessarily, the one will escape where the other has escaped.

Certain systematic writers prescribe a method intended, on the one hand, for reviving the animal heat, and on the other for restoring the movement of the circulation. It need hardly be remarked that the two form essentially but one and the same indication. If the circulation is restored the animal heat will revive, but not otherwise. The same treatment leads to both ends, and it consists partly, as already stated, in the use of stimulants, such as alcohol, camphor, coffee, ether, etc.; but their efficacy depends upon their being taken into the blood, and with it reaching the various nervous centres upon which the renewal of functional activity depends. Little, therefore, can be expected from them at the height of the disease—that is, in the stage of collapse—but as soon as any signs of reaction are manifested they tend to promote it, and hence may enable the functions to revive. For this reason they are adapted to persons who are feeble by reason of their tender or their advanced age, or who have previously suffered from ill-health. But if they act at all, and the more they tend to act, they must be employed with circumspection, lest they outrun the purpose of their administration and produce a violent or excessive reaction. Instead of, or in conjunction with, these internal remedies the local stimulants of the skin, already enumerated, may be used with the due precautions, and, in addition, baths at a temperature of 105° F. of water alone or with the addition of salt or mustard; but all such remedies are of little avail until reaction has commenced. Before that event there is reason to believe that the cold bath is preferable, or, still better, frictions of the whole body with cold water, or even with ice, after which the patient should be wrapped in dry and warm blankets. Yet the efficacy of this powerful agency is by no means comparable to that which it produces in the algid forms of malarial fever. The two conditions, although apparently analogous, are, in reality, very different. In the cold stage of fever the mechanism is indeed paralyzed, but none of its mechanical elements are wanting; but in algid cholera there is an actual subtraction of water from the blood, that turns it from a liquid capable of circulating through the narrowest channels into one that stagnates even in the largest vessels. In the one case force is wanting to circulate the blood; in the other there is no normal blood to circulate.

The treatment of the stage of reaction when it does not exceed a moderate degree, consists simply in strictly enforcing the rules for the patient's repose; that is to say, in intelligent nursing. Mental excitement must be forbidden, and neither medicine nor food allowed that is likely to interfere with the gradual and steady progress of convalescence. Of all articles of food, cool water is not only the most urgently desired, but is the most imperatively necessary for replenishing the emptied blood-vessels and restoring the normal functions. But unless great caution is observed it will be taken too freely and provoke a renewal of the discharges. If any food besides water is allowed, it should be of the simplest sort—of whey first, and then of milk in small quantities at a time, with lime-water if it provokes nausea or retching. Afterward thin broths may be given, also in great moderation, and by degrees farinacea in milk and in animal broths. Only when the strength is much improved should even the most [p. 764]digestible meats be permitted. In proportion as convalescence is marked or interrupted by symptoms of undue reaction is it necessary to prolong and render stringent this regimen; and if those symptoms unfortunately arise which oftener, perhaps, depend upon an over-zealous stimulant treatment than upon the natural reaction of the system, they must be combated by measures which will lessen the local congestions, especially of the brain and the lungs, and also by such as will tend to prevent the system from falling into a typhoid state. For the former dry cups applied to the back of the neck, and cold lotions and affusions upon the scalp, are to be recommended, and for the latter dry cups and warm stimulating poultices upon the chest near the affected region. It is probable that the general warm bath, with cold affusion upon the head at the same time, would prove as efficient as it does in analogous states of typhoid affections. If the urinary secretion is suspended or remains scanty, there is not usually an urgent need of using means for its restoration; for that will generally occur when the blood-vessels become replenished. It should, however, be mentioned that, according to Macnamara, if the patient does not pass any urine within thirty-six hours of reaction coming on, ten minims of the tincture of cantharides in an ounce of water should be given every half hour until six doses have been taken, and the patient encouraged to drink freely of water. If this treatment does not cause urine to pass, we must, after the sixth dose, discontinue the medicine for twelve hours, and then repeat it in precisely the same way. The dose here referred to is of the British preparation, and if the use of it were not recommended by so competent an authority its propriety might very properly be challenged.

After the cholera patient has become convalescent his restoration is very apt to be retarded by dyspeptic disorders, for which, perhaps, the best remedy is a judicious use of condiments with the food and of bitter tonics, especially quinine, colombo, quassia, etc., before meals. If there is constipation, it should be corrected by the cautious use of fruits, and, if these prove insufficient, of mild saline laxatives or small doses of castor oil or rhubarb. On the other hand, if there is a tendency to diarrhoea, it should be met by the use of a mild laxative, such as castor oil, magnesia, or rhubarb, followed by chalk or bismuth, and the use for a time of simpler food and in less than the usual quantities.

Having thus furnished a sketch of the plan of treatment of cholera which we regard as dictated by experience, it may be not without some interest to consider certain elements of the method a little more fully, and criticise, in passing, some other remedies which have from time to time been proposed. The first of these is venesection. There was a time when certain physicians, carried away by conceptions of the disease evolved from their inner consciousness, maintained that it consisted essentially of a spasm of the blood-vessels, and that the natural and legitimate cure for it was to be found in bleeding. No theory is so gratuitous or absurd but cases may be found which appear to justify it, and in this instance also examples were not wanting to illustrate at once the truth of the theory and its successful application. Longer experience, however, and a more correct conception of the disease, have long since condemned this method, which was almost as dangerous as it was irrational. If any additional argument against it were required, it would be found in the condition of the lungs after death. These organs, we have seen, are not [p. 765]only not engorged, but they are empty of blood, and death is due not to asphyxia, but to apnoea, when it takes place in collapse.

If ever there existed any reason for the administration of an emetic—and ipecacuanha has generally been used at the commencement of an attack of cholera—it must be looked for, not in any clinical experience of its virtues, but simply in the deplorable routine that required the administration of an emetic at the commencement of nearly all acute diseases, so that, whatever else was prescribed, the lancet and an emetic seldom failed to be so. In this case also the proofs of the successful administration of ipecacuanha were not wanting, and one might be tempted to suppose, in view of the alleged facts in its favor, that it was useful by causing an evacuation of the material cause of the disease. Physicians were even to be found, of high station and character, who contended that cholera is a species of fever, and to be treated by an emeto-cathartic composed of tartar emetic and epsom salts. If the treatment had been efficient, the absurdity of the reasons for it might have been overlooked; but the one was as disastrous as the other was false. But, as usual, the facts had been misstated or misinterpreted, and emetics ceased to form a part of the systematic treatment of cholera. The idea which possessed those who advocated the use of evacuants was that there was either a poison to be eliminated from the blood or one to be expelled from the bowels. Apparently, the method was not efficacious, for the latest phase of it, the use of castor oil in acute stage of cholera, was of short duration.

When cholera first appeared in Europe the tendency naturally arose to follow in its treatment the example of the British practitioners in India. It then appeared that one of the most eminent among them, Annesley, gave a scruple of calomel, with two grains of opium, at the commencement of the attack, and repeated the dose in six or eight hours, and again upon the following day. In the decline of the disease he ordered scruple doses of calomel for the removal of a "cream-colored, thick, viscid, and tenacious matter exactly like old cream cheese, which glues the gut together and obstructs its passage." Three, four, and even five, scruples of calomel were usually taken before this effect was produced. When it is added that this practitioner held depletion to be the capital element of the treatment, and that he was equally lavish of his patient's blood and of his own drugs, we can only wonder that any subjects of his heroic method survived. It is now conceded by all enlightened physicians that mercurials in large or in ordinary doses are worse than worthless in epidemic cholera. In 1832, Dr. Ayre of Hull, Eng., proposed another method of using calomel, to which he adhered in treating this disease. It consisted in the administration of very small doses of calomel at short intervals, and with each of the first doses a few drops of laudanum. Such a method, if not carried too far, certainly has the merit of sparing the patient a great deal of the perturbative treatment against which we have, in the preceding pages, protested. But that was not at all the notion of its proposer. He claimed for it positive and active virtues. He stated, as the fundamental ground of his plan, that "the primary and leading object of the treatment must be to restore the secretion of the liver." He did not in the least doubt that he was able to do this by the administration of mercury—not, indeed, by a direct action upon the liver [p. 766]itself, but indirectly and sympathetically through the stomach, and by the healthy and specific stimulus imparted to it, by which the due secretion of the bile is promoted. It is, indeed, difficult to conceive of any stimulus that calomel could impart to the stomach that would not be equally given by any other non-irritant and insoluble powder—subnitrate of bismuth, for example. Indeed, Ayre himself relates the case of a man who in an attack of cholera took during three days no less than five hundred and eighty grains of calomel, and recovered without any soreness of the mouth. But the plan which he finally elaborated was different. It was to give small doses of calomel repeatedly—in the premonitory stage one grain every half hour or hour for six or eight successive times, or, if this failed, every five or ten minutes—and in the stage of collapse one grain and a half every five minutes. In a few cases of extreme severity two grains of calomel were given every five minutes for an hour or two, and then the ordinary dose of one grain was resumed. But this was not all: with every dose of calomel was associated one, two, or three drops of laudanum, so that if these doses were repeated frequently the patient received a very efficient amount of the narcotic during the attack. Indeed, Ayre attributed to it the virtue of sustaining the vital powers under the depressing influence of the disease, and of removing or abating the cramps, as well as of detaining the calomel in the stomach.[64]From the preceding account it follows that the treatment of cholera by small doses of calomel with laudanum is founded on an erroneous assumption of the mode of action of calomel, and that whatever efficacy the plan of treatment may possess may with more justice be attributed to the opium, whose effects we know, than to the calomel, whose action, so far as it is known at all, has no conceivable relation to the disease for which it was given. However this may be, if the results of Ayre's treatment are compared with those of other plans, it exhibits very little if any superiority. In the report of the cholera committee of the College of Physicians, London, made in 1853, we find the statement that in 725 unequivocal cases treated on Ayre's plan the deaths were 365, or about 50 per cent., and also the following commentary: "In general, no appreciable effects followed the administration of calomel, even after a large amount in small and frequently-repeated doses had been administered. For the most part, it was quickly evacuated by vomiting or purging, or, when retained for a longer period, was passed from the bowels unchanged. Salivation but very rarely occurred, and then only in the milder cases. We conclude that calomel was inert when administered in collapse, and that the cases of recovery following its employment at this period were due to the natural course of the disease, as they did not surpass the ordinary average obtained when the treatment consisted in the use of cold water only."[65] It is of interest to compare the mortality of 50 per cent. above stated to have occurred under this sort of calomel treatment with the mortality noted at the London Hospital under various kinds of treatment, including the administration of calomel in doses varying "from five to ten and twenty grains every quarter, half, one hour, two, four, etc." Out of 509 cases, 281 were fatal, or 54.9 per cent.[66]

[64] *A Report on the Treatment of the Malignant Cholera*, Lond., 1833.
[65] Dr. Gull's *Report*, p. 177.
[66] *Lond. Hosp. Reports*, iii. 437, 441.

Every disease in which exhaustion and coldness occur is sure to be [p. 767]treated more or less actively with alcohol, but in the collapse of cholera, as in the cold stage of fevers, it is generally useless, and sometimes hurtful. We believe that the following protest of Macnamara is sustained by almost universal experience: "I would here enter an earnest protest against the use of brandy or any alcoholic stimulant in this [the second] stage of cholera. I believe these, both theoretically and practically, to be the cause of unmitigated evil. I simply, therefore, mention brandy, champagne, and the like in order to condemn their use most emphatically in cholera; according to my ideas and experience, it is almost impossible to hit on a more detrimental plan of treatment than that usually known as 'the stimulant' in this form of disease."[67] It is true that apparent dissidents from this judgment may be found, like Playfair, a deputy inspector of hospitals in Bengal, who even circulated printed directions for the treatment of the first stage of the disease by means of brandy or strong rum, cayenne pepper, and laudanum, and had entire confidence in the efficacy of the method.[68] Dr. Macpherson, inspector-general of hospitals, also, after comparing the results of a stimulant treatment with those of other methods, reaches the conclusion that the mortality-rate of cholera is affected neither by the moderate nor by the excessive use of alcohol.[69]

[67] *Op. cit.*, p. 456.
[68] *Edinburgh Med. Jour.*, xix. 471.
[69] *Med. Times and Gaz.*, Jan., 1870, p. 62.

Upon no other point in the treatment of cholera is the agreement of physicians more complete than upon the use of opiates in the early stage of the disease. The premonitory diarrhoea has always been treated by opiates alone or associated with astringents. Probably the best rule is to give from twenty to thirty drops of laudanum, or an equivalent dose of some other liquid preparation of opium, in a little brandy and water, and repeat the dose as often as a stool is voided. Opiates have also been generally employed to mitigate the symptoms of the fully-developed disease. But, like all other medicines introduced into the stomach or rectum, they are apt to be rejected, and even if they are not, their absorption is very doubtful, so that at the height of the attack they must be considered as nearly if not quite useless. When the vomiting and purging begin to subside and reaction is about to commence, small and repeated doses of opiates undoubtedly tend to lessen the evacuations; but great caution must be observed not to exceed the due degree of stimulation, lest a dangerous state of narcotism or collapse be induced. It might be supposed that the hypodermic use of morphia would be less open to objection than its administration by the stomach; but it is to be remembered that the suspension of gastric absorption is only a part of the similar condition affecting the whole circulatory system, and that the stagnation of the blood in the systemic veins prevents the absorption of medicines administered subcutaneously perhaps as completely as the state of the gastric blood-vessels interferes with their absorption from the stomach itself. In point of fact, the utility of opiates at any stage of cholera after the first is not easily determined, for nearly always they are associated with other medicines, and especially with astringents. In this disease, as in others that involve life, we are seldom at liberty to test the powers of individual medicines, but are bound to endeavor to save life by associating those which seem to be required for the purpose. Opiates, then, are nearly always given in conjunction with astringents or stimulants[p. 768]during the first (or diarrhoeal) stage of the attack, but after vomiting is added to diarrhoea and a tendency to collapse is manifested they are at least useless.

The patient, it has already been said, should be disturbed as little as possible, and hence, if he becomes restless, and especially if he is rendered so by pain, he should be tranquilized by means of anæsthetics. Chloroform has generally been employed, and is best administered on the first accession of cramps. Much pain, with muscular fatigue and depression, is thus saved, and the inhalation of the medicine may be repeated as often as the pain threatens to return. No doubt other anæsthetics, and especially ether, would answer the same purpose.

Camphor has been claimed to be a valuable medicine in cholera, but there is no clinical evidence that it is so. Indeed, the only series of cases in which it was mainly depended upon gave a large mortality.

Acids have been employed in cholera, but chiefly on theoretical grounds, "in the hope of destroying the specific cholera process going on in the intestinal canal" (Macnamara). It is hardly necessary to discuss so vague a reason. What specific process is going on? What relation to it has the administration of acids? And, after all, only the hope is held out of destroying the hypothetical morbid process. The reaction of normal stools is usually acid, but sometimes it is neutral or even alkaline. In other acute bowel complaints with profuse diarrhoea they are acid, as in cholera infantum, but in epidemic cholera they are alkaline, because they consist chiefly of the water of the blood. It is far from proven that mineral acids can be useful merely by reversing the reaction of the stools. Far more probable is it that, in so far as they are of use, it is because they act as astringents upon the digestive mucous membrane. This may be inferred from the fact that, according to the advocates of these medicines, it is always difficult, and is often impossible, to acidify the stools in cholera. Moreover, it must be remembered that, like other medicines, the greater part of them are rejected by vomiting. If, then, mineral acids tend to lessen the diarrhoea of cholera, they act by their astringency and not by their acidity. Diluted or aromatic sulphuric acid may be given in the dose of from two to thirty minims, at intervals of an hour, in acid water or carbonated water, or diluted nitric acid, in doses of from twenty to fifty minims, at the same or somewhat longer intervals.

Intravenous injections were used in England during the first epidemic of cholera in 1832-33, but their results were regarded as unfavorable; subsequently, in 1849, they were tried with somewhat better success, and in 1867 the effects were still more encouraging. The liquid employed on the last-mentioned trial consisted of chloride of sodium 60 gr., chloride of potassium 6 gr., phosphate of sodium 3 gr., carbonate of sodium 20 gr., alcohol 2 drachms, and distilled water 20 ounces. The alcohol was added only when the liquid was about to be used, and the temperature of the latter was not allowed to exceed 110° F. or fall below 100° F. The liquid was contained in a zinc vessel holding about eighty ounces, with a lamp underneath, a thermometer hanging within, and a tap near the bottom, from which proceeded an india-rubber tube four feet long, with a silver nozzle at its end. The fluid was allowed to enter the vein by the force of gravity. If difficulty was experienced in introducing the nozzle, the vein was freely exposed, supported on a probe, and incised longitudinally. It was found that the success of the operation depended greatly [p. 769]upon having an ample supply of the solution prepared, so as to repeat the injection as often as might be found necessary. Mr. Little, who practised this method in numerous cases, stated as follows: "When a patient has been long pulseless clots form in the heart, and, as I have seen, extend into the larger veins. In one case the fluid would not flow in, and only distended the veins of the arm injected. After death clots were found extending from the heart into the axillary vein."[70] Five out of twenty apparently hopeless cases recovered under this treatment. The first effect of the injection was to revive the pulse, which had ceased to be felt; the voice also was restored, the color and expression improved, the cramps were relieved, the temperature rose, and the patients became convinced that their recovery was assured. A profuse perspiration and a severe rigor accompanied these symptoms. The rigor was evidently a nervous phenomenon, and not a chill, for it occurred when the temperature was rising. Other cases might be cited which unquestionably owed their recovery to this mode of treatment. It is true, however, that much more frequently it failed of success; and probably not only because the injection could not reach the heart, but because, having permeated the blood-vessels of the whole body, it escaped, as the serum of the blood had done, from the damaged intestine. Nevertheless, it would seem that an expedient which in a certain proportion of cases has been quite successful might yet be rendered more certain in its results if the operative procedure were perfected.

[70] *London Hosp. Reports*, iii. 470.

Cramps in the limbs may be lessened by active friction and shampooing, but there is no clinical reason for believing that these measures tend to restore the circulation. Equally ineffectual are other means used for communicating heat to the algid body and thereby reviving its functions. It is true that some physicians found that warm baths, at from 90° to 104° F., gave relief to the cramps and restored the failing pulse. In most cases the calming influence of the bath was noted, but it does not seem to have been curative or to have diminished the mortality-rate.[71] It should not be forgotten that the patient has no perception of his coldness. In all analogous conditions, as has already been remarked, such as frostbite and the cold stage of periodical fevers, cold, and not heat, promotes reaction. Still more injurious, if possible, than hot applications are irritants and stimulants after the stage of collapse has set in. Not only are they absolutely futile for restoring the animal temperature, but they are liable, unless very cautiously used, to produce intractable sores upon the skin if recovery ensues. It should also be remembered that the cholera patient's exhaustion is exceptionally great, and is apt to be increased by the officiousness implied in the use of many stimulating agents.

[71] *Ibid.*, iii. 445; *St. Bartholomew's Reports*, iii. 190.

As early as 1832 a marked advantage was ascribed to the use of cold affusions in cholera.[72] One of the physicians of the cholera hospital of Berlin said: "In these living corpses which are struck with asphyxia, lying cold and powerless, external and internal medicines cease to stimulate; no steam apparatus, no warm bathing, no friction, no irritant, avails." The condition is comparable to that in approaching death by cold, in which friction with snow is well known to be the proper remedy. Cold affusions were employed in the second stage of the disease. If the pulse revived, the affusions were continued in a tepid bath, after which the patient was [p. 770]put to bed and gently rubbed with cold flannels. Internally, ice-water was freely administered. Labadie-Lagrave[73] refers to forty cases treated in this manner, with only seven deaths. Yet the cold-water treatment does not appear to have commended itself to physicians generally. Evidently it does not meet the prime indication, which is to restore the wasted waters of the blood and retain it in the blood-vessels.

[72] Ainsworth, *Pestilential Cholera*, 1832.
[73] *Du Froid en Thérapeutique*, 1878.

Cold water ought to be given as freely as possible to assuage the thirst that exists in every stage of cholera, and especially in collapse. Nor should it be withheld because it will presently be rejected, for not only does it produce a grateful sensation in the mouth and throat, but it renders the act of vomiting easier. Yet, to some extent at least, the thirst may be allayed by rinsing the mouth and throat with cold water. Iced water is preferable to ice used for the same purpose, for the latter, by its relatively intense coldness, irritates and dries the mouth. Fragments of ice swallowed whole allay the burning heat in the stomach.

On the hypothesis that the cholera poison consists of organic germs various antiseptics have been employed in this disease. Permanganate of potassium was fortunately excluded from the list, on account of its corrosive action, but, unfortunately, carbolic acid was conceived to possess virtues that rendered it an eminently suitable remedy, and creasote, which resembles it very closely, was presumed to possess corresponding virtues. Then sulphurous acid and the sulphites, which for a time were warranted to destroy every species of germ, were confidently appealed to to stay the progress of cholera, and it was at one time even a matter of dispute whether sulphite of sodium or sulphite of potassium was the more efficacious. In truth, all of these medicines were useless, even when they were not mischievous.

Cholera has never prevailed in any country without giving rise to extraordinary theoretical and practical divagations. One physician in the earliest American epidemic gravely proposed, as the best mode of checking the diarrhoea, to plug the anus with a soft velvet cork. Another, in England, suggested that the "blood may be kept circulating by putting the patient on his back on a board and keeping up a rocking, see-saw, to-and-fro movement from eighty to one hundred times a minute." Another had the revelation that the disease is essentially a "paralysis of the sympathetic nerve and want of performance of the organic functions, with deficient vitality of the mucous membranes," and that its proper remedies are "bleeding, turpentine, and cool drinks, without heat and stimulants;" and to this remarkable doctrine a well-known physician gives his adhesion, thus: "The cause, I firmly believe, is an union of the poison with the sympathetic."[74] Still another discovered that the disease is a spinal disorder, and is to be treated by the application of ice-bags to the spine. Were not the evidence so palpable, it would hardly be believed that such irrational ideas should have been published concerning a disease which had then been under observation by the whole medical profession in Europe and America for more than thirty years, and in Asia for a much longer period.

[74] *Times and Gazette*, Aug., 1866, p. 209; *ibid.*, Nov., 1866, p. 555.

The most important lesson to be drawn from this history of the treatment of epidemic cholera is, that the arrest of the disease in the diarrhoeal stage is comparatively easy, and that in the stage of collapse its cure by any means whatever is altogether an exceptional occurrence.

[p. 771]

THE PLAGUE.
BY JAMES C. WILSON, M.D.

DEFINITION.—An acute specific fever of short duration and very fatal, endemic in certain Oriental countries, and frequently epidemic; it is characterized by buboes, carbuncles, and petechiæ.

SYNONYMS.—([Greek: plêgê], *plaga*, a stroke); the Pest; Pestilence; the Bubonic, Glandular, Inguinal Plague; the Oriental, Levantine, Levant Plague; the Indian, Pali Plague; Máhámari; Septic or Glandular Pestilence; Pestilential Fever, Adeno-nervous Fever; Typhus Pestilentialis, Gravissimus, Bubonicus, Anthracicus, etc. *Gr.* [Greek: ho loimos]; *Lat.* Pestis; *Fr.* La Peste; *Ger.* die Pest, Beulenpest.

CLASSIFICATION.—The plague, pest, pestilence, and their equivalents in various tongues, are terms that have been used from the earliest historical times to designate every epidemic disease attended by great mortality. As knowledge of diseases becomes clearer the terms by which they are designated become more definite; those which did service for a class are restricted to particular groups, and new names are found for other maladies only allied to such groups by superficial resemblances. Hence by degrees the term plague has become more restricted in its use. To-day it is understood as designating exclusively the specific affection defined above, the bubo plague.

The student of medical history meets with insurmountable difficulties in attempting to classify the recorded epidemics which have been described under this term. Even when used in its more restricted signification, difficulties as to the propriety of its application to certain epidemics arise. Thus, nosologists are not in agreement as to whether the great plague—the black death—which swept over Europe in the fourteenth century and destroyed in three years twenty-five millions of inhabitants, was a modification of the bubo plague or an essentially different disease. A like difference of opinion exists in regard to the relationship between the Indian or Pali plague which has from time to time prevailed in North-western India during the present century and the true plague.

The black death of the fourteenth century and the Pali plague, though presenting many of the characteristics of bubo plague, differ from it, while they resemble each other, in one important particular. Among the earlier and more common symptoms of note are those dependent upon gangrenous inflammation of the lungs, a lesion, according to Hirsch,[1] extremely rare in bubo plague. This author informs us that recent observations have fully confirmed the early opinion that the Pali plague[p. 772]differs from that of the Levant chiefly in this modification, and cites Pearson and Francis as saying of the former disease that "the collective symptoms are more like those of plague than of any other known disease.... We believe it to be in all essential particulars identical with the plague of Egypt."

[1] *Handbuch der historisch-geographischen Pathologie*, Dr. August Hirsch, 1860.

The three forms of plague—(*a*) the grave (or ordinary), (*b*) the fulminant (pestis siderans), and (*c*) the larval or abortive, observed in epidemics and hereafter to be described—do not represent distinct varieties of the disease, but are merely expressions of differences in the intensity of the action of the infecting principle upon different groups of individuals in given communities—differences to be explained here, as in the other infectious diseases, in part by variations in the activity of the poison itself, in part by the individual peculiarities and susceptibilities of those exposed to it.

HISTORICAL SKETCH.—Upon the authority of Rufus of Ephesus, quoted by Oribasius,[2] it is stated that the bubo plague prevailed as an endemic, and at times as an epidemic disease, in Libya, Egypt, and Syria prior to the beginning of the Christian era.

[2] *Medicinalia Collecta.*

In the year 542 A.D., according to Procopius,[3] the plague appeared in Egypt, at Pelusium; extended westward to Alexandria; eastward to Palestine, Syria, and Persia; passed from Asia Minor to Europe, where it first invaded Constantinople, whence it spread in all directions with such fury that before the close of the sixth century one-half the inhabitants of the Eastern empire had perished, either of the plague itself or of the universal destitution that followed in its train.

[3] See Hirsch.

With this epidemic, known in history as the Justinian plague, this disease established itself for the first time in Europe, where it maintained foothold for more than a thousand years.

About the middle of the seventeenth century the wide prevalence of the plague in Europe began to draw to an end. In Spain it was epidemic for the last time from 1677 to 1681; in Italy the last general epidemic came to a close in 1656, although local outbreaks continued to occur till the beginning of the following century. In France it still prevailed in several provinces in 1668, although it had for the most part disappeared some years before. In Switzerland we encounter it for the last time in 1667-68; in the Netherlands in 1677; from England the plague disappeared with the great outbreak of 1665. In the early part of the eighteenth century two important epidemics occurred within the boundaries of Europe. The first spread from Turkey, through Hungary and Poland, to Russia, thence to Norway and Sweden, and along the shores of the Baltic Sea to the Low Countries. This epidemic came to an end in 1714. Six years later the last great outbreak of the plague on European soil took place. It prevailed with great fury in Marseilles in 1720-21, and overran the whole of Provence. From this date till the close of the century Europe remained free from the plague, with the exception of Turkey and the contiguous countries. During the second and third decades of the present century repeated epidemics occurred in the Balkan Peninsula and the regions bordering on the Lower Danube and the Black Sea. The plague appeared also in Malta in 1813, and prevailed till 1815, and in 1816 it reached certain of the Ionian Islands. [p. 773]Only twice has this pest shown itself during the present century in Western Europe—once, during the epidemic at Malta in 1815, at Noja, a town of the Neapolitan province of Bari; the second time, in 1820, at Majorca, whither it was carried over from the coast of Barbary.

Between 1552 and 1784 the plague prevailed twenty-six times in Tunis and Algiers. Some idea of the importance assumed by this scourge in the countries of North-western Africa may be found from the fact that many of these epidemics lasted continuously for years, that which came in 1784 not ceasing for fifteen years. Between 1816 and 1821 the plague again prevailed in Tunis and Algiers, and again in 1836-37.

During the first half of the present century a change took place in the prevalence of the disease elsewhere. Shortly before its complete disappearance from Europe it ceased to prevail in Western Africa (with the exception of the Nile countries), in Mesopotamia, and in Persia. It disappeared from Asia Minor, Syria, and Palestine in 1843, from Egypt in 1844.

For a short period the plague seemed to have disappeared altogether. Those who cherished this hope were, however, destined to disappointment. In 1853 an outbreak occurred in the Assyr country, Western Arabia; and from that time till the present unmistakable local epidemics of the bubo plague have occurred in isolated regions of Africa and Asia; thus, in 1858 at Benghazi in Tripoli; in 1857 in Mesopotamia; in 1863 in the district of Maku, Persian Kurdistan; in 1867 in the marsh district on the right bank of the Euphrates; in 1870 in Persian Kurdistan; in 1871-73 in the Yunnan province, Western China; in 1873 in the marsh district on the left bank of the Euphrates. During four years following the outbreak of 1873 the disease continued to prevail over an extensive area in the countries bordering on the northern banks of the Persian Gulf. In 1874 it reappeared also in the Assyr district, Western Arabia, and in Benghazi, Northern Africa. In 1876, whilst still infesting the regions about the Lower Euphrates, the plague appeared in South-eastern Persia, and during this and the following years it appeared at several isolated points on the borders of the Caspian Sea. Early in 1878 the disease was reported as prevailing in the district of Souj-Bulak, Persian Kurdistan, and it appeared in October of the same year at the Cossack village Vetlanka, on the Lower Volga, district of Astrakhan, Russia, after an absence from Europe of thirty-seven years. It has more recently prevailed in the Assyr district, Western Arabia, and there have been rumors of its reappearances in Persian Kurdistan.

The Indian or Pali plague (Máhámari) has prevailed in local epidemics of great severity on several occasions during the present century in the North-western provinces of India. This fever was first recognized in Kutch in May, 1815, after a season of great scarcity of food. It spread rapidly over an extensive territory, and appeared in the spring of the following year at various points in Guzerat, next in Merawi, later in Rhadenpur, spreading thence westward to Sindh. Not until the following year (1817) did the pest reach the British possessions. This epidemic continued to prevail until 1821. The disease did not reappear until July 6, 1836, when it broke out in Pali, the principal dépôt of traffic between the coast and North-western India. It spread with great rapidity to the[p. 774]adjoining provinces. Toward the close of the year 1837 the disease broke out anew in Pali, and raged until the spring of the following year. In 1834-35, again in 1837, there were outbreaks of this pest in Gurwal, and in 1846 and 1847 in Karmoun, provinces of the southern slopes of the Himalayas. This destructive pest has raged at an altitude of 10,300 feet, and we learn from Hirsch that it has never wholly disappeared from the mountain-districts of the Himalayas since 1823, and that its ravages in these regions have been so great that certain settlements have been wholly destroyed.

The fever was remittent in type, with a great tendency to become continued; it was characterized by rapidly developing extreme prostration, and was very fatal. In most cases there were glandular swellings in the groins, armpits, and neck. Carbuncles and petechiæ are not mentioned as having been observed. Dyspnoea, cough, and bloody expectoration were frequent symptoms. Vomiting, at first of bilious matter, later of dark, coffee-colored fluid, was likewise common.

The plague has never appeared in the western hemisphere.

ETIOLOGY.—1. Predisposing Influences.—Whilst the present views as to the causation of the specific diseases compel us to assume a specific infecting principle as the real cause of every outbreak of the plague, there are certain circumstances which are recognized as so favoring the development and action of that principle that they have come to be looked upon as indirect or auxiliary causes of particular epidemics. It is more in accordance with the facts to speak of them as predisposing influences. Chief among these circumstances is that combination of physical and social wretchedness which goes hand in hand with poverty and overcrowding. The plague has been termed by a recent observer (Cabiadis) miseriæ morbus, and he has thus reproduced in 1878 a name applied to the great plague of London in 1665—the poor's plague. All observers of recent epidemics unite in ascribing to poverty the foremost rank among the predisposing influences of plague epidemics. It is only necessary to enumerate the evils which form the train of poverty, whether in cities or in villages, to complete the list.

With poverty come ignorance and neglect of all sanitary laws; overcrowding and ill ventilation; personal filthiness; improper as well as insufficient diet; indifference as to the location of dwellings and their surroundings. The condition of the villages which have been the scene of some of the recent epidemics beggars description. All observers unite in testifying to such accumulations of filth in and around the houses as requires to be seen to be believed. In these communities latrines are unknown, and no such thing as organized scavenging has ever existed.

The accumulation of unburied or imperfectly buried corpses has been looked upon as the real cause of the plague, and some of the recent epidemics have followed the prevalence of distinctive epizoötics. Whilst it is not difficult to disprove that under ordinary circumstances the effluvia from exposed and rotting carcasses can give rise to outbreaks of the plague, it is more than probable that an atmosphere charged with such emanations (together with other causes) can so unfavorably influence a community as to increase its susceptibility to the specific cause of this or any other infective disease. There can be but little doubt that the [p. 775]dead bodies of the victims of the plague are capable of disseminating the disease, and that the reopening of graves containing such bodies, even after a long period of time, has given rise to fresh outbreaks of the disease.

The season of the year does not appear to exert any very marked influence upon the development of epidemics, if we base our deductions upon observations made in different countries. In northern countries the disease has prevailed as severely in mid-winter as in summer. The epidemics of London showed a rise during July and August, their furious prevalence in September, and a gradual decline during October and November. In Constantinople the disease has commonly remained dormant during the winter months, and become active as the weather grew hotter. In Egypt, on the contrary, the activity of the outbreaks has developed in winter, increased with the advance of spring, and suddenly abated upon the advent of the summer. Such also has been the case with the three general epidemics in Mesopotamia studied by Tholozan.[4] "Their beginning took place in winter, their development during the spring, their decline and their extinction in summer. Their recrudescences obeyed the same laws: after an incubation during the summer season ... revivification took place in winter and in spring." It is added in this writer's account that the exceptional hot weather of summer in that country, and especially that of the shores of the Persian Gulf, has always moderated or directed the course of epidemics of this pest. In Cairo the epidemics have usually ceased upon the recurrence of intense summer heat in June. Dampness, and particularly a thoroughly wet soil, are favorable to the development and spread of the disease. The marshy regions of the Lower Euphrates, the shores of the Caspian and the Black Seas, the valley of the Nile, have been the scenes of repeated visitations. On the other hand, the plague has maintained its foothold in the mountainous districts of Western Arabia, in Yunnan, on the slopes of the Himalayas at a great elevation, and upon a dry, non-alluvial soil even more firmly than in the low and humid plains of Mesopotamia.[5]

[4] *Histoire de la Peste Bubonique en Mesopotamie*, 2d Mémoire, Paris, 1874.
[5] Tholozan, *Histoire de la Peste Bubonique en Perse*, 1st Mémoire, Paris, 1874.

Individual predisposition to contract the disease seems to be increased by all depressing influences, among which may be mentioned excessive bodily or mental exertion, intense and prolonged anxiety, fear, and the like. Previous debilitating disease also increases the liability to the attack. Neither sex nor age exerts an influence in this respect, save that after the age of fifty few contract the disease. Occupation confers no immunity. Physicians, nurses, and others occupied in the care of the sick, and those who bury the dead, have especially suffered in recent[6] as well as in the older outbreaks. Oil-carriers and dealers in oils and fats, and to a less degree water-carriers and the attendants at baths, are said to enjoy a comparative immunity from attack. Those who have suffered from the disease and recovered also enjoy a relative immunity. Second attacks are usually of less intensity than the first.

[6] See summary of a report addressed by Dr. G. Cabiadis to the Constantinople Board of Health on the outbreak in Astrakhan in Russia, 1878-79, by E. D. Dickson, M.D., *Medical Times and Gazette*, 1881, vol. i. pp. 4, 32, 119.

2. The Exciting Cause.—The exciting cause of the plague must, in [p. 776]the present state of our knowledge, be assumed to be a specific infecting principle. Upon no other hypothesis can the continued existence of a disease so specific in its characters, unchanged through the course of centuries, disappearing when the influences favorable to its presence cease, reappearing in certain regions when they again arise, be explained. Capable of being transmitted by the vehicles of commercial intercourse, of control by quarantine and cordons sanitaires, of spreading from limited foci of contagion into overwhelming epidemics, the plague is the very type of the infective diseases. The nature of this infecting principle is wholly unknown. It is probably a microphyte capable of development within the human organism—capable also of a prolonged independent existence under favorable circumstances outside of the body, and of again giving rise to the disease. The plague is

properly to be classed as a contagious-miasmatic disease (Liebermeister) with cholera, dysentery, and enteric fever. It continues to exist by the continuous propagation of its cause, and it spreads by the transportation of that cause.

It is conceded on all hands that the plague has never arisen autochthonously in Europe, but has in every instance been conveyed thither. Those who regard its reappearance after long intervals of time in those countries where it still occasionally prevails as spontaneous are compelled to ignore difficulties in reasoning far greater than the supposition of an equally prolonged condition of quiescence or an inexplicable or unsuspected reintroduction of the cause.

As to the disputed question of the contagiousness of the plague, to set forth the arguments and examples adduced in favor of either view would far exceed the limits of the present article. All the facts are to be explained upon the theory that the exciting cause of the plague, like that of cholera and enteric fever, consists of a miasm that must undergo certain changes outside the body before acquiring its virulent properties, and that the time required for these changes is exceedingly brief. But what the physical properties of this miasm are, or how it finds access to the body, or how it is eliminated, are alike utterly unknown to us.

It is certain, however, that it is incapable of being freely transmitted to great distances in the air. Whether or not it is conveyed or retained by the discharges from the bowel is not known. The history of recently observed outbreaks, from which alone definite and trustworthy facts are to be obtained, goes to show that the exciting cause of the plague clings closely to the patients and their immediate belongings. The closer the relation between those sick and the healthy, the greater the risk that the latter will contract the disease. Those in the house with the patients are more liable to fall sick than those in the adjoining houses—those who are constantly in their presence than those who occasionally see them. Thus, nurses much more frequently contract the plague than doctors, though the latter have in all epidemics been largely numbered among the victims. Among 357 deaths in the outbreak in Vetlanka, already referred to, were a priest, his wife and mother, three doctors, six assistant medical officers, and two Sisters of Mercy. Dr. Cabiadis remarks that the information obtained "shows that the malady propagated itself, in the first instance, from the sick to their relatives and to those who lived with them or who assisted them during their illness. If, on the one hand, these facts showed its contagious character, on the other hand evidence is [p. 777]still wanting to prove whether this transmission of the malady was caused by contact with the sick and their clothing, or by breathing an atmosphere impregnated with the deleterious particles emanating from their morbid bodies."

The period of incubation is from two to seven days. In the report of the commission of the French Academy of Medicine, drawn up by Prus in 1844, the statement appears that the plague has never shown itself among compromised persons after an isolation of eight days. The recent outbreaks tend to confirm this conclusion. L. Arnaud concluded from observations made at Benghazi in 1874 that the mean duration of this period was five or six days, and that the maximum did not exceed eight days. Cabiadis sets this stage down as three days as the rule, but as occasionally not exceeding twenty-four hours. He found no data, however, to show the longest period to which it could extend. Hirsch, from information collected in his investigation of the same epidemic (that of Astrakhan), concluded that the minimum period of incubation observed was from two to three days, the maximum more than eight, and that the average was five days. He states that very short or very long periods were seldom observed.

SYMPTOMATOLOGY.—Individual cases of the plague, as of other epidemic diseases, differ in their onset and progress under different circumstances and at different periods of particular outbreaks. Besides the ordinary form, to which as a type the greater number of the cases more or less closely conform, there are, on the one hand, others so severe that death takes place before the characteristic manifestations have time to appear, and, on the other hand, cases so light that such manifestations are but partly developed, and the nature of the malady is only to be recognized in the light of the prevalent epidemic influence.

Hence among the cases three forms are recognized: (*a*) The grave or ordinary form; (*b*) the fulminant form; and (*c*) the larval or abortive form.

(*a*) Grave or Ordinary Form.—The plague in typical cases is a febrile malady of the most acute kind, with localizations in the form of buboes or carbuncles.

The course of the attack may, for convenience of description, be divided into four stages: 1, the stage of invasion; 2, the stage of intense fever; 3, the stage of fully-developed localizations; and 4, the stage of convalescence.[7]

[7] This formal division of the description is suggested in some of the older accounts. (See "*Loimologia; or, An Historical Account of the Plague in London in 1665*, by Nathan Hodges, M.D., and Fellow of the College of Physicians, who resided in the City all that Time, Lond., 1721.")

The appearance of the plague in France in 1720 was the occasion of a great number of curious and interesting publications on this subject.

1. The stage of invasion is marked by a feeling of lassitude, by pains in the loins and extremities. There is extreme bodily and mental weakness, headache, fulness and throbbing of the head, dizziness. The patient's expression is dull, stupid; he replies to questions slowly or awkwardly, his face is pale, his eyes languid, his gait feeble and staggering. The appearance in this stage has been compared by several observers to that of a drunken man. Shivering occurs, but if fever be present it is slight. Nausea, vomiting, and diarrhoea are symptoms sometimes [p. 778]observed. This stage begins suddenly. It is often imperfectly developed, and it may last only a few hours or a day or two.

2. The second stage is characterized by fever of the most intense kind. It is ushered in by a chill, sometimes slight, commonly severe. The lassitude continues, the headache increases, the dulness deepens to stupor or gives way to delirium. The temperature rises to 102°-104° F., or even to 107.6° F. The pulse quickly mounts to 120 or 130. The skin is hot and dry; the patient complains of burning inward heat and of great, sometimes unbearable, thirst. The eyes are sunken and injected; the tongue moist, pale, and thickly covered with a chalk-white or grayish pasty coating; the vomiting often continues. The delirium is commonly active or noisy, and accompanied by great restlessness; it may, however, be mild, tending to sopor or coma. The progress of the disease now rapidly advances. The patient falls into the so-called typhoid state. His tongue becomes dry, hard, and fissured; sordes collect upon the teeth and lips, bloody crusts about the nostrils. At this time the evidences of failure of the forces of the circulation become conspicuous. The pulse grows feeble, small, often irregular—sometimes it can scarcely be felt; the lips become bluish, the extremities cold. There is tendency to collapse. During the course of this stage buboes begin to make their appearance. Sometimes the enlargement of the superficial lymphatics is preceded by tenderness or pain of more or less intensity; often the glands are found to be enlarged only upon search.

The termination of this stage is marked by a sudden fall of the temperature to subnormal ranges (93.2° F. has been observed); at the same time copious strong-smelling sweat not infrequently occurs. The pulse grows feebler, and falls to 100 or below it, and the mind becomes clearer.

3. These changes lead up to the stage of fully-developed local manifestations. The enlarged lymphatics are most commonly situated in the groins or on the upper part of the thighs at a point below that commonly the seat of venereal buboes; less often they are to be found in the armpits or the region of the angle of the jaw; as a rule, they occupy only one or two of these positions in the same patient. They vary in size from a little mass or kernel, only to be discovered after careful search, to the bulk of a hen's egg or a mandarin orange. The swelling of the gland takes place at times with great rapidity. Suppuration is followed by the discharge of an ichorous pus, and not rarely by ulcerative destruction of the surrounding tissues. Suppuration occurs more frequently than resolution, but is comparatively rare in fatal cases. Hence it has come to be popularly regarded as a favorable prognostic sign, whilst the early subsidence of the swelling has been looked upon as an omen of grave import.

The time of the appearance of the buboes varies greatly. In the greater number of cases they have shown themselves on the second, third, or fourth day of the attack, occasionally within six or eight hours of the beginning of the attack, and occasionally they have been observed to precede the general manifestation of the disease; rarely they have appeared as late as the fifth day. In many cases they are absent altogether.

Carbuncles demand attention as being among the characteristic local manifestations of this stage. They are less common than buboes. Their usual position is upon the lower extremities, the buttocks, or the back of [p. 779] the neck. In favorable cases the gangrene after a few days becomes limited and the slough separates. Boils also occasionally appear.

Petechiæ occur in the worst cases, and often at an early period in the course of the disease. Their appearance usually indicates a fatal issue. They occupy at times extensive areas of the body or the greater part of its surface; at times they appear only in the neighborhood of the buboes. They vary in size from a mere speck to spots several lines in diameter. When very numerous they give a livid hue to the skin, and that appearance to the cadaver to which, together with the high mortality, was doubtless due the term black death by which severe epidemics were known in the Middle Ages.

Vibices and extensive ecchymoses sometimes appear shortly before death.

4. The stage of convalescence sets in between the sixth and tenth days. It is often protracted by prolonged suppuration of the bubonic enlargements. Both relapses and distinct second attacks have been noted by recent as well as the older observers.

In addition to the foregoing sketch of the course of the disease in its ordinary form it is necessary to describe certain other symptoms.

The attack has sometimes begun with a convulsive tremor, at other times with a prolonged shaking, which has lasted from six hours to three days, the patient remaining free from fever and not complaining of cold. This condition has terminated in coma, followed speedily by death.

Sometimes the attack has come upon the patient with great confusion of mind, so that he appears dazed, or else a curious distraction has befallen him in the midst of his ordinary avocations. If absent from home, such patients commonly at once set out to return, either trembling and staggering as though tipsy, or else rushing wildly through the streets with frantic gestures and outcries.

The vomited matters are usually at first gastric mucus with bile, afterward dark coffee-colored fluid; in certain cases blood is vomited. Bleeding from the nose, lungs, bowels, vagina, and urethra have also been observed. Cases attended by hemorrhages have in almost all instances terminated fatally.

Constipation has been, as a rule, present during the acute stages; later in the attack diarrhoea has occasionally occurred. It has been looked upon as a favorable symptom.

The urine has been diminished and suppressed in grave cases. Trustworthy observations, both as to its quantity and its chemical composition, are wanting. It has been observed to contain blood.

As has been already pointed out, the Máhámari of North-western India has been especially characterized by lung symptoms. Other regions also have been visited by epidemics in which acute pulmonary lesions formed a prominent part of the morbid complexus.

(*b*) The Fulminant Form.—Chiefly in the early days or weeks of epidemics, but to some extent also later, cases occur in which the intensity of the sickness is so great that the patient dies before its usual manifestations have time to develop. The duration of the whole attack, which ends fatally, is often not more than a few hours; its symptoms, which differ but little if at all from those of similar cases of other epidemic diseases—such, for example, as epidemic cerebro-spinal fever in its fulminant [p. 780] form—are of the most aggravated character, and the patient perishes overwhelmed by the infection as though struck by a thunderbolt. Profound disturbance of the nervous centres, convulsions, coma, the rapid formation of vibices and petechiæ, collapse, are the speedy forerunners of the fatal issue.

(*c*) The Larval or Abortive Form.—Toward the close of an epidemic the character of the disease usually undergoes a change. It becomes less malignant. The cases present the essential symptoms, but in diminished intensity. Some cases terminate in an early defervescence with rapid subsidence of beginning local manifestations; others present merely the evidences of a slight disturbance of the general health, without any characteristic symptoms of the prevalent disorder; others, again, are characterized by the appearance of buboes without pain or fever. These swellings undergo resolution in fourteen days or thereabout. Exceptionally they suppurate.

The duration of the plague is from six to ten days in typical cases running a favorable course; those of fatal cases from one to twenty days. Clot Bey[8] found the duration of the worst cases two or three days, of those next in point of severity five or six days, whilst in milder cases death did not occur until the second or third week. Of 534 fatal cases noted by W. H. Colvill, 126 occurred one day after the attack, 80 two days after it, 105 three days, 76 four days, 60 five days, 26 six days after the attack. After six days the number of deaths rapidly declined; on the nineteenth day 1 death, and on the twentieth day after the attack 11 deaths, occurred. It is said that death after the seventh day is commonly not in consequence of the disease itself, but of sequels. Of 16 fatal cases in the village Prischib in Astrakhan, noted in the report of Dr. Cabiadis, and of whom the names, as well as the day of their exposure, their falling sick, and their death are given, 1 died in one day, 4 in two days, 6 in three days, 3 in four days, and 2 in six days.

[8] *De la Peste observée en Égypte*, Paris, 1840.

The mortality of the plague is greater than that of any other epidemic disease. In all epidemics a large majority of those who contract the disease die. This is especially true of epidemics at their beginning, when it has often happened that for a time all the cases have perished. Of this, as of other epidemic diseases, it is true that the death-rate has varied in different outbreaks and at different periods of the same outbreak. Colvill states that in the epidemic of 1874 in Mesopotamia the mortality of stricken villages during the first half of the time was 93 to 95 per cent. of those attacked, but that afterward the majority of those attacked recovered. The same authority states that in Bagdad in 1876 the mortality was 55.7 per cent. of persons attacked. Arnauld gives the mortality at Benghazi in 1874 as 39 per cent. of attacks. The death-rate at Vetlanka was 82 per cent. of those attacked. In Toulon in 1721, of a population of about 26,000 human beings, about 20,000 were attacked, and of these 16,000 died. It has been by no means of rare occurrence that nearly half the population of towns have perished in an epidemic, or that small villages have been completely depopulated by this scourge.

COMPLICATIONS AND SEQUELS.—The appalling mortality of the plague on its approach, the rapidity of its spread, the popular commotion upon its appearance, its brief course, and the fact that its recent outbreaks have[p. 781]taken place in regions where trained European physicians have been, with a few exceptions, beyond reach, all unite in maintaining the gloom that has since the Middle Ages enveloped the clinical facts of this disease.

Of its clinical course, beyond the brief outline already given, little is accurately known, of its complications still less. In some of the recent epidemics, and particularly in the outbreaks of plague in India, the evidences of pulmonary lesions have been so conspicuous that they deserve to be classed among the essential manifestations of the disease rather than as complications; in others pulmonary congestion, hæmoptysis, the evidences of croupous or catarrhal pneumonia, have occurred in a small proportion of the cases. Aside from this, there is nothing to be said as to the complications.

Among the known sequels are protracted ulceration of the enlarged lymphatics, boils, superficial or deep abscesses, catarrhal pneumonia, pertussis, mental troubles, and the like. Extensive and deep cicatrices are not infrequently found in the site of the ulcerating local manifestations.

MORBID ANATOMY.—The existing knowledge of the morbid anatomy of the plague is but scanty. The observers of the early outbreaks contributed nothing; the recent outbreaks have taken place under circumstances in which anatomical investigations were impracticable. The knowledge which we possess is almost wholly due to the investigations conducted by the French in Egypt at the close of the last and the beginning of the present century, and again during the years 1833 to 1838.

The descriptions of Bulant,[9] Clot Bey, and others point to gross lesions, such as are found after death in the acute stages of the infectious diseases in general. The viscera were engorged with dark fluid blood; ecchymoses were often found in the mucous and the serous membranes, in the substance of the different organs, and into the connective tissue. The spleen was in almost all cases enlarged, softened, and of a dark color. Not rarely the kidneys were deeply engorged, and extravasations of blood into their substance, their pelves, and into the surrounding connective tissues were often encountered.

[9] *De la peste oriental d'apres les matérnaux recuillés à Alexandrie, à Smyrne, etc., pendant les Années 1833 à 1838*, Paris, 1839.

The only constant and characteristic changes relate to the lymphatic system. The lymphatic glands were, as a rule, enlarged and deeply injected with blood. Where no buboes existed the glands of the various cavities of the body showed evidences of acute inflammatory processes. In some instances the affection of the glands appeared to be general; less frequently it was most conspicuous in, or apparently limited to, one or more great groups. Thus, the bronchial, the mediastinal, the mesenteric, the lumbar, etc. were severally the seat of marked changes with or without enlargement of superficial groups, or several of these groups were at the same time implicated.

In no instance were symmetrical enlargements of the inguinal regions, the axillæ, or the throat met with.

According to Runnel,[10] in 2700 cases there were inguinal buboes in 1841, axillary in 569, maxillary in 231; inguinal buboes occurred 175 times on both sides, 729 times on the right only, 589 times on the left only; the axillary buboes were double 9 times, right only 185, left only [p. 782]163. Buboes of the neck only occurred 130 times, and of them 67 cases were children.

[10] *A Treatise on the Plague*, London, 1791.

The connective tissue surrounding the affected glands was the seat of an infiltration sometimes serous, sometimes cellular; it also very commonly contained more or less extensive extravasations of blood. Even where no buboes appeared on the surface of the body the glands were enlarged to twice their usual size or more. The substance of the glands in the larger swellings was at times uniformly red or violet, again whitish or marbled or pulpy or denser, or of the consistence of fat. It was also sometimes soft like jelly, and rarely it contained minute collections of pus. Some observers speak of dilatation of the lymph-vessels in the neighborhood of the enlarged glands.

DIAGNOSIS.—The difficulties attending the recognition of the plague at the beginning of an outbreak speedily subside. The rapid spread of the disease, its frightful mortality, the overwhelming intensity of the symptoms, the prompt occurrence of cases characterized by buboes, carbuncles, or petechiæ, are collectively considered diagnostic of this, and of no other disease whatever. In regions subject to the repeated visitations of this pest there exists a universal unwillingness to mention even the name of a disease whose suspected presence alone is followed by consequences of the most serious nature to the freedom of personal and commercial intercourse. To this unwillingness, rather than to any real likeness between the plague and other diseases with which it has been compared, are to be traced most of the difficulties as to the differential diagnosis that have been raised, especially in the regions bordering on the Mediterranean Sea.

It is not, therefore, necessary in this place to discuss the diagnosis between the plague and malarial and other pernicious fevers, malignant typhus, epidemic dysentery, lymphadenitis, syphilitic buboes, parotitis, and so forth.

TREATMENT.—Preventive.—The efficient treatment consists in prophylaxis. The history of this disease indicates with singular clearness the measures which, properly carried out, are capable of controlling the spread of the epidemic diseases. These measures arrange themselves into two groups, of which the first has to do with the removal of the conditions familiar to the development of the disease, the predisposing influences; and the second with the restriction of the disease to the locality in which it shows itself—isolation, quarantine.

The conditions favorable to the development of the plague have already been set forth under the heading Etiology. They relate to poverty and ignorance, and their attendant evils, in communities. They are those conditions which tend to disappear under the influences of civilization, and in truth it may be said that at the present time the plague occurs only in half-civilized countries.

Preventive medicine has achieved no other work comparing in magnitude and importance with the extinction of the plague in Europe. This was, to use the words of Hirsch, "a gradual process, and kept pace in great measure with the development and perfection of the quarantine system with reference to the Orient and the different countries of Europe." This author continues: "I cannot, in fact, understand how any one criticising the facts without prejudice, and having regard to the [p. 783]state of the plague in the East, can for a moment hesitate to attribute the chief cause of the disappearance of the plague from European soil to a well-regulated quarantine system." The European has by no means lost his susceptibility to the disease. He is liable to attack in the East. His protection at home lies in the restriction of the exciting cause of the disease to its present haunts.

Any extended notice of quarantine and quarantine laws is beyond the scope of this article. It may be said, however, that with reference to the plague measures quite unnecessary under ordinary circumstances assume the greatest importance when this disease makes its appearance in countries bordering upon Europe, and that no amount of hardship to individuals necessary to avert so great a calamity as a plague epidemic could be looked upon as excessive. Indeed, we can with difficulty realize the severity with which measures of isolation have been carried into effect at times when the devastation produced by the plague was still vividly remembered. Violation of the orders issued during an epidemic has been punished with no less a penalty than death. It is related that upon the appearance of the plague in the little town of Noja in Lower Italy in 1815, troops were despatched immediately to surround the place with a cordon. The town was encircled by two deep ditches, and opposite the gates three ditches were spanned by drawbridges, which served as a means for the introduction of provisions, but no other communication was allowed. Only letters were allowed to leave the city, and these were first dipped in vinegar. Cannons were posted at the city gates. The ditches were occupied by sentinels, who were ordered to shoot down any one who approached and failed to stand still the moment he was hailed. A plague patient who escaped while delirious and attempted to pass the lines was, in fact, shot dead. Outside this cordon two others were established. Those who disobeyed the orders were treated with the greatest severity. An inhabitant of Noja, who had thrown a pack of cards to the soldiers, together with the soldier who picked it up, was tried by court-martial and shot.[11]

[11] *Ueber die Pest zu Noja*, Nürnberg, 1818, quoted by Liebermeister in *Ziemssen's Encyclopedia*, article "Plague."

Lower Italy, possibly Europe also, owed its escape to the rigorous measures carried out in this instance; nor can it be doubted that the measures of isolation practised during the outbreak on the Volga 1878-79 restricted the disease to the district in which it appeared and brought it to a speedy end. On this occasion three efficient cordons were established to isolate the infected places. The first cordon was put around every place where plague prevailed, to prevent persons from entering or quitting that locality until forty-two days had elapsed after the last attack of the malady there. The second cordon was formed around the infected area, encircling all the infected localities. Its circumference extended 800 kilometres, and was guarded by pickets of soldiers stationed at intervals of five kilometres. This cordon had four quarantine stations. The third and outermost cordon was established round the whole province of Astrakhan. It served to control the functions of the inner cordons, inasmuch as all persons coming from within its area, who could not prove that they had undergone quarantine at the stations of the middle cordon, were stopped.

[p. 784]The complete disinfection of all clothing and other articles used in the service of the sick is to be included among measures of prophylaxis. It is no uncommon thing to destroy by fire the houses in which cases have occurred, along with their contents.

No efficient means of protection are known for those who during an outbreak cannot escape from the infected neighborhood. It would be without purpose other than to amuse the reader to reproduce the quaint fancies of the older physicians in this matter, or to dwell upon the amulets and incantations, the absurd costumes, the protective power of tobacco, according to Diemerhoeck, or the disbelief in its virtues on the part of Hodges, who preferred "canary, of the best sort, of which he frequently drank while he attended the sick."

Clinical.—"The treatment of individual cases must in the present state of knowledge be expectant and symptomatic. Notwithstanding our acquaintance with the symptoms that characterize plague, we are utterly ignorant of the treatment best suited to its cases" (Cabiadis).

Physicians who have written from personal observation unite in advising a treatment of the simplest kind. Ventilation, cleanliness, a liquid diet, abundant cool drinks, are to be ordered. The initial collapse and the evidences of failure of the circulation call for the use of stimulants, and especially of alcohol. Cold or tepid sponging, in accordance with the sensations of the patient, may be resorted to. If there be high fever an energetic antipyretic treatment might be carried out. Cold effusion is said to have been of use in many instances.

Purging, bloodletting, mercurials, blistering, emetics, have proved either positively injurious or altogether without effect upon the course of the disease.

Of drugs, ammonium chloride, salicylic acid, carbolic acid, quinine, have been administered without positive effect.

It is stated that the free inunction of oil from the very beginning of the attack was affirmed to exert a favorable influence.[12]

[12] See Griesinger, *Virchow's Handbuch der Speciellen Pathologie und Therapie*, ii. 2, s. 316.

In early times the buboes were often incised, or even excised, as soon as they began to swell. More recently they have been treated with leeches or inunctions of mercurial ointment. The treatment by poultices and the evacuation of pus as soon as it can be detected is at present regarded with greater favor. Carbuncles are likewise to be treated in accordance with accepted surgical procedures.

[p. 785]

LEPROSY.
BY JAMES C. WHITE, M.D.

DEFINITION.—Leprosy is a constitutional disease of chronic course and fatal termination, characterized by peculiar changes in the tissues of skin, mucous membrane, nerves, and most organs of the body.

SYNONYMS.—Elephantiasis of Greek writers; Lepra of Arabian authors; Anssatz (Germany); Spedalskhed (Norway). The local names in use among the numerous races in which it prevails are too numerous to be given here.

HISTORY.—Although great confusion has existed among the most ancient as well as later medical writers with regard to the definition of this disease, it having been confounded with several other affections (elephantiasis arabum, syphilis, psoriasis, morphoea, etc.), leprosy has prevailed in certain parts of the world from the time of the earliest records. The biblical accounts show that it existed among the Jews in Egypt, although it was not accurately distinguished from other diseases resembling it in some respects. It was recognized in Greece before the Christian era, and in the early centuries after Christ it had extended widely over Europe. In the seventh and eighth centuries special leper-houses were founded in Italy, France, and Germany. The disease reached its height in Europe in the twelfth and thirteenth centuries, when 19,000 lazarettos are said to have been in existence. Its spread was greatly increased by the constant intercourse kept up between Europe and the East during the Crusades. In the fifteenth century it began to diminish, and in the course of the seventeenth it had almost wholly disappeared from the most civilized states. It has lingered, however, in other parts, and exists to-day in France and Spain and Portugal, in Norway and Sweden, and in Italy, Greece, and Southern Russia. As in ancient times, it is widely spread along the coasts of Africa and prevails largely throughout Asia. It is found in many of the islands of the Indian and Pacific Oceans, in Japan, New Zealand, Madeira, the West Indies, extensively in some of the states of Central and South America and Mexico and the Hawaiian Islands.

It may be interesting to trace its history in the United States and adjacent districts more minutely. It is not known just when leprosy was introduced into North America.

According to the Louisiana historian, Gayarré, the Spaniards established leper hospitals in several of their colonies on the Gulf of Mexico during the last century. One existed in New Orleans as late as 1785. In 1776 the disease was reported as existing among the blacks in Florida. It seems to have died out, and with [p. 786]it all remembrance of its former existence amongst us, until within the last few years, when its occurrence in the Southern States has again attracted attention. In Louisiana the first case was discovered in 1866 in an old woman whose father came from the south of France; she died in 1870. In 1871 it appeared in one of her sons, in 1872 in two others, and in 1876 in a nephew. A sixth case developed in a young woman who was in constant attendance upon the first case. In addition to this group, other cases have been observed in several parishes, amounting to twenty-one in all, as collected by Salomon of New Orleans in 1878.[1] Two other cases, brother and sister, in Louisiana are known to the writer, one of whom has recently died under his care. In South Carolina the disease is reported by J. F. M. Geddings[2] to have been observed in sixteen cases since the year 1846; four were Jews, four negroes, and eight whites. In none was any hereditary taint to be traced. No new cases have developed since that report.[3]

[1] *New Orleans Med. and Surg. Journal*, March, 1878.
[2] *Trans. Intern. Med. Congress*, Philadelphia, 1876.
[3] See article on "Contagiousness of Leprosy" by writer, in *Amer. Journ. of Med. Sciences*, Oct., 1882.

In Minnesota and other North-western States leprosy has been known to exist for a considerable time among the Norwegian immigrants who have settled in them in large numbers. Holmboe in 1863 and Prof. Boeck later made visits to these colonies while in this country, and published reports concerning them after their return.[4] The latter found eighteen cases among his countrymen, most of which were leprous before emigration; in others the disease developed after arrival in America. It had not manifested itself in any person born in this country. The character and progress of the affection seem to have been little influenced by residence here. Since these observations other cases have been collected by the committee on statistics of the American Dermatological Association,[5] showing the continuance of the disease in these States. In 1879 there were fifteen cases in Minnesota. Its spread in this portion of our country is slow.

[4] *British and For. Med.-Chir. Review*, Jan., 1870, and *Nord. Medic. Ark.*, Bd. iii.
[5] See *Transactions*.

Since 1871, 52 cases of the disease have been inmates of the hospital for lepers in San Francisco, California. Of these, all, with one exception, were Chinese, and forty-five of them had been sent back to China. It is presumed to have shown itself after arrival in this country, as "unproductive labor would not be imported by the Six Companies."[6] No case of the disease known to have been acquired in this country has yet been reported upon the Pacific Coast. One case has developed in San Francisco after residence in the Hawaiian Islands.

[6] *Trans. Am. Derm. Assoc.*, 1881.

In Oregon, too, the disease has appeared among the Chinese immigrants, steps having been recently taken to re-ship five lepers from the poor-farm at Portland to China.

Since 1815, possibly earlier, leprosy has prevailed among the poor French settlements along the Miramichi River, near the Bay of Chaleurs, New Brunswick. It was first noticed in a woman whose mother came from Normandy, and has continued mainly in her descendants since. No measures were taken to control the disease until 1844, when a hospital was erected on Sheldrake Island. In 1849 the present lazaretto at [p. 787]Tracadie was established. During the first five years (1844-49) there were admitted 32 patients; from 1849 to 1863, 67 additional patients were received; and from the latter date to 1879, 30 more, making a total number of 129 up to the last report. The greatest number present at any one time was 37. In 1878 there were 16 patients in the lazaretto—6 men and 10 women. The total number of deaths in the hospital has been, up to 1878, 123. A. C. Smith, who resides near Tracadie, states that at the latter date but three cases were known to exist outside the lazaretto. Residence is not compulsory, and no sufficient measures are taken to remove patients from their homes before they may have inoculated other members of the family. The disease is more restricted in locality than formerly.

Within the last two years two or three small groups of the disease have been discovered in the island of Cape Breton, which are described in the *Canadian Journal of Med. Science*, Sept., 1881.

These are all the places north of Mexico where the disease exists in an endemic form. A considerable number of cases have been reported within the past few years from other parts of the United States, where it has manifested itself in persons who have formerly resided in leprous countries or in those who have wandered from the above infected districts. A very few instances have been recorded in which it has appeared in those who have never visited any infected locality or have been in apparent contact with lepers. Such cases, if authentic, establish the possibility of a sporadic origin of the affection. The fact of so many foci already established, and the penetration of a race so prone to the disease as the Chinese into all parts of the country, give the study of leprosy in America a special importance.

ETIOLOGY.—The study of the etiology of leprosy is intimately connected with that of its history and geographical distribution. From the earliest times it was regarded in all parts of the world as a contagious affection, and efforts were made by the sternest laws of Church and State to control its spread by segregation, by interdiction of marriage, etc. No disease has ever been regarded with an equal degree of abhorrence by mankind; none has received greater attention from physicians of every age. Within the present century it has come to be regarded, almost without exception, by the profession as non-contagious. Peculiarities of climate, soil, and modes of life have been looked upon as predisposing, exciting, or even essential influences in its causation; but the widespread distribution of the disease, with the consequent diversity of diet and customs of living, its prevalence upon the coast and in interior regions, in high altitudes as well as at the sea-level, in Iceland as in the tropics, show that these conditions, however they may affect the course of the affection, have no direct relation to its causation. The theory of heredity, as the most plausible explanation, has received its strongest support in the investigations of Boeck and Danielssen in Norway, where the disease can be traced for several generations in families. The same conclusions readily present themselves where the disease is studied in restricted localities, as in Louisiana and New Brunswick at the present time, where, as we have seen, it manifests itself closely in families in different generations. But this is a narrow point of view from which to study the etiology of leprosy. It often fails to manifest itself in the descendants of lepers in [p. 788]such communities, and affects persons in whose families it has never previously existed. Moreover, in countries where it does not prevail it not infrequently attacks individuals who have at some time visited regions where it was endemic, and in the latter places may develop in immigrants from parts of the world where it has never existed.

The same class of facts which seem to demonstrate its hereditary nature may be used in support of its infectious character. The proper field for observation in this regard would be a virgin region where its natural course could be studied independently of theories. Fortunately for science, such an opportunity is afforded in the history of the disease in the Hawaiian Islands. The exact date and mode of its introduction there are not definitely known. The islands have for years been the resort of the whaling-fleets manned by sailors coming from leprous regions. The natives also shipped as sailors, and after visiting such ports returned home. The absence of any restraint in the intercourse of crews and native women is well known. Isolated cases may have occurred as far back as 1830, but the disease made slow headway until about 1860, when it increased so rapidly that the government took stringent measures to control it, all cases discovered being sent to the leper segregation upon an island from which there is no escape. Since 1866, 2000 cases have been received there, and at last report the asylum contained 750 inmates. This by no means represents the extent of its prevalence in the islands, however. As the native population by recent census was only 44,000, it will be seen that the proportion affected is very large. This unwonted rapidity of spread cannot be accounted for on the ground of heredity. Transference from individual to individual by inoculation seems to be the only possible explanation, and all resident physicians believe that the disease is contagious in this sense. It affects almost exclusively those of native descent, and their habits of life are such as would greatly facilitate its wide dissemination in this way—viz. their great licentiousness and absence of all fear of the disease, which affords no bar to ordinary association or cohabitation; the crowding of large families in small huts and sharing the same mats and blankets; the eating of poi with the fingers from the same dish; passing a common drinking-vessel or pipe from mouth to mouth, etc.[7] Promiscuous and compulsory vaccination with impure virus, too, has been generally practised during recent epidemics of small-pox. It is evident that abundant opportunity has in many ways been presented for the inoculation of pus or blood into the circulation from infected to healthy persons. Where immunity from contraction has followed marriage with a leper, it may be assumed that the conditions of an abraded surface and the contact with pus or blood have not been fulfilled. The wide spread of syphilis among the natives, and a consequent cachexia, have no doubt contributed to these conditions and established a national lack of resistance to the ravages of the disease. Nor can we overlook the proclivity of all endemic diseases to extraordinary manifestations of virulence in insular nations not previously protected by gradual inoculation. Many reliable cases are cited by resident physicians where the evidence of direct communication of the disease seems to be reliable. Facts of the same nature may be collected in the study of the history of [p. 789]the disease in New Brunswick and in Louisiana, where, as above stated, much better fields for investigating this question exist than in the Old-World regions where the affection has been rife for centuries.

[7] Dr. G. W. Woods, U.S.N., in *Hygienic and Med. Reports* of Navy Department, vol. iv., 1879.

If we admit the fact of transference by inoculation in a single instance, there is no reason why we should not regard this as the principal if not the only means of extension of the disease, whether we accept or not the theory of its parasitic nature. It is not inconsistent with our knowledge of its laws and history to believe that leprosy is an affection communicated with difficulty, and after a prolonged period of incubation, from one person to another by contact with certain products of the diseased tissue; that it has in past and present time in this way spread from nation to nation; and that its progress as an endemic affection has been checked only by laws based upon this theory. All the negative facts so frequently urged against this doctrine of contagion apply as strongly to that of heredity, and may be interpreted in support of the former. The latest investigations into its pathology afford tangible evidence in its favor. It may at least be claimed that the question of contagion through inoculation must be reopened.[8]

[8] See article on the question of contagion in leprosy in the *American Journal of Med. Sciences*, Oct., 1882, by the writer.

Leprosy affects both sexes in about equal degree, and may first show itself in early childhood. It is apt to produce sterility, so that marriages between lepers are rarely fruitful. This result seems to limit the extension of the disease under the law of heredity if we admit its action. There can be no doubt that cohabitation may take place for years without communication of the disease where one party alone is leprous; and such immunity may be explained by the failure of favorable conditions for sexual inoculation, just as in syphilis. The disease would naturally be most dangerous in its ulcerative tubercular form.

SYMPTOMATOLOGY.—There are two well-marked forms of leprosy—viz. the tubercular and the anæsthetic—which are characterized by certain easily recognized external manifestations, and which are accompanied by symptoms indicative of disturbances of the general economy as well as of special organs. These forms are not always sharply defined, and often occur simultaneously or in succession in individual cases. Both are generally preceded by premonitory symptoms, consisting of unaccountable languor of mind and body, tingling sensations in the skin, rise of temperature in the evening, and various disturbances of digestion, or by the occasional outbreak of single or several blebs. This prodromal stage affords no indication of the type of disease to follow, and may last for days, months, or even years, with greater or less intervals and intensity.

TUBERCULAR LEPROSY.—This form may declare itself at once by the characteristic tubercles, but frequently an earlier manifestation is the appearance of macules or dull red spots, varying in size from a pea to two or three inches in diameter. They have an indistinct margin, a glazed and smooth surface, and become paler on pressure. The patches, although not at all or but slightly elevated above the general surface, are firmer, and penetrate more or less deeply into the cutaneous tissues. They may increase in size peripherally and undergo involution in the older central portions simultaneously. During the latter process the color changes from a more or less dull red to a brown, yellow, or grayish tint, and [p. 790]finally may become quite white. The spots also become thinner or even slightly depressed. Their seat is principally the trunk, but also the limbs, and less frequently the face. This condition of the skin may precede any other changes in its tissues for months or years, the patches appearing and disappearing or remaining as permanent stains. At last well-defined tubercular elevations show themselves, varying in size from a small shot to a filbert, flattened or semi-globular in form, generally smooth and firm to the touch, and of a dull red or brown color. They occur upon any part of the surface, but are especially abundant upon the face, where they may cause great deformity of the features. The forehead and eyebrows may become very greatly thickened by general infiltration, or thrown out into very prominent folds and protuberances by the massing of individual tubercles. The lips thicken, the nose broadens, and the ears stand out conspicuously with their increased bulk. All these changes in form, with the great darkening in tint which is often present, give at times a most repulsive expression to the face. The tubercles are sometimes to be felt imbedded in the skin, or considerable areas are found to be uniformly thickened and scarcely at all prominent. All forms are capable of involution after an existence of months, and may leave dark-colored atrophic patches to mark their seat. They are rarely painful, and occasionally slightly sensitive. They may be transformed into ulcers, especially upon prominent positions, as the knuckles, elbows, knees, as the result of pressure or injury, which are extremely indolent, although shallow, and may heal and break down repeatedly. Occasionally they give rise to serious complications—inflammation of the lymph-vessels, suppuration of the joints with loss of the attendant members, as the fingers and toes. Tubercles appear also upon the mucous membrane of the nasal cavities, the mouth, and larynx, often in great abundance, causing a very characteristic hoarseness or loss of voice. With these changes in the cutaneous tissues, which may be accompanied in their periods of greatest activity by febrile disturbances, there are developed after months or years, with gradual failure of strength, manifestations of changes in the internal organs, the lungs, intestines, and brain, which may prove fatal at any time, or the patient may die of slowly progressive marasmus. The course of the tubercular form is on the average between eight and ten years. At any period there may supervene manifestations of the anæsthetic type, which makes the so-called mixed variety, in which either form may predominate.

ANÆSTHETIC LEPROSY.—This variety is characterized by the loss of sensation in the skin over areas of varying extent, which occupy no definite positions in relation to nerve-distribution. The anæsthetic patches may appear upon the seat of old maculæ or former tubercles or of a preceding bullous efflorescence, or upon parts not previously affected in any way. They may follow a reddened and hyperæsthetic condition of the cutaneous tissues, or they may be surrounded by a serpiginous border of this character. The degree of anæsthesia in the affected parts is sometimes so complete that the skin and underlying tissues may be deeply pricked or cut or burned without the patient being aware of the injury. Such patches may possibly regain their sensibility. Their surface appears in later stages dry, wrinkled, shrunken, and of a brownish color, and atrophy, not only of the skin but of the muscles, is gradually developed, [p. 791]in consequence of which the expression of the face undergoes a marked change. The eyelids and lips droop, the hair falls, the hands contract, and the joints of the fingers and toes are laid bare, so that the phalanges, or even the whole hands and feet, drop off. Ulceration or gangrene of the parts may develop, and whole extremities may shrivel up. With these manifestations of local derangements of nerve-action the functions of the brain fail, the patient becoming stupid and incapable of action or motion, the temperature and pulse are lowered, and death comes slowly by marasmus or the most various complications—tetanus, disease of the lungs, pyæmia, etc. The average duration of this form is from eighteen to twenty years.

PATHOLOGICAL ANATOMY.—The structural changes which take place in the tissues of parts which are the seat of the appearances above described have received the special study of many excellent observers[9] in recent times, and are now well understood. A section through the thickened skin or a tubercle shows the corium and underlying connective tissue infiltrated with round cells, as in lupus and syphilis; in other words, converted into "granulation tissue." This change first takes place along the course of the cutaneous vessels and glands, penetrating more deeply and forming a firmer cell new-growth in proportion to duration, the cells being enclosed in a coarse meshwork of fibrous tissue, and encroaching upon the various structures of the skin, so as to produce atrophy and finally destruction of all its characteristic tissues. This cell-infiltration may of itself undergo later changes, as fatty degeneration and softening (ulceration). The lymph-glands and corpuscles assume a special fatty metamorphosis. An examination of the tubercles upon the mucous membrane reveals the same small-celled new-growth. In the nerve-tissues also marked structural changes are found, both in the central and peripheral systems, in the anæsthetic form of the disease. In many cases the posterior segments of the gray cornua and the fibres of the commissure, as well as the nerves of the extremities, have been found altered by inflammation, which will account for the disordered sensibility and the subsequent disturbances of nutrition, muscular atrophy, etc. The nerve-trunks are often to be felt beneath the skin, thickened and sensitive on pressure. The chronic cell-infiltration affects the fibrous structure of the outer sheath, the neurilemma, and the septa between the nerve-bundles, producing fatty metamorphosis and atrophy of the nerve-bundles. Similar cell-infiltrations are found also in the connective tissue of all the internal organs of the body, which lead to destructive processes in their respective structures.

[9] Boeck and Danielssen, *Traité de la Spedalskhed*, Paris, 1848; Virchow,*Die Krankhaften Geschwülste*; Kaposi in *Hebra's Lehrbuch der Hautkrankheiten*; Monasterski, *Vierteljahressch. für Derm. u. Syph.*, 1879, p. 203; Hansen, *Virchow's Archiv*, Band 79, 1880; Neisser,*Virchow's Archiv*, Band 84, 1881; Cornil et Souchard, *Annales de Derm. et de Syph.*, 1881, No. 4.

Within the last two years repeated observations have been made which confirm the statement published by Hansen in 1873, that a peculiar bacterium occurs in leprous tissues, which, it is claimed, establishes the parasitic nature of the affection. These examinations have been carried on with leprous material derived from many parts of the world, and the results have been uniform. Within the round cells which characterize the cutaneous neoplasms, both in the distinct tubercles and the diffused[p. 792]infiltrations, small agglomerations of minute rod- or staff-like bodies (bacilli) are found, arranged in parallel rows or placed end to end. Their length is one-half or three-fourths the diameter of a red blood-globule, and their breadth is one-fourth their length. With them minute granular particles are seen in the cells. They occur in greatest numbers in the cells of the upper layers of the true skin, which are considerably swollen by their presence. They never penetrate the epithelial layer, nor are they found in epithelial cells in any position. When the protoplasm of the cell is interfered with by the later tissue-changes of the disease, the bacillus perishes. They are found not only in the leprous cells, but also in those of the connective tissue running between the agglomerated masses of the former. Between the leprous cells and the filaments of connective tissue but few free bacilli are seen. The neoplasms of the mucous membrane and of many organs of the body have been found to contain them also. In the blood they have been detected by some observers. Their presence in the nerve-tissues is of importance as throwing light upon the question of the specific or inflammatory nature of the morbid processes above described as affecting them. If we regard the bacteria as pathognomonic of leprous tissue-changes, their occurrence, recognized in the cells penetrating between the fibres of the peripheral nerves, would seem to make all primary structural changes identical, and the anæsthetic as much as the tubercular form the direct result of their presence. Neisser draws the following conclusions from his investigations: "Leprosy is a real bacterial disease, caused by a special kind of bacterium. The bacilli appear in the tissues as such, or more probably as spores, and remain for a longer or shorter time in a state of incubation, according to circumstances, in dépôts, perhaps in the lymph-glands. This period, much longer than in other infective diseases, is in proportion to the physiological resistance of the human organism compared with the feeble developing power of the bacilli. It, as well as the course of the disease, is more rapid in tropical countries than in Europe. From these dépôts the disease extends throughout the body in those portions of the skin most exposed, the face, hands, elbows, knees, and into the peripheral nerves. The other organs are less freely invaded. The bacilli excite inflammation, and by a specific action transform the migrating cell into the leprous cell. Leprosy is probably an infectious disease, and its specific products are contagious—viz. the leprous cells of the tubercles, the tissue-fluids, and the pus containing bacilli or viable spores. On the other hand, the pus may not always be infectious, as the fluid contained in the bullæ is not."

It must be said that the bacterial nature of leprosy, if established in accordance with the above observations, furnishes a satisfactory basis of explanation of all facts, historical, clinical, and pathological, which have so long been awaiting solution. The inability of the parasite to penetrate the epithelial layer of the skin and mucous membrane explains why contagion is so difficult, and why the ulcerative tubercular form would be more favorable to such transference than the anæsthetic variety.

DIAGNOSIS.—Leprosy in some of its early appearances may be readily confounded with vitiligo, morphoea, pemphigus, lupus, and syphilis. In some cases its prodromal manifestations cannot be positively diagnosticated until other symptoms have developed, which by concurrence establish their true significance. Such are the pemphigus-like bullæ, the [p. 793]pigment-changes, and the smaller tubercular efflorescences. In regions where the disease occurs only by importation, and in the so-called sporadic cases, it is not at all strange that it should fail of recognition, even in well-advanced forms, unless the observer is acquainted with its whole symptomatology. On the other hand, there is no disease which presents more strikingly characteristic features in its advanced stages.

PROGNOSIS.—Leprosy is almost uniformly a fatal affection, and its course toward this termination varies but slightly under the most diverse conditions of life. Its development and progress are naturally more rapid under circumstances of least individual resistance, where food is poor and scanty, where extremes of climate are most felt, where the constitution of the individual or nation is debilitated by previous disease, as that of the Hawaiians by syphilis, or where no proper professional care is employed. It has been believed that a change of residence from infected to non-leprous regions would retard its advance or avert its appearance in those supposed to be hereditarily disposed; but the former effect follows probably only so far as the general condition of the patient is affected by the change, as in other constitutional disorders, and the latter is necessarily a matter wholly of conjecture. No case of leprosy in the Norwegian colony in our North-western States has ceased to progress after arrival toward its fatal ending, even if this has been somewhat delayed in individual cases under more generous ways of living. If it could be known that a child born in Norway had escaped leprosy by removal to America, we should not, if we accept the bacterial origin of the disease, consider that climate or other mysterious influences had overcome its inherited tendencies, but that it had been taken away from the chance of direct inoculation. It is stated that very rarely cases cease to progress beyond certain stages even in countries where the disease is endemic. The course, as has been stated, varies according to the clinical form, the duration of the tubercular variety being on an average but one-half that of the purely anæsthetic type. Leprosy may be called the slow disease, its period of incubation, so far as this can be determined, extending from one to several years, its prodromal stage lasting often several more years, and its well-developed forms requiring at times more than twenty years to destroy the patient. Cases sometimes prove fatal, however, in a single year.

TREATMENT.—In a disease which affects so many of the races and such great numbers of mankind, which has been for centuries the object of special attention on the part of physicians, and of late years of government commissions and of eminent pathologists, it is evident that every remedy which the materia medica includes, as well as those of merely popular reputation in the widely-diverse geographical regions in which it prevails, must have been employed in its treatment. None of them exert any specific action upon it; it remains incurable. Every year some new article is employed with the usual claims of success which accompany the introduction of new remedies, but they merely swell the long list of failures in the therapeutics of the affection. Still, leprosy is influenced somewhat by medical care; life may be prolonged and made more comfortable. To this end we may employ remedies which are capable of improving and maintaining the constitutional powers of resistance to the disease, such as are found of service in other chronic wasting affections.[p. 794]The patient is to be put in as healthy ways of living as possible, removed from debilitating localities, and given generous diet and tonics, as iron and quinia. Several new drugs which seem to stimulate the nutrition and produce temporary improvement in the local and general symptoms have lately been widely employed, as Gurjun balsam and chaulmoogra oil, but they have wrought no cure. Digestion is to be aided, diarrhoea to be checked, and disturbances of respiration to be alleviated. Local treatment is also of service. The tubercles may sometimes be made to disappear—partly, at least—by stimulating applications, and ulcers made to heal by cauterization and other well-known methods of dressing. These ulcers and their secretions should be regarded as possible sources of infection by attendants and members of the patient's household. For the anæsthetic alterations in the tissues but little can be done locally. If the bacterial origin and causation of the disease be eventually established, its future extinction must be based upon studies directed to the nature and mode of protection against this organism. Collectively, the disease should be treated by every nation by thorough segregation, and importation should be prevented by the most rigid quarantine laws.

[p. 795]

EPIDEMIC CEREBRO-SPINAL MENINGITIS.
BY ALFRED STILLÉ, M.D., LL.D.

DEFINITION.—A febrile, and often malignant, but non-contagious disease of unknown origin; usually occurring as a local epidemic; confined hitherto to the North American and European continents, and to the vicinity of the latter; characterized by its rapid and irregular course, and usually by a tetanic rigidity or retraction of the neck, a tendency to disorganization of the blood, and the formation of inflammatory exudates beneath the membranes of the brain and spinal cord.

SYNONYMS.—Spotted fever; petechial fever; malignant purpuric fever; malignant purpura; pestilential purpura; black death; typhus petechialis; typhus syncopalis; febris nigra; febbre soporoso-convulsivo; tifo apoplettico tetanico; fièvre cérébro-spinale; typhus cérébro-spinale; phrenitis typhodes; epidemic meningitis; epidemic cerebro-spinal meningitis; malignant meningitis; typhoid meningitis; méningite cérébro-spinale épidémique; méningite cérébro-rachidienne; Genickkrampf; Genickstarre.

The names which have been given to this disease convey more or less distinctly one or the other of two ideas: 1st, that the disease is essentially a blood-disorder; and 2d, that it is an inflammation of the cerebro-spinal meninges. Under the first head belong the following names: Malignant purpuric fever; malignant purpura; pestilential purpura; petechial fever; spotted fever; febris nigra; black death, etc. Under the second head belong epidemic cerebro-spinal meningitis; epidemic meningitis; malignant meningitis; typhoid meningitis, etc. As partaking of the qualities of both categories may be cited the names cerebro-spinal fever and fever with cerebro-spinal meningitis. In regard to all those of the first class it is sufficient to repeat the criticism made by the early American writers who described this disease after having largely studied it. One only of them need be cited, because he expresses the opinion of all. Miner, writing in 1822, said: "It is quite unfortunate that a single symptom (petechiæ), and one, too, that is wanting in a great majority of cases, should have been seized upon to give it the odious and deceptive name of spotted fever, as that name has been applied by European writers to a very different kind of fever." Among the names given to the disease, cerebro-spinal fever is perhaps the least suitable and the least in harmony with the principles of scientific nomenclature. It is one of those terms which may be pardoned when used by the laity, but which educated physicians ought not tolerate. Parallel examples may be found in such compounds as brain-fever, lung-fever, gastric-fever, and, most unfortunate of all, enteric fever. The first three of these are [p. 796]inflammations, pure and simple, of the brain, lung, and stomach; and, after their example, cerebro-spinal meningitis would be, what it is not, merely an inflammation of the membranes of the brain and spinal marrow. The name of the remaining disease has only to be turned into English and called intestinal fever to demonstrate its defects. It is evident that other diseases—and dysentery in particular—are equally entitled to be called enteric fever. Moreover, there are cases of enteric fever in which death takes place so early that the intestinal lesion is undeveloped, and the fatal issue must be attributed to the fever-poison in the blood or else to the changes it has wrought in that fluid. Analogous illustrations abound in the history of the eruptive fevers. The disease we are studying presents another affection in which the septic element sometimes so far overrides the inflammatory as to destroy life before the latter has developed characteristic tissue-changes. There may be no valid objection against classing it among the fevers, but there can be no excuse for denominating it cerebro-spinal fever. The very reasons that militate against its being regarded as a meningitis forbid its being considered as a meningeal fever. But if it is a meningitis, inchoate or complete, then the prefix epidemic denotes its constitutional nature and its probable blood origin, and a term is employed which is descriptive and accurate, and not misleading. Moreover, the term epidemic indicates, or at least implies, the characteristic type of the disease, which is asthenic and sometimes more or less typhoidal, just as other inflammatory diseases become so in their epidemic form—*e.g.* pneumonia, bronchitis (influenza), dysentery, etc.

There ought to be no doubt whether epidemic meningitis should be classed with general diseases or with inflammations. It is excluded from the latter class by the total absence of any tangible external cause from its causation, as well as by its frequent fatal termination before the characteristic signs of inflammation have had time to form, or because the peculiar type of the disease prevents their development. It belongs to the former class because it is epidemic in the largest sense, its outbreaks occurring simultaneously in remote parts of the earth and independently of all cognizable celestial or terrestrial influences. In this as in other elements of its pathology the disease stands absolutely alone. While the acute affections of the pulmonary and digestive organs, which were just now alluded to, affect large districts, and even sweep over a whole continent, epidemic meningitis breaks out in limited localities, and may for years prevail in a populous city within a hundred miles of another still more populous which during that time may altogether escape its ravages. Of this curious fact the cities of Philadelphia and New York present a striking illustration. Since, then, we are ignorant of the circumstances under which the disease arises, and since, as will more distinctly appear later on, its several forms really include quite various morbid conditions, we are compelled to consider it as occupying a peculiar and exceptional nosological position.

HISTORY.—Previous to the present century the existence of this disease can hardly be demonstrated. And yet Dr. B. W. Richardson believed that some faint traces of it could be discovered, as in the following statement:[1]"The great plague which visited Constantinople in 543, and which Procopius and Enagrius described, the plague of [p. 797]hallucination, drowsiness, slumbering, distraction, and ardent fever, with eruption on the skin of black pimples the size of a lentil,—this plague, which usually killed in five days, and left many who recovered with withered limbs, wasted tongues, stammering speech or such utterance of sound that their words could not be distinguished,—this plague, which had passed into mythical learning under the name of cerebro-spinal meningitis, has also in our time reappeared." The concluding statement in regard to the name of the plague is quite erroneous, and there is nothing in the description which distinctively applies to the disease we are examining. On the other hand, we know that Procopius wrote a history of the Oriental plague, which invaded Europe for the first time at the very date above given. It had as a distinctive symptom the well-known inguinal bubo, and there is no mention whatever, in the descriptions of it that have survived, of the tetanoid symptoms belonging to epidemic meningitis. In 1802 an epidemic occurred at Roetlingen in Franconia which had a certain resemblance to the subject of this article, for it was characterized by lacerating pains in the back of the neck. According to Hecker, this was the sweating sickness which had ravaged various parts of Europe during the Middle Ages, and of which limited outbreaks still recur. In 1880 such a one took place at l'Ile d'Oléron in France, and many of the patients were affected with tonic or clonic spasms, both general and local, but not, apparently, opisthotonic.²

[1] *Diseases of Modern Life*, p. 16.
[2] Pineau, *Archives gén. de méd.*, tom. i., 1882, pp. 25, 169.

If epidemic meningitis occurred before the nineteenth century, it must have been confounded with other affections, but when we consider its characteristic symptoms such an error seems improbable. The comparatively rare resort at that time to post-mortem examinations, particularly of the cranial and spinal cavities, may in part account for such a confusion of ideas; and even when dissections were made, the skill to interpret the discovered lesions was possessed by few. It has been thought that in the latter part of the last century some cases of this disease were seen and described, although their nosological value was unrecognized. Thus, Stoll[3] speaks of a young soldier who was seized with a pain in the back of the head and neck, and who was affected with opisthotonos before he died. On examination pus was found between the arachnoid and the pia mater. The first clear and unquestionable description of epidemic meningitis was published in 1805, first by Vieusseux and directly afterward by Mathey.[4] The disease appeared at Geneva in the spring of the year, in a family composed of a woman and three children, of whom two of the latter died within twenty-four hours. A fortnight later four children in a neighboring family died of it after fourteen or fifteen hours' illness, and a young man in an adjoining house, being attacked, died the same night, with his whole body of a violet color. The disease ceased during the spring, after having destroyed thirty-three lives. Its distinctive features were an abrupt attack during the night, bilious vomiting, excruciating headache, rigidity of the spine, difficult deglutition, convulsions, nocturnal paroxysms, petechiæ, and death in from twelve hours to five days. Vieusseux calls it "a malignant non-contagious fever," and Mathey gives as the lesions revealed by dissection a gelatinous [p. 798]exudation covering the convex surface of the brain, and a yellow puriform matter upon its posterior aspect, upon the optic commissure, the inferior surface of the cerebellum, and the medulla oblongata.

[3] Quoted by Boudin, *Hist. du typhus cérébro-spinal*, p. 5.
[4] *Journ. de Méd., Chirurg. et Pharm., etc.*, an. xiv., tom. xi, pp. 163, 243.

After its first appearance at Geneva the disease does not seem to have extended in any direction from that place as a centre, but we next hear of it at two points remote from it and from one another—Germany and the United States. From the former it extended to the conterminous countries, Bavaria, Holland, and the east of France, where, however, it prevailed neither extensively nor fatally, and soon died out; while in America it first appeared at Medfield, Mass., in 1806. The European epidemic was faintly felt in England the following year, and between that time and 1816 it prevailed at several places in the east of France, and slightly at Paris, while during the corresponding period it had extended through New England into Canada, New York, Pennsylvania, and several Western and South-western States. It is a noteworthy fact that on both sides of the Atlantic it ceased in the same year (1816). During the six following years we can discover no trace of its existence, but in 1822-23 it reappeared at Vesoul in France, and at Middletown, Connecticut, and does not seem to have extended beyond those places. Again, after an interval of five years, in 1828 it was heard of in Trumbull co., Ohio, two years later at Sunderland in England, and three years afterward (in 1833) at Naples.

After four years of quiescence the disease entered upon a wider and more destructive career than ever before, which was almost uninterrupted from 1837 to 1850. During the first two years of its recurrence in Europe it was confined almost wholly to France. It began in the southern departments, with Bayonne as a centre, and extended gradually westward and northward, in some places attacking only military garrisons and in others only civilians. Elsewhere the predilection was reversed, or, again, civilians and soldiers were equally affected. As Boudin has pointed out, "it located itself in certain districts; in garrison-towns it seemed to affect certain barracks only, and in them only certain rooms. In one place it broke out in a prison and spared the soldiers; in another its victims were among the soldiers and the citizens, while the prisoners were untouched." Thus the disease spread over the whole of France, and was more fatal almost everywhere else than in Paris itself. Almost at the gates of the capital, at Versailles, and among the garrison, it was very destructive in 1839, causing a mortality among those attacked of from 50 to 75 per cent. About the same time it occasioned a great mortality at other military posts, especially at Rochefort and Metz, and in 1840-41 at Strasbourg. In 1843 the disease had almost ceased to prevail in France, but in 1846 it reappeared at Lyons, and in the following years, and until 1849, affected the garrisons of Orléans, Cambrai, Saint-Étienne, Metz again, Lunéville, Dijon, Bourges, and Toulon. In some of these places the military experienced five, and even seven, successive epidemics. Meanwhile, the disease spread to Algeria (1839-47), and to Italy in the former year—not, however, on the confines of France, but at Naples and in the Romagna, whence it extended to Sicily and Gibraltar, and did not cease there until 1845. In 1839 it first showed itself in Denmark, and remained for about three years, while in 1846 it "appeared in the [p. 799]majority of the workhouses of Ireland," and in the spring of the same year it occurred in England, at Liverpool and Rochester.

While the disease was thus spreading throughout Europe, it again, in 1842, appeared in the United States, but at places as remote as possible from Transatlantic communication and hundreds of miles distant from one another—*e.g.* in Louisville, Kentucky, in Rutherford co., Tennessee, and in Montgomery, Alabama. In the following year it prevailed in Arkansas, Mississippi, and Illinois. In 1848 it occurred again at Montgomery, Ala., and simultaneously, in Beaver co., Pa.; in 1849 it existed in Massachusetts and in Cayuga co., N.Y., and in 1850 at New Orleans.

Between 1850 and 1854 epidemic meningitis ceased to be heard of, but in the spring of the latter year it began to appear in the southern provinces of Sweden, whence it rapidly spread over the greater part of the kingdom, reaching an extreme degree of fatality in 1858, and not finally disappearing until 1861. It is said to have caused more than four thousand deaths. It was not until the height of the Swedish epidemic in 1858 that it invaded Norway, where it seems to have been even more malignant and extensive. Between 1850 and 1860 local outbreaks of the disease took place in Ireland, and isolated cases were observed in various parts of England, but in that country it has never prevailed as a general epidemic. This fact alone is sufficient to defeat all the attempts that have been made to trace the origin of the disease to any of the conditions associated with a crowded population. In Scotland, where such conditions exist in their greatest intensity and fulness of development, it has never occurred as an epidemic. During the decade under consideration (in 1856 and 1857) epidemic meningitis again appeared in the United States, and, as before, at points very remote from one another. In the former year it occurred for the first time in North Carolina, and in the latter year in the central portions of New York and Massachusetts.

Hardly had the disease subsided in the Scandinavian peninsula and in the United Kingdom when it reappeared in Holland during the winter of 1860-61. In the following year and at the same season it occupied a large extent of Portuguese territory, including the cities of Oporto and Lisbon, and now for the first time it spread over Germany. Beginning slightly during the summer of 1863 in Prussia, it acquired new vigor during the succeeding winter, and in the two following years it devastated almost every part of Northern Germany, and in 1864-65 extended throughout Bavaria except in its southern and western provinces. Strange to relate, the disease appears to have passed almost wholly by Austria proper, and to have prevailed, although not extensively nor fatally, in Hungary, and in the latter part of the decade in Istria, Greece, Turkey, and Asia Minor.

The American counterpart of this epidemic first appeared in Livingston co., Missouri, in the winter of 1861-62, and during the same season it invaded Indiana and Kentucky in the West and Connecticut in the East. From about the same date, and until 1864, it prevailed in Ohio, and during the last-named year in Illinois. Cases occurred at Newport, Rhode Island, in 1863, and in Vermont in 1864. In the winter and spring of the latter year it broke out at Carbondale, Pa., and in a population of 6000 caused the death of 400, principally among children and [p. 800]very young persons.[5] In the winters of 1863-64 and of 1864-65 it prevailed in the U.S. army, and in the early part of this period in the Confederate army which at the time was stationed near Fredericksburg, Va. In North Carolina also, from 1862 to 1864, the disease assumed a very malignant type, and affected citizens and soldiers equally, and the latter in the Union and Confederate armies alike. During the winter of 1864-65 a limited but very fatal epidemic of the disease prevailed at Little Rock, Arkansas. About the same time it existed as an epidemic in Maryland, Alabama, and other Southern States, and throughout the Civil War affected both whites and negroes, but showed, as in France, an exceptional gravity among the military.

[5] Burr, *Trans. Med. Soc. State of N. York*, 1865, p. 40.

The first appearance of the disease in Philadelphia took place in 1863, and from that date until the present (1884) it has never failed to appear among the causes of death in the reports of the Health Office. A table compiled by Dr. C. F. Clark, and printed in a paper on the subject by Dr. James C. Wilson,[6] exhibits the difficulties of obtaining accurate statistics, even from official reports, on this subject. The medical profession of the city, having had but little knowledge of the disease either by reading or observation, reported deaths from it which occurred in their practice under various denominations. At first it was spotted fever, which continued to be used by many for a year or two, when it was superseded almost entirely by cerebro-spinal meningitis. There can be no doubt that both of these terms were used to designate the same disease, and therefore no error will be committed in merging the deaths charged to each of them, and in estimating by their annual totals at least the relative mortality of the disease in the successive years of the period. But in the Health Office reports there are at least three other rubrics that suggest doubt. One is typhus fever, which seems to have presented a sudden and remarkable increase of mortality during the first years, and the most fatal, of the existence of cerebro-spinal meningitis. It should also be observed that typhus fever is applied by many German physicians in this country, as in their native land, to typhoid fever. A second is malignant fever, and a third is congestive fever, neither of which has claimed many victims in the health reports of Philadelphia except while meningitis was epidemic. It seems probable, therefore, that nearly all of the deaths charged under these heads belong to the disease under consideration.

[6] *Phila. Med. Times*, xiii. 88.

Deaths in Philadelphia from Cerebro-Spinal Meningitis from 1863-82.

Year	Deaths	Year	Deaths
		Brought over	136
1863	9	1873	46
1864	84	1874	2
1865	92	1875	3
1866	2	1876	5
1867	09	1877	6
1868	5	1878	0
1869	7	1879	2
1870	6	1880	8
1871	9	1881	0
1872	33	1882	41 to Sept. 23d.

Total

If to these deaths are added those charged to malignant fever, 111, and to[p. 801]congestive fever, 279, we obtain a total of 2439 deaths, nearly all of which may be set to the account of epidemic meningitis. It may also be remarked that up to the date at which this computation was made (May, 1883) hardly a week passed in which the Health Office did not register several deaths from this cause. Hence it would appear that the disease continues to linger in this locality longer than has been reported of any other place from which information has been obtained.

In the city of New York it appears to have been much more limited both in extent and duration. The first recorded death from it was in 1861; in 1866 the deaths were 18; in 1867 the deaths were 32; in 1868 they were 34; in 1869, 42; in 1870, 32; in 1871, 48. In 1872 the disease became epidemic, and "from January 6 to May 31, inclusive, 632 cases were reported to the City Sanitary Inspector, and 469 deaths to the Bureau of Records of Vital Statistics" (Clymer). After this period the disease seems to have declined very rapidly, and not to have reappeared, since no notice is taken of its recurrence by the medical journals of New York.

It was mentioned above that about 1870 some traces of the disease were observed in Asia Minor, and in 1872 several cases are said to have occurred at Jerusalem,[7] but beyond that time and place it does not appear to have extended as an epidemic. In 1879, Cheevers said: "I am not aware of the existence of any report of an outbreak of the disease in India." He refers, however, to several cases occurring in Calcutta as possibly representing this affection.[8]

[7] *Berlin klin. Wochensch.*, May, 1872.
[8] *Times and Gazette*, Aug., 1879, p. 121.

In 1867-68 sporadic cases occurred at Little Rock, Ark., and in the former year in Madison co., N.Y., thirty-three cases were reported.[9] In Chicago, between February and April, 1872, Dr. Davis reported forty cases observed in his own practice in seventy-two days. In the same year the disease occurred at Elizabethtown, Ky.,[10] and at Louisville, Ky., in December of the same year. It existed in Michigan between 1868 and 1874, but only in the latter year epidemically, and not to a very great extent.

[9] *Trans. Med. Soc. State of N.Y.*, 1868, p. 251.
[10] *Richmond and Louisville Journ.*, Nov., 1872, p. 555.

Of later occurrences of the disease the following may be mentioned: Several cases were reported in London in 1867, 1871, 1876, and 1878.[11] In 1870 four cases were observed in Providence, R.I.[12] In 1882 cases were met with in Boston, New York, Philadelphia, Pittsburg, Western Ohio, Indianapolis, Detroit, Louisville, Memphis, New Orleans, Richmond, Milwaukee, St. Louis, Salt Lake City, San Francisco, etc., but in none of these places did the disease become epidemic.

[11] *Times and Gazette*, July, 1867, pp. 58, 59; Nov., 1867, p. 511; *Guy's Hospital Rep.*, 3d Ser., xvii. 440; *St. Bart's Reports*, xii. 267; *Times and Gaz.*, Aug., 1878, p. 167.
[12] *Boston M. and S. Jour.*, Oct., 1870, p. 261.

ETIOLOGY.—Epidemic meningitis has occurred in Europe and America in every portion of the temperate zone, but its greatest prevalence and mortality have undoubtedly been in the northern rather than in the southern portions of that region. One of its most interesting features consists in its appearing simultaneously at points very remote from one another and having no connection with each other save through the atmosphere. Of this statement several illustrations have already been presented. Another [p. 802]peculiarity of the disease consists in its occurring with hardly any relation to external natural conditions or to those of its victims. It affects localities as diverse as possible in their geological, meteorological, and sanitary states, the rich and the poor, the old and the young, and both sexes, and (as it is certainly not in a strict sense contagious) its rise and spread must necessarily be attributed to some occult cause pervading the atmosphere.

It is evident that the prevalence of the disease has some relation to meteorological agencies, for not only is it greater, on the whole, in *cold* than in warm climates, but it is also greater in cold than in warm seasons. Thus, if we examine the epidemics in Europe and

America we shall find that they almost invariably were most severe in the winter and spring. Yet the rule presents several exceptions on both continents. In France, out of 216 local epidemics, more than one-fourth took place during the warm months of the year, and in Sweden the proportion was about the same. It is evident, therefore, that cold is not an essential cause of the disease. Among the problems that remain unsolved in regard to this disease none is more obscure than the apparent immunity of Russia from its ravages, although the climate seems adapted to favor it, and the domestic habits of no people are fitter to intensify it if individual conditions entered into the etiology of the disease; but, in truth, no such causes are related to epidemic meningitis. Localities of every sort, high and low, dry and moist, those saturated with marsh miasmata and those fanned by pure mountain-breezes, have been alike visited by this disease. It has passed by large cities reeking with all the corruptions of a soil saturated with ordure and populations begrimed with filth, as Vienna, Berlin, Paris, London, and New York, to devastate clean and salubrious villages and the families of substantial farmers inhabiting isolated spots.

By far the greatest number of the subjects of epidemic meningitis are young persons. In Sweden, according to Hirsch, of 1267 fatal cases of the disease, 889 occurred in persons under fifteen years of age, 328 between sixteen and forty years, and 50 in persons of forty years and upward. In 1866, in the Kronach district (Germany), of 115 cases, 75 occurred under the seventh year, 22 between the seventh and twelfth years, and 10 between the thirteenth and twentieth years (Schweitzer). During 1865 a local outbreak of the disease in Bavaria affected 53 persons, of whom 22 were children under ten years of age, 18 between ten and twenty years, and 11 between twenty and thirty years. Under the fifth year few were attacked (Orth). Dr. J. L. Smith[13] found that, according to the reports of the Board of Health of the city of New York, out of 975 cases, 771 occurred in persons under fifteen years of age, the greatest number for any quiquennial period being 336 in children under five years. Of the 469 deaths occurring in this epidemic, 216 were of children under five years of age, and the next largest number for an equal period was 99, which represented the deaths between the ages of five and ten years. Of adults or persons beyond the age of twenty, the whole number was but 39. The peculiar liability to the disease of the young recruits in the French army has already been alluded to. The proportion of male victims to this affection is rather larger than that of females in the civil population, but in France especially the excess was greatly on the side of males, owing to the prevalence of the disease in the army. In other places, as [p. 803]in Sweden and Germany, the number of deaths among females equalled, or even exceeded, that of males, and in Leipsic the garrison remained exempt while the disease prevailed among the citizens. In 1847 a fatal epidemic of it affected the second regiment of the Mississippi Rifles, and was entirely confined to that corps (Love). During the Civil War of the United States the disease affected particular corps or regiments in the South or in the North, yet it never became epidemic in the army, even when the disease prevailed among the adjacent civil population.

[13] *Amer. Jour. of Med. Sci.*, Oct., 1873, p. 320.

Various depressing or debilitating causes, such as lowness of spirits, home-sickness, mental or bodily strain, over-eating, drinking alcohol, the action of excessive cold or heat, checking perspiration, etc., have been enumerated as causes of this disease. It is unnecessary to dwell upon such gratuitous assumptions. All of these influences are constant, but epidemic meningitis is the rarest of epidemic diseases, and the agencies referred to have no further operation than to lessen the resistance of the body to morbid influences of every description. If there be one peculiarity about this disease which is more surprising and inexplicable than another, it is that its peculiar victims are not the feeble and delicate, but the vigorous and active—not the old and decaying, but the young and stalwart.

No one of authority has claimed that this disease can be propagated by *contagion*. All of its early American historians are of the same opinion upon this question, and nearly all European authorities are in perfect accord with them. The apparent exceptions to this all but universal judgment are so insignificant in number and weight as not in the least to diminish its validity. A case has been published in which a pregnant woman at full term died of the disease after giving birth to an apparently healthy child. "Two hours later the infant presented symptoms of meningitis, followed rapidly by death."[14] Supposing the concluding statement to be accurate, the case only shows that the cause of the disease which destroyed the mother's life infected the system of the child also. If there is one point in the history of the disease established by the concurring testimony of American and European writers, it is the extreme rarity of its attacking either the physicians and nurses in attendance upon patients affected with it, or those laboring under other diseases and occupying beds adjacent to persons ill with epidemic meningitis. That, nevertheless, there is a material morbific principle which inheres in certain localities, so that those who occupy them successively are liable to suffer from this disease, and that also this principle may be carried from place to place so as to render certain houses (barracks) infectious, seems to be demonstrated by the history of the disease in the French army. Between 1837 and 1850, when the disease prevailed in various parts of France, it did so not indiscriminately, but it usually followed the ordinary routes of communication, and especially the movements of the military in their transfers from one post to another, and the course of navigable streams. Strangely, also, it attacked soldiers much oftener than civilians. The most curious fact of all is one already referred to—viz. that although the disease prevailed in almost every part of the provinces, and although then as ever an incessant stream from them was flowing into the capital, neither its civil nor its military population was generally affected, nor,[p. 804]indeed, at all so, until near the close of the period mentioned. Meanwhile, however, the disease extended to several countries conterminous with France or in close and frequent intercourse with it—to Italy (1839-45), Algeria (1839-47), England, Ireland, and Denmark (1845-48). These events seem to point to a certain transmissibility of the disease until we examine the negative facts that bear upon the question. They are such as these: The epidemic did not spread at all from France into two of the adjacent countries, Belgium and Switzerland, with which the first-named country maintained an incessant intercourse by travel and traffic, but, on the other hand, it broke out at an early date within the period mentioned at places very remote and absolutely independent of all influence emanating from France or any other European source—in the south-western portions of the United States. It is by numerous facts of this description that we are compelled to remove the disease from the category of endemic and even epidemic diseases, and relegate it, along with influenza, to that of pandemic affections.

[14] *Med. Record*, xxii. 547.

There seems to be some reason for thinking that the epidemic cause of this disease may affect the lower animals as well as man. It was stated by Gallup in 1811 that during the epidemic of meningitis in Vermont "even the foxes seemed to be affected, so that they were killed in numbers near the dwellings of the inhabitants;" and of the epidemic in 1871 in New York, Dr. Smith relates that "it was common and fatal in the large stables of the city car and stage lines, while among the people the epidemic did not properly commence until January, 1872." It would be desirable to learn more precisely the characters of these vulpine and equine epidemics before associating them with the disease we are studying, the more so that we have been unable to discover a similar relation between any epizoötic and other epidemics of meningitis. In this connection may be recalled the statement of Dr. Law of Dublin, that while he was attending a lady suffering from cerebro-spinal meningitis "nine rabbits, out of eleven which her son had, died, all in the same way: their limbs seemed to fail them, they fell on their side, and then worked in convulsions, and died." On examination of the bodies of several of them congestion of the vessels of the base of the brain was found, and also "vascularity of the membranes of the spinal marrow, indicating inflammation."[15]

[15] *Dublin Quarterly Journ.*, May, 1866, p. 298.

TYPES.—No disease presents a greater variety—and, indeed, dissimilarity—of symptoms than epidemic meningitis. Some of its epidemics are sthenic and even inflammatory in their type, while others have the malignant aspect of rapid blood-poisoning. These contrasts have been exhibited on a large scale, for while upon the continent of Europe the disease for the most part has presented sthenic phenomena, it has been more generally asthenic and adynamic in Ireland. One might be inclined to attribute the latter peculiarity to the permanent prevalence of typhus fever in the latter country, or rather to the special causes producing typhus, were it not that in the United States both types of the disease have been observed at different times and in different places. Such contrasts of type are, however, not unusual in other diseases that occur as epidemics, including not only the eruptive fevers, but inflammations, or affections involving inflammation, such as pneumonia, dysentery, [p. 805]diphtheria, etc. Hence it is evident that certain epidemics, and certain cases in each epidemic, may exhibit on the one hand a predominance of inflammatory, or on the other of adynamic or ataxic, symptoms, and each of them in every conceivable degree and combination. It is this variation of type that has led to such different conceptions of the nature of epidemic meningitis, many physicians regarding it as a fever, and many others as an inflammation, while, as we believe, it is both the one and the other, and acquires from either element, according to its ascendency, the typical character of the particular epidemic under observation.

As illustrative of these statements we may mention in this place the several *forms* of the disease as they have been seen and interpreted by different observers. Forget classified them as follows: (*A*) CEREBRO-SPINAL; 1, *Explosive (foudroyante)*; 2, *Comatose-convulsive;* 3,*Inflammatory;* 4, *Typhoid;* 5, *Neuralgic;* 6, *Hectic;* 7, *Paralytic.* (*B*) CEREBRAL: 1, *Cephalalgic;* 2, *Cephalalgic-delirious;* 3, *Delirious;* 4,*Comatose.* In the first of these divisions three-sevenths belong to the first and fourth varieties. But "there were slight and severe cases; violent and hectic forms; cerebral symptoms predominant in some and spinal in others, etc."

In his excellent paper on the epidemic of 1848 in New Orleans, Ames arranged his cases in two categories—the *Congestive* and the*Inflammatory,* subdividing the former into the *Malignant* and the *Mild.* Malignant congestive cases were distinguished by prostration, coma or delirium, or both; opisthotonos; and a pulse varying extremely in its degree of frequency. In *mild congestive* cases a good degree of strength was preserved; the pulse was below 90; there were marked pain in the head and tenderness of the spine, but no coma, delirium, or stiffness of any muscles besides those of the neck. The purely *inflammatory* cases were, in general, distinguished by a temperature of the skin above that of health and a full, firm pulse, but the *malignant inflammatory* were marked by the early occurrence of delirium or coma, great irregularity of pulse, opisthotonos, convulsive spasm, strabismus, and occasional amaurosis, with vomiting and a rapid and fatal course; the *grave*, by a slighter development of the same symptoms, except coma and delirium; and the*mild*, by a lower grade of febrile excitement, the preservation of a good degree of strength, a tendency to become chronic, and by the absence of coma, drowsiness, delirium, and a cold stage.

Wunderlich adopted the simple plan of arranging the cases in three categories: 1, the *gravest* and most rapidly fatal cases; 2, the *less grave,*and 3, the *lightest.* The arrangement of Hirsch had more significance, as well as a clinical foundation—viz. 1, the *abortive;* 2, the *explosive* (*m. siderans,* the same as *m. foudroyante* of Tourdes); 3, the *intermittent;* 4, the *typhoid.*

Dr. Bedford Brown,[16] who observed the epidemics in North Carolina from 1862 to 1864, arranged the cases under the following heads: 1, the*inflammatory* form, in which the fever is high, the pain very acute, and the delirium furious, but which is exceedingly rare; 2, the *neuralgic* form, which is stated to be the most frequent and protracted, with moderate fever and a pulse but slightly accelerated, and giving a favorable prognosis; 3, the *ataxic* form, in which great nervous depression is[p. 806]associated with a low and busy delirium, and the temperature "is generally much reduced below the natural standard.... This is always a dangerous form;" 4, the *paralytic* form, in which stupor and insensibility are early and prominent features, with a very slow and feeble pulse, blanched skin, and death by syncope.

[16] *Richmond Med. Jour.*, ii. 1.

Dr. Purcell of Cork[17] furnished a classification which is one of the best for practical and clinical purposes—viz. 1, the *rapid* variety, attended with purple blotches, embarrassed respiration and circulation, followed by sopor, insensibility, and coma; 2, the *cerebro-spinal* form, with retraction of the head, pain and cramps of the muscles, hyperæsthesia of the skin, delirium, etc., accompanied by fever, herpetic eruptions, etc. These two forms are apt to be more or less associated in the same case.

[17] *Dublin Quarterly Jour.*, Aug., 1870, p. 243.

Of the various forms admitted by different authors, and of which we have seen examples, we would class together—(*a.*) The abortive, in which the characteristic phenomena are often faintly defined, and yet to the practised eye distinctive. (*b.*) The malignant, in which the symptoms, of whatever kind, are exaggerated, the attack sudden, the course short, and the issue fatal. (*c.*) The nervous, including 1, the *Ataxic*—viz.—1, the *delirious;* 2, the *cephalalgic;* 3, the *neuralgic;* 4, the *convulsive;* 5, the *paralytic;* and 6, the *adynamic* (*comatose* and *typhoid*). (*d.*) The inflammatory. (*e.*) The intermittent. Of these the *abortive* and *intermittent* call for a brief explanation. Abortive meningitis is observed only during the prevalence of the disease in a more characteristic form. Thus, the mother of a boy who had died of the fully-developed disease "complained of the head and back and limbs, and of chilliness, and presented a petechial eruption. After active purgative and counter-irritant treatment she was about her work on the second day."[18] The late Dr. Burns of Frankford, Philadelphia, while attending patients affected with the disease suffered from headache, severe pains along the spine and in every joint of the body, and a general languid feeling.[19] Kempf during the decline of an epidemic observed "a great number of individuals, especially adults, who complained of headache, malaise, neuralgic pains in various parts of the body, and pain in the nape of the neck or other parts of the spine."[20] In a case observed by the writer (June, 1867) most of the characteristic symptoms were present in a mitigated form, and the pulse was at 60. Within five days restoration was complete.[21] The *intermittent* and *remittent* types are apt to be quotidian or tertian, and in fatal cases the former has been taken for malignant intermittent fever, which it resembles by a periodical febrile movement, with pains, cramps, delirium, etc. This type sometimes first manifests itself during the decline of an attack.

[18] Sargent, *Amer. Jour. of Med. Sci.*, July, 1849, p. 35.
[19] *Amer. Jour. of Med. Sci.*, April, 1865, p. 339.
[20] *Ibid.*, July, 1866, p. 55.
[21] *Epidemic Meningitis*, p. 42.

SUMMARY OF THE SYMPTOMS.—Like other fatal epidemic diseases, meningitis is sometimes sudden and sometimes gradual in its development. In the former case the patient, who has gone to bed apparently in perfect health, awakes suddenly from a sound sleep about the small hours of the night to find himself in a severe chill. In the case of young children a convulsion attends the awakening. Or the patient, while[p. 807]pursuing his ordinary avocations, may be seized with a chill, prostration, vomiting, and headache, of which symptoms the last is often intensely distressing. In this, as in other epidemic diseases, such violent seizures are most common during the earlier periods of its prevalence, but later in its course premonitory symptoms are more frequently observed. They may last for an hour or two, or may extend to several days; and, in general, it may be stated that the longer their duration the milder will be the subsequent attack. But the symptoms in either case are essentially the same—prostration, chilliness, feverishness, and sometimes vomiting and sharp pains in the head, back, and limbs. The character of the vomiting, as well as the absence of all gastric lesions in fatal cases, proves that it is occasioned by an irritation of the central nervous system.

In the cases which are regularly developed these phenomena more or less gradually assume a graver aspect or usher in a heavy chill, which in its turn is followed by alarming symptoms, and especially by an excruciating pain in the head, a livid or pale and sunken countenance, and extreme restlessness. The pulse is as often slow as frequent, and the skin is rarely hot, and, indeed, is generally but little, if at all, warmer than natural. The vague pains that began with the attack are now concentrated, and seem to dart in every direction from the spine, which is also, at its upper part, the seat of severe aching; and in some cases hyperæsthesia of the skin is very marked. In a large proportion of cases the spinal muscles become more or less rigidly contracted, so that the head is drawn backward or the whole trunk is arched as in tetanus. Trismus is not uncommon, and clonic spasms frequently affect the limbs. Even general convulsions are occasionally observed. As these phenomena grow more decided delirium of various degrees is often manifested, from mere wanderings and hallucinations during the sleepless watches of the night to violent maniacal ravings or incoherent mutterings, or the stertor of coma. Frey and others have noted a remission of the symptoms occurring on or about the third day in cases of a regular type. The rigidity of the cervical muscles becomes relaxed, the headache subsides, and the mental condition improves. But this amelioration lasts but a short time, and then the normal course of the symptoms is resumed.

As the attack advances the pulse gradually or rapidly rises above the normal rate, and sometimes becomes very frequent, and the skin, although it grows warmer, does not often acquire the temperature observed in idiopathic fevers or sustain it as they do. In many cases eruptions appear upon the skin. During some epidemics the only one observed is herpes labialis; in others the eruption resembles roseola, measles, or the mulberry rash of typhus, or from the first it consists of petechiæ, vibices, or extensive ecchymoses. The tongue presents the characters which belong generally to the typhoid state. At first moist and coated with a whitish fur or a mucous secretion, it afterward, if life is prolonged, grows red and shining or brown and fuliginous. There is usually a complete loss of appetite, and the thirst is not commonly urgent. One or two liquid stools at the commencement are generally followed by constipation, which continues throughout the attack, although in very grave and protracted cases diarrhoea may persist, and even become colliquative. When the attack tends to a fatal issue the patient generally, but by no means always, sinks into a soporose condition, in which [p. 808]muscular relaxation, debility, and tremulousness, such as are common in the typhoid state of fevers, are associated with paralysis of the sphincters and of other muscles. But we have seen rigid opisthotonos continue until within a few hours of death in a case of more than the average duration.

In cases that tend toward recovery the typhoid condition is rarely so grave, but patients have often survived very severe nervous symptoms. It is true that the return to health may be tedious and uncertain, and not unusually a perfect restoration of all the functions is very long delayed, or, it may be, is never attained.

INDIVIDUAL SYMPTOMS.—Pain in the head is one of the most characteristic symptoms of epidemic meningitis. It is always present, except in those malignant cases in which the morbid poison seems to spend its fatal power upon the blood. In some, however, of a less rapid but still malignant type, in which after death no exudation is found, but only an extreme venous congestion of the membranes, or it may be an effusion of blood beneath them, this symptom may be more or less marked. It is generally an excruciating pain, sometimes darting apparently through the head from the nuchæ to the forehead, extorting cries and groans, and is variously described by the sufferers as throbbing, boring, lancinating, sharp, or crushing, "as if the head were in a vice or nails or screws were being forced into the brain." Its paroxysms arouse the patient from his apathetic stupor or his coma, and cause him to become restless or violent or to shriek with agony. Even when this evidence of anguish is wanting the patient often attests his suffering by contortions or cries, or by frequently carrying his hands to his head. That it depends upon mechanical pressure upon the sensitive ganglia within the cranium and upper part of the spine is shown by the relief which revulsive and counter-irritant measures afford when applied to the occipital region and the back of the neck. Identical in cause and quality with this pain is the spinal pain proper. No better description of it has been given than that of Fiske in 1810. It is in these words: "Its bold and prominent features defy comparison.... In some a pain resembling the sensation felt from the stinging of a bee seizes the extremity of a finger or toe; from thence it darts to the foot or hand or some other part of the limbs, sometimes in the joints and sometimes in the muscles, carrying a numbness or prickling sensation in its progress. After traversing the extremities, generally of one side only, it seizes the head, and flies with the rapidity and sensation of electricity over the whole body, occasioning blindness, faintings, sickness at the stomach, with indescribable distress about the præcordia—a numbness or partial loss of motion in one or both limbs on one side, with great prostration of strength. The horrible sensation of this process no language can describe."[22] These spinal pains are always aggravated by pressure made on either side of the spinous processes of the vertebræ, and, like the cephalic pains, are more or less mitigated by revulsive applications. Accompanying the pains is a hyperæsthesia or morbid sensibility of the skin, rendering it painfully sensitive to the slightest touch; in the advanced stages of the disease, when the spinal phenomena predominate, the irritation of the nerves by the pressure of the exudation on their roots is exchanged for numbness or [p. 809]absolute insensibility, due to the increase and continuance of that pressure. Moving the limbs or separating the closed eyelids will sometimes provoke resistance, and even extort cries; and especially is this true of attempts to straighten the rigidly bent spine or the flexed extremities. Lewis states that such outcries were so often excited by slowly introducing the thermometer into the rectum that he was forced to believe that the anal and perhaps the rectal surface was hypersensitive.

[22] North, on *Spotted Fever*, p. 176.

The physical causes that give rise to the pains which have just been described likewise occasion the spasmodic and tetanoid phenomena that are so peculiar to this disease. In general terms, they are most marked in cases attended with inflammatory exudation, and least so when, instead of this lesion, there is only vascular congestion of the meninges of the spinal cord. But the rule is, of course, not absolute, for individuals are so differently constituted that one will remain impassive under an irritation that will throw another into convulsions. There is no doubt that spinal rigidity may be produced by mere congestion of the cord, and, on the other hand, that it may be absent even when plastic exudation is abundant. This symptom is, however, more than any other one, characteristic of the disease. It existed in the original epidemic at Geneva, attracted the attention of the earliest American observers of the disease, and elsewhere has marked a greater or a smaller proportion of the cases in every epidemic. It was described by such terms as these: "a drawing-back of the head;" "a corpse-like rigidity of the limbs;" "the form of tetanus called opisthotonos;" "spastic rigidity of the muscles of the lower jaw and the posterior muscles of the neck;" "rigidity of the posterior cervical muscles, retracting the head considerably backward." The historians of the disease in Europe are, if possible, still more emphatic in their elaborate descriptions of this phenomenon, and, on the Continent at least, it seems to have been more uniformly present than it was in Ireland or in this country. Tourdes, in describing the epidemic of 1842 at Strasburg, said: "The decubitus of the sick was distinguished by a backward flexion of the head and spine; most frequently the neck alone was affected, but sometimes the whole trunk was arched." And again: "The contraction often involved all of the extensor muscles of the spine, and the trunk formed an arch opening backward and resting upon the occiput and sacrum." In Ireland, Gordon says of a patient, "Her spine presented a most wonderful uniform curve concave backward; her head was also curved backward on the spine of the neck." During an epidemic at Birmingham in 1875 in one case "the retraction was so marked that a slough formed from the occiput pressing between the scapulæ."[23] In some cases rigid flexion of the body forward or laterally has been noticed. The rigidity persists, as a rule, until death, but sometimes ceases a short time before that event. If recovery takes place, this symptom gradually subsides, and disappears within a few days; but, on the other hand, more or less stiffness of the spine may last for several weeks. In one case it continued for more than two months, and in another until death on the forty-ninth day.

[23] Hart, *St. Bart's Rep.*, iv. 141.

The same physical cause that occasions rigidity, when acting less intensely or when a special susceptibility of the nervous system exists, also excites clonic convulsions. They are oftenest observed in patients of the [p. 810]age especially liable to spasmodic affections—in children before the completion of the first dentition. They vary in degree from twitching or subsultus affecting particular muscles, as of the eyes, the face, a limb, etc., to general epileptiform convulsions with loss of consciousness. They may be associated with paralysis, as where the two halves of the body are, the one convulsed and the other paralyzed. A case occurred in Dublin which "presented the very striking phenomenon of continued and violent convulsions during the whole of the brief course of the illness."[24] These convulsions, like others occurring at the commencement of acute diseases, are by no means always fatal, even when they are general. In the case of a robust adult convulsions occurred repeatedly during the first two days, and less frequently during the two following days, but the patient ultimately recovered.[25]

[24] *Dublin Quart. Jour.*, xlvi. 187.

[25] *Boston Med. and Surg. Jour.*, Feb., 1884, p. 121.

Paralysis, it may be inferred from the statements already made, is an incident of this disease, for an excess of the action causing tonic or clonic spasm must induce paralysis. Paralysis of an arm or leg or of the muscles of deglutition was long ago noticed among even the initial symptoms of the attack. In Dublin (1865) it was said of a patient, "All his members seemed to be paralyzed; he could move neither arms nor legs." Wunderlich describes the case of a man who "on the second day of the disease lost both sensibility and motility in the lower limbs and over the greater part of the trunk, while his left arm also was partially paralyzed." In another case complete paralysis of the right side occurred on the third day, the left side being rigid.[26] Baxa relates the case of a soldier in whom paralysis of the left side persisted after recovery from the disease,[27] and that of a woman in whom paralysis of the left lower limb continued along with right ciliary paralysis. Ptosis, strabismus, paralysis of the bladder and rectum, of the muscles of deglutition, and even general paralysis, have been observed. Aphasia also has been recorded by Hirsch and by Hayden.[28]

[26] *Dublin Quart. Jour.*, 1867, p. 431.
[27] *Wiener med. Presse*, No. 29, p. 715.
[28] *Dublin Quart. Jour.*, xlvi. 187.

The condition of the eyes and of vision in this disease is directly due to pressure of the exudation at the base of the brain upon the nerves and blood-vessels that supply these organs. One of the most striking peculiarities of the countenance of a patient at the beginning of an attack is the diffused and uniform redness of the conjunctivæ. In children it has a light tint, but a darker one in adults, and in some cases the eye becomes suffused with an extravasation of blood. The conditions of the pupil are also very peculiar. Very long ago it was observed to undergo sudden changes from contraction to dilatation, or the reverse. Dilatation is, however, its ordinary condition, especially in the fully-formed attack. Very often the pupils of the two eyes are in opposite states. In cases of long duration, with great exhaustion, they are almost invariably dilated. Photophobia is not uncommon, and oscillation of the pupils and spasmodic movements of the eyeball have frequently been observed. Strabismus is a symptom of very ordinary occurrence, particularly when other paralytic or spasmodic phenomena exist. It may be convergent or divergent, but most commonly is the former, and may be either a transient or a [p. 811]permanent symptom. Like other individual symptoms, it may be present rarely or frequently in a particular epidemic.

Blindness has been repeatedly observed. At first it seemed to be noticed as a transient symptom only. Fish (1809) states that it was sometimes the first deviation from health, and then was followed by paralytic spinal symptoms. He also observed that sight was sometimes restored in a few hours, and in no case did he know it to be permanently lost. American as well as European physicians, however, have met with many cases in which the sight was seriously and permanently impaired or altogether destroyed. In 1873 the changes affecting the eye were more fully and accurately described, especially those which tend to the structural injury of the organ. The abnormal appearances included cloudiness of the media, discoloration of the iris, irregularity of the pupils, and their obstruction with exudate. In exceptional cases the cornea ulcerated, and the globe collapsed after losing its contents. Ordinarily, however, says Lewis, "no ulceration occurs, and as the patient convalesces the oedema of the lids, the hyperæmia of the conjunctiva, the cloudiness of the cornea and of the humors gradually abate, and the exudation in the pupils is absorbed. The iris bulges forward, and the deep tissues of the eye, viewed through the vitreous humor, which had a dusky color from hyperæmia, now present a dull white color. The lens itself, at first transparent, after a while becomes cataractous, and sight is lost totally and for ever."

Impairment or loss of hearing has been occasionally observed during the successive epidemics of this disease, even from the beginning of its history, and it was early noticed that the symptom was often quite independent of any cognizable lesion of the ear itself. It was also observed that the sense of smell sometimes became impaired or was lost at the same time with that of hearing. More recently, Collins reported a case in which the patient lost the sight of one eye and became permanently deaf in both ears. Knapp states that in all of thirty-one cases examined by him the deafness was bilateral, and, with two exceptions of faint perception of sound, complete. Among twenty-nine cases of total deafness only one seemed to give some evidence of hearing afterward.[29] This surgeon holds that the deafness results from a purulent inflammation of the labyrinth, and his judgment has been confirmed by Keller and Lucas. When the impairment of hearing occurs simultaneously, or nearly so, in both ears, it is probable that the chief cause of the deafness is the pressure of the plastic exudation in which the auditory nerve is imbedded. Such deafness is rarely permanent. When the loss of hearing, whether complete or partial, does not improve, there is reason to believe that the internal ear has suffered great and incurable changes of structure. Sometimes this follows a distinct attack of suppurative inflammation of the middle ear; but as complete and permanent deafness sometimes occurs without being preceded by any such affection, it must be inferred that atrophic changes have taken place in some portion of the nervous apparatus of hearing. It is stated by Moos that of sixty-four cases of recovery from cerebro-spinal meningitis, which showed disturbance of hearing as a sequel, one-half manifested in addition a more less disordered equilibrium. Of these twenty-nine were totally deaf on both sides, two totally deaf on one and hard of hearing on the other side, and one case had merely [p. 812]impaired hearing in both ears. The disturbance of locomotion had existed for periods varying from three weeks to five years from the inception of the disease, and was chiefly characterized by a staggering or waddling gait.[30] In the deaf-mute institutions at Bamberg and Nürnberg it is said that out of 91 pupils, 80 owed their infirmity to this disease (Ziemssen). Salamo states that some awake out of sleep totally deaf, and remain so for a long time, or, it may be, permanently (Moos).

[29] Smith, *loc. cit.*
[30] *Mening. Cerebro-spinal epid.*, p. 11.

The expression of countenance in this disease is peculiar. When the pain in the head is severe and paroxysmal the features are apt to be violently distorted; when it is more persistent the face assumes a fixed or rigid expression, or is at the same time dull, particularly after a long continuance of the pain. In the apoplectic form the expression may be set and stupid, but the features have neither the dark, dull, swollen, and duskily-flushed aspect of typhus, nor the languid, sleepy expression, and circumscribed flush on the cheek which are so characteristic of typhoid fever. Except during absolute insensibility in rapidly fatal cases there is a look of greater intelligence than belongs to either of the diseases mentioned. Indeed, in the beginning of the attack in regular cases the distinctive facies presents pale and sunken features, with paleness of the skin over the whole body.

Delirium in this disease exhibits a great many degrees and varieties. It may occur among the earliest symptoms in certain rapid cases not of the congestive type, but is more apt to arise on the second or third day in those more typically developed. It may be mild, reasoning, hysterical, or maniacal, or it may change from one to another of these forms during the same attack. Fish states that it is apt to be violent if it comes on at the commencement of the illness, but that when it begins at a later period it is milder, and sometimes playful, the patient being sociable and humorous. All good observers have furnished similar descriptions of this symptom; some have added that the mental condition is often desponding and apprehensive, and others that certain patients remain sombre and silent; and it sometimes happens that the delirium comes on abruptly, as when a patient "woke suddenly in the middle of the night and began to hum tunes, to fancy that people were conversing with him," etc. (Gordon).

Coma is met with sooner or later in nearly all fatal cases, but rarely in a marked degree until the approach of death. If anything is surprising in epidemic meningitis, it is the absence of that deep and prolonged stupor that characterizes the typhoid state, notwithstanding the pressure of the exudation upon the brain in most cases, and in others such a profound alteration of the blood that it exudes through the tissues as water passes through a porous body. Another striking phenomenon of the disease is that the patient after recovery has generally a complete oblivion of all that happened to him between the beginning of the attack and convalescence. This is true even of cases in which the brain symptoms are far from being conspicuous.

Another symptom closely related to the local lesion and the blood-change in this disease is vertigo. As originally described by Miner in 1823, it occurred from the very commencement of the attack, and was even then regarded as denoting a deficient supply of the blood to the [p. 813]brain, so that when the patient rose to an erect posture it was felt along with uneasiness in the stomach, acceleration of the pulse, dimness of sight, nausea, and fainting. Tourdes, speaking of it as it occurred in the Strasburg epidemic, says that it confused the mind and rendered walking impossible. In two cases patients were seized with a giddiness which compelled them to whirl around, when they fell and did not rise again. According to Moos (1881) unilateral affections of the labyrinth give rise to vertigo, and bilateral lesions to a staggering gait. Bilateral hemorrhage or acute suppuration of the ampullar terminations of the auditory nerve occasions paralysis and staggering. Children, and those who at the same time have the sight impaired, are apt to remain affected for a long time. Otherwise, prolonged and systematic muscular exercise may remove the tottering walk.

To the same causes must doubtless be attributed the debility which is so early and so conspicuous a symptom in this disease, and which gave it one of the names, typhus syncopalis, by which it was first known in this country. It was manifested by the vertigo already noticed, by a sense of sinking in the epigastrium, by a quick, frequent, feeble, and irregular pulse, and by a sudden and extreme loss of muscular power, so that the patient found himself unable to raise his hand before he was sensible of being ill. This state of asthenia is conspicuous throughout the whole of the disease, and is the immediate cause of the slow and irregular convalescence which is characteristic of it.

Of the symptoms peculiar to the digestive apparatus hardly any belong to it directly. They are nearly all the effect of reflex influences. The condition of the tongue is for the most part quite unlike that which belongs to the typhoid state. The fuliginous condition of the tongue, gums, cheeks, and lips which characterizes that state is seldom met with in epidemic meningitis. The older writers agreed that even when the tongue does grow dry and brown the condition is not of long continuance, and later observers have confirmed their statements. Thus, J. L. Smith (1872) says, "Occasionally, in cases attended with great prostration, the fur of the tongue is dry and brown, but only for a few days, when the moist whitish fur succeeds." We have generally found it moist, whitish in the centre and at the tip and edges.

Nausea and vomiting are very constant among the initial symptoms of the disease, and, as already pointed out, are due to irritation of the cerebro-spinal ganglia. Very often the vomiting is not preceded by nausea, and is brought on by the patient's raising himself, etc. The stomach itself undergoes no change. Both symptoms are usually accompanied by faintness or giddiness, and are more decided in the initial than in the later stages of the attack. The matters vomited, varying with the contents of the stomach and the urgency and duration of the symptom, consist of ingesta, mucus, serum, or bile, and in some grave cases of a dark grumous matter taken to be altered blood. In some epidemics, apparently, more than in others, this symptom is very distressing, as it was at Birmingham in 1875.[31] The inability of the stomach to retain food necessarily leads to a rapid wasting of the flesh, which is aggravated by the patient's suffering, restlessness, and want of sleep. Nevertheless, no sooner is the vomiting appeased than a desire for food is felt, and when [p. 814]it is retained it generally undergoes digestion. Indeed, in no other disease is the return of a good appetite and digestion so prompt and complete. It is true that the recovery of flesh and strength is not always in proportion to the appetite. As might be expected in a disease in which fever plays so subordinate a part, there is seldom urgent thirst. But epidemics differ in this as in so many other respects. In that which we witnessed in the Philadelphia Hospital in 1866-67 the patients were clamorous for liquids. Constipation is the rule among patients with this disease, as, indeed, might naturally be expected, for no lesion affects the bowels and little or no food is retained by the stomach. Yet in a few cases diarrhoea accompanies persistent vomiting.

[31] Hart, *St. Bart's Rep.*, xii. 112.

The fauces appear to have been more or less inflamed in some epidemics; swelling of the parotid glands is an occasional occurrence, and sometimes they undergo suppuration. Aphthæ have also been met with.

The secretion of urine is not affected in any uniform manner. Sometimes it is diminished and sometimes increased in quantity. The latter symptom has occasionally long survived the disease. It retains its normal acidity. In rare cases either albumen or sugar has been detected; the former may have been due to the action of blisters of cantharides used in the treatment of the disease.

One of the most curious and unintelligible phenomena occasionally met with in this disease is a peculiar affection of the joints, which first was observed in this country. Jackson (1810 and 1813) wrote: "In some cases swellings have occurred in the joints and limbs. They have been very sore to the touch, and their appearance has been compared to that of the gout. The parts so affected feel as if they had been bruised. These swellings arise on the smaller as well as on the larger joints, and are often of a purple color." So Collins[32] reports: "The joints sometimes become swollen, red, and tender; at other times red and painful without any swelling; while, again, intense pain and rapid enlargement from effusion have occurred unattended with redness. The joints most usually attacked are the knee, elbow, wrist, and the smaller articulations of the fingers and toes." In an epidemic which occurred in Greece in 1869 articular swellings similar to those of inflammatory rheumatism were observed.[33] These descriptions, which apply to some cases in most epidemics, are of more than casual interest, for they demonstrate conclusively, as we think, the truth which the whole history of the disease confirms—viz. that it is a systemic and not a local affection, and is dependent for its existence upon a specific poison which is absolutely unlike every other morbid poison known to pathology.

[32] *Dublin Quart. Jour.*, Aug., 1868, p. 170.
[33] *Archives générales de med.*, Mai, 1883, p. 622.

The act of respiration is variously modified in this disease, as might, indeed, be expected from the seat and nature of the cerebro-spinal lesions. It is sighing, labored, and interrupted. Burdon-Sanderson describes its differences from the so-called Cheyne-Stokes respiration; it is, he says, "marked by a slow, labored inspiration, followed by a quick expiration and a long pause." When opisthotonos is very great and persistent, it necessarily interferes with the dilatation of the lungs, and leads to oedema of those organs, and even to sanguineous effusions into them. [p. 815]Pneumonia is not an unusual complication of the disease when it prevails in cold weather.

The distinguishing characters of the pulse are diminished force and volume, and a tone so much impaired that slight causes produce extreme variations in its rate and rhythm. If the disease be a fever, as is by some maintained, then it is the only fever in which the pulse-rate is often far below the normal, and at the same time neither full nor tense, unless transiently and in altogether exceptional cases. In no other disease attended with inflammation do the rate and quality of the pulse vary so greatly within short intervals. It may be said, in general terms, to be variable in rate and strength even in the most sthenic cases of the disease, and in those which tend to a fatal issue to be small, thready, weak, intermittent, or imperceptible for a longer or shorter time before death. It is no uncommon thing for the pulse-rate at the beginning of an attack to fall as low as 40, or even 27, and afterward rise to 120 or even more, in a minute, without necessarily indicating a fatal issue. Muscular exertion, rising from a recumbent posture, etc., will sometimes double its frequency, besides producing irregularity. Read, describing the pulse as he observed it in Boston in 1873-74, speaks of cases in which "both the rhythm and the force of the beats are entirely destroyed; ... one moment, while beating very fast, it will suddenly drop to a much lower rate.... These conditions also may outlast apparent convalescence." Some fatal cases are attended by distressing palpitations of the heart.

Nothing is more remarkable in the early histories of this affection than their unanimous statement that it is not distinguished by a febrile temperature. It is true that the observers of those days had not the advantage of using clinical thermometers, but they were too nearly agreed in their judgments and harmonious in their descriptions to permit any serious doubt of the substantial accuracy of their conclusions, which were expressed in such terms as these: "A diminution of heat may be considered as among this most striking symptoms of this disease" (Strong); or, "the temperature never exceeded the standard of health in more than three or four cases, ... and a great majority of the patients had no fever at all" (Miner); or, again, "A high febrile movement took place only in a limited number" (Gilchrist); or, "The heat of the surface was less in all cases than is usually observed in acute diseases" (Jenks). It will be observed that these statements, and very many others which agree with them, were founded upon the perception of the patients' temperature by the hand, which was of course applied to the most accessible parts of the body—the face, neck, arms, and hands—but they have more real value and significance than the more recent measurements taken in the mouth, axilla, rectum, or vagina, for we know that, however valuable the temperatures of these parts may be for comparative studies, they do not really indicate the condition of the individual who presents them. It is a familiar fact that the difference of temperature in cholera when taken in the rectum and the axilla may be 4° F., or even more than this.

Since the thermometer has been used in the study of epidemic meningitis greater accuracy of results has been attained, and yet the general statements of the earlier observers have been confirmed. Thus, Githens has shown that the temperature of the body in this disease is lower than that recorded of any other fever or inflammatory affection; the average,[p. 816]indeed, of his cases was lower by four or five degrees than that of typhus or typhoid fever, pneumonia, etc. In 2 cases only did the thermometer in the axilla reach 105°. The highest temperature in 15 cases was between 104° and 105°; in 12, between 103° and 104°; in 7, between 102° and 103°; in 6, between 101° and 102°; and in 2 it was below 100°.[34] Tourdes, Niemeyer, and others have noted the slight rise of temperature during the first and second days of the attack, and Wunderlich found fever of very unequal degrees and with very variable maxima, but the highest temperatures were observed by him as well as others in fatal cases and immediately before death. In one instance it reached 107.5° F. Burdon-Sanderson and others have found that an increased temperature always attended exacerbations of pain. Von Ziemssen gives the average temperature as varying from 100.4° to 103° F., but with variations between higher and lower points, and particularly notes the persistence of a normal temperature while the other symptoms are undergoing a variety of changes, as well as the fact that, unlike other febrile affections, this disease has no representative temperature curve. In his clinical observations Hart found for several successive days as much as six degrees of difference between the morning and evening temperatures. A morning rise for several days was noticed in four cases, and usually there was no relation between the pulse and the temperature, nor any uniformly between the temperature and the gravity of the attack.[35] But not rarely it has been noticed that the daily exacerbations, if any, did not occur in the afternoon, but with great irregularity, so that the maxima and minima might occur on successive days and at the same hour of the day. Dr. J. L. Smith, whose thermometric observations in this disease seem to have been carefully made, used the thermometer in the rectum, and thus obtained temperatures higher that the average of other observations, such as $105.^4/6°$ to $107.^2/6°$ in several cases. Yet he found the fluctuations of rectal temperature remarkable, though less so than the surface temperature, of which he states that sometimes it rose above or fell below the normal standard several times in the course of the same day.

[34] *Amer. Jour. of Med. Sci.*, July, 1867, p. 38.
[35] *St. Bart's Reports*, xii. 112.

Nothing can be more irregular, uncertain, or various than the eruptions and other cutaneous symptoms that have been met with in this disease. When it first appeared in New England a large proportion of the cases, and especially of the grave cases, exhibited petechial eruptions and ecchymotic spots, whence the disease presently received the name of spotted fever. Yet even then, North and the other historians of its epidemics were careful to state that spots on the skin were by no means characteristic of the disease, and very often were not present at all, especially in cases that terminated favorably. Woodward, for example, wrote (1808): "An eruption on the skin so seldom appeared that it could no longer be considered a characteristic symptom of the disease." In various American local epidemics an eruption of some kind seems to have existed in about one-half of the cases. In one that we observed in the Philadelphia Hospital no eruption whatever was observed in thirty-seven out of ninety-eight cases. In the epidemic at Chicago in 1872, N. S. Davis says:[36] "About one-third of the cases presented some red erythematous spots" between the third and the seventh day. In mild cases they were few and [p. 817]bright red; in grave cases, darker and larger, with some swelling of the skin; and in the worst cases, purple spots one or two or more inches in diameter. In that of Louisville,[37] Larrabie states that the eruption "was generally herpetic in its character, and accompanied by sudamina; but in several instances an urticarious eruption suddenly appeared and disappeared." Nothing is said of petechiæ or ecchymoses. In the New York epidemic of 1873[38] the skin in grave cases presented dusky mottlings, especially when the animal temperature was reduced; also a punctated red eruption, bluish spots a few lines in diameter, and large patches of the same color. Herpes also was common. It is chiefly in cases of a malignant type and rapid and fatal course that ecchymoses have been observed. Of this statement illustrations will be given in the paragraph relating to the duration of the disease.

[36] *Louisville Med. Jour.*, June, 1872, p. 705.
[37] *Louisville Med. Jour.*, Dec., 1872, p. 782.
[38] *Amer. Jour. of Med. Sci.*, Oct., 1873, p. 329.

In continental European epidemics of meningitis the proportion of cases in which a general eruption existed seems to have been smaller than it was in this country. In the Geneva epidemic of 1805 a considerable number of cases at the point of death presented purplish spots, some earlier than this, and some after death only. In the Neapolitan epidemic of 1833, and in that which occurred in Dublin in 1867-68, ecchymoses were often present, and in a very marked degree. Stokes and Banks mention that in some rare instances the spots ran together and coalesced over some portions of the body, so as to cover a large extent of the skin and render it completely black, as though it were wrapped in some dark shroud. The entire right arm and half of the right side of the chest in one case, and in the other the whole of the lower portion of one leg and foot, were thus affected.[39] In Strasburg, on the other hand, only three cases of petechiæ were observed by Tourdes; at Rochefort and Versailles, in 1839, they were rarely noticed; at Gibraltar, in 1844, they do not seem to have been observed; in 1848-49, at the Val de Grâce Hospital (Paris), they appear not to have attracted attention; and at Petit Bourg they were not noticed, although the state of the skin was fully described. In Prussia, in 1865, neither Burdon-Sanderson nor Wunderlich mentions petechiæ or vibices as occurring during life; and Hirsch, after noting their occasional presence, is obliged to draw upon American authors for an account of them.

[39] *Dublin Quart. Jour.*, xlvi. 199.

Of the eruptions other than petechiæ and ecchymoses, several of which have already been mentioned, it is necessary to take some notice here. They are, chiefly, and in general terms, exanthems, including erythema, roseola, and urticaria, and in addition herpes, particularly of the lips. The last has no special relation to this affection, as it is met with in almost every febrile disease, but it has sometimes extended to the whole face in this one. The former may be connected pathologically either with the altered condition of the blood or with the irritation produced by the exudation in the spinal nervous centres. They have frequently been compared to measles and to scarlatina, but sometimes they have assumed the form of bullæ. Thus, in the case of a child four years old, described by Grimshaw,[40] an eruption of pemphigus occurred over the whole body. Jackson long before had mentioned, as one of the eruptions belonging to this disease, "large bullæ, as if produced by cantharides." Jenks [p. 818]described "large elevated spots of a very dark color, presenting outside of the dark color a blistered appearance." In some cases gangrene of the skin has been observed when the spots have been exceptionally dark, and occasionally has been produced by pressure.

[40] *Jour. of Cutaneous Med.*, ii. 37.

The cause of death in many of the more rapid cases is coma, which is often preceded by convulsions, especially in children; but in many others, even when attended with all the marks of dissolution of the blood, consciousness may be but slightly impaired until the actual imminence of death. In many other cases, which are fatal in the midst of an attack with spinal symptoms, death is due to asphyxia, partly owing to pressure on the medulla oblongata, and partly to the interference with the respiratory act due to this pressure, and occasioning excessive bronchial secretion. Again, death may occur through a gradual exhaustion of the powers of life, without marked spasm, blood-change, or complication. In these cases also the intelligence remains unimpaired almost until the moment of dissolution. Death is not very rarely due to pneumonia, and when the disease is greatly prolonged or the convalescence from it is imperfect a fatal termination by dropsy of the brain is still among its dangers.

Hirsch once declared that the duration of epidemic meningitis "is between a few hours and several months," and, however hyperbolical the phrase may seem, it is quite accurate. Such inequalities are more characteristic of acute blood diseases than of inflammations, and in this case the coexistence of elements of both kinds doubtless accounts for the extreme irregularity of the symptoms and duration of the attack. The early American writers insisted strongly on this as a characteristic feature of the disease. They record an unusually large proportion of cases that were fatal within the first day, and even after an illness of five hours, although they agree that the most usual date of death was between the fourth and seventh days—a result that has been confirmed by subsequent observation. Dr. N. S. Davis gives the duration of the disease, as seen by him, as between twenty hours and twenty-eight days. Out of 469 fatal cases in the city of New York in 1872, 334 are said to have terminated within eleven days, and of this number 270 were fatal in the first six days of the attack, including 52 who died on the first day, and 51 in from one to two days. It is perhaps worthy of note that while from the eleventh to the fourteenth day only 11 deaths occurred, 20 took place on the fourteenth and fifteenth; and while from the fifteenth to the twenty-first day only 16 died, yet from the twenty-first to the twenty-second 12 deaths were reported. This would seem to indicate a peculiar danger on the days represented by multiples of seven. Of cases that recover, the duration is even more indefinite than that of fatal cases, owing to complications that occur in many, and especially such as involve the cerebro-spinal centres. When death takes place within a few hours it usually, if not always, is attended with symptoms that denote a disorganization of the blood. In 1864 we attended a young man previously in perfect health, but who died in twenty-one hours after the first seizure. His mind was unclouded throughout his brief but fatal illness. Within seven hours of death a purpurous discoloration of the skin began, and about an hour before that event the surface everywhere assumed a dusky hue. The forearms and hands were almost uniformly purple and the face turgid; many ecchymotic spots on the trunk and lower limbs were nearly black and measured [p. 819]one or two inches in diameter.[41] In the case of a child of five years death in convulsions took place after an illness of ten hours, the skin presenting purpurous spots, some of them very large and of a deep bluish livid hue. On post-mortem examination there was not the slightest appearance of any meningeal lesion, except a few dark spots like sanguineous effusion under the arachnoid. The heart was full of dark blood in a semi-coagulated state, and the white corpuscles were three times as numerous as the red.[42] A case is reported by Gordon[43] in which the entire duration of the illness until death was five hours. This is probably the shortest case on record. A lady aged twenty-two years died in sixteen hours, the skin covered with livid ecchymoses, some of them measuring an inch or an inch and a half in diameter.[44]

[41] *Amer. Jour. of Med. Sci.*, July, 1864, p. 133.
[42] *Dublin Quart. Jour.*, 1867, ii. 441.
[43] *Loc. cit.*
[44] *Med. Press and Circular*, May, 1866. For other cases see *ibid.*, pp. 296, 298-300.

The character of the convalescence from epidemic meningitis must evidently be affected by the causes that determine its duration, the grade of the disease, the development and extent of the lesions, etc.; but it is certain that, except in those imperfect and, as it were, shadowy cases which denote a very slight action of the morbid cause, its subjects do not recover rapidly. The essential lesion of the fully-formed disease requires time for its removal, just as in typhoid fever the intestinal ulcers are often slow of healing, and hence become a cause of tardy recovery and even of unlooked-for death. The convalescence, then, from the disease we are now studying is slow and irregular, is attended often with debility and emaciation, and sometimes with persistent headache, neuralgia, convulsions, stiffness of the neck and pain in moving it, hyperæsthesia of portions of the skin, palpitation of the heart, dyspepsia, etc. Relapses are very far from being uncommon.

Among the causes of tardy convalescence in this disease are those lesions and disorders which may be embraced by the term sequelæ. Impaired vision, due to various affections of the eyes, has already been considered among the symptoms proper of the disease, but they are not infrequently developed after the acute attack has subsided. Thus, in a case reported by Larrabie:[45] "Just as convalescence seemed beginning the left eye became affected in all its parts, with entire loss of vision and also complete deafness. After a short remission hydrencephaloid symptoms appeared, followed by the same changes in the hitherto sound eye, complete blindness and deafness, general cachexia and marasmus, rigid flexion of the right limbs, and death by exhaustion at the end of sixteen weeks." The impairment of hearing, which also was described as a symptom of the acute attack, is apt to become more marked after the acute stage has passed by, and, as before stated, is very often permanent. Occurring in young children, it then involves deaf-mutism. It is in many cases associated with defective vision, weakness or loss of memory, mania, impairment of intelligence, persistent pains in the head or chronic hydrocephalus. Sometimes to one or more of these symptoms is added more or less general paresis or complete paralysis. Southhall[46] mentions the case of a child two years old whose attack was followed by incomplete paralysis, and death at the end of eight months with softening[p. 820]of the brain. Gordon thus describes the conclusion of a case: "The man has gradually passed into a state of almost organic life; he eats, drinks, and sleeps well; he passes solid feces and urine without giving any notice, yet, evidently, not unconsciously; ... he seems to understand, but cannot answer; ... he can draw up his legs and arms, but he cannot use his hands at all." Hirsch has remarked that disorders of speech are met with, due apparently to an inability to articulate certain sounds. Von Ziemssen regards chronic hydrocephalus as not a rare consequence of epidemic meningitis, and as one not absolutely or immediately fatal. Its symptoms include severe paroxysmal pain in the head or neck or extremities, with vomiting, loss of consciousness, convulsions, and involuntary evacuation of excrements. Between the paroxysms, which sometimes occur periodically, the patient generally suffers from neuralgic pains, hyperæsthesia, and various motor and even mental disorders; but in other cases the intervals are free, or nearly so, from all morbid manifestations. Davis (1872) and many others speak of severe neuralgic pains following this disease; according to Dr. D., they are most frequent at the heads of the gastrocnemii muscles, in the abdomen, and the head; a very fretful disposition, variable appetite, and disturbed sleep are often observed. Relapses have been noticed in almost all the epidemics, and it seems probable that they are often due to the influence of accidental exciting causes, mental or physical, in renewing the inflammation around the cerebro-spinal lesions. Miner (1825) remarked that they were most apt to occur within the first week, but that when the disease had once run its course there were very few relapses during convalescence. But, he adds, there were several repeated attacks after the most perfect recovery, and several of the patients had had the disease the preceding year.

[45] *Richmond Journal of Med.*, Dec., 1872, p. 779.
[46] *Ibid.*, Aug., 1872, p. 141.

Like other epidemic diseases, meningitis presents itself with every possible degree of gravity between that of a slight indisposition and that of a malignant and deadly malady. The mortality in a number of epidemics compared by Hirsch varied between 20 per cent. and 75 per cent. It changes with the locality. Thus, nearly at the same time that the death-rate from this disease in Massachusetts was 61 per cent., it was but 33 per cent. in the Philadelphia Hospital. In 1872 the whole number of deaths caused by it in Philadelphia was 133, while at St. John's College, Little Rock, Ark., 21 cases out of 29 were fatal (Southhall). It differs, also, at different periods; for while ten epidemics in various places, occurring between 1838 and 1848, presented an average mortality of 70 per cent., a similar number, occurring between 1855 and 1865, gave an average mortality of only 30 per cent. It must, however, be confessed that such statistics cannot be relied upon as accurate, for in private practice many cases occur that are never reported unless they end fatally.

MORBID ANATOMY.—The lesions found after death from epidemic meningitis consist essentially of congestion or inflammation of the cerebro-spinal meninges, but they also include in many cases hemorrhage, serous effusion, plastic exudation, and tissue-changes in the brain and spinal marrow, and in many other cases an impaired constitution of the blood. As the signs of the latter, and not the former, alterations are met with in the more malignant cases, it is evident that, looking at the disease as a [p. 821]whole, it must involve a toxic element of whose operation the various post-mortem lesions are only effects. These lesions, on the whole, vary with the type of the disease, and also with its duration, but some are chiefly met with in cases of a malignant and others in cases of an inflammatory type.

The exterior of the body after death in the early stages of this disease almost always presents the marks of transudation of the contents of the blood-vessels. The dependent parts of the body exhibit large livid patches or a uniform discoloration of the same hue. In acute cases the muscles are more deeply colored than natural, and when the attack is prolonged they are said to have their cohesion impaired by fatty degeneration. Congestion of the brain is an unfailing accompaniment of the first stage of the disease; its blood-vessels are all distended with dark blood; the sinuses of the dura mater are usually filled with coagula of the same hue, though sometimes very dense. Serum abounds in the arachnoid cavity and in the ventricles of the brain; it may be clear or milky, and sometimes it is quite purulent. It is alleged by one reporter that no less than three pints of turbid serum escaped in a case in which, however, death did not occur until the thirty-fifth day. Craig found eight and twelve ounces of a limpid fluid in two cases; and Tourdes found pus in more than one-half of his cases, either unmixed or forming a milky liquid. J. L. Smith refers to the case of an infant who had the disease at the age of five months, and two months subsequently great prominence of the anterior fontanelle, and other symptoms which indicated the presence of a considerable amount of effusion within the cranium. In a case in Dublin,[47] there was no meningeal lesion except in a "few dark spots like sanguineous effusion under the arachnoid." White[48] mentions the case of an adult that terminated fatally in thirty-six hours, in which the vessels of the pia mater were very much congested, and sanguineous effusions existed above and below the cerebellum, and a clot of blood three inches long and external to the theca extended downward from the lowest portion of the medulla oblongata. In all of these instances, then, congestion, the first stage of inflammation, existed. That such was its real nature is proved by what follows.

[47] *Dublin Jour.*, July, 1867, p. 441.
[48] *Med. Record*, iii. 198.

The most characteristic lesion is a fibrinous or purulent exudation in the meshes of the pia mater. American physicians described it as early as 1806 in such terms as these: "The dura mater and pia mater in several places adhered together and to the substance of the brain; ... between the dura mater and the pia mater was a fluid resembling pus" (Danielson and Mann). In 1810, Bartlett and Wilson found "an extravasation of lymph on the surface of the brain;" and in the same year Jackson and his colleagues, after describing the congestion and serous effusion found within the cranium "in those who perished within twelve hours of the first invasion," state that the arachnoid and pia mater present an effusion between them of "coagulated lymph or semi-purulent lymph" both on the convexity and at the base of the brain. These descriptions correspond in all respects with those of Mathey relating to the epidemic at Geneva in 1805, for he says: "The meningeal blood-vessels were strongly injected. A jelly-like exudation tinged with blood covered the surface of the brain; ... on its lower surface and in the ventricles a [p. 822]yellowish puriform matter was found." Such lesions have been described by a long line of observers—by Wilson in 1813, Gamage in 1818, Ames and Sargent in 1848; by Squire, Upham, and a host of others since 1860 in the United States, and by Tourdes, Gilchrist, Ferrus, Wilks, Gordon, Banks, Gaskoin, Niemeyer, Burdon-Sanderson, and many more in Europe.

It is evident, therefore, that in a certain number of fatal cases only sanguineous congestion of the membranes of the brain and spinal cord are found, and in certain others—constituting, it may be added, nine-tenths of the whole number—evidences exist of cerebro-spinal meningitis. Hence the natural conclusion is that the congestive lesions represent the first stage of a process which if prolonged and perfected occasions the lesions peculiar to inflammation. For the development of the latter two factors would seem to be essential—not only a fibrinous condition of the blood, but also sufficient time for exudation to occur. But when we come to study the actual results of examinations post-mortem, it is found that the duration of the attack does not determine absolutely the nature of the lesions. On the one hand, in a case which terminated fatally after a week's illness there was found reddish serum between the arachnoid and the pia mater and in the lateral ventricles, with intense injection of the pia mater of the base, medulla oblongata, and upper part of the spinal cord, but no exudation of lymph.[49] And, on the other hand, numerous cases have been published in which, although death occurred within twenty-four hours from the onset of the attack, coagulated lymph and also pus were found upon the brain and spinal marrow. For example, during the winter of 1861-62, in the army, that then lay near Washington, D.C., a soldier was attacked with a chill, severe fever, and headache, followed by opisthotonos and repeated convulsions before his death, which occurred in about twenty-four hours. No eruption or discoloration of the skin is mentioned in the history. On examination there was found beneath the arachnoid a thin layer of lymph and abundant exudation over the posterior lobes of the cerebrum, and also at the base of the brain and on the medulla oblongata.[50] In a case reported by Gordon[51] the entire duration of the illness was under five hours, and after death the cerebral arachnoid was more or less opaque, and in some spots had a layer of very thin purulent matter beneath it. And, again, not only may the symptoms belonging to blood-dissolution be consistent with a certain prolongation of life, but also with decidedly inflammatory tissue-changes. Thus, in another case of Gordon's the duration of the illness was at least six days, and the patient presented all the characteristic symptoms of the disease, including "a most wonderful and uniform curve of the spine and head backward," "spots black as ink," "bullæ which rapidly became opaque and dusky," "herpetic eruption, etc." After death the body had a very frightful appearance. It was still prominently arched forward. It was of a dusky blue color, with a copious eruption of black spots of various sizes, and one or two of them were gangrenous.... When the theca vertebralis was opened purulent matter flowed out, and a purulent effusion was found in patches on the brain. [p. 823]The cerebral arachnoid was all opaque, the lateral ventricles were filled with serum, and the blood in all the cavities was very fluid and dark colored. From all that precedes, therefore, it must be inferred that the nature of the lesions in this disease depends not on the type alone, nor on the duration merely, of the attack—that a very brief course is compatible with marked inflammatory lesions, and a prolonged one with profound alterations in the condition of the blood. In other words, it seems that there must be something besides the appreciable lesions that influences, if it does not determine, the issue of an attack of this affection. While bringing forward prominently this proposition, and the facts on which it rests, we have no intention of under-estimating the relative significance of the two most conspicuous types of the disease, the purely inflammatory and the adynamic, or calling in question the fact that the evolution of the former is most usually comparatively slow and regular, and of the latter rapid and irregular. In the one, when death takes place early, congestive changes are found, and when later these have merged into exudative lesions; in the other or adynamic cases congestion and liquid transudation prevail, and the results of complete inflammation are seldom seen. When the disease has been very much prolonged the exudation becomes tough, adherent, and shrivelled.

[49] Davis, *Richmond Med. Jour.*, June, 1872, p. 709.
[50] Frothingham, *Amer. Med. Times*, Apr., 1864, p. 207.
[51] *Dublin Quart. Jour.*, May, 1867, p. 409.

The brain-tissue has generally been found softer than natural, and, although in some cases this diminished consistence might be attributed to post-mortem changes, yet on the whole it must be associated with the inflammatory lesions of the meninges. As a rule, it is greater the longer the attack has lasted, and is by no means equally diffused, but is more marked where the meningeal alterations are greatest. Ames found softening in nine out of eleven cases, and chiefly in the cortical substance, but also in the fornix and septum lucidum; and Chauffard states that in protracted cases "the interior surface of the ventricles, the fornix, and septum lucidum, were reduced to a pultaceous and creamy consistence." But it is by no means true that softening is met with in all cases of long duration.

The lesions of the spinal marrow and its membranes correspond with those of the brain. The dura mater is often very dark, its blood-vessels engorged, its arachnoid cavity distended with serum more or less bloody, turbid, or purulent. Two ounces of pus have been removed from it through a puncture. Fibrinous and purulent exudation fills the meshes of the pia mater, and is usually most abundant in the cervical and dorsal portions, and generally upon the posterior rather than upon the anterior surface of the organ; but sometimes large accumulations of lymph and pus are found at the lower end of the cord. Gordon[52] relates of a case that "when an opening was made into the lower part of the theca vertebralis purulent matter flowed out, and the entire surface of the pia mater was covered with a coating of thin purulent matter, which, like a thin layer of butter, remained adherent to it." Occasionally the cavity of the spinal arachnoid contains blood. Softening of the spinal cord has been often noticed. Chauffard states that in some cases of particularly long duration it was reduced to a mere pulp, and he adds, "in the place of portions of the spinal marrow, completely destroyed, was found only a yellowish liquid, or the empty membranes fell into contact where it was [p. 824]wanting." Similar disorganization has been described by Ames, Klebs, and others. Fronmüller reports the case of a girl aged fourteen years in whom the central canal of the spinal cord was distended with pure pus.

[52] *Dublin Quart. Jour.*, xliii. 414.

The lesions of the internal auditory apparatus consist of softening in the fourth ventricle and of the root of the auditory nerve, yet such lesions are said to have been found even when no defect of hearing had existed. In other cases in which deafness did occur the lesions consisted of inflammatory changes in the cavity of the tympanum and suppuration of the labyrinth. They probably arose from an extension of inflammation from the pia mater along the trunk of the auditory nerve (Von Ziemssen). In like manner, the inflammatory and destructive changes in the eye which have been elsewhere described arise from an analogous cause affecting the optic nerves.

It is unnecessary to dwell upon the condition in which other organs are found after death from epidemic meningitis. In cases that present a typhoid type, and even in such as are rapidly fatal with ecchymotic discoloration of the skin, the various organs present no distinctive tissue-change, but only such engorgement as is common to all diseases of a similar type. It deserves to be particularly mentioned that in this affection the spleen is not enlarged, as it always is in a greater or less degree in diseases whose primary stage involves an altered condition of the blood. This fact becomes all the more important in view of the remarkable contrast which the constitution of the blood presents in epidemic meningitis and in various typhous affections.

The state of the blood in this disease is one of peculiar interest, dominating as it does its whole pathology and determining its nosological position. It is the blood of a phlegmasia rather than of a pyrexia. This fact was early established by American physicians who observed the disease, and the opportunities for doing so were not wanting, since venesection was used by every one who treated it. In 1807-09 a rapidly fatal case or two was found in which the "blood was darker and had a larger proportion of serum than usual," but in others "it did not present any uncommon appearance, and no inflammatory buff, nor was it dissolved" (Fish). In 1811, Arnell stated that "the blood drawn in the early stage appeared like that of a person in full health; there was no unusual buffy coat, neither was the crassamentum broken down or destroyed." In the epidemic studied by Mannkopff (1866) he found that blood obtained by venesection gave a clot with a thick buffy coat. Andral, seeking to establish the law that in every acute inflammation there is an increase in the fibrin of the blood, remarks that in a case of cerebro-spinal meningitis it was very marked.[53] Ames states that "the blood taken from the arm and by cups from the back of the neck" "coagulated with great rapidity." "Its color was generally bright—in a few cases nearly approaching to that of arterial blood; it was seldom buffed; in thirty-seven cases in which its appearance was noted it was buffed in only four." Analyses were made in four cases, "the blood being taken early in the disease from the arm, and was the first bleeding in each case. They furnished the following results:

[p. 825]

	Fibrin.	Corpuscles.
	6.40	140.29
I	5.20	112.79
II	3.64	123.45
V	4.56	129.50

The first was from a laboring man thirty-five years old; the second from a boy twelve years old, while comatose; and the two others from stout women between thirty and thirty-five."[54] Tourdes, whose analyses follow, states that "blood drawn from a vein was rarely buffed; if a buffy coat existed, it was thin, and generally a mere iridization upon the surface of the clot."[55]

	Fibrin.	Corpuscles.
	4.60	134.00
I	3.90	135.54
II	3.70	143.00
V	5.63	137.84

Maillot gives, as the result of an analysis of six cases, an increase of fibrin to six parts and more in a thousand. This summary represents, as far as is known, all of the analyses of blood taken from living patients in this disease, and it shows that in every case the proportion of fibrin exceeded that of healthy blood, and corresponded exactly to that observed in the blood of inflammatory diseases, while the proportion of red corpuscles varied within the normal limits. How different is this condition of the blood from that of typhus fever, in which there is a marked diminution of fibrin, and a falling off in the red corpuscles as well, or from that of typhoid fever, in which neither element declines until the disease affects the body by inanition! (Murchison).

[53] *Path. Hæmatology*, p. 73.
[54] *New Orleans Med. and Surg. Jour.*, Nov., 1848.
[55] *Epidemie de Strasbourg*, p. 160.

In regard to the condition of the blood after death the historians of the disease are not so well agreed; nevertheless, the preponderance of the testimony is in favor of the statement that the blood presents appearances resembling those belonging to the continued fevers rather than to the inflammations. It is true that even in this the agreement is neither general nor complete. Tourdes, for example, states that in an autopsy "the blood was remarkable for the abundance and toughness of the fibrinous clots," but the greater number have reported it as being dark and liquid. Such was its condition in the epidemic which we studied at the Philadelphia Hospital in 1866-67, and it has been correctly described by Dr. Githens as follows: "The blood was fluid, of the color and appearance of port-wine lees; under the microscope the corpuscles were shrivelled and crenated, and there was a space apparent between them as they were arranged in rouleaux. There were in two cases white, firm, fibrinous heart-clots extending through both ventricles and auricles and into the vessels leading to and from the heart."[56] It may be added that the red corpuscles are often crenated and shrivelled when the case has been protracted, and it has been stated—from limited observation, indeed—that "the white corpuscles are three times more numerous than the red."[57] The blood has been scrutinized to discover, if possible, some of those bodies which are judged by Koch and his disciples to differentiate [p. 826]general diseases, but it is stated that the investigation has been without definite result.[58]

[56] *Amer. Jour. of Med. Sci.*, July, 1867, p. 23.
[57] *Dublin Quart. Jour.*, May, 1867, p. 441.
[58] Jaffé, *Phila. Med. Times*, xii. 599.

It does not seem difficult to reconcile the conflicting statements now given of the condition of the blood in epidemic meningitis. One of them points to an excess and the other to a loss of the spontaneously coagulable element of the blood. It is evident that venesection, which was necessary for procuring the living blood for analysis, would only be performed when the type of the disease authorized it—that is, when the type was sthenic; whereas the blood examined after death had necessarily undergone changes which tended to, if they did not actually, occasion death. Hence we find among the former cases, when fatal, the most extensive and massive exudation, and always among the latter less evidence of inflammation, but, on the other hand, a greater or less manifestation of those appearances which denote a loss of the vitality and organization of the blood. In the one case death may fairly be attributed, above all other causes, to the pressure upon, and the disorganization of, the cerebro-spinal organs essential to life; in the other, primarily, to the death of the vital elements of the blood produced by the specific cause of the disease. It is probable that the post-mortem fluidity of the blood exists under two conditions. In the one the morbid cause is powerful enough from the very commencement rapidly to destroy the life of that fluid, and in the other it acts less violently, but continuously, to exhaust the powers of life.

Our conception of the pathology of epidemic meningitis is implicitly contained in the foregoing discussion. Of its essential cause and of the conditions that call it into existence nothing whatever is known. The disease is most probably due to some atmospheric agency that is capable of acting at the same time upon widely separated localities. Its specific cause appears to enter the blood first of all, and doubtless through the lungs, and to be capable of destroying life by its action upon the blood alone. Failing this effect, its force is spent upon the cerebro-spinal pia mater, and it may become fatal by the mechanical interference of the products of inflammation with the nutrition of those parts of the central nervous system which are essential to life. An inflammatory and a septic element together constitute the fully-developed disease; either may be in excess and overshadow the other. According to the relative predominance of one or the other, the disease assumes more of a typhoid or more of an inflammatory type, and it is doubtless this diversity in its physiognomy, as well as in the lesions that attend it, which has led to the most opposite doctrines respecting its nature and its nosological affinities.

DIAGNOSIS.—The most distinctive phenomena of epidemic meningitis are suddenness of attack and rapidity of development of the following symptoms: acute pain in the head, neck, spine, and limbs; faintness, vomiting; stiffness or spasm of the cervical or spinal muscles; hyperæsthesia of the skin; delirium, alternating with intelligence and merging afterward into dulness or coma; occasional convulsive spasms; paralysis of the face or of one side of the body. The evidences of associated blood-poisoning are, the epidemic prevalence of the disease, various eruptions upon the skin (herpes, roseola, petechiæ, etc.), ecchymoses, debility out of proportion to the evidences of local disease, redness of the eyes, [p. 827]foulness of the tongue and mouth, and more or less of the other conditions which characterize the typhoid state. To these features must be added the rate of mortality, which is greater in most epidemics of meningitis than that of any disease with which it is liable to be confounded.

It is distinguished from sporadic meningitis by the fact that the latter disease is never primary, but is always either an epiphenomenon of some other and previous malady (various fevers and chronic blood diseases) or is traumatic in its origin. The thermometer readily distinguishes it from various functional nervous affections, chiefly hysterical, in which the temperature remains normal.

From typhoid fever it differs as widely as possible by its rapid onset, the exquisite pain in the head, the neuralgic pains, the opisthotonos, and the convulsions. The alternate delirium or coma and clearness of mind in meningitis contrast with the persistent hebetude, stupor, or muttering delirium and the muscular relaxation in typhoid fever. The sordes on the tongue, the diarrhoea, the meteorism, the intestinal hemorrhage of the latter, instead of the moist or merely dry tongue and the transient vomiting and torpid bowels of the former; high or continuous fever on the one hand, slight or variable increase of temperature on the other; diffluence of blood in the one and an increase in the proportion of its fibrin in the other; in the one suppurative inflammation of the cerebro-spinal meninges, in the other specific lesions of the intestinal and mesenteric glands,—these, as well as the very different modes of origin of the two affections, draw a broad and manifest line of distinction between them.

It would scarcely be necessary to point out the contrasts between epidemic meningitis and typhus fever were it not that, notwithstanding the abundance of instruction on the subject in medical treatises and lectures, a large number of physicians confound typhus fever, typhoid fever, and the typhoid state of inflammatory diseases with one another. The confusion was intensified at one time by designating the disease we are studying as spotted fever—a term originally applied and properly belonging to typhus fever (typhus petechialis). It is true that New England physicians soon became aware of their error, which was distinctly pointed out and condemned by North, Strong, Miner, Foot, Fish, and others in the early part of this century. A similar error was at first committed both in Ireland and England, but was corrected by maturer experience. In order to contrast the two diseases as strongly as possible, we place their distinctive features side by side in the following table:

[p. 828]

EPIDEMIC MENINGITIS.	TYPHUS FEVER.
A pandemic disease. Occurs simultaneously in places remote from one another and without intercommunication.	An endemic disease, due to local causes and spreading by intercommunication.
Attacks all classes of society. Is never primarily developed by destitution, squalor, or defective ventilation.	Attacks the poor, filthy, and crowded alone.
Is not contagious.	Contagious in a high degree.
Attacks more males than females.	Both sexes equally affected.
Attacks more young persons than adults.	More adults than young persons.
Generally occurs in winter.	Epidemics irrespective of season.
Eruptions are absent in at least half of the cases; they occur within the first day or two.	Eruption rarely absent, and appears about the fifth day.
The eruptions are various; they include erythema, roseola, urticaria, herpes, etc. Ecchymoses are common.	Eruption always roseolous, and then petechial. Ecchymoses are rare.
Headache is acute, agonizing, tensive.	Headache dull and heavy.
Delirium often absent; often hysterical, sometimes vivacious, sometimes maniacal. Generally begins on the first or second day.	Delirium rarely absent; usually muttering. Rarely begins before the end of the first week.
Pulse very often not above the natural rate; often preternaturally frequent or infrequent. Is subject to sudden and great variations.	A slow pulse exceedingly rare. Its rate usually between 90 and 120.
"The temperature is lower than that recorded in any other typhoid or inflammatory disease." It is also very fluctuating.	The temperature is always elevated, and does not fall until the close of the attack. "The skin is hot, burning, and pungent to the feel."

The body has no peculiar smell.	The mouse-like smell is characteristic.
The tongue is generally moist and soft, and if dry is not foul. Sordes on teeth rare.	The tongue is generally dry, hard, and brown, and the teeth and gums fuliginous.
Vomiting is an almost constant and urgent symptom, especially in the first stage.	Vomiting is rare and not urgent.
Pains in the spine and limbs of a sharp and lancinating character are usual.	The pains, if any, are dull, and apparently muscular.
Tetanic spasms occur in a large proportion of cases and within the first two or three days. They are due to an exudation on the medulla oblongata and spinalis.	Tetanic spasms are unknown in typhus. Convulsions sometimes occur, due to pyæmia.
Cutaneous hyperæsthesia is a prominent symptom.	The sensibility of the skin is generally blunted.
Strabismus is common.	Strabismus is rare.
The eyes, if injected, have a light red or pinkish color.	The blood in the conjunctival vessels is dark.
The pupils are often variable and unequal.	The pupils are equal and contracted.
Deafness and blindness are often complete and permanent.	Deafness almost always ceases with convalescence. Blindness never follows typhus.
Duration very indefinite, but generally from four to seven days.	Duration from twelve to fourteen days.
Relapses are common.	Relapses are rare.
The blood is often fibrinous.	The blood is never fibrinous.
The lesions, except in the most rapid cases, consist of a plastic or purulent exudation in the meshes of the cerebro-spinal pia mater.	In typhus no inflammatory lesions exist.
Mortality from 20 to 75 per cent.	Mortality from 8 to 40 per cent.

PROGNOSIS.—In the section relating to the mortality of epidemic meningitis it has been seen that its death-rate varies at different times and places between widely remote extremes. This fact must be borne in mind in estimating the influence of various circumstances in controlling the issue of the disease. The relative as well as the aggregate mortality is far greater in childhood than in adult life. After the age of thirty or thirty-five it decreases rapidly until old age, when recovery from the disease is quite exceptional. A sudden or rapidly developed attack is generally unfavorable, especially when the symptoms are adynamic and there is a purplish discoloration of the skin. Indeed, even apart from evidences [p. 829]of blood-change, cerebral are, on the whole, of graver importance than spinal phenomena, and the more so the more typhoidal their type. Of still more serious significance is a want of perception of the gravity of the situation or unconcern about its issue. A preternaturally slow and compressible pulse implies danger, and so does coolness of the skin, especially if it grows purplish from a diffusion of blood beneath it or even from venous stasis. The various eruptions that have been described including petechiæ, are not necessarily dangerous signs. Profuse sweats during a soporose state, bullæ and gangrenous spots, obstruction of the bronchia with mucus or serum, pneumonia or pericarditis,—these are all grave indications. So, too, are a dry, fissured, shrivelled, and pale tongue or a fuliginous state of the mouth, swelling of the parotids, obstinate vomiting, and profuse diarrhoea at an advanced stage of the disease. Among the most unfavorable nervous symptoms are great restlessness, rigid retraction of the head, spasms of other than the spinal muscles, general convulsions, extensive hyperæsthesia, deep coma, dilatation and insensibility of the pupils or their rapid change from a dilated to a contracted state, retention or incontinence of urine, and all cerebral paralyses, including that of the muscles of deglutition. The favorable indications comprise a general mildness of the symptoms, a moderate loss of strength, a slight degree of pain and muscular stiffness, the absence of petechiæ or vibices (although in many grave epidemics they are of rare occurrence), a desire for food and the ability to digest it. Yet it is imprudent to make an absolute prognosis in any grave case of this disease. Recovery has sometimes occurred when it appeared impossible, and some have died when the period of danger seemed to have passed on the sudden accession of cerebral or spinal nervous symptoms.

TREATMENT.—The difficulties that attend the solution of therapeutical questions regarding diseases which are comparatively regular in their evolution, and are produced by definite causes acting in an intelligible manner, are very numerous and often insuperable. They become multiplied in relation to a disease which, like this one, stands alone in many respects; whose causes, phenomena, and lesions—in a word, whose laws—are specific; and whose varieties of type are as numerous as can be formed by the combination, in a constantly varying proportion, of a special (hypothetical) alteration of the blood, deranging the molecular actions of the economy, and at the same time of an inflammation of the cerebro-spinal meninges, and even of the substance of the great nervous centres. These reasons are sufficient to account for the diverse and often opposite methods of treatment that have been applied to the disease. As in almost all other cases, the methods have consisted in using remedies to counteract certain symptoms—now a stimulant or tonic regimen to combat the debility which conferred the name of "sinking typhus" on the disease; now an antiphlogistic course to allay the inflammation of the brain and spinal marrow denoted by the neuralgic pain and the tetanoid phenomena; and, again, large doses of narcotics to blunt the pain and subdue the spasm. Still other medications have been used with a similar purpose, and some, as we shall see, with more or less theoretical views. It may be said, with Von Ziemssen, "that we are far from having it in our power to decide whether a rational treatment of the symptoms has cured the disease or lessened its mortality;" but a review of the methods [p. 830]that have been employed and their results leads to no doubtful conclusion that some are mischievous and others more or less salutary.

Emetics were among the first medicines used in the treatment of this affection, and were probably suggested by the vomiting which is one of its most constant initial symptoms. But we can readily understand why they failed to afford relief. The vomiting and retching are not gastric symptoms at all, but, as already stated, are due to the irritation of the congestive or inflammatory process at the base of the brain. These medicines may therefore be omitted. The employment of purgatives is even less rational; they debilitate without affording any relief.

Venesection was probably employed as a part of a routine treatment which neither sound reason nor clinical experience justified. It was generally found to fail of its curative purpose, and often induced, especially in young persons, dangerous exhaustion. No better illustration is needed to show that the disease we have been studying is far more than a local inflammation of the cerebro-spinal meninges. On the other hand, local depletion is often of marked utility. Our own experience would lead us to conclude that in the more sthenic cases scarified cups, applied to the nape of the neck and along the cervical vertebræ, are of essential service in mitigating—and generally, indeed, in wholly removing—the neuralgic pains which form so prominent and severe a symptom in many cases of this disease. When any abstraction of blood appears to be contraindicated by the patient's debility, even dry cups will afford him signal relief. Leeches have been applied to the parts mentioned, and over the mastoid processes have sometimes been used with advantage, but their depletory surpasses their revulsive action, and is, so far, injurious. Cold to the head and spine is among the most efficient means of relieving certain symptoms. In the Massachusetts Medical Society's Report of 1810 we read: "Cold water, snow, and ice have been applied to the head when there was violent pain in that part with heat and flushed face, and when there was violent delirium. They afforded great comfort to the patient, and mitigated or removed those important symptoms." It is probable, however, that the value of the remedy is almost entirely restricted to the forming—or at least the early—stage of the attack, when the pain in the head is most intense. Its soothing influence is then very marked, as well as its indirect action in promoting sleep. Heat of head is not an essential condition for its use, for even in the most violent cases it is rarely extreme, and is often entirely wanting. Pain calls more distinctly for the application, and when that symptom has subsided cold is apt to be more annoying than grateful to the patient. Cold is best applied to the head in the form of pounded ice enclosed in a bladder or rubber bag; but cold affusions are also very valuable, especially for children. For the application of cold to the spine the most efficient apparatus is the long, flat rubber bag, either single or double.

From the earliest history of epidemic meningitis in this country blisters formed a conspicuous element in the treatment. They were used, as they had been in other forms of meningitis, to relieve the pain and diminish the congestion in the cerebro-spinal centres. The results of their use were by no means uniform, for not only were they employed in many of the cases which must almost necessarily have been fatal before inflammation could be established, but even in the inflammatory cases [p. 831]they were often applied when time enough had elapsed to allow the exudation to be fully formed, and when, therefore, they were too late to be useful. Again, they were sometimes used so as to vesicate too deeply, and thus by the pain they caused at first, and by the exhaustion that resulted from the excessive discharges they maintained, the patient was more injured than benefited. Our own experience proves that in the early stage of the inflammatory form of the disease blisters applied below the occipital ridge and upon the back of the neck, and only allowed to vesicate superficially, not only remove the pain in the head, but diminish the delirium, spasms, and coma, and therefore contribute as directly as other remedies, if not more so, to the favorable issue of the attack. But such salutary effects are not to be looked for when the disease assumes a malignant type nor after its constitution has become definitely fixed. The application of stimulant and even vesicating agents to the spine below the neck has not been generally practised because, probably, the seat of the spinal lesions was known to be chiefly at the upper part of the organ. Still, the neuralgic pains felt in the spinal nerves may be mitigated by stimulant and anodyne liniments applied with friction to the spinal column.

American physicians early recognized coolness of the skin among the most striking phenomena of the disease; and this probably suggested their use of diaphoretic remedies, among which were the external application of moist heat in baths and warm wrappings, as well as "bottles of hot water or billets of wood heated in boiling water and wrapped in flannel," or the patient "was wrapped in flannel wrung out of boiling water, sinapisms were applied to the feet, while hot infusions were administered, made from the leaves of mint, pennyroyal, and other similar plants, and also wine-whey, wine and water, wine, brandy, and other ardent spirits more or less diluted, camphor, sulphuric ether, and opium. It was not generally thought useful to excite profuse sweating, but important to maintain the activity of the skin from twenty to forty hours, and even longer in some instances. Soup and cordials were at the same time administered. Under this treatment most commonly the violent symptoms, and not very rarely all the appearances of disease, have subsided" (Jackson). Beyond all doubt, this method was a rational one, for it tended to promote an elimination of the morbid poison, while it depleted the blood-vessels and acted revulsively upon the local inflammation of the cerebro-spinal meninges. Yet it seems not to have been revived during the more recent epidemics of the disease, unless, partially, by Gordon (1867), who says:

"What I have seen most useful in the stage of collapse is external warmth applied to the entire surface by means of flannel bags containing roasted salt, applied along the spine, along the chest, inside the arms, and to the feet and legs and between them."

Except typhus fever, there is no disease in which a due administration of alcoholic stimulants may become more important. In cases of the inflammatory type they are rarely needful, and are frequently hurtful, but in those which exhibit signs of blood disorder with nervous exhaustion they are often indispensable. Nothing demonstrates their necessity more clearly than the extraordinary tolerance of alcohol exhibited in some cases of the disease. Among the earlier American authorities may be found many illustrations of this statement. Woodward (1808) [p. 832]observed that very large quantities of wine or ardent spirits may be given without injury. Arnell said: "In some cases I have given a quart of brandy in six or eight hours with the happiest effect." Haskell maintained that "the bold and liberal use of diffusible stimuli is the only safe and efficacious mode of treatment." In Ireland the habitual use of alcohol in the treatment of typhus fever no doubt suggested its liberal employment in this disease, but such stimulants have never been in vogue among the physicians of France or Germany. This difference may in part be accounted for by the generally asthenic type of the disease in the first-named country and its more inflammatory character in the others. Similar contrasts of type mark different epidemics, and individual cases during the same epidemic. We have no doubt that while these agents are indispensable in the treatment of cases of the former type, they must even then be exhibited discreetly, for their too lavish exhibition entails the gravest peril by intoxicating the patients and oppressing instead of arousing their vital energies. In 1866, on taking charge of the medical wards in the Philadelphia Hospital, we found that the patients were using as large quantities of alcohol as are given in typhus fever, but a very short period of observation showed that this use of the stimulant was excessive; consequently the dose of it was first reduced, and finally it was omitted altogether unless special indications for it arose. This change was followed by a manifest improvement in the general aspect of the sick and the subsidence of symptoms which, it then became evident, were due to a lavish use of stimulants rather than to the gravity of the disease. Alcohol is no more essential to the treatment of epidemic meningitis than of any other acute affection; it is a cordial to be held in reserve to meet those signs of failure of the heart and nervous system which may arise in all acute diseases attended with changes in the condition of the blood.

The use of opium in the treatment of this disease was strongly advocated by nearly all of the early American writers upon the subject, and by many of them enormous doses were given. It was observed not to produce narcotic effects in ordinary doses. In one case, marked by excruciating pain in the head and maniacal delirium, sixty drops of laudanum were given every hour until nearly half an ounce had been taken within eight hours (Strong). Haskell states: "We have been obliged frequently to exhibit ten grains of opium for a dose in some of the violent cases attended with strong spasms, and have never known it to produce stupor in a single instance." Miner relates that "a few cases imperiously required half an ounce of the tincture of opium in an hour, or half a drachm [of opium] in substance in the course of twelve hours, before the urgent symptoms could be controlled, and even some cases required a drachm in the same time. All these patients recovered." In Europe, Chauffard administered opium in doses of from three to fifteen grains, and Boudin frequently prescribed from seven to fifteen grains at a single dose at the commencement of the attack, and subsequently one or two grains every half hour, until the patient grew sleepy or his symptoms subsided. This tolerance of the drug is remarkable, and so is the fact that it does not cause constipation. These and many similar statements agree entirely with our personal experience. We were in the habit, during the epidemic above referred to, of prescribing one grain [p. 833]of opium every hour in very severe and every two hours in moderately severe cases, and in no instance was narcotism induced, or even an approach to that condition. Under the influence of the medicine the pain and spasm subsided, the skin grew warmer and the pulse fuller, and the entire condition of the patient more hopeful. It seemed probable, however, that the benefit of the opium treatment was most decided in the early stages of the attack, and hence in those in which the inflammatory and spasmodic elements predominated. The hypodermic injection of morphia is to be preferred before the internal administration of other preparations of opium, not only on account of its prompter action, but because it avoids the rejection of the medicine by vomiting. On the whole, Von Ziemssen is within the bounds of truth when he says, "Beyond all doubt morphia may be considered the most indispensable medicine in the treatment of epidemic meningitis."

There is no evidence sufficient to show that epidemic meningitis has ever been cured by quinia alone. In the early prevalence of the disease it was treated by large doses of cinchona, but unavailingly, and subsequently smaller doses were given during the convalescence, as it was in that of other acute diseases. In some parts of this country where miasmatic diseases prevail, and epidemic meningitis, like all other acute, and especially febrile, disorders, displayed more or less of a periodical or paroxysmal type, quinia was used in large doses, but the expected result was not realized. Upham states that in some instances it was given to the extent of sixty, or even eighty, grains within twelve hours from the beginning of the attack, but without effect. In Europe it was extensively tried and unanimously condemned. It may very properly be left out of the list of medicines suitable for this disease, particularly since it is no longer probable that any physician would be rash enough to employ it in the so-called antipyretic doses with or without their usual associates, cold baths. According to Karl Jaffé, the medicinal antipyretics (quinia, salicylic acid, and also sodium benzoate) may be entirely discarded, because they ruin the already weakened digestion.[59]

[59] *Phila. Med. Times*, xii. 600.

Common sense has also proved stronger than theory in excluding mercurials from the treatment of epidemic meningitis. At one time they were extensively used, especially when it was learned that the disease in its full development included a paramount inflammatory element. But it was soon found that the results of their use were far from uniform, and farther still from being demonstrably beneficial. In this, as in many other similar cases, it is quite impossible to reach a definite judgment unless it were known what was the type of the cases in which the medicine was given, whether they were asthenic or inflammatory, and again whether it was used during the active or during the declining stage and toward convalescence. In the absence of any trustworthy testimony upon the subject it is only possible at present to state that in the treatment of this disease mercurials should not be used. This conclusion is all the more imperative because the medicine is not an indifferent one. If it is not necessary—and it certainly is not—it is too dangerous in its immediate and ultimate effects for its employment to be warranted.

Since belladonna and ergot were shown to diminish vascular action in the cerebro-spinal axis by contracting its capillary blood-vessels, they have[p. 834]been put forward as having a specific virtue in this disease. If the fact be so, how is that other fact—a clinical one, moreover—to be disposed of, which is that opium, the physiological antagonist of belladonna and ergot, is more efficient than they are in curing the disease? It is possible, indeed, that they may have that curative power, and that opium possesses it also, and that the explanation given of the action of all of these agents is erroneous. Upham states that, in 1863, Haddock recommended ergot upon theoretical grounds, and that during an epidemic at Newbern, N.C., several cases treated by it recovered. Three cases recovered in which it was prescribed by Borland. Read used it in 1873-74 at Boston, Mass., and out of 19 cases 16 recovered and 3 died.[60] This mortality of about 15 per cent. is not more than half of that which has generally been met with, and if it can be attributed to the treatment would go far to prove the efficacy of the latter. One grain of ergotine, with one-tenth of a grain of extract of belladonna, was administered every three hours. Considering the exiguity of the dose of belladonna, it is not surprising that, except in one case, it did not dilate the pupil; and the dose of ergotine is likewise far smaller than the average medicinal dose of that preparation. Moreover, all of the cases except the fatal ones appear to have presented the disease in a subacute, and certainly not in an aggravated, form.

[60] *Philadelphia Med. and Surg. Reporter*, Jan., 1875, p. 68.

In 1872, Dr. S. N. Davis,[61] moved by the success of Calabar bean in tetanus, employed it in this disease. A mixture of one ounce of tincture of Calabar bean with one and a half ounces of fluid extract of ergot was administered in doses of half a teaspoonful every two hours, and with better results than had followed other remedies. Here, again, it is to be noticed that the analogy suggesting the use of physostigma is not a logical one. That drug indeed relieves the spinal spasms of tetanus—a disease in which there is an irritation of the spinal axis, but no exudation from its meningeal vessels, as in the affection we are studying. Moreover, it is a disease of extraordinary power, as shown not only by the spasms, but by the exceptionally high temperature, and thus again is in direct contrast to epidemic meningitis. If, therefore, Calabar bean benefits that disease, it cannot do so in the manner suggested by the author.

[61] *Richmond and Louisville Med. Jour.*, xiii. 711.

Bromide of potassium and hydrate of chloral have also been employed to allay the spasmodic symptoms; but the former is too feeble for the purpose, and the depressing action of the latter upon the heart renders it dangerous. Bromide of potassium has been given to children of two and five years in doses of four and six grains every two hours; but these doses appear to be quite too small even for the purpose in view—viz. to prevent convulsive attacks. Whatever remedies may be suggested hereafter, none should be employed that tend to reduce the power of the heart, which, as we have seen, is dangerously depressed by the disease.

During the decline and convalescence of the affection it is probable that iodide of potassium may be advantageously used to promote the removal of the exudation-matter on the brain and spinal marrow, and probably to prevent the hydrocephalus which sometimes follows the attack, and is attributable to the pressure of effused lymph upon the cerebral veins.

DIET.—The mildly febrile character of epidemic meningitis, and the[p. 835]remarkable debility which characterizes so many cases of the disease, and which, as was before pointed out, conferred upon it the name typhus syncopalis, plainly justify what experience has taught, that appropriate food for the subjects of this affection is at once the most digestible and nutritious that can be taken. It is true that this regimen is interfered with by the vomiting, but, as that symptom is of cerebral and not of gastric origin, it is more apt to be allayed by suitable food than by abstinence. It has been our custom to observe in this disease the same rules respecting diet that are recognized as the most suitable in typhus fever. In doing so, indeed, we did, without at the time knowing it, follow the example of the early American physicians. Strong, who wrote in 1811, advised "soup made from chicken, veal, mutton, and beef, richly seasoned with pepper and savory herbs." These articles were prescribed by him during the height of the disease. Later on he says: "The stomach soon begins to crave something more solid than soup; oysters, beefsteak, cold ham, or neat's tongue are received with peculiar relish. Often I have seen convalescents, when they had hardly strength enough to raise themselves in bed, make a hearty meal of the above-mentioned articles, which were received with great satisfaction, sat well upon the stomach, and were well digested and assimilated." This method is substantially the same that was found successful in the earlier, as it has been in the later, epidemics in this country, and we have no hesitation in attributing to it and the appropriate use of opium and blisters the degree of success we enjoyed in the treatment of the disease in the Philadelphia Hospital and elsewhere.

During convalescence from epidemic meningitis the patient should carefully abstain from physical exertion and mental excitement, and before this state is fully established he should even very cautiously change his position from a recumbent to an erect posture. And, finally, he should return to his ordinary occupations, mental or physical, as late as possible, on account of the danger of a relapse, which has already been described.

[p. 836]

PERTUSSIS.
BY JOHN M. KEATING, M.D.

HISTORY.—A careful study of this disease from the various writings since the time of Hippocrates leaves little doubt in the mind of the reader as to its antiquity, so little indeed has it changed in its various characteristics. Whether the affection passed to continental Europe from Africa, or whether its starting-point was India, are questions difficult to solve, and, except for the medical historian, of little import. Desruelles probably truthfully asserts that the many differences which mark the descriptions of the disease, especially by the early Grecian writers, may be due, not to the non-existence of the disease as we know it, but to the influence which climate exerted then as now, and to the unrecognized fact that it is only fatal in its complications. The writings of Hippocrates, Galen, and Avicenna, though undoubtedly referring to the many affections in which paroxysmal cough is a prominent symptom, contain many expressions that would point clearly to the existence of a specific disease. Dr. Watt believed that the disease was not known to the Greeks, and other writers claim that it came from the north and spread southward over Europe about the sixth century; nevertheless, it first appears on record as a distinct affection, disentangled from the confused mass with which it was involved for centuries, about the middle of the seventeenth century. Steffen mentions the first well-established accounts as coming from Baillou in the year 1600, and Schenck in 1650, and Ettmüller in 1685. Sydenham casually mentions it in 1670. Since the time of Willis the definition of the disease has remained unaltered, and so accurate was the description then given of it that we can but naturally conclude that for many centuries at least it has varied but little.

In studying affections of this kind, occurring in epidemic form especially, and which are increased in intensity by whatever means the contagious element, whether gaseous or parasitic, is made more virulent, much allowance is to be made for the climate, customs, and habits of the people whence our data are derived. Thus, most of the diseases of antiquity, the descriptions of which have reached us, have been drawn from types modified by mild climates where the people have led an out-door life, and though the disease we see at the present day is one and the same so far as its causation is concerned, the indoor life and close confinement, the bad ventilation, and the artificial existence in our large cities must weaken the individual, intensify the poison, and exert an influence on the disease.

DEFINITION AND DESCRIPTION.—Whooping cough has been[p. 837]characterized as an acute contagious affection, occurring usually in childhood, though it may occur at any age, and lasting several weeks. It is manifested usually by malaise, catarrh of the respiratory tract, and subsequently by a convulsive cough occurring in paroxysms, the peculiarity of which consists of a series of forcible expirations, followed by a sonorous inspiration or whoop, which may be repeated several times.

At the beginning of these paroxysms of coughing, there are evidences of slight laryngeal irritation, attended by an effort at suppressing the cough; then follow gradually increasing and more audible inspirations, which become more and more difficult. The child is agitated, the face becomes pale, and the countenance has a mingled expression of supplication and fear. If it is old enough it will seize the nearest object for support. As the spell advances, the eyes become suffused and prominent and the loose tissue surrounding the orbits appears puffy and congested. Finally, the paroxysm reaches its height; the child, with a livid countenance, with veins standing out like cords, gives a succession of violent expiratory efforts, followed by a long inspiratory whoop. The same is repeated several times, until finally almost complete cyanosis takes place; the spasm relaxes, a glairy, tenacious mucus runs from the mouth, the contents of the stomach are vomited, and the child falls back exhausted. The lividity of the countenance is succeeded by a deathly pallor; the face still appears swollen and puffy beneath the eyes; the tears course down the cheeks, and frequently hemorrhage occurs from the eyes, nose, ears, or throat, owing to the terrific strain upon the circulation. As soon as the child has recovered from the fatigue of the paroxysm all is apparently over, and were it not for the characteristic expression of the eye, which is pathognomonic in a well-advanced case, nothing would be noticed to even suggest the disease when uncomplicated. The voice is clear; there is little or no elevation of temperature.

The paroxysms which have given the name to this disease can only be likened to an epileptic convulsion, which by gradually increasing cyanosis is self-curable, the carbonized blood finally bringing about an anæsthetic effect. The severity of the paroxysms is by no means in proportion to the local catarrh, which latter may be superficial and slight, not to be detected during life by the most careful laryngeal examinations, and only after death by the aid of the microscope. The frequency and intensity of the paroxysms are dependent in a measure upon the degree of excitability of the nervous system, which of course differs in individuals. It is evident that the success of treatment must be powerfully influenced by this circumstance, and it is partly owing to it that there are so many opinions as to the value of remedies in this disease.

The complications are usually dependent upon outside causes, and have nothing to do with the poison proper of whooping cough, as far as we can tell. There are some which depend on an inflammation of the mucous membrane, which may be limited to any portion of the respiratory tract or may extend throughout it. Complications may arise from mechanical obstruction to inspiration by the swollen mucous membrane or from plugs of tenacious mucus, which may cause pulmonary collapse and favor the development of catarrhal pneumonia, and later even of phthisis; or from impediments to free and easy expiration, whether from spasm of the bronchioles, from forcible compression of the thorax through reflex[p. 838]nervous irritation, or from other obstructions, all of which tend to produce emphysema. Disturbances of the circulation, in the brain or elsewhere, may proceed from thrombi or emboli and give rise to complications which will render fatal an otherwise mild form of the disease. The invariable disturbance of nutrition which accompanies every disease affecting the nervous system is apt to show itself in the breaking down of products which are simply inflammatory. Vomiting may be a most serious complication, both from its immediate and remote effects. It may be due to gastric catarrh, or more frequently to irritation of the pneumogastric nerve.

ETIOLOGY.—Very numerous theories have been advanced as to the nature of this interesting disease. Hufeland, Lebenstein, Pinel, Jahn, Todd, Cullen and a host of others have regarded it as essentially a neurosis. By many others it has been supposed to be due to a lesion of the brain or of its membranes, but careful investigation has established the fact that there is no lesion in whooping cough at all constant or characteristic. By still others, and especially by Gueneau de Mussy, it has been regarded as essentially an affection of the tracheo-bronchial glands, a bronchial adenopathy, causing irritation of the pneumogastrics and of their bronchial branches by pressure of the enlarged glands. We have, however, seen many post-mortem examinations of the bodies of children who have died of measles, where marked enlargement of these glands was constantly found, but where no symptoms of whooping cough had been present. There are indeed many features of the disease which seem inexplicable on any other theory than that the essential cause of whooping cough is a specific poison, and such is the view now generally adopted. This poison is capable of being carried by fomites, though as it is highly infectious it is often communicated through the atmosphere, and is most frequently conveyed from individual to individual. Dolan,[1] who has recently published a very interesting and valuable monograph on this affection, quotes Linnæus, who ascribed it to the irritation of insects, as the author of the modern view that whooping cough is due to the presence of a peculiar microbe, though it must be conceded that as yet it has not been discovered. Most observers hold that the contagium is not in the blood, but that it resides in the secretions of the respiratory passages, and is most virulent during that stage of the disease when the secretion is abundant. Letzerich states that he has [p. 839]succeeded in producing whooping cough in rabbits by inoculating the trachea with the sputa of the human subject. Dolan obtained similar results by injecting the nasal secretions, and also by compelling rabbits to inhale air impregnated with decomposing sputa and vomit of patients suffering with the disease.

[1] Dolan, Thos. M., *Whooping Cough*, London, 1882.

The following brief statement of his conclusions may be quoted as presenting the most important facts concerning the pathology of the disease:

1st. Pertussis depends on a specific poison or contagion; this is universally admitted.

2d. This contagion is active and highly infectious; this is also granted.

3d. The contagion is analogous to the contagia which produce splenic fever, measles, scarlatina, variola, etc.

4th. It has a peculiar determination to the lungs.

5th. Like all other contagia, it has its period of activity and decline.

6th. The period of greatest activity is in the first and second stages.

7th. Pertussis runs a regular course like measles, scarlatina, variola, etc., and rarely attacks a person but once.

8th. It may thus be classed among zymotic diseases.

9th. The fact that there is no primary pathognomonic morbid change supports this view.

10th. There are various secondary lesions which are characteristic, as ulcerations of the frænum linguæ.

11th. The mode of death harmonizes with this view.

I do not, however, feel entirely satisfied in adopting the view that the contagium of whooping cough resides alone in the mucous membranes of the air-passages.[2] Children have been known to be born with the disease, the mother having suffered from it some time previous to confinement. The following case occurred under my own observation: Mrs. F———, the mother of two children, was in her eighth month of pregnancy; the two children had at the time a very severe attack of whooping cough, which required the constant attendance of the mother. She, though an extremely intelligent woman, belonged to the poorer classes, and had no one to assist her at this trying time. One day she complained that the movements of her child in utero had entirely changed. Suddenly, without any previous motion, the child would become very active; the force of its movements was such as to make hazardous any attempt on her part to walk in the street. The suddenness with which the movement would come on would oblige her to seize the nearest object for support. This continued until the child was born. Shortly after labor my attention was called to the infant, which had a curious attack, it became deeply cyanosed, seemed asphyxiated, as it were, for a moment, had no convulsions, and within a few seconds resumed its normal breathing and the circulation seemed once more established. I saw the child in several of these attacks; its health did not seem to be impaired, and without treatment, within a few weeks they disappeared altogether. The mother insisted upon the fact that the child had whooping cough, and the absence of the characteristic whoop was the only thing that prevented the diagnosis from being positive. This would show—and there are enough cases on record to warrant our basing an opinion upon them—that the contagium of whooping cough is found not alone in the matters expectorated, notwithstanding the statement of Dolan and others that their experiments failed to show its existence in the blood.

[2] Colson, *Lancet*, July 2d.

It must not be forgotten, in reference to cases which seem to have arisen without any exposure to the specific poison, that the characteristic whoop is not always present, and that consequently the true nature of mild cases of the disease which may infect other individuals may have been overlooked. Childhood probably acts as a predisposing cause, though the disease occurs at all periods of life, and as it usually occurs but once in the same individual, it is clear that the apparent diminution of susceptibility in later years may be largely due to the fact that most persons have had the disease in childhood. More children are attacked from one to five years, and the disease is more prevalent in summer and fall months. Causes which, like exposure to inclement weather, give rise to irritation of the bronchial mucous membrane, or diseases which, as measles, are accompanied with catarrhal symptoms and susceptibility of the bronchial mucous membrane, also may serve as predisposing causes. Sex appears to exert some positive influence. Of 360 cases of pertussis by Dessau,[3] the total number of males were 154, that of females 206. Girls are more[p. 840]frequently attacked than boys, in proportion of 2 to 1.50; this seems true at all ages; this statement is substantiated by Unruh of Dresden, based on an analysis of 1952 cases.

[3] *N.Y. Jour. of Obst.*, 1881, xiv. 490-503.

SYMPTOMS.—The disease begins usually with an ordinary catarrh, preceded by malaise and slight laryngeal irritation, which may be overlooked; in fact, during the first stage there is nothing to attract special attention, unless a direct history of exposure be known and suspicion be aroused on that account. Meigs and Pepper state that the earliest period at which they have known the distinctive whoop of the disease was three days, though in a great many instances it was delayed as late as three weeks. The same authors state that the ordinary duration of a paroxysm or kink is from one-fourth to three-fourths of a minute. They mention a case where the paroxysm lasted fifty-five minutes. Ordinarily they number about thirty-five or forty during the twenty-four hours at the height of the disease, differing greatly in individuals. Their number is most frequent in the course of the third or fourth week, after which they remain stationary, and then gradually decline. The paroxysms may occur spontaneously, or they may follow some irritation, either direct or reflex, or they may be induced by nervous excitement. Toward the end of the attack, after the catarrhal irritation has greatly subsided, or in fact has entirely disappeared, the paroxysmal kinks may be provoked by irritation of the fauces, and also by nervous excitement; and there is no question but that at this time they can be controlled by will-power. In many cases a distinct relapse occurs after the disease has been apparently cured.

Dolan believes the phenomena of the cough or kinks to be due, as suggested by Laennec, to a "spasmodic condition of the muscular or contractile fibres of the bronchi and their branches." He remarks that the lungs are supplied from the anterior and posterior pulmonary plexuses, formed chiefly of branches from the sympathetic and pneumogastrics. The filaments from these accompany the bronchial tubes upon which they are lost. Irritation of these nerves is said to have the effect of producing contractions of the bronchial canals sufficient to expel a certain quantity of air. If this theory is true, it helps us in explaining why the large, mediate, and smaller bronchi are closed during the expiratory stage of the paroxysmal cough of pertussis. The general opinion seems to be that the pneumogastric nerve is not inflamed, as has been asserted by some.

The highly sensitive condition of the nervous system, which is probably in a great measure intensified by the anæmia, and by the interference with nutrition due to the disturbance of the circulation by the cough, will show itself in many ways, and even when no secondary nervous affections complicate the attack or follow it. Some time will elapse after the disease has passed away before the child will recover its self-control, or its nutrition will show the influence of a healthy nervous system. The total duration of the affection is said to vary from six weeks to three months in ordinary cases; though probably, if active treatment could be instituted early enough and kept up with thoroughness, there is no specific disease more capable of being shortened in its course than the one under consideration; this remains, however, for future statistics to decide.

During the second stage of the disease the symptoms are sufficiently[p. 841]marked to attract attention and render a diagnosis easy to make. Frequently the catarrh seems to extend to the bronchioles, and gives rise to symptoms that are alarming; and the intensity of the paroxysm will cause the engorgement of the blood-vessels to get relief in profuse hemorrhage; this is the period for caution. Complications may arise, the strength may fail, the secretions may become too abundant, and asphyxia may ensue; emphysema may show itself, or catarrhal pneumonia may gradually supervene.

The period of decline is very gradual; the secretions become less in quantity and more viscid, the paroxysmal cough is less frequent, but may at times be equally severe, the child's strength is usually exhausted, and its nutrition is greatly impaired. The expected paroxysm throws it into a state of intense nervous excitement; it is sleepless—in fact, worn out. Probably at this period of the disease treatment will show the most marked results, and the long lists of sedatives, tonics, etc. which are presented to us by their zealous advocates owe much of their popularity to their value at this stage of the disease. The catarrhal symptoms are the first to subside; the nervous disturbances remain for some time, and gradually fade, and the constitutional symptoms, or those from exhaustion, are the last to leave the patient.

Strange as it may seem, the heart appears to suffer but little in the long run from the great strain upon it; the palpitation and irregularity of its actions are not followed by structural changes as a rule, though we may state that feebleness of the circulation has remained in most of our bad cases for some months after recovery.

As regards the ulceration of the frænum linguæ, which has given rise to so much discussion as to its exact value as a symptom of this disease, our own experience leads us to believe that though it is nearly always present in the severe cases, its almost invariable absence before dentition and in milder cases shows it to be of traumatic origin. Roger's exhaustive report before the French Academy supported this view, and showed how clearly it is caused by the violent rubbing of the frænum on the free border of the incisors. On the other hand, Delthil of Paris and Blake of England believe that it is a pathological feature of the disease. The former reported cases in which it occurred before dentition. The ulcer is not always found on the frænum linguæ, but is found on either side of it. Bouffier noted severe cases of ulceration in children who had no teeth, but he attributed it to the injury produced by the mother in detaching the mucus with the finger.

Examinations of the urine have been carefully made by many observers. The appearance of sugar, about which so much has been said, does not seem to be constant, or even very frequent. Out of 50 cases, Dolan found traces of it in but 13. This coincides with our experience also, for we have frequently tested the urine in seven cases with negative results. Since, as is well known, irritation of the pneumogastric centre may cause glycosuria, it was at one time attempted to show that the paroxysms in whooping cough were due to congestion of the pneumogastric nerves, a condition which is said to have been occasionally found in this disease. Dolan says he has never seen hemorrhage from the kidneys during the course of whooping cough, nor blood in the urine.

MORTALITY.—It is an extremely difficult matter to reach, with any [p. 842] degree of certainty, the true mortality of this affection. Meigs and Pepper say: "Of the 208 cases observed by ourselves, 143 were simple, all of which recovered;" and, again, "Some form of complication occurred in the 65 of the 208 cases observed by ourselves; of these 65, 12 died." The mortality seems greater under five years; thus: Of the 9008 deaths attributed to it in the United States during the census year ending June 1, 1870, the number of persons under one year of age was 4424, and 8396 were under five years. There were 1784 deaths from it recorded in Philadelphia from 1860 to 1876; of this number, 1724 were under five years of age. The census of the United States for 1880 gives a return of 11,102 deaths from this disease.

Females seem more liable to die of it than males; of the 1784 deaths in this city, 766 were males and 1018 females. As we have already seen, females are more liable to the disease than males.

Robt. J. Lee, M.D.,[4] says that from the Registrar-General's report of 1876 it is seen that in a total mortality in England of 510,315, whooping cough was returned as the cause of death in 10,554 cases, or nearly 2 per cent.

[4] In a paper in the *British Med. Jour.*, 1879, vol. i. p. 307.

As for the time of year, we quote the following: "Thus, according to the census statistics, most deaths occur in the spring, there being a rise up to the middle of May. From the middle of May the number lessens largely until August, when a rise occurs and continues until October, when a decline sets in and continues until December, when a rise begins and goes on increasing until the middle of May. This rise in mortality from August to October is attributed to the wear and tear of a hot summer and the intestinal troubles then so prevalent."

The mortality statistics of this disease are uncertain. It is fatal in its complications or by inducing a debilitated condition which invites degenerative processes. The severity of the symptoms is no guide for prognosis as far as uncomplicated cases are concerned, and there is no doubt but that at present we are able to greatly reduce the mortality-rate by care and medical treatment, as well as to shorten the attack. Sporadic cases are apt to be neglected until they become complicated. When the disease occurs in epidemic form, measles is often prevalent simultaneously, and in consequence children who become affected by both diseases have a greater tendency, from debility, to become the victims of those affections of the respiratory organs which are such frequent and fatal complications of both maladies.

Instead of surprise at the mortality of this affection, the marvel is that so large a percentage of recoveries take place, when we consider that we are dealing with a disease whose lesion is a catarrh of the air-passages which seldom lasts less than two months, with a tendency to involve the lungs in one way or another, and then witness the carelessness with which, among the lower classes, the child is often treated—exposed to all weathers, underclothed, under-fed, and probably allowed to pass through the whole attack without medical treatment. Taking this into consideration, the probability is that the mortality of this disease could be reduced to a very small figure by careful management, even if the investigations of those now seeking the microbe of pertussis do not lead to any plan, in accordance with Pasteur's teachings, which will still further lessen the gravity of the disease. Until [p. 843]then, we can but insist upon a rigid quarantine of schools, a registration of all cases, and the seclusion of them, as we have done to-day in the case of variola and scarlatina.

MORBID ANATOMY.—Although whooping cough is a serious disease, the cause of death is generally found to be dependent upon its complications, and there is no lesion at all characteristic of it. The chief complications and sequelæ are—bronchitis, which may become capillary; lobular collapse, which, according to Alderson,[5] is frequently found; emphysema, usually marginal, probably due, as suggested by Jenner, to violent expiratory exertions; rupture of air-vesicles, with subcutaneous emphysema; catarrhal pneumonia, pleurisy, phthisis, acute tuberculosis, croup, cerebral apoplexy, meningitis, etc. As any of these complications, and others which may arise from debility, may be the cause of death, independent of the action of the specific poison itself, it is usual to divide the post-mortem appearances into those that are the result of the extension of the catarrh itself and those produced by the interference with the circulation and with nutrition from mechanical violence. Of the former, the usual causes of death are pneumonia, gastritis and enteritis. Of the latter, we have thrombosis of the cerebral sinuses, hemorrhages, emphysema, and exhaustion following constant vomiting.

[5] *Medico-Chir. Trans.*, pp. 90, 91, 1830.

Tubercular disease of the lungs or of the brain is apt to be a cause of death. Convulsions carried off 5 of the 12 fatal cases reported out of 208 by Meigs and Pepper. This may be due to congestion of the brain, especially in teething children. Spasm of the glottis with sudden death is occasionally found. In such cases there is found intense congestion of the brain, also of the liver and kidneys, and at times of the mucous membrane of the stomach and intestines, as well as of that of the respiratory tract.

In all cases, especially at the teething age, sudden death may occur because effusion into the ventricles of the brain or the formation of heart-clot has taken place. It is important to know this, that active treatment applied early enough may save the patient.

PROPHYLAXIS.—Should the interesting and seemingly conclusive statements of Dolan and the microscopic investigations of Carl Bruger[6] receive the endorsement of future workers, the subject of prophylaxis will assume a degree of importance which hitherto it has only maintained with the medical profession. No one has doubted that the disease was contagious, and yet there is no affection which has attached to it a corresponding fatality that is so carelessly dealt with as pertussis.

[6] Bruger of Bonn, in the *Berliner klinische Wochen.*, describes at length the special micro-organisms of pertussis. They appear as small elongated elliptical bodies of unequal length, the smallest being double as long as broad. High powers show subdivisions in the largest specimens. They are generally isolated, but may appear in groups. They bear some resemblance to *Leptothrix buccalis*, the spores of which are often found in whooping-cough sputa. Occasionally the bacillus is seen inside the mucous corpuscle in the sputum. They stain in the usual way, fuschin and methyl violet. This bacillus is not found in any other kind of sputum, is very abundant in pertussis, and increases in direct proportion to the severity of the disease.

Within the past few days we have heard on two occasions in crowded railway-cars the characteristic paroxysm of the third stage of the disease, and yet people will endeavor to convince themselves that unless contact with the child takes place the danger is little.

[p. 844]The atmosphere in school-rooms, railway-cars, and places of amusement which are badly ventilated, is an excellent medium for the propagation of the contagious matter, and many extraordinary cases are on record of momentary exposure being sufficient to contract the disease. Believing that the contagium or virus resides in the mucus and air thrown off by the child, and also in the vomited matters, which contain a large amount of ropy mucus, and also that it gains entrance by means of the respiratory organs, protection from contagion divides itself as follows: thorough disinfection of the exhaled air, of the mucus remaining within the bronchial tubes and air-passages, and of the clothing, together with exposure to fresh air and thorough cleansing of all furniture and household utensils, including cups, silverware, and toys, used by the child. Oxygen is said to have this effect, and thorough, constant ventilation, with the breathing of fresh air by the child, the thorough washing of its surface, and disinfection of its clothing, are the first indications; while the impregnation of the atmosphere with the spray of well-known germicides by means of the steam or other atomizer and the frequent inhalation of such materials by the patient are no less important. Every case of whooping cough should be compelled to use two or three times daily the spray impregnated with a substance of this sort, either carbolic acid, the oil of eucalyptus, a solution of quinia, or thymol. Chlorine (from chloride of lime) used thus has of late been followed by excellent results, and the spray of a solution of corrosive sublimate or of ammonium chloride has been found very useful. The protective treatment should be applied to those exposed to contagion. Such children should be guarded from exposure to colds; their diet should be simple and nourishing, their clothing warm; they should be kept as much as possible in the open air. The breathing of air impregnated with such substances as above mentioned will no doubt act upon the virus before it comes in contact with the mucous membranes so as to be absorbed, and probably the severity of the attack might be mitigated by modifying the germ of the disease.

TREATMENT.—As can be readily imagined, a disease which is so universal, so distressing, and at the same time so obscure in its pathology, as the one under consideration, would have in its literature a mass of recommendations for treatment from zealous advocates, based upon theory or experience, as numerous as the authors themselves. It would be impossible for us to dwell at length upon all of these, but we will confine ourselves especially to the consideration of a few of the most important. It will be convenient to consider first those remedies which have been used with the view of relieving the congestion and irritability of the respiratory mucous membrane and of promoting more free secretion. It will also be observed that many of these remedies may now be regarded as of value for destroying the special germ which is thought to be the essential cause and real virus of pertussis. Allusion has been made above to the importance of inhalations as a prophylactic for those who have been exposed to the contagion, as well as for the purpose of rendering the secretions less contagious; and so too we find that the inhalation of various substances has received favor with many as a method of treatment. Thus, hyoscyamus, belladonna, ammonium bromide have been used. Helenke and Serbaud say that bromide of [p. 845]potassium is best for inhalation. Letzerich recommended the insufflation of quinia twice daily, using the quinia muriate with potassium bicarbonate and gum-arabic. Forchheimer[7] reports 97 cases of whooping cough treated by the insufflation of the quinia muriate; of the 97 cases, 52 were females, 45 males—the youngest three weeks, the oldest nine years old. Five cases gave no results, while in the others benefit was shown by a shortening or amelioration of the disease. The vapor of benzole has been used with good results. The vapor of carbolic acid has of late been highly recommended, either administered with the atomizer several times daily, or used by saturating flannels in carbolic acid solution and placed around the child's bed at night. It is said that the inhalation of the vapor of a few drops of carbolic acid on some hot coals will ensure a night of freedom from violent coughing. Probably in this way we may account for the belief that proximity to gas-works is beneficial to a child with this disease. As is well known, Niemeyer and others in the north of Germany believed in the value of the inhalation of oxygen, and the experience of every one who has had much to do with this disease favors an out-door life. We may here also mention the value of a small quantity of chloroform or ether, by inhalation, in allaying the severity of the paroxysms of cough. We have also tried the nitrate of amyl, but without marked result.

[7] *New York Jour. Obstet.*, 1882.

Others have recommended the use of solutions of various substances, applied directly by a brush to the interior of the larynx. Quinia has been used in this way also by Hagenbach; but the most satisfactory results have been obtained by the application of very weak solutions of nitrate of silver, as first recommended by Watson in 1849.

After the secretions have been fully established and the characteristic whoop has appeared, the indications in the treatment are to relieve the respiratory tract of its burden by occasional emesis with alum or ipecacuanha, to give freely antispasmodics and sedatives, as belladonna, chloral, the bromides, hydrobromic acid, or, as recommended by some, digitalis; to give quinia freely, and to use counter-irritants to the neck and chest with liniments composed of oil of amber, croton oil, or turpentine.

The value of emetics has been long recognized in this affection, although we are told by Vogel that the continuous use of emetics in the early stage for several days causes harm. Copeland ordered an emetic every third day in ordinary cases. All writers agree that the milder emetics should be used by preference; that tartar emetic should be avoided, except as an external application where a counter-irritant is desired; and that ipecacuanha is the safest, though alum is also safe and as an astringent useful. Trousseau preferred the sulphate of copper. In the earlier stages of the disease emetics are not, as a rule, indicated; it is only when the secretion has become extremely tenacious, and the paroxysms so frequent and severe as to greatly strain the patient and endanger his lungs, that they are of value. There seems to be a close connection between the amount and tenacity of the secretion and the severity of the paroxysm. The potassium carbonate has been recommended as an active agent in the amelioration of this affection; it is probably valuable in rendering the secretion less tenacious. Alum has been used with success, as has tannin, probably owing to their local action on the mucous membrane. Macartan[8] says that in the East[p. 846]Indies the disease is treated in the first stages by astringent and tonic gargles.

[8] *Dictionnaire des Sciences Méd.*, 1813, vol. vi.

Belladonna certainly receives the endorsement of the greatest number of writers. Vogel considers it superior to all other drugs, and regards dilatation of the pupil as the only sure guide in its administration. He says it does not cut short the attack, but mitigates the paroxysm. Trousseau was also an advocate of this form of treatment. When combined with alum[9] it is considered by Meigs and Pepper to be one of the most valuable drugs recommended. They also advise the use of potassium carbonate. Seiner trusted belladonna more than any other remedy; so also Rilliet and Barthez. William Lee, in an interesting paper in the *New York Medical Journal,* 1883, advocates the use of atropia hypodermically; he believes that atropia chiefly acts in these cases on the laryngeal branches of the pneumogastric nerves, and that it is probable that it has a decided effect also on the medulla oblongata itself, and renders it less capable of exciting reflex action. Kroon's experiments led him to conclude that the valerianate of atropia was the most useful. Evans[10] gave the 1/120 of a grain of atropia to a child aged three years until the pupils were dilated, then reduced the dose; this stopped the paroxysm in twenty-one days. At the commencement of the treatment the child had twenty-three paroxysms in the day, and twenty-seven at night. Case No. 2 under same circumstances recovered in fourteen days. In case No. 3 the paroxysms were reduced from twenty-six to two or three a day. Arthur Wiglesworth[11] used a solution of sulphate of atropia, administered in the morning fasting; the dose he advises for children from one to four years is gr. 1/120, given only once a day except in some cases. The results are as follows: There is a steady diminution in the number of paroxysms; a change in the character of the whoop as if the vocal cords were not so closely approximated. If atropia is withheld, the beneficent effect derived from it subsides.

[9] Golding Bird, *Guy's Hosp. Rep.*, April, 1845.

[10] *Glasgow Med. Jour.*, 1880.

[11] *Lancet*, April 12, 1879.

West advises dilute hydrocyanic acid, and many writers agree with him, ranking it next to belladonna.

Harley and others are strong advocates for the bromide of ammonium; it is supposed to have a local anæsthetic action on the pharyngeal and laryngeal mucous membrane. Fordyce Grinnell[12] during four months treated 223 cases with this remedy, and highly recommends it. The doses were in accordance with those of Dr. Kormann—¾ to 4 grains, as indicated by age, three or four times a day and at night when the paroxysms were severe. No other treatment was used in these 223 cases, except camphorated oil to the throat and chest in some cases. Potassium bromide has been recommended by Helenke, Beaufort, Erlenmeyer, and others. Henry Field[13] recommends sodium bromide.

[12] *Med. News*, 1882.

[13] *Brit. Med. Jour.*

Probably next to belladonna in the treatment of this disease we should place chloral hydrate.

Hebner, after an elaborate study of the relative value of potassium bromide, quinia, salicylic acid, chloral, and belladonna, says: "Salicylic acid and chloral tend to relieve the paroxysms—belladonna and quinia to shorten the disease." Kennedy[14] writes: "I cannot doubt [p. 847]its specific effects on the cough. Chloral seems to me to yield the best and most constant results. The advantage of chloral hydrate seems to exist in producing sleep; it should be given in from 2- to 5-gr. doses, at night." If there is much irritability or fretfulness, or any premonition of eclampsia, it should be associated with potassium bromide.

[14] *Dublin Jour. M. S.*, 1881.

Croton chloral has received much praise from those who have used it; we have had no experience with it.

We have already alluded to the value of quinia, which has been used largely in this disease, both internally and as a local application. Originally recommended in the latter manner on account of its power of controlling the development of low organisms, it has not proved so satisfactory or valuable as when given internally. Binz in 1870 was perhaps the first to recommend quinia given frequently and in solution, and Dawson in 1873[15] reports excellent results from the sulphate or muriate of quinia given in full and frequent doses, and in such solutions as will not prevent its acting on the mucous membrane in its passage through the pharynx. Breidenbach[16] gives the quinia muriate in larger doses—one and a half to fifteen and a half grains per diem. The effects were surprising as soon as the proper dose for each person had been determined; this, he says, is the keynote of success. To prevent complications he continued it for a long time in small doses.

[15] *Am. Jour. Obstetrics.*

[16] *Practitioner*, Feb., 1871.

Our own experience favors the view that quinia, when given in solution or suspended in mixture, is valuable in many cases of this disease; it can be ordered in powder, and given in a spoonful of simple syrup or of the preparation known as the syrup of yerba santa, which makes an excellent vehicle. Liquorice also disguises the taste of quinia admirably for children.

Albrecht[17] has found from an experience of ten cases of whooping cough in children between the ages of one and a half and nine years, all of a marked scrofulous type, much benefit from the muriate of pilocarpine, given in small doses after every fit of coughing. To prevent collapse, he advises that it should be given in a mixture containing a little brandy. After twenty-four hours of its administration an obvious change for the better takes place in the appearance of the mucous membrane of the throat, velum palati, and uvula, which becomes paler, less swollen, and more moist; laryngoscopic examination shows a similar improvement. During the catarrhal period cold compresses to the neck and sweetened milk containing potassium chlorate are used instead of the pilocarpine, which is to be resumed as soon as a whoop recurs.

[17] *London Med. Rec.*, March 15, 1882, p. 110.

Dr. Tordeus, of the Hospice des Enfants Assistés, Brussels, states that he has found the sodium benzoate useful in whooping cough, diminishing the frequency and violence of the paroxysms, and by its action on the pulmonary mucous membrane preventing those pulmonary complications which so frequently supervene and constitute the danger of the disease.

Sulphur has been largely used by the Germans in two- or three-grain doses, and is said to be greatly esteemed by them. Cantharides has been recommended, and it is stated that when strangury is produced the whoop will cease; we should consider this rather severe treatment. The [p. 848]fluid extract of castanea is used by many with undoubtedly good results, though this also has been somewhat of a disappointment in the way of treatment, as at one time it was looked upon almost as a specific. Many claim that an infusion of the fresh leaves gives a better result. Dewar[18] regards ergot with great favor in the treatment of pertussis. Certainly in those cases where, from violent straining, hemorrhages have taken place we have found it to be highly valuable. We have had no experience with it in the treatment of ordinary cases, though Dewar claims that it shortens the attack. The ammonium picrate, and recently resorcine, have been used with success.

[18] *The Practitioner*, London, May, 1882.

Counter-irritation to the neck and chest has always been found useful in the treatment of this disease. Autenreith[19] recommends tartar emetic to the epigastrium till vesicles appear and even ulcerate. Milder forms of counter-irritation over the chest seem equally efficacious if continued for some time. The oil of amber, when used in liniment with camphor or turpentine, is by some considered almost a specific. Great care should also be observed in the dress of children with whooping cough. Warmth about the chest is always indicated, while there should be nothing close or tight about the throat allowed.

[19] *Dict. des Sciences Med.*, 1813.

In the third stage, when there is the nervous element remaining, tonics, such as cod-liver oil, iron, the phosphates and hypophosphites, are required.

The diet should be nutritious, easy of digestion, and abundant, and the bowels should be kept regular by fruits or laxatives. Over-feeding should of course always be avoided, and the attempt at weaning a babe with this disease would certainly meet with unfavorable results.

Bicarbonate of soda or lime-water should be given freely with the milk taken by children with this disease. Milk certainly should form the basis of the diet of children with pertussis, and reliable meat-extracts are to be recommended in this disease even for older children, who from the severity of the attack would vomit more solid food. If the vomiting be so severe as to affect nutrition, the child should be sustained by peptonized milk, soup, or gruel, given by the bowel.

The importance of a proper regulation of the temperature of the air which the patient breathes is especially recognized in France. If the attack occurs in mid-winter and the seashore be inaccessible or inexpedient, the child should be restricted to a well-ventilated nursery or suite of rooms, the temperature of which should be kept uniform.

Salt air is recognized to be of great value in advanced cases of this disease; this has been attributed partly to the effects of stimulation of the mucous membrane in rendering less viscid and more copious the bronchial secretions, and also to the balmy softness and great purity of the atmosphere at the sea-shore. But probably there is another element in the local action of the chloride of sodium, either in establishing a resistance on the part of the patient or in modifying the germ of the disease.

The most serious complication of whooping cough is pneumonia. It occasionally happens that an attack of croupous pneumonia may develop during the course of whooping cough, but in the vast majority of cases the disease is of the catarrhal type. When, indeed, it is remembered that a bronchial catarrh, which is the invariable precursor or accompaniment [p. 849]of catarrhal pneumonia, is a constant factor in whooping cough, and, further, that all conditions of debility, and especially of enfeebled or embarrassed respiration, dispose to this form of pneumonia, it is not surprising that this complication should be of such frequent occurrence. It is not impossible that in aiming at securing sufficient fresh air and out-door exercise to maintain the general health, an injudicious degree of exposure may be permitted which will aggravate the existing bronchitis and induce an extension of inflammation to the alveoli. But usually the catarrhal pneumonia develops in a subacute and more or less insidious manner, and without being traceable to any such exposure. It may happen occasionally that in the violent inspiratory efforts at the close of the paroxysms irritating secretions may be sucked from the bronchioles into the alveoli, and there excite inflammation. Or, again, it doubtless happens frequently that, with the existence of swelling of the bronchial mucous membrane and of viscid secretions in the bronchial tubes, collapse of portions of lung tissue is developed by the forcible expulsion of air during the paroxysms of cough, which cannot be replaced owing to the relative weakness of inspiration and to the ball-valve action of the plugs of mucus in the obstructed bronchioles. The intimate relation between pulmonary collapse and catarrhal pneumonia is familiarly known. It is not to be considered that the mere occurrence of collapse will induce pneumonia in the areas affected, but certainly it will aid in rendering effective the other irritating causes. As a consequence, it usually happens that when catarrhal pneumonia occurs in whooping cough it is associated with more or less collapse. When, then, especially in children of debilitated or rachitic constitution, or in those who are subjected to unfavorable hygienic influences, such as overcrowding, bad air, and the like, there is a rather gradual development of dyspnoea, with increasing debility, emaciation, and evidences of impaired oxygenation of the blood, it is to be feared that this serious complication has developed. The physical signs are often difficult of interpretation, but if careful examination of the chest be conducted, together with thermometric observations, the approach of this danger or its actual presence may be detected. The result is fatal in a large proportion of cases, so that suitable treatment—for the details of which reference is made to the appropriate section— must be instituted without delay.

Our investigations of this disease have led us to the conclusion that we have to deal with an affection caused by a specific germ, which is usually, after a period of incubation, made manifest by a catarrh of a portion of the air-passages; that this catarrh, existing for an indefinite period, is capable of being influenced by medication, applied either by means of inhalation or by acting on the mucous membrane after absorption by the stomach. In this way we have known the administration of quinia and of alum diminish the number of paroxysms, to all appearance checking the excessive secretion to a marvellous extent. The other element of the disease, the neurosis, which soon follows the initial catarrh, and seems to last for an indefinite time after the mucous membrane has regained its normal appearance, is also capable of being controlled by the use of drugs, especially belladonna, chloral, the bromides, and hydrocyanic acid, not to speak of the other antispasmodics and sedatives, and by the [p. 850] analgesic effect of carbonic acid gas, or by the spray of bromide of ammonium, carbolic acid, and other substances upon the larynx.

Vogel tells us in his classical work on children, "If now, as a résumé, I would give an explanation of my views, it would go to show that there never has been, and most probably never will be, a remedy by which whooping cough may be abridged, any more than we are able to cut short the acute exanthemata or typhus fever or pneumonia." And yet the experience of many whom we have quoted in this article tends to support the view that by a form of treatment calculated to act on the two elements of the disease which we have just noted, the affection can be greatly modified in its intensity, and probably the attack be somewhat shortened. Certain it is that the recent studies of this disease give us hope that the day is not far distant when the cause, whatever it is, will be definitely known, and if it is found to reside in the secretions from the larynx, that treatment by inhalation or atomization will modify or destroy it, and prevent its dissemination.

[p. 851]

INFLUENZA.
BY JAMES C. WILSON, M.D.

DEFINITION.—A continued fever, occurring in widely-extended epidemics, and due to a specific cause; it is characterized by early catarrh of the mucous membrane of the respiratory tract, and in many cases also of the digestive tract; by quickly oncoming debility out of proportion to the intensity of the fever and the catarrhal processes; and by nervous symptoms. There is a strong tendency to inflammatory complications, especially of the lungs. Uncomplicated cases are rarely fatal except in feeble and aged persons. An attack does not confer immunity from the disease in future epidemics.

SYNONYMS.—Febris catarrhalis; Defluxio catarrhalis epidemicus; Catarrhus a contagio; Rheuma epidemicum; Cephalalgia contagiosa; Epidemic catarrhal fever; Tac;

Horion; Quinte; Coqueluche; Ladendo, also written La Dando; Baraquette; Générale; Coquette; Cocotte; Allure; Follette; Petite poste; Petit courier; Grenade; La Grippe; Ziep; Schaffhusten and Schaffkrankheit; Huhner-Weh; Blitz-Katarrh; Mödefieber; Mal del Castrone. There are also several names indicating its supposed origin; thus it has been called in Russia, Chinese catarrh; in Germany and Italy, the Russian disease; in France, Italian fever, Spanish catarrh, and so forth.

It is a remarkable fact that in two instances at least the popular name for the disease under consideration has found its way widely into medicine and medical literature, almost to the exclusion of the studied terms by which science has sought to designate it; these are influenza and la grippe.

Such obsolete and now meaningless terms as Peripneumonia notha (Sydenham, Boerhaave), Peripneumonia catarrhalis (Huxham), Pleuritis humida (Stoll), have been omitted from this list of synonyms as being of interest rather to the student of medical history than to the student of medicine.

Febris catarrhalis, Defluxio catarrhalis epidemicus, Rheuma epidemicus are terms which no longer retain the place given them in the literature of influenza by the older medical authorities.

Catarrhis a contagio (Cullen) and Cephalalgia contagiosa are derived from a view of the nature of the disease, which has been the cause of no little controversy.

Epidemic catarrhal fever is, with its Latin equivalent, the most satisfactory of the so-called scientific names by which the disease is at present known.

In the popular names for the affection there is to be noted an [p. 852]indication of the national character of some of the peoples who have suffered from its frequent visitations.

Among the English it is known as cold or epidemic cold, or, in deference to medical authority, as catarrh or epidemic catarrh; and at present, both among the folk and the doctors, as influenza. Englishmen are neither quick to see in the disease a resemblance to some common circumstance or thing, nor are they disposed to make a joke about it.

The Germans find obvious resemblances. In the labored respiration and the character of the cough they find a suggestion of a common epizoötic affecting the sheep, hence Schaffhusten and Shaffkrankheit; or, because the cough is like the crowing of a cock and the disturbance of respiration and rapid prostration suggest some resemblance to a common disease of the domestic fowl, it has been called Huhner-Weh (chicken disease, whooping cough), and Ziep, which is about equivalent to pip. They call it also, from its rapid invasion, Blitz-Katarrh, and from its diffusion, Mödefieber.

The French are disposed to make a jest of everything, and the more serious the subject the better the joke. Hence they have found a new name for almost every great epidemic, and each more trivial than the last. Thus, tac (rot); horion (in jest, a blow); quinte, because the spells occur at intervals of five hours (sic); coqueluche (a hood or cowl), from the cap worn by those suffering from the malady; and so on through the long list given above.

La grippe is said to be derived from the Polish Chrypka (Raucedo); it may, however, be derived from agripper (to seize).

Influenza is of Italian derivation. It is said that the disease received this name because it was attributed to the influence of the stars, or from a secondary signification of the word indicating something fluid, transient, or fashionable.

HISTORICAL SKETCH.[1]—Epidemics of influenza have been clearly recorded only since the beginning of the sixteenth century. There are numerous accounts of earlier epidemic diseases resembling it, but they are not sufficiently particular to warrant us in inferring its undoubted existence. It is supposed to be referred to in the writings of Hippocrates, who, however, gives no exact description.[2] An outbreak in the Athenian army in Sicily (415 B.C.), recorded by Diodorus Siculus, has been supposed to have been influenza. Despite these statements, and those of others to the effect that it is a disease known from a remote antiquity, it may be said that no accounts can be confidently established, as referring to the disease now known as influenza, in the writings of classical antiquity.[3]

[1] See also *The Continued Fevers*, by the author of this paper, New York, 1881.
[2] Parkes, *Reynolds's System of Medicine*, vol. i., 1868.
[3] Zuelzer, *Ziemssen's Cyclopædia of Medicine*, vol. ii., 1875.

As early as the ninth century several epidemics of catarrhal fever, Italian fever, and the like, which were probably influenza, were made matter of history. In the year A.D. 827 a cough which spread like the plague was recorded. In 876 there appeared in Italy a similar epidemic, which spread with great rapidity over all Europe. It is related that dogs and birds suffered with symptoms not unlike those characterizing the affection in man. In 976, Germany and all France suffered from a fever of which the chief [p. 853]symptom was cough. No further epidemic is noted until two centuries later, when, in 1173, a widespread malady, of which the symptoms were chiefly catarrhal, raged throughout Europe; while less important epidemics of a like character are recorded as having occurred during the following century (1239-99).

In the medical writings of the fourteenth century there are to be found records of six epidemics, and in the fifteenth seven great visitations of influenza are described (Parkes).

Aitken[4] speaks of a very fatal prevalence of influenza throughout France in 1311, and of an epidemic in 1403 in which the mortality was so great that the courts of law in Paris were closed in consequence of the deaths.

[4] Aitken's *Practice of Medicine*, vol. i., 1872.

Influenza is mentioned in the *Annals of the Four Masters* as having prevailed in Ireland in the fourteenth century, and a disease characterized by similar symptoms is alluded to in early Gaelic manuscripts under the name of Creatan (creat, the chest). The disease is described also in an Irish manuscript of the fifteenth century under the terms Fuacht and Slaodan.[5]

[5] Theophilus Thompson, *Annals of Influenza*, 1852.

The earliest epidemic that prevailed in the British Isles of which any accurate description remains is that of the year 1510. The disease came from Malta, and invaded first Sicily, then Italy and Spain and Portugal, whence it crossed the Alps into Hungary and Germany as far as the Baltic Sea, extending westward into France and Britain. Its track widened over the whole of Europe from the south-east to the extreme north-west, and it is said that not a single family and scarce a person escaped it. It was attended by a "grievous pain in the head, heaviness, difficulty of breathing, hoarseness, loss of strength and appetite, restlessness, retchings from a terrible tearing cough. Presently succeeded a chilliness, and so violent a cough that many were in danger of suffocation. The first day it was without spitting, but about the seventh or eighth day much viscid phlegm was spit up. Others (though fewer) spat only water and froth. When they began to spit, cough and shortness of breath were easier. None died except some children. In some it went off with a looseness, in others by sweating. Bleeding and purging did hurt."[6] Blisters were commonly employed— two each upon the arms and legs, and one to the back of the head. The description is sufficiently clear to place the nature of this epidemic beyond all doubt.

[6] Thomas Short, *A General Chronological History of the Air, Weather, Meteors, etc.*, London, 1749; quoted in the *Annals of Influenza*.

The epidemic of 1557, starting westward from Asia, spread over Europe, and then crossed the Atlantic to America. The malady broke out in England, after a season of unusual rain and great scarcity of corn, in the month of September. "Presently after were many catarrhs, quickly followed by a more severe cough, pain of the side, difficulty of breathing, and a fever. The pain was neither violent nor pricking, but mild. The third day they expectorated freely. The sixth, seventh, or at the farthest the eighth day, all who had that pain of the side died, but such as were blooded on the first or second day recovered on the fourth or fifth; but bleeding on the last two days did no service." "Some, but very few, had continual fevers along with it; many had [p. 854]double tertians; others simply slight intermittent. All were worse by night than by day; such as recovered were long valetudinary, had a weak stomach, and hypped." Gravid women either aborted or died. This epidemic spread with frightful rapidity. Thousands were attacked at the same time. The entire population of Nismes, with scarcely an exception, fell ill of it upon the same day. It was extremely fatal. In Mantua Carpentaria, a small town near Madrid, it broke out in August, and so fatal were the bloodletting and purging which constituted the treatment at first, that, of the two thousand persons who were bled, all died. The disease raged in some parts till the middle of the following year (1558), and carried off, in Delft alone, five thousand of the poor. In all cases mild treatment was called for, with warm broths and speedy immersals, "to recall the appetite and keep the vessels of the throat open."

In 1580 a great epidemic of influenza spread from the south-east toward the north-west over Asia, Africa, and Europe. From Constantinople and Venice it overran Hungary and Germany, and reached the farthest regions of Norway, Sweden, and Russia. It spread into England, and has been described by Dr. Short. In Italy it prevailed during August and September, in England from the middle of August to the end of September, and in Spain during the whole summer. In most places its duration was about six weeks. As a rule, the termination was favorable, although the disease ran a somewhat protracted course. In the account of Dr. Short it is stated that "few died except those that were let blood of or had unsound viscera." In some places, on the contrary, the course of the disease was very severe. In Rome two thousand died of it, according to the author just cited, but Zuelzer informs us that the victims of this epidemic in the Eternal City were not less than nine thousand, and adds that Madrid must have been almost depopulated by it. This high mortality has been attributed to the bloodletting practised in the treatment of the disease. The symptoms were similar to those of the previous epidemics, with a greater shortness of breath, which continued in many cases for some time after the disappearance of the catarrhal trouble. There was great sweating at the end of the attack. The plague, measles, and small-pox prevailed also, and with considerable violence, during the year 1580.

Influenza, unfelt for several years, reappeared in Germany in 1591; an epidemic extending from Holland through France and into Italy occurred in 1593. In 1610 catarrh is said to have prevailed throughout Europe. In 1626-27 epidemic catarrhal fever made its appearance in Italy and France; in 1642-43 in Holland; in 1647 in Spain and in the colonies of the Western World; and again, in 1655 in North America. According to Webster,[7] this epidemic of 1647 was the first catarrh mentioned in American annals.

[7] Noah Webster, *A Brief History of Epidemic and Pestilential Diseases*, London, 1800.

In 1658 and 1675 it again visited Austria, Germany, England, etc. The first of these two epidemics is described by Willis,[8] and the second by Sydenham,[9] as they occurred in England, and the accounts are to be [p. 855]found in the *Annals of Influenza*. It is about this period that the disease began to be known as influenza, and it is not without interest to observe that the influence of the stars suggested itself, in connection with its sudden appearance and wide prevalence, to the minds of the physicians of this date. Willis writes that "about the end of April (1658), suddenly a distemper arose, as if sent by some blast of the stars, which laid hold on very many together; that in some towns in the space of a week above a thousand people fell sick together."

[8] Dr. Willis, *The Description of a Catarrhal Fever Epidemical in the Middle of the Spring in the Year 1658: Practice of Physick*, 1684.

[9] *The Epidemic Coughs of the Year 1675, with the Pleurisy and Peripneumony that supervened:* from the *Works* of Thomas Sydenham, M.D.

Epidemics are recorded as having occurred in Great Britain and Europe in 1688, 1693, and in 1709. The disease raged in 1712 widely over Europe from Denmark to Italy.

In 1729-30 a widespread epidemic swept over Europe. In five months it extended over Russia, Poland, Germany, Sweden, and Denmark. In Vienna sixty thousand persons fell ill of it. In the autumn it spread to England, and reached France and Switzerland; from there it extended to Italy, and by February it had reached Rome and Naples. Spain did not escape its ravages, and it is said to have found its way to Mexico. The symptoms did not differ in any important respect from those already described as characterizing previous epidemics. Pains in the limbs and fever marked the onset of the attack; catarrh, oppression, hoarseness, cough followed. In some cases delirium, drowsiness, and faintings occurred. A petechial eruption was observed, in some instances, between the fourth and seventh days. This renders it probable that typhus or cerebro-spinal fever prevailed at the same time. Turbid urine, copious sweats, bilious stools, and nose-bleeding were often noted. In Switzerland only children and old persons died. The disease was not very fatal.

Two years later (1732-33) an epidemic, starting from Saxony and Poland, overran Germany, Switzerland, and Holland, and invaded Great Britain in the month of December. Toward the end of January it spread in a south-easterly direction to France, Italy, Spain, and westward to North America, thence southward to the islands of the West Indies, and on to South America. The course of the disease in this epidemic was favorable. The attack terminated in from three to fourteen days, with sweating, bleeding from the nose, or an abundant discharge from the nasal passages. The aged and those suffering from chronic pulmonary diseases mostly perished. In Scotland three forms of the affection were described—namely, the cephalic, the thoracic, and the abdominal. The epidemic slowly spread over Eastern Europe and in a south-easterly direction, and may be said to have lasted till 1737.

Concerning this epidemic John Huxham of Plymouth wrote as follows:[10] "About this time a disease invaded these parts which was the most completely epidemic of any I remember to have met with; not a house was free from it; the beggar's hut and the nobleman's palace were alike subject to its attacks, scarce a person escaping either in town or country; old and young, strong and infirm, shared the same fate." The malady had raged in Cornwall and the western parts of Devonshire from the beginning of February; it reached Plymouth on the 10th, which was on a Saturday, and that day numbers were suddenly seized. The next day multitudes were taken ill, and by the 18th or 20th of March scarcely [p. 856]any one had escaped it. "The disorder began at first with a slight shivering; this was presently followed by a transient erratic heat and headache and a violent and troublesome sneezing; then the back and lungs were seized with flying pains, which sometimes attacked the heart likewise, and though they did not long remain there, yet were very troublesome, being greatly irritated by the violent cough which accompanied the disorder, in the fits of which a great quantity of a thin, sharp mucus was thrown out from the nose and mouth. These complaints were like those arising from what is called catching cold, but presently a slight fever came on, which afterward grew more violent; the pulse was now very quick, but not in the least hard and tense like that in a pleurisy; nor was the urine remarkably red, but very thick, and inclining to a whitish color; the tongue, instead of being dry, was thickly covered with a whitish mucus or slime; there was an universal complaint of want of rest and a great giddiness. Several likewise were seized with a most racking pain in the head, often accompanied by a slight delirium. Many were troubled with a tinnitus aurium, or singing in the ears; and numbers suffered from violent earaches or pains in the meatus auditorius, which in some turned to an abscess. Exulcerations and swellings of the fauces were likewise very common. The sick were in general very much given to sweat, which, when it broke out of its own accord, was very plentiful and continued without striking in again, and did often in the space of two or three days wholly carry off the fever. You have here a description of this epidemic disease such as it prevailed hereabouts, attacking every one more or less; but still, considering the great multitude that were seized by it, it was fatal to but few, and that chiefly infants and consumptive old people. It generally went off about the fourth day, leaving behind a troublesome cough, which was very often of long duration, and such a dejection of strength as one would hardly have suspected from the shortness of the time.

"On the whole, this disorder was rarely mortal, unless by some very great error arising in the treatment of it; however, this very circumstance proved fatal to some, who, making too slight of it, either on account of its being so common or not thinking it very dangerous, often found asthmas, hectics, or even consumptions themselves, the forfeitures of their inconsiderate rashness."

[10] *Observations on the Air and Epidemical Diseases, translated from the Latin*, London, 1758.

Arbuthnot also described this visitation of the disease.[11] He regarded the uniformity of the symptoms in every place as most remarkable, and tells us that during the whole season in which it prevailed there was "a great run of hysterical, hypochondriacal, and nervous distempers; in short, all the symptoms of relaxation."

[11] *An Essay concerning the Effects of Air on Human Bodies*, London, 1751.

During the years 1737-38 influenza again swept over England, North America, the islands of the West Indies, and France; in 1742-43 it prevailed in Western Europe and the

British Isles; in 1757-58 in North America, the West Indies, France, and Scotland. In 1761 it overran the North American colonies and the West Indies.

The epidemic of 1762 extended very generally over Europe and Great Britain. In Germany nine-tenths of the population were attacked by the disease.

Widely extended epidemics prevailed in Europe and America in 1767 [p. 857]and 1775; in 1772 it raged in North America; in 1778-80, in France, Germany and Russia. Noah Webster found influenza prevalent in North America in 1781; the next year one of the most remarkable epidemics of this disease (described as the epidemic of 1782) appeared in Europe. It came from the East, from Asia into Russia. From St. Petersburg it spread during the winter and spring over Sweden, Germany, Holland, and France. In the autumn it was in Italy, Spain, and Portugal. The crews of Dutch and English ships were taken ill with the disease upon the high seas.

In Vienna three-fourths of the population fell ill of it with such suddenness that it got here for the first time its name of "Blitz Katarrh" (lightning catarrh). It was characterized by great pain in the back, breast, and throat, and by extraordinary enfeeblement. Relapses occurred, and inflammation of the lungs and bowels was common. Children remained relatively exempt from its seizure. This epidemic broke out in England about the end of April and raged until the end of June. "The duration of the malady in some was not above a day or two, but it usually lasted near a week or longer. In a few the symptoms seemed to abate in two or three days, but some returned and raged with more violence than at first."[12] The disease was not regarded as in itself fatal, and few could be said to have died of it "but those who were old, asthmatic, or who had been debilitated by some previous indisposition."

[12] *An Account of the Epidemic Disease called the Influenza of the Year 1782. Collected from the Observations of several Physicians in London and in the Country, by a Committee of the Fellows of the Royal College of Physicians in London. Read at the College, June 25, 1783.*

Numerous recurring outbreaks took place in Europe and America during the years 1788-90. One of these, as it occurred in America, is well described by Dr. John Warren[13] of Boston in a letter to Lettsom. This letter is dated May 30, 1790, and among other matters of great interest respecting the disease it is stated that "Our beloved President Washington is but now on the recovery from a very severe and dangerous attack of it in that city" (New York).

[13] *Memoirs of the Life and Writings of J. Coakley Lettsom*, Thomas Joseph Pettigrew, 1817.

Webster mentions an epidemic in America in 1790, one in Europe in 1795, and another in Europe in 1797, but there seems to have been no general epidemic of sufficient importance to attract the attention of other writers upon the subject until 1798, when the malady again broke out in Russia and spread over the greater part of Europe, continuing to prevail in various regions till 1803, when it again appeared in England, and is described by several writers of that country.

From 1805 to 1827 influenza prevailed (according to Zuelzer, who tells us that few years during this interval were free from it) in frequently-recurring epidemics in Europe and America. Thompson mentions no visitation in England between 1803 and 1831.

In the year 1830 began a series of epidemics remarkable for their wide diffusion and the rapid succession with which they followed one upon another. The disease began in China; in September it reached the Indian Archipelago; it swept into Russia, and invaded Moscow in November; in January, 1831, it was raging in St. Petersburg; March found it in Warsaw; April in Eastern Prussia and Silesia; in May it prevailed in Denmark, Finland, and a great part of Germany, and in [p. 858]the same month it fell upon Paris; in June it affected England and Sweden; it was still creeping about Middle Europe and lingering in Great Britain at the end of July; in the early winter it swept southward into Italy, and westward across the Atlantic to North America, and was still harassing the inhabitants of certain regions of the United States in January and February, 1832. Meanwhile it continued in the East, spreading to Java, Farther India, and the Indian Archipelago. It continued in Hindostan after it had died out in Europe. But in January, 1833, it again visited Russia, and rolled thence southward and eastward over the most of Europe. It is recorded that by February it had reached Galicia and Eastern Prussia; in March it was in Prussia, Bohemia, and Warsaw, and had extended to Syria and Egypt; in April to many parts of Germany and Austria and to France and Great Britain. Midsummer found the disease yet prevailing in some districts of Germany and Northern Italy, and in the early autumn it was in Switzerland and Eastern France; in November it visited Naples.

Epidemics so frequent, so widespread, and so unsparing of individuals wherever the disease appeared could not fail to excite a deep and general interest. From this period the literature of the subject has been voluminous.

A brief period of repose ensued. For three years no epidemic occurred which was of sufficient importance to attract the attention of medical historians.

In December, 1837, influenza reappeared, and first, as so often before, in Russia; Sweden and Denmark were almost simultaneously affected; in January, 1837, it broke out in London, and rapidly swept over all England and into France and Germany. In January it appeared in Berlin, and shortly afterward in Dresden, Munich, and Vienna. The disease spread by February into Switzerland, and into Spain as far as Madrid by the end of March. In London almost the whole population was attacked, and the mortality was enormous. It is stated that the deaths were quadrupled during the prevalence of the disease. Large populations suffered most. This epidemic spread into the southern hemisphere, and prevailed at the same time, and consequently at exactly the opposite season that it prevailed north of the equator, in Sydney and at the Cape of Good Hope.

From 1837 to 1850-51 numerous epidemics of influenza occurred. Few years were exempt from them. The epidemic of 1847-48 has been described by many writers, and more particularly, as it occurred in London, by Peacock[14] with great exactitude. It is estimated that one-fourth of the entire population of that city were more or less affected by the disease. The epidemic prevailed in London for six months, and, although the deaths registered for the entire period as from influenza amounted to only 1739, it is stated in the report of the registrar-general that during the six weeks the epidemic was at its height not less than five thousand persons died, in the metropolitan districts, in excess of the average mortality of the period, the excess showing itself in nearly every class of disease, the local maladies which had been the predominant affections being doubtless in many cases assigned as the cause of death. This[p. 859]epidemic affected between one-fourth and one-half of the population of Paris, and in Geneva the proportion of those attacked was not less than one-third of the entire population.

[14] *On the Influenza, or Epidemic Catarrhal Fever of 1847-48*, Thomas Berill Peacock. M.D., 1848.

More or less widespread epidemics of influenza are recorded as having occurred in 1857-58 and 1860; in 1864 in Switzerland; in 1867 in Paris in the spring; and at various times in the United States and Canada.

A mild epidemic occurred in 1874 in Berlin.

Influenza prevailed over a wide area in the United States during the early months of 1879. The characteristics of this visitation have been well described by Da Costa.[15]

[15] "The Prevailing Epidemic of Influenza—Its Characteristic Phenomena—Pulmonary, Gastro-intestinal, Cerebral, and Nervous—Its Wide Distribution, Mortality, and Treatment," *Medical and Surgical Reporter*, Philadelphia, March 8, 1879.

The disease, since the great epidemic of 1847-48, has affected a smaller proportion of the inhabitants of the localities visited, and has run a less dangerous course, than in the earlier epidemics. It has for this reason occupied a less conspicuous place in the medical literature of recent years. It is nevertheless true that even in the mildest epidemics, when a relatively small number of persons are seized and the symptoms are in most cases almost insignificant, cases do here and there occur which are of a serious or even fatal character, and that the death-rate from other diseases is for the time considerably increased.

Catarrhal affections have often prevailed among the domestic animals when influenza has been epidemic. Horses, dogs, and cats are subject to these disorders; neat cattle, goats, and sheep have been less commonly affected; chickens and pheasants have suffered, and it is stated by some of the older writers that birds, and particularly the sparrow, have deserted localities in which influenza was prevailing, and that migratory birds have taken flight earlier than usual.

These epizoötics have sometimes preceded the appearance of influenza among men by a period of some weeks or days; in other instances they have appeared at the same time; and in a widespread outbreak among horses in the United States in 1872, in which the symptoms and morbid anatomy, accurately observed, were undoubtedly those of influenza, the disease did not affect man except to a very limited extent. A want of fulness of description, and the inaccuracy of diagnosis too common in the consideration of the general diseases of the lower animals, leave the precise nature of most of the epizoötics described by the earlier writers doubtful.

An extensive influenza of moderate intensity prevailed as an epizoötic, chiefly affecting horses, during the latter part of the summer and the autumn of 1880 in Canada and the United States east of the Mississippi River. Dogs were also affected, but less generally, and human beings to a still slighter extent. In several localities where this invasion was observed by the writer the horses were first affected, the dogs next, and after the lapse of some weeks, as the animals were recovering, the disease became epidemic; but those persons who took care of horses and were much in contact with them neither suffered earlier nor more severely than others not so exposed.

ETIOLOGY.—1. Predisposing Influences.—There are no [p. 860]well-established facts pointing to the existence of individual peculiarities that can be regarded as predisposing influences. When the disease appears a large proportion of the population is attacked without distinction of age, sex, social condition, or occupation. Previous illness, whether acute or chronic, local or constitutional, affords no protection. Aged and infirm persons and those of nervous temperament are peculiarly liable to attack, but the robust possess no immunity. All races and dwellers in every climate are the victims of influenza. In a community invaded by the disease females are apt to be the first attacked, adult males next, and children last. It has been observed that in some epidemics children are but little liable to contract the disease.

An attack confers no exemption from the disease in another epidemic, and independently of relapses, which are not infrequent, persons have been known to experience a second attack during the prevalence of the same epidemic.

Persons dwelling in overcrowded and ill-ventilated habitations and in low, damp and unhealthy situations have, in certain epidemics, especially suffered, and the increase of deaths by influenza is proportionately much greater in districts in which there is ordinarily a high mortality than in healthier places.

Influenza appears at all seasons of the year and affects the inhabitants of every latitude. It has no connection with known atmospheric conditions. Many of the earlier writers sought to establish a relation between low temperatures and sudden variations of temperature and influenza, and by reason of the confusion among the people between these diseases and common "colds" there has always existed an opinion that such a relation obtains. There is, however, no evidence to sustain this view; neither low temperature nor abrupt changes give rise to the affection. It has prevailed in hot and dry seasons, in the West Indies, on the coast of Java, in India, in Egypt, at the Cape of Good Hope, on the Riviera in summer.

The condition of the air as regards moisture, or dryness, does not influence the spread of the disease. It has occurred at sea, on low sea-coasts, and in the dryest climates, as, for example, in Upper Egypt.

Its spread is not much influenced by local winds. It does not travel with the same velocity, and even sometimes advances against them. In several well-authenticated instances a dense and foul fog has preceded and attended the local outbreak of epidemics. The much greater number of epidemics that have occurred altogether without such manifestations make it in a high degree probable that this has been a coincidence. Ozone in large quantities artificially produced may give rise to the symptoms of ordinary catarrh, but it is not a cause of influenza. The disease is not in any way connected with the condition of the soil, elevation, volcanic eruption, or any other local cause. The history of every epidemic may be adduced in proof of this statement.

Before taking up the consideration of the exciting causes of influenza, it is important to review the known facts concerning the march of epidemics and the spread of the disease in affected localities. It has prevailed with greater or less frequency in almost every region of the globe. Epidemics recur at irregular periods. It was at one time supposed that the course of the disease was cyclical, with a return at intervals of about one hundred years. This view was long ago proved to be unfounded. About every[p. 861]twenty-five or thirty-five years great epidemics have swept over vast areas of the globe, and influenza may be said to be, at such times, pandemic. Less-widely extended epidemics have taken place with greater or less frequency in the intervals between the great outbreaks. But it is not possible to establish anything like a regular periodicity in the returns of the disease.

It has been supposed in some instances to prevail within restricted localities, as, for example, in a single city. Such local epidemics are without doubt due to local causes, and are of the nature of simple ordinary catarrhal fever, rather than true influenza.

The epidemics have extended over great areas, usually in a direction from the east or north-east toward the west and south. At other times they take the opposite course, and in some years they have appeared to radiate in various directions from several centres. It is in consequence of these facts that two views have arisen concerning the origin of the affection. The first of these is, that each epidemic starts out from some single unknown source, and spreads thence from point to point, invading more distant localities successfully as it advances, until at length it dies out in regions remote from the starting-point. This opinion is in accord with the popular belief. Thus, the Italians have called it the German disease; the Germans, the Russian pest; the Russians, the Chinese catarrh. The geographical relation of these nations indicates the usual track of the great epidemics, as shown in the foregoing historical sketch. The other opinion is, that it arises not from some single particular place, but that it may start anywhere, and that widespread epidemics are due to the successive outbreaks of the disease at many distinct points of origin.

The evidence that the great epidemics of influenza are due to some general and pandemic influence is conclusive. The point of origin of the great epidemics has not yet been indicated with precision, and must remain beyond conjecture until further facts bearing upon the question of their source are brought to light. When it has prevailed over a large portion of the earth's surface its progress from place to place has usually been rapid. In this respect, however, the epidemics show a great diversity. It sometimes travels exceedingly slowly. It is said to have overrun Europe in six weeks, and it has again taken six months to do so. It sometimes attacks places widely remote from each other within short intervals of time, and it has appeared at the same time in different quarters of the globe. It does not follow the great lines of travel and commercial intercourse.

When influenza enters a city it continues to prevail, as a rule, from four weeks to two months, but exceptionally it remains a longer time; for example, the epidemic of 1831 was prevalent in Paris for the greater part of the year. It in all instances finally disappears, and sporadic cases do not occur in the intervals between the epidemics.

In rare instances the epidemics are heralded by scattered cases. But as a rule this disease attacks simultaneously great numbers of the inhabitants of affected districts, so that, when the epidemic is severe, the sick are in a short time to be counted by thousands and business is paralyzed as by a blow. Epidemics rapidly reach their height, and subside almost as suddenly as they began. In a large city the disease frequently, perhaps always, makes its appearance nearly at the same time in several [p. 862]different localities, affecting certain streets and quarters solely or more generally than others for a time, and spreading thus from several centres through the entire community. Large towns and cities are generally affected earlier than the villages around them, and the latter, though closely adjacent, sometimes escape for weeks. The crews of ships upon the high seas, not sailing from an infected port, are said to have suffered from the seizure, and epidemics have many times crossed the Atlantic from the Old World to the New, and more than once in the opposite direction.

2. The Exciting Cause.—Large as has been the place in medical literature occupied by the histories of epidemics of influenza, the nature of the "epidemic influence" which gives rise to the disease is still unknown.

The question of the contagiousness of influenza is one of grave interest, and has been the subject of much controversy. The great rapidity of the spread of epidemics, the vast area they overrun, the fact that they do not follow the lines of human intercourse, the suddenness with which great numbers of the inhabitants of an invaded district or city are seized, the fact that the most complete seclusion from intercourse with affected persons, or even the shutting up of houses, affords in most instances no protection whatever,—all go to show that the disease spreads, in the main, independently of direct contact. This opinion has been almost universally entertained. There is evidence, however, to show that the disease is to some extent contagious; and so convincing have the facts bearing upon this point appeared to some that they have believed it to be propagated entirely by human intercourse. Haygarth[16] declares, as the result of his observations during the epidemics of 1775 and 1782, that the influenza spreads "by the contagion of patients in the distemper;" and Falconer,[17] writing of the epidemic of 1803, says, "I have no doubt that it is contagious in the strictest sense of the word." Watson[18] regards the instances in which the complaint has first broken out in those particular houses of a town at which travellers have arrived from infected places as too numerous to be attributed to mere chance. Very often those dwelling near the invalids are attacked next in the order of time, and when the disease affects a household all do not usually manifest the symptoms at the same time, but one member after another is stricken down with it.

[16] John Haygarth, M.D., F.R.S., *On the Manner in which the Influenza of 1775 and 1782 spread by Contagion in Chester and its Neighborhood*.

[17] William Falconer, M.D., F.R.S., *An Account of the Epidemic Catarrhal Fever, commonly called the Influenza, as it appeared at Bath in the Winter and Spring of the Year 1803*, Bath, 1803.

[18] *Principles and Practice of Medicine*.

In a few rare cases the isolation or seclusion of a community has appeared to give protection, as in cloisters, prisons, garrisons, and the like; at all events, there are instances on record where segregated communities of this kind have escaped attack.

The following observation, conducted under unusual circumstances, establishes the fact that influenza may be brought from an infected city in such a way as to give rise to a localized outbreak in a remote community. Drs. Guitéras and White[19] narrate that, influenza prevailing in Europe, and particularly in Paris and London, an American gentleman in bad health contracted the disease in London, improved, suffered a relapse [p. 863]shortly afterward in Paris, and died there at the end of December, 1879. His body was embalmed and sent home. Following the exposure of the remains of this person to the view of his family in Philadelphia there was an outbreak of influenza with characteristic symptoms, which affected, in the first place, members of that family; afterward, friends living in close intercourse with them; next, the medical attendant of some of them; and finally, the housekeeper and a patient or two of one of the physicians who wrote the paper, the whole number affected in Philadelphia being eighteen at the time of the publication of the account. Subsequently two or three other cases were developed, but the disease did not extend beyond the immediate circle of those in direct communication with the invalids.

[19] John Guitéras, M.D., and J. W. White, M.D., "A Contribution to the History of Influenza, being a Study of a Series of Cases," *Philadelphia Medical Times*, April 10, 1880.

It was at one time thought that influenza developed at once, without a period of incubation, persons in perfect health being struck down with it as by lightning-stroke. It is, however, now known that a period of incubation, varying from a few hours to several days, and usually without subjective symptoms, exists. Many instances are recorded in which persons coming into an infected city have remained well for one, two, or three days, but have eventually shared the sufferings of those into whose midst they have come. There are cases also in which the period of incubation could not have been less than two or three weeks.

There is no sufficient evidence of a causal relation between influenza and any other epidemic disease. The statement that other prevalent diseases abate in frequency and intensity upon its outbreak is not sustained by well-observed facts. Graves[20] holds that those suffering with acute diseases are less liable during the febrile stage, but that they are attacked as convalescence sets in.

[20] *Clinical Medicine*.

The facts in reference to the spread of epidemics of influenza and the course of the disease in infected localities are comprehensible upon no other theory than that of a specific infecting principle as its exciting cause. What this principle may be is not yet known; where it originates is equally unknown; and our knowledge of the influences that from time to time call it into activity and send it forth in definite directions over the earth is no less negative.

So general a disease can only be disseminated by the most general medium, the atmosphere, and its exciting cause must be capable of reproducing itself in that medium, otherwise it would be lost by dispersion in traversing distances measured by the boundaries of continents and oceans. The rapid diffusion of influenza, sweeping over continents in a few weeks at one time, its slow migration, creeping about a city and its environs for months, at another, are to be most easily explained upon the theory of a living miasm capable of being transmitted by the air, and possessing at the same time an independent existence. Such an entity would find certain localities more favorable to its growth, reproduction, and prolonged existence than others. From this point of view influenza is a miasmatic disease. The infecting principle of this disease is also, to a slight extent, capable of being reproduced in or about the human body and transmitted by personal intercourse, as well as conveyed from place to place by the persons or clothing of those affected or those travelling from localities in which the disease prevails. We are thus led to the conclusion that it is also contagious, though feebly so.

[p. 864]CLINICAL HISTORY.—Influenza, in individual cases, presents the greatest variation as regards intensity, from the most trifling indisposition to an illness of the gravest kind, terminating in death. These variations are dependent upon—1st, the previous health of the individual, his age, and the power of resisting depressing influences which he possesses; 2d, the energy and the amount of the specific cause of the disease to which he has been exposed—in other words, the dose of the fever-producing poison; and 3d, the character of the prevailing epidemic.

It is important to observe that cases of very great severity are occasionally encountered during the prevalence of mild epidemics. In every epidemic, on the contrary, a considerable part of the community suffers from influenza in the mildest, or what has been called the rudimentary, form. This is characterized by general malaise, an easily oncoming weariness upon bodily and mental effort, a disinclination for business, some inability to fix the attention, and slight mental confusion; to these nervous disturbances are added catarrhal symptoms, as coryza, sore throat, a tickling cough, and the like; but the indisposition is subfebrile—it does not amount to a fully-developed fever. Other cases present the symptoms of an ordinary attack of acute coryza, laryngitis, bronchitis, pharyngitis, with unusual constitutional disturbance, distressing headache, and pains in the back and limbs. The fever in this class of cases does not range high, yet the patients are ill enough to betake themselves to bed.

In severe cases the onset is usually abrupt. The attack begins with shivering or a chill, or with fits of chilliness alternating with heat. Fever is rapidly established. It is usually moderate; sometimes it reaches a high grade. It shows a tendency to morning remissions. Sensations of chilliness occur; they are called forth by slight changes in the external temperature. They are often followed by flushes of heat, and are, in many cases, attended by annoying sweats. The febrile outbreak is sometimes preceded by intense frontal headache, with pain in the orbits and at the root of the nose. In other cases these pains quickly follow the chill. Sneezing, redness of the eyes and edges of the nostrils, a more or less abundant thin discharge from the nose, and lachrymation, now occur. In some instances there is bleeding from the nose. The throat becomes sore; there is a tickling sensation in the upper air-passages; a dry cough sets in, attended by more or less hoarseness and shortness of breath. The cough is paroxysmal, hard, distressing. It sometimes causes vomiting, like that which occurs in the paroxysms of whooping cough. Chest-pains, stitches in the side, frequent sneezing, loss of the sense of smell and of taste, attend the development of the general catarrhal manifestations.

The fever is attended by great depression, pains in the limbs, loss of appetite, thirst, constipation, and diminished secretion of urine. The pulse is full, but, as a rule, only moderately increased in frequency. There is in many cases slight, or even decided, blueness of the lips and finger-tips. The patient is distressed by restlessness and want of sleep. At the end of four or five days the febrile symptoms decline, at times gradually, oftener rapidly, with copious sweats or spontaneous flux from the bowels. The fever continues, however, when severe complications have taken place, ten or twelve days. The defervescence is marked by [p. 865]an increased flow of sedimentary urine and considerable amelioration of the subjective symptoms. The catarrhal symptoms outlast the fever two or three days, but cough and expectoration may not disappear for some time.

With these symptoms are associated the evidences of functional disturbance of the nervous system. There is remarkable nervous depression; loss of strength and lowness of spirits are combined with mental weakness, or even stupor and delirium. In some cases slight convulsions take place. Cutaneous hyperæsthesia occasionally occurs, and areas of burning pain in the skin are to be met with. Neuralgia, muscle-pain, and aching referred to the bones are very common and often severe.

In other cases abdominal symptoms are prominent, while those referable to the head and chest are less urgent. The disease assumes the guise of a more or less severe catarrh of the gastro-enteric mucous membrane, with disturbance of the functions of the liver. The fever and the peculiar nervous depression are, however, the same. Cases likewise present themselves in which but little of the usual tendency to localization of the catarrhal processes is to be observed; there is fever of varying intensity, with great depression, and simultaneous and equal implication of the head and the organs of the chest and abdomen.

Many writers have sought to arrange the foregoing different forms of influenza in definite categories. It would be a useless task to reproduce their views upon the subject, or even to enumerate the varieties that have been described. In practice, the various described types merge so gradually into each other, and are so modified by the individual peculiarities of the sick, and by the complications which arise in the course of the attack in consequence of such peculiarities or of previously existing diseases or tendencies to special forms of disease, that, in point of fact, particular cases cannot usually be referred to theoretical categories. Hysterical persons and those of a nervous constitution are prone to suffer especially from the peculiar nervous symptoms of influenza. The disease is also modified by the age of the subject of the attack; children manifest in a high degree the signs of cerebral congestion, while old persons are subject in a peculiar manner to dangerous pulmonary complications, and those of a gouty or rheumatic constitution suffer more than others from muscular pains.

The duration of the mildest form of influenza is from two to three days; in well-developed cases without complications convalescence sets in between the fourth and tenth days; while severe cases with complications last much longer, several weeks often elapsing before recovery is complete.

SYMPTOMATOLOGY.—ANALYSIS OF THE SYMPTOMS.—For the purpose of separate consideration it is convenient to take up the symptoms belonging to the fever first, then those of the special catarrh, and finally those more particularly referable to the nervous system; but we encounter in the present state of our knowledge of the pathology of influenza—or our ignorance of its pathology—no little difficulty in deciding under which of these headings particular symptoms are properly to be classed, by reason of the close interdependence of the chief processes of the disease and the anomalies of its phenomena viewed as a whole.

The Fever.—The fever is of the sub-continuous or remittent type, [p. 866]but its range is very irregular. Irregularity of temperature is characteristic of influenza and may assume diagnostic importance.

The intensity of the fever is variable. As a rule, it is moderate or slight; occasionally it is severe. I observed in several cases during the epidemic of 1879 in Philadelphia an evening temperature of only 39° C. (102.2° F.). Da Costa in the same outbreak found the febrile movement not high; the highest temperature he observed was 40° C. (104° F.). Biermer found a temperature of over 39° C. in moderate cases of catarrhal fever, and does not doubt that under certain transient conditions the temperature may reach the height of that of pneumonia or typhus. In weakly persons and the aged the fever is adynamic.

The pulse has no constant characters. Its frequency is moderately increased; it is apt to be less forcible than in health, is generally compressible, sometimes full, often irregular, changing in character in the course of a few hours.

The urine is usually diminished; sometimes its secretion is temporarily suppressed; as a rule, it shows little change, and is rarely, as in other fevers, concentrated and high-colored. It deposits on cooling a sediment of urates, which toward the close of the fever is often very abundant. The defervescence is in many instances attended by a copious secretion of urine. Albumen is not present except as a result of some complication.

At first the skin is hot and dry; later, frequent sweats occur; sweating generally attends the febrile remissions and the defervescence not rarely sets in with copious, acid, ill-smelling sweats. In some cases a tendency to sweat shows itself early and continuous throughout the attack. Sudamina occur in great numbers.

The face is often flushed, and irregular mottlings of the skin, especially upon the neck and chest, have been frequent in some of the epidemics. An outbreak of herpes about the lips is occasionally seen.

Disturbances of the digestive tract are more or less prominent in almost all cases. Only in a rudimentary and sub-febrile form are they absent. In many cases they are such as are usually seen in febrile disorders—namely, loss of appetite, thirst, impaired taste, pasty tongue, tenderness in the epigastrium, and constipation. Nausea and vomiting sometimes usher in the attack. In other cases (the so-called abdominal form) all the above symptoms are more severe, and diarrhoea, colicky pains, and vomiting are superadded. In certain epidemics the intestinal catarrh has shown a tendency to run into dysentery.

The expression of the countenance is changed, in part by the appearance characterizing an ordinary attack of coryza of considerable or great severity, and in part by anxiety and depression. It is pale. Where the pulmonary catarrh is excessive and dyspnoea great the lips become bluish. The facies sometimes suggests that of typhoid fever.

The Catarrh.—A more or less extensive hyperæmia of the mucous membrane of the respiratory tract is invariably present, and may be said to characterize the disease.

There is cold in the head, more severe in most cases than ordinary simple coryza. The eyelids are swollen and reddened, there is lachrymation, sneezing is frequent, and the discharge from the nose is abundant. Epistaxis is not rare. Sore throat, with tickling sensations and difficulty [p. 867]in swallowing, is due to inflammation of the pharynx and neighboring parts. In many instances the catarrhal symptoms are due to a pharyngitis and tonsillitis only, the lower air-passages escaping. Hoarseness is common.

Cough is a prominent symptom. It is apt to be frequent and distressing—sometimes paroxysmal from the beginning of the sickness, almost always so at some period of its course. Its spasmodic character in some of the older epidemics led to the confounding of epidemic catarrhal fever with whooping cough. It is apt to be worse toward evening and at night, but the sick are often tormented day and night by the loud racking cough. It often leads to vomiting, and by its violence and persistence gives rise to pain and soreness in the muscles of respiration (myalgia), and occasionally to hernia. It is at first dry or attended with a scanty muco-serous expectoration; later on the sputa become opaque and muco-purulent, and in consumptive or full-blooded persons or those having mitral disease they are sometimes streaked or mingled with blood. Toward the close of the attack the cough becomes less urgent and loses its spasmodic character. In some epidemics cough is not a prominent symptom, and a few cases are encountered in most epidemics in which well-developed influenza runs its course without unusual, peculiar, or excessive cough. If the cough be due to bronchitis, we find on auscultation the physical signs of that affection. They are of course wanting when it is due simply to laryngo-tracheal irritation. Hence we frequently detect sonorous and sibillant or mucous and subcrepitant râles upon both sides of the chest in the course of the attack, as in non-epidemic acute bronchitis; and, on the other hand, cases occur where the auscultatory signs are but little or not at all altered from those of health. It is scarcely necessary to add that there are no special physical signs that can be regarded as diagnostic of influenza.

Many patients suffer from dyspnoea. Although due in some instances to complications, it occurs with remarkable frequency in those in whom none of the objective signs of any pulmonary lesion can be discovered. It is here of nervous origin. Graves assumes a direct disturbance in the function of the vagus as its cause. This view is sustained by the observation that the dyspnoea is now and then intermittent, or shows rhythmically recurring remissions, which are unattended by alteration of the physical signs. To Biermer it appears more probable that the congestions so common in influenza, not attended by marked physical signs until they lead to oedema, are to be regarded as the cause of the dyspnoea. It varies greatly in intensity. In many patients it goes on to marked oppression, great shortness of breath, precordial pain, and the like. In certain epidemics orthopnoea and suffocative attacks were very common. Stitches in the side and pain under the sternum are observed without appreciable physical signs.

Symptoms Referable to the Nervous System.—Great prostration of muscular strength is a very early symptom, and constitutes, in most epidemics, one of the remarkable features of the disease. Patients from the onset feel extremely weak, and are exhausted by the slightest bodily effort. The ordinary strength is not regained until convalescence is far advanced.

Headache is a constant symptom. Severe frontal pains are scarcely [p. 868]ever absent. They extend across the brow and deeply about the orbits and at the root of the nose, having their seat in the Schneiderian mucous membrane and its prolongations lining the frontal sinuses and the nasal ducts. Sometimes the pain is referred also to the region of the antrum of Highmore and to the Eustachian tube and the middle ear. It occasionally extends over the whole head. Cutaneous hyperæsthesia of the head and neck and stiffness of the neck-muscles are also met with. The headache is often most intense; it lasts commonly till the end of the attack, and may even outlast it. It increases in severity with the fever and mental agitation toward evening. The occurrence of epistaxis affords some relief.

Among the more constant symptoms of influenza are very severe pains in the limbs. Patients experience sensations of soreness and bruising, such as follow the most severe and unaccustomed muscular effort. Dull, tearing, and burning pains are felt sometimes in particular muscles or tendons; sometimes they are diffused over the whole body. Distressing pains of a dragging or boring character in the loins and calves of the legs are complained of. These pains are neither relieved nor aggravated by gentle movement or by moderate pressure. A sense of contraction of the chest and precordial distress also occurs, and stitches in the side (pleurodynia), substernal pain, and pains in the throat and nape of the neck are common. When the attack is severe the patient is usually restless, sleepless, and anxious. Dizziness and a tendency to faint occur on rising, particularly in women. Mild delirium is not uncommon, but the more intense forms are occasionally observed. Active delirium was thought to be a mortal symptom in some of the older epidemics.

The inability to sleep bears no direct relation to the intensity of the fever. It is seen in some cases where fever is slight or even absent.

Somnolent states also occur. Great hebetude and torpor have marked some epidemics. That of 1712 was called the sleepy sickness, by reason of the prevalence of these symptoms.

In grave cases painful muscle-cramps, subsultus tendinum, twitchings of particular muscles, and tremblings of the hands occur.

The mental power is enfeebled, and the acuteness of the special senses is diminished.

COMPLICATIONS AND SEQUELS.—The most important complications of influenza are inflammatory diseases of the lungs. The hyperæmia and intense bronchitis already described as occurring in the severer cases cannot properly be looked upon as complications. They constitute rather essential processes of particular forms of the disease. But capillary bronchitis, catarrhal pneumonia, and less frequently croupous pneumonia, arise as complications in the course of the disease. Satisfactory statistics are wanting, but Biermer estimates that from 5 to 10 per cent. of the whole number of patients suffer from inflammatory lung-complications, and holds that the bloodletting so frequently practised by the older physicians was due to a desire to combat inflammation. The comparative frequency of chest complications in different epidemics varies greatly, but the estimate of Biermer may be accepted as an approximate average.

Owing to the masking of the physical signs in the early stages and the pre-existing pulmonary oedema, it is not always easy to recognize at once [p. 869]the occurrence of capillary bronchitis. This complication is attended with increasing dyspnoea, decided lividity of the face and extremities, and great prostration. Crepitant and subcrepitant râles at the lower portions of the posterior dorsal regions, rapidly spreading to all parts of the chest, without dulness at first and with increased resonance later, instead of the signs of consolidation which are met with in pneumonia, are the signs which attend its appearance.

Catarrhal pneumonia occurs insidiously, with gradual intensification of the bronchitic symptoms about the fourth or fifth day, but it may set in as early as the second day, or much later, during convalescence. It is, as a rule, developed without chill or great increase in the fever.

Old persons and those of feeble constitutions are most liable to the foregoing complications.

Lobar pneumonia is less common. It is a late complication, occurring toward the close of the attack or even when the patient is beginning to get about. It is easily recognized, and differs in no wise from acute lobar pneumonia occurring under other circumstances.

In October, 1880, influenza being prevalent in Philadelphia, both epizoötic and epidemic, but very mild both among horses and men, I attended a medical student who, having had what he regarded as a cold for about a week, had kept at his work without treatment, until, upon the occurrence of a chill followed by grave thoracic symptoms, he was obliged to betake himself to bed. I first saw him the following day in the hospital of the Jefferson College. There were the symptoms of acute lobar pneumonia, with the signs of extensive consolidation of the left lung and pleurisy of the right side. Moreover, there were delirium and jaundice. The urine was non-albuminous. The next evening he died. At the same time many members of the class suffered from influenza, and a careful inquiry into the history of the case of this young gentleman satisfied me that the pneumonia had arisen as a complication in a neglected and moderate severe catarrhal fever. Until the eighth day before his death he was in excellent health. No examination of the body was permitted.

Graves[21] thought that a kind of paralysis of the lungs, with great oedema, takes place in some cases, and attributed it to an affection of the vagus. It was his conviction "that the poison which produced influenza acted on the nervous system in general, and on the pulmonary nerves in particular, in such a way as to produce symptoms of bronchial irritation and dyspnoea, to which bronchial congestion and inflammation were often superadded."

[21] *Annals of Influenza.*

It is certain that localized collapse of the lung often occurs. White and Guitéras attributed the consolidations of the lung to congestive collapse due to enlargement of the tracheal and bronchial glands and "disturbance of the great nervous tract about the root of the lung." They were enabled to satisfy themselves of the existence of glandular enlargement—adenopathie bronchique—in nine of their eighteen cases by percussion practised in the method of M. Geneau de Mussy,[22] who was the first to call attention to the importance of percussing the spinous processes of the vertebræ over the course of the trachea. Following this line in the healthy subject, a distinct tubular (high-pitched and slightly [p. 870]tympanitic) sound is elicited by percussion down to the point of bifurcation of the trachea on the level of the fourth dorsal vertebra. Opposite the fifth and downward we get the lower-pitched pulmonary resonance. When the tracheal and bronchial glands are enlarged, the tubular sound over the upper dorsal vertebræ is replaced by dulness, which may contrast sharply, above with the tracheal, and below with the vesicular resonance.

[22] *Chirurgie médicale*, Paris, 1874.

Some well-recognized peculiarities of the so-called pneumonias of influenza give weight to the view that the consolidations are not, in the beginning, pneumonic at all. Thus, we have at first weakness of the vesicular murmur, then its absence; the respiration soon becomes bronchial, without being preceded by dulness or the crepitant râle; the extension of those consolidations from one part of the lung to another is very irregular; the process is more apt to involve both sides than one; the disappearance of the consolidation is frequently very rapid.

The relations of cause and effect between collapse and catarrhal pneumonia are so close that it is not difficult to see how the condition spoken of may lead to secondary lobular or catarrhal pneumonia. In truth, this is a frequent result of collapse from any cause.

White and Guitéras do not adduce any post-mortem facts in support of their theory. Peacock, however, observed in the epidemic of 1847 softening and enlargement of the bronchial glands in several cases, and in one instance where there was no antecedent disease of the lungs, and where the physical signs corresponded to some extent with those of the cases upon which White and Guitéras base their views.

Gangrene of the lungs must be named as one of the less common complications.

These complications are the chief cause of the danger of influenza in the aged, the debilitated, and those suffering from previous disease of the thoracic organs.

Pleurisy is rare except where there is coexisting inflammation of the lungs. It may be associated with pericarditis. In old persons serous effusions into the pleural sac are now and then encountered.

Troublesome laryngitis and chronic bronchitis may follow the attack. In consequence of the extension of the catarrhal processes along the Eustachian tube an actual inflammation of the middle ear is, in rare instances, set up. Parotitis with salivation sometimes occurs, likewise aphthous inflammations of the mouth.

Herpes labialis occasionally occurs toward the end of the attack; it is then a favorable indication.

Phthisis may be developed in consequence of an attack of influenza, and if phthisis be already established it is apt to run a more rapid course. Emphysematous affections are aggravated; diseases of the heart are unfavorably influenced; chronic nervous affections are made worse, and, in particular, neuralgias are aggravated. Old neuralgias, that have long ceased to give trouble, occasionally reappear during the convalescence.

Persons subject to latent or chronic Bright's disease are especially liable to the more serious manifestations of influenza. The fatal termination of such cases not unfrequently occurs in consequence of an attack.

Many of the older observers speak of the intermittent character of[p. 871]influenza in certain epidemics, and its tendency to run into intermittents, particularly of a certain type, during convalescence. This has not been observed in the outbreaks of later years, and it is probable that in such instances an endemic malaria has modified the epidemic catarrhal fever, or the former has broken out as the latter passed away.

Pregnant women are in danger of aborting.

PATHOLOGY.—Our knowledge of the pathology of influenza is as yet very imperfect. Biermer has described it as the sum of a series of catarrhal manifestations developed under a common epidemic influence. The close association of the various local affections arises from their almost simultaneous occurrence as results of primary pathological processes common to them all. Each of the three groups of symptoms which make up the clinical picture of the disease—namely, the fever, the catarrh, and the symptoms referable to the nervous system—constitutes a distinct factor of influenza, and is a direct outcome of the action of the infecting principle. There is no constant interdependence among these groups, either in the order of their succession or in their intensity. Thus, while all three groups are commonly present from the beginning of the attack, any one of them may be the first to appear or have an intensity out of all proportion to each of the others. The fever is not a result of the catarrhal inflammation, nor are the nervous symptoms the result of both the others. They all spring directly from the action of the same cause.

This view is at variance with the opinion—based upon the fact that ordinary acute local inflammatory diseases, tonsillitis, bronchitis, and the like, sometimes run their course in a similar way to influenza, with fever, nervous depression, and a serious sense of illness—that influenza is a simple epidemic catarrhal inflammation.

The sudden onset of influenza, its not infrequent abrupt termination, which suggests crisis, its unsparing seizure of great numbers of the population, the severity of the nervous symptoms, and the amount of laryngo-bronchial irritation, often out of measure with the lesions of the mucous membranes,—all point to the action of a morbid agent affecting the body at large. The severity of the symptoms also, in many cases, is much greater than in similar acute non-specific local affections, while the complications, and in particular the recrudescence of fading neuralgias and the tendency to abortion, and the sequels, as cough, weakness, headaches, flying pains, which often remain long after convalescence, are evidences of its belonging to the group of infectious diseases rather than to that of simple acute inflammatory diseases.

In conclusion, it must be urged that the similarity of the symptoms in many epidemics, occurring during the course of several centuries and under different social conditions, and even different degrees of civilization, forcibly demonstrates the specific and definite character of the causes which give rise to influenza.

Very little light is thrown upon the pathology of the disease by the anatomical changes found after death. Uncomplicated influenza is rarely fatal. As a rule, the unfavorable termination is due to lung complications. The essential lesions are congestion and catarrhal swelling of the mucous membrane of the upper air-passages and the bronchial tubes. These changes may be restricted, in the lungs, to the trachea and larger [p. 872]bronchi, or they may extend to the finest twigs. They may amount to great thickening and deep capillary injections of the mucous lining of the tubes, which contain clear, frothy mucus or thick, viscid masses of muco-purulent secretion unmixed with air.

More or less congestion of the gastric mucous membrane, and more rarely of that of the intestine, is also met with. The solitary and agminate glands of the intestine are not affected, save as the result of special complications. A few observations relate to the finding of enlarged and softened bronchial glands. More extended researches are needed, not only upon this point, but also in the whole domain of the pathological anatomy of the disease.

Hyperæmia, oedema, hypostatic congestions, splenization, catarrhal pneumonia, and hepatization affect the lung-tissue in cases fatal by the complications which are associated with such changes. The tissue-changes of diseases existing prior to the attack of influenza, such as old consolidations, tubercle, brown induration, emphysema, and so forth, are of course frequently discovered.

DIAGNOSIS.—The discrimination of influenza from other affections having some points of resemblance to it is, under ordinary circumstances, unattended with difficulty. The march of the epidemic, the number of persons attacked, the prominence of the nervous symptoms, the rapidly developed debility, and the character of the cough, usually severe out of proportion to the physical signs, distinguish it from all other epidemic diseases.

It is to be differentiated from non-specific catarrhal affections attended by fever, malaise, weakness, severe headache, and pain in the extremities by a due regard to the causative relations of the two affections. Simple catarrhs not rarely present the group of symptoms which characterize epidemic catarrhal fever, but they occur almost constantly as the result of great and sudden changes in the weather, and are therefore met with in greatest frequency in bad seasons, and are particularly common at the end of winter and in the spring. Influenza is not in any way dependent upon the vicissitudes of the seasons, and may occur, as has been shown, at all times of the year, in wet or dry, mild or cold seasons equally, and in every variety of climate. It is of course diagnosticated without difficulty from the sporadic catarrhal fevers, which lack the characteristic depression, neuralgic and rheumatoid pains, the irritative cough, dyspnoea, and so on.

Cases of influenza are met with that bear a strong resemblance to beginning enteric fever. The malaise, headache, obtunded hearing, mental depression, high fever, coated tongue, tender belly, diarrhoea, are symptoms to be observed in both affections. But influenza lacks the temperature curve, the splenic enlargement, and the eruption of enteric fever, and the progress of the disease will in a few days clear up the most doubtful case.

PROGNOSIS AND MORTALITY.—Death is rare in uncomplicated cases. The very young bear influenza badly; the old bear it more badly still. Nevertheless, children have in some epidemics enjoyed a considerable proportionate immunity. Healthy persons in the middle periods of life bear it well. Certain pre-existing diseases modify its course unfavorably; among these are chronic bronchitis, emphysema, fatty heart, and Bright's disease. [p. 873]The debility of advanced phthisis and other exhausting diseases renders influenza dangerous. Death takes place, in by far the greater number of cases, as the result of the complication of the attack, either by some pre-existing affection or by an acute disease arising in its course. The commonest of the latter are inflammations of the parenchyma of the lungs.

Patients presenting very severe symptoms generally recover if they be not the subjects of complicating maladies or very young or very old.

Relapses are not uncommon; independently of relapses, second attacks have been known to occur during the continuance of an epidemic; it is often the case that an individual in the course of his life passes through several epidemics of influenza, and is the subject of the disease in each of them.

The prognosis is greatly modified by the character of the prevailing epidemic. In some epidemics the deaths are few, and the mortality from other diseases does not appear to be greatly augmented. In others many die of the epidemic disease, and the death-rate of certain endemic affections is much increased. In some of the older epidemics the high mortality was doubtless due to injudicious measures of treatment, among which bloodletting and other depressing agencies were conspicuous. Some of the older accounts also warrant the suspicion that a coexisting typhus had to do with the high death-rate. It is estimated that in the epidemic of 1837, which was a very severe one, 2 per cent. of those attacked died. The proportion of fatal cases in particular epidemics varies in different countries, and even in different quarters of the same city.

TREATMENT.—Efficient measures of prophylaxis are as yet unknown. Unfavorable hygienic surroundings, overcrowding, a damp, unhealthy locality, appear to increase the prevalence and severity of influenza. The opposite conditions of living do not, however, secure immunity from the attack. During an epidemic aged persons, those enfeebled by chronic diseases, and in particular those subject to chronic bronchitis, consumption, emphysema, fatty heart, and Bright's disease should be cared for with unusual diligence and solicitude, since they constitute the classes most prone to the graver complications of the disease, and from which its fatal cases are almost wholly derived. Such individuals should be warmly clad; they should shun, so far as possible, the vicissitudes of the weather, even, if practicable, keeping within warmed and well-ventilated apartments; they should exercise unusual prudence in diet and lead a carefully regulated life, with long hours of sleep. It is true that these measures are not preventive of the attack. Families not quitting the house, living in the greatest seclusion, even the bedridden, do not always, or even as a rule, escape. Yet it has frequently been observed that those whose occupations are carried on in the open air are attacked earliest and in greatest numbers. On the other hand, in rare instances, persons isolated from the community with strictness—in prisons, cloisters, hospitals—have remained free from the disease prevailing around them. It therefore appears probable that, under certain favorable circumstances not as yet perfectly understood, the avoidance of the open air and of the direct influences of the weather may confer some degree of immunity from the attack, and it is desirable that the class of persons most liable to the graver consequences of the disease should avail themselves of even the most uncertain precautions.

[p. 874]The treatment of influenza is expectant and supporting. Not only is the epidemic self-limiting, tending to exhaust the susceptibility of a community, in most instances, in the space of a few weeks, but the attack is also of definite duration, and the perturbations set up by the action of the influenza-poison upon the individual subside spontaneously in three or four, or at most ten or twelve, days. The susceptibility of the individual is also, for the time being, exhausted, for second attacks in the same epidemic are not very common. In cases where the duration of the attack is prolonged beyond the period indicated, it is kept up by complications, and we have to do not so much with the pathological processes of influenza as with secondary diseases that the influenza has excited either by the intensity of its action or by reason of some peculiarity of the subject of the attack.

By far the greatest number of cases are light and unattended by danger. The treatment is therefore, for the most part, an extremely simple one. These lighter cases seldom require medical measures. The patients are uncomfortable and anxious, easily fatigued, and unfitted for business. It is best that they keep the house, and, if willing, the bed or sofa, for the space of two or three days. The diet should be restricted to a few simple and easily-digested dishes. Meat should be avoided. The common custom of taking hot beef-tea is an extremely bad one; it often increases the headache and languor. Moderate quantities of cold drinks may be taken. The fruit-syrups, lemonade, raspberry vinegar, a weak solution of citrate of potash or of cream of tartar, and barley-water with lemon, are useful. Very weak wine-whey is often liked. The effervescing mineral waters or Apollinaris are preferred by many persons. The best of such drinks is a mixture of equal parts of Seltzer-water and milk, iced. If the stomach be irritable, koumiss will be found an excellent beverage and food. In the mild cases stimulants are not necessary. Sound claret, with or without Seltzer-water, is not contraindicated. In all cases the amount of fluid taken should be moderate.

Quinine in moderate doses should be taken from the onset. The head-pains are not increased by it. Dover's powder, if well borne, should be administered at night. Some form of opiate may be required, even in mild cases, to counteract wakefulness. A compressed pill, containing extract of opium 0.030 gramme (gr. ½), camphor 0.15 (gr. ij), and ammonium carbonate 0.15 (gr. ij), will be found useful when Dover's powder cannot be employed. During convalescence iron and barks are often requisite.

The coryza, tonsillitis, laryngitis, bronchitis are to be treated according to general principles, if they require treatment at all. In most mild cases the catarrhal symptoms call for no special measures of treatment.

Free inunctions of fatty substances about the brow and over the bridge of the nose are of use as regards the coryza. For this purpose animal fats, washed lard, simple cerate, cold cream, and the like are to be preferred to cosmoline and vaseline.

Morphine dissolved in cherry-laurel water, one part in fifty or sixty, is useful for the relief of the head-pains associated with the coryza. A few drops may be snuffed up from time to time. These pains are mitigated to some degree by wearing a flannel cap or wrapping the head in a silk handkerchief. Warm applications sometimes give comfort, while cold almost invariably add to the distress.

[p. 875]Distress in the upper air-passages and the tickling cough call for steam inhalations, and the air of the apartment may be rendered moist by the evaporation of water kept boiling in a broad, shallow vessel. Gargles of potassium chlorate, or potassium chlorate with sumac, exert a soothing influence upon the congested tonsils.

Severe cases call for more energetic measures of treatment. The most prominent indications are the control of the fever; the diminution of the hyperæmic fluxion to the mucous tracts; measures of support; the mitigation of pain and the induction of sleep; and, finally, the prevention of the pulmonary congestion, to which the depression leads by enfeeblement of the circulation. The last indication is especially urgent in infants, the very old, and those previously debilitated from any cause.

Inflammatory complications require special treatment or modifications of treatment.

The febrile movement is not, as a rule, high; grave nervous symptoms and serious catarrh may be associated with moderate fever.

An anti-febrile regimen is to be observed. The moderate duration of this fever, as compared with enteric fever, renders it less important that large amounts of fever-food should be given, while the tendency to depression makes it of the utmost importance that the administration of food be systematic and carefully looked after by the medical attendant. The disinclination to take food is so great that it is often with difficulty that a sufficient quantity can be given in the early days of the attack, and it is to be doubted whether benefit follows anything in excess of the most moderate amount. It is necessary to observe regular hours, as in the management of all the low fevers. As soon as convalescence begins the patient should be urged to eat; the quantity of food taken at one time is to be augmented, and the intervals between the meals may be longer.

A favorable action upon the excretory function of the skin and kidneys will result from the moderate drinking of water or of the beverages already spoken of. At least enough fluid should be taken to relieve thirst.

Diaphoretics have been much used, upon the theory that by determination to the skin they correspondingly diminish the tendency to hyperæmia of the affected mucous tracts. Dover's powder, solution of the acetate of ammonia, and other mild diaphoretics are to be selected. Jaborandi should be employed with caution. The wet pack and other hydrotherapeutic measures have been employed to act upon the skin and to effect a direct reduction of temperature in influenza. For old and feeble persons warm packs are employed.

A profuse sweating at the onset of the attack is said to occasionally cut it short. Early diaphoresis often brings about a rapid and lasting amelioration of the symptoms. It is to be borne in mind that the fever is rarely excessive, and that sweating is not infrequently a troublesome symptom. In some epidemics it has been a very troublesome one.

General bloodletting is not to be resorted to in influenza. Its danger was apparent to some of the early writers. As has been pointed out, the high mortality of some of the older epidemics is to be explained by the venesections practised at the beginning, and even during the course, of the attack. It has no favorable effect upon the catarrhal processes, and but little upon the subjective symptoms. The fever is not relieved by it; the[p. 876]nervous depression is increased and the risk of lung-congestion is augmented. Bleeding is not likely to be practised in epidemic catarrhal fever while the present views of its place in therapeutics continue to influence practice. Cautious local bloodletting for the relief of local inflammatory trouble is spoken of in most of the modern books. The occasions for its employment are so rare in the treatment of this disease that even this statement should be henceforth omitted. In influenza, as it is known to medical men of the present from the descriptions of the old and personal experience of the few recent and milder epidemics, bloodletting, either general or local, is clearly uncalled for.

Emetics hold a high historical place. It was of old customary to begin the treatment with a vomit. As late as the epidemic of 1837, Lombard of Geneva believed that they shortened the attack and lessened the intensity of the symptoms when administered at the beginning. In cases attended by early gastric disturbance and nausea they are said to be especially of use. They sometimes set up great irritability of the stomach, with vomiting that it is difficult to control. On the whole, the cases in which an emetic would do good are extremely rare.

Purgatives were formerly regarded as important in the treatment. This view no longer prevails. In case of constipation gentle purgation, ex indicatione symptomaticâ, is a necessary part of the proper management of the case. For this purpose the laxative mineral waters, as Friederichshalle, Hunyadi, Pullna, are excellent. Castor oil may be given, and calomel is in some cases, and particularly in childhood, of great service. Simple enemata of warm water or soap and water will often suffice. The tendency in some cases to exhausting and troublesome diarrhoea, and the fact that diarrhoea occurs spontaneously some time in the course of most cases, should inspire caution in the use of purgatives. Repeated purgation during the progress of the attack is not only useless—it is also positively injurious.

In the severe cases quinine is to be given early and in full doses. It exerts at the same time a powerful influence upon the temperature, upon the tendency to local hyperæmias, and upon the nervous symptoms, and in particular the headache. Rawlins,[23] as early as 1833, found that excellent results followed its administration, the effect being the better the earlier it was given. It has even been lauded as a specific for influenza.

[23] *London Medical Gazette*, May, 1833.

The mineral acids may be given with a view to realizing their tonic effects.

For the most part, the foregoing measures, directed against the fever, will exert a favorable influence upon the catarrhal processes. Expectorants are of advantage; ipecac is useful. The preparations of antimony are inadmissible by reason of their tendency to depress. Ammonium chloride is indicated in the earlier stages of the bronchitis. Among recent drugs, yerba santa (Eryodiction glutinosum) and the oil of eucalyptus are of use in mitigating the symptoms in epidemic catarrh, as they do in certain forms of simple sporadic catarrh.

The peculiar dry, racking cough so often present in the early days of the attack should be relieved. It is not useful in removing bronchial accumulations, being, as has been shown, in most instances out of proportion to the lesions of the bronchial mucous membrane; on the other[p. 877]hand, it tends to increase the hyperæmia of the upper air-passages by the mechanical violence of the cough-paroxysms. Further, it is distressing and exhausting, and contributes to the muscular and nervous prostration. Benefit will be derived from keeping the air of the apartment moist, and from the occasional inhalation of the steam from hot water, either used alone or poured upon the compound tincture of benzoin, a pint to the teaspoonful, or upon paregoric, a pint to the tablespoonful, in a proper vessel or inhaler.

No drugs are more potent to this end than opium and its derivatives, and in particular morphia and codeia. The hypodermic use of the morphia salts, judiciously resorted to, constitutes our most valuable therapeutic resource in fulfilling the threefold indication of relieving cough, alleviating both the head-pain and the pains in the extremities, and in procuring sleep. The old-time dread of opium in influenza was not well founded. The administration of this drug in moderate doses is attended with advantages that far outweigh any danger of increasing the tightness across the chest and retarding expectoration. It is necessary to observe the same caution in giving it to infants and aged persons in influenza that is necessary under other circumstances. The influence of carbolic acid in restraining cough makes it a useful addition to soothing draughts in this disease.

The substernal and other chest-pains may be combated with sinapisms, turpentine stupes, repeated inunctions of fatty substances containing extract of belladonna, and the like. Pleurodynic stitches call for similar measures; a long strip of machine-spread belladonna plaster, about five centimetres (two inches) in width, applied very firmly to the side of the chest from the spine in a direction downward and forward parallel with the ribs, and reaching to the median line in front, affords great relief to the lateral chest-pains.

The control of the debility must be regarded as the most important indication in old and feeble persons. Wine, spirits, milk-punch, ammonia, spirits of chloroform, are to be used, not in accordance with fixed rules, but as occasion may require. In many cases wine or whiskey will be indicated from the beginning, the quantity being determined rather by the effect upon the circulation and the general condition of the case than by rule. Women and others unaccustomed to the use of alcoholic drinks often take wine and brandy in considerable quantities, with striking benefit and without flushing or other evidences of its disagreeing.

Chloral is inadmissible as a hypnotic by reason of its depressing effect upon the heart. Paraldehyde may be used, or the bromides in connection with opium if the latter alone is not well borne.

Diarrhoea must be managed in accordance with general principles. If slight, it does not require special treatment. It is apt to occur at one period or another in the course of most cases, and not infrequently marks the beginning of convalescence. Colic may be treated with warm fomentations and carminatives; if it be due to constipation, mild laxatives are to be combined with them.

Severe cases of influenza demand the careful attention of the physician, who must be on the alert to detect the inflammatory lung complications which so often lead up to the fatal issue as early as possible. Their treatment must be regulated by the circumstances of the case, the nature[p. 878]of the particular complication, the age of the patient, and so on, in accordance with general therapeutical indications.

Finally, all measures, of whatever kind, that tend to depress the general nervous system or the functional activity of the respiration, and especially the heart-power, are to be sedulously avoided in the management of influenza. During the convalescence unfavorable influences of the weather are to be guarded against. It is important to warn the patient that a severe attack of influenza renders him liable for some time afterward to pulmonary disorders. The sequels, and in particular those implicating the respiratory tract, are to be appropriately treated. After severe cases a course of tonics is commonly of advantage, and a change of climate often necessary to re-establish the health.

As bearing on what is stated in the foregoing pages on the causation of influenza, reference may be made to the investigations of Seifert,[24] who claims to have found in the mucus expectorated by patients with influenza numbers of a peculiar micrococcus. It is evident, however, that no conclusions can be based upon these observations until the results have been subjected to careful examination in other epidemics.

[24] *Volkmann's klinische Vorträge*, No. 240, June 20, 1884.

[p. 879]

DENGUE.
BY H. D. SCHMIDT, M.D.

SYNONYMS.—Break-bone fever, Dandy fever.

HISTORY.—The history of this disease dates only from the second half of the last century, though it appears very probable that previous to this time dengue existed in the tropical regions of Africa and Asia, whence it was carried to Europe and America.

In Spain the disease has been known since 1764, when, up to 1768, it prevailed in Cadiz and Seville under the name of la piadosa or la pantomina.[1] In 1780 it appeared in the form of an epidemic in Philadelphia, where it was first noticed and described by Rush under the name of bilious remitting fever, commonly called break-bone fever on account of the violent pains attending it. Next it prevailed in Calcutta in 1824, and two years afterward it made its first appearance on the southern coast of the United States, in Charleston and Savannah, where it prevailed to 1827. Toward the close of 1827 another dengue epidemic broke out in the West Indies, whence the disease proceeded to the American continent, reaching New Orleans in the spring, and visiting Charleston and Savannah in the summer and autumn of 1828.[2] In 1844 it showed itself in Mobile, and in 1848 in Natchez, whilst in 1850 it reappeared along the Southern seacoast, particularly in Charleston, from which it proceeded even to inland towns, such as Augusta, Ga.[3] In 1865 dengue appeared in Teneriffe and other Canary Islands, whilst at the same time and through the years 1866 and 1867 it prevailed in Andalusia and in some other Spanish provinces.[4]

[1] R. H. Poggio, *La calentura roja observada in sus apariciones epidemicas de los anos 1865 y 1867*, Madrid (reported in *Virchow und Hirsch's Jahresbericht für das Jahr 1871*, vol. ii. p. 200).

[2] G. B. Wood, *Practice of Medicine*, 4th ed., vol. i. p. 444.

[3] S. H. Dickson, *Elements of Medicine*, 2d. ed., p. 747.

[4] R. H. Poggio, *Virchow und Hirsch's Jahresbericht für das Jahr 1871*, vol. ii. p. 200.

One of the most extensive epidemics of dengue prevailed from July, 1870, to January, 1871, in Zanzibar,[5] on the East Coast of Africa, whence it extended to Aden in Arabia and Port Said in Egypt. In December, 1871, the disease appeared simultaneously at Bombay and Calcutta,[6] to which place it had been carried by transport-ships from Aden. Proceeding from Bombay in a northern direction along the railroad, it spread [p. 880]over the central regions of the North-western Provinces, the Rajputana states, Cashmir, and the Punjaub. From Calcutta it passed over Assam and Bhotan to Thibet, and thence downward into Burmah and to all the large cities along the coast; while it also extended along the coast of Malabar over Visigapatam to Madras and Pondichery, finally arriving at Mysore. Thus the disease had actually spread over the whole Peninsula from Cape Tutikorin to the foot of the Himalayas, attacking equally all races or nationalities without regard to age, occupation, or position. Forty years previously, however, an epidemic of dengue had prevailed in Burmah. In 1873 it appeared on the island of Mauritius, to which it had been carried from India by an emigrant ship. In the same year a considerable number of cases of dengue were observed in New Orleans. In 1877 it appeared again in Egypt, where it prevailed in Ismailia.

[5] J. Christie, "Remarks on Kidniga Pepo, a peculiar form of exanthematous disease epidemic in Zanzibar, East Coast of Africa, from July, 1870, to January, 1871," *Brit. Med. Journal*, July 1, 1872, p. 577 (reported in *Virchow und Hirsch's Jahresbericht für das Jahr 1872*, vol. ii. p. 203).

[6] *Virchow und Hirsch's Jahresbericht für das Jahr 1873*, vol. ii. p. 208.

Finally, in 1880, dengue, in the form of a very extensive epidemic, prevailed once more along the Southern coast, visiting equally Charleston, Savannah, and New Orleans. A number of valuable observations concerning the nature and symptoms of the disease were made during this epidemic by Drs. D. C. Holliday of New Orleans, J. G. Thomas of Savannah, and F. T. Porcher and J. Forrest of Charleston.[7] At the same time it prevailed at Alexandria[8] (Egypt) to such an extent as to affect nearly the whole population.

[7] The papers of Drs. Holliday, Thomas, and Porcher were read before the American Public Health Association at its annual meeting, December, 1880, and published in the *Proceedings* of the Association. Dr. Forrest's paper was published in the *American Journal of Med. Science*, April, 1881.

[8] A. Vernoni, "Le Dengue à Alexandrie d'Égypte en 1880," *Gaz. hebd. de méd. et de chir.*, 41, 42 (reported in *Virchow und Hirsch's Jahresbericht für das Jahr 1880*, vol. ii. p. 5).

Dengue has been known under various popular names which it received from the people of the particular localities where it appeared in epidemic form. Even the designation, dengue, itself, by which the disease is at present generally known to the medical profession of the leading civilized nations, is of popular origin,[9] for it is supposed to be a Spanish corruption of the word dandy, the name of dandy-fever having been jocosely conferred on the disease by the negroes of St. Thomas from the stiff carriage of those affected with it. At Zanzibar it received the popular name of kidniga pepo, signifying spasmodic pains.

[9] G. B. Wood, *Practice of Medicine*, 4th edit., vol. i. p. 444.

DEFINITION.—Dengue is a peculiar febrile disease, generally appearing epidemically in tropical or semi-tropical regions, and characterized by a single paroxysm with or without remissions, severe pains, and stiffness in the joints and muscles, a peculiar exanthematous eruption, and almost never terminating fatally.

SYMPTOMS, COURSE, AND DURATION.[10]—Dengue never commences with a decided chill, though in many cases the attack of the disease is preceded by a feeling of general uneasiness and depression, vertigo, and headache, or even by a slight chilliness—a condition which may last from a few to twelve or even eighteen hours. In the majority of cases, however, the disease appears suddenly, very frequently at night, and announces itself at once by pains and a feeling of stiffness in the muscles, joints, back, and loins; in severe cases the pain may even extend to the [p. 881]bones.[11]The larger and smaller joints are equally affected, either simultaneously or successively, and frequently swollen, those of the hands and feet generally before the others. The pain in the joints is increased by motion, and is therefore justly regarded by most authors as rheumatic in nature. The same may be said of the muscles. Sheriff even observed redness of the skin covering the joints. According to the degree of severity of the case these pains may be more or less intense. In some cases hyperæsthesia of the skin of the palms of the hands and of the soles of the feet has been observed.

[10] Judging from the various accounts rendered by a considerable number of observers, it appears that the clinical symptoms of dengue had been the same in all the different localities on the globe where it has hitherto prevailed epidemically.

[11] M. Sheriff, "History of the Epidemic of Dengue in Madras in 1872,"*Med. Times and Gazette*, Nov. 15, p. 543 (reported in *Virchow und Hirsch's Jahresbericht für das Jahr 1873*).

Simultaneously with the affection of the joints and muscles the fever commences; its duration is from four to five days on the average, with one or, in exceptional cases, even more remissions. The temperature of the body during the first and second days of the fever rises to 102, 103, or even to 105° F; it then declines, to return to the normal standard on the fifth day. According to the measurements made by the late Dr. D'Aquin[12]of New Orleans, the temperature curves of dengue showed a continuous and steady rise until the highest point was reached on the first, second, or third day of the attack; then comes a short stadium of a few hours, and then a remission, soon to be followed by another rise of temperature, which, however, never reaches the maximum point of the first. The pulse rises with the temperature of the body, generally to from 80 to 120 beats a minute, and subsequently declines with the temperature. Delirium is very rarely observed in adults, but frequently in children, though without aggravation of the other symptoms. The face is generally flushed, the eyelids swollen, and the eyes injected and watery. The tongue in the beginning of the disease is covered with a white fur; its edges are red and its body swollen. As the disease advances the coating increases in thickness and assumes a dirty yellow color. The appetite is lost, without excessive thirst. In many cases there is slight irritability of the stomach, accompanied sometimes with nausea, though vomiting rarely takes place. The condition of the bowels is variable. The urine is small in quantity, and highly colored in some cases, whilst in others it has been reported to be pale and copious, and rich in phosphates in the beginning of the disease; it seldom shows any sediments and very rarely contains albumen. The disease generally reaches its acme on the third or fourth day, when the fever commences to subside, and an amelioration of the other symptoms takes place, so that the patient feels greatly relieved. This, however, is only of short duration, for not many hours afterward the fever rises again, while the other symptoms also increase in severity. At this time an exanthematous eruption appears upon the upper part of the body, the face, neck, breast, and shoulders, which in the course of two days extends over the whole body. Simultaneously with the appearance of the eruption the lymphatic glands of the back of the head and those of the neck, axillæ, and groins commence to swell; in severe cases the mucous membranes of the nose, mouth, and pharynx also become congested. The eruption, which is attended with much heat, itching, or even pain, is not uniform in character; for while in some cases it may [p. 882]represent a simple rash or erythema, it resembles in others the eruptions of scarlatina, rubeola, lichen, or urticaria. Frequently it is very light and evanescent, showing itself only for a few hours, and perhaps in the majority of cases it does not appear at all. In the severer cases it generally remains two days, when it commences to fade and disappear with desquamation, while at the same time the fever subsides and disappears entirely, though the stiffness and soreness in the joints and muscles, together with the inflammatory condition of the superficial lymphatic glands, may persist for many weeks. In exceptional cases the eruption, after an intermission of a few days, reappears, generally with greater intensity and with an aggravation of the other symptoms. In others, again, it has been observed to remain a whole week.

[12] D. C. Holliday, "Dengue or Dandy Fever," read before the Amer. Publ. Health Assoc. at New Orleans, December, 1880.

Hemorrhages from the nose and gums are also occasionally observed. Holliday even observed the occurrence of black vomit in the cases of two female children, aged respectively six and twelve, in the same family, who had suffered from yellow fever in 1878; they both recovered from the attack of dengue, though they were extremely ill and much prostrated. In female patients an attack of dengue not unfrequently causes the reappearance of the menstrual flow, while the pains attending the disease equally predispose to premature labor in pregnant women.

In severe cases of dengue the prostration following upon the subsidence of the fever is very great, for the patient is affected with a general weakness both of body and mind, indicating a great loss of nervous energy. In some cases observed by Slaughter the memory for names and words, as well as the ability for correctly writing even short sentences, was lost for one or two weeks after the commencement of convalescence. In children also cases are reported in which the mind remained affected for a short time after the attack. The convalescence in dengue, therefore, is comparatively slow, particularly as the pains in the muscles and joints, as already mentioned, pass away only gradually.

The duration of the disease, including the stage of convalescence, of course depends upon the degree of intensity of the attack, and accordingly varies in different cases. In a great number of cases dengue manifests itself only in its milder form. The average duration of the disease is from three to six days.

PATHOLOGY.—The pathological changes taking place in the different organs during the course of dengue are unknown, on account of the almost constantly favorable termination of the disease. From the peculiar features of some of the clinical symptoms accompanying the disease, however, we may speculate to a certain extent upon the nature of the pathological processes to which they are due. The sudden appearance of the characteristic pains in the muscles and joints, but particularly those in the head, neck, and loins, accompanied by a comparatively high fever, evidently point to the presence of an infectious poison in the system, though the question whether the noxious influence of this poison primarily affects the blood or the nervous system will be difficult to answer. But, judging from the early appearance of the pains, as well as from the physical and mental depression of the patient, we may presume that the nervous system is involved from the very beginning of the disease, and that the pains depend upon a hyperæmic condition of the affected parts, probably caused by a vaso-motor paralysis. The great resemblance of the painful [p. 883]affection of the muscles and joints in dengue to that of acute articular rheumatism leads to the supposition that the pathological condition in these joints is the same in both diseases; this view appears to be held by the majority of medical observers. In dengue, as in rheumatism, the pain due to the pressure of the hyperæmic and swollen tissues upon the irritated sensory nervous filaments is increased by motion—a phenomenon generally absent in neuralgia. The persistent headache, restlessness, and want of sleep, as well as the delirium and loss of memory observed in the severer cases, furthermore indicate a hyperæmic condition not only of the pia mater, but even of the brain-substance.

It is to be regretted that the literature of dengue within our reach shows no record of a quantitative analysis of the urine, from which we might have learned the quantity of urea secreted during the different stages of the disease, and which might have enabled us to form some idea of the extent of the destruction of the albuminous substances during the febrile stage, though, judging from the high grade of fever observed in the severer cases, we may well presume that the interchanges of matter are considerably augmented during this stage; while, on the other hand, the great nervous prostration of the patient directly after the subsidence of the fever, as well as the tardy convalescence, sufficiently shows that a large part of this waste is derived from the nervous tissues. The exanthematous eruption, representing a hyperæmia, or even an inflammation, of the skin, furthermore contributes to depress the nervous system by the pain and itching which it causes. This eruption, together with the inflammation and swelling of the superficial lymphatic glands, we are inclined to associate with the final elimination of the infectious poison from the organism.

Very little also is definitely known about the condition of the remaining organs, such as the kidneys, liver, and alimentary canal. The examinations of the urine in dengue recorded in literature are very few in number, and appear too unreliable for drawing any definite conclusions from them with regard to the condition of the kidneys. As albuminuria is met with in other infectious diseases, it is not impossible that it has also occurred in severe cases of dengue; though from the favorable termination of the disease it appears quite improbable that organic changes take place in these organs. In the same way may the liver be functionally deranged, or, judging from the destruction of matter during the febrile stage, a slight fatty infiltration of the organ may even occur—conditions which are apt to pass away with the exciting cause. The gastric irritability, whenever present, may be of nervous origin, though the vomiting, and particularly that of black hemorrhagic matters, observed in exceptional cases, evidently depends upon a hyperæmia of the stomach.

ETIOLOGY.—There is nothing positively known of the origin of dengue, but in perusing the accounts given by a number of medical observers from the different localities of the globe where it prevailed, we may presume that it existed in some parts of Asia and Africa long before it appeared in Europe and America. Perhaps the earliest record of dengue is the one dating from Cadiz and Seville, and concerning the epidemics prevailing in the cities in 1764 and 1768, when it was believed by the people that the disease had been imported from Africa. In Zanzibar (Christie), during the epidemic of 1870, the older native inhabitants [p. 884]remembered that fifty years before the disease had prevailed in this place. The Arabians living at this island also had known the disease in their own country, while the inhabitants hailing from the East Indies had never seen it. From the accounts of other writers we may presume that dengue has been known in Arabia for many generations. But, leaving aside its origin, it is authentically known that wherever dengue has appeared it has almost always been in the form of an epidemic, spreading from place to place and from family to family, without respect to race or nationality, to age, occupation or position, until every one susceptible to the disease was affected. Slaughter reports from India that even domestic animals, especially dogs and cats, were not exempt, as they appeared to suffer from rheumatoid affections of the joints.

Although toward the end of the last century dengue once prevailed epidemically in the temperate zone, at Philadelphia, it must nevertheless be considered as a disease especially at home in the tropical and semi-tropical regions, where it prefers to haunt low lands, particularly along the sea-coast, leaving almost untouched more elevated places. Though nothing definite is known about its special cause, its history and symptoms evidently show that it is not only infectious, but also highly contagious, in its nature, and in consequence must be caused by the entrance of a specific poison into the system. This view is held by the great majority of physicians residing in the various localities of the globe where the disease has prevailed. But, contagious as it may be, it greatly distinguishes itself from other contagious diseases by almost never proving fatal. As dengue generally prevails in the summer season and disappears with the approach of cold and rainy weather, its cause is apparently subject to the influence of certain meteorological conditions.

DIAGNOSIS.—When dengue appears epidemically, it is distinguished from other diseases without difficulty. The only disease with which it might be confounded when appearing in a sporadic form is acute articular rheumatism. But even from this affection it may be distinguished in its earlier stage by the pains not being limited to the joints, as is generally the case in articular rheumatism, but being also present in the head, back, and loins. Dengue is, moreover, characterized by a general physical and mental nervous depression, while in rheumatism the mind almost always remains clear. In the latter stage the peculiar eruption and painful swelling of the superficial lymphatic glands in dengue decides the question.

It has frequently been stated that dengue resembles yellow fever, and some physicians have even regarded it as a mild form of this disease. In examining attentively, however, the temperature of the patient during the febrile stage, it will be found that while it steadily rises in yellow fever, it is remittent in dengue. There is, furthermore, a difference observed in the state of the pulse, which in yellow fever generally falls on the third day, while the temperature continues to rise; in dengue, on the contrary, the pulse rises with the temperature. In the condition of the stomach also dengue considerably differs from yellow fever, for while in the latter disease this organ is almost always irritable, and vomiting is very frequently present, it is but rarely affected in dengue. The urine in yellow fever very frequently contains albumen as soon as the third day; in dengue, almost never, so far as the analyses recorded enable us [p. 885]to judge. Finally, the absence of jaundice and the appearance of the eruption on the fourth or fifth day remove all doubt about the nature of the disease. There are a number of other points by which dengue may be distinguished from yellow fever, which we, however, forbear to enumerate, for the reason that those already mentioned will suffice for a correct differential diagnosis.

PROGNOSIS.—Dengue, as has been stated before, scarcely ever terminates fatally unless it is complicated by some intercurrent disease. The prognosis, therefore, is highly favorable.

TREATMENT.—Nearly all authors recommend a symptomatic treatment in dengue, beginning with a mild cathartic, mercurial or not, and followed by a mild diaphoretic. To relieve pain and procure sleep opium—either uncombined or in the form of Dover's powder—belladonna, camphor, assafoetida, valerian, etc. have been recommended by different physicians; liniments containing camphor or chloroform have also been used with advantage for the same purpose. Foot-baths have been recommended to relieve the headache. To relieve the stiffness of the muscles and the articular pains after the subsidence of the fever iodide of potassium appears to be a favorite remedy in the East. Colchicum combined with aconite is also recommended for this purpose, as well as artificial sulphur baths and massage. The nervous depression during convalescence is to be combated with tonics and with regulation of the diet. Quinia appears to be generally discarded as a remedy in dengue.

[p. 886]

RABIES AND HYDROPHOBIA.
BY JAMES LAW, F.R.C.V.S.

SYNONYMS.—Canine Madness, Rabidus Canis, Canis Rabiosa. *Greek*, Lyssa, Lytta, Lyssa Canina, Cynolyssa, Hydrophobia, Pantephobia, Ærophobia, Phobodipsia, Erethismus Hydrophobia, Clonos Hydrophobia, Dyscataposis. *French*, Tetanus Rabien, La Rage, Toxicose Rabique.*German*, Wuth, Hundswuth, Tollwuth, Wuthkrankheit, Hundtollheit.*Italian*, Rabbia, Arabiata. *Spanish*, Rabia, Rabiosa. *Swedish*, Hundsjuka.*Roumanian*, Turbarea.

DEFINITION.—Canine madness is an acute infectious disease, supposed to arise spontaneously in the genus Canis (dog, wolf, fox, etc.) and Felis (cat, etc.), but transmissible by inoculation to the other Mammalia and to birds. It is characterized by a long period of incubation, by exaggerated reflex excitability, by disorder of the intellectual, emotional, and other nervous functions, by change of habits, by extreme irritability of temper, by optical and other delusions, by spasms of the muscles of the eyeballs and throat, by paralysis, and by more or less fever. The disease runs a short and almost without exception fatal course.

HISTORY.—Plutarch claims that hydrophobia was first recognized by the Asclepiadæ, and Homer's allusions to the malign dog-star and to Hector's acting like a raging dog have been quoted as implying a knowledge of rabies. We find no certain reference to the affection, however, until we come to Democritus and Aristotle, in the fourth century B.C. The latter clearly describes the disease and uses the name lytta, but, singularly enough, claims for man an exemption from the general susceptibility to the infection by inoculation.[1] From that date to this the successive outbreaks, sufficiently noteworthy to secure a place in history, are so numerous and widespread as to show a continuous prevalence of the malady in the Old World, and, since the early part of the eighteenth century, in the New.

[1] *Historia Animalium*, lib. viii. cap. 22.

GEOGRAPHICAL DISTRIBUTION.—Rabies is more prevalent in temperate regions than in the tropics and Arctic Circle, but this is common to all animal plagues propagated solely or mainly by contagion, and is manifestly due chiefly to the density of population, the activity of commerce, and the free movement of men and animals in the temperate zone. That a hot or cold climate is incompatible with rabies is disproved by its prevalence under the tropics in Southern China, India, Abyssinia, the West Indies, Peru, Chili, and Brazil, and in the Arctic Circle in Northern Greenland, Lapland, Siberia, and Kamtchatka. On the other hand, many [p. 887]islands and secluded regions in the temperate zones maintain a continued immunity or have been invaded only recently by the introduction of infected dogs. We may instance the Hebrides, Australia, Tasmania, New Zealand, South Africa, West Africa, the Azores, St. Helena, and, until the last half century, La Plata, Malta, and Hong-Kong. The disease is well known throughout North Africa, Arabia, Syria, Turkey, and Asia generally, in Ceylon and other of the East Indian islands. It is also notorious that even when unusually prevalent its progress is often abruptly arrested by a considerable river, and Schrader and Virchow both notice that though it ravaged both banks of a river, yet the islands in the river escaped, as was notorious of the islands in the Elbe during the great Hamburg epizoötic in 1852-53. While, therefore, rabies prevails most extensively in the more civilized countries and in large cities, yet we can point to no geographical area in which the contagion has failed to spread among those bitten by rabid animals, nor to any locality in which the disease has been shown to arise spontaneously from unwholesome conditions of climate, soil, or general environment.

ETIOLOGY.—We know of but one efficient cause of rabies—namely, infection. Yet as many conditions are believed to favor its extension, or even to determine its spontaneous eruption, it is necessary to speak of them shortly.

As shown above, climate cannot be charged with the generation nor diffusion of rabies. Many countries formerly thought exempt are now known to suffer. The following may be named: The East and West Indies, Syria, Egypt, Cyprus, Siberia, the lands north of the Baltic, and South America. Others manifestly maintain their exemption only because the morbid germ has not yet been introduced.

Certain seasons undeniably show a far wider extension of the disease than others, but such epizoötics are not limited to a particular season or year, and, unless cut short by human intervention, cover a succession of years of the most varied climatic character, spare inaccessible or secluded islands in the very centre of the outbreak, and the cycles of prevalence will succeed each other, in place of occurring simultaneously, in closely adjacent countries subject to the same climatic vicissitudes, but separated by narrow seas. Even a broad river destitute of bridges usually abruptly arrests an epizoötic, and protects the land beyond lying under precisely the same general influences. In this connection may be quoted the recent great epizoötic of 1856-72 in England, which succeeded, but did not accompany, that of 1851-56 in Germany. Prof. Röll reports the extraordinary prevalence of rabies at Vienna in 1814, 1815, 1830, 1838, 1842, and 1862—years remarkable for diversity rather than uniformity of climatic characters.

Popular opinion refers rabies to the extreme heats of summer, and each year dogs are muzzled or otherwise confined by order of municipal authorities during the dog days, though left at liberty throughout the rest of the year. In 1780, Andry observed that the coldest and hottest months furnished the least number of cases, and later Hurtrel D'Arboval claimed that in France dogs suffered most in May and September, and wolves in March and April. Bouley claims that the majority of dogs suffer in March, April, and May. The following statistics are interesting in this connection:

[p. 888]

Cases of Rabies in

	WINTER.	SPRING.	SUMMER.	AUTUMN	
	Dec., Jan., Feb.	March, April, May.	June, July, Aug.	Sept., Oct., Nov.	
ogs	755	857	788	696	(Bouley).
en	17	25	42	13	(Boudin).

The increase of cases of rabies canina in the spring and summer months, as shown by the above statistics (7-15 per cent.), cannot reasonably be attributed to the influence of the weather, since even the strongest advocates for spontaneity would at once decline to claim any such ratio of spontaneous developments. The increase must therefore be mainly, if not altogether, due to the increased number of inoculations; and these latter are provided for in the jealousies and quarrels in the troops of males that follow each rutting bitch in spring, the principal period of oestrum in the canine female. The infection spread in this way in early spring tends to remain more prevalent throughout the hot summer months.

With regard to the greatly enhanced mortality in man during the summer months, as shown in Boudin's statistics for France, in the absence of any genuine hydrophobia in man apart from inoculation from a rabid animal, it may be attributed to three principal causes: 1st. The bites sustained from rabid dogs in spring and early summer, when the disease is most widely spread among these animals, will give rise to hydrophobia weeks or months later. 2d. In the warm season the body is more thinly clad and the hands and other portions are more frequently left bare, so that the teeth are less likely to be cleansed of the virulent saliva by passing through the clothes before entering the skin. 3d. The languor, fever, and nervousness attendant on extreme heat tend not only to hasten the activity of any disease-germs actually present in the system, but also strongly favor the increase of that nervous fear which so often generates a fatal pseudo-hydrophobia (lyssophobia) in persons that have been bitten by dogs.

Hunger, thirst, and spoiled food are invoked as causes of rabies, yet in the East, where the dogs are the scavengers of the cities and often suffer severely from hunger and thirst, eat the most offensive carrion, and drink the foulest water, the disease has a very restricted prevalence, while in South Africa and Australia the outcast and sheep-dogs, often the victims of starvation and thirst, entirely escape. Bourgelat, Dupuytren, Majendie, Breschet, and others have cruelly destroyed dogs by privation of food and water and by exposure under a broiling sun, but no rabies, nor anything resembling it, was produced. Dogs perspire little and suffer severely from heat, but there is no evidence that this can develop canine madness. It is claimed that Rossi of Turin developed rabies in cats by withholding food and drink, but, as he furnishes no inoculation-tests confirmatory of its virulence, the claim cannot be endorsed. Experiments with an exclusive diet of salt meat, putrid meat, and water only have failed to produce rabies.

The large preponderance of male dogs attacked with rabies has been constantly remarked by writers. Of 1990 rabid dogs reported by different authors, 1746 were males and 244 females—a ratio of more than 7 to 1. This excess of males attacked is much higher than the ratio of males in the dogs of the districts drawn upon. Thus, Bourrel found a [p. 889]ratio of 6 rabid males to 1 rabid female, while in his patients generally the proportion was 4 to 1. Leblanc found that 14 per cent. of the male dogs went mad, while but 1 per cent. of the females suffered. That sex is no protection against inoculated virus is shown by the frequent inoculation of castrated dogs of both sexes. The excess of male subjects may be attributed mainly to the frequency with which these bite each other when following a female in heat, and the respect of all alike for the latter sex. Even in the rabid dog the sexual instinct rises above the propensity to bite in the early stages of the malady.

Toffoli claims that he has caused spontaneous rabies by shutting up several dogs in a loose box with a bitch in heat and allowing them to fight for the prize. Weber and Leblanc have noticed similar occurrences. But Greve and Menecier have repeated the experiments with a contrary result; so that it remains probable that when successful the victims had already been inoculated before they were shut up. Moreover, the seclusion of male canine animals for a lifetime in menagerie cages, often adjoining those of their corresponding females, has never been known to induce rabies.

The bite of the violently enraged dog, and the bites mutually given when following a rutting bitch, are popularly supposed to cause rabies; but if this were the case, the disease must have been universally prevalent. The idea that the bite of a dog will cause hydrophobia should that dog at any subsequent period go mad is a similar delusion. Men doubtless occasionally develop lyssophobia under such an influence, but animals do not contract genuine rabies.

Dogs are alleged to have gone mad from violent suffering after an operation, and cats from being scalded or robbed of their kittens, but all such causes are continually operating without such effect, and when in a solitary case rabies develops, it can only be looked on as a coincidence.

Much popular prejudice exists against certain breeds, and the Pomeranian has been virtually ostracised on account of its supposed liability to rabies; but statistics show that the liability to contract the affection bears a relation to the exposure rather than the special breed. Eckel, Pillwax, and Hertwig found that dogs kept as house- or watch-dogs, and most pampered and confined, are the most liable, while St. Cyr and Peuch found the greatest number of cases among those running at large and allowed the freest exercise.

There is a popular belief that the bite of the skunk (*Mephitis mephitica*) is always rabific. Rev. H. C. Hovey describes a number of cases of infection from this animal,[2] and John G. Janeway has reported other instances.[3] Both claim that the disease is spontaneous in the skunk, and Mr. Hovey holds, on very insufficient grounds, that the affection is a distinct variety of rabies (rabies mephitica). The facts seem to warrant only the conclusion that skunks in certain districts of Michigan and Kansas have had rabies communicated to them, and follow the rabid impulse to bite other animals and men. The Mephitinæ abound in the Eastern States, but we never hear of them stealing up and biting men or dogs, nor of the latter contracting rabies from skunk-bite. Eastern dogs frequently kill skunks and sustain bites, but do not thereby contract rabies. Even in Kansas this evil [p. 890]influence of the skunk-bite was unknown until 1870, showing that it is not inherent in the climate nor soil, but has been presumably imported. The spontaneity of the affection is assumed, not proved.

[2] *Amer. Jour. of Science and Art*, May, 1874.
[3] *New York Medical Record*, March 13, 1875.

In the above epitome of alleged causes we find nothing proving the spontaneous evolution of rabies. The prevalence of the affection in wolves, foxes, jackals, cats, skunks, etc. proves nothing for spontaneity, more than its existence in the dog. In all these species of animals the malady develops the dread propensity to bite, and thus in all alike provision is made for the perpetuation and propagation of the malady. Unless a previous attack by a rabid animal has been observed, owners usually insist that their dogs have contracted the malady spontaneously, yet a rigid scrutiny will almost always reveal a strong probability, at least, of inoculation. The rabid dog wanders far from home, and sometimes accomplishes wonderful feats of leaping to reach his victim, so that his presence in a district is not even suspected, and animals thought to be safely secluded inside high walls suffer from his fangs. He is more inclined to bite and rush on than to stay and devour, and thus small animals, like the skunk, when bitten may survive to propagate the disease in places to which a dog could not possibly find access. Much circumstantial evidence makes strongly against the theory of spontaneity. Thus, the immunity of the islands of the Elbe in the very midst of a severe and protracted epizoötic, the continued immunity of the Hebrides and of Malta, each famed for its indigenous race of dogs, for long centuries, during which the malady prevailed at frequent intervals on the adjacent mainlands, and the continued exemption of South Africa and of the Australasian and other islands, in the face of the counter-fact that the affection persisted after importation in the West Indies and South America, speak strongly for the doctrine that the introduction of a pre-existing germ is an essential condition of the evolution of the disease. The following statistics of cases which entered the Berlin Veterinary College furnish further corroborative evidence. There entered the college,

In 1845-53, 9 years, inclusive, 78 rabid dogs.

In 1854, rabid dogs.

In 1855, rabid dog.

In 1856, rabid dog.

In 1857-61, 5 years, inclusive, rabid dog.

The average for each of the first nine years was a fraction less than 31. In the two last of the nine the cases rose to 68 and 82, and this led early in 1854 to an order for the muzzling of all dogs, which was rigidly enforced by the police. The disease was promptly suppressed, the two cases in the two succeeding years being probably due to infected kennels or to importation from without. The results in Eldena (Fuertenberg) and Holland (Van Capelle) are equally conclusive. The inefficiency of some orders for the muzzling of dogs makes nothing against these facts. A law on the statute-book is not always a law in force, as I saw in Alfort and Lyons in 1863; the dogs wore their muzzles only in honor of the periodic visits of the commissionnaire of police, and rabies prevailed.

The great majority of competent observers of to-day deny, or at least strongly doubt, the occurrence of the disease apart from inoculation. Without assuming to decide the question for all times and places, it may[p. 891]be safely asserted that there is no sufficient proof of such an occurrence in any recent time.[4]

[4] Mr. Sâzé, a former student, informed me that boys in Japan produce what is believed to be canine rabies by administering to dogs a fungus (bukeryo) found growing on a coniferous tree. The dogs do not all seem to die, but are usually killed by way of precaution. The symptoms are those of delirium, with a propensity to bite, and the disease is assumed to be communicable, though no facts are given to show that it is so. This popular fancy has all the air of a popular fallacy, but as the counterfeit attests the genuine, it shows the familiarity of the Japanese with true rabies.

The contagion of rabies is usually resident in the saliva, but is by no means confined to that product. Paul Bert found the bronchial mucus virulent in dogs in which the saliva was non-virulent. The flesh has conveyed the disease when eaten, though probably only because of sores or abrasions on the alimentary tract. Smith records the death of negroes in Peru from eating rabid cows;[5] Schenkius, that of persons who ate of a rabid pig; and Gohier and Lafosse have infected dogs by feeding the flesh of rabid dogs and ruminants; Rossi and Hertwig have separately induced rabies by inoculating sound animals with portions of nerves from rabid ones. No absolute proof can be adduced that the disease has been conveyed through consumption of the milk. Cases quoted to show its virulence are open to the objection that the dam probably licked the offspring. A similar uncertainty attaches to the spermatic fluid. Women are alleged to have acquired hydrophobia by coitus, but no such case can be adduced among animals, though rabid males have often had connection with healthy females. The alleged cases in women were therefore probably the result of an excited imagination or caused by virus introduced through some other channel. The breath and perspiration seem incapable of becoming media for the transmission of the disease. The blood was supposed to be non-virulent by Breschet, Majendie, Dupuytren, Blaine, Youatt, etc., but has been shown by Eckel and Lafosse to be rabific. Eckel successfully inoculated the blood of a rabid he-goat on a sheep and that of a rabid man on a dog. Lafosse accomplished the same in one of three attempts by inoculation from dog to dog. The blood is probably only virulent in the advanced stages of the disease, and its virulence implies the virulence of all vascular tissues.

[5] *Peru as it Is*.

The saliva of rabid Herbivora and Omnivora, long held to be harmless, is now known to be virulent. Berndt has successfully inoculated it from an ox to four sheep; Eckel from a goat to a sheep; Rey from sheep to sheep; Lessona from an ox to two horses and a sheep; Tombaro from a heifer to a sheep, a horse, and two dogs; Youatt from horse and ox respectively to dogs; Ashburner from an ox to fowls; King from a cow to fowls; and Majendie, Breschet, Eckel, Hertwig, and Renault from man to dog; and Earle from man to rabbits. Besides these are a series of accidental cases, as from horse to man (Youatt), from a sheep to its shepherd (Tardieu), and from man to man (Aurelianus, Enaux, Chaussier).

Experiments by Hertwig and Eckel seem to show that saliva loses its virulence on the supervention of cadaveric rigidity or putrefaction in the dead body. Haubner even believed dried saliva to be innocuous. Yet Count Salm successfully inoculated the dried saliva of a rabid dog, and Schenkius reports a case of hydrophobia produced by a scratch of a hunting-knife that had been used to kill a mad dog some years before. A veterinary student at Copenhagen cut his finger while dissecting [p. 892]the body of a rabid dog twelve hours after death, and died of hydrophobia six weeks later. These cases in man may, it is true, have resulted from fear, but the same cannot be said of the infection of hound after hound placed in empty infected kennels, as recorded by Blaine, Youatt, and others. In the face of this it would require very strong negative testimony, indeed, to prove that the virus of rabies is devitalized in drying—a process which prolongs the vitality of other virulent matters.

Up to the present time the germ of rabies has not been demonstrated. That it is a particulate living organism may be reasonably deduced from its power of indefinite increase—a quality possessed by no mere chemical nor mechanical agent, also from the saliva proving non-virulent after filtration through plaster, while the solid residue left on the filter was virulent (Bert). But, although bacteria have been found in the saliva, those demonstrated up to the present are manifestly ordinary aërial bacteria, such as in Pasteur's experiments produced septicæmia rather than rabies. It still remains, therefore, for some future observer to discover that germ of which we cannot doubt the existence.

The point of election of this germ appears to be mainly the nervous tissue. Pasteur found the brain-matter of rabid animals invariably infectious, and has preserved the moist brain in an infecting condition for three weeks at a temperature of 12° C. He found that by direct inoculation in the brain-substance the period of incubation was abridged, rabies often showing itself in six, eight, or ten days. In the face of Rossi's successful inoculation of nerves and Pasteur's results with brain-matter it is difficult to account for the unsuccessful inoculation of nerve-tissue in six successive experiments by Hertwig. It seems to show that though the virus is concentrated in the brain, and especially in the medulla and pons, yet it does not equally permeate the entire nervous system. This election of the poison for the nervous tissue led Dr. Douboue in 1851 to advance the theory that it is propagated from the seat of inoculation to the brain through the medium of the nerves—a position now assumed by Pasteur. This, we fear, is not well founded. The poison, advancing for a month or more along the lines of the nerves, would probably derange and abolish their functions, as it does so speedily and effectually that of the nerve-centres after it has gained a seat in them, whereas, in reality, the local paralysis only appears in the last stages and after the symptoms of cerebral disorder are well established. Furthermore, a common premonitory symptom of rabies is congestion, swelling, and irritation of the inoculation wound, showing a sudden extraordinary activity at that point as a herald, if not a condition, of the general infection, whereas under a slow propagation along the nerves from the first this irritation would probably have been greatest in the wound at the outset, and would have thereafter kept pace with the progress of the virus along the nerves. Again, the blood is not always infecting. Blaine, Youatt, and others of the older observers had no fear of the blood. Hertwig obtained rabies in two cases only out of eleven inoculations with the blood of rabid subjects. The blood in this, as in some other diseases (variola equina, v. ovina, lung plague of cattle), proves to a certain extent inimical and destructive to the poison. Galtier inoculated nine sheep and one goat by intravenous injection of the saliva of mad dogs, in no case with fatal results nor indeed with any manifestation of rabies, but with the effect of fortifying the system so, [p. 893]that subsequent inoculation into the tissues of the saliva of rabid animals was harmless. Test inoculations made in the tissues of other animals with the same virus used in his intravenous injections, and his subsequent inoculations of the animals so treated, invariably determined rabies. Pasteur repeated these intravenous injections in dogs with the result of rapidly inducing rabies in a fair proportion of cases. One of his cases produced in this way recovered, and thenceforward resisted all further inoculation with the virus. Others that did not perish from intravenous injection afterward died of rabies after inoculation in the brain. Unfortunately, neither Galtier nor Pasteur have reported how much virulent saliva was injected in any one case, so that we have no data as to whether the difference was due to the varying quantity of the virus introduced in the various cases. Lussana, an Italian physician, had already in 1878 experimented on two dogs by injecting into their veins the blood of a physician who died of hydrophobia. The blood was drawn by leeches and cupping-glasses, and five grammes were injected into each dog. One died on the twenty-fourth day, presenting the symptoms and post-mortem appearances of rabies. The second at the end of one hundred and forty days developed symptoms of rabies which lasted a month, when the animal was sacrificed, and nothing special found at the autopsy. The data do not warrant a very positive conclusion, yet they seem to imply that the receptivity on the part of the dog is greater than that of the small ruminants. They suggest, further, a greater relative potency in the battle for life of the blood-globules of the small ruminants with this unknown rabific germ. This antagonism between the blood of the ruminant and the germ of rabies finds a parallel in the case of other disease-poisons in their relations to the nuclei of the tissues. Thus animals may prove refractory to a small dose of the poison of anthrax, yet Chauveau has shown that this virus will overcome all native or acquired insusceptibility when administered in excess. The same is true of the poison of chicken cholera, which Salmon dilutes until it is non-fatal, though still affecting the system and conferring an immunity from its attacks in the future. So with the lymph of variola ovina, which Peuch diluted to 1/50 and injected with the effect of producing slight fever and immunity without vesiculation.

This view would imply that in ordinary cases (inoculation with a moderate amount of the poison) the virus is for a time localized in the vicinity of the wound; and this is further supported by the fact that thorough excision and cauterization of the wound some time after it has been received is still often protective. It is weakened by the fact that bites of dogs in the stage of incubation sometimes produce rabies, but it must be borne in mind that there is still a period between the passage of the living germ to the salivary glands and brain and the growth of the germ in the nerve-centres, so as to produce pathognomonic symptoms, during which both blood and saliva must be virulent.

The ratio of successful inoculations to the bites is very varied. Thus, out of 555 dogs reported to have been bitten by rabid dogs, 188 contracted rabies; out of 183 experimentally exposed till bitten or inoculated, 91 became mad; out of 73 cattle bitten, 45 became rabid; out of 121 sheep bitten, 51 succumbed; and of 890 persons bitten, 428 took hydrophobia (48 per cent.). Of 440 bitten by rabid wolves, 291, or 66 per cent., took the disease. Such statistics are, however, far from satisfactory. Of dogs[p. 894]reported mad, some have only suffered from epilepsy, convulsions, or colic, while of those bitten by the really mad dog, some have sustained simple bruises without any real abrasion; in other cases the teeth have been wiped clean by passing through thick wool, hair, or clothing, or even the flesh of other animals just bitten; in other cases the bite has been inflicted at a time when the virulence of the saliva was at its minimum, or in a subject which was naturally insusceptible. The protective effect of clothing was well illustrated in a case which came under my notice in London. Six animals bitten by a rabid dog all contracted rabies, whilst a man bitten a few hours before through the coat-sleeve, and who did not have the wound cauterized for a full hour after the bite, escaped. Bouley found that in 32 persons bitten in the face, 29 died of rabies (90 per cent.); of 73 bitten on the hands, 46 died (63 per cent.); of 28 bitten on the arms, 8 died (28 per cent.); of 24 bitten on the lower limbs, 7 died (29 per cent.); of 19 bitten on the body (usually multiple wounds), 12 died (63 per cent.). The high mortality from the bites of rabid wolves and skunks is mainly due to this habit of attacking the face and hands. As illustrative of insusceptibility may be quoted the poodle of Hertwig, which was inoculated nine times with unquestionably rabic virus without effect; also the pointer of Rey, which was seventeen times bitten by rabid dogs without harm; also the acquired immunity of Galtier's sheep and rabbits, above referred to.

INCUBATION.—In the dog this varies from 6 days (Pasteur) to 240 days (Bollinger). In the majority of cases it ends in from 20 to 50 days. Pasteur, by inoculating into the brain substance direct, reduced the incubation from 20 days to 6 days. In the horse the limits of reported cases are from 15 days to 92 days. In the ox incubation varies from 20 to 30 days; in sheep, from 20 to 74 days; and in swine, from 20 to 49 days in recorded cases.

In man incubation is believed to be often much more prolonged. In 6 per cent. of all cases it is from 3 to 18 days; in 60 per cent., from 18 to 64 days; and in 34 per cent. it exceeds 64 days (Hamilton, Thamhayn). Quite frequently symptoms of hydrophobia appear from three to six months after the bite; in a few the period is prolonged to one or two years, and in rare instances to seven (Schule), and even twelve years (Chabert). But all such cases of prolonged incubation in man are at the least extremely doubtful. Man often contracts a pseudo-hydrophobia as the result of fear, and is curable by moral suasion alone; and as no such protracted incubations are noticed in the lower animals, and as no one of these abnormally deferred attacks in man has been verified by successful inoculation on animals, it is prudent to reserve a full assent until they are supported by better testimony. A specimen of such cases is that recorded by Chirac, in which a cadet bitten at Montpellier afterward spent ten years in Holland, and then, returning and hearing that his fellow-cadet bitten by the same dog had died of hydrophobia, he also manifested the disease and died. Another is the case of a man who, after having been bitten, spent two years in prison, and then developed hydrophobia and died. A mind naturally erratic and rendered weaker and more susceptible by prolonged confinement would prey upon itself and exaggerate the danger when the subject had been forcibly presented. In all such cases the attending physician should feel bound in the interests of humanity to [p. 895]inoculate a dog or other animal and ascertain whether or not the disease is virulent. The value of such results in dealing with future cases of the same kind cannot be overestimated.

The period of incubation appears to be relatively shorter in the young (average 45 days) than the old (average 70 days), and is believed to be shortened by constitutional excitement from violent passion, fever, the heat of the weather, or electrical disturbances.

During incubation no sign of the disease can be detected; it is even said that the wounds heal with unusual rapidity; but it is certain that toward the end of the latency the cicatrix, alike in man and animals, tends to become sensitive, itchy, congested, and even the seat of papular eruptions. The vesicles (lyssi) which, according to Xanthos, Marochetti, and Magistel, appear near the opening of the sublingual glands within a few days (6 to 20) after inoculation, have not been found by any recent observer.

SYMPTOMATOLOGY.—Three forms of rabies in the dog are recognized—the furious, the paralytic, and the lethargic. The prodromata are, however, the same in all, so that these may be conveniently considered before the different types are noticed.

The premonitory symptoms are by far the most important, as if these are recognized the dog may be safely secluded or destroyed before there is any disposition to bite. Any sudden change in a dog's habits or instincts is ground for suspicion. Bouley well says that a sick dog is always to be suspected. In some cases there is unusual dulness and apathy, in others great restlessness, watchfulness, and nervousness. A morbid appetite, in house-dogs a tendency to pick up and swallow straws, thread, paper, pins, and other objects, or to devour their own dung and urine, is highly characteristic. A desire to lick cold smooth objects, as a stone, a boot, a piece of metal, or the nose of another dog, is often seen. Smelling and licking the anus or generative organs of another dog and the exhibition of sexual desire are frequent manifestations. An increased fondness for the owner, shown by fawning and licking, is occasionally seen, though more commonly there is a change from a formerly amiable temper to a morose, sullen, retiring, and resentful disposition. If a naturally quiet dog flies into a violent passion at the sight of another dog or a cat, and attempts to bite it, he should be carefully watched. If a social dog seeks seclusion and darkness, or if while crouching and shrinking from a blow (hyperæsthesia) he yet bears it without howl or whine, he is to be strongly suspected. Barking without object, constant moving, searching, and scraping, a disposition to tear wood, clothing, etc. to pieces, and, above all, an absence from home for a day or two, should beget grave apprehensions. The rabid bark or howl which is often heard early in the disease is hoarse, low, and muffled, partaking of the nature of both bark and howl, the first running into the second, and consists of one loud howl followed by three or four others progressively diminished in force and uttered without closing the mouth. Some rub the chaps with the forepaws as if to dislodge an offending body from the mouth; others reject bloody matter by vomiting; and others turn the head and eyes as if following imaginary objects, and snap at them. Finally, a tendency to bite, rub, or gnaw the wound is significant, and usually draws attention to the fact that the wound, long healed, is still red, sensitive, and swollen, [p. 896]or even papular. The conjunctivæ are usually congested, there is an increased nasal defluxion, and the skin of the forehead and over the eyes is drawn into wrinkles. This stage lasts from a half to two or three days.

Following one or more of the above symptoms, paroxysms of wicked fury come on, alternating still with periods of quiet, in which prodromata only are observed. The red congested eyes assume a fixed stare, often squint or roll as if following an imaginary object, at which the dog presently snaps. A paroxysm is ushered in by increasing uneasiness, frequent change of position, and a desire to escape, shown in rushing at the door, tugging at the chain, or gnawing the post and walls of the kennel. The tendency to bite and gnaw is further shown by seizing the straw or tearing to pieces wooden and other articles within reach, or even by the victim lacerating its own body.

The rabid howl becomes more frequent, and the rage and disposition to bite strange animals and persons merge into a mischievous desire to worry all that come in the way, the respect for former companions and friends being steadily lost as the paroxysm increases in violence. Yet for a considerable time the voice of a loved master recalls the suffering animal to some degree of self-control. If free to escape during such paroxysms, the dog expends his excitement in wandering, making long journeys of five, ten, or twenty miles, and flying at every animal or man he meets, especially if they increase his excitement by any noise or outcry. If the victim escapes destruction during one of these wanderings, he returns during a lucid interval exceedingly dangerous, for, though he may recognize or even fawn upon his friends, yet the demon of mischief is even more potent within him, and may be roused to sudden violence by any noise or excitement. The intervals of quiet are attended by a prostration proportionate to the violence of the previous paroxysm, and the animal usually seeks seclusion and darkness, where he may lie dull and torpid, but he may be roused at any time to a renewed paroxysm by any noise, disturbance, the presentation of a stick, or, above all, by the approach of another animal. During the paroxysm the animal is manifestly the subject of acute delirium, has hallucinations, snatches and bites at unreal objects, turns on his best friends, even his master, seizes and holds on to a stick or iron bar until the teeth are detached and the gums lacerated, bites his own body, even amputating tail, testicles, or toes with his teeth; a bitch deserts her puppies or worries them, and all follow the unconquerable impulse to wander and to wound living beings. The victim will sometimes manifest incredible strength in breaking his chain and scaling high walls. Twitchings of the muscles of the face, and even general convulsions, are sometimes seen. Food is usually rejected, or if swallowed is soon vomited. In the course of two or three days the furious stage merges into the paralytic one, first shown by paresis of the hind extremities and a swaying motion in walking, then by paralysis of the lower jaw, which hangs pendent and allows the escape of a viscid saliva. The palsy gradually extends over the whole body—a sure precursor of approaching death, which is rarely delayed beyond eight days, and never more than ten, from the onset. In this last stage the animal has become extremely emaciated, with dry withered hair, hollow flanks, and small weak pulse; he may at first rise on his fore limbs when [p. 897]disturbed, and even attempt to snap, but there is now little danger of a bite. Convulsions may alternate with the paralysis. The result is invariably fatal.

The peculiarity of dumb or paralytic rabies in dogs is that the last or paralytic stage supervenes at once on the prodromata, without any intervening period of acute delirium and fury. The animal is throughout dull, quiet, and depressed, and shows little tendency to bite, to wander, or to restless movement. The excitement of the sexual passion is the same as in the furious forms, and the howl is still emitted, though much more rarely. Soon the lower jaw drops from paralysis, allowing the saliva to drivel from the mouth, and the animal can only succeed in closing it momentarily under the greatest provocation to bite. Paralysis of the hind limbs and of the whole body speedily follows, and death ensues in from two to three days. As soon as the jaw is paralyzed the subject is unable to drink, eat, bite, or bark, and emaciation advances with extraordinary rapidity.

The lethargic or tranquil form of rabies in dogs is manifested neither by furious madness nor by palsy of the jaws, but the nervous prostration is shown in a profound lethargy and apathy. The patient curls himself up, and will not be roused by his master's voice, by any noise, disturbance, or even punishment; he makes no response to the caresses of his friends, and pays no attention to the food or drink they bring him, but remains in his place, growing daily more emaciated and lethargic, until relieved by death toward the tenth or fifteenth day of the illness.

Besides the three typical forms there are intermediate varieties, which are classed with one or other according as the symptoms of that type seem to predominate. The same virus, inoculated, will produce different types in separate individuals, the result seeming to depend more on the susceptibility of the subject than any special quality in the poison. With many notable exceptions it may be stated that, on the whole, furious rabies predominates in hounds, bull-dogs, and other less domesticated or naturally vicious and courageous breeds, while the paralytic and tranquil types attack especially house and pet dogs.

POPULAR FALLACIES.—It is a dangerous delusion to suppose that mad dogs have a dread of water and polished surfaces, that they will not eat or drink, that they froth abundantly from the mouth, and that they run with the tail drooping between the hind limbs. There is no hydrophobia in the dog or other domestic animal. The rabid dog drinks freely in the early stages of the disease, lapping even his own urine; later, he still laps, and even plunges his nose in water, though often unable to swallow; and in his wanderings he swims rivers without the slightest reluctance. The appetite is not entirely lost, though greatly impaired and usually depraved, all sorts of unsuitable, noxious, and disgusting objects being picked up and swallowed with avidity. Frothing from the mouth is exceptional in rabies, and the flow of saliva is rarely seen unless when the jaw is paralyzed and pendent. Carrying the tail between the legs is a symptom of all diseases attended by abdominal pain, and is by no means constant in rabies. During the paroxysms the tail is usually carried erect.

Foxes, jackals, and badgers attacked by rabies lose their natural [p. 898]shyness, enter villages, follow and bite other animals and men, and, like rabid dogs, die in an unconscious and paralytic condition. Wolves are affected like foxes, but are more dangerous because of their power, the ferocity of their attack, and their habit of flying at the face and hands. Rabid cats are more retiring than dogs, and show less disposition to attack, but when they do, use both claws and teeth, and especially on bare portions of the body. The cry is hoarse like that emitted during the period of rut. They usually die about the third or fourth day.

The rabid horse is the subject of violent excitement, nervousness, and fear. There are trembling, loss of appetite, rubbing and eversion of the upper lip, neighing, sexual excitement, and inclination to bite and kick. Delirium may be suspected, but during the paroxysms the true nature of the disease is betrayed by the unconquerable desire to bite, kick, and otherwise injure those about him. He will even gnaw the manger and kick the stall to pieces, or lacerate his fore limbs and flanks with his teeth. In the early stages there is the same tendency to lick and rub the wound, which becomes red and irritable, the same red glaring or squinting eyes, and the same jerking of the muscles, as seen in the dog, and the affection winds up in the same way, in paralysis and death in four or five days.

Rabid cattle lose appetite, become very restless and excitable, grind the teeth, lick the cicatrix, evert the upper lip, and otherwise show sexual excitement, bellow often in a loud, terrified manner, as if still apprehensive of the attack of the dog, paw and scrape the ground with the fore feet, butt and kick viciously, have twitching of the muscles, and finally paralysis and death in from four to seven days. When paralysis is coming on the hind feet are often drawn forward as in inflammation of the feet. The pulse and breathing are accelerated during the paroxysms, but I have not found the temperature raised.

Rabid sheep and goats present the same general symptoms, bleat hoarsely, but viciously, have sexual excitement, nibble the cicatrix, have muscular weakness, emaciation, and paralysis, and die in from five to eight days.

Rabid swine show much fear, restlessness, and excitability, hide under the litter, start violently at noises, grunt hoarsely, champ the jaws, show a great disposition to bite and to gnaw and tear objects to pieces, have dark red, glaring eyes, gape and yawn, and become weak and paralytic. Breathing is often labored, and the mucosæ and white skin assume a dull red or leaden hue. Death ensues as early as the fourth or fifth day.

In Herbivora and Omnivora a paroxysm is usually induced by the sight of a dog—a fact of importance in diagnosis.

Rabid skunks have naturally received but little study. They tend, however, to steal up to men and animals and bite some exposed part of the body, like the finger, ear, or nose, and as stealthily retire. It is claimed that their odorous secretion is suppressed.

Symptoms of Hydrophobia in Man.

In some cases the prodromata are altogether omitted, the disease setting in suddenly with spasms of the pharynx and inability to swallow. More commonly, the premonitory symptoms last from one to three days. The first symptom is often an itching, prickling, or more or less violent [p. 899]aching in the seat of the bite, and even of an aura, a numbness, or shooting pain extending from that point toward the heart. In such cases the wound is red or bluish, and even swollen. In other cases there is chilliness, a general feeling of headache, malaise, and prostration, with lack of appetite or nausea, gloomy forebodings, taciturnity, nervous excitability, and restlessness. That restlessness which in patients cognizant of the consequence of the bite often induces insomnia during incubation, now often shows itself in an inability to keep quiet or to remain in one position or place—the exact counterpart of the initial restless stage shown in the canine patient. The sleep is now even more broken and unrefreshing and disturbed by fearful dreams. The restlessness soon merges into intense nervous irritability. Though devoured by thirst, the patient is afraid of water, and the attempt to drink will cause slight spasms with a sensation of filling of the throat and difficulty of deglutition. Even the air blowing upon his surface produces nervous irritation and apprehension, and a sudden glare of sunshine or other strong light is still more injurious. The pulse is increased in frequency, hard, and small; the breathing accelerated, oppressed, with at times yawning, sighing, or sobbing; there is some redness of the fauces, vascular injection of face and eyes, with, in some cases, dilated pupils; nausea or oppression at the epigastrium, sometimes vomiting; and usually constipation, which cannot, as in dogs, be referred to the earth, sand, and unsuitable materials swallowed. Intelligence is unimpaired.

With or without some or all of the premonitory symptoms above described the patient is sooner or later seized with constrictive spasms of the pharynx and respiratory muscles, the immediate occasion being an attempt to swallow liquid or some sudden fright or excitement. So great is the agony produced by this attack that, though consumed by thirst, the patient will rarely afterward attempt to drink, and the mere sight or offer of water, the noise of liquid flowing from one vessel to another, or even the sight of the vessel in which liquid was contained, suffices to bring on a violent paroxysm. This hydrophobia is peculiar to the human being suffering from this disease, being rarely seen in rabid animals; and it serves to enormously enhance the agony and horror of the affection. During a paroxysm the dyspnoea is usually extreme; there is a gasping or sighing respiration, and shrill, inarticulate sounds or screams are emitted which have been likened to the bark of a dog. These are manifestly due to the threatened suffocation rather than to an attempt to bark. The sensations have been described as a rising of the stomach into the throat, while others felt as if the throat had turned into bone and could not admit nor pass on the liquid. The abdominal contractions are often well marked, and retching and vomiting ensue. This reflex irritability of the nerves of deglutition and respiration is followed or attended by a condition of the most intense hyperæsthesia and a great exaltation of the special senses. A deaf and dumb child is said to have heard distinctly at this stage. There are, besides, during a paroxysm, general muscular trembling and clonic spasms of the muscles of the trunk and extremities. The facial muscles are contracted, the nostrils dilated, the face and eyes red and injected, and the pupils dilated, producing a spectacle of the most intense agony. Even in the intervals the hyperæsthesia is so extreme that the slightest touch of an attendant, a [p. 900]current of air, the approach of a candle, or even the ordinary tones of conversation, produce extreme agitation and may precipitate a violent convulsive paroxysm. The duration of the paroxysms and of the intervals varies much, but in general terms the former increase rapidly in number and severity, while the latter are correspondingly shortened. Restraint serves to aggravate the paroxysm, while, according to Hunter, the earlier and lighter ones may be relieved by running. The intense excitement sometimes becomes manifest in the persistent talking, and it is noticeable that the patient is free from mental delusions. As it is impossible to swallow, the patient spits out the now viscid saliva on all sides—a feature, like the fear of water, peculiar to man. As the disease advances the paroxysms are marked by the most perfect hallucinations and delirium, which impel the victim to acts of insane violence toward every one and every thing about him. In these fits he will use every available means of offence, even to the snapping of the jaws, though on the subsidence of the fit he will often express the greatest regret and warn his victims to be on their guard when he finds another paroxysm coming on. In some few instances the delusions continue even during the remissions, and the patient remains possessed of a sense of suspicion and horror of all about him, and yet the fear of being left alone is usually greater still. The convulsions may become tetanic (as opisthotonos). They are habitually more severe in men than in women and children. During a convulsion the victim will at times become black in the face, and may die from suffocation, apoplexy, or nervous exhaustion.

Should he survive this danger the final paralytic stage sets in. The spasms gradually become weaker, reflex irritability is lessened, and a period of quiet, and even comparative composure, may ensue, during which the former sights and sounds fail to produce a paroxysm, and some patients even recover the power of deglutition; but muscular weakness and prostration become more extreme, the lower jaw may even drop, and the viscid saliva drivel from the lips; finally, stupor supervenes, and the patient dies in a state of profound coma or complete exhaustion. This last stage lasts from one to eighteen hours.

Cases are met with in the human subject, as in the dog, in which the paroxysmal stage is omitted in greater part or entirely. The patient complains only of oppressed breathing, and sighs deeply when he attempts to swallow, and paroxysms, if they occur at all, are very mild. Decroix indeed claims that if a person suffering from hydrophobia is kept in a dark room and perfectly quiet, no paroxysms appear. The malady is, however, none the less fatal.

DIAGNOSIS.—The diagnosis of rabies and hydrophobia is not usually difficult if the disease has progressed to its paroxysmal stage. The most pathognomonic features are the fact of a bite by a rabid animal and the evidence of lesions and an extraordinary irritability of the medulla oblongata, inducing severe reflex spasms of the muscles of deglutition and respiration under the influence of any peripheral irritation. The clonic nature of the spasms and the entire absence of trismus serve to distinguish it from tetanus. From pharyngeal anthrax and diphtheria attended with spasm it is diagnosed by the extreme exaltation of the special senses and the absence of any marked febrile reaction; from acute mania by the difficulty of breathing and deglutition, the more rapid heart-beats during [p. 901]a paroxysm, and by the marked hyperæsthesia and exalted reflex susceptibility, as well as by the perfectly lucid intermissions; and from epilepsy, in that the latter is not associated with the same hyperæsthesia, that the paroxysm is not developed by noise, movement, attempts to swallow, sight of water, etc., that the spasms are more universal, and that they do not recur often, nor can they be roused by the causes immediately producing those of hydrophobia. Hysterical cases can usually be recognized by the imperfection of the symptoms; the subject, not knowing all the manifestations of hydrophobia, naturally fails to produce them.

The most difficult to distinguish from the genuine disease are those cases in which hydrophobia occurs as a disease of the imagination, the result of fear—the lyssophobia or hydrophobie non-rabique of the writers. In these there is always the history of a bite; the cicatrix even may have become the seat of congestive redness, itching, or neuralgic pains, and these, acting on a susceptible brain, develop a disease which is hardly distinguishable from true hydrophobia, and which is quite as fatal if left to run its course. These cases have usually less reflex susceptibility than genuine hydrophobia; the attack mostly occurs shortly after some conversation on the subject, and especially about the effects of the bites on others; and the victim is seen to have a nervous organization, and may even be known to have been subject to hysteria or other nervous disorder. At the same time, the concentration of the mind on this subject sometimes produces even structural changes in the medulla, and the reflex susceptibility in co-ordination with the other symptoms may be almost perfect. In a case reported a few years ago by Hammond the symptoms appeared perfectly characteristic, and at the necropsy circumscribed points of congestion were found near the roots of the vagus; yet the dog that bit this man was said to be alive and well, and in the absence of any successful inoculation from biter or bitten the case must be presumed to have been lyssophobia.

Many cases with a more favorable issue are recorded. Bellenger had a patient who had been bitten by his cat, and manifested violent paroxysms of hydrophobia, but was instantly cured by the sight of the animal in good health. Bouardel records that a man was bitten by his dog, which afterward disappeared. He was seized with severe hydrophobia, which continued for two days, when the lost dog was found and presented to him, and the symptoms disappeared. Trousseau speaks of a magistrate whose hand had been licked by his hound, which immediately after attacked a flock of sheep, so that many of them died of rabies. The master then manifested hydrophobia, but as death was deferred beyond the usual time, he concluded it was not genuine and recovered. Prof. Dick was called to visit a man who had been bitten by a favorite dog while suffering from distemper, had manifested severe hydrophobic symptoms, and had been given up by the attending physicians. He succeeded in convincing the subject that as the dog had had distemper, and as no two great diseases could coexist in the same system, it could not have had rabies. In spite of the false premises, this reasoning had the desired effect and the patient recovered. A few years ago a boy twelve years old in Ithaca, N.Y., was bitten by a dog supposed to be rabid, and in due time manifested hydrophobia, which advanced rapidly until he was having a violent paroxysm every half hour, and it was pronounced impossible for him to survive another day. At this time I saw him, observed that he [p. 902]had a nervous organization, and was somewhat lacking in the hyperæsthesia of rabies, learned that he had recently been gorging himself with Christmas delicacies, and was now very costive; and, as there was no satisfactory history of the dog, I at once suspected lyssophobia. The friends and strangers who had come to condole with the parents and feast on the horror were excluded, and the boy's attention fully engaged in amusing pictures and conversation; the paroxysms were omitted, and in two hours the patient, overcome by weariness, went to sleep. Next morning he was still kept secluded and quiet, and two enthusiastic students took up the rôle of keeping his attention constantly engaged on whatever would interest him. The prima viæ was relieved by medicine, and under a course of tonics the boy quickly recruited, and at the end of a week went back to school.

In doubtful cases the test by inoculation may be tried. Inoculation with the saliva of a man suffering from hydrophobia is manifestly useless, since he must die before we can hope for the development of the disease. But in the case of a dog having bitten one or more people the inoculation of the virus on the brain of one or two other dogs would ensure the development of the affection in the course of one or two weeks, provided the first was rabid. The non-success of this operation when practised on two dogs would provide the best possible medicine for the diseased mind of the person bitten.

PATHOLOGICAL ANATOMY.—Post-mortem lesions are rather remarkable for their inconstancy than for their specific characters. Hardly a single lesion can be specified which may not be absent in particular cases, yet some are so characteristic that, when taken along with the symptoms during life, they very materially assist in diagnosing the disease. Of the pathological appearances common to man, dog, and other animals the following may be named: The body is greatly emaciated; the rigor mortis is normal or nearly so; decomposition usually sets in early; a white skin is livid, cyanotic, or petechial; the cicatrix is often hardly noticeable even after the animal has been shaved; the superficial veins, especially those of the neck and head, are filled with black inspissated blood; the external mucous membranes are of a dark livid hue, those of the mouth and nose being covered by a tenacious mucous or muco-purulent secretion (in dogs they are usually covered with earth or dust); the fauces, pharynx, and tonsils are usually of a dark livid hue, and sometimes swollen; in other cases the dark red hue and manifest swelling that obtained during life disappear after death; similar lesions are found in the larynx, and I have seen extensive erosions; the bronchial mucous membrane is reddened and coated with a muco-purulent secretion (and in dogs with earth and foreign bodies); the lungs are usually congested, often to the extent of showing death by asphyxia; the heart and large blood-vessels are filled with a black thick, venous blood, and the muscles, charged with the same blood, have a dark reddish-brown hue; the stomach is usually congested, sometimes to a port-wine hue, and is the seat of blood-extravasations and even erosions; this congestion is often present, though to a less degree, in the intestines; the mesenteric glands and those in the vicinity of the pharynx are not unfrequently enlarged and congested; a very constant feature is the entire absence of proper food in the stomach and of chyme in the small intestine; the liver is usually hyperæmic, [p. 903]exuding on pressure the characteristic dark blood, and it may be the seat of some granular degeneration, but it usually retains its normal consistency; the spleen is normal; the kidneys are hyperæmic and leaden or bluish gray, and slightly cloudy on the surface (in dogs fatty degeneration of the inner cortical layer is common even in health); the urinary bladder is usually empty or contains a little turbid, yellowish, slightly albuminous urine, while the mucous membrane is often covered with dark reddish-brown petechial spots; the brain is usually hyperæmic, and, together with its membranes, slightly oedematous, yet the lesions are not constant either in kind or degree; the medulla oblongata usually shows a similar condition, and even minute points of acute congestion, but neither these nor the hyperæmia and oedema of the spinal cord can be found in every case.

Some conditions are especially pathognomonic in the dog. In nearly all cases of furious rabies the stomach is gorged with foreign bodies, such as hay, straw, wood, coal, leather, portions of textile fabrics, fæces, earth, sand, stones, pieces of iron, lead, etc., and the same materials are usually found in the small intestine, while the large intestines are empty. Portions of these foreign bodies are often found in the bronchia as well, giving rise to circumscribed lobular pneumonia. The significance of such matters when found in large amount in the stomach of a dog which has been given to biting or other symptom of rabies is very great, and if the stomach contains none of the natural food of the animal and the duodenum no chyme, it may be held pathognomonic of rabies. If, however, the materials are small in quantity and mingled with natural food, and if the duodenum contains chyme, the dog was probably not rabid. Dogs frequently chew and swallow fresh leaves of grass, and those in detention gnaw and swallow pieces of wood, cloth, horn, etc.; but these are used either as an emetic or a teething-ring, and virtually imply that digestion is not entirely abolished. Their presence, therefore, along with food does not indicate rabies.

PROPHYLAXIS.—In view of the almost or quite constantly fatal issue of rabies in man and animals, the main attention should be given to the question of prevention. As the disease is perhaps never in our time developed except as the result of contagion, we have the most perfect guarantee that by suitably devised measures it may be absolutely suppressed and excluded from any country. Even if we allow that a rare case is at long intervals developed spontaneously, it is none the less certain that the disease can be practically abolished, as nothing can be easier than to nip the disease in the bud in the locality where it first shows itself. Thus in Australia, Tasmania, and New Zealand rabies has not yet appeared, though prevailing in the same latitude and climate in both hemispheres. It reached Mauritius in 1813, and has prevailed uninterruptedly since, while in Bourbon, immediately adjacent and almost identical in geology, climate, flora, and fauna, it is still unknown. The same truth is told in the entire extinction of rabies in Berlin by the universal muzzling of dogs, as recorded above. The immunity lasted for nine years, during which muzzling was enforced. A more recent example of the same kind is found in Holland. In 1875 universal muzzling was made obligatory in all communes where rabid animals had been and in adjoining communes. From 1877 on the disease was unknown save on the borders of [p. 904]Belgium and Prussia and in a very few dogs recently imported. Nearly all cases of hydrophobia in man and animals being due to bites by rabid members of the canine fraternity, a fundamental condition of all success in prevention is the prohibition of its diffusion by dogs. For this reason the following measures are requisite: 1st. All dogs should be registered and heavily taxed. The number of useless dogs kept in every community affords the greatest opportunity for the speedy diffusion of the rabid germ whenever that has been introduced. Whatever tends to reduce this number directly tends to the restriction and extinction of rabies. 2d. Every dog should be made to wear a collar with plate bearing the name and residence of his owner. All stray dogs without such badge should be summarily shot by the police. This will secure the payment of the taxes and the destruction of superfluous and dangerous dogs. 3d. In all cities and counties where rabies has existed within a year, and in the counties adjoining them, every dog should be muzzled except when securely shut up or tied. All dogs found at large without a muzzle should be promptly shot by the police. The objection to muzzles is satisfactorily met by the use of the wire muzzle, which impedes neither breathing nor drinking. 4th. Dogs and cats suspected or known to have been bitten by rabid animals should be at once destroyed, or if considered sufficiently valuable may be confined in a secure cage for six months under veterinary supervision. 5th. Dogs which have bitten and are supposed to be rabid should be similarly caged and placed under veterinary supervision. If rabid, the symptoms will be fully developed in a few days, whereas if destroyed at once the bitten party is liable to develop lyssophobia. 6th. Dogs imported from countries where hydrophobia is known to exist should be subjected to a period of quarantine of six months. 7th. Foxes, wolves, badgers, martens, skunks, must be indiscriminately destroyed in localities where they have become infected with rabies. 8th. The disinfection or burning of the kennels where rabid dogs have been is a natural corollary of the above.

Other measures less thorough and efficient are often advocated and resorted to, but should be discarded whenever it is possible to practise a method of absolute extermination. Among these may be named the flattening of the teeth, and especially of the canines, with a file, as advocated by Bourrel, and later by Fleming. While this is a measure of protection, it does not remove the desire to bite, nor the power of wounding the skin when that is delicate or tender. Another method is to hang a block of wood from the neck, so that it may impede the movements of the forelegs and prevent a rush and sudden attack. The futility of such a resort need hardly be remarked upon. The emasculation of dogs is another preventive measure advocated. The single advantage of this is that it does away with the host of suitors that follow a rutting bitch, and the mutual worrying and biting that ensue. But it is not yet proved that the disease is produced by privation of the generative act, while if it were it is still certain that cases of spontaneous rabies are extremely rare; that the rabid dog bites the castrated one as readily as the perfect male; that the emasculated one contracts rabies as readily as others when bitten, and that he communicates it no less persistently. Galtier's method of intravenous injection of the rabic saliva, which seems to have proved effectual in sheep and rabbits, utterly failed in the hands of Lussana and[p. 905]Pasteur in dogs. Besides this objection, that it is useless for the animal which is beyond all comparison the main propagator of rabies, it has the serious disadvantages that its practice would necessitate the maintenance of a constant succession of cases of rabies, that great danger attends this production and handling of the virus, and the expense and risk of a general application of the measure must absolutely forbid it.

More recently Pasteur has found that the virus when transmitted through several monkeys in succession becomes so weak as to be harmless to the animal inoculated, and yet protects the animal against the more virulent poison. This fact he utilizes by inoculating this mitigated ape-virus on the brain of the animal just bitten, so as to render that refractory to the disease when the poison from the bitten wound shall reach it by its ordinary slow channel. At the time of writing, the method is being attempted on a man bitten by a mad dog.

Another precautionary measure which is always in place is the diffusion among dog-owners of correct information as to the premonitory symptoms of rabies, and the necessity for careful seclusion when any such symptoms are manifested.

TREATMENT OF BITES.—The treatment of bites by animals supposed to be rabid consists mainly in seeking the elimination of the poison or its destruction by caustic. The first object should be to prevent absorption of the poison. If the bite has been on a limb, a tourniquet should be instantly placed above it. A stout cord or handkerchief is always at hand, and may be tied around the limb and twisted with a piece of wood until circulation is arrested. Sucking the wound is usually effective in withdrawing the poison, and can convey no additional danger to the person bitten. If the patient cannot reach the wound with his own mouth, another may volunteer to suck it, though in these days of diseased teeth and gums the act is pregnant of danger. This may be largely obviated by alternately sucking and rinsing the mouth with a solution of carbolic acid, or, better, by applying such a solution to the wound before sucking, or finally by sucking through a tube. Cupping over the wound is highly commendable, though less effective than sucking. When cupping can be combined with wringing of the wound, there is an approximation to sucking. Cupping is especially valuable in wounds of the trunk, where a tourniquet cannot be applied. Intermittent squeezing and wringing of the part and steeping in warm water is an excellent resort when no better measure can be had. Cutting the wound open to its depth, while it may in certain cases be necessary to allow of the thorough application of a caustic, is objectionable as multiplying the points of infection and absorption. Drinking of liquids to excess temporarily retards absorption by overfilling the vascular system. Ammoniacal, alcoholic, and other stimulants are resorted to for the same purpose, being held to cause plenitude, not only by quantity, but by rarefying the animal fluids.

No such measures should, however, be allowed to delay for an instant the use of caustics. This is the one effectual means of destroying the poison, and the choice of caustic is of less consequence than its thorough application. The hot iron in the form of a skewer, nail, poker, or other available instrument, at a white heat, may be brought in contact with all parts of the wound to its utmost recesses.

Of chemical caustics, solid sticks of nitrate of silver, chloride of zinc, [p. 906]and potassa, or the crystals of cupric or ferric sulphate, are to be preferred to the liquid forms (mineral acids, butter of antimony, etc.), because of the greater thoroughness with which they can be brought into contact with all parts of the wound. Lastly, the galvano-cautery may be used if within reach. If the liquid caustics are employed, they may be introduced into the depth of the wound by means of a pipette, a piece of porous wood, or a pledget of tow. For a great number of small wounds a bath of corrosive sublimate has been recommended.

In some cases the amputation of a badly-lacerated member or one with a compound fracture offers the only measure of protection.

But although nothing should be allowed to delay cauterization, yet the impossibility of an immediate application should not be accepted as a reason for its neglect at a later date. On the presumption that the virus is localized in the seat of inoculation until it has increased largely and is poured into the blood in sufficient quantity to subjugate the blood-globules to its influence, it is logical to excise the cicatrix and cauterize the wound, though days or even weeks have elapsed.

If it should be shown by further experiment that Galtier's intravenous injection of virulent saliva is harmless and protective to sheep, rabbits, and it may be other Herbivora, it would be logical to employ this in these animals just after they have been bitten, as there will be ample time to establish the systemic influence of the intravenous injection before the poison shall have accomplished its recrudescence in the cicatrix. The constantly fatal result of rabid bites in these animals would at least warrant such an attempt, the main precaution being that the liquid shall be most carefully preserved from contact with any of the tissues, including even the coats of the injected vein.

In addition to the local treatment of the sore, certain general medication has usually been resorted to, though its real value may well be questioned. Thus, the elimination of the poison has been sought by profuse perspiration induced by warm, Turkish, and Roman baths, and by the use of medicinal agents, sudorifics, sialogogues (mercury), laxatives, and diuretics (cantharides). The neutralization of the poison has been attempted by ammonia, the sulphites and hyposulphites, chlorine, etc. Besides these are used nerve-sedatives and tonics, such as venesection, belladonna, prussic acid, tartar emetic, sulphates of copper and zinc, arsenic, strychnia, etc.

What is probably of greater importance is a sound hygiene. Stimulating food eaten to excess is injurious alike to man and beast, and by inducing digestive disorder and cerebral congestion will tend at least to precipitate the attack. Costiveness or biliousness from sedentary habits and lack of exercise in the outer air and sunshine, exposure to intense heat or cold and over-exertion, are all to be guarded against.

Finally, psychical treatment is of the highest importance. Those about the person who has been bitten should preserve a calm, equable, and cheerful demeanor and avoid all allusion to the occurrence. The patient should be protected against all sources of excitement, and should not be allowed to see that he is an object of solicitude. If the matter is referred to incidentally, he should be impressed with a conviction of the efficacy of the treatment adopted.

THERAPEUTIC TREATMENT.—Almost every agent in the [p. 907]Pharmacopoeia has been employed as a remedy for hydrophobia, but, up to the present, it must be acknowledged, with no measure of success. The agents supposed to be prophylactics are those also resorted to as therapeutic remedies. To these may be added the potent nerve-sedatives and anti-spasmodics—chloroform, chloral hydrate, ether, bromides of potassium, sodium, and ammonium, curare, Calabar bean, and the sialogogue diaphoretic pilocarpine.

Chloroform is one of the most appropriate, as it may be taken by inhalation, though with much excitement to the patient, and it at once relieves the oppressed breathing and pharyngeal and other spasms, while it acts as a cerebral sedative and anæsthetic; and if it cannot be held up as a curative agent, it at least secures euthanasia. Chloral given as an injection, so as to induce its soporific action, is equally soothing, though nothing more. Curare injected hypodermically overcomes the spasms, but does not usually, if ever, retard death. Three cases of hydrophobia in man treated in this way recovered, but we have no proof that even these exceptional cases were rabies. Pilocarpine has been used in a number of cases, but, with the exceptional case of a young man reported by Denis Dumont, all terminated fatally. The committee of the Paris Academy of Medicine reported in 1874 that in three experimental cases "it hastened death by the fits it brought on." Morphia is often of great value in calming the excitement and giving rest and sleep during the intervals of the paroxysms. Daturia and atropia, administered hypodermically, are somewhat less effectual. Inhalation of oxygen is said to arrest the convulsions and delirium, but not to retard death. Vaccine virus and the venom of the viper have each been tried, but with no good effect.

Of non-medicinal therapeutic measures the following are among the most promising: Perfect seclusion, quiet, and darkness serve to abate the hyperæsthesia, the painful acuteness of the senses, and the convulsive and delirious paroxysms. It can no longer be doubted that a very few cases of genuine rabies recover, but those that do so have almost all had special advantages in the way of quiet and seclusion, and few have had the excitement of medicinal treatment. Eight cases of the recovery of rabid dogs are reported by Menecier, Decroix, Laquerriere, Rey, Harold Leiney, and Pasteur. The two first were attested by successful inoculation on other animals; Decroix's second case was caused by inoculation with the saliva of a hydrophobous man; the next three had been bitten by dogs undoubtedly mad; while Pasteur's was inoculated with the brain-matter of a rabid cow. All in due time presented the characteristic symptoms of rabies, yet all recovered, without any record of medicinal treatment. Pasteur's case, when again inoculated, resisted the disease. A certain number of recoveries of men from pronounced hydrophobia under medicine and without it are on record, but in the absence of successful inoculations it is impossible to tell how many were cases of infecting rabies. The parallel between rabies and tetanus in the intensity of the reflex excitability would demand darkness and quiet as a sine quâ non of any rational treatment. Faradization has produced a temporary relief, but no permanent improvement. Warm baths, steam baths, and hot-air baths serve to abate excitability and spasm, and have been lauded as specific in hydrophobia, but have proved useless in the lower animals.

[p. 908]Intravenous injection of warm water (two pints) in a hydrophobous man reduced the pulse from 150 to 86 and restored the power of deglutition. Life was prolonged for nine days, but in great agony, from the supervention of suppurative arthritis (Majendie). In another case the dread of water disappeared, but death ensued in fifty-four hours. In the hands of Youatt and Mayo it proved equally unsuccessful in dogs. A cold bath with submersion to unconsciousness is an old remedy now abandoned. Venesection to fainting, with or without mercury, mitigated the symptoms, but seemed to hasten paralysis and death. The excision and cauterization of the cicatrix, or the cutting of the nerves proceeding from it, has been useful in delaying, or even absolutely preventing, the paroxysms. When, therefore, the premonitory symptoms of hydrophobia have set in, and when an aura or shooting pain is felt proceeding from the seat of the wound toward the heart, one or other of these measures may serve to prevent the immediate occurrence of reflex convulsions. When the poison has actually invaded the brain, this can be looked on as a palliative measure only, but in the many cases of lyssophobia it may put an instant stop to the affection.

[p. 909]

GLANDERS (EQUINIA GRAVIOR, FARCY).
BY JAMES LAW, F.R.C.V.S.

SYNONYMS.—*Greek*, [Greek: malis]. *Latin*, Malleus, Equinia Nasalis, E. Apostimatos, Farcinia. *French*, Morve, Farcin. *German*, Rotz, Lungenrotz, Hautrotz, Wurm, Hautwurm. *Italian*, Morva, Moccis, Cimurro. *Spanish*, Cimorro, Lamparones.

DEFINITION.—An infectious, bacteridian disease occurring in the horse, ass, or mule, and communicated by inoculation to various other animals, including man. It is usually ushered in by rigors, followed by articular pains, lameness, and the formation of a specific deposit in the lymphatic system of some part of the body, with a tendency to destructive degeneration and ulceration. In the form known as glanders these deposits and ulcers take place mainly in the nasal mucosa, in the lungs, and in adjacent glands, while in that known as farcy the deposits occur in the cutaneous and subcutaneous lymphatic plexuses and the dependent glands.

HISTORY AND GEOGRAPHICAL DISTRIBUTION.—Under the name of malis Aristotle describes a fatal disease of asses, supposed to have been identical with the malleus humidus of Vegetius Renatus and other writers of early Christian times, and with the cymoira of other early Roman writers. This malady was characterized by swelling of the submaxillary glands and discharge from nose and mouth. From the fourteenth century onward glanders is reported from different parts of Europe at frequent intervals; thus in 1320 in England (Rogers); in 1640 in Badajoz, brought by Portugese horses (Villalba); in 1686 at Treves (Eggerdes); again in 1776 in Southern France (Lafosse); in 1794 in Bavaria (Plank); in 1796 in Franconia (Laubender); and in 1798 in Piedmont (Toggia). At the beginning of the present century this affection was very widely prevalent in Great Britain, the chronic cases being habitually worked in stage-coaches, but of recent years, when it has been made criminal to expose or use a glandered horse, the malady has to a great extent disappeared. To-day glanders is almost coexistent with the distribution of the domesticated equine family, yet its prevalence bears a direct relation to the facilities for infection (horse-traffic, war, preservation of the diseased, confinement in close stables, ships, etc.), and some countries appear to be entirely free from the affection. Thus, Krabbe gives the yearly losses per 100,000 horses for the principal countries of Europe and Algiers as follows: Norway, 6; Denmark, 8.5; England, 14; Sweden, 57; Wurtemberg, 77; Prussia, 78; Saxony, 95; Belgium, 138; [p. 910]France (army), 1130; Algeria (army), 1548. The losses in Prussia more than doubled after the Franco-German War; thus, in 1869-70 they were 966, and in 1873-74, 2058. In Bavaria they rose in the same period from 173 to 390 (Hahn). In Lisbon, Portugal, glanders was unknown for the thirty years preceding the Peninsular War, whereas after the war it proved a veritable scourge (Saunier). Charles Percivall, during an eight years' residence at Meerut and Cawnpore, Hindostan, saw not a single case of glanders, and so late as 1275, Fleming claims an entire immunity for India; yet in 1877 complaints were numerous of the very general prevalence of the disease in Upper India especially, while in 1879 the campaign in Afghanistan was seriously affected by its ravages. Climate appears to have little influence. The disease is virtually unknown in the island of Bornholm with 7000 horses, and in the Faroes and Iceland with 35,000, while it is quite frequent in Sweden. It is unknown in Australia, but is very prevalent in China, South Africa, Abyssinia, and Algiers, and but little known in Asia Minor, Arabia, and Egypt.

In the United States as in Europe the disease has mainly concentrated itself in the large cities in times of peace, and spread widely on the advent of war. It is alleged that it first entered Mexico in 1847 with the American cavalry, though with the horses kept in the open air it failed to gain a wide extension. The horses and mules drawn into the Union armies in 1861 brought infection with them, and soon the disease was most prevalent and destructive, not only in the ranks, but in every State in which the armies operated. John R. Page says the first case he saw in the Confederate army was a captured Federal troop-horse on the retreat from Manassas, and that the breaking down of the Confederate cavalry in the last two years of the war was mainly due to glanders. At the close of the war the sale of army horses distributed the infection widely through all the States, North as well as South. Every year in a country district in Western New York I see several cases of glanders, and occasionally a whole stud is carried off through an infected purchase. In other States the case is no better. In Pennsylvania, Ohio, Illinois, and Michigan cases are constantly seen in the country districts, and in the three last-named States five human victims have been reported within a short period. In Connecticut the same is true, and the disease made one human victim in Waterbury in 1879. In the large cities the case is still worse. Liautard of New York in 1878, in a single visit to one car-stable, condemned 8 horses, in another stable 18, and in a third, at two visits, 45, while a fourth had lost no fewer than 200 horses in the course of one year from glanders. In the Troy (N.Y.) car-stables the malady prevailed from 1875-77, most of the subjects suffering from chronic farcy, until in the latter year, by my advice, these propagators of contagion were destroyed. In Springfield, Mass., in 1879, the disease assumed such alarming proportions that it was vigorously suppressed by a city ordinance enjoining summary slaughter. These are but indications of what is happening all over the country, entailing losses of many hundreds of thousands yearly as well as an enormous risk to humanity.

The following table gives the number of cases occurring in the equine family in two of the principal countries of Europe in the last few years:
[p. 911]

Cases of Glanders in—	Great Britain.	Germany.
1878	888	2753
1879	1367	
1880	2048	1941

1881	1710	17 / 74
1882	1389	18 / 38

As both countries systematically suppress this disease through their veterinary sanitary officials, it cannot be doubted that the figures for America, if obtainable, would be relatively higher.

Glanders prevails especially in horses, asses, mules, and other solipedes, and is communicated by inoculation to all domestic animals except the genus Bovis. In the sheep and goat the receptivity is considerable, and the disease may prove fatal in fifteen days (Gerlach) or it may be delayed for seven weeks (Bollinger). The Carnivora (dogs, cats, lions, polar bears) contract the affection by eating diseased flesh, as do some rodents (prairie-dogs, rabbits, guinea-pigs, mice), and, by administration, solipedes. Swine contract the disease by inoculation (Gerlach, Spinola), though in these and in the dog the constitutional symptoms are usually slight and recovery may follow the local affection.

The susceptibility of man is doubtless less than that of the solipedes, judging from the few cases of glanders compared with the frequent exposures, yet when once established in the system it can hardly be said to be less malignant or fatal.

ETIOLOGY.—The one known cause of glanders is contagion, and the recent experiments of Capitan and Charrin in France and of Schütz and Löfler in Germany, demonstrating that the bacillus of the glanderous deposits is the one essential cause of the disease, effectually dispose of any claim of its spontaneous origin. Glanders can no longer be considered spontaneous, further than that its germ is now proved capable, like that of anthrax, of survival and multiplication out of the animal economy, so that infection may come from other objects than a sick animal; and it may even yet appear that the bacillus, living at times as a harmless saprophyte out of the animal body, may acquire deadly properties under certain conditions of the environment. At the same time, the most extensive acquaintance with glanders and the broadest generalizations from known facts do not warrant the assumption of the extension of the disease by the growth of the bacillus out of the living body, unless it be on the rarest possible occasions, while the soundness of extensive countries (Australia, New Zealand) for a century or more speaks strongly against any frequent development from a harmless saprophyte.

To the same effect speak the experiences of the English army. At the beginning of the century, under the teaching of Coleman, most cases were attributed to lack of stable care, and extensive experiments were made in the treatment of the disease, with the result of a very high mortality from this cause. Now, when contagion is looked on as the main or sole cause, and all suspected horses in the army are promptly destroyed, the disease is only seen in recently-purchased animals or after the inevitable exposures of a campaign.[1] In the French army the doctrine of the [p. 912]non-contagiousness of chronic glanders led to a greater prevalence of this disease than in any other country of Europe. Prior to 1836 it was about 90 per 1000 per annum, whereas now, under the doctrine of contagion and a corresponding practice, glanders kills but 2 per 1000 per annum (Rossignol).

[1] Wilkinson, *Jour. of Roy. Agr. Soc.*, No. 50.

But while the essential cause of glanders is the specific bacillus, an individual susceptibility is no less requisite to an attack. This may be innate or acquired. As we have seen, it varies according to the genus, being greatest in the solipede. But many solipedes show a strong power of resistance. Of 138 horses similarly exposed by cohabitation with glandered horses, but 29 (21 per cent.) suffered. Of 28 inoculated with glanders virus, but 9 (32 per cent.) succumbed (Lamirault, Bagge, Tscherning). The accessory causes which predispose the system to the reception of glanders may be included under one general term—low condition and ill health. Three of these causes, however, deserve especial mention: 1st. Impure and rebreathed air. Prior to 1836 the yearly losses per 1000 of the French army horses were from 180 to 197. At the date named the ventilation of the stables was greatly improved, and the mortality fell to 68 per 1000 per annum, one-half from glanders. Later improvements have reduced the 34 cases to 2. During the Italian War, in

1859, 10,000 of these horses were kept for nine months in open sheds, with but one case of glanders.[2] In the expedition to Quibéron during the Napoleonic wars, a cavalry contingent, believed to be healthy, shipped on new transports, encountered a storm, and had the hatches fastened down, so that several horses were suffocated. Among the survivors, landed at Southampton and placed in stables hitherto unchallenged, many soon developed glanders in its worst form. Similar results followed the English expeditions to Varna in 1854, and that to Abyssinia in 1867. In badly-ventilated mines and stables, especially cellar stables, glanders, once started, is always most virulent.

[2] Larrey, *Hyg. des Hop. Mil.*, 1862, p. 63.

2d. Cold, damp, draughty stables greatly favor the progress of glanders. Leblanc reports the case of a stud of 240 horses that had had no glanders for eight years, but which lost half their number in three months after removal into a new stable, very lofty, but dark and damp, and subject to cold draughts. It is worthy of notice that they had also been subjected to double work, and were consequently emaciated, but there was not known to be any unusual exposure to contagion. In a Boston street-car stable, where glanders had long prevailed, Thayer cut it short by destroying the infected animals and by improving the ventilation by windows hung at the bottom and opening inward, so that the air entered in an upward direction, and cold draughts on the horses were avoided.

3d. Debility from ill-health, low feeding, or overwork.—The nervous and nutritive debility consequent on chronic disease, overwork, and exhaustion lessens the power of resistance to specific poisons, but in such circumstances there is always the added predisposition of an excess of waste material in the blood, a specially abundant food for the disease-germ. So notorious is this that it used to be held that the specific poison of glanders was generated in connection with the excess of creatine, creatinine, and lactic acid resulting from muscular action. Of the effect of[p. 913]low diet we have a striking example, furnished by Bouley, of a stud of 120 horses, 60 of which were attacked within a year after they had been placed on a food insufficient to repair the body-waste, and from which the disease disappeared after the slaughter of the infected and improvement of the ration. So long as glandered horses were preserved for work, the then nearly ubiquitous germ attacked nearly all that were run down by chronic diseases; hence glanders was looked upon as the natural winding up of exhausting diseases in the horse, as tuberculosis was thought to be in the human subject. Modern discovery shows that without the germ all such debilitating causes are impotent, but it can never disprove the great potency of these in laying the system open to attack, nor the value of vigorous health and sound hygiene in fortifying the system against it.

The channel of infection manifestly varies in different cases. In direct inoculations the morbid process develops first at the point of insertion, and secondly in the nearest lymphatic glands and internal organs. When contracted in the ordinary way, the lesions are usually first seen in the posterior nasal passages, the larynx or the lungs, or in the superficial lymphatics, especially of the hind limbs. This susceptibility of the deeper portions of the air-passages seems to imply that the bacillus, borne on the air, is lodged on different parts of the respiratory mucous membrane, and first sets up the morbid process in the thinnest or most susceptible portion. That it can be thus borne on the air is shown by the experiments of Viborg and Gerlach, who separately collected the particulate elements from the exhalations of glandered horses and successfully inoculated them. That the virus is not usually carried far on the air in a virulent form is attested by the many instances in which horses have stood for months in the same stable with a glandered animal without becoming infected. That infection may also take place through the ingestion of infected matters is undoubted, as glanderous products mixed with food, or even made into balls and enclosed in paper and administered to horses in this form, have produced the disease. The virulence is said to be lost by passing through the digestive canal of man (Decroix), dog, pig, and fowl (Renault), but even to Carnivora the infection may be conveyed in the food.

While the virus is concentrated in the material of the special glanderous deposits and the discharges from these, yet no part of the body can be considered as free from the poison. Viborg, Coleman, Hering, and Chauveau have communicated the disease by transfusion of blood from a glandered horse to a healthy one; hence every vascular organ must be liable to infect. The secretions of the diseased body (tears, saliva, mucus, sweat, urine, and milk) have each been successfully inoculated, and the conveyance of the disease to the foetus in utero and to the female by coition imply that even the generative secretions are virulent. Failures to convey the disease by inoculation with the blood and secretions have often occurred, however, and they must be held as less virulent than the products of the local disease-processes.

The claims that inoculation with pus, ichor, and other irritants have produced glanders must be entirely discredited. The deposits and ulcers in the lungs and elsewhere resulting from such inoculations have been either septicæmia, mistaken for glanders in the earlier days of pathological anatomy; or the septic and other inflammations set up by these[p. 914]inoculations have merely served as fertile spots for the planting and growth of the glanders bacillus accidentally present, and which to a healthy system might have proved harmless.

In 1882, Chauveau had demonstrated the particulate nature of the glander germ by his unsuccessful inoculations with the liquids filtered from dilutions of pus taken from a pulmonary glanderous ulcer. The filtrate and the liquid mixture formed by mixing the pus with five hundred times its own weight of water retained their virulence undiminished. In 1868, Christol and Kiener discovered in glanderous products a bacillus which they figured as made up of a chain of nearly globular elements apparently enclosed in a common sheath. In 1881-82, Bouchard, Capitan, and Charrin cultivated these microphytes in a neutralized extract of meat through five successive cultures, using in each case a milligramme of the previous culture, or less than 1/1000 part of the culture-liquid. Counting that the milligramme of pus would give to each centigramme of the first culture-liquid 1,000,000,000 bacilli, it follows that the second culture would, on the principle of dilution, contain 1,000,000, the third 1000, the fourth 1, while for the fifth it was as 999 to 1 that it would receive nothing unless the germ were multiplied in the culture-liquid. Inoculation of a cat with this fifth culture, started originally from a nasal ulcer of a glandered horse, led to a fatal result in twenty-five days, with suppurating tumor of the left testicle and inguinal glands. The products of the first cat were inoculated on a second, those of the last on a third, those of the third on a guinea-pig, and those of the guinea-pig on an ass, producing in every case specific lesions of glanders, including miliary nodules and abscesses, and death respectively on the following days: 16, 7, 31, and 10.

In September, 1882, and the two succeeding months, a similar course of experiments was conducted by Schütz and Löfler at Berlin. The virulent matter used for starting the culture was procured from a pulmonary deposit and spleen of a glandered horse; the cultivation was continued through eight successive culture-fluids. One horse was successfully inoculated with the product of the eighth culture, and a second with both the fifth and eighth. The first died on the fifty-eighth day, and the second, now very weak, was sacrificed on the fifty-ninth. Both showed the most extensive lesions of glanders alike in the skin, the lymphatic glands, the pituitary and laryngeal mucous membrane, and the lungs. To demonstrate the bacillus they take a thin layer of the infecting liquid on a cover glass, dry it, stain with methyl violet, wash with dilute acetic acid, dehydrated by absolute alcohol, and clear by oil of cedar. Like other pathogenic microphytes this may be preserved for months or years if thoroughly dried, but in the moist condition it is easily destroyed by heat (133° F.; Viborg, Hofacker, Renault), chlorine, and the disinfectant chlorides and sulphites.

SYMPTOMS.—Acute nasal glanders in horses has a period of incubation lasting from three to five days in inoculated cases. Where in infected subjects the incubation appears to have extended over months or a year, there have usually (or always) been deposits in internal organs which passed without recognition until the lesions appeared in the nose. At the outset there is fever, which appears before any local lesions are recognizable, even post-mortem (Chauveau), and soon with languor, [p. 915]and loss of appetite, there is a serous nasal discharge, often from one side only. By the sixth day this has become yellowish, the margin of the nostril is often swollen, and upon the pituitary membrane may be detected elevations of various sizes of a general yellowish tinge, dotted with minute red points and surrounded by a bright-red or purple and slightly elevated areola. These may be simple, pea-like nodules or more or less extensive patches, which in certain cases extend over nearly the whole pituitary membrane. At the same time the submaxillary lymphatic glands on the same side become the seat of a hard nodular painless enlargement, feeling like a conglomerate mass of peas, and often showing a tendency to become more closely adherent to some adjacent part (bone, skin, base of tongue); but they only ulcerate exceptionally. Extensive hot, painful engorgements also often appear on other parts of the body, and if on the limbs or joints cause lameness. Soon the swellings on the mucosa become eroded and are gradually destroyed, forming large unhealthy, chancrous-looking ulcers, tending to become confluent and to eat deeply through the mucosa into the subjacent tissues. These are mostly reddish gray or yellowish gray, with raised ragged red or yellowish-red margins. They bleed readily, and may be black from hemorrhage, or greenish or of some other shade from decomposition. The discharge is always somewhat glutinous and sticky, but it may vary in color from simple white to yellowish, greenish, brownish, or red, according to the destruction of tissue, the septic changes, or the effusion of blood.

By the sixth to the fifteenth day the acme has been reached. The alæ of the nostrils are glued together by the drying discharge, and this, with the general swelling of the nasal passages, renders the breathing snuffling and difficult. The lymphatics on the side of the face are usually inflamed and corded, and the same is true of the cutaneous lymphatics of the hind limbs of some other part of the body (farcy). Death usually ensues from suffocation, preceded by the most painful dyspnoea.

Chronic glanders in horses often sets in insidiously, but frequently also it first shows itself by constitutional disturbance, which gradually subsides as the local lesions are formed. Among frequent premonitory symptoms may be mentioned intermittent or continued lameness, oedema of one or more limbs, infiltration of the testicle, cough, and bleeding from the nose. The general health may appear good, and if in good hygienic condition the digestion and nutrition may be sufficient, the body plump, and the skin shining; but there is usually some dulness of the eye, dryness of the coat, lack of endurance, and a tendency to sweat easily and to run down rapidly under hard work or debilitating conditions. The discharge, at first clear, becomes turbid, grayish, sticky, and purulent, tending to agglutinate the hairs and edges of the alæ nasi, and is expelled by snorting in masses. The nasal mucosa, and especially over the septum, is the seat of the peculiar elevations, ulcers, and firm white, condensed deposits resembling cicatrices, usually low enough down to be seen or felt. The submaxillary lymphatic glands are the seat of the nodular enlargement described in acute glanders, and, as in that affection, there may be pulmonary or skin deposits shown by cough or oedema, with swelling and cording of the cutaneous lymphatics with nodules and ulcers.

These cases often maintain this indolent type for years, spreading the[p. 916]infection widely, but they tend sooner or later to develop the acute type, especially under some debilitating conditions.

When the mucous membrane of the larynx and bronchi is first attacked the nasal lesions may be delayed for a time, but the cough, the variously colored tenacious expectoration, the excessive tenderness of the larynx, and the nodular enlargement of the adjacent lymphatic glands, with the general ill-condition, suggest that which is later confirmed by the specific lesions in nose and skin.

When the affection is confined to the bronchia and pulmonary parenchyma, there are the usual signs of bronchitis, disturbed breathing, with hard, soft, mucous, or dry husky cough, and blowing, mucous or sibilant râle, at points crepitation, and at others some diminution of murmur and resonance. The breath is mawkish or fetid, and expectoration more or less sticky and charged with bacilli; but all these symptoms are at times equivocal, and inoculation alone can attest the true nature of the disease. This should be practised by preference on a donkey or an old horse in poor condition but with general good health. Then the disease shows itself in the acute form in six days. If solipedes are not available, rabbits or guinea-pigs may be used for inoculation.

In acute cutaneous glanders or farcy, premonitory symptoms resemble those of ordinary acute glanders, which indeed is usually present as well, and always supervenes before farcy terminates in death. The local lesions consist in inflammation of the lymphatic vessels, which become like firm cords, the appearance at intervals along these cords of rounded glanderous nodules varying in size from a pea to a hickory-nut, and with a marked tendency to ulceration and the formation of hot, painful oedematous swellings. The swelling of the lymphatics appears by preference in the lower part of a hind limb, and the first nodules may be near the fetlock or tarsus. The ulcers forming about the sixth day have a yellowish-white appearance with red points and raised irregular borders, and the discharge is grumous and viscous, with a yellowish or reddish tinge. The disease extends toward the body, the upper air-passages become involved, and death speedily follows.

Chronic cutaneous glanders, chronic farcy, usually begins by a local swelling, mostly of the fetlock, in the midst of which a careful examination detects a small glanderous nodule. This tardily softens, ulcerates, and discharges the characteristic ichor, the lymphatics leading up from it become thick and rigid (corded), and new nodules appear. Though very indolent, these finally tend to ulcerate, and in time oedematous swellings appear in the vicinity or at distant parts of the body, with nodules at intervals. This will go on for months, or even for years, and recoveries occasionally take place, while in other cases, and especially when the conditions of life are bad, acute glanders supervene.

MORBID ANATOMY.—The lesions consist essentially in a cellular growth in the connective tissue, determined by the presence of the specific poison, and in destructive changes in the elements of such growth—softening, fatty degeneration, ulceration, and discharge. In certain cases of nasal glanders at the earliest stage there is merely an increased proliferation of the mucous corpuscles, which become more granular or purulent. Soon, however, the fibro-vascular layer is involved, the affected part being the seat of dark bluish congestion, and [p. 917]of the proliferation of small rounded lymphoid cells, comparable to those of the early stage of tubercle, and enclosed in more or less dense fibrous areolæ. The common nasal nodule or patch has a soft velvety surface, dirty gray or grayish yellow, and the lymphoid cells are so circumscribed in nests that when soaked in water the cells are washed out and the fibrous reticulum is left hollowed out like a honeycomb. In this fibrous reticulum are many spindle-shaped and a few rounded cells. Its vascularity is easily demonstrated by injection. The centre of each nest is the palest part of the mass, and unless stained by extravasation it contrasts with the reddish areola. These islets of lymphoid cells, at first isolated and each the size of a pin's head, may enlarge and become confluent, forming the larger nodules. With this increase the centre of each becomes turbid, and the cells are found to have become granular and fatty, and to have in part broken up into a granular débris. This characterizes the period of ulceration, and erosions and ulcers follow in ratio with the extent of the neoplasm and the rapidity of its growth. If the growth is tardy, the ulcer, with irregular eroded and everted edges, may remain for some time stationary or even recede, while if rapid, new tubercles form around the margin of the first, and by the disintegration of their elements the ulcer is continuously extended. The lesions are especially common on the septum nasi and turbinated bones. Similar lesions may be found in the nasal sinuses or larynx.

The nodules found in the lungs strongly resemble miliary tubercles, but are usually less numerous. As in the nose, they have a punctiform, central, grayish, turbid portion, encircled by a more translucent ring, surrounded in its turn by a vascular area. They are also composed of the same granular rounded cells, though they may, especially in the chronic forms, have undergone caseous, fibrous, or calcareous degeneration. The acute tubercles are often surrounded by circumscribed pneumonia with considerable exudation. They are distinguished from genuine tubercle by their vascularity and by the absence of giant-cells.

The cutaneous deposits are composed of the same histological products imbedded in the dermis or in the subcutaneous connective tissue, and extending in some cases deeply between the muscles, with no clear line of demarcation from the sound tissue. Not only the chains of nodules (farcy-buds), but the connecting lymphatic trunks, are the seat of the characteristic cellular product, and in chronic cases there is the enlargement of the adjacent lymphatic glands as well. In these there is a special tendency to early disintegration and ulceration.

In the diffuse glanderous swellings (infiltrated glanders, inflammatory glanders) the affected tissues are the seat of an inflammatory process with profuse exudation throughout, while in the interstices of the connective tissue are numerous granular glander-cells. The same tendency to necrobiosis is shown as in the other forms of glanderous neoplasms, and such diffuse swellings become the seats of very extensive, deep, and irregular ulcers, or frequently of fibroid growth and induration, forming the so-called cicatricial deposits. These are hard, firm, and resistant, and histologically consist of a dense fibrous stroma interspersed with the spindle-shaped cells. They are especially common in chronic cases, and such an appearance on the nasal mucous membrane is always suspicious, as this dense fibroid appearance rarely follows a simple traumatic lesion.

[p. 918]Diffuse glanderous infiltrations in the nose may implicate the entire mucosa of one or both nasal chambers, and the ulcers are liable to be greater than from the nodular form of the disease. They are also especially associated with thrombosis of the veins, which occurs to a less extent in the nodular form and conduces to the dark-blue tint of the mucosa.

Glanderous infiltration of the lungs is inflammatory in its nature (pneumonia malleosa), attacking an area of two or three inches in diameter at or near the margin of the lungs, and proceeds to caseous necrobiosis, suppuration, calcification, or fibroid induration. In the skin such infiltrations also frequently terminate in induration, while ulceration and abscess tend to appear when the proliferation of glander-cells is most abundant (farcy-buds).

The glander-nodules are not uncommon in muscles, intermuscular connective tissue, spleen, liver, kidneys, and testicles. Leukæmia is also a constant feature, the irritation of the lymphatic glands manifestly stimulating the production of the lymph-cells.

DIAGNOSIS.—The diagnosis of glanders usually rests on the viscid nature of the discharge, the painless nodular swelling of the submaxillary glands and the indisposition to suppurate, the characteristic appearance of the nodules, elevations, ulcers, and indurations of the nasal mucosa, and the presence of the specific bacillus. The diagnosis of farcy rests mainly on the nature of the nodules and corded lymphatics, of the ulcers and their discharges, on the extension of the affection toward the trunk, and the tendency to implicate the respiratory organs. Usually, there are several victims, the earlier ones chronic cases, the later ones acute, or there is a history or presumption of exposure. Yet in many cases, and especially in the more chronic internal forms (laryngeal, pulmonary, etc.), the diagnosis is difficult, and inoculation of a horse, goat, sheep, or rabbit may be the only available means of reaching a decision. Auto-inoculations are unreliable, as parts not yet the seat of active disease will often resist inoculation.

PROGNOSIS.—This is always unfavorable. The constancy of internal deposits and the viability of the germ in such products render it impossible to eliminate the poison from the system in the great majority of cases. In external glanders only is there any reasonably good hope, and even this is confined to the chronic cases. In stating this much, it is not denied that recoveries even of chronic nasal glanders do occur, yet these are few, and the majority of those that do apparently recover usually succumb as soon as they are subjected to hard work or specially trying conditions of life, so that but little faith can be placed in most of the alleged recoveries.

TREATMENT.—Considering the great danger of multiplying and preserving the germs of a disease so fatal alike to man and beast, the treatment of glanders is never commendable. The danger is least in the case of chronic farcy, not only because the processes are less active, but because the virus is not being thrown out and diffused with the tidal air of respiration, sneezing, and coughing. The unbroken farcy-buds and swollen lymphatics may be actively treated by compound iodine ointment, and the ulcerous nodules freely cauterized with corrosive sublimate, biniodide of mercury, chloride of zinc, sulphate of copper, or iodized[p. 919]phenol. Local inflammations may demand fomentations and astringent antiseptic lotions. Meanwhile, the system must be supported by a tonic regimen and medication, abundance of pure air, a liberal and wholesome diet, and the maintenance of the various bodily functions in a healthy condition. Of medicinal agents the most pronounced tonics have the best reputation—sulphate of copper and iron, biniodide of copper, arsenic, and, above all, arsenite of strychnia. Next to these the sulphites rank, and a combination of the two last named is perhaps to be preferred.

PREVENTION.—The glandered horses and all animals attacked with acute or obstinate farcy should be destroyed and their bodies be burned or deeply buried. Every State should legally interdict the use of a glandered horse or his exposure in any public or other place where infection is likely to reach other animals by contact or through fodder, litter, stable utensils, or any other objects employed about animals. No less imperative should be the perfect disinfection of all stables, harness, and other objects with which glandered animals have come in contact. The value of such measures is sufficiently attested by what has been stated above as to the prevalence of this disease in the French army so long as the doctrines of non-contagion dominated in its management, and the comparative disappearance of the disease so soon as a change of theory and method had been inaugurated; the absence of the disease in the English army, where the doctrine of contagion and its extinction has long prevailed; and the entire absence of the disease from Australia, New Zealand, etc., into which it has never been imported, though prevailing in a corresponding latitude and climate at the Cape of Good Hope.

Glanders in Man.

Up to 1812 the communication of glanders to man failed to be recognized. Then Lorin, a French surgeon, published a case of the kind in which inflammation of the hand was induced by inoculation from a horse suffering from farcy, and Waldinger and Weith drew attention to the dangers of infection about the same time. In 1821, Muscroft in England and Schilling in Germany simultaneously reported cases of infection from the horse in which the true symptoms of glanders in man were recognized. Rust, Sedow, and Weiss soon followed with additional cases; then Forozzi (1822), Seidler (1823), Wolff, Grossheim, Eck, Brunslow, Lesser, Travers (1826), Kries, Grubb, Brown (1829), Neumann (1830), Vogeli (1831), Alexander (1832), and Elliotson (1833). Though the disease was now well recognized, yet its nature has been elucidated by a series of later writers, including especially Rayer, Tardieu, Virchow, Leisering, Gerlach, and Korányi.

ETIOLOGY.—Man is rarely infected from any other source than the horse. In a very few instances the contagion has been derived from infected men. The modes of infection, immediate and mediate, are the main points to notice in this connection. Those employed about horses are usually infected by direct contact of the poisonous discharges, blood, or tissues with abrasions on the skin or mucous membranes. The inoculation received in giving medicine, examining the nose, performing operations with effusion of blood, dressing cutaneous ulcers, slaughtering, [p. 920]skinning, making a necropsy, burying, etc., is not uncommon. Again, direct infection is sustained through snorting of the horse, so that particles of the virulent discharge are lodged on the mucous membrane of the eye or nose. Closely allied to this is infection by inhaling the exhalations of glandered horses, and this doubtless accounts for some few cases which have been recorded as communicated through the unbroken skin. The bite of the glandered horse is a rare means of infection. From infection by eating glandered animals man is usually saved by the cooking of his food and by his inherent power of resistance, yet with instances of this kind on record, as recorded by Ringheim, and the well-known conveyance of the disease to animals in this way, it would be folly to ignore the risk to man from eating the flesh of glandered horses, sheep, goats, and rabbits.

Among the mediate forms of contagion may be named drinking from the same pail or trough after a glandered horse, using a knife that has been employed to open a glanderous abscess, wiping a wound with an infected blanket or handkerchief, handling infected harness, wagon-pole, or manger with wounded hands, sleeping over glandered horses or in a stall or on litter previously used by such horses.

Conveyance of glanders from man to man has taken place through using or handling the same dishes, towels, or handkerchiefs, through dressing the wounds, or, as in the case of the veterinarian Gerard, through making an autopsy of a victim of the disease.

Fortunately, the susceptibility of man is slight, but few out of the multitudes handling glandered horses becoming infected. It is essentially an industrial disease, 114 cases being distributed as follows among the different occupations: hostlers, 42; farmers and horse-owners, 19; horse-butchers, 13; coachmen and drivers, 11; veterinary surgeons and students, 10; soldiers, 5; surgeons, 4; gardeners, 3; horse-dealers, 2; policemen, shepherds, blacksmiths, employés at veterinary school, and washerwomen, 1 of each.

A condition of ill-health doubtless predisposes to this as to other invasions of infectious disease, yet men in apparently the most vigorous health have succumbed to the poison.

SYMPTOMS.—The incubation of acute glanders in inoculated cases usually varies from one to four days. In cases in which the mode of entrance is not so manifest it may apparently extend over one, two, or even three weeks. If the disease has occurred by external inoculation, the seat of the wound shows the first symptoms, consisting of tense swelling, pain, and a dark or yellowish erysipelatoid redness, while the edges of the wound are puffy and everted, the matter escaping is sanious, and the surrounding lymphatics are swollen and red and the lymphatic glands enlarged and tender. After a few days constitutional disorder sets in—languor, extreme weakness and prostration, aching in the limbs (muscles and joints) and in the head, rigors alternating with fever or a continued fever after the first violent chill, and in some cases nausea, vomiting, and even diarrhoea. In cases not resulting from external inoculation the febrile symptoms are the earliest to be noticed, and the muscular and articular pains may be at first mistaken for acute rheumatism. In other cases, in which the gastric and intestinal disorders are the most prominent and the prostration and weariness extreme, the symptoms at first strongly [p. 921]suggest typhoid fever. Soon, however, with a sense of formication a local yellowish or livid erysipelatoid inflammation appears, by preference on the softer parts of the face, the nose, eyelids, cheeks, or on one of the principal joints, the shoulder, elbow, or knee. In the midst of the phlegmonous swelling, or even antecedent to it, there appear small firm red spots or nodules, sometimes as small as those of variola, at others like a pea or as large as a walnut or larger. These gradually blanch in the centre, soften, and change into pustules or abscesses, and, bursting, discharge a slimy, thick, sanguineous pus, often emitting a mawkish or fetid odor. The sores thus formed are ulcerous and unhealthy, with puffy, ragged, everted borders and a grayish or yellowish red base, which often extends deeply between the muscles and exposes tendons and bones. When several deposits of this kind are closely aggregated, they tend to combine in one slough, which may involve a great extent of tissue. In all cases there are the swollen, reddened, tender condition of the connecting lymphatics and the tumefaction of the lymphatic glands. At times the deposits and abscesses are deeply seated in the interstices of the muscles, and at other times the joints are enlarged by exudation.

In nearly one-half of the cases glanders supervenes on the cutaneous symptoms. At first a viscid, whitish nasal catarrh appears from one or both nostrils, mixed with striæ of blood; then upon the pituitary membrane appear ulcers like those already described in the horse; the same form on the buccal, pharyngeal, and laryngeal mucous membranes, and by physical examination they may even be found to have invaded the lungs. The margins of the nostrils become adherent through the drying of the tenacious mucus; the meati are blocked or narrowed by the swelling of the mucosa, the detachment of sloughs, and the accumulation of the discharges; the breathing becomes snuffling and difficult; the voice altered or lost; the cough weak, with a mucous and bloody expectoration, and the breath offensively fetid. The submaxillary lymphatic glands are inflamed and enlarged, and may even go on to suppuration and ulceration. The conjunctiva is usually involved, and at times the specific formation and ulceration extend to the stomach and intestines, and nausea, vomiting, indigestion, irregularity of the bowels, and fetid diarrhoea ensue. There is complete anorexia, but thirst is ardent, especially with diarrhoea. With the advance of the disease dyspnoea supervenes, and nervous disorder is shown by the extreme weakness, anxiety, sleeplessness, troubled dreams, nocturnal delirium, dilated pupils, and even coma. The temperature, though at first unaltered, may later rise to 104° F., and the pulse to 110 to 120 beats per minute. The diagnosis is confirmed by detection of the bacillus in the discharges, and, above all, in the liquids of freshly-opened pustules (Wassilieff).

The duration of acute glanders in man may be no more than three days, though usually it is protracted to fourteen or twenty-one, and exceptionally to twenty-nine days. The almost constant termination of this form of the disease is in death.

Chronic glanders occasionally appears in man, and is in most respects the counterpart of that of the horse. The morbid process shows itself in the integumental or other tissues of the body, and only attacks the nose and air-passages later, when the constitutional symptoms become more intense. The general malaise, languor, prostration, aching of [p. 922]limbs and joints, and inappetence are usually present, complicated by a local swelling in the seat of inoculation (face, hands, etc.), with small nodules progressing to pustules, congestion of the lymphatics, and swelling of the lymphatic glands. These lesions may subside even before suppuration, and the disease is manifested for a week or two only by a general feeling of weariness and ill-health; but sooner or later the local symptoms reappear in the same or another seat, and the neoplasms, though indolent for an indefinite length of time, finally degenerate, soften, burst, and form ulcers. These ulcers have the general characters already described—a livid grayish or yellowish hue, with red, puffy, irregular edges, and a viscid greenish, yellowish, dirty white, or bloody discharge. They tend to increase, or they may appear to heal by the peculiar firm cicatricial formation, but on the swollen margins new deposits, abscesses, and ulcers tend continually to form. Sometimes these are of considerable size and seated deeply among the muscles, but when opened they show the same unhealthy serous or bloody pus, and manifest a tendency to extension rather than to healing. When the disease extends to the respiratory organs, often two or three months after the onset, there is cough and sore throat, blocking of the nose by the tenacious discharges and swollen mucosa, and in the pharynx, fauces, and nose the characteristic ulcer may be detected. The attendant constitutional symptoms are also much more marked—indigestion, nausea, vomiting, diarrhoea, rigors, profuse perspiration, high temperature, excited breathing and pulse, a yellowish or earthy hue of the skin, rapid emaciation, and great prostration. Though great emaciation, debility, and hectic ensue on the indolent chronic processes, yet the disease usually assumes all the characters of the acute type before terminating fatally.

In cases that recover the fever diminishes, exacerbations cease, ulcers granulate and cicatrize, vesicles dry up, the nodules and enlarged glands diminish, the erysipelatoid swellings of skin and nose subside, and a very tardy and imperfect convalescence is established.

The duration of chronic glanders, nasal or cutaneous (farcy), is exceedingly indefinite, varying from three months to ten or eleven years. One of the most protracted cases is that recorded by Bollinger of a veterinarian who, after an eleven years' illness, recovered with cicatricial contraction of the nose and larynx and a decided cachectic appearance.

MORBID ANATOMY.—Besides the lesions above mentioned as occurring in the skin and mucous membranes of the nose, mouth, and pharynx, the frontal sinuses, the larynx, and less frequently the lungs, are the seats of the specific glanderous processes. In the lungs there are then the nodules, hard, caseous, or purulent according to their age, and varying in size from a millet-seed and pea upward to the involving of the greater part of a lobe. Beneath the pleuræ may be seen ecchymoses, hard, fibrous nodules, and yellow elevations, which on being incised furnish grumous pus. The spleen is usually enlarged, gorged with blood, gray or black, and is the seat of suppuration. The liver is enlarged, softened, and may be the seat of glanderous processes, with ulcers in the bile-duct or gall-bladder. The joints, like other serous cavities, become the seat of specific suppuration. The bones are often implicated in adjacent deposits, especially in the face, cranium, and hands, so that the compact tissue may become reduced to the merest shell, while the medulla and periosteum [p. 923]abound in the specific products. The cerebral meninges and brain-tissue are frequently the seat of specific growths and minute abscesses. It is noticeable that the enlargement of the lymphatic glands is usually less than it is in the horse, though they are never entirely free from lesions. Indeed, the tendency in man to the formation of considerable glanderous neoplasms is much less than in the solipede.

The microscopy of the lesions is essentially the same as in the horse. O. Wyss describes the cutaneous nodules as formed by a great proliferation of round cells (like pus-cells) in the upper layer of the corium just beneath the papillary layer. In a more advanced stage the corium and papillæ are filled with pus-cells, and, becoming disorganized, give rise to the formation of pustules and small abscesses. Lagrange describes in a chronic ulcer of the palm, a layer about 2 mm. in thickness of embryonic cells closely packed with an amorphous intercellular substance. The nuclei appeared larger than in ordinary ulcers or tubercles. Extending into this layer were capillary vessels packed with red globules and with blind extremities, or in some instances minute ruptures and hemorrhages. Beneath this superficial cellular layer was a stratum of striated muscle, especially noticeable for the excess of condensed connective tissue making up the intermuscular septa, and the great multiplication of nuclei with large, clearly-defined nucleoli, not only inside the sarcolemma, but also between the fibrillæ and separating them widely. At some points the muscular tissue had undergone a vitreous degeneration, while at others were many fusiform cells. At one point, where the ulcer extended to the phalanx, the compact layer of the bone was attenuated to the thinnest shell and perforated, so that the medulla was continuous with the ulcer. The medulla contained a great number of white globules, medulla-cells, and minute embryonic nuclei. The vessels were remarkable by the extensive fibroid thickening of their coats. On section of the ulcer many orifices stood widely open because of the rigidity of their walls. The internal coat was plicated, as if too large for the lumen. The external fibrous layers were at points abundantly interspersed with, and even replaced by, groups of embryonic cells, the active proliferation of which meant the destruction of the perivascular fibrous layer. These embryonic cells even invaded the lumen of the vessel and partly blocked it, so that the remnant of the tube remained as the centre of a disintegrating mass, or later a caseous or purulent focus.

DIAGNOSIS.—Acute glanders, when well developed, is unmistakable. The presence on or near the skin of the characteristic nodules, pustules, phlyctenæ, and ulcers, the oedema or erysipelatoid condition of the adjacent skin, the redness of the lymphatics, the presence of the neoplasms and ulcers in the nose, and the sticky, fetid, variously colored nasal discharge, with the acute fever, prostration, and pains in the limbs and joints, make a tout ensemble that is pathognomonic. In the initial stage only it may be confounded with rheumatism, but the arthritic pains are not usually attended by the same amount of redness and swelling of the joints, the prostration is far more profound, and there are in most cases an irritable, unhealthy-looking wound and a history of exposure to infection from glandered horses.

In chronic glanders, and especially in the external form (farcy), the diagnosis is often more difficult. From pyæmia and septicæmia it is[p. 924]usually to be distinguished by the comparative absence or the slightness of the chills, by the less healthy character of the pus, and by the implication of the nasal mucosa, the larynx, and lungs. When the nose, larynx, or lungs are but slightly affected, there may be a strong resemblance to syphilis or miliary tuberculosis, but a close attention to the character of the lesions, the absence of any concomitant history or symptoms of syphilis, and deductions drawn from the occupation of the patient and the presumptive exposure, will greatly assist in reaching a diagnosis.

The detection of the bacillus is not conclusive, as in tuberculosis and some forms of septicæmia there are similar organisms, agreeing with the microbe of glanders even in the matter of size. In cases of doubt a little delay will usually allow the development of new and more characteristic symptoms.

The final resort, however, is to inoculation. Auto-inoculation, as practised by Poland, is rarely satisfactory, as the system has acquired a partial tolerance of the disease and local lesions are not so certainly developed as in the healthy subject (St. Cyr). Inoculation on a healthy goat, sheep, or rabbit can always be availed of, and if practised on more than one subject can be relied upon, as the virus loses nothing of its power in passing through the human system, but usually determines an acute form of the disease in the animal inoculated.

PROGNOSIS.—Acute glanders is almost constantly fatal to man. Of chronic cases, and especially the external form (farcy), from one-third to one-half of the subjects recover. When both internal and external (farcy—glanders), the issue is usually fatal. Kütner claims that cases caused by external inoculation are more favorable than those caused by the inhaled poison. This accords with the general principle, that a poison viable in the comparatively vitiated air of the lungs or on the surface of the intestinal canal is better fitted by its habit of life for survival in the blood and plasma, and is consequently more redoubtable. The greater the duration of the disease in any particular case, the more favorable is the prognosis.

TREATMENT.—In the treatment of glanders in man the same principles must guide as in animals. In external, inoculated cases the wounded tissues should be early destroyed by potent caustics—fuming nitric acid, corrosive sublimate, iodized phenol, chlorine, sulphate of copper, carbolic acid, or the hot iron. The erysipelatoid swellings may be treated by leeching, followed by solutions of carbolic acid, iodine, or chlorine-water, by ice, and internally by laxatives and iodide of potassium. The first two antiseptics may be freely used by hypodermic injection. Abscesses and tumors should be laid open and cauterized as above, and then treated by weaker solutions of the same agents. Nasal ulcers may be treated by insufflation of iodoform and injections of creasote, carbolic acid, nitrate of silver, or permanganate of potash solutions. Of the greatest importance is a general tonic and stimulating regimen. A nutritious diet (including beef-tea), abundance of pure air, alcoholic stimulants, quinia, tincture of the chloride of iron, and, above all, arseniate of strychnia, have been used with advantage. Various anti-ferments, such as the bisulphites in full doses, carbolic acid, and iodide of potassium, have apparently proved beneficial, and deserve a further trial. As in the horse, a great [p. 925]variety of other agents, mostly of a tonic nature, have been employed, but with very variable results.

PREVENTION.—The first step toward the prevention of glanders in man is the systematic restriction and extinction of the affection in animals. This has been already sufficiently referred to above. Further measures of prophylaxis embrace the following: the avoidance of contact with glandered and suspected horses by all persons having any wounds, abrasions, or ulcers on their skins; the cauterization with nitrate of silver of all such sores on persons necessarily brought in contact with glandered or suspected animals or their products; the general diffusion of information as to the danger from glandered animals; washing of hands and face in a solution of carbolic acid or chloride of lime after handling infected or suspected animals or their carcases or products; the thorough disinfection or destruction (preferably by fire) of harness, clothing, racks, mangers, wagon-poles, buckets, troughs, brushes, combs, litter, and fodder that have been exposed to infection; and, finally, the exclusion from the markets of all meat derived from suspected or infected animals. It is generally held that the flesh of the horse alone demands inspection, but with the known susceptibility of sheep, goats, and rabbits it can easily be conceived how the infection may reach man through his food, though horse-flesh is never consumed. That glanders has never been recognized as arising from the consumption of diseased sheep or rabbits does not prove that it has never reached man by this channel, any more than the absence of all recognition of the infection of man from the horse would prove the non-occurrence of such infection until the beginning of the present century. The knowledge that the animals used for food in this country are liable to contract and convey this disease is an additional reason for the systematic and universal suppression of the disease among the equine population.

[p. 926]

ANTHRAX (MALIGNANT PUSTULE).
BY JAMES LAW, F.R.C.V.S.

SYNONYMS.—*Latin*, Ignis Sacer, Anthrax Epizoöticus, Pustula Maligna, Pustula Pestifera, Erysipelas Carbunculosum, Carbunculo Contagioso, Glossanthrax, Angina Carbunculosa, Anthrax Hæmorrhoidalis, Mycosis Intestinalis, Apoplexia Splenitis, etc. *English*, Black Erysipelas, Malignant Vesicle, Anthrax Fever, Splenic Apoplexy, Splenic Fever, Inflammatory Fever, Carbuncular Fever, Black Quarter, Blood-Striking, Bloody Murrain, Blain, etc. *French*, Pustule maligne, Charbon, Fièvre putride, Typhohémie, Pélohémie, Mal de Rate, Splenite Gangréneusé, etc.*German*, Karbunkelkrankheit, Contagiose Karbunkel, Milzbrand, Milzseuche, Milzbrandfieber, Brandbeulenseuche, Rothlauf, etc. *Russian*, Jaswa (boil-plague). *Italian*, Antrace. *Spanish*, Carbunculo, Lobado.*Swedish*, Boskapssjukan. *Mexican*, Calentura del piojo.

DEFINITION.—Anthrax is an acute, infectious, bacteridian disease, occurring mostly in the Herbivora and Omnivora, but communicable to other mammals (including man), to birds, and even fishes. Its local manifestations are exceedingly varied in kind, but the malady is characterized by the presence in the tissues or blood, or both, of specific spherical and linear bacteria (micrococcus and bacillus anthracis), leading to arrest of hæmatosis, to disintegration of the blood-globules, to sanguineous engorgement of the spleen, to capillary embolism, and to a spreading gangrenous inflammation.

HISTORY AND GEOGRAPHICAL DISTRIBUTION.—While ancient history is not clear as to the specific diseases of animals, yet there is the strongest presumption that nearly all great plagues that attacked indiscriminately animals and man were of this nature. Thus, the plague of murrain, with boils and blains breaking out on man and beast, in the days of Moses, was probably of this kind (Gen. ix. 3.); also that which at the siege of Troy extended from animals to man, and many later epizoötics in all parts of the world. No infectious disease of man and animals, with the single exception of tuberculosis, has been more widely diffused, and none can be considered as more cosmopolitan. Heusinger, in his classic work on *Milzbrandkrankheit*, traces the ravages of the disease from the highest to the lowest latitudes in the northern and southern hemispheres and in the Old World and the New. He adduces outbreaks in Siberia, Astrakan, Lapland, and Finland, in Russia, Prussia, Poland, Silesia, Bavaria, Holland, Belgium, France, Spain, Portugal, Italy, Switzerland, Austria, Hungary, Greece, Turkey, Egypt, East and West Indies, [p. 927]North and South America, etc. We can now add all the great English, French, and other European colonies not included in the above (South Africa, Australia, New Zealand, Algeria, etc.), together with China and Japan. We find, moreover, that the disease is always most prevalent where agriculture is in its most primitive condition, so that there can be little doubt of the prevalence of the affection in the less-civilized countries as well. But while the disease is prevalent in all parts of the world, its ravages are largely subordinate to the nature of the soil. Wherever this is close, impervious, marshy, or charged with an excess of organic matters, the gaseous emanations of which drive out most of the oxygen, the anthrax-germs, once introduced, tend to be preserved indefinitely. Thus, in drying up basins with no natural drainage, on lake and river margins, on deltas, in forests, in mucky, mossy, or peaty soils, and on those that are habitually over-manured, the germs of anthrax are especially liable to be perpetuated. It has long been noticed that herbivorous animals are the most susceptible to anthrax, while the purely carnivorous, and to a less extent the omnivorous, have relatively a far higher resisting power. That the immunity is largely due to the food is manifest from the experiments of Feser on rats. Those fed on vegetable aliment contracted anthrax readily from inoculation, while those kept on an exclusive diet of flesh successfully resisted. The same rats that escaped while on a flesh diet were afterward placed on a vegetable diet, and then perished after inoculation.[1] Davaine found the same to be true of foxes kept on meat and vegetables respectively, and inoculated with the virulent blood of the allied disease, septicæmia. He found, moreover, that guinea-pigs were much more susceptible to anthrax than rabbits. One-thousandth of a drop of virulent anthrax blood invariably killed the guinea-pig, while it left the rabbit unharmed.[2] Klein has never found a rabbit insusceptible. It has recently been claimed that pigs are insusceptible, but I have known of many instances in which the offal of anthrax cattle, when devoured by pigs, has determined fatal anthrax in the latter. Chickens too prove much less susceptible to anthrax than the Herbivora. Inoculations made by Cohn and others proved invariably unsuccessful, while Pasteur has showed that they can be infected easily after the body has been cooled by partial immersion in cold water.[3] Pasteur attributes this immunity to their normally high temperature, yet rabbits, sheep, pigs, wolves, and foxes, though maintaining a correspondingly high temperature, are still subject to anthrax. Even the herbivorous mammal suffering from acute anthrax fever has its temperature raised to that of the chicken, yet the disease progresses none the less surely to a fatal result. Again, anthrax liquids inoculated under the skin of a fox proved harmless, while if thrown into the warmer peritoneal cavity they proved fatal. It may well be suspected that the relative insusceptibility of chickens is in part due to the large amount of animal food consumed by them, and that the chilling process increases the receptivity by deranging sanguinification and nutrition.

[1] *Wochenschrift f. Thierheilkunde und Thiersucht*, Nos. 24 and 25, 1879.

[2] *Rec. de Med. Vet.*, Mar. 15, 1879.

[3] *Ibid.*, Mar. 15, 1880.

The insusceptibility to anthrax is often characteristic of certain individuals or families or of the animals living in a particular district. Thus, Chauveau found that some French sheep, and nearly all Algerian ones, [p. 928]resisted inoculation with a moderate amount of anthrax virus, while the introduction of a maximum amount proved fatal to these as to others. In the same way, it is often noticed that animals living in an anthrax region escape the evil effects of the poison, while strange animals brought in either fall ready victims or for a time do badly until they have become habituated to the locality. In view of the subsequent protective effect on the system of a first and non-fatal attack of anthrax, it is probable that all these examples of immunity in the Herbivora depend on a previous mild attack of the same disease or on the extinction of the more susceptible races. Even in the case of the animals that do badly on first coming into an anthrax district, and recover better health with immunity later, we may well infer that a mild form of the anthrax infection has been passed through.

ETIOLOGY.—The one essential cause of anthrax is the introduction into the system of a specific bacteridian germ (bacillus anthracis or its spores). This is not, as a rule, carried far on the atmosphere, but demands for its propagation contagion, immediate or mediate. Unless, therefore, it meets in the soil the conditions necessary to the preservation and propagation of the germ, it is transmitted with some uncertainty from animal to animal, and thus the disease does not spread widely and rapidly, like an ordinary plague, but tends to become localized in particular districts as an enzoötic.

But its dangers are none the less real nor its existence less to be dreaded. In predisposed localities, where the disease-germ has gained a footing, the animal mortality may exceed that caused by the great plagues, while the risk to human beings is incomparably greater than from any other acute infectious disease of the lower animals. Thus, in San Domingo, in 1770, 15,000 people perished in six weeks from eating the carcases of anthrax animals, and the mortality was only arrested when the meat was legally interdicted. In the worst anthrax years on some of the Siberian steppes as many as one-fourth of the whole human population suffer from the malady. The prevalence and death-rate, however, vary greatly in different localities and seasons. Sometimes only one or two solitary cases of the affection are observed; at other times the disease becomes moderately prevalent, but a lack of virulence in the poison or a previously acquired insusceptibility of the individual protects the great majority of the animals exposed, while at others, still, the poison attacks nearly all exposed to its contagion.

The animal products that mainly convey the disease are the blood, the liquid exudations, portions of the diseased carcase, and the bowel dejections. The virus is most potent when derived from an animal still living or only recently dead, yet under certain conditions (with spore-formation) it may long retain its virulence under the most extreme changes of climate, temperature, dryness, and humidity. Russian hides tanned in England or America frequently convey anthrax, which is known especially as a tanner's malady, and wool and hair sent from Buenos Ayres have repeatedly produced malignant pustule (woolsorter's disease) in Britain and the United States. The preserved scabs of malignant pustule have been often successfully inoculated on the lower animals, so that, like other forms of poison, this seems to be preserved indefinitely by desiccation.

The simple contact of the virus with the slightest abrasion will suffice [p. 929]to convey the disease. It has often been communicated where no lesion of the epidermis could be found, yet the presumption is that even in such cases the cuticle had been in some way wounded. Eating the flesh of animals killed while suffering from anthrax has often conveyed the disease. In an outbreak in Swineshead, Lincolnshire, England, in 1863, I found a dog and a number of swine suffering from eating the bodies of dead bullocks. In 1864 an East Lothian (Scotland) farmer fed his pigs with the offal of a slaughtered anthrax bullock, and lost nearly the whole herd. The carcase of the bullock had been sent to market. About 1860 cattle, and even horses, died yearly on a swampy meadow at Brighton, Mass. On one occasion the owner, John Zoller, fed the offal of a dead bullock to his pigs, which were speedily attacked with anthrax, and as speedily killed to save their bacon (Dr. Thayer). Even when cooked the flesh is not always safe. Of this we have the undoubted case in San

Domingo above noticed, the alleged death of 60,000 people in the vicinity of Naples from the same cause in 1617 (Kircher), and the thousands that die on the Russian steppes every anthrax year from eating the sick horses (Rawitch). But in all these, and in the ever-recurring cases in which families suffer from eating anthrax meat, there is the possibility, if not the probability, of the contamination of the meat subsequently to cooking by the knives, forks, tables, and dishes used. The San Domingo slaves had few appliances for cleanliness, much less disinfection, and the Tartars eat their meat from the same board on which it has been chopped up raw.

In accurate experiments it has been found that the bacilli are destroyed by a temperature of 145° F. maintained for five minutes, but the spores are capable of surviving the boiling temperature for five or even ten minutes. The varying power of resistance may be compared to that of the green stalk of the pea and the dry flinty seed. The first is destroyed by a very moderate heat, while the second will sprout after having had boiling water poured over it. The resisting bacillus-spores are never found in the living animal, but may be developed in the blood and tissues after death, and may account for the occasional extraordinary viability of the poison when exposed to a boiling temperature.

Milk, though often used with impunity, conveyed the disease when inoculated by Bollinger, and the same was true of the vaginal mucus. Innocent in the early stages of the disease while the germs are still localized, they become virulent after the bacilli swarm into the blood.

Healthy men and animals often carry the poison, though themselves insusceptible. The question of its conveyance by insects has been much debated, but the constant occurrence of malignant pustule on the uncovered parts of the body goes far to settle the question. Bourgeois long ago noticed that it was most frequent on the face, hands, neck, and arms, and rare on the trunk. In sixty cases recorded by A. W. Bell of Brooklyn, all occurred on the face except two on the hands, one on the wrist, and one on the forearm. The bite of a fly or mosquito had in many of these cases proved the starting-point of the malady. Bollinger has shown the presence of the bacillus in the stomach of such flies as fed on flesh and blood (horse-flies, bluebottles, etc.), and, together with Raimbert and Davaine, has produced anthrax by inoculations with the stomachs, legs, and proboscides of these insects.

[p. 930]Surgical instruments occasionally convey anthrax. At Cockburnspath, East Lothian, Scotland, a yearling heifer contracted anthrax, and the whole herd was bled, commencing with the sick one. Next morning seven were found dead, the disease in each case extending around the fleam-wound. At Brunt, in the same county, a shepherd skinned an anthrax bullock, and after washing and taking a turn among his sheep, on the same day castrated several litters of pigs, all of which perished. In St. Lawrence Co., N.Y., in 1870, a surgeon inoculated himself while opening a vesicle on the hand of a farmer.

Harness, stables, stable utensils, vehicles, fodder, and litter are frequent bearers of contagion. At Geneseo, N.Y., in 1877, three horses and a cat died in midwinter after licking the blood from a stone-boat which had conveyed the skin of an anthrax bullock to market. Green fodder or hay harvested from ground formerly occupied by anthrax victims or from their graves often convey the poison, but probably only by the adherent earth and dust containing the anthrax-germ.

That the anthrax bacillus and its spores may be long preserved in earth is abundantly proved. At Avon, N.Y., nine months after any cases of the disease, the liquid leaking out on the river-bank near to the grave of a victim of the year before was licked by six cattle, and in two days they all perished. On the same pasture victims were seized yearly for seven years, but with a rigid seclusion of these, their products, and their graves the malady has finally disappeared. The persistent deadly effect of some soils on animal life, apart from the presence of the carcasses, seems to show that in certain soils we find the normal home of the anthrax bacillus, while the migration into the animal economy is but an accident of its existence. The soils that are especially subject to anthrax are the dense clays, the limestones, and the rich alluvials. Among the essential conditions are the exclusion of oxygen, excepting a limited amount bearing some relation to what is found in the animal fluids, and the abundance of some alkaline agent (lime, potash, soda, ammonia), so that the earth is either neutral or only very slightly alkaline or acid. An acid vegetable infusion is inimical to the germ, which soon disappears from such a medium. The requisite paucity of air is found in all the dense, less pervious soils (clays, etc.), in soils habitually waterlogged (swamps, deltas, river-bottoms, low meadows, natural basins, drying lakes and ponds), and in soils rich in decomposing organic matter (peat, alluvial, over-manured). The antacid is often found present as lime or potash, or is constantly being produced in the form of ammonia, etc. by organic decomposition. Such places are known to farmers as "dead lots," because no stock will live on them. The bacillus in the buried carcase does not produce spores (Bollinger), though it may in the soil at any temperature between 59° and 110° F. In the graves, therefore, at a lower temperature, the poison can only be preserved by a continuous generation of the bacillus.

Pasteur, who successfully inoculated the casts of earth-worms taken from anthrax graves, attributes to these an important rôle in bringing the germs to the surface. A more important agent, however, is probably the rise and fall of water in the soil. By this means the bacilli and spores are washed up toward the surface, and when the superficial layers dry out they are easily carried by the winds. Hence it is that anthrax is usually prevalent in late summer and when the soil is dried and heated to its [p. 931]greatest depth. Thus it is, too, that wet seasons followed by specially dry and hot ones are, above all, productive of anthrax in herds. Wet seasons fulfil the further purpose of carrying off the germs into rivers and depositing them on the banks or on inundated meadows, where after the subsidence of the flood the disease appears, for the first time perhaps.

There is, however, good reason to believe that the effect of a warm season is not confined to its influence on the soil and its germs. The high temperature deranges the vital functions of the animal economy, and, inducing a febrile disturbance, lessens the power of resistance to the anthrax virus, just as the cooling of the warm-blooded bird lays it open to infection. On this account, and because of the frequently recurring electric storms, the hot dry season is especially the season of anthrax. The hottest, driest autumns of Siberia always coincide with the anthrax years, and in the last fifteen years in the United States I have noticed the wide extension of anthrax whenever the season has been unusually hot and dry. In Corsica the herdsmen confidently pasture their stock in the close still valleys throughout spring and early summer, but whenever the surface soil is dried out they make all haste to remove it to the hills, well knowing that delay means devastation and ruin.

Plethora is undoubtedly an important predisposing cause of anthrax, and so is the alternation of cold nights with hot days. The febrile condition induced in the animal economy is perhaps the main factor at work in each case. Finally, youth is on the whole more liable than age, but whether because of the greater receptivity of the growing system and its tissues, or because it has not yet acquired some immunity by exposure to the milder effects of the poison, is not certainly determined. Sex is without influence.

It is not a little remarkable that the bacillus germ has not yet been found in the placental liquids nor foetal blood of sheep, goats, or rabbits, though swarming in that of the mother. Bollinger attributes this to the action of the placenta as a "physiological filter"—a conclusion seemingly at variance with the passage of the bacillus through all the other animal membranes, including those lining the mammary glands and the vagina. Two other possible explanations remain: first, that the secretions of the uterine glands are inimical to the bacillus; and, second, that the foetus, being in some sense a carnivorous animal, possesses the immunity characteristic of Carnivora. Bacilli have recently been found in the foetal guinea-pig.

The bacillus anthracis was first observed by Pollender and Branel in 1849 (Birch-Hirschfeld), but it was only publicly claimed as the cause of the disease in 1855 by Davaine. Branel discarded Davaine's theory, because blood in which he had failed to find bacillus produced anthrax with bacillus in the blood of two foals inoculated. Later observations by Bollinger and others have shown that cultures of bacillus can always be made from such infecting blood, and that in most cases the presence in the infecting blood of spherical bacteria can be demonstrated by the microscope. That the bacillus is the true pathogenic element is proved by the following facts: 1st. That the bacillus is the only ectogenous, particulate, organized structure constantly found in the anthrax blood and fluids; in cases in which it is apparently absent cultures show its actual presence. 2d. After cultivation in pork or beef infusion to the [p. 932]hundredth generation the virulence is unimpaired, though it must be assumed that all non-organized poisons derived from the infected animal body must have been diluted or decomposed to extinction. 3d. That filtration of the anthrax liquids through a plaster or other efficient filter renders the filtrate innocuous, while the solids retained in the filter remain infecting (Chauveau, Bert, Toussaint). 4th. That the clear filtrate injected to excess killed by virtue of its contained chemical products in twelve hours, while the solids filtered out and containing the bacillus or its spores only killed after thirty hours.[4] 5th. Anthrax blood from the living animal or one just dead, and destitute of spores, when subjected to compressed oxygen (50 atmospheres), is non-infecting (Bert). 6th. The same anthrax liquid, destitute of spores, after boiling is completely innocuous. 7th. The same liquid, if kept in a closed tube apart from oxygen for eight days, shows the bacilli broken down by granular degeneration, and proves absolutely harmless when inoculated in small quantity. 8th. The same sporeless anthrax fluid when treated with absolute alcohol loses its virulence. 9th. The anthrax liquid which has been cultivated with free access of air in a temperature varying from 25° C. (77° F.) (Klein, Löffler) to 41° C. (105.5° F.) forms spores, and then remains infecting, though it may have been subjected to compressed oxygen, boiling for several minutes, absolute alcohol, dilution with water, putrefaction, or the exclusion of oxygen.

[4] Bert, *Compt. Rend. de la Société Biol.*, p. 355, 1879.

The bacillus anthracis, as found in the blood and animal fluids, is in the form of fine rods, straight (rarely bent or angular), motionless, and 0.007 to 0.012 Mm. in length. Smaller forms are seen to be minute ovoid or oblong bodies, and the smallest absolutely spherical (micrococcus); but in all cases, as seen under the highest powers of the microscope, they have clear-cut, even margins, linear or curved, which easily distinguish them from the irregular normal granules of the blood and tissues. Under the highest powers of the microscope the bacillus is seen to be made up of a series of oblong (Koch) or cubical (Klein) cells enclosed in one common sheath. This is rendered more manifest if they are first swollen by the addition of water. The motionless form of the anthrax bacillus is of especial value in distinguishing it from the motile bacteria of putrefaction (saprophytes).

Within the living animal body the development never goes aside from these forms. The growth appears limited to micrococcus and bacillus rods, while spores or bacillus threads are never found. This finds its counterpart in the micrococcus poisoning caused by the inoculation with the spores of common moulds (Grawitz); and in septicæmia also micrococcus and bacillus forms only are found, the filamentous never.

When grown in organic infusions out of the animal body the anthrax-germ develops from micrococcus or bacillus into a long, branching, filamentous product, which in the presence of oxygen develops into spores. Apart from oxygen or when the proper nourishment of the bacillus is exhausted the protoplasmic elements within the filamentous sheath undergo granular degeneration, and finally the empty envelope disintegrates and disappears. The spores appear at intervals in the protoplasm of the filament as clear, brightly refrangent bodies, at first spheroidal, afterward larger and oblong. Unlike the micrococcus and bacillus, [p. 933]they do not stain. Under favorable circumstances the primary cell is capable of forming one, or if extra long, two spores (Koch, Klein). Cossar-Ewart claims to have seen the formation of motile flagellate organisms aggregating themselves into zooglæa masses, but as these were not found in the carefully-conducted cultures of Koch and Klein, they are supposed to have been aërial microphytes accidentally introduced.

The great tenacity of life in the spores in heat and cold, dryness and wet, excluded from air and under several atmospheres of oxygen, in the midst of putrefaction and in pure watery fluids, well accounts for the persistence of infection in buildings and localities where the poison has gained a foothold. In order to their destruction in a natural manner it seems necessary that they should germinate and develop into the anthrax micrococcus, bacillus, or mycelium. This germination may take place in the presence of moisture, oxygen, and suitable nourishment, whether in the soil, the animal body, or elsewhere, and then the exhaustion of the aliment, the exclusion of the oxygen by putrefaction, the submergence in a medium unfavorable to development, or exposure to a very high temperature, may suddenly destroy the poison.

There is reason to believe that a too free exposure to oxygen proves destructive to the virulence, if not to the life, of the poison, and thus in all porous, well-drained soils the anthrax poison, even when introduced from without and concentrated by the death and burial of many victims, soon disappears. This feature, which is common to many zymotic diseases the germs of which live and multiply outside the animal body (typhoid, yellow fever, tuberculosis, swine plague, chicken cholera, diphtheria, etc.), offers countenance to the claims of Buchner that he had by prolonged culture, in the presence of air, metamorphosed the bacillus anthracis into a harmless mycrophyte, and that, conversely, by continuous cultivation under the surface of a suitable beef infusion he had changed the harmless bacillus subtilis of hay into the deadly bacillus anthracis. Koch, Klein, and others have discredited Buchner's results, on the ground that he had not, in their opinion, taken due precautions against impure cultures, and that his alleged transitions took place too abruptly; yet further observation must determine whether he has been condemned too hastily. The diminished virulence of Pasteur's attenuated virus, which is unaffected by the next subsequent culture or by the formation of spores, shows plainly enough that the bacillus anthracis is capable of physiological changes under the influence of varying conditions of growth, and that such changes are not at once undone by a return of the former conditions.

How anthrax-germs enter the body is partly known and partly conjectured. Direct inoculation on a sore by contact, by insects, by harness, by accidents, etc. is an undoubted method. The sound cuticle is probably an efficient barrier, since bacteria habitually inhabit, without hurt, the surface and gland-ducts of the skin; yet the entrance of these saprophytes through the shell and membranes of the egg leaves a doubt as to the efficiency of the cuticular obstacle. The mucous membranes are manifestly frequently penetrated by the parasite. Hence the local affections in the mouth and throat (glossanthrax, anthrax angina) and in the lungs (pulmonary anthrax). Cohn claims that the gastric juice of Carnivora especially is destructive to the anthrax poison, yet the constant recurrence of intestinal anthrax (mycosis) seems to imply that the germs often escape destruction [p. 934]in the stomach. Pasteur supposes that anthrax-infected food is only injurious when there are inoculable sores in the mouth or pharynx, but it seems as if in that case the disease would be first shown at these points and in the nearest lymphatic glands rather than in the bowels, the rule for the inoculated anthrax being to develop first in the tissues and thence to reach the blood-vessels through the lymphatics.

The anthrax poison expends its fatal energy especially on the blood and blood-vessels. The bacilli in the blood use up the available oxygen, so that the circulating liquid becomes venous, dark, and unfitted for the maintenance of the normal functions of life. What is even worse, the ability of the blood to absorb oxygen is greatly impaired. In men and dogs suffering from anthrax the consumption of oxygen was found to be reduced in one instance even by two-thirds, probably in part by reason of the action of the chemical products of the bacillus. A third condition constantly found is embolism of the capillaries by the bacillus and the occurrence of local gangrene.

SYMPTOMS.—Anthrax shows itself in three principal forms: 1st, the apoplectiform; 2d, anthrax fever without local external lesions; and 3d, external localized anthrax. The two last forms correspond in the main to the acute and subacute forms.

The period of incubation varies according to the dose of the poison and the receptivity of the animal. In some cases infection is at once followed by illness. In these it is probably the chemical products that produce the first effect, while the disease caused by the propagation of the bacillus appears later should the animal survive. Such incubation is shortest for the smaller animals (mice, rabbits, guinea-pigs, cats), in which illness usually sets in in from twenty-four to forty-eight hours. In sheep and goats incubation may be extended to three or four days, while in horses and cattle it may last a day longer.

The apoplectiform type attacks animals which a few minutes before seemed in fine health, appetite, and spirits, striking them down as if by lightning, and the victims struggle convulsively for some minutes, expel blood perhaps by the nose or anus, and expire. In the less suddenly fatal cases there may be muscular trembling, unsteady gait, excited breathing, accelerated pulse, tumultuous heart's action, bleeding from some natural orifice, and death in from one to several hours. Occurring as these cases often do in summer, the sudden death is probably hastened by insolation.

In anthrax fever or acute internal anthrax there is loss of appetite, and, in ruminants, of rumination, suppression of milk, dulness, languor, staring coat, or even a rigor, and thirst. Then follows the hot stage, in which the temperature may rise to 106° or 107° F.; there are acceleration of pulse and breathing, petechiæ or a brown or yellowish tinge of the mucous membranes and white parts of the skin, tenderness of the spine, often jerking or clonic spasms of the muscles of the extremities, and much prostration and weakness, the patient hanging back on the halter, leaning against a wall, or swaying when made to move. The feces are usually more or less mingled with blood-clots, or may be at once liquid and bloody. Bloody urine and the discharge of blood from other natural channels are frequent. Some cases are manifestly delirious, and in others the skin crackles on being handled. Remissions are not uncommon, [p. 935]during which the animal remains dull and prostrate. As the disease advances and the blood is robbed of its oxygen, the temperature descends below the natural standard, great weakness and stupor set in, the pupils are widely dilated, and death from asphyxia occurs in one or two days from the onset.

In localized external anthrax the local swellings may be first seen. There are usually some tenderness of the skin, erection of the hair, and the formation of a little nodule, like a hazel-nut or walnut, adherent to the deeper parts of the skin, firm and comparatively painless even when cut. Sometimes the swelling is diffuse, with a dropsical or erysipelatoid aspect, and crackles like parchment when handled. Whether the affection attacks the tongue, the throat, or some part of the head, body, or limbs, the tendency is to gangrene of the part, and, if the subject survives long enough, to an extensive sloughing and unhealthy sore. The sloughs and sores have either a black sanguineous appearance or they are lardaceous and intermixed with streaks of dark red. If fever is not present at the outset, it sets in early, and passes through the same stages as in the acute internal anthrax, the animals being suddenly plunged in prostration and stupor, with dusky yellow or blood-stained mucous membranes, dyspnoea, dilated pupils, convulsions, and death. On the mucous membranes (gloss-anthrax, anthrax angina) the engorgement is usually complicated with bullæ with red or yellow contents, and which on bursting leave unsightly gangrenous ulcers. In all such cases the morbid liquids of the swellings teem with bacilli.

MORBID ANATOMY.—The most characteristic changes are usually met with in the blood. This is black, thick, tarry, uncoagulable or coagulates only in loose diffluent clots, which are redissolved before squeezing out the serum; the fibrin is diminished (often by two-thirds), the red globules are not adherent in rouleaux, and are crenated and broken down and the hæmatin diffused through the liquid, so that it stains the hands or paper deeply; the white globules are increased, probably by reason of the early irritation of the lymphatic glands and spleen by the poison; and it reddens slowly and but slightly on exposure to the air, and speedily passes into decomposition. The blood can scarcely be made to flow in a full stream, but often trickles down the hair and skin by reason of its thick, consistent character. The microphytes above described are usually found in the blood, and always in the affected tissues if examined just after death.

Next to the blood, the spleen presents the most constant lesions, being enlarged (by one-third, one-half, or to double, triple or quadruple its normal size) and gorged with blood (sometimes even to rupture). The lymphatic glands, and especially those adjoining the local anthrax swellings of the tissues, are always enlarged, marked with petechiæ, friable, easily reduced to a pulp, and swarming with bacilli and micrococci. Next to the glands of the affected parts the central ones, the axillary, prepectoral, thoracic, sublumbar, and abdominal, are the most constantly affected. The lymph is reddish and opaque.

Decomposition sets in early, and the resulting gases cause a puffy, emphysematous condition of the connective tissue. The fat and other white tissues are dusky brown or yellow, and petechiated; the muscles are soft, flabby, and dark red or brown, with occasional blood [p. 936]extravasations; the blood-vessels, especially the veins, and the right heart are gorged with black, uncoagulable blood, and have their inner coats blood-stained. The serous membranes present numerous petechiæ, and contain more or less of a reddish serum. The intestines, and sometimes the stomach, are dark red throughout, marked by petechiæ, and are often the seat of thickening from sanguineous or transparent colloid infiltration. The lesions are especially extensive on the small intestines and rectum. The vagina and womb are also the frequent seats of sanguineous infiltration. The liver and kidneys are enlarged, congested, softened, and friable, and the ganglia of the sympathetic are enlarged, congested, and softened. The swellings are of two kinds, sanguineous and colloid. The former, when cut into, present one or more loose clots of black blood or a grumous mass of blood-elements, separating the tissues and often mixed with fetid gases. The colloid exudations are glairy, semi-solid, jelly-like masses, infiltrating the tissues. The tissues affected and the skin covering them are the seat of bacterial embolism and gangrene, and there is no tendency to suppuration. These products swarm with the specific microphytæ.

DIAGNOSIS.—The differential diagnosis of anthrax from other affections due to the propagation of microzymes in the system is not always easy—so much so that a variety of bacteridian and allied diseases (septicæmia in its various forms, erysipelas, swine plague, chicken cholera, poisoning by the micrococci of fungi, black quarter from bacteria, milk sickness, and Texas fever) have been erroneously confounded with this affection. These all show the same dusky or cyanosed mucous membranes, disintegrating blood-globules, loose blood-clots, petechiæ, blood-extravasations, sudden and great prostration, and enlargement and congestion of the lymphatic glands or spleen. In some of these the duration of incubation (in swine plague six to fourteen days and in Texas fever one month) serves to distinguish, while in the majority the microzyme is globular (Texas fever, micrococcus of fungi-poisoning, chicken cholera); in swine plague the cocci are arranged in pairs; in black quarter the microbe is a refrangent ovoid, single or in chains of two or three and a motile linear body with a refrangent nucleus in one end; and in milk sickness the germ is a spirillum. The germs are far more likely to be detected in the local lesions and lymphatic glands than in the blood. The specific nature of the symptoms and lesions can usually be relied on, but in cases of doubt the inoculation of a small animal (rabbit, guinea-pig, sheep) will be a material guide.

PROGNOSIS.—True anthrax leads to a very high mortality. The apoplectiform cases are fatal almost without exception; the acute cases of anthrax fever in many outbreaks perish to the extent of 75 or 80 per cent., and the more tardy ones to the number of 50 per cent. In a general outbreak the earlier cases are usually the most fatal, while later, when the less susceptible animals are attacked, the mortality is often decreased. Again, the mortality is often at once arrested by the emigration of the herd to a more healthy soil, a large proportion of those already attacked recovering.

PROPHYLAXIS.—In prophylaxis the soil demands the first attention. If this is damp and calcareous or rich in organic matter, the remainder of the herd should be at once removed to a drier and more porous soil, where the germ is less likely to be preserved and increased. In an [p. 937]enzoötic in Livingston County, N.Y., in 1875, 40 bullocks out of 200 had perished in ten days, yet after removal to an adjacent dry pasture and the use of antiseptics with the food and water the attacks abruptly ceased and 48 out of 50 head already sick recovered. The drainage of anthrax soils leads to a steady reduction of the poison, favoring as it does the germination of the spores and the destruction or modification of the germ. When drainage is impossible, the mortality may be reduced by driving the stock to drier grounds during the hot, dry season, by stabling them morning and night when the dews are on the grass, also in wet times, when they are likely to pull up the plants by the roots, or, better still, by cutting the fodder and soiling the stock in stables or yards. Yet in all these cases the germs will at intervals find access to the animals in the green food or hay, so that badly infected soils must be secluded from live-stock, and either be abandoned or devoted to other cultures. A point of the very first importance is the safe disposal of the products and carcases of the sick. These should be thoroughly burned, or, failing this, deeply buried (4 feet) and the graves covered with coal tar and fenced in from all other stock for from five to ten years. Contaminated litter and fodder should share the same fate. Stables and yards where the sick have been, and all vehicles and implements used for them or their products, should be thoroughly disinfected. In the epizoötic in Livingston County, above referred to, these measures seem to have eradicated the disease in the course of six years, though the land was neither drained nor subjected to cultivation, and the dangerous meadows are now again pastured with impunity.

In the case of sick animals the greatest care is requisite to keep them from common drinking- or feeding-troughs; to exclude all other animals, even the smaller quadrupeds and birds, which may become the bearers of the poison; to avoid the chance of the drainage of infected excreta into other yards and pastures, and to carefully disinfect and guard the human attendants against contamination. The sale of animals out of an infected herd, and, above all, for the meat-market, and the use of the milk or other products of such animals, until attested sound, are highly reprehensible.

Finally, there are the different methods of protecting the system by inoculation with modified virus. The first of these is that of Burdon-Sanderson, Dugnid, and Greenfield, who in 1878 and 1879 inoculated six cattle with the blood of guinea-pigs dead of anthrax, all of which survived except an old, emaciated, worn-out, and pregnant cow, and all the survivors would only afterward contract anthrax in a mild form. The anthrax blood of the guinea-pig inoculated on the sheep proved fatal. The second mode is that of Pasteur, who cultivated the anthrax-germ artificially in flasks of meat-infusion, and after the nourishment in the latter had been used up left the bacilli to degenerate until their virulence had been so far decreased that the liquid could be safely inoculated on animals, so as to produce a mild anthrax infection and thereafter secure immunity from this poison. For all the larger domestic animals he found that the eighth day of the culture sufficed, provided there had been no formation of spores; and the method has now been applied on many scores of thousands of domestic animals. Klein, however, has found that cultures in pork-broth of the same age are invariably fatal to rodents, [p. 938]and that a guinea-pig which survived inoculation with culture a month old did not possess immunity against fresh virus. The third method, that of Toussaint, consists in heating the fresh virus, so as to lessen its activity, and then inoculating it on the animals to be protected. He found that a temperature of 55° C. (131° F.) maintained for one hour rendered the virus non-fatal, without impairing its prophylactic powers on animals inoculated. In spite of a partial failure at Alfort from insufficient heating of the virus, the method has now been firmly established as at once easy and effective.

The great value of these discoveries can hardly be overestimated, yet it is to be feared that the éclat of their reception has led to a far too general adoption of the methods. No one of the methods professes to destroy the life of the bacillus nor to impair its power of self-propagation. The bacillus, therefore, is likely to be planted in the localities where it is being employed, and, if the soil is favorable, to be perpetuated there. It follows also, from the susceptibility of the bacillus to change under varying conditions of life, that the modification impressed on it by the methods of Pasteur and Toussaint may be reversed under a reverse state of the environment, and that the harmless virus sown by our inoculators may in favorable soils produce the more deadly types. The methods secure the safety of the individual herd inoculated, at the expense of planting in the pasture a seed most perilous to all future uninoculated herds that may roam there. The only place for such protective inoculations is on pastures already charged with the anthrax bacillus, and from which that cannot be eradicated. On the dry, healthful soils where the bacillus cannot survive the inoculation is useless, while on the dense, damp, rich soils favorable to its preservation, but as yet uninfected or nearly so, this inoculation is but sowing deadly seed to secure a very temporary and questionable advantage.

TREATMENT.—Bloodletting and laxatives have been largely used in the treatment of anthrax, though both are mostly useless in acute cases, their possible good effects being anticipated by the early death. When of service at all, it is probably mainly in reducing that plethora which serves often to enhance the virulence and severity of the malady. Apart from these, the agents resorted to are more or less of an antiseptic nature, and probably exert their action mainly on the bacilli undergoing development near the surface of the skin or intestinal mucous membrane. In extensive outbreaks I have had the best results with the administration thrice daily of carbolic acid, nitro-muriatic acid, or bichromate of potassium, and hypodermically of iodide of potassium and sulphate of quinia. Alcoholic stimulants, chlorate of potassium, and muriate of iron are equally indicated, especially when the period of prostration has set in. If the local anthrax can be detected when there is as yet but a hard nodule, there should be no hesitation in cauterizing it to its depth and treating the resulting sore and surrounding parts with tincture of iodine or iodized phenol. After crucial incision the nodule may be treated with powerful caustics (potassa, nitric acid, chloride of zinc), to be followed by iodized phenol, with or without poultices or fomentations.

[p. 939]

Anthrax in Man (Malignant Pustule or Vesicle, Anthrax Intestinalis, Mycosis Intestinalis).

Fournier in 1769 first traced the communicated anthrax of man to the consumption of the flesh of diseased animals and the handling of their wool. Until quite recently, however, the form which originated as a local external affection was the only type recognized, while internal anthrax was confounded with a multitude of other affections.

ETIOLOGY.—That anthrax in man is almost invariably derived from the lower animals by infection is now undoubted, while for the direct infection of man, as of animals, by the germs propagated in the soil, there is no absolute proof. The latter mode of propagation has only been recognized in the Herbivora, which are so much more exposed to contamination from the soil; yet, abstractly, there is no reason to suppose that man is less susceptible to the earth-grown bacillus than to that produced in the animal, if only he were as frequently exposed to its infection. The spontaneous development of anthrax apart from the pre-existent bacillus in animals or soil is a chimera. The principal modes of infection may be considered as direct and mediate. Among the direct are included infection from handling the sick animals, their carcases, their wool, hair, bristles, hides, fat, and guts; the inoculation of physicians, surgeons, and nurses from their patients; and the infection of men by the meat, milk, and cheese eaten. As attested modes of mediate infection may be cited the inoculation by insects (mosquitoes, bluebottles, and other bloodsuckers), and the introduction by water into which anthrax products have drained or been washed; there are also hypothetical cases in which anthrax-germs from the earth have entered the system in the air, drink, or food (raw vegetables). The direct inoculations are especially common in certain classes (shepherds, farmers, butchers, knackers, tanners, veterinarians, and workers in hides, hoofs, glue-factories, fat-rendering works, in hair, wool, bristles, and catgut, and in felting and paper-making). In such cases the disease usually begins as a local one, and occurs on uncovered portions of the body. Three such cases occurred in 1875 on one farm at Avon, N.Y., where the victims had assisted in burying forty dead cattle, and a number of other similar instances can be adduced in different parts of the same State, in one of which a physician was accidentally inoculated in dressing a farmer's hand. Physicians whose practice includes large tanneries become very familiar with the disease and recognize it very readily.

Infection through food is much less frequent in men than in animals, the process of cooking combining with the action of the gastric juice in destroying the poison. Yet it is by no means unknown. The records above given of infection in St. Domingo, Naples, and the Russian steppes can be easily supplemented. Dr. Keith of Aberdeen, Scotland, records the case of a family that suffered, two of them fatally, after partaking of broth and meat which had been boiled for hours, one member of the family (a vegetarian) having alone escaped. Infection through milk, butter, and cheese is less common, the gravity of the disease in animals leading to an early suppression of the mammary secretion. In all such cases the infection enters through sores in the mouth or from the bowels.

Those cases in which the bacillus enters the system with the inspired [p. 940]air are probably the least numerous. Yet the germ may reach the lungs in fine dust, and then find in the delicate respiratory mucous membrane the most accessible of all channels into the system.

The proportion of men affected is much greater than that of women and children, doubtless by reason of their greater exposure to infection, and, as in the lower animals, the summer months are most productive of anthrax. The susceptibility of the human race appears to be less than that of the Herbivora, and doubtless varies, as in these animals, with the nature of the food. It is at least temporarily exhausted by a first attack, though in exceptional cases and under a strong dose of the poison a man may be affected a second time.

SYMPTOMS.—Symptoms usually set in within twenty-four hours after inoculation of the poison, though it is alleged that the incubation may be extended to twelve or fourteen days. Itching draws attention to a small red spot like a mosquito bite, but with a black central point. This speedily increases to a small rounded swelling (papule), and in fifteen hours is surmounted by a minute vesicle with dark-red or bluish contents. From the size of a millet-seed this increases to that of a pea, and in thirty hours bursts spontaneously or under friction and forms a dark-red, indurated, comparatively painless nodule (parent nucleus, Virchow). The adjacent skin shows a swollen areola livid and red, on which there appear vesicles similar to the first, which pass through the same stages, burst, and leave a livid, hard, or doughy gangrenous surface. By this time the surrounding skin is red, shining, and puffy, and the disease continues to spread by the same method of extension. The diseased part now becomes the centre of an oedematous swelling which may invade the entire arm, face, or neck, and is attended with more or less constitutional symptoms. The affected part may be cold or hot, and it may show the red lines of lymphangitis and the swelling of the adjacent lymphatic glands.

The pyrexia, at first slight, often reaches a high grade, attended with occasional chilliness, pains in the back and loins, great prostration, languor, dulness, and even delirium, with cold sweats, anxiety, dyspnoea, and at times muscular spasms. As in beasts, there are the dusky skin and mucous membranes, petechiæ, and cyanosis, and in bad cases there may be sudden collapse and death. The symptoms vary much, however, according to the extent of the local lesion, to the amount of poisonous chemical products thrown into the blood, to the degree of the invasion of the blood by the bacillus, and to the complication (not infrequent) of the affection with septicæmia. In the very mildest cases the affection never proceeds beyond a local slough, the size of a quarter or half dollar, the germs do not enter the blood in sufficient numbers to survive, the constitutional symptoms are few or absent, and the sore heals by granulation.

The disease usually lasts from six to ten days, and for the first forty-eight hours the symptoms are generally purely local.

Malignant anthrax oedema (oedeme maligne) was first observed by Bourgeois as occurring in the eyelid, and has since been recognized in other parts of the body (arm, forearm, head). It differs mainly from malignant pustule in the absence of the preliminary vesicle, of the hard nodule (parent nucleus), and of the early circumscribed gangrene. It has this further peculiarity, that the local disease often appears as a [p. 941]sequel rather than a precursor of the constitutional disturbance. It corresponds in the main to the diffuse erysipelatoid anthrax of the lower animals, and has been attributed to the anthrax poison introduced by inhalation. It has been observed to follow eating of anthrax flesh (Leube, Müller). Inasmuch as the active disease is often delayed a week or ten days after exposure to infection, it may reasonably be supposed that the bacillus has been imprisoned on the mucous membrane, or, entering the blood in small quantity only, has been held in check by the antagonism of the blood-globules until some elements, escaping into the connective tissue, have started the local disease. The symptoms are usually first languor, sleeplessness, restlessness, with some sense of chill, debility, and headache, and finally, after a few days, the formation of the specific oedema at one point or more. This has a pale, semi-translucent, slightly yellowish or greenish aspect, pits on pressure nearly equally at all points, and tends to a rapid extension, with concomitant aggravation of the constitutional symptoms, and in many cases nausea and vomiting. Gangrene sets in—not progressively, as in malignant pustule, but simultaneously over a more extensive surface—and is followed by great prostration, stupor, dyspnoea, cyanosis, collapse, and death.

Anthrax intestinalis may be looked upon as the counterpart of the internal anthrax or anthrax fever of animals, described above. As in animals, the constitutional symptoms may result early in a fatal issue, with scarcely any local lesion save in the blood and spleen (Carganico, Leube, Müller, Winkler, Lorinser). As in animals too, the sanguineous engorgement of the spleen and the intestinal anthrax are often complicated by external anthrax oedema or malignant pustule (Heussinger, Virchow, Buhl, Waldeyer, etc.). In this form pyrexia and other constitutional disturbances are first seen. There is a general feeling of languor and depression, with some chilliness, fever, pains in the limbs, back, and head, vertigo, and ringing in the ears. Even at this early stage there is noticed a dusky hue of the skin and visible mucous membranes, which goes on increasing to a brown or yellow tinge, to petechiæ, or, with the supervention of dyspnoea, to cyanosis. Digestive derangement is early shown in abdominal pain, nausea, vomiting, tenderness, some swelling, and finally diarrhoea, often bloody and sometimes profuse and exhausting. In acute cases the symptoms become rapidly worse, and then follow discharge from the mouth and nose of uncoagulable blood, dyspnoea, cyanosis, small pulse, dilated pupils, great anxiety or drowsiness, and stupor, or there may be tonic spasms of the trunk or extremities. Death usually results from asphyxia or collapse, as in animals. These cases are almost invariably fatal within a period of thirty-six hours, though some linger six or seven days.

Allied to the intestinal anthrax is anthrax angina, a not unknown occurrence in man. This begins as a bad sore throat, with an especially dark-red hue of the pharyngeal mucous membrane. As it advances the shade becomes increasingly darker, the power of deglutition is lost, serous phlyctenæ with gangrene and deep ulceration set in, but without any tendency to the formation of false membrane as in diphtheria. There are early superadded the constitutional symptoms above described, and the patient dies in a state of collapse or asphyxia.

MORBID ANATOMY.—The lesions closely agree with those already[p. 942]described for animals in general. The blood presents the same dark-red or black, tarry, incoagulable, or only slightly coagulable condition in the worst cases, yet this is less constant in man, as the bacteria are less constant or numerous in the blood, in keeping with the more prolonged localization of the external anthrax in man, and the more pronounced antagonism between the blood and the bacillus which results from feeding exclusively or largely on flesh. The red globules do not tend to adhere together, and the white globules are in excess and very granular. The spleen is less extensively enlarged than in animals, but is highly charged with blood, bacilli, and micrococci. The lymphatic glands too are enlarged, hyperæmic, cloudy, hemorrhagic at points, of a dark grayish, deep red, or blackish color, and highly charged with the bacillus. The surface of the skin and mucous membranes (mouth) presents hemorrhagic spots and patches, with serous vesicles and eschars. The malignant pustule when cut into presents a central slough and a surrounding hard indurated mass, both of a dark blood-red, with similar prolongations downward into the adipose tissue, and around all the characteristic oedematous infiltration, often streaked with blood. The bacillus is found in tufts or dense groups at intervals in the rete mucosum, the dermis, and the subcutaneous connective tissue. The serous membranes present the same general lesions as in animals. The walls of the stomach and bowels are the seat of cloudy red infiltration, with at intervals small hemorrhagic foci, and on the mucous surface distinct sloughs. Jelly-like exudations are also found in these membranes in the mesentery and in the retro-peritoneal tissue. The liver and kidneys are usually congested or are infiltrated with an oedematous exudate, and in these, as in all the local anthrax lesions, the characteristic bacilli are found.

DIAGNOSIS.—Malignant pustule is distinguished by its commencing from a minute red point with dark centre, and by its progressive extension from this point by a dark-red, puffy, and vesicular areola, with steadily advancing induration and gangrene. The bites of insects have a yellowish central point with red areola. A boil lacks the dark centre and the rapidly rising elevated red areola. Carbuncles and plague-boils tend to appear on clothed parts of the body, respectively on the back of the neck and shoulders and on the trunk and extremities. In carbuncle several boils rise and burst simultaneously, though they may finally slough into one sore, while in anthrax the extension is from one point. The plague-boil is usually multiple and much more painful than anthrax. The glanderous nodule is usually multiple, situated at intervals on the course of a lymphatic, the intervening portion of which is inflamed, hard, and cord-like. It is also usually associated with the specific glairy discharge from the nose, the nasal ulcers and nodules, and the enlarged painless, nodular, and indolent submaxillary lymphatic glands. As a last resort the detection of the bacillus in the indurated nucleus and the inoculability of the disease on the lower animals (rabbit, guinea-pig), may be appealed to.

Malignant anthrax oedema is less easily recognized, but may be inferred from the sudden swelling with a dusky yellow or greenish hue and a tendency to vesiculation and gangrene, the whole preceded and attended by the constitutional symptoms of anthrax, and, above all, from the presence of the bacillus in the exudate.

[p. 943]In both of these forms much may be deduced from the known liability of the district to anthrax, from the occupation of the subject as being exposed to infection (worker in hair, wool, bristles, hides, catgut, etc.), or from his having eaten meat which was open to suspicion.

Internal anthrax is less certainly diagnosed because of the absence of local symptoms until the constitutional disorder is well advanced. Yet the reasonable suspicion of infection and the sudden and violent eruption of the disease (headache, nausea, vomiting, bloody diarrhoea, extreme anxiety, debility, dyspnoea, cyanosis, convulsions, collapse, with petechiæ, and local discharges of diffluent blood) serve to identify it. The bacillus is not always to be detected in the blood under the microscope, but its presence can usually be demonstrated by inoculation.

PROGNOSIS.—The prognosis of malignant pustule energetically treated in its early stages is good. The disease is as yet a local one, and the germs can be extinguished by local treatment. In anthrax districts, where the disease is feared and early recognized, the mortality may be from 5 per cent. (Nicolai) to 9 per cent. (Lengyel, Koranyi). Even this mortality is mainly due to delay in treatment. In districts, on the other hand, where the malady is infrequent, and where efficient measures are applied too late, the mortality is often 30, 40, or even 50 per cent. After internal infection, and where local symptoms only appear after general infection, the case is very hopeless.

PROPHYLAXIS AND TREATMENT.—The prophylaxis of anthrax in man is to a large extent identical with that for animals. All considerations as regards soil, culture, drainage, sick and dead stock, cremation, burial, disinfection, etc. have a most important if only a secondary bearing on the protection of man. Still more important is the free use of carbolic acid, chloride of lime, or tincture of iodine for the hands of those dressing unhealthy sores in animals or handling suspicious cases of sickness or cadavers, and of those working in hides, wool, hair, horns, hoofs, guts, etc. Similarly, all products of animals with anthrax should be withheld from general use.

In external anthrax of man, before the system has been contaminated, the thorough destruction by caustic of the diseased part with its contained poison is most effectual. Where there is as yet but the preliminary papule it may be incised and thoroughly destroyed by a stick of chloride of zinc, caustic potassa, or nitrate of silver, or, if more convenient, by fuming nitric acid, muriatic or sulphuric acid, or, perhaps preferably to all others, iodized phenol. Should the parent nucleus have already formed, it should be excised with the knife or deeply incised in a crucial direction, and then thoroughly cauterized with one of the more potent escharotics (caustic potassa, strong nitric acid) or with the iodized phenol. The latter agent may be further applied on the sound skin adjacent, especially if there is the slightest swelling or redness. Should the peripheral oedema persist or reappear after the cauterization, the latter should be repeated until this tendency is overcome. Hypodermic injections of a solution of iodine and iodide of potassium may be made into the entire swelling. After the caustic has done its work the eschar may be softened and its separation favored by a warm poultice containing a small amount of carbolic acid or iodized phenol. This treatment is often highly beneficial, even after constitutional symptoms have set in, by arresting the [p. 944]propagation of the bacillus and checking its introduction and that of its chemical products into the circulation.

Constitutional treatment is not to be forgotten. Carbolic acid may be profitably given to the extent of fifteen drops daily, iodide of potassium ten to twenty grains thrice a day, and sulphate of quinia ten grains at the same intervals. The strength should be sustained by iron (tincture of the chloride) and wine or other alcoholic beverage, both being, like the agents already named, calculated to retard if not to limit the propagation of the bacillus. The diet throughout should be nutritious and easily digested.

When a person is known to have eaten anthrax meat an emetic will be indicated, followed by a smart oleaginous purgative combined with five drops of carbolic acid, and subsequently by the constitutional treatment above recommended. In case of extensive anthrax oedema, incisions may be made into the part as far as the yellow exudate extends, and a poultice containing carbolic acid may be applied. Or, preferably, the swelling may be freely injected with a weak solution of iodized phenol (1:100 water), and then painted with the same agent or with tincture of iodine.

[p. 945]

PYÆMIA AND SEPTICÆMIA.
BY B. A. WATSON, M.D.

HISTORY.—There is little to be learned from existing literature of the views which were maintained by the ancients, prior to the birth of Christ, in regard to the morbid conditions now designated pyæmia and septicæmia; although it is certain they were recognized by the "Father of Medicine," who reports a well-marked case of puerperal fever terminating fatally on the twentieth day of the disease, and also a case in which death was unquestionably caused by septic poisoning, as is clearly shown in the following:[1] "Criton, in Thasno, while still on foot and going about, was seized with a violent pain in the great toe; he took to his bed the same day, had rigors and nausea, recovered his heat slightly; at night was delirious. On the second, swelling of the whole foot, and about the ankle, erythema with distension and small bullæ (phlyctænæ); acute fever; he became furiously deranged; alvine discharges, bilious, unmixed, and rather frequent. He died on the second day from commencement." Additional confirmation of the fact that Hippocrates was familiar with the phenomena of these diseases may be found in his dissertation on empyema and fevers. Prof. C. Heuter says, under the head of septic fever,[2] "Hippocrates and Celsus observed the fever in cases of injuries which proved so dangerous that this danger could not have originated from the inflammation or from the wound alone." Jacotius, a commentator of Hippocrates, has even mentioned putrid fevers, the same as Adrianus Spigelius, who spoke of fevers which arise from putrefaction; but both authors, as well as their followers, did not discriminate between septicæmia arising from the putrescence of wounds and pyæmia. In the mean time both varieties were regarded as intermittent fever.

[1] *Works of Hippocrates*, trans. by Adams, vol. i. p. 377.

[2] Pitha und Billroth, *Handbuch der Chirurgie*, 1 Band, 2 Abth., 1 Heft, 1 Liefg., S. 6.

"Aretæus lived during the middle of the second century of the Christian era. In his remarks on pneumonia he observes that the subjects of this disease die mostly on the seventh day. 'In certain cases,' he says, 'much pus is formed in the lungs, or there is a metastasis from the side if a greater symptom of convalescence be at hand. But if, indeed, the matter be translated from the side to the intestine or bladder, the patients immediately recover from the peripneumony.' He speaks of a metastasis to the kidneys and bladder being peculiarly favorable in empyema. He ascribes suppuration of the liver to intemperance and protracted disease,[p. 946]especially dysentery and colliquative wasting. The symptoms described by him resemble those of chronic pyæmia."[3]

[3] Braidwood on *Pyæmia*, p. 2.

Galen and some of the other ancient physicians recognized the existence of septic poisoning, as is shown by the opinions expressed on the subject of putrid fevers. According to Galen, putrid fevers may either arise from the conversion of ephemerals, or originally from putrefaction of the fluids within the vessels.

Aetius states that they arise from constriction of the skin or viscidity of the humors, whereby the perspiration is stopped, and the quantity of vital heat so altered as to give rise to putrefaction, first of the fluids, and afterward of the fat and solid parts. When these corrupted fluids are contained within the vessels they occasion synochous fevers, but when distributed over the body they give rise to intermittents. Synesius and Constantinus Africanus give a similar account. Alexander gives an interesting and ingenious disquisition on the origin and nature of putrid fevers, one of the most common causes of which he holds to be the conversion of ephemeral fevers, and the inseparable symptoms being want of concoction in the urine and quickness of the pulse with systoles. This is the account of them given by most of the other authorities, both Greek and Arabian, so that we need not enter into any circumstantial exposition of their views. We shall merely give the brief account of those furnished by Palladius. There are, he says, two kinds of synochous fevers, the one being occasioned by effervescence, and the other by putrefaction of the blood; of these the latter are the more protracted and dangerous. In them the pulse is contracted, the heat pungent, and the urine white and putrid.[4]

[4] Paulus Ægineta, trans. by Adams, vol. i. p. 236 (Sydenham Soc., 1844).

A new era in the literature of this subject dawned during the sixteenth century. Ambrose Paré and Bartholomew Maggi each published a work in which they pointed out the old errors and announced new truths. Paré's *Treatise on Gunshot Wounds* was published in Paris in 1551, while Maggi's treatise appeared a year later at Bologna. Paré gained his first experience in the treatment of gunshot wounds in 1536, which is described as follows: "The storming of the small mountain-fortress Villane, near Susa, probably gave him for the first time full occupation, and he followed in all things the example of older colleagues. Like them, although hesitatingly, he poured into the gunshot wounds boiling oil of elder to destroy the poison, but the oil fell short, and then he was compelled to dress the other wounded men with an ointment of oil of roses and turpentine. Fearing that the latter would soon become victims of the wound-poison, he passed a sleepless night, got up early to see the ill consequences, but was greatly surprised to find those that he had half given up free from pain and without inflammation or swelling, while those who had been treated with boiling oil lay in a state of fever, with great pain and much swelling. He therefore determined, as he tells us, never again to burn the poor subjects of gunshot wounds so cruelly."[5] It will be seen that Paré's treatise on gunshot wounds was published fifteen years after this impressive experience at the fortress of Villane. In this work he sought to correct the prevailing idea that [p. 947]gunshot wounds were poisonous, and was ably supported in his effort by Bartholomew Maggi; but it required all the respect which Paré enjoyed in riper years to gradually obtain consideration for the new view. The idea that gunshot wounds were poisonous is supposed to have originated in the fact that in every war there are cases of acute sepsis, developed after the infliction of these injuries, which agree in all their essential points with the results of the bites of poisonous snakes. We are even informed that during the late Franco-Prussian War there were cases which even excited suspicion among the laymen that the enemy had used poisoned missiles.

[5] *German Clinical Lectures*, 2d series (New Sydenham Soc., 1877), p. 65 *et seq.*

The nature of the error which Paré and Maggi endeavored to correct is shown by the declaration made by Johannes de Vigo at the commencement of the sixteenth century, who expressed in dogmatic form the views then firmly held by physicians. "A gunshot wound is a contused wound, he says, for the bullet is round; it is burnt, for the bullet is heated; it is poisoned, for the powder is poisonous. The poisoning is the essential condition; therefore the treatment must be directed above all to counteract this."

The next step was that a poisonous substance may develop itself or settle in the wound, and especially in gunshot wounds—a substance which has nothing to do with powder or lead. Paré himself adopted this view. When he took part in the siege of Rouen many wounds sloughed and had a cadaverous smell, and on opening the bodies of those who died numerous collections of pus were found in different parts full of greenish ill-smelling ichor. Besiegers and besieged believed themselves to be wounded with poisoned bullets. Paré looked for the cause in a deterioration of the air by the large quantity of decomposing substances, and he appears to have assumed, as is done at this day, a direct action of the so-called deteriorated air upon the wound itself.

The evil influence of air vitiated by the products of decomposition, not upon wounds only, but upon the organism generally, has never been lost sight of by physicians since that time. That rotten straw, decomposing bodies of men and animals, surfaces saturated with excrement, and overcrowding of badly-ventilated hospitals give rise to infectious fevers and unhealthy state of wounds is not a result of modern observation only. That it was a question of the processes of fermentation which became communicated to the body by means of the exciters of fermentation contained in the air was a view frequently adopted. "To quote one only out of many; John Pringle, in his *Observations on the Diseases of the Army*, published in 1775, devotes a chapter especially to 'Diseases resulting from Bad Air,' and his forty-eight experiments on septic and antiseptic substances contain numerous hints at attempts resembling those made at the present day to determine the antiseptic power of certain things. No advance was made, however, beyond vague surmises concerning the nature of the exciters of putrefaction, and they were for the most part looked for amongst the volatile, ill-smelling products of decomposition, and were believed to be extremely subtle gaseous matters."[6]

[6] *German Clinical Lectures*, Second Series (New Sydenham Soc., 1877), p. 67 *et seq.*

Ambrose Paré (1582) first taught that secondary abscesses in surgical cases, "which he had observed in the spleen, lungs, liver, and other viscera, were due to a changed condition of the fluids produced by some[p. 948]unknown alteration in the atmosphere and determining a purulent diathesis."[7] The following quotations force the conclusion that in the early history of medicine there was supposed to be some important relation between wounds of the head and multiple abscesses. "Nicholas Massa (1553) mentions a case of abscess of the left lung, following an injury of the head."[8] "Valsalva (1707) was induced by his own observation to say that the viscera of the thorax were sometimes affected in wounds of the head." "Desault (1794) considered abscesses of the liver to be a very frequent sequence of head injuries."[9] The fact that wounds of the head were frequently followed by abscesses of the lungs, liver, and other organs probably led to the opinion expressed by Desault, Barthez, Brodie, W. Phillips, Copeland, and others, that the disease had its origin in a nervous agency.[10] "Bertrandi and Audouille (1819) sought for a mechanical explanation of the occurrence of hepatic abscesses after head injuries and in cases of apoplexy." Morgagni (1740) somewhat obscurely hinted at the doctrine of the reabsorption of pus—a doctrine which was afterward elaborated by Quesnay in 1819. Morgagni, after quoting a great number of instances of wounds of the head followed by visceral abscesses, opposes the idea of a mechanical transportation of pus thither, and states that abscesses are not confined to the liver and that they may follow wounds and ulcers of other parts besides the head. He ascribes their formation to particles of pus (not always deposited in the form of pus) resulting from the softening and suppuration of small tubercles, which, having been mixed with the blood and disseminated, are arrested in some of the narrow passages, perhaps of the lymphatic glands, and by obstructing and irritating these, as happens in the production of venereal buboes, and by retaining the humors therein, distend them and give origin to the generation of a much more copious pus than what is carried thither; and by this means, he says, we may also conceive how it is that much more pus is frequently formed in the viscera and cavities of the bodies than a small wound could have produced.[11]

[7] Braidwood on *Pyæmia*, p. 2 *et seq.*
[8] *Ibid.*, p. 2.
[9] *Ibid.*, p. 3.
[10] *Ibid.*, p. 10.
[11] *Ibid.*, p. 3 *et seq.*

Cheston (1766) believed that the translation of matter from one point to another was a frequent occurrence after amputations of the larger limbs. John Hunter (1793), and after him Velpeau, demonstrated the existence of pus in the blood. Hunter believed that the pus was derived from the interior of the inflamed veins. He described three forms of inflammation of these vessels—viz. adhesive, suppurative, and ulcerative. Pyæmia he considered to be an aggravated form of phlebitis. Arnott (1829) concluded from his observations—1, That death does not result from the extension of the inflammation of the veins to the heart; 2, that the dangerous consequences of phlebitis have no direct relation to the extent of the vein which is inflamed; and, 3, that the presence of pus in the veins, though the principal, is not the sole, cause of the secondary affection. He accordingly opposes the idea of Abernethy, Carmichael, and others that the constitutional affection is owing to the extension of the inflammation to the heart. The publication of Arnott's and Dance's treatises led to the general opinion being held in England and in France that phlebitis and purulent infection were identical affections, or, at least, that the latter was invariably caused by the former.[12]

[12] *Ibid.*, p. 14.

[p. 949]Cruveilhier (1829), admitting the doctrine of the formation of secondary abscesses being due to capillary phlebitis, further laid down an axiom, since proved untenable, that the foreign body introduced into the veins, whose elimination by the emunctories is impossible, will produce visceral abscesses similar to those which occur after wounds and operations, and that these abscesses are the result of capillary phlebitis of those viscera.[13]

[13] Braidwood on *Pyæmia*, p. 14 *et seq.*

During the early part of the present century it was generally admitted by the best authorities that the symptoms and lesions in pyæmia were entirely due to the presence of pus in the blood, but whether absorbed from the wound or developed by an inflammation of the veins was at that time a disputed question.

Haller made the first experiments on animals with putrefying substances in the latter part of the eighteenth century, and was convinced that nothing destroys the animal fluids more powerfully than putrefaction. Gaspard (1822) published a complete work based upon his experimental research in regard to the action of putrefying substances on living organisms. He, having produced septic infection in animals by injecting into their blood pus or other putrefying substances, thus prepared the way for other experimenters, by whom he was quickly followed. Ernst R. Virchow repeated the experiments of Gaspard, and discriminated with greater precision between the surgical diseases—septicæmia with its sharply-defined group of symptoms, the opposite of pyæmia. Furthermore, "he showed that the changes in the veins which had been regarded as due to phlebitis were caused by the coagulation of the blood and by subsequent degenerative changes in the thrombi thus formed; that the infarctions and abscesses seen in the viscera were due to emboli which had become detached from softened thrombi; that, as the white blood-globules and pus-globules were identical in appearance, they could not be distinguished; and that it was improbable that pus-globules made their way into the blood."[14]

[14] *The International Encyclopædia of Surgery*, ed. by Ashhurst, vol. i. p. 204.

Panum (1855) conducted a series of important experiments, and endeavored to separate the infectious substance and determine its real nature. He concludes that the real poison is not identical with any of the chemical combinations or any of the single substances which have until now been isolated by chemical analysis from the products of nitrogenous decomposition, but adds that it is probably a concealed ferment belonging to the so-called extractive matters—carbonate of ammonium, leucin, tyrosin, fatty acids, acetic acid, etc. Furthermore, that the putrid poison is stable, fixed, and non-volatile; that it is neither decomposed by boiling nor by evaporation to dryness; that it is insoluble in absolute alcohol, but soluble in water; that the albuminous substances found in putrefying liquids become venomous only because they are impregnated with the septic poison; and that washing these substances in a large quantity of water renders them innocuous; and that the energy of these putrid poisons can only be compared to the venom of serpents, curare, and other vegetable alkaloids.

The prize offered by the Faculty of Medicine at Munich for the best essay on the action of putrefying substances in the animal organism was awarded to Hemmer in 1866. His essay was distinguished for its [p. 950]accurate delineation of the pertaining literature and for the number of experiments reported, while his conclusions bear a striking resemblance to those of Panum.

Bergmann in 1868 sought to determine the poisonous element contained in decomposing animal substances, and for this purpose chemically treated putrid fluids, hoping to find the agent that would excite all symptoms of septic poisoning. He obtained a body of this nature from decomposing yeast, which he called sepsin, although we have no proof that either he or any one else has ever found the same in pus or any decomposing animal matters; and even if it had been found in these, it would then become necessary to demonstrate the fact that no other substance contained in the putrefying liquids could produce septic poisoning. Many other experiments, similar to those which have just been mentioned, were made in the mean while by Magendie, Stich, Billroth and Hufschmidt, O. Weber, Duprey, Learet, Urfrey, Saltzman, Fischer, Frese, Muller, and others. Bergmann had extracted the sepsin from yeast, but Schmidt and Petersen (1869) were able to obtain it from putrefied blood. In 1869, Zuelzer and Sonnenschein claimed, on the contrary, to have separated a new, unnamed septic alkaloid, which was not the sepsin, and the action of which resembled that of atropine and hyoscyamine. Nevertheless, the separation of the sepsin or of the alkaloid of Zuelzer seemed to demand a talent in the manipulator which is not possessed by everybody, and rare are the chemists who possess it—so rare that these substances are not yet either officially recognized or classified. The attention of the medical profession had now become thoroughly fixed on the chemical character and the physiological action of these newly-discovered substances. It is therefore only natural that we should find during the next few months that the medical societies were much occupied with discussions on these subjects, although no important progress seems to have been made.

Political events now gave a new direction to thought, and the Franco-Prussian War filled the hospitals of both nations with wounded in which there was opened a grand field for the practical study of purulent infection in all its various forms. Humanity now demanded the best efforts of the medical profession. Neither the mechanical nor chemical theories had ever yielded practically any beneficial results; consequently, something better was demanded in this emergency. It was during this important epoch that the germ theory began to assume form and to attract some general attention in the medical profession, although Schroeder and Dusch had shown in 1854 that the filtration of the air through cotton was sufficient to prevent the putrefaction of albuminous substances which had been previously boiled. Pasteur also demonstrated the existence of germs in the air in 1863, and likewise showed their agency in the process of fermentation.

Lister began the antiseptic treatment of compound fractures in 1865, although he did not publish his report until 1867. The cotton-wadding treatment of wounds, which is based on the fact that the air passed through cotton is freed by it from all germs, was first employed by Alphonse Guérin, who refers to it in the following language: "In the latter part of 1870 I had the idea that the cause of purulent infection existed in the germs or ferments which Pasteur had discovered in the air. It was at the end of the war; all the cases of [p. 951]amputation had succumbed to the purulent infection, and not a single large wound escaped the scourge. The studies which I had made from the month of September to the end of December in 1870 had confirmed me in the opinion that purulent infection is neither due to phlebitis nor to the absorption of pus. I believed more firmly than ever that the miasms emanating from the pus of the wounds were the real cause of this frightful malady to which I had been compelled to see the wounded succumb, whether they were treated with charpie or cerate, whether with the lotions of alcohol or of carbolic acid applied several times a day, and which was soaked up by the linen which remained in contact with the wounds. But this miasmatic theory remained, nevertheless, useless, since from 1847, when I professed it, the cases of amputation in my service succumbed to purulent infection in about the same proportion as those who were cared for by my partisan colleagues did from the absorption of pus or the inflammation of the veins. In my despair, seeking constantly a means to prevent this terrible complication of wounds, I had thought of the miasm of which I had admitted the existence, because I was not otherwise able to explain the production of the purulent infection, and which was not only known to me by its deleterious influence, but which appeared to consist of living corpuscles of the nature of those that Pasteur had seen in the air; and then the history of the miasmatic poison possessed for me a new clearness. So, said I then, the miasms are the ferments. I am able to protect the wounded against their fatal influence by filtering the air, as Pasteur had done, while maintaining, in opposition to Pouchet of Rouen, that there is no spontaneous generation. I thought then of the cotton-wadding treatment, and had the satisfaction of seeing my anticipation realized. It was from this time that dates in reality the theory of germs or of ferments as a cause of purulent infection."[15]

[15] *Nouveau Dictionnaire de Médicine et de Chirurgie pratiques*, t. xxx. p. 265.

A series of important experiments were made in 1872 by Coze and Feltz, which consisted in injecting into the jugular vein and the subcutaneous cellular tissue putrid liquids;

and they record, among other interesting results observed by them, that the blood of the animal thus destroyed always contained infusoria. These experiments have been repeated and their results confirmed by several observers, and in particular by Davine in 1872.

Another series of experiments were made by Behier and Lionville, which absolutely confirmed those of Coze and Feltz; they likewise found in the blood rounded and rod-shaped corpuscles possessed of movements more or less energetic. Vulpian also confirmed the results obtained by Davine and Behier. He says: "It will not do to deny to the immovable or movable vibriones and corpuscles found by Coze, Behier, and Davine a very important rôle, because they are not the essential contagion of the poisonous blood; it is at least necessary that they should be there in order to produce the alterations which have occurred in this fluid." Chauveau has experimented extensively, and likewise admits the action of the septic vibriones of Pasteur.

Pasteur has made known the result of his investigation in communications to the Academy of Medicine in 1877, 1878, and 1879. There exist, according to him, two principal vibriones—the pyogenic, or the [p. 952]producer of pus, and the septic, the producer of the properly so-called septicæmia. But the latter is not a unique disease, and, as we have seen from the outset, there are confounded under this name different states, light or grave, corresponding with as many forms of vibriones.

The questions of greatest practical importance in regard to this whole group of diseases seem to us to be, as expressed by Dr. Budd, where and how the specific poisons which cause them breed and multiply; and all who have closely followed the scientific investigations bearing on these points which Prof. Tyndall has conducted during the past few years, and who have repeated even a portion of his experiments, cannot fail to be powerfully impressed with the value of the views which he embodied in his work entitled *Floating Matter of the Air.*

NOMENCLATURE.—The want of a systematic classification of the various morbid conditions arising from septic infection has long embarrassed alike authors and students, and even at the present time the vague manner in which the terms pyæmia and septicæmia are used leads to much confusion. The Pathological Society of London appointed, in 1869, a committee to investigate the nature and causes of those infectious diseases known as pyæmia, septicæmia, and purulent infection. This committee, having spent ten years in the study of these affections in connection with nearly all the large hospitals of London, report the following: "Summary.—It would seem, from a careful study of all the cases here collected, that it is probable that the diseases commonly known clinically as pyæmia and septicæmia may be grouped as follows: 1. Septic intoxication.—The effects of poisoning by the chemical products of putrefaction. A non-infective disease. 2. Septic infection.—A general infective process arising from the introduction of some peculiar constituent of putrid matter into the blood-stream. It is supposed by some to be due to the multiplication of living organisms in the blood, and by others to the effect of a non-organized ferment. It terminates fatally without secondary inflammations. 3. Pyæmia (for want of a better name).—An infective process probably, similar in nature to septic infection, but differing from it by giving rise to local inflammation and suppurations, often complicated by thrombosis and embolism, probably due to the blood condition. 4. Thrombosis with softening and decomposition of the thrombus and embolism, causing local abscesses in the viscera wherever the septic emboli lodge, but without the development of any general infective process. 5. Various combinations of one or more of the foregoing conditions in the same subject. 6. Infective periostitis or acute necrosis. 7. Infective endocarditis or ulcerative endocarditis. 8. Infective myositis. 9. A group of obscure cases in which it is impossible to form any idea as to the exact nature, often called spontaneous septicæmia or pyæmia."[16]

[16] *Trans. Pathological Soc. of London*, vol. xxx. p. 38.

It will be observed that the earlier writers on medicine, although aware of the existence of septic diseases, wholly failed to discriminate between pyæmia and septicæmia until 1848, and even since that date these terms have been only partially adopted by authors, by whom frequently the meaning of the same word has been so modified as to refer to essentially different conditions. Custom having fully sanctioned the use of these terms, it is now thought that a separate consideration of their [p. 953]nomenclature may be advantageous, and consequently we shall pursue this course.

NOMENCLATURE OF PYÆMIA.—In Dunglison's *Medical Dictionary* the definition given to pyæmia is, "Pyohæmia," and the latter word is defined as follows: "Pyohæmia, Pyæmia, Pyohémie (F.), from *pyo*, and [Greek: haema], 'blood;' alteration of the blood by pus, giving occasion to the diathesis seu infectio purulentia."

The committee appointed by the Pathological Society of London in 1869 report on this subject as follows: "The most common definition of pyæmia is, no doubt, that adopted by the College of Physicians in the nomenclature of diseases. It is as follows: 'A febrile affection resulting in the formation of abscesses in the viscera and other parts.'"

Birch-Hirschfeld includes under the name pyæmia "all cases in which any general infective process is set up as a secondary consequence of a wound."[17] Virchow has proposed the name ichorrhæmia. O. Weber uses the name embolhæmia for the condition in which emboli are found in the blood. Hueter in pure cases of purulent infection without metastasis calls the disease pyohæmia simplex; in cases with metastasis, pyohæmia multiplex; and when complicated with septicæmia he designates it as septo-pyohæmia. The term hospitalism has been applied to this disease by Erichsen and Sir James Y. Simpson, and the former remarks that "the term pyæmia is used in a very wide and elastic manner, and by many is made to include various forms of blood-poisoning."[18] Billroth says: "Pyæmia is a disease which we believe to arise from the taking up of pus, or of the constituent parts of pus, into the blood." Koch employs the term pyæmia merely to denote a general affection accompanied by metastatic inflammation and suppuration.

[17] *Trans. Pathological Soc. of London*, vol. xxx. p. 22.

[18] *On Hospitalism*, p. 73.

The French definition and nomenclature of pyæmia, according to Guérin, is as follows: "Purulent infection, or pyohæmia, purulent fever, surgical typhus." The purulent infection is a poisoning of the blood, which terminates by the formation of multiple abscesses, which have been improperly known under the name of metastatic abscesses.

From 1820 to 1870 surgeons admitted that these abscesses were the result of a phlebitis having its origin in a wound exposed to the air. Therefore, this disease was variously designated under the name of phlebitis, pyohæmia, or purulent infection. Tessier called it purulent diathesis; "in 1847, I compared it to the typhus, and, as the poison is absorbed from the surface of the wound in the purulent infection, I gave it the name of surgical typhus or purulent fever."[19]

[19] *Nouveau Dict. de Méd. et de Chir. pratiques*, t. xxx. p. 222.

Having given enough on this subject to answer our purpose, we will consider the nomenclature of another septic complication.

NOMENCLATURE OF SEPTICÆMIA. The term septicæmia was first employed by Piorry, and was applied for a considerable time to all those diseases in which the blood was submitted to a septic influence. Therefore, the term was made applicable to the morbid conditions existing in anthrax, glanders, typhus and typhoid fevers, variola, and also all forms of purulent and putrid infections. Guérin now adds: "Fortunately, for several years the most competent authors seem to have wished to [p. 954]reserve the name of septicæmia for what surgeons call putrid infection, and for the morbid state that the experimenters produce by the injection of putrid material into healthy animal tissues; it is consequently the experimental septicæmia which we aim at first and foremost."[20]

[20] *Nouveau Dict. de Méd. et de Chir. pratiques*, t. xxx.

Dunglison defines septicæmia with a single word, septæmia. The same authority gives the following derivation and definition to septæmia: "From [Greek: sêptos], 'rotten,' and [Greek: haema], 'blood.' A morbid condition of the blood produced by septic or putrid matters."

Sanderson says: "What I mean by septicæmia is a constitutional disorder of limited duration, produced by the entrance into the blood-stream of a certain quantity of septic material. It must, therefore, be regarded less as a disease than as a complication, differing from pyæmia not only in the fact that it has no necessary connection with any local process, either primary or secondary, but also in the important particular that it has no development."[21]

[21] *British Medical Journal*, Dec. 22, 1877.

Both Davine and Koch designate as septicæmic all cases of general infection from wounds in which no metastatic changes occur. "Birch-Hirschfeld limits the term septicæmia much in the same way as Sanderson. He describes as septicæmia those cases in which the disease results merely from the absorption of the products of putrefaction, and regards it merely as a process of poisoning, such as might arise from the injection of any other noxious chemical substance into the blood. Pyæmia, on the other hand, he considers a truly infective process, probably due to the entrance of specific organisms into the body. He would therefore include many of the cases described by Koch as septicæmia under pyæmia."[22]

[22] *Trans. Pathological Soc. of London*, vol. xxx. p. 9.

Billroth defines septicæmia as an "acute general affection which arises from the taking up of various kinds of putrid substances into the blood, and it is believed that these putrid substances so change the quality of the blood that it can no longer fulfil its physiological functions."[23]

[23] *Lectures on Surgical Pathology and Therapeutics* (trans. from 8th ed.), vol. ii. p. 41.

Heuter defines septicæmia as a fever caused by the entrance into the circulation of the products of putrefaction from local centres of decomposition. He draws no clear distinction between an infective and a non-infective form, but the affection he describes as pyæmia simplex or pyæmia without metastasis seems to include many cases which Davine, Koch, and others would include under septicæmia.[24]

[24] *Trans. Path. Soc. of London*, vol. xxx. p. 9, 1879.

Having before us the views of some of the prominent authors who have written upon the nomenclature of pyæmia and septicæmia, we observe that the use of these terms is based either on known or imaginary morbid conditions of the body, more especially of the blood. It therefore seems that the first step toward determining the proper limit within which these terms can be employed consists in learning their accurate meaning, which is fortunately clearly shown by their derivation. The next step consists in the application of these terms to the morbid conditions which are described more or less completely by these words. It may be here added that there will be frequently required for a full and definite expression certain modifying words, and consequently we may [p. 955]properly employ such phrases as puerperal septicæmia, spontaneous pyæmia, etc.

Having carefully examined the terms employed by various authors in connection with the morbid changes which are known to occur in certain cases of septic contamination, we give our preference to the following nomenclature: Septicæmia, septo-pyæmia, pyæmia simplex, and pyæmia multiplex.

The term septo-pyæmia is applied to a morbid condition possessing certain peculiarities of both septicæmia and pyæmia, and it is supposed to arise from the absorption of both poisons; the term pyæmia simplex is applied to a pyæmic condition in which there is no metastasis; while the name pyæmia multiplex is given to that form of disease which is characterized by the existence of metastatic abscesses. It may be well to add here that this nomenclature is not intended to cover all cases of septic poisoning, but to be applied to those cases only in which the morbid changes give to the terms a certain degree of appropriateness.

Septic poisoning may be justly regarded as a single chain composed of many links. Take, for example, a case of amputation of the thigh, followed within a few hours by traumatic fever, later by septicæmia; afterward there may be developed secondary fever; formation of ichorous pus, with absorption and its concomitants; pyæmia, accompanied by embolism, thrombosis, abscess in the lungs, liver, etc. To these may also occasionally be added phlebitis and inflammation of the joints, terminating speedily in suppuration. This chain may in this case be further lengthened or varied with traumatic erysipelas or with hospital gangrene. In fact, the variations in these cases are very numerous, and all these conditions, together with many others, are due to septic blood-poisoning.

ETIOLOGY OF PYÆMIA.—Four theories have been advanced at different times to explain the etiology of pyæmia, and they have been designated as follows: the mechanical, the nervous, the chemical, and the germ theories respectively; and their action is based on the following hypotheses: 1, that pus enters the blood, circulates in it, and acts as a poison; 2, that an irritation is excited in certain visceral organs in sympathy with inflammation of the fibrous membranes of the cranium or the bones of the upper or lower extremity, and there is thus produced a metastasis to these organs of an ichorous miasm or of a fluid which is more or less acrid; 3, that a chemical poison is generated from the pus in the wound, and when it is absorbed produces pyæmic manifestations; 4, that the putrefaction of pus in wounds is caused by a microscopic organism which enters the circulation and produces pyæmia.

The first hypothesis was somewhat modified, as we have already mentioned, by John Hunter and others, who advanced the idea that pyæmia consisted essentially of a phlebitis, and that the pus found in the circulation had its origin within the veins. However, it has since been shown conclusively that pyæmia cannot be produced by the injection of healthy pus into the cellular tissue or veins. This fact having been generally admitted by the profession, it is thought unnecessary to adduce here either the experiments or the arguments which have been accepted as conclusive on this important point. It is not even necessary to bring forward the disputed question of the possibility of the entrance of pus into the blood, since laudable pus does not produce pyæmia. In fact, we have reached a point in the [p. 956]progress of medicine when the discussion of either the first or second hypothesis ceases to be interesting to medical men. Consequently, our chief interest in the study of the etiology of pyæmia centres in the third and fourth hypotheses; and we believe that it may be safely asserted that the origin of this disease has been fully demonstrated by an almost unlimited number of experiments.

The injection of pus into living animals produces local, remote, and constitutional symptoms. The character of these symptoms depends principally on the kind of pus, laudable or ichorous, the quantity injected, and the site of the injection. It will be readily perceived that in cases where the pus is thrown directly into a vein the local symptoms would be unimportant, while the danger of remote trouble—metastatic abscesses in the lungs, liver, etc.—would be very great; but should the injection be made into the connective tissue, then the relations would be reversed. Constitutional symptoms may exist in both cases, but will differ in character and degree.

In regard to the character of the pus, and its agency in the production of this disease, Billroth says: "The old view, that pyæmia is only induced when decomposed pus (ichor) is reabsorbed, is entirely erroneous. There are cases where decomposed, putrid pus enters the blood, and which present a combination of the symptoms of septicæmia and pyæmia (septo-pyæmia of Hueter)."[25] Dupuytren failed to produce metastasis by injections of pus into the veins of dogs; these results were confirmed by Boyer, who only obtained metastasis when he used ichorous pus in his experiments. The same results are recorded in the works of Günther and Sedillot, based on numerous experiments. Beck made fourteen experiments very carefully, but did not succeed in producing metastasis in a single case. The same results are recorded by a commission of the Physiological Society of Edinburgh. O. Weber has recently shown by extended experiments that carefully filtered pus will not produce metastatic abscesses in the lungs. Therefore, it may be considered as proved that fluid pus injected into the veins of an animal produces no metastatic points of inflammation.

[25] *Surgical Pathology*, p. 344.

It should not be supposed, however, that because injection of fresh (non-ichorous) pus failed to produce metastatic abscesses, it was therefore without results, as the earlier experimenters thought. Billroth and O. Weber have shown by their recent experiments that these injections are uniformly followed by fever, and, if subcutaneous, by abscess; and further, that injections of fresh pus produce even a higher temperature than do those of ichorous pus; but the pus taken from cold abscesses has apparently very slight effect. The fresh non-ichorous dried pus was found to possess in a similar degree the power to excite inflammation and suppuration; even the removal of the albumen did not change its character or power. It will be observed that these injections caused not only local inflammations, but severe constitutional symptoms, as high temperature, etc. Experiments have thus far completely failed to show the agent that excites the inflammation, although it is generally admitted that it at least exists in the molecular bodies.

Virchow and Panum have shown conclusively by their experiments on living animals that the introduction of foreign bodies into the [p. 957]veins—as powdered coal, wax balls, and quicksilver—fail in all cases to produce metastatic abscesses in the visceral organs or symptoms of pyæmia. These foreign bodies were frequently found blocking up the terminal branches of the pulmonary artery, in some cases encapsulated, frequently resembling miliary tubercles, and occasionally surrounded by evidences of slight local inflammation, but in every instance without suppuration. The same experimenters, however, observed that the introduction of ichorous pus and decomposing animal tissue into the veins was attended with the formation of metastatic abscesses and other symptoms of pyæmia. They therefore conclude that the introduction of putrid animal substances into the veins, and the further transport of the same to the branches of the pulmonary artery, produce metastatic abscesses, and that the origin of these deposits is independent of the mere stopping up of the branches of this artery.

The occlusion of the blood-vessels in this diseased condition is a subject which has given rise to much discussion. Some of the earlier writers supposed this phenomenon constituted the disease pyæmia, while others believed it to be the essential cause. Roser says: "But the thrombus is, as can be easily proved, not the cause, but only a symptom, of pyæmia. If a surgical patient—e.g. one suffering with an injury of the head—is attacked by inflammation, and occlusion of a large vein, as of the common iliac vein, for instance, then there are three different theories for the inflammation of the occluded vessel—viz. Hunter's, Rokitansky's, and Virchow's. According to the old Hunterian phlebitic theory, the coagulation of the blood should be the result of the inflammation of the vein. On account of the circumstances under which the coagulation of the blood in the vein has occurred, one might suppose that the cause must be the oozing of coagulable exudation from the inflamed wall of the vein, but pathological dissections, especially Rokitansky's, would not accord with it. Large veins were found plugged up without the existence of corresponding indications of inflammation, and perfectly clear indications were often present that occlusion had preceded the inflammation. Consequently, the occlusion of the vein was the primary condition, and this must be explained in some other way than by its inflammation. Rokitansky in his theory recognized an independent disease of the blood. Yet it does not appear, on examination of the morbid conditions, that this theory can account for them. If it is recognized as correct that a primary disease of the blood is to be admitted, yet the coagulation of the blood in a large vein has not been traced back to it. It remained wholly unexplained why a single vein, especially one so large and strong as the common iliac, should become the seat of the local coagulation. The necessity of finding a local basis for the local coagulation could not be denied. For that reason it was greeted as a highly desirable advance when Virchow pointed out that the occlusion of such large veins could be dependent on the coagulation of the blood in the concave spaces behind the valves of the veins, or through the coagulation in the small branches—e.g. the hypogastric veins, which is gradually carried forward until it reaches the common iliac, and by continual increase this vein may also be filled up. At the same time, it was demonstrated that not infrequently, much oftener than [p. 958]was formerly supposed, the coagulated masses of blood are broken up and carried farther on in the circulation, in this manner producing occlusion of the pulmonary artery or its branches."[26]

[26] *Archiv der Heilkunde*, Erst. Jahrg., Erst. Heft, S. 4.

The examination of this subject finally brings Roser to this conclusion: "Contamination of the blood is essentially the primary cause of pyæmia; thrombosis is only a result of this morbid contamination, and cannot, therefore, be regarded as the cause of pyæmia, but only as an apparent part, as one of the symptoms of the same."[27] The opinion here expressed by Roser I believe to be the one generally entertained by the profession at this time.

[27] *Ibid.*, S. 43.

In cases of pyæmia there are recognized two principal sources of contamination of the blood—viz. the wound itself, and the vitiated condition of the atmosphere surrounding the patient—contamination, in the first place, directly from the wound through the blood-vessels; and in the second, by the passage of disease-germs or of the poisonous elements into the blood along the respiratory tract. E. Wagner says: "The latest examinations in regard to the vegetable parasites have made it very probable not only that these are the active agents, but also—what has been clinically quite generally accepted—that septicæmia and pyæmia owe their origin to different plants (the first to rod bacteria, the latter to globular bacteria); and, finally, that both may combine."[28] These germs may be generated in the wound or be received into it from the surrounding atmosphere. The character of the wound and the conditions surrounding the patient thus become important subjects for the consideration of the surgeon.

[28] *Manual of General Pathology*, p. 593.

It has been observed, and is now generally admitted, that wounds complicated with a fracture of the long bones of the extremities, opening large medullary cavities and accompanied by extensive laceration of the soft parts, always increase the danger of blood-poisoning. This fact may be more thoroughly understood by a brief consideration of the condition of the parts. Frequently in open fractures large quantities of pus constantly remain in contact with the surface of the wound, while detached fragments of bone, which become speedily necrosed, move about with every motion of the injured limb, lacerating more or less the surrounding tissues, and thus exciting inflammation and suppuration. The periosteum becomes inflamed; a widespread suppurative periostitis is the result; necrosis of the bone from insufficient nutrition follows, while mechanical pressure on the pus aids in its absorption. The medulla frequently takes on suppurative inflammation, and here the surgeon fails to receive prompt warning of danger; slowly the suppuration progresses, without pain or other symptoms unless the disease has extended to the other tissues; the medullary cavity at the fractured end of the bone may be completely or partially occluded by a new osseous formation; and in such cases the absorption of pus by the comparatively large venous vessels of this cavity is greatly facilitated.

The soft parts may also be the seat of dangerous trouble. The same force that produced the wound and fracture may have also contused the soft parts, destroying in a greater or less degree their nutrition, thus giving rise to gangrenous sloughs, or in other cases to the formation of abscesses, etc. I will also call attention to the fact that the laudable pus [p. 959]in these cases is most favorably situated for a rapid change into that commonly called ichorous. The heat of the parts and the contact of the pus with the atmosphere will not fail to effect its rapid decomposition.

ETIOLOGY OF SPONTANEOUS PYÆMIA.—It is unquestionable that cases of true pyæmia have been observed in which the etiology was not traceable to a wound; and it is equally certain that this failure to discover such a source of contamination in the majority of cases is no proof that it did not exist. When it is remembered that a large portion of the alimentary canal, the respiratory and the genito-urinary tracts, are so situated that the existence of a contaminating wound might be absolutely undiscoverable, we are compelled to admit the possibility of a local centre of contamination in all these cases. But the question may be asked here with propriety, "Is fatal pyæmia, independent of a wound, ever produced by breathing vitiated air?" The answers to this question must generally be a negative, although it is certainly true that poisoning of the blood does take place to a certain degree, as is abundantly shown by the different symptoms arising in patients thus exposed who are not suffering with wounds. It is said that dogs exposed in this way are found to rapidly emaciate and suffer from severe and constant diarrhoea. The various symptoms arising in patients confined in overcrowded and pus-infected wards, among which may be mentioned loss of appetite, with diarrhoea and emaciation, are too well known to require an enumeration here. Therefore it appears highly probable that living in and breathing a vitiated atmosphere may act as a strongly predisposing cause, only requiring a slight scratch or abrasion of the skin, in which the infection may be said to act as an exciting cause of pyæmia.

In reference to such complications the following questions are asked by Roser: "Is it a specific deleterious material, a miasmatic or contagious disease-poison, or, as it is generally expressed, a zymotic agent? Must we regard each particular typhus-like fever, with its remarkable changes of blood, with its various localizations in all the organs and membranes, with its chills, furred tongue, petechiæ, delirium, etc., as we regard typhus, scarlatina, variola, etc.? or, as Virchow teaches us, is this pyæmia, so greatly feared by all surgeons, only an ontological idea? Is the word pyæmia only a general name for three different conditions—

viz. leucocythæmia, thrombosis, and embolism, or ichorrhæmia and septicæmia? or are there, as many have supposed, two ways in which pyæmia may originate? Is there one primary miasmatic pyæmia analogous to the other epidemic, so-called zymotic diseases? and again, a secondary pyæmia arising from suppurative inflammation, wherein the poison is formed in the patient's own body, which is infected by a single organ?"[29]

[29] *Loc. cit.*, S. 39.

That this disease is caused by a specific deleterious material in the large majority of cases is no longer a question for discussion. The only question to consider is, whether it always arises from the same cause. Is it possible for pyæmia to originate spontaneously? Are there any cases of sporadic origin, or are they always due to endemic or contagious influences? No definite answer can be given to these questions, although, undeniably, the weight of the argument is strongly opposed to a sporadic origin. The term miasmatic, as [p. 960]used by Roser, probably refers to the vitiated condition of the atmosphere, as seen in the overcrowded surgical and obstetrical wards of hospitals. In no other sense can the word be appropriately used in connection with the subject of pyæmia. It is true, pyæmic diseases are found to prevail at certain seasons and in certain localities much more extensively than under other circumstances. The same, however, is true of cholera, typhus fever, scarlatina, variola, and other contagious diseases. That pyæmia is contagious has been frequently demonstrated. I therefore conclude that the prevalence and spread of this disease must be explained by the same rules as are applied to the existence and propagation of these allied affections.

This inquiry into the etiology of pyæmia brings before us again the four hypotheses which have been given in explanation of the same number of theories. The first and second have been already abandoned by the medical profession, after it was satisfactorily demonstrated that they were based on false theories, and consequently there remain for our consideration only the third and fourth.

The third hypothesis assumes that a chemical poison is developed in the wound-secretions, which when absorbed produces pyæmia. An examination of the subject does not justify us in asserting that this proposition has been proved, although it is certain that the results of experimental inquiry demand for it a more extended investigation. In all the analyses which have thus far been made the investigators have entirely failed to give us an adequate knowledge of this poison, and not a word has ever been said in regard to the agency by which it is produced, although it is universally admitted to have been only obtained from decomposing animal substances. It is therefore pertinent to the continuation of this inquiry to ask, By what agency is the putrefaction of animal substances produced? It has now been fully shown that there can be but one answer given to this question—viz. the putrefaction of albuminoid substances can only be effected by living organisms. We therefore conclude that the fourth hypothesis brings us at least one step nearer the correct explanation of the etiology of pyæmia than the third, since we justly assume that if there is a chemical poison in decomposing albuminoid substances, it is produced through the agency of living organisms.

ETIOLOGY OF SEPTICÆMIA.—The first question which arises in the discussion of the etiology of this morbid condition is entirely dependent on the scope which we give to the word septicæmia. Sternberg says: "The view which is entertained by high authorities, upon clinical and experimental evidence, is that there are two forms of septicæmia—the one a septic toxæmia due to the effects of a chemical poison or poisons evolved during the putrefactive decomposition of certain organic substances, especially of nitrogenous animal products; the other an infective disease produced by the rapid multiplication in the body of the infected animal of a parasitic organism. The best-studied and most widely known form of septicæmia, due to the presence of a parasitic organism, is the disease known as anthrax—charbon of the French, milzbrand of the Germans—but several other varieties are now well established, in which similar symptoms and pathological results are produced by organisms morphologically different from the bacillus anthracis. Among these may[p. 961]be mentioned the form of septicæmia in the mouse, so well studied by Koch, which is due to a minute bacillus, and the form of septicæmia in the rabbit, produced by the subcutaneous injections of human saliva, due to micrococci, which has been studied by Pasteur, Vulpian, and myself independently."[30]

[30] *Amer. Jour. Med. Sci.*, July, 1882, p. 70.

The terms septic toxæmia and septic intoxication are applied indiscriminately to the same disease, and the committee appointed by the London Pathological Society to investigate the nature and cause of those infectious diseases known as septicæmia, etc. further report that "ordinary wound-fever is merely septic intoxication in a very mild form, and it is only necessary for the dose absorbed to be sufficient in quantity for fatal consequences to ensue. Septic intoxication is, therefore, of the commonest possible occurrence as a complication of severe surgical injuries, but it is in so mild a form as to bear but little resemblance to that experimentally produced on animals."[31] The question which now arises is, Shall septic intoxication be classified with septicæmia?

[31] *Trans. Pathological Soc. of London*, vol. xxx. p. 14.

We have been long accustomed to speak of this complication as a surgical or traumatic fever; and consequently any change in this classification must necessarily lead to confusion. Furthermore, it is now generally supposed there is much difference in the etiology of these morbid conditions. It is claimed that septic intoxication arises from the absorption of a chemical poison evolved through the agency of living organisms during the process of putrefaction in a wound, and that the conditions are unfavorable for their development within the blood or tissues of a living animal; but in true septicæmia the organisms are developed in the wound during putrefaction, and then find their way into the blood and tissues of the body, where they rapidly multiply. Consequently, the former condition tends to a rapid recovery—unless the quantity of poison primarily admitted to the system has been excessive—while the latter tends to a fatal termination.

Septic intoxication is regarded as a non-infective disease, and true septicæmia as an infective malady. The only etiological similarity between these morbid conditions is found in the fact that they take their origin in putrefaction, which is effected by the action of different organisms possessing marked morphological differences and requiring essentially different surroundings for the maintenance of life and reproduction. Thus, it is supposed that in cases of septic intoxication the organism by which putrefaction is caused in the wound-secretions can only live in the open air, and that its life is commonly only of a few hours' duration. The brevity of bacterial action in this instance may be due to a failure of the absorptive power or to a changed condition in the wound-fluids, rendering them unfit to support the organism.

It is now a well-recognized fact that all septic absorption ends so soon as the wound-surfaces are covered with healthy granulations, but that septic absorption, which produces septic intoxication, is most commonly of a much shorter duration, and, consequently, that the wound complication, which I prefer to designate traumatic fever, is essentially an acute disease, and can only be lengthened out by unusually favorable circumstances for the continuance of the absorption of the poison by which it is produced.[p. 962]The severity and danger of the disease will necessarily depend on the amount of poison absorbed and the resisting power of the patient; but since there is no multiplication of the materies morbi within the body, a rapid elimination by the natural emunctories may be reasonably expected under favorable circumstances.

It should be observed here that the etiology of septicæmia differs from that of traumatic fever, since the organisms in the former condition are first formed in the wound-secretions, but quickly enter the body, where they rapidly multiply; consequently, Chauvel has defined surgical septicæmia as follows: "The particular intoxication which results from the penetration and multiplication in the body of a specific microbe designated by Pasteur under the name of septic vibrio." The bacterial origin of this disease is now generally accepted, and the only question in the professional mind seems to be whether the organisms are the direct or indirect cause of the malady.

There are also some other interesting questions which have arisen in connection with the study of this subject, and are thought to be of sufficient importance to merit mention here. It has long been known that dissecting wounds are most dangerous when made while examining the body very soon after the death of the subject. Recent observations seem to justify the conclusion that the greatest activity of the septic agent is often, if not always, attained before the odor of putrefaction has become fairly perceptible; and even before this odor has reached its maximum degree of offensiveness the danger from septic poisoning has generally disappeared. In some cases septic intoxication is promptly followed by a slight inflammation in and about the wound, which may entirely disappear within a few hours, but only to reappear after a lapse of eight to fifteen days, with the first vigorous physical exercise of the patient. Two cases of this kind have recently come under my observation. In both instances the wounds were located in the hands, and the exercise which developed the septicæmia consisted in rowing a boat, and while thus engaged the local symptoms reappeared with such severity as to cause the patients to quickly discontinue the labor. The reappearance of the local inflammation in both these instances was quickly followed by a rigor and the rapid development of other constitutional symptoms, although prior to the recurrence there was no pus, nor even marked inflammatory action, in any part of the hands.

Professional attention was first called to the above-stated facts by Panum in 1855, who discovered that the maximum toxic action of putrid substances is generally developed during the first hours of bodily activity. In this stage of incubation in cases of surgical septicæmia, if we admit the bodily action as an etiological factor, we observe a striking resemblance to one of the leading characteristics of all the infectious diseases, which unquestionably depend on some sort of septic poison. Furthermore, this analogy becomes most striking if we contrast the effects arising from dissecting wounds with those of the bites of poisonous serpents and rabid animals.

Further investigation is required to settle the perplexing questions of etiological and pathological differences in these allied morbid conditions, for although much has been accomplished during the last two decades, still much more remains to be done. It has only recently been discovered[p. 963]that the septic material in septicæmia is absorbed by the lymphatics, while in pyæmia the poison enters the body through the veins.

ETIOLOGY OF SEPTO-PYÆMIA.—It is now generally admitted that remittent fever and typhoid may be associated, and this morbid condition is commonly designated by the term typho-malarial fever. The etiology is unquestionably dependent upon the action of the two distinct and entirely dissimilar poisons. Scarlatina is likewise frequently complicated by diphtheria, and here we have the combined action of two poisons, each commonly designated as septic and supposed by many physicians to be similar.

In a like manner, it is believed that septicæmia and pyæmia may be associated, and take their origin in dual poisons; but since the etiology of both these morbid conditions has been already described, it is not deemed necessary to dwell longer on septo-pyæmia under this division of our subject.

PATHOLOGY OF PYÆMIA.—The study of the pathology of pyæmia is advanced by adopting the following classification, which is based on recognized post-mortem lesions. The pathological appearances in these forms of the disease differ widely, although the clinical symptoms are often similar. In pyæmia simplex the pathological conditions are essentially more negative. This variety of the disease can only destroy life by the height and duration of the fever which is maintained in connection with the continued existence of ichorous pus. There is found, as an essential basis of this form of disease, extensive suppuration in the subcutaneous tissues.

The arguments in favor of the admission of pus-corpuscles into the blood are as follows: 1. The blood in pyæmia is known to contain more white granular spherical bodies than are normal. The question has been raised, Are they pus-cells or white blood-corpuscles? The answer is difficult, and has not yet been attained. Virchow, in the mean time, has proved that we cannot differentiate, morphologically, between the blood- and pus-corpuscles. 2. Cohnheim has demonstrated the existence of the wandering corpuscles in cases of inflammation. Therefore it appears probable that in cases of pyæmia the blood may contain the pus-corpuscles, but further investigation is needed to establish this fact. However, the establishment of this point would still leave the more important undetermined.

There are often important changes observed in the blood of patients dead of pyæmia, to which I now desire to direct attention. The red corpuscles of the blood, even in the early stage of the disease, in many cases show signs of disintegrating into molecules, and are observed to be accumulated in masses without showing the slightest tendency to form rouleaux. There is a steady increase in the number of pus- or white corpuscles in the blood of pyæmic patients during the whole course of the disease in fatal cases. The condition of the red corpuscles, already mentioned, becomes more and more marked toward the fatal termination.

In all cases of pyæmia multiplex the increased coagulability of the blood may be observed in the early stages of the disease, and steadily increases as the disease progresses.

In pyæmia simplex this condition is less marked, although generally present, "while we know septicæmia diminishes or destroys the[p. 964]coagulability of the blood. Hereby the possibility is given, at least on the cadaver, to differentiate between pyæmia simplex and septicæmia, although cases occur of the more fatal septic infection in which the post-mortem condition is a complete or almost complete negative. Therefore, in these cases the differential diagnosis on the cadaver must be limited to this, that we are able to demonstrate the existence of a purulent or ichorous deposit." It will be readily observed that the difference in diagnosis mentioned above relates to pyæmia and septicæmia, and not to the different varieties of the former disease.

The following facts should be constantly kept in mind by the surgeon to enable him to differentiate between the two forms of pyæmia: In pure cases of purulent infection, without metastasis, the disease is called pyæmia simplex, and in cases with metastasis, pyæmia multiplex. The various conditions on which the metastasis may depend are shown by Hueter, who says: "The metastatic abscesses of pyæmia multiplex met with in the lungs, liver, spleen, and other internal organs are regarded, with the greatest probability, as a result of the embolic process. The metastatic inflammation of the serous membranes, of the cellular tissues, and of the parotid glands, and probably also a few metastatic inflammations of the internal organs, are at present supposed to arise from a general inflammatory diathesis."[32] It has already been shown by numerous experiments on animals that metastatic abscesses in the lungs, liver, and other visceral organs only arise after the introduction of ichorous pus, while healthy pus has uniformly failed to produce these results.

[33] Billroth's *Handbuch der Chirurgie*, S. 88.

It now remains to be shown how the introduction of ichorous pus acts in the production of pyæmia multiplex. The ichorous pus, having found its way into the venous circulation, gives rise to the formation of thrombi in the veins; these clots become more or less broken up, and are carried forward by the blood to the right auricle; from this auricle to the right ventricle; from this ventricle to the pulmonary artery, and through its ramifications to every part of the lungs. In the minute ramifications of this vessel are found wedge-shaped clots of various sizes in different conditions, some softened and others still firm. The possibility of these clots ever passing through the lungs, and afterward being arrested in other visceral organs, has been demonstrated on animals. It has been shown that fine particles of foreign matter injected into the veins have passed through the lungs and subsequently lodged in the liver. This theory enables us to account, upon a mechanical basis, for the existence of the metastatic abscesses in the liver which have apparently originated as the result of primary infection.

In other cases these abscesses are supposed to arise from secondary infection. Thus, ichorous pus, having found its way into the venous circulation, produces primarily venous thrombi, which, as in other instances, break up, the clots being carried in the same manner into the terminal branches of the pulmonary artery, where they are designated as emboli. The first action of the emboli is the mechanical closure of these vessels, thus depriving the surrounding parts of nutrition to a greater or less extent. It will be proper now to recall the fact that the composition of these emboli is such as to favor rapid suppuration; this commonly commences [p. 965]in the clot and surrounding tissues, having been preceded by a brief stage of congestion and inflammation. There is also occasionally found around these points more or less extravasation. The metastatic abscess thus formed in the lungs is favorably situated for the production of secondary infection. From this abscess thrombi arise in the pulmonary veins, which become disintegrated, and are carried to the auricle, thence to the left ventricle, and finally through the aorta, and find lodgment in the terminal branches of the arteries of the various organs, where they produce the characteristic lesions.

The organs which most frequently become the seat of this secondary infection are the liver, spleen, kidneys, brain, and eyes.

Let us now briefly examine this mechanical theory. Do metastatic abscesses arise from a single cause or from a combination of causes? I am inclined to the opinion that the proximal cause of metastatic abscesses in the visceral organs is the existence of emboli in the terminal branches. The vitiated atmosphere surrounding the patient, the existence of a wound, and the formation of ichorous pus are conditions which should not be lost sight of. These are the elements acting on the blood, producing in it morbid changes, and may therefore be regarded as predisposing causes. The morbid conditions of the blood, the increased number of white blood-corpuscles (possibly pus), the disintegration and other changes in the red corpuscles, may be regarded as the exciting causes of metastatic abscesses. It is thus readily observed that emboli may form in the lungs and liver at the same time, or the origin of those in the lungs may precede the formation in other organs.

Is the formation of emboli in the terminal branches of arteries always dependent on the disintegration of thrombi? The answer to this question must, I think, be a negative, although in surgical practice it rarely happens that the emboli take their origin from any other cause. In the large majority of cases, unquestionably, the thrombi primarily exist in the vicinity of the wound in which ichorous pus is generated; but it not infrequently happens during the process of disintegration that broken-up clots are carried forward by the current of blood, receiving accretions on the way, until finally they fill a large venous trunk. In confirmation of these facts relating to the primary origin of thrombi, it is said to have been observed in epidemics of puerperal fever, which were complicated with metastatic abscesses of the visceral organs, that the thrombi occurred in the pelvic veins. In case of wounds of the lower extremity the clot is frequently found in the common iliac vein, although probably it should always be regarded as a secondary formation. In rare cases the only thrombi discovered at the autopsy are found situated far away from the injury.

Observation fully establishes the fact that, after death from pyæmia, pathological changes are much more frequently met with in the lungs than in any of the other organs. This certainly strengthens the embolic theory. Billroth mentions eighty-three cases of true pyæmia multiplex, in which the metastatic abscesses occurred as follows: seventy-five times in the lungs, seventeen times in the spleen, eight times in the liver, and four times in the kidneys. Sedillot remarks that in one hundred cases of pyæmia we find the lungs affected in ninety-nine, the liver and spleen in eight, the muscles in seven, and the heart and peripheric [p. 966]cellular tissue in five cases. The brain and kidneys are comparatively seldom involved.

The theory previously mentioned as the embolic relates to the aggregation of fibrin into clots; but another theory has been recently advanced by E. Wagner, who found in many cases the capillaries in the lungs filled with fat, and was inclined, from the direction it extended in these vessels, to explain a certain number of the pyæmic cases by the fat emboli; but it has been shown that the existence of the fat emboli in pyæmia is purely accidental and possesses no significance. Pyæmia multiplex very frequently occurs without fat emboli, and vice versâ; either process may complicate the other, and so the fat emboli may acquire special importance by obstructing the respiration, and probably also in their way the embolic fat may serve as a carrier of putrid material.

MORBID ANATOMY.—The external appearance of the body varies greatly. The skin, in those cases in which the patient was jaundiced before death, will be found in every part of the body to be of a dark orange or dirty icteric tinge, but in other cases it may present a pale or anæmic appearance. There are also sometimes found circumscribed ecchymoses or purpuric patches, while the edges of ulcers or open wounds are generally of a blackish or dirty yellow color. The lips and finger-nails present a livid appearance; epithelial defects are observed in the cornea, but these had their origin there before the death of the patient.

The eyes in some cases are sunken deeply in their sockets, and where the disease has been protracted there is often very great emaciation. Rigor mortis is commonly well marked after a few hours. When death occurs from puerperal pyæmia there are generally found some indications of the recent parturition, although the principal lacerations or injuries may be confined to the womb. All fluids disappear from external wounds before the death of the patient, and they remain dry afterward.

In some cases the cellular tissue is the seat of diffuse suppuration. The pus formed is thin, fetid, and unhealthy. This suppuration is limited to certain parts of the body, as an injured extremity, or, as frequently happens, it may be found on the trunk and limbs at the same time. The pus in this form of suppuration is exceedingly apt to burrow, on account of the peculiarities of the tissue in which it occurs, and also the condition of the surrounding structures, especially the relaxed and flabby condition of the skin. These abscesses in some instances are superficial, in others deep-seated.

There are few changes which occur in the muscles, and these are not uniform or constant. They are occasionally the seat of abscesses, which have been observed in the heart, tongue, and other organs. The muscles may be of a light-brown or greenish color when they have been covered a considerable time with pus, and are sometimes softened and pultaceous. Suppuration may also take place beneath the fascia of the tendons.

The brain and its membranes are frequently found in a perfectly healthy state after death from pyæmia, although when the diseased process has extended during the life of the patient to the lungs and pleura, giving rise to great dyspnoea, there will generally be observed some congestion of the membranes, an increased quantity of fluid in the brain-substance and ventricles, and also an increased fulness of the meningeal veins and sinuses. Occasionally there have been observed suppurative [p. 967]meningitis, blood extravasations on the surface of the brain, lymph-deposits on the membranes, softening of the cerebral tissues, and circumscribed abscesses in the substance of the brain, which in some cases have been traceable to embolism of its vessels. The changes in the spinal cord and its membranes are probably similar to those found in the brain, but these parts appear to have been rarely examined.

Virchow found emboli of the retinal and choroidal vessels. Heiberg found these vessels occluded with colonies of micrococci. There have also been observed opacity of the cornea, sloughing of the conjunctival epithelium, suppurative infiltration into the periphery of the vitreous body, and deposits of pus in Petit's canal and in the anterior and posterior chambers. Pyæmic ophthalmia has been observed somewhat frequently in puerperal cases, especially when preceded by endocarditis, with deposits on the semilunar or mitral valves. In surgical cases it is rarely seen.

Toynbee "relates several cases of purulent infection following suppuration of the ear. Cases of disease in the mastoid cells terminate fatally, he says, from two different causes: first, from purulent infection, arising from the introduction of pus into the circulation through the lateral sinus; second, from disease of the cerebellum or its membranes. Cases of purulent infection, he further remarks, have not been met with where the disease occurs in the tympanic cavity."[34]

[34] Braidwood on *Pyæmia*, pp. 168, 169.

Numerous lesions of the osseous system have been noted in pyæmia, probably from the fact that this disease results very frequently in cases of bone-lesions, but these changes have very little diagnostic importance. The following have been observed: thickening or infiltration of the periosteum, which may be found to separate readily from the bone after the death of the patient, or there may be pus found between the periosteum and the bone. In the bone-structure there were found caries and necrosis, "while in other cases the whole thickness of the compact tissue is perforated in a honeycomb-like manner by minute cavities filled with thickish pus or caseous matter of a pinkish-white color."[35] "To sum up, the chief morbid alterations met with in the bones are congestion, dilatation of the Haversian canals and cancellated tissue, tending to abscess formation, and the excavation of the cavities by the unhealthy pus."[36]

[35] *Ibid.*, p. 192.

[36] *Ibid.*, p. 194.

The pathological lesions of the joints commence with marked congestion of the synovial membranes and increase in the synovial fluids, and afterward the fluid is mixed with pus; these conditions are followed by erosion of the cartilage and ligaments, the former thus becoming separated from the bone. Both the small and large joints are occasionally the seat of morbid changes.

The parotid gland is occasionally the seat of a secondary inflammation during the progress of pyæmia, and this may endanger life by interfering with respiration and deglutition. The lymphatic glands are only secondarily affected, and even this takes place very rarely. The changes in the glandular system, when observed, are similar to those which happen in other tissues of the body—viz. congestion, inflammation, and suppuration.

The arteries are usually found empty after death from this disease, and the coats are sometimes apparently thickened. The veins, on the contrary, are commonly found filled, or even distended, with firm fibrinous clots. They are sometimes also found inflamed or altered, although more [p. 968]commonly healthy. The distended condition of the veins gives rise to the cord-like feeling often mentioned by different observers. In some cases of phlebitis there may be pus deposited between the coats of these veins. The most important pathological changes are found in the blood. These changes occur early in the disease, become more marked toward its fatal termination, and may be always studied after death. It is generally admitted that pus is frequently found in the blood of these patients; but it has been shown by numerous experiments that healthy pus never produces the pathological changes which characterize this disease. Pyæmia is only produced by the presence in the blood of ichorous pus or some other decomposing animal substance, or some material having its origin in the decomposition of the same, and no decomposition in these substances is ever effected except through the agency of living organisms. It therefore follows that the discovery of living organisms in the blood of those sick and dead of this disease has given a renewed interest to the study of its pathology. The recent investigations made by Pasteur, Koch, Birch-Hirschfeld, and the London Pathological Society show conclusively that in all cases of pyæmia and septicæmia organisms are present in the blood during the entire course of the disease, and that in the former there is found the globular, and in the latter the rod bacteria. It has further been observed in each morbid condition that the severity of the disease is always increased in proportion to the increase of the organisms in the blood, and that the bacteria found within the body are of the same species as those in the wound from which they have gained admission. The micrococci found in the blood of pyæmic patients are surrounded by the decomposed products of the red and white corpuscles, which appear in the blood-plasma in the form of pale granular bodies. There is likewise in this disease an increased coagulability of the blood, and it steadily increases as the disease progresses. In this condition there may be found in the blood-vessels both thrombi and emboli. The thrombi are occasionally observed as firm fibrinous clots, but they may be likewise found in the rapidly fatal cases to have undergone suppurative changes. These changes begin in the centre of the clots, which often contain true pus or a greenish or puriform fluid.

The pericardium may contain a small amount of serum tinged with blood, but it is seldom covered with recent lymph. Both the lung-tissue and pleuræ are commonly inflamed in this disease. The costal and visceral layers may be agglutinated by old adhesions, but are more commonly united together by recently formed lymph. The pleural cavities often contain some opaque, muddy, sero-purulent fluid, mixed with blood and having masses of lymph floating in it.

The lungs are more frequently the seat of metastatic abscesses and other morbid changes in pyæmia multiplex than any other organs of the body. There may be found emboli in the branches of the pulmonary veins, and in the lung-tissue metastatic abscesses surrounded with capillary congestion and other evidences of inflammation; "The smaller vessels, trying to overcome this afflux of blood, may produce ecchymosis or extravasation beneath the lining membrane of the air-vesicles, but the minute capillary congestions are generally observed as red points studded over the pulmonary surface, which by and by exhibit yellowish-white or bluish-white centres. While one part, generally the lower half of the [p. 969]lung, is thus hepatized, solid, and of a dark greenish color, the remainder of the lung is emphysematous and more or less oedematous. A section of the former presents the same appearance as is observed in the lungs of pneumonic patients. Whether these incipient abscesses are developed from the minute points of congestion before mentioned, by the breaking down of the thrombic clots in their centres, or whether the pus is developed out of the serum exuded by the walls of the engorged capillaries, cannot be easily determined, and has as yet not been decided. These secondary abscesses vary in size from that of a hemp-seed to that of a hen's egg."[37] These are generally situated on the periphery of the lungs and in the lower lobe, although in some cases they are found imbedded deeply in the pulmonary tissue. The contents of these abscesses are similar to those found in other parts of the body in this disease. The bronchial mucous membrane is commonly of a bright pink color, while its secretion is increased in quantity, and may be clear and frothy. These changes are the result of acute bronchial catarrh. Lobular pneumonia has been frequently observed as a complication of pyæmia, and is supposed by some authors to be caused by the vitiated condition of the blood; but probably it is more frequently occasioned by infarctions and embolic abscesses, which have been previously mentioned in this connection.

[37] Braidwood, *op. cit.*, p. 173 *et seq.*

Billroth and Sedillot observed pathological lesions involving a solution of continuity in the spleen, liver, and kidneys, in the order in which they are mentioned; other authors, however, assert that the liver, next to the lungs, is the most frequent seat of purulent deposits. Enlargement of the spleen is frequently met with in cases of pyæmia multiplex. The metastatic abscesses found in the spleen and kidneys are much smaller than those found in the lungs and liver, but in other respects are of a similar character. The capillary congestion and the accompanying infarctions require no special attention here. The liver, like the spleen, is sometimes enlarged, and at other times is found to have undergone fatty degeneration to a greater or less degree; in which condition its tissues are generally soft and friable. Abscesses in the liver are so much like those in the lungs as to need no separate description. The same may be said of other pathological changes found in this organ in pyæmia multiplex. The abscesses found in the kidneys vary from the size of a hemp-seed to that of a bean, and are surrounded by the usual zone, marking more or less definitely the extent of the inflammation. The capsule is generally healthy. There are also, in very rare cases of this disease, abscesses found in the stomach and intestines, involving the thickness of the mucous membrane; and it is further supposed that these abscesses may be found occasionally on any portion of the mucous membrane lining the alimentary canal. Post-mortem examinations in pyæmia multiplex have established the fact that there is no organ in the body that may not become the seat of pathological lesions in this disease; but there is unquestionably a vast difference in the relative frequency of these changes in the various organs. In some instances of this disease peritonitis is developed, with its concomitant changes in this membrane and the abdominal fluid, which is generally increased in quantity and sometimes slightly tinged with blood, but more frequently remains clear. [p. 970]This inflammation is commonly dependent on an extension of the inflammatory process from a metastatic abscess, which may be situated near the periphery of some organ covered with peritoneum, although it is claimed that pleuritis occasionally occurs in connection with pyæmia independent of metastatic abscesses in the lungs.

The careful study of the pathology of pyæmia multiplex renders it exceedingly probable that the immediate agency in the production of all these lesions is the presence in the blood of a particular species of living organism, and that all the morbid changes which occur in the visceral organs are secondary to those which take place in the blood, but that the former are only dependent on the latter in a minor degree. The pathological changes effected by these organisms seem to be as follows, and to occur in the following order: viz. disorganization of the blood, especially a destruction of the red and white blood-corpuscles; the formation of granular bodies around the organisms out of this débris; the production of an increased coagulability of the blood; the lodgment in the blood-vessels of these granular bodies, which are increased in size by a deposit of fibrin; these obstructions occur most frequently in minute ramifications of the pulmonary arteries; nutrition is effected locally by these infarctions, and generally by the vitiated condition of the blood, which enables the organisms under these favorable circumstances to penetrate the adjacent tissues and produce the metastatic abscesses and other accompanying lesions.

The pathological changes in pyæmia simplex are of the same kind as those which have just been described as characterizing pyæmia multiplex, with the exception of the metastatic abscesses, which are always absent. Furthermore, the disease in both instances is believed to have its origin from the same causes, and the dissimilarities in the pathological lesions are equally susceptible of a rational explanation, as are those of scarlatina simplex and scarlatina maligna.

There were reported by the committee of the London Pathological Society some interesting details pertaining to this form of pyæmia. Their report shows that among the one hundred and fifty-five cases classed as pyæmia there were twenty-four cases without visceral abscesses; and furthermore it shows that in twenty-three of these cases there was no suppuration, although local inflammations affected many of the different tissues, since these patients suffered with arthritis, cellulitis, pleuritis, meningitis, pericarditis, and carditis. It is also added that "the post-mortem appearances, in addition to the local secondary inflammation before noted, were in many cases those changes common to all forms of blood poisoning. Out of the twenty-four cases, the following are noted: Swollen spleen, nine times; congestion of the lungs, ten times; swollen liver, six times; cloudy swelling of the kidney, fourteen times."[38]

[38] *Trans. London Pathological Soc.*, vol. xxx. p. 26.

In this form of pyæmia it has been supposed by some authors that the materies morbi occasionally produces death before the metastatic abscesses have had time to develop, but this is not always the case. The same committee report on the above-mentioned twenty-four cases, on this point, as follows: "The duration of the cases before the fatal termination was very various. It is tolerably accurately recorded in eighteen cases: of these five died in the first week, five in the second, [p. 971]four in the third, and the remaining four survived to the thirtieth, forty-ninth, fifty-second, and sixty-second days."[39]

[39] *Trans. London Pathological Soc.*, p. 25 *et seq.*

The pathology of pyæmia multiplex having been already fully described, and since the only essential difference in these morbid conditions consists in the complete absence of the metastatic abscesses in cases of pyæmia simplex, it is therefore thought unnecessary to dwell here longer on this subject.

The morbid anatomy of septicæmia has been carefully studied of late, and it is now known that the most characteristic lesions are found in the blood and the alimentary canal.

As a manifestation of the general poisoning of the blood, it might be expected that putrefaction would follow rapidly after the death of the patient. In fact, Davine defines septicæmia as "putrefaction of a living body." Observation has now thoroughly confirmed that which was formerly an anticipation. Panum, Hemmer, and Bergmann have each called attention to the fact that rapid decomposition follows the death of all animals in which septicæmia has been produced for experimental purposes. It has also been observed that putrefaction in the human cadaver begins much sooner, and progresses much more rapidly, under similar circumstances, when the death has been produced by this disease than when it has occurred from any other cause. Furthermore, this rapid decomposition is not limited to the internal organs, but may be frequently strongly marked on the surface of the body after the lapse of twelve hours, although it has been kept in a comparatively dry and cool atmosphere. In those cases where the septicæmia has originated in an external wound it has been uniformly observed that putrefaction goes on most rapidly in the vicinity of the wound after the death of the patient.

In every case of fatal septicæmia the post-mortem examination will show that the coagulability of the blood has been diminished or destroyed. In fact, it has been abundantly shown that in all cases of true septicæmia the coagulability of the blood is more or less diminished. The few imperfect clots of blood found after death are of a deep-black color. The putrefaction of the soft tissues is greatly hastened by the presence of this blood; and, consequently, this process goes on most rapidly in the most dependent portions of the body, especially along the course of the large veins. The septicæmic blood possesses a peculiar putrefactive odor, and it is occasionally found to be acid in its reaction, according to Vogel and Scherer, making it highly probable that it will end in the formation of the carbonate of ammonium. The chemical examinations of septicæmic blood which have heretofore been made have completely failed to give satisfactory results in regard either to the existence or nature of the materies morbi in this disease, although, without doubt, there has occasionally been found, principally in the blood of those who have died of acute septic intoxication, a poisonous substance, which Bergmann designated sepsin. Microscopic examinations have shown that in the blood and also in various organs of those who have died of septicæmia there are always present, under these circumstances, a large number of the rod bacteria; in fact, they are more numerous than after death from any other infectious disease. Furthermore, they are found in the blood, lymph-glands, and cellular tissues during the whole course of the disease.

[p. 972]There are no pathological changes in the central nervous system which arise directly from septicæmia, although in some cases, when there has been some cardiac complication or very severe dyspnoea from any cause immediately prior to the death of the patient, there may be found hyperæmia of the membranes of the cerebro-spinal axis. The brain and spinal cord remain unchanged.

The endo- and pericardium occasionally present a somewhat mottled appearance resembling ecchymosis, which is evidently a deposit from the blood, and may be washed off with water. The inner surface of the ventricles presents a similar appearance from the same cause. In addition to those changes which have been mentioned there are occasionally found some slight traces of an inflammatory process in these parts; but it never extends to the formation of pus or ulceration, which frequently happens in cases of pyæmia. The quantity of pericardial fluid is sometimes increased in septicæmia, and is generally somewhat thickened, cloudy, and slightly tinged with blood. The changes in the pleural surfaces are the same as those which have been noted in the pericardium, but any increase of the fluid within the pleural sacs is an exception to the general law, and is very rarely seen. The lungs are generally found slightly congested, but there may be some ecchymosis in exceptional cases. Pus is never found in the lungs or within the pleural cavities in pure unmixed septicæmia. The pathological changes in the liver resemble those in the lungs. This organ is commonly found in a state of passive congestion, while the color of its tissues is slightly darkened. The congestion of the kidneys and spleen in this disease is much more marked than that of the lungs and liver. The parenchymatous tissue of the kidneys is commonly found in an oedematous condition, and the tubuli uriniferi are more or less affected by a catarrhal inflammation, which is manifested by the exfoliation of granular epithelium. The same catarrhal condition, but in a milder form, is found to affect the mucous membrane of the bladder. In females the ovaries, uterus, and vagina are in a state of hyperæmia, with more or less catarrhal inflammation of the latter organ. Septicæmia invariably causes pregnant females to abort. There is commonly softening of the spleen. The alimentary canal is almost constantly affected by acute intestinal catarrh, with enlargement of the intestinal follicles and mesenteric glands, while there are frequently hemorrhages from the serous and mucous membranes. The various muscles of the body and the extremities are found to be of a dark brownish-red after the death of the patient, instead of possessing their natural pale-red color. It may now be stated, finally, that the pathological changes in septicæmia are less marked than those of pyæmia multiplex.

The semiology, etiology, and pathology of septo-pyæmia consist in a blending, in different degrees, of the essential parts of pyæmia and septicæmia; and since the pathology of both these diseases has been presented separately, it is deemed unnecessary to enter into a consideration of this combination.

SYMPTOMS OF PYÆMIA.—Pyæmia very rarely, if ever, develops except in connection with an open suppurating wound, and consequently it must generally be regarded as a wound complication or as a secondary diseased condition. Those open wounds are unquestionably the most favorably situated for the development of this disease which involve the medullary[p. 973]cavities of the long bones, owing to the liability of unhealthy suppuration, the difficulty of complete drainage, and the favorable anatomical conditions for absorption.

Every form of pyæmia is frequently preceded by a distinctly marked prodromal stage, which varies in duration from four days to two weeks. In fact, the ordinary precursor of this disease, in all those cases in which the bones are involved, is an attack of osteo-myelitis; but in other cases the patient often complains of malaise, giddiness, headache, pain in the limbs, weakness, and loss of appetite, while the experienced surgeon will be deeply impressed with the patient's rapid emaciation and cadaverous face. These symptoms are soon followed by jaundiced skin, etc. The commencement of an attack of pyæmia is commonly manifested by a chill. The importance which will naturally be attached to this phenomenon in connection with an open wound must depend to a certain degree on the circumstances attending its occurrence; and therefore the following question will present itself: Is the chill associated with suppuration? A negative answer to this question, based on the fact that insufficient time has elapsed since the occurrence of the injury to render suppuration possible, can never fail to be a source of satisfaction to the surgeon, whose experience has taught him to dread pyæmia.

Billroth has observed in 83 cases of true pyæmia multiplex that 62 commenced with a chill, and 21 without; in 81 cases of septicæmia and simple pyæmia 24 commenced with a chill and 57 without. The number of chills in each individual patient occurred according to the following table:

Number of patients	9	1	4	5						
Number of chills									0	3	4

In one patient during three weeks sixteen chills were observed, and probably the longer the duration of the disease the greater is the number of chills. Still, there are chronic cases with a single chill, and acute cases with many. It rarely occurs that a patient has more than one chill in twenty-four hours. Billroth noticed among his patients only sixteen who had two chills, and only six who each had three chills, in one day. The experience that fewer chills occur during the evening and night than in the morning and afternoon has been confirmed by statistics. Among 287 chills, 220 occurred from 8 A.M. to 8 P.M., while during the night, from 8P.M. to 8 A.M., only 67 were observed. By this arbitrary division of the twenty-four hours Billroth desired to take into consideration the daily exacerbation in connection with the usual daily irritation of the wound, the bandaging, and other manipulations. He saw, for example, a chill occur three times from the introduction of a sound, and twenty times after the opening of an abscess. The time which elapsed from the first injury to the first chill is shown in the following table:

First chill began, times	4	9	5				
Length of time after injury, in weeks							

Patients who had fever before the operation were more inclined to early chills than recently-injured healthy individuals. Billroth's experience was to have only the first chill before the end of the first week. It may be further stated that nervous, irritable patients suffer much more [p. 974]frequently from chills than those of a phlegmatic temperament. This fact has given rise to the opinion that the absorption of pus acts especially on the central nervous system.

The chills in pyæmia are supposed by Billroth to be associated with inflammation, and he says: "It must be mentioned, as a matter of observation, that chills occur almost exclusively in the commencement of an acute inflammation, and are intermittent only in intermittent fever and reabsorption of pus, while they do not occur in acute septicæmia."[40] But the fever in pyæmia rarely intermits entirely; it is generally lower, however, in the morning than in the afternoon. This symptom is even more important than the rigors in enabling the surgeon to make a correct diagnosis. Let it, however, be remembered that the temperature frequently becomes very high within a few hours after the receipt of an injury or the performance of a surgical operation; that this high temperature may be due to septic absorption, and that this diseased condition is what we designate as septicæmia. Another condition, less marked, with an elevated but somewhat lower temperature, is usually spoken of as traumatic fever. In this condition the fever may gradually increase for a few days, and then disappear.

[40] *Surgical Pathology*, p. 344.

One important peculiarity of the temperature in pyæmia are the sudden and great changes; thus, at one hour the temperature may be slightly raised above the normal, and at the next the thermometer may mark 105° F. These sudden changes of temperature are of frequent occurrence, are not observed to the same extent in any other disease, and therefore supply a very important diagnostic indication. It is impossible to know, or even to anticipate with any degree of certainty, when the highest temperature will exist; consequently, Billroth and other writers have suggested the desirability of having a thermometer constantly kept in a position to indicate every change in the heat of the body, and a careful attendant to note the same; but, thus far, I am not aware that this has been attempted, probably on account of the inconvenience to the patient and the additional labor in nursing it would entail. It has been further observed that during the existence of a chill the temperature continues to steadily increase, and the maximum seen during the whole course of the disease is attained during the hot stage which immediately follows the rigors. "This condition is followed by profuse cold perspirations. The perspirations which accompany this disease are most profuse, like those of advanced phthisis. They never precede the rigors, but may occur independently of them. They are either continuous in their duration, or exhibit more or less distinct exacerbations. They are occasionally accompanied by sudamina, and they do not abate with the use of any known remedy.... Occasionally perspiration is scanty; but before death a cold clammy sweat and a tawny discoloration of the skin occur."[41]

[41] Braidwood, *op. cit.*, p. 112.

Besides the sudamina there are frequently observed on the skin vesicles, pustules, and boils, purpuric patches, and various discolorations. There is frequently observed to arise in the neighborhood of the wound a reddish erythematous blush, which soon extends to the whole limb, and commonly begins to disappear in the early part of the second week. This recently occurred to a patient under my care, and was speedily followed by an abscess of the knee-joint. The wound was situated at the hip-joint,[p. 975]and the first change in the color of the integument took place around its lips. The redness extended rapidly downward until it covered the foot, and even the toes; but the extension upward was slight, not much above the nates, on which there was situated at the time a bed-sore. It observed the same order in passing off as in coming on—*i.e.* where it first made its appearance it first disappeared. The superficial veins leading from the wound were inflamed and cord-like. This condition of the integument and the abscess of the knee-joint were followed by diarrhoea, on which medicines had no beneficial effect. It continued, with occasional vomiting, until the death of the patient.

The pulse in pyæmia may be nearly normal as regards frequency, while at other times very rapid. It has been remarked in some cases that the pulse seldom rose above 90 per minute until near death. The pulse, although only moderately accelerated at the commencement of the disease, always becomes more rapid, quick, feeble, and irregular toward the termination of the unfavorable cases, while in cases of recovery it returns gradually to the normal standard.

In all cases in which the blood has been examined during the progress of pyæmia the examiners have agreed in regard to its extreme coagulability, the diminution of the number of red corpuscles, and the increase of the granular spherical bodies. The red corpuscles, even in the earlier stages of the disease, show evident indications of disintegrating; and these become more and more marked as the disease progresses, while there is a steady increase in the number of pus- or possibly of white blood-corpuscles. Epistaxis occasionally occurs, and also venous oozing from the wound.

The condition of the tongue in pyæmia may be regarded as an important symptom, indicating the state of the alimentary canal—not, however, during the prodromal stage, but after the disease has progressed a few days. It is then observed that the tongue has become peculiarly smooth, dry, and often excessively red. This smoothness is caused by the collapse of the papillæ, and the dryness by a diminished secretion. The organ now frequently appears as if covered with a thin layer of collodion which had been caused to dry on the surface, so as to present a glazed look. Again, the tongue may be covered with brown crusts and the teeth with sordes. These brown crusts and sordes are usually seen in advanced cases, following the first condition described. Much importance is attached to these brown crusts by many experienced surgeons, and although there may be very marked improvement in all other symptoms, still they insist on a very guarded prognosis until the tongue has assumed a healthy appearance. Aphthæ on various parts of the mouth and pharynx are frequently present in the more chronic cases, but are usually absent in acute cases. Herpes of the lips sometimes occurs in the commencement of the disease.

Vomiting is comparatively rare, but there is, even in the early stages, a complete failure of the appetite, with great thirst. Singultus is rarely present in genuine pyæmia, but frequently so in septicæmia, and occasionally in septo-pyæmia. Diarrhœa is not so frequent or the stools so copious in pyæmia as in septicæmia. Billroth observed in one hundred and eighty cases of pyæmia thirty-two cases of diarrhœa. It is impossible to determine whether those cases in which the diarrhœa [p. 976]occurred were pure or mixed pyæmia. The stools are often of a pappy consistence, and passed involuntarily in bed. There are, however, severe cases of pyæmia with high fever, and accompanied by obstinate constipation.

Examination of the heart may, in rare cases, show the existence of pericarditis, although usually the only indications of disease are the too feeble sounds. Auscultation and percussion of the lungs may yield unsatisfactory results when the metastatic abscesses are small and scattered, for the same reason as in miliary tuberculosis. The large deposits in the lungs are by these means readily determined. There may be a sensation of suffocation, the pneumonic sputa, the friction sound of pleurisy, or the signs of pleuritic effusion; and the existence of these symptoms or signs would naturally aid in the diagnosis of metastatic abscesses.

Enlargement of the liver and spleen may be determined before death, and in connection with other symptoms would aid in diagnosing deposits in these organs.

The urine in the first stage of this disease is scanty, high-colored, contains a large amount of salts, and is of a high specific gravity. Epithelial, fibrinous, and blood casts, and also albumen, are occasionally found in it during the course of the disease. Billroth mentions a case in which there was complete suppression, with uræmia.

In many cases of pyæmia suppuration of the joints, one after another, takes place with great rapidity and with comparatively little pain, but occasionally some swelling, redness, etc. are present. In most cases these suppurations are easily diagnosed. Instead of suppuration taking place in the joints, there are cases in which it occurs in the cellular tissue; and I have recently seen a case where abscess after abscess formed with such rapidity that within a single week the patient was literally covered with abscesses from the crown of his head to the soles of his feet.

Delirium generally exists during some stage of the disease, more frequently the last, and is then mild in its character, although active delirium has been observed in the first stage. Patients are low-spirited and very apprehensive of death. The face at the beginning of the attack may be flushed or pallid, but toward the end it always becomes careworn and haggard. The breath occasionally has a sweetish or purulent odor.

The changes in the wound are in some cases very marked, even in the first stage of the disease. The suppuration, which has been previously free and healthy, may be suddenly checked, the wound becoming dry. The discharge, if it continues, becomes scanty, thin, ichorous, or greenish. The granulations, if previously healthy, may soon slough. These changes may not always appear in the first stage, but should they not then take place they may be expected later in the disease.

SYMPTOMS OF SEPTICÆMIA.—These are commonly developed within twenty-four hours after the receipt of an injury or the performance of a surgical operation, and they may be sketched as follows: Frequent pulse; tongue, lips, and throat dry; skin hot and the temperature of the body high. The patient replies accurately to questions, but with some hesitation. He is much inclined to sleep, has entirely failed to take nourishment, drinks frequently when aroused from his lethargic condition, and has vomited everything taken into his stomach since the receipt of the injury or the performance of the operation. If [p. 977]the dressings are now removed from the wound, the foul odor of putrefaction greets the attendants. In cases of amputation-wounds considerable discoloration of the flaps may be observed, the edges being blackened. Above these blackened edges the integument is reddened and slightly oedematous. The wound having been closed with sutures, which are now removed, there escapes a few drachms—possibly ounces—of highly offensive fluid, the decomposed remains of blood, etc. A further examination of the flaps on their inner surfaces show that their capillary circulation has ceased. The tissues, instead of presenting a life-like appearance, are now of a very dark color and occasionally mottled with dull grayish spots, although the movements of the ligature at the point where it embraces the femoral artery, for example, show that the blood still rushes against the artificial boundary.

Let us now leave our patient, without further comment, for the next forty-eight hours, when we will resume the examination. We now find the same dryness of the mouth that was previously noticed; the pulse is more frequent, and has become very feeble; he complains of much thirst, has vomited frequently, and has taken very little nourishment, and that only at the earnest solicitations of the attendants. The temperature is higher than at the former examination, and has been steadily increasing; in the morning it is lower, however, than in the evening of the same day. The patient is lethargic, and is suffering with a profuse diarrhoea. The odor of the stools is highly offensive; they are properly described as rice-water evacuations. The abdomen is tympanitic; the body bathed in perspiration; the respirations rapid; the urine scanty, high-colored, and contains albumen. The examination of the stump shows that gangrene has extended rapidly, involving not only the flap, but a portion of the adjacent tissues. The stench arising from the wound is almost stifling. The decomposing fluids are continually forming. That portion of the thigh not already gangrenous is now very oedematous, and the integument covering it is much discolored, being of a dark, icteric, or reddened hue.

We now allow twenty-four hours to elapse, and then make our final examination. The patient's tongue is more moist; the body still bathed in perspiration; the eyes dull; the conjunctivæ icteric, and the same hue extends to the body, though in a less marked degree; the pulse has become very frequent, feeble, and not easily counted; the temperature is below normal. Singultus is now present, and has been so during the last twenty-four hours. Bronchial symptoms, combined with marked oedema of the right lung, have appeared; the diarrhoea continues the same; the gangrene is still extending.

It must be admitted that the report here offered shows only the symptoms that are found in a single class of cases. The symptoms vary greatly in different cases, but they are especially marked in the acute sepsis mentioned by Massanneuve under the head of *gangrène foudroyante*. In these cases there appears, immediately after the receipt of an injury, enormous oedema about the wound, which extends rapidly in every possible direction, followed by the death of the patient within a few hours unless prompt measures are adopted. The puncture of the cellular tissue or of the blood-vessels involved in the oedema prior to the death of the patient gives rise to the escape of a highly offensive gas. Roser mentions a case of this disease in which he promptly amputated [p. 978]the limb of the patient through the healthy parts, without even waiting for the administration of an anæsthetic, and his patient recovered.

The symptoms of septicæmia must necessarily depend greatly on the condition of the patient and the amount of septic material introduced, but it is not deemed necessary to dwell longer on this subject.

DIAGNOSIS.—It is thought that a brief presentation of the etiological, pathological, and semiological differences may be advantageous to busy physicians who desire to obtain, with the least expenditure of time, an accurate knowledge of the chief points of distinction between these morbid conditions. This effort at differentiation is merely intended to place the most important characteristics in marked contrast; and consequently it should be remembered that it is not our intention to give here the complete etiology, pathology, or semiology of either of these morbid states, but only their essential differences. Furthermore, it is thought that the following arrangement will facilitate the object which we desire to accomplish:

[p. 979]

ETIOLOGY.	
PYÆMIA..	SEPTICÆMIA.
1. Pyæmia generally commences with the putrefaction in an open wound of the secondary wound-fluids—pus, etc.—in which there are developed globular bacteria, which enter the blood and certain tissues of the body, where they multiply and produce constitutional disturbances.	1. Septicæmia generally commences with the putrefaction in an open wound of the primary wound-fluids—blood, serum, etc.—in which there are developed rod bacteria, which enter the blood and certain tissues of the body, where they multiply and produce constitutional disturbances.
2. Pyæmia is commonly preceded by some local inflammatory wound-complication, such as suppurative periostitis, osteo-myelitis, etc., and is rarely developed before the end of the second week after the receipt of the injury.	2. Septicæmia is commonly a primary wound-complication, which is generally developed within forty-eight hours after the receipt of the injury.
PATHOLOGY.	
1. Increased coagulability of the blood.	1. Diminished coagulability of the blood.
2. There are metastatic abscesses in various parts of the body, especially in the lungs, liver, and kidneys: serous cavities frequently contain sero-purulent deposits; similar deposits are often found in the joints; abscesses in the cellular tissue; and also abundant evidence of the existence during the life of the patient of pyæmic endo- and pericarditis.	2. Complete absence of purulent or ichorous deposits in all cases of unmixed septicæmia. Post-mortem appearances may be completely negative, with the exception of the condition of the blood, although there is often some oedema of the lungs.
SEMIOLOGY.	
1. Pyæmia commonly commences with a chill.	1. Septicæmia commonly commences without a chill.
2. Fever variable, but rarely entirely intermits.	2. Fever steadily increases, but is lower in the morning.
3. Sudden and great changes in temperature, followed by profuse perspiration.	3. The temperature is high at the beginning of the disease, increases until near the fatal termination, when it falls below the normal. The skin is moist, but without profuse sweatings.
4. Pulse variable; toward the fatal end rapid, feeble, and irregular.	4. Pulse rapid, and gradually increases in frequency toward the fatal end.
5. Facies at the beginning flushed or pallid, toward the end careworn.	5. Facies expressive of a dull, listless condition throughout the whole course of the disease.

6. Tongue smooth, dry, and excessively red, later brown-coated, and even the teeth coated with sordes.	6. Tongue, lips, and throat dry at the commencement, toward the end moist. Thirst is marked.
7. Diarrhœa with stools of a pappy consistence.	7. Rice-water evacuations, very offensive; obstinate vomiting.
8. Epistaxis.	8. Epistaxis rarely occurs.
9. Mild delirium toward the fatal end.	9. A lethargic condition from the beginning, increasing toward the fatal end.
10. Aphthæ in the mouth and throat, sudamina, vesicles, pustules, and purpuric patches.	10. Icteric hue of conjunctivæ; singultus often present.

The differences in the local manifestations occurring in and around the wound, during the progress of these diseases, may be summed up as follows:

At the commencement of this disease the suppuration is commonly checked, the wound becoming dry, and if a discharge continues, it becomes scanty, thin, ichorous, greenish, etc. The granulations, when previously healthy, soon slough, and venous oozing sometimes takes place. There occasionally appears in the later stages of this disease around the wound a reddish erythematous blush, which soon extends over the whole limb.	The odor of putrefaction is commonly very marked within twenty-four hours after the receipt of the injury, the integument slightly reddened about the wound, and the surrounding parts somewhat oedematous. The wound-tissues soon assume a dark-brown color, and are occasionally mottled with dull grayish spots, while the edges of the wound are at the same time blackened, although the movements of the ligature, when arteries have been tied, show us that the blood still rushes against its artificial boundary.

TREATMENT.—It must be admitted that the management of either pyæmia or septicæmia, when fully developed, is always unsatisfactory, and generally unsuccessful; consequently, the success which has attended the use of the prophylactic measures employed in connection with the treatment of wounds during the last ten years has given much satisfaction to the medical profession. The committee of the London Pathological Society reports as follows on this subject: "The accumulation of septic matter in the uterus after labor, in contact with the raw surface left by the separation of the placenta, would also present the conditions favorable to acute septic intoxication. In the present day, when the necessity of thorough drainage of wounds is so thoroughly understood, and the means at the surgeon's command for carrying it out are so efficient, it can only be under peculiar circumstances that a sufficient quantity of putrid serum or pus to yield the fatal dose of the septic poison is allowed to accumulate in the wound. Moreover, the antiseptic treatment of wounds, now so largely adopted, by preventing decomposition of course renders septic intoxication impossible. Ovariotomy would seem to furnish conditions most favorable to septic intoxication, and a large proportion of the deaths occurring in the first forty-eight hours [p. 980]have always been attributed to it. The proportion of fatal cases from this cause has, however, of late been greatly diminished by drainage, and more especially by the employment of the antiseptic treatment."[42]

[42] *Trans. Path. Soc. of London*, vol. xxx. p. 15.

We cannot repeat too frequently or too emphatically the fact that the treatment of pyæmia and septicæmia, when fully developed, is almost invariably unsuccessful, and that consequently he who desires to save the greatest number of lives must make every exertion and use all available means to prevent their development—a task which fortunately has now been brought within the scope of possibility in the large majority of cases. Every surgeon will readily admit that, were it possible to secure union by first intention in all cases of wounds, then it would be impossible for either septicæmia or pyæmia to occur in surgical practice. Therefore, it follows that the character of the wound, the method of operation, the surroundings of the patient, the character of the treatment, become proper points to consider in this division of the subject. The character of the wound and its relations to pyæmia and septicæmia have already been briefly referred to under the etiology of these diseases. The various methods of operating, with their respective advantages and disadvantages, are of course not suitable topics for discussion in this work.

The surroundings of the patient form a subject of vast importance in a prophylactic view, and should never be lost sight of in the construction of hospitals. I desire here to express my firm conviction that surgical pyæmia is essentially and almost wholly a hospital disease. The question of surroundings for the patient presents to my mind the following demands as a sine quâ non for obtaining the best possible results in surgery: (1) Absolute cleanliness. This demand should be strictly enforced in regard to the wound, the patient's body, the bedding, and everything else, including nurses and instruments. (2) Absolute purity of the atmosphere. (3) Moderate and equable temperature, containing a proper amount of moisture. (4) Proper quantity of nutritious and easily digestible food, with suitable drinks, etc. (5) Cheerful and pleasant surroundings, especially in companions, nurses, and other attendants. It may be objected to these conditions that they can never be attained. I must confess that perfection in every detail cannot always be attained, but I am thoroughly convinced that he who makes a determined effort in this direction will succeed far better than that person who is constantly looking about for some excuse for negligence.

The question of treatment brings up the entire subject of antiseptics. The favorite remedies of this class are carbolic and salicylic acids, permanganate of potassium, chloride of zinc, bichloride of mercury, and liquor sodæ chlorinatæ. There is no doubt that good results may be obtained with any of these remedies. The surgeon should never forget that he uses medicines merely as agents to enable him to accomplish certain objects; and, keeping this in mind, he need very seldom fail with his antiseptic when the object is to prevent putrefaction in an open wound. Therefore it appears certain that each method of treatment may possess special advantages in particular cases, and probably the same may be said of the antiseptic itself. The importance of this subject may be more fully appreciated when it is remembered that it is generally admitted by the best surgical authorities [p. 981]that more lives are lost from septic infection than from all other causes combined during a war. The further consideration of this subject may be arranged for convenience under the heads of local and general treatment.

The local treatment of the wound should, if possible, be of such a character as to prevent the absorption of either putrid substances or pus. It therefore becomes highly important, in cases of amputation and other operations, that all tissues injured to such a degree as to be likely to excite either putrefaction, irritation, or inflammation should be removed. The same care is necessary in removing all foreign bodies from the wound in cases where no operation is to be performed. The amputation of the injured limb may be necessary to prevent the development of these diseases, or it may be resorted to in certain rare cases after the origin of pyæmic symptoms; however, in the latter instance great care should be taken to remove all the tissues already infiltrated with serum, otherwise nothing will be gained. The use of the surgeon's knife at the proper time may be the best prophylactic against both pyæmia and septicæmia, but it should be directed by an intelligent mind and the instrument guided by a practiced hand. Again, it is found that opening a large medullary cavity may be attended with danger to the patient. This fact teaches us an obvious lesson.

The wound existing or the operation having been performed, the surgeon now turns his attention to the prevention of putrefaction and inflammation. The first source of danger requiring attention from the surgeon is the fluid escaping from the wounded surface. Do not allow it to undergo putrefaction in contact with the wound. It should not be forgotten that pyæmia is an infectious disease, having its origin in a local nidus, an open wound, in which putrefaction of pus or other wound-fluid is taking place. The question of amputation, or of the extirpation of the parts for the relief of this disease, should only be entertained when the surgeon is confident that he can remove the whole of the infiltrated tissues. In other words, the performance of these operations after the disease has become constitutional can never be advantageous to the patient. Even in those cases where infiltration is limited to the lymphatics, unless all these glands so affected are removed the operation will be unsuccessful. It has been further recommended in the treatment of this disease, in order to prevent the formation of metastatic abscesses, to ligate the veins in which thrombi have formed or may be reasonably expected to form, at some convenient point between the heart and these obstructed points. The value of this proceeding has never been fully determined, and may be reasonably questioned. The formation of metastatic abscesses in various parts of the body within the reach of the surgeon's scalpel demands his attention; and we have been taught by experience that they should be speedily opened, which generally lowers the temperature and diminishes the danger from septic absorption. In the performance of this operation Lister's antiseptic system of wound-treatment should be strictly adhered to, since it unquestionably gives the best results which can be obtained under the circumstances. When the metastatic inflammation which occasionally appears in the thyroid and parotid glands during the course of this disease terminates in the formation of pus, this should be speedily evacuated. This prompt action is often required, particularly for the relief of the grave symptoms which are apt [p. 982]to arise in connection with respiration and deglutition. The accumulation of pus within the joints in pyæmic cases should, it is now thought, be treated in the same manner as abscesses in the cellular tissues—*i.e.* the articulations should be opened and thoroughly disinfected, and afterward kept in a perfectly aseptic condition, and also rendered absolutely immovable during the treatment.

Having directed attention to the more important local measures, we may now briefly enter on the consideration of some of the constitutional remedies. In the general treatment of pyæmia there have been recommended at various times a great variety of drugs, but the general want of success attending their use leaves comparatively few to be mentioned here. The mineral acids are still employed, and are found to be at least agreeable drinks, and as such can be still recommended. The sulphites of magnesium, sodium, potassium, and lime were recommended by Giovanni Polli for the treatment of typhus fever, scarlet fever, small-pox, septicæmia, and pyæmia. He further suggested that the medicine should be given until the whole quantity taken bore to the weight of the patient's body the proportion of 1 to 1000. The experiments made on animals with these salts seem to confirm their value in the treatment of septic diseases. It is certainly true that animals treated with these salts are not so easily affected by septic poison as those which have not received this treatment. Further, it has been shown that putrid substances when mixed with either permanganate of potassium or the sulphite of sodium, and then injected, are harmless, although the same quantity of putrid matter injected without either of these salts destroys life.

Brandy and other alcoholic stimulants have been strongly recommended on account of their well-known antiseptic properties. The sulphate of quinia is certainly, in most cases of pyæmia, a valuable agent. In large doses it enables the surgeon to reduce the temperature of the patient, and in smaller doses it frequently serves a valuable purpose as a tonic. It has also considerable value as an antiseptic.

Lattin has recommended the use of large doses of ergotine in infectious fevers, but this substance, when employed in the treatment of pyæmia, should be given in the formative stage of the disease. The use of drastic cathartics should be avoided, as should that of sudorifics, on account of their prostrating effects. In some cases hypnotics may be required to secure sleep.

Tonics are always more or less useful. The free use of stimulants and nutritious food is also indicated. Brandy, wine, and whiskey may be advantageously used as stimulants. Musk, ammonia, and camphor are occasionally required. However, it should not be forgotten that in cases where the disease has become fully developed the usual termination is death, few recoveries being recorded. In the early stages of this affection, by the removal of the patient from an overcrowded hospital ward to some place where pure air and proper hygienic arrangements can be obtained, recovery may take place, but under other circumstances the prognosis is exceedingly grave.

The treatment of septicæmia in most particulars is the same as that of pyæmia. The first effort should be to prevent the development of the disease, and the second to care for the patient in cases where the affection has already developed. It is not, of course, in our power to limit or in any way [p. 983]regulate the primary injury, for we are obliged to take the patient as he is. The amount of injury to living tissue may be great or small. The question of an operation, the character of the same, and the subsequent management must be determined in accordance with the circumstances of each particular case.

The primary death of the parts is generally due chiefly to the injury itself; the secondary, frequently to bad surgical management. Let us now take a case in which the primary injury has been severe, greatly diminishing, but not destroying, the circulation in the injured parts. Here the immediate application of ice would be injurious, but a warm application might assist nature. It is humiliating to the profession that we are obliged even at this date to admit that the treatment of septicæmia is largely symptomatic. The profuse choleraic diarrhoea which generally accompanies this disease may be regarded as an effort of nature to eliminate the septic poison; but, nevertheless, it is so prostrating in its effects that it requires to be controlled with properly selected astringents, and these remedies may be still further aided by the use of stimulants and tonics.

The treatment of septicæmia may be summarized as follows: (1) A strict adherence to the five rules given under the head of the prophylactic treatment of pyæmia. (2) The avoidance of all putrefaction in contact with the wound, especially prior to the development of sufficient granulations to completely cover its surface. This object is to be accomplished by the removal of all necrotic tissues, the avoidance of putrescent fluids by cleanliness, and the proper use of antiseptic agents. (3) Free use of the alkaline sulphites and hyposulphites. These drugs should be used in all cases where there is reason to anticipate the development of septic diseases, as soon after the receipt of the injury as practicable, but should not be neglected even after the disease has become fully developed. (4) Sulphate of quinia should be used in all cases where the temperature is above 100° F., and its persistent use in large doses may be necessary to prevent the fever from rising still higher. It will be remembered in this connection that experience has taught us that "a temperature of 108.5° F. is the limit beyond which life can no longer exist,"[43] and even a much lower temperature is not without dangers. "The essential danger of fever in acute diseases consists, then, in the deleterious influence of a high temperature on the tissues."[44]

[43] Liebermeister, *New Sydenham Soc. Trans.*, vol. lxvi. p. 278.
[44] *Ibid.*, p. 280.

The treatment of puerperal septicæmia, although requiring the application of the same principles as any other form of this disease, may be briefly described as follows: The womb should be maintained in a firmly-contracted state by the proper use of ergot, even as a prophylactic measure, and also during the whole course of the disease; the uterus and vagina should be kept in an aseptic condition by the efficient use of antiseptics; sulphate of quinia should be given in large doses, and repeated as often as may be necessary in order to lower the temperature; and morphia or some form of opium should be employed for the relief of the pain.

[p. 984]

PUERPERAL FEVER.
BY WILLIAM T. LUSK, M.D.

DEFINITION.—Puerperal fever is an infectious disease, due, as a rule, to the septic inoculation of the wounds which result from the separation of the decidua and the passage of the child through the genital canal in the act of parturition.

To maintain this definition it is, however, necessary to group by themselves cases of childbed fever dependent upon causes which are operative in the non-puerperal condition, though the latter imparts to these causes oftentimes an exceptional activity and virulence. In this category are to be placed especially scarlatina, typhus, typhoid, and malarial fevers. It is to be borne in mind that the zymotic fevers may provoke in the puerperal woman the same inflammatory lesions commonly associated with puerperal fever.[1] This is in accordance with the well-known surgical experience that a febrile paroxysm from any cause exerts an unfavorable influence upon a wounded surface.

[1] Hervieux, *Traité clinique et pratique des maladies puerperales*, pp. 1073 *et seq.*

Like all brief statements, the writer is well aware that the foregoing definition is necessarily imperfect, and stands in need of further limitations to meet the requirements of exactness. Exceptions, however, either apparent or real, will be noted hereafter in their proper connections.

FREQUENCY.—In a careful search through the records preserved by the Health Department of New York City, I found that from 1868 to 1875 inclusive the total number of deaths for nine years was 248,533. Of these, 3342 were from diseases complicating pregnancy, from the accidents of child-bearing, or from diseases of the puerperal state; or, in other words, 1:75 of all the deaths occurring during that period was the result of the performance of what we are in the habit of regarding as a physiological function.

The deaths from miscarriage, from shock, from prolonged labor, from instrumental delivery, from convulsions, from hemorrhage, from rupture of the uterus, and from extra-uterine pregnancy, and deaths from eruptive fevers, from phthisis, and from inflammatory non-puerperal affections complicating childbirth, made a total of 1395, or about 42 per cent. of the entire number. The remaining 1947 cases, variously reported as puerperal fever, puerperal peritonitis, metro-peritonitis, phlebitis, phlegmasia dolens, pyæmia, and septicæmia, represent the very serious sacrifice of life resulting from inflammatory processes which have their starting-point in the generative apparatus. If we apply the general term, puerperal fever, to this class of cases, it will be seen that the malady is the cause of nearly one [p. 985]one-hundred-and-twenty-seventh of all the deaths occurring in the city. The actual number of births for the nine years in question was roughly estimated at 284,000[2]—an estimate erring upon the side of liberality. The total number of deaths to the entire number of confinements was, then, at least in the proportion of 1:85, or, from puerperal fever alone, in the proportion of 1:146. Garrigues[3] examined the records of the various city institutions during the period in question, and from them estimated the number of births which took place in hospitals at 10,572. The recorded deaths were 420. Deducting these from the totals given above, the general death-rate in civil practice from puerperal causes in New York City was in the proportion of 1:94. Max Boehr[4] in his now-famous statistics reckons that one-thirtieth of all married women in Prussia die in childbed. The Puerperal Fever Commission[5] appointed by the Berlin Society of Obstetrics and Gynæcology arrived at the conclusion that from 10-15 per cent. of the deaths occurring in women during the period of sexual activity were due to childbed fever, and that this disease destroyed nearly as many lives as small-pox or cholera. But puerperal fever differs from either small-pox or cholera in that the latter presses largely upon the aged and the very young, while the former gathers its victims exclusively from a selected class—viz. from women in adult life, the mothers of families, whose loss, as a rule, is a public as well as a private calamity.

[2] This estimate was based upon the assumption that the natural birth-rate is 33 to the 1000—a proportion believed by the statisticians of the Board of Health to be approximatively correct, though probably somewhat in excess of the reality. P. Osterloh has recently stated that my statistics were computed in so arbitrary a manner as to render deductions from them valueless. In this, however, he is mistaken. The most conscientious care was taken in their preparation; wherever the possibility of error existed the fact was distinctly indicated, and all calculations were made in such a way that whatever corrections might be required would strengthen the conclusions.

[3] "On Lying-in Institutions," *Trans. Am. Gyn. Soc.*, vol. ii., 1878.

[4] "Untersuchungen über die Haüfigkeit des Todes im Wochenbett in Preussen," *Zeitschr. f. Geburtsk. und Gynaek.*, vol. iii. p. 82.

[5] *Zeitschr. f. Geburtsk. und Gynaek.*, vol. iii. p. 1.

For those who regard statistics with habitual distrust it may perhaps be well to state that the foregoing frightful picture is no exaggeration, but is less sombre than the actual truth.

Before proceeding to consider the nature of puerperal fever it is desirable to first recall the anatomical lesions with which it is associated. These, it will be found, are for the most part inflammatory processes having their starting-point in injuries of the genital passage produced by parturition, complicated in many cases by septic changes in the blood, by secondary degeneration of parenchymatous organs, and at times by phlegmonous and erysipelatous affections in remote as well as in the adjacent serous and cutaneous tissues.

MORBID ANATOMY.—The primary lesions connected with puerperal fever are so various that the student will find it convenient to classify them according as they are situated in the mucous membrane of the utero-vaginal canal, the parenchyma of the uterus, the pelvic cellular tissue, the peritoneum, the lymphatics, or the veins. Not, indeed, that such an arrangement is strictly in accordance with clinical experience—as a rule, the inflammatory processes are rarely limited to a single tissue—but because the prognosis and treatment [p. 986]are determined in great measure by the tissue-system which is predominantly affected. The significance of puerperal inflammations, wherever seated, likewise depends upon whether they are local and circumscribed or whether they present a spreading character.

Personally, I have found the following classification of Spiegelberg[6] of great utility as a means of keeping in mind the principal points to which inquiry should be directed in estimating the significance of the febrile conditions of childbed:

1. Inflammation of the Genital Mucous Membrane.—Endocolpitis and endometritis.

a. Superficial.

b. Ulcerative (diphtheritic).

2. Inflammation of the Uterine Parenchyma, and of the Subserous and Pelvic Cellular Tissue.

a. Exudation circumscribed.

b. Phlegmonous, diffused; with lymphangitis and pyæmia (lymphatic form of peritonitis).

3. Inflammation of the Peritoneum covering the Uterus and its Appendages.—Pelvic peritonitis and diffused peritonitis.

4. Phlebitis Uterina and Para-uterina, with formation of thrombi, embolism, and pyæmia.

5. Pure Septicæmia.—Putrid absorption.

[6] "Ueber das Wesen des Puerperalfiebers," *Volkmann's Samml. klin. Vortr.*, No. 3.

ENDOCOLPITIS AND ENDOMETRITIS.—In the superficial, catarrhal form of inflammation the mucous membrane of the vagina is swollen and hyperæmic, the papillæ are enlarged, and the discharge is profuse; in the vaginal portion of the cervix the labia uterina are oedematous and covered with granulations which bleed at the slightest touch; in the cavity of the body there are increased transudation of serum and abundant pus-formation. The deep structures of the uterus are usually not affected. Sometimes the inflammation extends to the tubes—*salpingitis*—or, passing outward through the fimbriated extremities, it may spread over the adjacent peritoneum.

The small wounds at the vaginal orifice are at times converted into ulcers with tumefied borders. These so-called puerperal ulcers are covered with a greenish-yellow layer. They are associated usually with oedematous swelling of the labia. Under favorable sanitary conditions the deposit, which consists in the main of pus-cells, clears away and the surface heals by granulation. The ulcerative form of inflammation is very rare outside of crowded hospitals.

Diphtheritic ulcers are situated with greatest frequency in the neighborhood of the posterior commissure or around the vaginal orifice. In rarer instances they are found upon the anterior wall and in the fornix of the vagina, in the cervix, and upon the site of the placenta. The borders are red and jagged; the base is covered with a yellowish-gray, shreddy membrane; the secretion is purulent, alkaline, and fetid; and the adjacent tissues are oedematous. From the vulva they may extend to the perineum or pursue a serpiginous course down the thighs. In the uterus and about the cervix they vary as regards size, and are either of a rounded shape or form narrow bands. The intervening portions of tissue which have not undergone destructive changes swell and stand out in strong [p. 987]relief. Where the entire inner surface has become necrosed, it is often covered with a smeary, chocolate-brown mass which, when washed away with a stream of water, leaves exposed either the deepest layer of the mucous membrane or the underlying muscular structures.

The difference between the superficial ulcerations of the genital canal and the diphtheritic form involving destruction of the deeper tissues is due to the presence in the latter of minute organisms termed micrococci, the relations of which to puerperal infection will be considered in a subsequent division.

METRITIS AND PARAMETRITIS.—In ulcerative endometritis, and even in the extreme catarrhal form, the parenchyma of the uterus likewise becomes involved. The changes which are designated under the term metritis consist in the first place of oedematous infiltration of the tissues. As a consequence, the organ contracts imperfectly and becomes soft and flabby, so that sometimes, upon post-mortem examination, it bears the imprint of the intestines.

In diphtheritic endometritis the gangrenous process may attack the muscular tissue, and give rise to losses of muscular substance—a condition known as necrotic endometritis or putrescence of the uterus.

Inflammatory changes are rarely lacking in the intermuscular connective tissue, which exhibits in places serous or gelatinous infiltration, with afterward pus formation, and with here and there small abscesses. The sero-purulent infiltration of the connective tissue is specially marked beneath the peritoneal covering of the uterus either behind or along the sides at the attachment of the broad ligaments. In the same situations the lymphatics, which normally are barely perceptible to the naked eye, are sometimes enlarged to the size of a quill, and are characterized by varicose dilatations occurring singly or presenting a beaded arrangement. In the substance of the uterus the dilated vessels are liable to be mistaken for small abscesses. The pus-like substance contained in the lymphatics is composed of pus-cells and of micrococci. From the cellular tissue surrounding the vagina, or that beneath the peritoneal covering of the uterus, the inflammation may spread by contiguity of tissue between the folds of the broad ligament, and thence pass upward to the iliac fossæ. Usually the process is unilateral. After the inflammation has crossed the linea terminalis it may take a forward direction above the sheath of the ilio-psoas muscle to Poupart's ligament, or it may creep upward, following the course, according to the side affected, of the ascending or descending colon, to the region of the kidney. It is rare for inflammation of the cellular tissue to travel around the bladder to the front. In such cases it pursues its course between the walls of the bladder and the uterus, and along the round ligament to the inguinal canal. In a few cases the cellulitis mounts above Poupart's ligament, between the peritoneum and the abdominal wall.

The course of the inflammation is not simply fortuitous, but follows prearranged pathways in the connective tissue. König[7] and Schlesinger[8] have shown that when air, water, or liquefied glue is forced into the cellular tissue between the broad ligaments the injected mass has a tendency to invade the iliac fossæ. In Schlesinger's experiments, if the canula of the syringe was inserted into the anterior layer of the broad ligament, [p. 988]the glue spread between the folds to the abdominal end of the Fallopian tube; thence, following the track of the vessels, it passed to the linea terminalis; and finally mounted upward along the colon or swept forward to Poupart's ligament until the advance was stopped at the outer border of the round ligament. If the injection was made to the side of the cervix through the posterior layer at the junction of the cervix and the body, the posterior layer gradually bulged out, the peritoneum was lifted from the side wall of the pelvis, and the glue passed beyond the vessels to reach the iliac fossa. If the injection was made to the side of the cervix through the anterior layer, the glue passed between the bladder and the uterus, and forward along the round ligament to the inguinal canal, while another portion of the fluid passed between the layers of the broad ligament, and reached the peritoneal covering of the side walls behind the round ligament. If the injection was made in the median line in a peritoneal fold of Douglas's cul-de-sac, the fluid travelled forward upon one side along the round ligament and thence to the posterior wall of the bladder.

[7] *Arch. der Heilkunde*, 3 Jahrg., 1862.

[8] *Gynaekologische Studien*, No. 1.

The term parametritis, introduced into use by Virchow, is, properly speaking, limited to inflammation of the connective tissue immediately adjacent to the uterus, the older one of pelvic cellulitis furnishing a more comprehensive designation for cases where, as a consequence of a progressive advance from the point of departure in the genital canal, the remoter regions have likewise been invaded. Connective-tissue inflammation presents, as the first essential characteristic, an acute oedema, the fluid which fills the gaps and interspaces consisting of transuded serum rendered opaque by the presence of pus-cells or possessing a gelatinous character. In the mild, uncomplicated cases the oedema disappears rapidly. Where the cell-collections are of moderate extent the entire process may vanish without leaving a trace of its existence. If the cell-elements, on the other hand, are present in great abundance, they, as a rule, first undergo fatty degeneration, and, after the absorption of the fluid portion, form a hard tumor composed of a fine granular detritus, which under favorable circumstances likewise after a few weeks becomes absorbed. In rare cases abscess-formation in the tumor results.

In the cellulitis resulting from septic infection, especially in cases complicated by diphtheritis, the tissues seem as if soaked with dirty serum, and contain scattered yellowish deposits, which soon present, even to the naked eye, the appearance of pus-collections. This sero-purulent oedema is always associated with lymphangitis, the lymphatic vessels possessing varicose dilatations and beaded arrangements similar to those already described in the uterine tissue. The foregoing changes are most distinct in the firm connective tissue adjacent to the uterus and at the hilum of the ovary, while they are less clearly traced in the looser structure of the broad ligament (Spiegelberg).

In favorable cases the inflammation is circumscribed, or at least is limited, by the nearest lymphatic glands. In cases of intense infection it spreads rapidly, and justifies the title bestowed upon it by Virchow of parametritic malignant erysipelas.

PELVIC AND DIFFUSED PERITONITIS.—Inflammation of the pelvic peritoneum may result from severe attacks of catarrhal endometritis, the inflammatory process either traversing the uterine tissue or passing[p. 989]through the Fallopian tubes to the adjacent serous membrane; or it may proceed, secondarily, from the stretching and irritation occasioned by an associated parametritis.

As a rule, pelvic peritonitis is not attended with much exudation. The latter is situated upon the folds of the peritoneum limiting the cul-de-sac of Douglas, upon the ovaries, and upon the broad ligaments. In favorable cases it consists of fibrinous flakes and fluid pus. If the latter is abundant, it may become encysted by the formation of adhesions between the pelvic organs.

General peritonitis may result from the extension of a pelvic peritonitis, or from the transport of poison through the lymphatics into the peritoneal sac. In the first case the entire peritoneum is injected, and the contents of the abdominal cavity are loosely bound together by pseudo-membranes, composed of pus and coagulated fibrine. The intestines are at the same time distended and the diaphragm is pushed upward. In the so-called peritonitis lymphatica the inflammatory symptoms are at the outset lacking. The abdominal cavity is found filled with a thin, stinking, greenish or brownish fluid composed of serum and micrococci. The intestines are lax and oedematous, and the muscular structures are paralyzed, with resulting tympanitic distension. The peritoneal covering of the intestines is devoid of lustre, and covered with injected patches, or is stained of a dark-brown color. Death often ensues before the occurrence of exudation.

Septic forms of pelvic inflammation are often associated with oöphoritis, the dilated lymphatics either extending to the substance of the ovaries, where they may lead to the production of small abscesses, or, as a result of blood-dissolution, the organs become soft, pulpy, and infiltrated with discolored serum, and present hemorrhagic spots distributed over the surface.

PHLEBITIS AND PHLEBO-THROMBOSIS.—The formation of thrombi in the uterine and pelvic veins is sufficiently common during the puerperal period. The coagulation may result from compression or from enfeeblement of the circulation. A predisposition to its occurrence is created by relaxation of the uterine tissue. A normal thrombus is in itself harmless. In time it becomes organized, and the occluded vessel is converted into a connective-tissue cord, or a channel may form through it which permits the passage of the blood-stream. When, however, pus or septic matters obtain access to a thrombus, it undergoes rapid disintegration, and the particles get swept away into the circulation until arrested in the ramifications of the pulmonary artery. Wherever these poisoned emboli happen to lodge inflammation is set up in the adjacent tissues, and abscesses result (pyæmia multiplex). Sometimes countless collections of pus may form in the lungs. Less commonly abscesses are found in the liver or spleen, originating either from emboli which have already made the pulmonary circuit or from thrombi in the pulmonary veins.

Inflammation of the veins (phlebitis) sometimes occurs when the vessels have to traverse tissues in or near the uterus infiltrated with purulent or septic materials. The endothelium then undergoes proliferation, and thrombosis is produced. Phlebitic thrombi do not necessarily break down, and may in that case act as a barrier to the progression of septic germs into the circulation (Spiegelberg). As a rule, however, [p. 990]under the influence of inflammation and infection, they become converted into puriform masses.

The thrombi grow by accretion in the direction of the heart. They may extend from the uterus through the internal spermatic, or through the hypogastric and common iliac veins, to the vena cava. Sometimes the thrombus may be traced back to the placental site.

SEPTICÆMIA.—From these local conditions, sooner or later, secondary affections develop in distant organs. The general affection is, in great part at least, likewise of local origin. Sometimes, however, where the poison, which enters the system through the lymphatics and veins, is very active and abundant, death may follow from acute septicæmia before the changes in the sexual organs have had time to develop. The fatal result in these cases is probably due to paralysis of the heart. After death post-mortem decomposition rapidly sets in, the blood is sticky, and swelling is found in the various parenchymatous organs.

The secondary affections consist in the metastatic abscesses already noticed as produced by infected emboli, in circumscribed purulent collections due to the conveyance of septic materials into the blood-current through the lymphatics, in ulcerative endocarditis, in inflammations of the pleura, the pericardium, and the meninges, and in purulent inflammation of the joints.

A study of the nature of puerperal fever will best show how intimately these seemingly distinct processes are linked together.

EARLIER VIEWS CONCERNING THE NATURE OF PUERPERAL FEVER.[9]—According to the teachings of Hippocrates, Galen, and Avicenna, of Ambrose Paré, of Sydenham, and of Smellie, the fevers of puerperal women were attributable to the suppression of the lochia. For twenty centuries this doctrine was accepted almost without dispute, the best clinical observers confounding a symptom which is often lacking with the cause of the disease itself.

[9] For data given, and for a great variety of historical information, vide Hervieux, *Traité clinique et pratique des maladies puerperales.*

In 1686, Puzos[10] taught that milk, circulating in the blood, is attracted to the uterus during pregnancy and to the breasts after confinement, but that milk metastases may form in other parts, and produce the symptoms of malignant or intermittent fever. In 1746, A. de Jussieu, Col de Villars, and Fontaine advanced in support of this theory the fact that they had found, on opening the abdomen in women who had died from an epidemic which raged that year in Paris, a free lactescent fluid in the lower portion of the abdominal cavity and clotted milk adherent to the intestines. This doctrine, which seemed to be based upon, and to accord with, observation, found many adherents in France. It lost ground, however, when, in 1801, Bichat pointed out the true nature of the abdominal effusions of women who had died in childbed, and demonstrated that they were to be found likewise in peritoneal inflammations occurring in men and in non-puerperal women.

[10] *Premier Mémoire sur les Dépôts lacteux.*

While, during the second half of the eighteenth century, the doctrine of milk metastasis held full sway in France, in England and Germany the dominant leaders in medicine referred the causes of puerperal fevers to inflammations of the womb and of the peritoneum. With the advances made in pathological anatomy in the beginning of the present century, France taking the lead, stress was likewise laid upon inflammations of the veins and of the lymphatics. The vitality of the doctrine of local inflammations is well shown by the records kept by the Health Board of this city, where a large proportion of the deaths returned from childbed fever are entered under the head of metritis, of peritonitis, of metro-peritonitis, and of puerperal phlebitis.

In opposition to the doctrines of the so-called localists, the theory that puerperal fever is an essential fever, and as much a distinct disease as typhus fever, typhoid fever, or relapsing fever, has been strenuously advocated by some of the most distinguished clinical teachers who have devoted their attention to obstetrical science.

Fordyce Barker, the most recent exponent of the essentiality of puerperal fever, in his classical work upon the *Puerperal Diseases*, states the arguments against the local origin of the diseases as follows: 1st, that puerperal fever has no characteristic lesions; 2d, that the lesions which do exist are often not sufficient to influence the progress of the disease or to explain the cause of death; 3d, that there may be inflammation, even to an intense degree, of any of the organs in which the principal lesions of puerperal fever are found, and yet the disease will lack some of the essential characteristics of puerperal fever; 4th, that the lesions are essentially different from spontaneous or idiopathic inflammations of the tissues where these lesions are found; 5th, that puerperal fever is often communicable from one patient to another through the medium of a third party, and that this is not the fact in regard to simple inflammations in puerperal women.

However, neither Barker, nor those who entertain views similar to his, question the local origin of many febrile affections in childbed, but claim that purely local inflammations have each their characteristic symptoms, which differ from those of true puerperal fever, that puerperal fever is a zymotic disease of unknown origin, and that local lesions, where they coexist, are not the primary source of trouble, but are secondary to changes in the blood.

In 1850, James Y. Simpson[11] published a short paper "On the Analogy between Puerperal and Surgical Fever." This article may well be regarded as the foundation of the modern doctrine concerning puerperal fever, and is well worthy of perusal at the present day; for, though in the then existing state of pathology many of the links were wanting which have since raised the argument to nearly a mathematical demonstration, the paper furnishes a brilliant example of the scientific foresight which is able to discern the truth even where the evidence lacks completeness.

[11] *Edinburgh Medical Journal.*

In 1847, Semmelweis, who was at that time clinical assistant to the Lying-in Hospital at Vienna, made the startling assertion that "puerperal patients were chiefly attacked with puerperal fever when they had been examined by the physicians who were fresh from contact with the poisons engendered by cadaveric decay; that fever ensued in the practice of those who after post-mortem examination washed their hands in the usual manner, whereas no fever or but few cases of disease followed when the examiner had previously washed his hands in a solution of chloride of lime." In the face of insult, ridicule, and abuse Semmelweis maintained this position for years, almost unaided, with fanatical persistency. It was easy for his opponents, for the most part managers of the great lying-in asylums, to show from clinical experiences the weakness of so one-sided a theory. But the employment of the equivocal demonstration *falsus in uno, falsus in omnibus*, served only as a temporary defence against the laxity which prevailed in hospital management only a quarter of a century ago. Though Semmelweis died with no other reward than the scorn of his contemporaries, it is impossible at the present day to so much as contemplate the abuses he attacked without a shudder.

In 1860, Semmelweis published the result of his ripened experience in a treatise entitled *Die Aetiologie der Begriff und die Prophylaxis des Kindbettfiebers*, in which, abandoning his earlier exclusive position, he maintained that puerperal fever arises from the absorption of putrid animal substances, which produce first alterations in the blood, and secondly exudations. He distinguished between cases in which the infection was introduced from some external source, and which he believed to be the most frequent variety, and those where the poison was generated in the system. The sources from which the infection is derived he believed to be—1st, from the dead body, regardless of age, sex, or disease, no matter whether the latter is of puerperal or non-puerperal origin, the virulence depending upon the stage of decomposition; 2d, diseased persons, whose malady is associated with decomposition of animal tissue, no matter whether the affected person suffers from childbed fever or not, the decomposing matter alone furnishing the product from which infection is derived; 3d, physiological animal substances in the process of decomposition. As carriers of infection he regarded the fingers and hands of the physician, midwife, or nurse, sponges, instruments, soiled clothing, the atmosphere, and, in brief, anything which, after being defiled with decomposing animal matter, was brought into contact with the genitals of a woman during or subsequent to parturition. Absorption takes place from the inner surface of the uterus or from traumata in the genital canal. Infection seldom occurs in pregnancy, because of the closure of the os internum, the absence of wounded surfaces, and because of the rarity with which examinations are made; during dilatation infection is common, but exceptional during the period of expulsion, because the inner uterine surface is at that time rendered inaccessible by the advance of the child; in the placental and puerperal period infection occurs from utensils and instruments, but chiefly through the access of atmospheric air when the latter is loaded with decomposing organic matter. In rare instances auto-infection may result from spontaneous decomposition of the lochia, of bits of decidua, of coagula of blood, of necrosed tissue, or in consequence of severe instrumental labors. In a word, puerperal fever was according to Semmelweis no new specific disease, but a variety of pyæmia.

I have been thus particular in giving prominence to the labors of Semmelweis partly from justice to a man who was hated and despised in his lifetime, and partly because I believe that few outside of Germany are really cognizant of the immense service he rendered to humanity, or that to him is really due a large part of what is now current doctrine concerning the nature and prophylaxis of puerperal fever.

THE NATURE OF PUERPERAL FEVER AS REGARDED FROM THE[p. 993]STANDPOINT OF MODERN INVESTIGATION.—The older beliefs in the suppression of the lochia and the metastases of milk have long since been relegated to the domain of old nurses' lore, and do not call for serious discussion. The localist theory, that puerperal fever is a metritis, a peritonitis, a phlebitis, or an inflammation of the lymphatics, is, as mortuary records show, still adhered to by many practitioners, and, as we have seen, is justified by the fact that puerperal fever is, with rare exceptions, associated at some period of its progress with certain inflammatory processes which have their starting-point in the generative apparatus. But the localist theory leaves out of view the existence of blood-poisoning, and yet the coexistence of a blood-poison with the local lesions is an essential feature of puerperal fever. It was this defect which gave to the advocates of the specificity of puerperal fever their real importance. The outcome of modern investigation tends, however, to prove that the puerperal poison is of a septic nature, and that the usual points of introduction of the poison are the lesions of the parturient canal. This does not, indeed, exclude other points of entry, for clinical experience renders it probable that, under certain conditions, the poison may be primarily introduced into the blood through the respiratory and digestive organs. Puerperal fever is really a surgical fever, modified, however, by the peculiar physiological conditions which belong to the puerperal state. The argument against its septic origin is based chiefly upon mistaken ideas concerning the nature of septicæmia. So long as the symptoms of the latter were derived for the most part from the effects observed as a consequence of injecting putrid materials into the veins of dogs, a confusion arose from the fact that the results obtained were commonly those of putrid intoxication, and not those of true septicæmia. Under such circumstances it was not difficult to formulate definitions of septicæmia which could be shown to be at variance with the phenomena which ordinarily exist in puerperal fever.

The argument that the infectious diseases of childbed are of a septic nature can best be understood by presenting the proofs in their orderly sequence.

1st. *It is demonstrable that septic poisons are capable of producing the lesions ordinarily associated with puerperal fever.* Thus, it is a matter of ordinary experience that the retention of a small bit of the membranes within the uterus will produce fetid lochia, and, as the result of infection, a febrile condition, which, as a rule, subsides with the expulsion of the offending body and the use of disinfectant washes. A virulent form of fever is not unfrequently occasioned by retained coagula or placental débris which have undergone decomposition. I was once sent for to see a puerperal patient suffering from fever on the fourth day following her confinement. On entering the room I found the stench intolerable; turning down the sheets, I discovered that the patient was lying in a decomposing mass, and learned that her doctor had forbidden, after the birth of her child, the removal of the soiled linen and blankets. The patient died in the third week from pyæmia multiplex.

Haussmann[12] reported a case of auto-infection in the rabbit which terminated fatally. A portion of the membrane, retained in the left cornu,[p. 994]led to diphtheritic losses of substance in the lower portion of the vagina, to hemorrhagic enteritis, and to peritonitis. The same author produced death from septicæmia by injecting into the gravid uterus of one rabbit serum from the abdomen of another which had died from infection. The postmortem examination showed the muscles filled with granules and the peritoneum injected, but no fibrino-purulent exudation. Injections into the uterus of pus from the abdomen of a woman who had died from infectious puerperal disease produced no effect upon rabbits two weeks gravid, while in the second half of pregnancy premature delivery and death occurred, in one case in one and a half, in another in two and a half, days. In the animal which died in thirty-six hours there was commencing perimetritis and peritonitis, while in the one that died after the lapse of sixty hours the abdomen was found to contain fibrine and pus.[13] D'Espine injected into the uterus of a rabbit which had just produced her young pus from the abdomen of a woman who had died from puerperal disease two days before. This was subsequently followed by other injections of fetid fluids during the four days following. On the twelfth day the animal died. The autopsy revealed peritonitis, most marked in the pelvic cavity, inflammatory alterations in the vagina, uterus, and tubes, small abscesses in the body of the uterus, softened clots in the veins of the broad ligaments, and infarctions of the liver.[14] Schüller found that subcutaneous injections of septic material in female animals during pregnancy produced a diphtheritic ulcerative process on the uterine surface, which determined the separation of the placenta; diphtheritic patches, likewise, were found in the cornua of the uterus.[15]

[12] "Entstehung der übertragbaren Krankheiten des Wochenbettes," *Beitr. zur Geburtsk. und Gynaek.*, Bd. iii. Heft 3, p. 345.

[13] *Contribution à l'étude de la septicémie puerpérale*, Paris, 1873, p. 28.

[14] *Ibid.*, p. 394.

[15] "Experimentelle Beiträge zum Studium der septischen Infection,"*Deutsch. Zeitschr. für Chir.*, Bd. vi. p. 141.

Thus we find that in the human subject and in experiments made upon animals septic poisons introduced into the system following or near delivery produce lesions similar to those found in puerperal fever. As a further coincidence, we notice that, as in puerperal fever, the lesions from direct septic poisoning have nothing characteristic about them, producing in one case pyæmia, in another partial peritonitis, in another general peritonitis, in another diphtheritis, while in others the lesions are comparatively trivial, these differences being due to variable facta, such as the qualities of the septic poisons, the points of entry into the organism, and the resistance offered by the invaded tissues.

2d. *Septicæmia is a disease characterized by the invariable presence in the organism infected of minute bodies generally termed bacteria.*[16]

[16] In 1865, Mayrhofer (*Mon. Schr. f. Geburtsk.*, vol. xxv., p. 112, 1865), at that time clinical assistant to the Lying-in Service of Braun in Vienna, stimulated by the researches of Pasteur, maintained that septic endometritis was the result of putrid fermentation within the uterine cavity, and drew attention to the vibrios—a term which he applied to the round as well as to the rod-like bacteria—as the source, and not the product, of putrefaction. He

claimed that while in puerperal processes vibrios are always present, in healthy women they never occur before the second, third, or fourth day, and not always even then. The chief progress that has been made as regards our knowledge of puerperal fever in the last ten years has been in the direction of strengthening Mayrhofer's argument by careful experiment, and by defining the action of microscopic fungi in the production of septic morbid processes.

Until very recently the whole subject of septicæmia has been in a state of wellnigh hopeless confusion. From Gaspard and Panum, through a long list of experimenters, hardly any two arrived at precisely similar [p. 995]results. Something like an approach to order has, however, been produced since it has begun to be understood that the effects produced by septic fluids vary with the quality of the poison and the method of experimentation, and that to obtain identity in the result there must be identity in all the conditions. Thus, Samuel has shown that the same organic substance produces different effects at different stages of decomposition; again, that the enteritis which is commonly quoted as characteristic of septic poisoning occurs, as a rule, in animals when the septic fluid is injected directly into the blood, and is rare when it finds its way into the circulation through the lymphatics, as is the case usually in clinical experiences.[17] There is one experimental point of extreme practical importance too in connection with puerperal septicæmia—viz. that if the injection of a septic fluid be made directly into a vessel, toxic effects speedily follow, but are transitory, unless the amount of the fluid be large, or its virulence exceptional, or the animal very young;[18] whereas very small amounts injected subcutaneously, by developing rapidly-spreading phlegmonous inflammation, resembling malignant erysipelas in man, are capable, after a period of incubation, of producing fatal results; or they may, if injected into a shut cavity or underneath a fascia, lead to the development of an inflammation of an ichorous character. In other words, the eliminating organs suffice, under ordinary conditions, to remove from the blood the same amount of septic fluid which would prove fatal if injected into the tissues.[19] To produce similar results the injections into the blood need to be repeated at intervals. This experience leads us to the conclusion that in the tissues septic poison possesses the capacity of self-multiplication, and that in the local inflammation set up a reservoir is formed from which poison is continuously poured into the circulation.

[17] *Loc. cit.*, p. 349.

[18] "Traube und Gescheidlen, Versüche über Faülniss und den Widerstand des lebender Organismus," *Schles. Ges. f. vaterländische Cultur*, Feb. 13, 1874.

[19] In some instances in which absorption from the tissues is very rapid the effects of subcutaneous injections may be similar to those produced by injections made directly into the circulation, and the local lesion be insignificant.

This capacity of self-multiplication which septic fluids possess has recently been found to be coincident with the presence of certain parasitic bodies, generically termed bacteria. All carefully-made experiments serve to show that if a septic fluid be deprived of these organic bodies by boiling or filtration while it continues capable of producing inflammation, the inflammation is usually of diminished intensity and remains local in its character;[20] whereas the bacteria retained upon the filter possess all the virulent properties of the original fluid.[21] This does not alone necessarily prove that the virus resides in the bacteria, for it does not exclude the possibility that both the virus and the bacteria remain upon the filter.

[20] In filtration through porous earthenware cylinders the filtrate possesses no phlogogenic properties.

[21] Tiegel, *Correspondenzblatt für Schweizer Aertze*, 1871, S. 1275; Klebs,*Archiv für exp. Pathol. und Pharmakol.*, Bd. i. Heft. 1, S. 35.

So far, attempts at isolating the microspores of septicæmia and cultivating them separately in vehicles composed of water holding in solution inorganic constituents, or sterilized fluids containing organic matters, or of the semi-solid gelatinous substances recommended by Koch, have been only partially successful in proving them to be the sole source of[p. 996]infection. Some earlier experiments of Tiegel and Klebs[22] were attended with positive results, and more recently confirmatory evidence has been furnished by Pasteur and Doléris.[23] Hiller, rarely quoted now, arrived at different conclusions. He found that bacteria washed in pure water were innocuous.[24] But pure water had long before been proven by observers to be inimical to the well-being of the organisms in question. Schüller says that Hiller's experiments prove apparently that while a putrid fluid may be in the highest degree poisonous, its component parts—viz. either the fluid or the bacteria singly—are neither deadly nor poisonous.[25] The fact is, that isolation experiments are subject to what has hitherto been in most experiments an unavoidable source of error. As Davaine noted early in his observations, the physiological action of bacteria is very dependent on the constitution of the medium in which they are developed, which is in entire harmony with what is known of organisms much higher in the scale. "Many plants," says Burdon-Sanderson,[26] "containing active principles, become inert when transplanted from an appropriate soil." Bucholtz, in a series of experiments designed to test the influence of antiseptics upon the vitality of bacteria, found not only a difference between those taken directly from the infusion and those cultivated in artificial fluids, but between bacteria derived from the same source and cultivated in modifications of the nutrient medium.[27] Then, too, it is not always safe to transfer to the human species the results of experiments made upon the lower animals. Indeed, among animals, not only in different species, but in varieties of the same species, differences in the susceptibility to septicæmic poisons are found ranging from gradations as to the intensity of the effect produced to absolute immunity. In anthrax, a disease analogous to the one in question, the bacterial origin has been established beyond dispute by the inoculation of isolated bacilli, which multiply in the blood and permeate in enormous numbers the lungs, liver, kidneys, spleen, and glandular structures. If the same unequivocal testimony has as yet not been obtained from isolation experiments as regards septicæmia, it is reasonable to suppose that this is due to the defects in the technique, for which it is presumable the ingenuity of investigators will in future find the remedy.

[22] *Archiv für exp. Pathologie und Pharmakologie*, "Beiträge zur Kenntniss der Pathogenen Schistomyceten," Band iv. Heft 3, S. 241 und ff.; Tiegel, *loc. cit.*

[23] In this connection may be mentioned some very interesting experiments by Dr. George Gaffky (*Experimentellen Erzengte Septicæmie, Mittheilungen aus den Kaiserlich, Gesundh. Amte*), in which micrococci from the blood of septicæmic mice were successfully cultivated in a gelatine preparation, and produced, when inoculated in small quantities, the symptoms identical with those obtained by inoculating the blood itself.

[24] "Exp. Beiträge zur Lehre von der organisirte Natur der Contagion und von der Faülniss," *Archiv für klinische Chirurgie*, Bd. xvii. Heft 4, S. 669 u. ff.

[25] "Exp. Beiträge zum Studium der septischen Infection," *Deutsche Zeitschrift für Chirurgie*, Bd. vi. S. 162.

[26] "Lectures on the Relations of Bacteria to Disease," *British Med. Journal*, March 27, 1875. See also Klebs, "Beiträge zur Kenntniss der Pathogenen Schistomyceten," *Arch. für Pathol. und Pharmakol.*, Bd. iii. S. 321.

[27] "Antiseptica und Bacterien," *Arch. f. exp. Pathol. und Pharmakol.*, Bd. iv., Heft 1 und 2.

It is, however, from the constant presence of the bacteria in infected wounds, and their distribution through the tissues, that the argument in favor of connecting septic symptoms with the bacteria has been mainly deduced. Here the ground is sufficiently solid, and, judged by ordinary laws of scientific evidence, the pathological importance of the microspores [p. 997]may be regarded as established. To be sure, we find them in tongue-scrapings of healthy individuals, but tongue-scrapings are poisonous if injected into the tissues. That they do not ordinarily prove so in the mouth is no more singular than that woorari can be swallowed with impunity. Tiegel[28] has endeavored to show that round bacteria are found normally in the internal organs of the body; but Koch[29] states that he has on many occasions examined normal blood and normal tissues by means which prevented the possibility of overlooking bacteria, or of confounding them with granular masses of equal size, and that he has never in a single instance found organisms.

[28] *Arch. f. Path. Anat. u. Physiol. u. f. klin. Med.*, vol. lx. p. 453.

[29] On *Traumatic Infective Diseases*, New Sydenham Soc. publication p. 15.

It is stated that bacteria are sometimes absent from the blood withdrawn during life in septic diseases. As, however, their constant presence has been confirmed in the vessels and glomeruli of the kidneys, it is fair to assume that those organs, acting as filters, must have received the colonies observed in them from the general circulation.

The difficulty of obtaining bacteria from the blood in many cases during life in septic diseases does not, however, as was once supposed, invalidate the theory of their pathogenic importance. Septicæmia is at present employed as a collective term for a number of processes which may occur singly or in combination with one another. When a relatively large quantity of a putrid fluid is injected into the veins of an animal, death follows from the action of a chemical poison (sepsin). The blood during life rarely displays the presence of bacteria, the latter disappearing in the circulation. In animals thus poisoned blood does not possess infectious properties. This form is termed putrid intoxication. That the poison in these cases is, however, produced by the bacteria is shown by experiments of Gutmann,[30] who demonstrated that bacteria from a drop of putrid blood cultivated in Cohn's solution developed in the fluid a poison which, when injected into the veins of dogs, occasioned death with all the symptoms of putrid intoxication. Still more conclusive were the experiments of Koch. This observer injected four drops of putrid blood beneath the skin of mice. The latter died in from four to eight hours. There were no bacteria in the blood, and the blood was not infectious. When, however, a single drop was injected, the mice often remained unaffected, but in a third of the cases they became ill after twenty-four hours, death occurring in from forty to sixty hours. The blood during life communicated the same disease to other mice, and bacilli were always present in large numbers. In these cases the dissolved poison in the fluid injected was too small in amount to destroy life, and death resulted only after a period of incubation as a consequence of the multiplication of bacilli in the blood and in the tissues.

[30] Vide Semmer, "Putride Intoxication," etc., *Virchow's Arch.*, vol. lxxxi. p. 109.

In another class of cases Koch experimented, not with putrid blood, but with a fluid produced by macerating a piece of mouse-skin in distilled water. Of this he injected a syringeful into the back of a rabbit. The result was peritonitis, swelling of the spleen, gray wedge-shaped patches in the liver, and in the lungs were found dark-red patches the size of a pea, devoid of air—all appearances in harmony with what is designated as pyæmia. Oval micrococci were found in great numbers [p. 998]everywhere throughout the body. But the point of special interest in the present connection is the fact that wherever these micrococci come in contact with the red blood-corpuscles the latter stick together and become arrested in the minute capillary network. The thrombi thus formed are further enlarged by the deposition of micrococci, which multiply, block up individual capillary loops, and invade contiguous tissues. In the blood-current itself, however, the micrococci do not increase in numbers, and cannot always be found in the circulation upon a single examination, but Doléris[31] assures us that in puerperal fever by repeated trials, especially after a chill, he has never failed to demonstrate their presence.

[31] *La Fievre Puerperale, etc.*, p. 120.

As to the exact manner in which these minute bodies exercise their pernicious influence, whether they operate mechanically, or whether they produce a virus in the process of nutritive activity, or whether, as is probable, both suppositions are correct, must be decided by future investigations. It is enough for us to note that the connection between sepsis and bacteria is intimate and vital.

3d. *Pathogenic bacteria are invariably associated with puerperal fever, and to them the infectious qualities of the disease are due.* I have been explicit regarding the evidence concerning bacteria in septic diseases, because it places the question of the infectious group of puerperal fever cases in the following position: Experiences occurring clinically, as well as those produced upon animals, teach us that certain lesions and symptoms, similar to those we are accustomed to regard as characteristic of puerperal fever, results from septic poisoning. In a large class of cases, however, the connection between childbed fever and sepsis has been deduced rather from analogy than direct proof. For those who chose to regard such as due to a specific poison peculiar to the puerperal state there was really no objection. If, however, bacteria are characteristic of septic poisoning, the question presents itself in a different light, and we have to inquire whether, in the less obvious cases, bacteria are present in puerperal fever in the proportions and groupings that we find them in other diseases due to putrid infection. Now, it is precisely proof of this nature that has recently been abundantly rendered.

Waldeyer,[32] Orth,[33] Heiberg,[34] and Von Recklinghausen[35] found the tissues and lymphatics of the parametria filled with pus-like masses, which consisted, in addition to pus-cells, chiefly of bacteria. Bacteria swarmed in the fluid of the peritoneal cavity. In one case examined by Waldeyer six hours after death, while the body was still warm, the peritoneal exudation was like an emulsion, and furnished an abundant deposit which consisted almost entirely of bacteria. Orth injected ten minims of peritoneal fluid from a woman dead of puerperal fever into the abdomen of a rabbit. As the animal was dying he broke up the medulla oblongata, and found in the peritoneal fluid enormous quantities of these [p. 999]organisms. In puerperal fever round bacteria have been likewise found, though in less quantities, in the lymphatics of the diaphragm and in the fluids of the pleura, the pericardium, and the ventricles of the brain. In post-mortem examinations of fresh subjects the serous fluids, withdrawn under proper precautions, do not contain round bacteria except in cases of septic infection.[36] Orth found in the purulent contents of the vessels of the funis, in children who died of sepsis, precisely the same formations as existed in the exudations of the mother.

[32] "Ueber das Verkommen von Bacterien bei der diphtheritischen Form des puerperal Fiebers," *Archiv für Gynaekologie*, vol. iii. p. 293.

[33] "Untersuchungen über puerperal Fieber," *Virchow's Archiv*, vol. lviii. p. 437.

[34] *Die puerperalen und pyæmischen Processe*, Leipzig, 1873.

[35] For the views of Von Recklinghausen I am indebted to his pupil Steurer. Vide the writer's paper on "The Nature, Origin, and Prevention of Puerperal Fever," *Trans. of the International Med. Congress*, Phila., 1876.

[36] Klebs, "Beiträge zur Kenntniss der Pathogenen Schistomyceten,"*Archiv für exp. Pathol. und Pharmakol.*, vol. iv. p. 441 *et seq*.

Doléris, in a remarkable essay already referred to, published in 1880,[37]furnishes not only conclusive evidence of the presence of bacteria in the various tissues and serous cavities of women dying of puerperal fever, but has added the evidence of their pathogenic character by cultivating them apart in sterilized fluids, and by reproducing in animals, by means of subcutaneous injections of the isolated bacteria, the infarctions, the blood-changes, and the suppurative processes of the original disease.

[37] *La Fievre Puerperale et les Organismes Inférieurs*.

So far, the generic term bacteria has been employed to indicate the disease-germs which are the active agents of infection in puerperal fever. It is not, however, intended to assume that the germs of septic processes are all identical, or that they all produce precisely the same pathological conditions. Koch, indeed, maintains that a distinct specific bacterial form is found in such closely-allied affections as pyæmia, septicæmia, gangrene, and erysipelas, the different forms possessing, however, this link in common—viz. that they are alike generated in putrefying media. Singularly enough, the bacterium termo and the bacterium commune—to which the fetidity of matters undergoing putrefaction is due—are in themselves harmless. They are rapidly destroyed in the circulation, and are not inoculable. Fetid discharges from wounds are not therefore necessarily dangerous. The putrid odor serves a useful purpose, as it gives warning of the existence of conditions which favor the development of life-destroying organisms; but the latter may develop without the concurrence of the forms which give rise to putrefaction—a fact of considerable importance in view of the common belief that septic infection is excluded by the absence of fetid odors.

In puerperal fever Doléris found the prevailing pathogenic organisms consisted of bacilli or rods, and micrococci or round bacteria in the varieties of micrococci, simple points; diplococci, double points; and chains or wreaths. The bacilli he regarded as the source of acute, rapid septicæmia, while pus-production was associated with the multiplication of the round bacteria, and especially of the diplococci.

4th. *The presence of germs in puerperal fever serves not only to fix cases hitherto doubtful in the category of septic diseases, but affords the most satisfactory explanation of the protean phenomena of puerperal fever itself.*

We have seen, from both Koch's and Gutmann's experiments upon animals, that death may occur independently of bacteria by the rapid absorption of a chemical poison developed in a putrefying fluid. Clinical experiences, such as the speedy death sometimes observed when retained coagula or portions of placenta undergo decomposition within the uterine cavity, renders it probable that similar cases of putrid intoxication are [p. 1000]not unknown in puerperal women, though, so far, the anatomical demonstration of the fact has not been furnished.

In cases, however, where puerperal fever has a distinct period of incubation, and progresses step by step to the fatal ending, bacteria are always found invading the tissues of the genital canal. In rare cases they pass by the Fallopian tube to the peritoneal cavity and excite salpingitis and peritonitis. More commonly from local lesions they enter the canalicular spaces of the connective tissue forming the framework of the genital canal, which is continuous with the subperitoneal connective tissue of the pelvis. From the canalicular space they enter the lymphatics. Cellulitis is excited by their presence, and the lymphatic glands become inflamed and enlarged. In pernicious forms they produce a sero-purulent oedema, which spreads rapidly with a wave-like progress after the manner of erysipelas; or in milder cases the progress of the disease-germs is arrested by the lymphatic glands or the resistance offered by the tissues themselves, and the ordinary circumscribed phlegmon is produced. By the lymphatics which accompany the vessels of the Fallopian tubes they reach the ovaries (puerperal ovaritis), and by the broad ligaments they pass to subperitoneal tissues of the iliac and lumbar regions. Through the same system they are conveyed to the great serous cavities of the body. In the peritoneum they give rise, unless death occurs too speedily, to pyæmic peritonitis, which, unlike the traumatic form, is attended with but little pain, and for which the claim has been set up that it is peculiar to puerperal fever. The wide stomata upon the abdominal surface of the diaphragm allows the facile entrance of the organisms into its lymphatics. Waldeyer found in diaphragmitis the lymphatics of the diaphragm filled with bacteria. And thus, following the lymphatic system, if we only admit that bacteria are the active agents of sepsis, the frequency, in severe types of puerperal fever, of inflammation of the serous membranes of the peritoneum, the pleuræ, the pericardium, the meninges, and the joints finds an easy explanation. Nor is it altogether accident which determines in different cases the precise serous membranes which are affected. The widespread ramifications of the lymphatic system would naturally give rise to eccentric inflammations in place of those following the apparent continuity of tissues.

The ductus thoracicus is the principal channel through which the bacteria enter the blood. It is possible that they may further obtain access into the circulation through the radicles which furnish the communications between the capillaries and the lymphatics. We have seen that bacteria are found with difficulty in the blood during life. A few hours after death they swarm in that fluid. That they do, however, enter the general circulation during life is incontestable. Steurer writes: "As the kidneys are the great filters of the human system, I never neglected to examine them, and almost invariably found micrococci filling the arterioles and glomeruli." This is in correspondence with what occurs in other septic diseases, and accounts for the albuminuria and interstitial nephritis which often supervene in the advanced stages.

The action of the bacilli upon the blood differs materially from that of the round bacteria. So soon as the latter come in contact with the red corpuscles, the corpuscles stick together and form larger or smaller clots in the blood. They then are no longer able to pass through the minute[p. 1001]capillary networks, but are arrested in the larger or smaller vessels (Koch). The micrococci in the resulting infarctions multiply, and migrate into the vessels and cellular tissue of the neighborhood. Thus fresh foci of infection are formed. Or by their destructive action they may, when situated near the serous surfaces, penetrate into the serous cavities, and in this way indirectly occasion peritonitis, pleurisy, meningitis, and purulent inflammations of the joints. When the micrococci enter directly into the circulation, they sometimes, in passing through the heart, adhere to the endocardium and the valves, where they cause exudation and ulceration, and give rise to the so-called endocarditis ulcerosa puerperalis.[38] The red globules of the blood undergo changes of shape, assume a stellate aspect, and rapidly disappear. The white globules are greatly increased in numbers, and the blood itself becomes nearly colorless. A certain amount of light is thrown upon these blood-changes by Doléris, who added micrococci to the fresh blood of a frog and watched the ensuing changes under the microscope. The micrococci could be seen in the act of penetrating the red globules, which thereupon lost their color and became shrunken, and, following the discharge of the organisms, which meantime had multiplied in an astonishing manner, little or nothing of the original globules remained.

[38] Heiberg, *Die puerperalen und pyæmischen Processe*, Leipzig, 1873, pp. 22 and 34, with references to cases reported by Wiege and Eberth.

In the bacillar form of septicæmia the blood is dark and has a semi-gelatinous appearance, compared by French writers to partially-cooked gooseberry jelly. The red globules, though they exhibit the various stages of deformation, are not diminished in number. The disease is further characterized by ecchymoses and minute apoplectic effusions, and by the absence of pus-formation. In the artificial septicæmia produced by Koch in mice by means of bacilli the rod-like organisms were found to enter the white corpuscles and to compass their destruction. They did not cause the red globules to adhere together, and there was no clogging of the capillary circulation. All the principal structures of the animals subjected to experiment were infiltrated with bacilli. The distribution of the latter was apparently accomplished by the blood-vessels, and not by the lymphatics, the bacilli probably effecting their entrance into the vessels by virtue of their penetrative power, in place of traversing preformed pathways. Possibly it is this action of the bacilli which causes the weakening of the vessel-walls, as evidenced by the large number of red corpuscles which pass out from them.

In puerperal fever it is rare to find either round bacteria or bacilli acting singly as the agent of infection. As a rule, both forms exist together in varying proportions, the predominant form, however, determining in general the character of the symptoms.

Thrombosis of the veins may be a physiological phenomenon, or may be due to an alteration of the blood, to weakness of the heart, or to local influences. So long as the clot remains firm its influence is limited to disturbances of the circulation. The pyæmic symptoms—viz. suppuration of the coagulum, the separation of emboli, and the formation of metastatic abscesses—are always dependent upon the presence of round bacteria. In phlebitis the latter are found in the endothelium and in the sheaths of the veins. The inflammation of the veins is followed by [p. 1002]thrombosis. According to Doléris, micrococci derived from the blood are deposited upon the central extremities of the clots; beyond these dépôts a fresh inflammation is set up, followed by fibrinous coagulation. Thus the micrococci become imprisoned between two plugs. The same process may be repeated until a series of abscesses are formed. For a time no mischief may ensue. Finally, however, the resistance of the outworks is overcome, an embolus becomes detached, and an infectious abscess is opened into the blood—an event which is announced by an intense chill and the familiar systemic derangement.

In septic diseases death takes place from apnoea, partly from the inability of the blood-corpuscles to carry oxygen to the tissues, and partly from paralysis of the nerve-centres.[39]

[39] Schüller, "Exp. Beiträge zur Studium der Septischen Infection,"*Deutsche Zeitschr. f. Chir.*, vol. vi. p. 149 *et seq.*

In hospital epidemics of puerperal fever diphtheritic patches situated upon the lesions of the vulva and in the course of the utero-vaginal canal are sometimes observed. Steurer found these patches were always associated with loss of substance, and were composed of disintegrated fibrin, white and red blood-globules, and colonies of round bacteria in great abundance. Morphologically, these so-called diphtheritic patches are identical with those which appear in the throat. Pallen[40] has reported an instance of the simultaneous occurrence of puerperal diphtheritis in the mother and throat diphtheritis in the two-weeks' old child. In lying-in hospitals it is the genital organs, as the locus resistentiæ minoris, and not the throat, which are the usual points of attack.

[40] *Trans. N.Y. Obst. Soc.*, 1876-78, p. 78.

The question as to the extent to which erysipelas and puerperal fever are cognate diseases is in a fair way to be solved by recent investigation. Orth took the contents of a vesicle from an erysipelatous patient which contained bacteria in great abundance, and employed the same for injections under the skin of rabbits. In this way he succeeded in producing in these animals a species of erysipelas malignum. In the subcutaneous oedema and affected portions of the skin he found enormous masses of bacteria, so far exceeding in quantity the amount introduced as to prove an abundant new production.[41] Samuel produced similar results by the injection of ordinary putrid fluids containing round bacteria. An affection resembling simple erysipelas he obtained most frequently by the application of fluid to a wound torn open after the second or third day.[42] Lukomski found that erysipelas could be produced by fluid containing micrococci even when putrefaction did not exist. The contents of erysipelatous vesicles containing no micrococci excited no morbid manifestations. Where the erysipelatous process was fresh and progressing micrococci were found in great abundance in the lymphatics and canalicular spaces. Where the process was retrogressive, there were no micrococci to be found, even in cases in which inflammation existed to an intense degree.[43] Doléris submitted to the culture-process of Pasteur fluid obtained from vesicles which developed in the course of facial erysipelas in a man of forty years. Micrococci in chains were found in the liquids employed identical with those he had discovered in puerperal fever. In many cases I have seen an erysipelatous inflammation start from a puerperal diphtheritic ulcer [p. 1003]upon the introitus vaginæ, and extend outward over the buttocks, the thighs, and the lower portion of the abdomen.

[41] "Untersuchungen über Erysipel.," *Arch. für exp. Pathol. und Pharmakol.*, Bd. i. S. 81.
[42] *Arch. für exp. Path. und Pharmak.*, Bd. i. S. 335, u. ff.
[43] "Untersuchungen über Erysipel.," *Virchow's Archiv*, Bd. lx. S. 430.

Virchow[44] has so far given in his adhesion to the new school as to say: "Especially in this connection are to be mentioned the diphtheritic process and the erysipelatous, especially erysipelas malignum. The granular deposit in diphtheritically affected tissues, of which I formerly spoke, has more and more proven to be of a parasitic character. What we formerly regarded as simple, organic granules, as infiltration or exudation, has since proven to be a dense aggregation of micro-organisms which penetrate into the tissues and cells to compass their destruction."

[44] *Die Fortschritte der Krieg's Heilkunde*, Berlin, 1874.

Thus we find in surgical fever, in puerperal fever, in diphtheria, and in erysipelas the presence of a common element which links them together, and which establishes the relationship which has long been recognized as existing between these various processes.

4th. *The differences between surgical and puerperal septicæmia are due to differences partly structural and partly physiological in the wounded surfaces exposed to septic contamination.*

A certain amount of misapprehension has arisen from the circumstance that along with many coincidences in the symptoms of puerperal and surgical fever there are observable differences which, from a purely clinical point of view, would justify a separate classification of the two affections. It will not do, however, to ignore the fact that the conditions which prevail in the parturient canal subsequent to labor have no strict analogue in the lesions which the surgeon is called upon to treat, and that therefore a complete identity as to all the clinical features of puerperal and surgical fever would hardly be within the range of possibility.

In the puerperal state it is necessary to take into account the blood-changes induced by pregnancy, the effects of shock and exhaustion in protracted labors, the frequency of hemorrhage, the deep situation of puerperal wounds, the presence of clots, decidua, and dead tissue in a state of disintegration or decomposition, the ease with which deleterious matters are absorbed by the wide lymphatic interspaces, the serous infiltration of the pelvic tissues, the exaggerated size of the lymphatics and veins, and the proximity of the peritoneal cavity.

Samuel,[45] in speaking of the immunities and dispositions to septic poisoning, says: "The statistical frequency of septic puerperal disease is due to the length of the parturient canal, to the fact that through this long passage there must pass all the pathological and physiological excretions, and to the soiling of these parts with fingers, instruments, and secretions which have become the bearers of sepsis." He found, on the other hand, that it was extremely difficult to produce a progressive ichorous condition by daily painting an open stump with a septic fluid,[46] though the same was readily obtained when an infinitesimal quantity of septic fluid was injected underneath a fascia.

[45] "Ueber die Wirkung des Faülniss Process auf den lebenden Organismus," *Arch. f. exp. Pathologie*, vol. i. p. 343.

[46] *Loc. cit.*, p. 339.

5th. *In the present state of our scientific knowledge it is necessary to admit that there is a limited number of febrile and inflammatory disturbances occurring in puerperal women, the bacterial origin of which may be fairly questioned.* As illustrations of this class may be [p. 1004]mentioned: 1. Cases of catarrhal endometritis due to errors of diet and exposure. Indeed, I have frequently, in hospital practice, been able to trace severe cases of cellulitis, pelvic peritonitis, and general peritonitis occurring in the winter season to the patient getting out of bed dripping with perspiration, and clad only in a night-dress, and going thus barefooted over a cold, uncarpeted floor to the water-closet. 2. Cases of puerperal disorders proceeding from emotional causes, the nervous system furnishing the first impulse to the disturbed action. 3. Cases of excessive vulnerability in non-pregnant women; individuals are sometimes found so susceptible that a parametritis follows a simple application of the tincture of iodine to the cervix. 4. Cases of pelvic peritonitis starting from old intra-peritoneal adhesions. 5. Cases of peritonitis and retro-peritoneal inflammations secondary to ulcerative processes in the cæcum or the descending colon. This condition is apt to be masked during pregnancy, but starts into activity during childbed as a consequence of fecal accumulation or of excessive purgation.

It is by no means easy to decide as to the precise nature of local inflammations following lacerations of the cervix and the bruising or crushing of the soft parts in long or instrumental labors. The marvellous absence of heat, pain, redness, and swelling in wounds treated in strict accordance with the principles of Lister, the very slight reaction when the atmosphere is pure, and the severity of these symptoms in overcrowded hospitals, tend indeed to strengthen the belief that even the simplest inflammations proceeding from wounds owe their origin in great part to septic germs. But, on the other hand, in hospital practice it is not uncommon to observe puerperal inflammations and febrile conditions which possess this distinctive peculiarity—that they in no wise visibly affect the health of puerperal patients in their vicinity. The symptoms of blood-poisoning too are either absent or present to a subordinate extent. Probably the difficulty is best solved by assuming with Genzmer and Volkmann[47] that there is such a thing as an aseptic surgical fever due to the absorption of the products of physiological tissue-changes at the seat of injury. In surgical cases, even where the precautions of Listerism have been faultlessly observed, febrile movements of considerable intensity, but of no prognostic signification, are of frequent occurrence. While in puerperal women we can never exclude the possibility of the septic infection of puerperal wounds, it is in accordance with clinical experience to assume that a high fever belonging to the aseptic class may coincide with a septic process of insignificant proportions.

[47] Genzmer and Volkmann, "Ueber septisches und aseptisches Wundfieber," *Samml. klin. Vorträge*, No. 121.

GENERAL SYMPTOMS.—As in other infectious diseases, there is, from the time of the entry of the poison into the system up to the outbreak of fever, a distinct period of incubation. The first febrile symptoms usually occur within three days of the birth of the child. An attack coming on a few hours after childbirth is indicative of infection during or previous to labor. The third day is the one upon which ordinarily the beginning of the fever is to be anticipated. After the fifth day an attack is rare, and at the end of a week patients may be regarded as having reached the point of safety. Apparent exceptions to this rule are probably referable to cases of mild parametritis, in which the initial [p. 1005]fever and the pain were insufficient to attract attention to the existence of local inflammation.

The symptoms of puerperal fever vary with the character of the local affections and with the extent to which the general system participates in the disturbed action. The different groups of puerperal processes possess the following pathognomonic symptoms— viz. increased temperature, enlargement of the spleen, disturbed involution, and sensitiveness of the uterus upon pressure (Braun).

In most cases the fever is ushered in by chilly sensations or by a well-defined chill. This symptom, however, does not possess much prognostic importance. A chill is significant of a sudden change between the temperature of the skin and that of the surrounding medium. It may, therefore, be absent in pernicious forms of fever, provided only that the temperature changes are inaugurated slowly, whereas it may follow a trifling increase of the body-heat if, as sometimes happens in sleep, the moist skin is exposed to cool currents of air. Repeated chills indicate phlebitis and pyæmia.

In order to grasp the many symptoms of puerperal fever, it is necessary to keep separately in mind the clinical features of each of the local processes, although in fact the latter rarely occur singly, but to a greater or less extent in combination with others.

The symptoms of ENDOMETRITIS AND ENDOCOLPITIS.—The uncomplicated catarrhal inflammation of the uterus and vagina is the most frequent and the mildest of the diseases of childbed. In endometritis the uterus is large, flabby, and sensitive upon pressure; the after-pains are often unusually severe, involution is retarded, and the lochia become fetid, remain sanguinolent for a longer period than usual, and at the outset may be temporarily suspended. Sometimes the large intestine is distended with flatus. In endocolpitis the vaginal discharge is thin and purulent, the patient experiences pain and burning in the acts of defecation and urination, and, where the wounds of the vulva and vagina assume an ulcerative character, there is often found at the same time inflammatory oedema of the labia.

The fever in these cases is ushered in frequently, but not always, by chilly feelings, and the temperature reaches its height usually upon the evening of the third or fourth day, is remittent, almost intermittent in character, and rarely exceeds 102° to 103° F. In mild forms the occurrence of the fever is often overlooked or is referred to disturbance produced by the secretion of the milk. In severer attacks the febrile symptoms may continue from three to seven days. At the end of a week the swelling of the labia subsides, the discharge becomes thick, and ulcers, if present, begin to assume a healthy granulating appearance.

In diphtheritic ulcerations, and in endometritis due to decomposing remains of the ovum, the load condition is often complicated by the invasion of the neighboring tissues.

The symptoms of PARAMETRITIS and PERIMETRITIS (Pelvic peritonitis[48]).— The symptoms of these two affections, as would be naturally [p. 1006]expected from the proximity of the peritoneum to the pelvic connective tissue, for the most part overlap. It must be very rare for one form to occur entirely independent of the other. For this reason it will be found convenient to consider first the symptoms common to both morbid processes, and subsequently to direct attention to what are believed to be points of distinction between them.

[48] The following clinical history, together with the statistical details, is borrowed in great part from the description of Olshausen ("Ueber puerperale Parametritis und Perimetritis," *Volkmann's Samml. klin. Vortr.*, No. 28), the exactitude of which I have had abundant opportunity to verify.

During the period of incubation there are usually no prodromic symptoms. Elevations of temperature in the course of the first twelve hours following labor are equally frequent under perfectly normal conditions. Suspicious symptoms are disturbed sleep, excessively painful after-pains, and a pulse of 80 to 90.

The beginning of the fever occurs in 90 per cent. within the first four days of childbed; most frequently upon the second or third day, and taking place upon the fourth day in scarcely 12 to 15 per cent. of the cases. If five days have elapsed without fever, the period of danger, with very rare exceptions, may be regarded as having passed.

At the outset the fever, especially in perimetritis, is ushered in by chilly sensations or by an intense chill. The temperature rises rapidly, though the highest point is usually not reached before the second, and in rare cases not before the third, day. In most cases the heat in the axilla exceeds 103°, and may even mount up to 105°. The decline occurs gradually, the fever ending in 70 per cent. in the course of a week, in 20 per cent. in two weeks, and only in 10 per cent. extending beyond that period. Protracted cases indicate abscess formation.

The fever does not, however, always pursue a regular course. In place of progressively declining until the termination is reached, the high temperature of the second day may be attained upon one or more occasions. The morning remissions are at first slight, but become marked as the disease approaches its close. In cases of long duration the morning hours are often free from fever, a circumstance calculated to mislead a physician who sees his patient but once a day. A pulse of 80 to 90 beats, a disturbed sleep, lack of appetite, and sensitiveness to pressure upon the sides of the uterus are, however, symptoms which should serve as a warning of some disturbing cause, and should lead the physician to renew his visit in the latter part of the day.

If, from a mistaken notion that the morbid process has come to an end, the patient is allowed prematurely to resume her household duties, the pains across the abdomen and along the hip and thigh return, and an examination reveals the existence of exudation in the pelvic cavity or upon an iliac fossa.

Errors of this kind are most frequent in cases of parametritis associated with slight peritoneal inflammation, as the local pain is then insignificant, and the initial chill, happening on the third or fourth day, is apt to be ascribed to engorgement of the breasts.

Relapses after the complete disappearance of febrile disturbance occur in 15 to 20 per cent. They are usually shorter, but sometimes more obstinate, than the original attack. As a rare exception may be mentioned cases with evening remissions and morning exacerbations.

In circumscribed pelvic inflammations the pulse rarely exceeds 120 beats to the minute. A pulse of 140, of more than half a day's duration, betokens severe septic complications, and is therefore of evil omen. In [p. 1007]some cases the slow pulse observed after labor makes its influence felt in the first day or two of the fever, so that the curious phenomenon may be witnessed of a temperature of 104° coinciding for a time with a pulse ranging between 50 and 70 beats to the minute.

As regards other symptoms, headache and sleeplessness are rarely absent. Profuse sweating follows the first febrile attack, and frequently recurs during the course of the disease.

Pain is present at the onset in the majority of cases, and is then usually most violent. The spontaneous pain, which is due to the affection of the peritoneum, subsides in great part in the course of one or two days, but the sides of the uterus remain sensitive to pressure. In the rare cases of pure parametritis, however, this symptom may be absent altogether. The pain, like that from the inflammation of serous membranes, is of a lancinating character. Sometimes it is associated only with the contractions of the uterus. After-pains occurring under unusual circumstances, as in primiparæ or after the third day, are to be regarded with suspicion.

Vomiting occurs occasionally, but is comparatively rare unless the peritonitis becomes diffused and spreads to the region of the stomach. The appetite is lost, and only returns, as a rule, with the departure of the fever. The tongue is coated and moist, and constipation is common. In other cases there is diarrhoea with rumbling in the bowels, but without pain or tenesmus. The urinary secretion is rarely interfered with, and when this is the case it indicates the extension of the inflammation to the peritoneum covering the bladder.

Most cases of perimetritis and parametritis terminate in five or ten days, the fever and other symptoms gradually subsiding. When, as may happen in exceptional instances, the temperature falls suddenly from a high degree to one below the normal level, the body grows icy cold, the pulse becomes small and irregular, and symptoms of collapse develop. But in twelve to twenty-four hours the symptoms of collapse subside, and the disease reaches its end with a disappearance of the alarming manifestations.

If the fever subsides within a week exudation is somewhat rare. Its continuance beyond that date should lead to a careful exploration of the pelvic organs. The exudation is usually demonstrable in the course of the second week or at the beginning of the third week. It is recognized, according to its location, by external or by internal examination, or, where the deposit is considerable, by both methods. In most cases the deposit is extra-peritoneal, and is situated between the folds of the broad ligament, above and to the sides of the vaginal cul-de-sac. It has generally a rounded form, though with less convexity than fibrous and ovarian tumors. Sometimes, however, the tumor is flat below, like a board. It seldom exceeds in size that of a large apple. In fresh exudations the sensation produced is often that of a hard tumor surrounded by a softer layer, due to continued succulence of the soft parts.

In a few weeks they may reach or exceed the hardness of a fibroid tumor. The older the tumor, unless suppuration sets in, the less sensitive it becomes. Often the exudation extends to the pelvic walls. The uterus, as a rule, is fixed, and in cases of large tumors becomes pushed toward the opposite side, while as a consequence of later shrinkage the fundus may be drawn permanently toward the affected side.

[p. 1008]The cul-de-sac of the vagina is rendered broader and flatter by the pressure of the deposit, or, when the tumor is deep enough, the vaginal surface may be rendered convex. Behind the uterus the exudation is as it were flattened antero-posteriorly, and in some cases it may be felt in the form of rigid bands between the posterior ligaments which enclose the cul-de-sac of Douglas. The ante-uterine tumors have a spherical shape and depress the vagina anteriorly.

Tumors situated in the iliac fossa have a more or less convex form, and may be of such considerable size that the swelling may be recognized by the eye through the abdominal walls. As the exudation between the broad ligaments may in these cases have been slight from the beginning, or may have subsequently disappeared by absorption, the iliac tumors have often apparently a spontaneous origin.

Sometimes the uterus is surrounded by exudation, and the entire pelvis appears as though it were a mould filled with a solid mass. The fornix is then often pressed downward, and irregular rounded masses are to be felt through the vaginal walls.

The recognition of parametritic tumors through the abdominal coverings is possible when they are situated above Poupart's ligament, in the upper portion of the broad ligaments, and in the iliac fossæ.

The pain and the functional disturbances in the pelvic organs depend upon the size and situation of these inflammatory deposits. Of the functional troubles may be mentioned frequent and painful micturition, obstinate constipation and difficult defecation, contractures of the ilio-psoas muscles when the exudation is seated beneath the sheath or between the muscle and the pelvic bones, disturbances of motility in the abductor muscles, paresis of the lower extremities, and radiating pains in the upper portion of the thigh and in the renal and lumbar regions, produced by pressure upon the obturator, the crural, the cutaneous, and the sciatic nerves.

So long as fever is present the exudation rarely diminishes. If absorption takes place in one point, growth almost certainly follows in some other direction. When, however, the apyretic period is reached, the exudation, as a rule, disappears rapidly, so that often in the course of six weeks no trace of its existence remains. In a smaller number the solid mass may persist for months or even years.

After the fever has departed the patient usually feels well. The sleep and appetite return, the night-sweats disappear, the pulse often falls to 50 or 60 beats, and the temperature is in many cases for a time subnormal in character.

Where the fever persists for from five to six weeks there is always a suspicion of abscess formation. With the exception of afternoon fever and night-sweats the patient may feel very comfortable. Then the exudation becomes sensitive, the spontaneous pains recur, sleep is lost, and locomotion, defecation, and urination occasion acute suffering. The fever becomes violent, chills announce the presence of pus, and finally, about the seventieth or eightieth day, perforation of the abscess takes place. The usual seat at which the pus is discharged is just above Poupart's ligament; next in frequency perforation takes place into the colon, and in rare instances into the bladder, the uterus, and vagina. Fortunately, of very rare occurrence is the discharge of pus into the peritoneal cavity, which is[p. 1009]naturally followed by acute peritonitis. Another likewise unfrequent but most dangerous accident is the septic infection of the abscess—an occurrence referred to by Olshausen to the diffusion of intestinal gases through the walls of the tumor.

In suppuration of parametritic exudations the pus commonly forms in small scattered collections, and rarely gives rise to large abscesses.

Although parametritis and perimetritis are usually found associated together, there are always cases in which the one form of inflammation so far predominates over the other as to justify an attempt to establish a clinical distinction between them.

In the beginning of the attack, sharp pain, high fever, and tympanitic distension of the lower abdomen are symptomatic of inflammation in the pelvic peritoneum. Whether the cellular tissue is simultaneously implicated can only be determined by a digital examination after the abdominal sensitiveness has subsided. The absence of the objective signs of cellulitis would then contribute to prove that the case had been one in which the peritoneum had been in the main affected. On the other hand, moderate fever, pain elicited only on pressure, and tympanitic distension confined to the colon, coinciding with exudation between the folds of the broad ligament, would be indicative of a nearly pure cellulitis.

A palpable exudation is by no means the necessary product of peritoneal inflammation. Indeed, in many cases, the distinctive symptoms of the latter may be present for from four to eight days, and may then subside without leaving a trace of its existence at the pelvic brim.

The demonstration of a fluid effusion by noting the change of level upon shifting the position of the patient is rarely possible, either because the quantity is too small or because it quickly becomes confined by pseudo-membranous adhesions between the intestines.

Bandl[49] mentions as a sign of local peritonitis, sometimes noticeable, a number of resistant points or tumors near the pelvic brim or above one of the iliac fossæ, due to a matting together of the intestines or to their adhesion to the uterine appendages. They are distinguished from solid tumors by their emitting a tympanitic sound upon percussion and by their changing position in consequence of an accumulation of urine in the bladder or of feces or gases in the bowels. Again, all tumors may be reckoned as intra-peritoneal which very rapidly form behind or to the side of the uterus from enclosed exudation-products, and which at the same time rise far above the level of the pelvic brim. If, however, they start from the cul-de-sac of Douglas, and do not much exceed the linea terminalis, or if they occupy an iliac fossa, it becomes very difficult to decide whether they are of intra- or extra-peritoneal origin. The peritoneal exudation, however, long remains soft and fluctuating. It arises, as a rule, behind the uterus, and does not exhibit a tendency to spread to the sides or to the anterior or posterior pelvic walls.

[49] *Handbuch der Frauenkrankheiten*, red. Von Billroth, 5te Abschnitt, p. —.

Still more difficult is it to decide as to the seat of exudations met with beneath the abdominal walls. When diffused and continuous with a pelvic deposit the diagnosis is uncertain. It is only safe to assume the peritoneal origin of extravasations of a rounded form, of a fluctuating consistence, and when they are situated high up and are disconnected from exudation at the pelvic brim. An opening of the abscess through the [p. 1010]navel would indicate a peritoneal source, while the discharge through the abdominal parietes would point to a seat in the connective tissue.

After the perforation of an abscess the fever and pain subside; the wound, if external, either closes in the course of one or two weeks, or fistulas form which become the source of protracted suppuration.

In psoas abscesses the exudation extends beneath the sheath of the muscle or between the iliacus and the bone. In puerperal patients they proceed from an inflammation originating in the broad ligament. They are situated too deep to be easily palpated. The pains they occasion are referred rather to the hip or knee than to the abdomen. The contracture of the psoas muscle furnishes a diagnostic sign which distinguishes this form from the superficial abscesses of the iliac fossæ. The pus eventually is discharged beneath Poupart's ligament, in the lower portion of the inguinal fossa, at some point upon the crest of the ilium, or exceptionally along the thigh. Often the discharge is maintained for months.

The symptoms of GENERAL PERITONITIS.—This form generally begins with the usual symptoms of pelvic inflammation, but the tenderness, which at first was limited to the side of the uterus, gradually spreads over the entire abdomen. The abdominal pain is of a tearing, lancinating, sometimes colicky character. It is increased by the slightest bodily movement, by jarring of the bed, or even by the weight of the bed-clothes.

As a consequence of the peritoneal inflammation and of the accompanying exudation, the muscular walls of the bowels become paralyzed, and tympanitic distension results from the accumulation of gases. In the dependent portions of the peritoneal cavity it is often possible to demonstrate by percussion the presence of fluid exudation, though distinct fluctuation is rarely to be made out. The size of the abdomen is due much more to the tympanites than to the amount of effusion. Sometimes the liver, with the diaphragm, is pushed by the swollen bowels to the level of the fourth or third rib, and exercises such a degree of compression upon the posterior portion of the lungs as to place the patient in danger of suffocation. The respirations are jerky and attended with a moaning sound.

The loss of muscular power in the intestines permits the contents of the middle portion to pass unchecked toward the duodenum, and thence, upon accidental contractions of the abdomen, they may pass to the stomach and be ejected by vomiting. The first vomited matter has a dark-green color, and that ejected afterward presents the color of intestinal matter. Constipation at the outset may be subsequently followed by colliquative diarrhoea.

The fever begins, as a rule, though not always, with an intense chill, the temperature rises to 104°, and the pulse becomes small, hard, and resistant. Its frequency rapidly increases, varying from 120 to 160 beats to the minute. The skin is sometimes dry, sometimes dripping with perspiration. In fatal cases, as the end approaches, the temperature frequently falls, while the pulse becomes more rapid, the face assumes a pinched, anxious expression, sweat gathers upon the forehead, the extremities grow icy cold, and the patient dies in collapse. The duration of peritonitis averages not more than from four to six days.

In cases of recovery the pulse improves, the vomiting ceases, and the tympanites disappears. The diffuse exudation then becomes converted[p. 1011]into circumscribed tumors, which on palpation are felt on the side of the pelvis and extending upward to the level of the umbilicus. Upon internal examination the uterus is often found depressed by the weight of the fluid, which likewise may bulge the cul-de-sac of Douglas into the pelvic cavity. Sometimes the exudation may become encysted above the pelvis and leave the contents of the latter free. In still other cases the uterus may become attached high up to the abdominal walls, so that the vaginal portion disappears and the os is reached with difficulty.

The peritoneal exudation may, as in pelvic inflammations, become absorbed and disappear. When, however, it is surrounded by loops of intestines it is apt to undergo purulent and septic changes, and the abscesses may then become discolored and filled with stinking gases. The patient, whose previous improvement has been watched with delight, now loses appetite, the pulse becomes frequent, the strength fails, and death may follow from septic fever or from rupture of abscess into the abdominal cavity.

In the pyæmic form—a still more deadly variety of peritonitis—the symptoms differ materially from those which have been recounted. As, however, it constitutes only a single one of the pathological changes connected with the poisoning of the blood through the lymphatic system, its consideration belongs properly to the study of the septic infection.

The symptoms of SEPTICÆMIA LYMPHATICA.—The symptoms of blood-poisoning in the infectious diseases of childbed vary to a considerable extent according to the channel through which the septic germs enter the general circulation. In the murderous epidemics which prevail in lying-in hospitals the lymphatics are, as a rule, the vessels primarily invaded. It is to this form that the cases already described belong, where, with diphtheritic patches upon the utero-vaginal canal and sero-purulent oedema of the parametrium, there are associated pyæmic peritonitis and deformation of the blood-corpuscles; or where, following the migrations of the round bacteria, the serous cavities become successively involved, septic vegetations gather upon the heart, and the glomeruli of the kidneys become choked with micrococci. The lymphatic form of septicæmia develops soon after labor, and is always ushered in by a chill. The temperature rises to 104° or even higher, and the pulse is thin and frequent. The abdomen swells rapidly, without being especially painful. Indeed, painless distension of the intestines is one of the characteristics of an acute invasion of the lymphatics. Peritoneal effusion is absent in cases which run a rapid course, and is distinctly recognizable only in a peritonitis of long continuance. The effusion is not so much due to exudation as to a transudation of serum with which micrococci are commingled. At the same time the tongue is moist, but slightly coated, and at times quite clean. Sometimes there is diarrhoea due to catarrh or to a diphtheritic affection of the colon. When the bowels have been constipated the administration of a purgative may provoke discharges which it may be found difficult to arrest. The skin is bathed in perspiration. At the beginning and during the course of the disease bleeding at the nose is of not infrequent occurrence.

Toward the end the pulse runs up to 140 to 160 beats, while in many cases the temperature falls. Immediately after death the heat of the body may for a short time exceed the highest point reached during life. The [p. 1012] respirations are superficial and jerky. In many instances the face, the neck, and the fingers are blue from defective oxygenation of the blood. At the same time the skin becomes clammy and the extremities cold.

The sensorium, in cases which run a rapid course, is usually affected at an early period. The patients appear somnolent, are restless in bed, have light delirium, and respond only when spoken to loudly. As a rule, they make but little complaint, and, were it not for the dyspnoea, would have nothing to disturb their sense of comfort. Very few, even as death approaches, have any idea of the danger that threatens them. Now and then, in place of stupor, great restlessness, and even a maniacal condition, is developed. Albumen is usually found in the urine.

Pleurisy, so frequently associated with lymphatic septicæmia, is frequently double, more rarely single, and begins, as a rule, with sharp pain in the side and an aggravation of the previous dyspnoea. Pericarditis is less frequent, and occurs usually without symptoms toward the close of life. The joint affections are characterized by redness and swelling, and by pain, which is sometimes so great that touching the inflamed part suffices to arouse the patient from sopor. Sometimes fluctuation is felt, but death occurs before perforation and discharge of the pus.

The most frequent ending is death, which follows in from two to twenty-one days, and, as a rule, between four and seven days. Recovery is, however, possible.

The symptoms of SEPTICÆMIA VENOSA (phlebitis uterina, pyæmia metastatica).—The putrid infection of a thrombus at the placental site may take place within twenty-four to forty-eight hours after labor. Usually, however, the approach is insidious, and the disease develops from an apparently insignificant endometritis or parametritis; or the patient, with the exception perhaps of a tired feeling, of slight chilly sensations, and of profuse perspiration, may not have been conscious of any indisposition for days preceding the attack, or even until the first getting up from childbed. The initial chill in typical cases is characterized by its violence and duration. In some cases it may last for hours. It is accompanied and followed by high temperature, the febrile attack ending with profuse perspiration as in intermittent fever, with which it is apt to be confounded. The fall in temperature often assumes the form of a prolonged remission.

In many cases the pulse rises and falls with the variations in the body heat, while in others it remains permanently above the average. A frequent pulse is always a suspicious symptom in childbed, even where the other symptoms are apparently normal.

Erratic chills announce the lodgment of emboli in distant organs. With the formation of metastatic abscesses in the lungs and other parenchymatous organs the typical character of the disease changes. In place of chills occurring at irregular intervals, followed by remissions and periods of apparent improvement, the fever is continuous, the pulse becomes small and rapid, while sopor, slight delirium, a dry skin, a dry, brown, cracked tongue, and a moderately tympanitic abdomen, give the case the appearance of one of typhus fever.

Peritonitis is present in hardly one-third of the cases. The abdomen is therefore flat and soft, and often is not sensitive upon pressure. Icterus, due to disintegration of the blood-corpuscles, is an ominous symptom.

Death usually occurs in the second or third week. In the [p. 1013] typhus-like cases, however, it may follow the first attack speedily. Recovery is possible where the organs secondarily affected are not of too great importance.

A combination of the lymphatic and venous forms of septicæmia is not uncommon in cases running a protracted course.

The symptoms of PURE SEPTICÆMIA.—Under the title of pure septicæmia should be placed cases in which the absorption of putrid materials into the blood gives rise to symptoms of intense blood-poisoning without the development of local lesions. A common example of this form is met with in the fever which results from the presence in the uterus of decomposing coagula or portions of retained ovum, the fever subsiding with the removal of the disturbing cause. In like manner we sometimes meet with cases of intense septic poisoning followed by speedy death, in which the post-mortem examination reveals only changes in the blood and softening of the parenchymatous organs. The symptoms are often similar to those produced by the injection of putrid materials containing rod-like bacteria into the vessels of animals. As the long bacteria do not possess the capacity of self-reproduction in the blood, to produce fatal results the quantity of putrid fluid injected must be large or be frequently repeated. This form is said not to be inoculable.

CAUSES.—The effects of a poisoned state of the atmosphere as a cause of puerperal fever is best observed in the so-called nosocomial malaria of hospitals. In days gone by, before I had learned by experience that the safe conduct of a lying-in service depends upon the fastidious exclusion of every source of contamination, I had frequent occasion to witness febrile outbreaks among puerperal women in the Bellevue Hospital, which were instantly arrested by the simple transfer of the inmates of the affected ward to a wholesome locality, though no changes were simultaneously made in either the personnel or the utensils of the service. In these instances it seems fair to assume that the previous unhealthy condition was not due to the direct transfer of an inoculable matter from patient to patient by the attendants, but by something residing in the air of the vacated apartment. In the inquiry as to the production of this condition it can be assumed that it is not caused by aggregation alone. The medical wards of Bellevue, always crowded, have often furnished in times of need safe receptacles for puerperal patients. It is certainly not due to the presence of the ordinary constituents of the atmosphere. We must therefore look for some additional element capable of unfavorably affecting the economy. What this element really is, is demonstrated by a familiar clinical experience. When the disturbance produced by nosocomial malaria is not at an early stage arrested by change of locality, the secretions of patients affected become inoculable. Then the epidemic spreads rapidly, and assumes continuously a more and more severe type. If during an epidemic the external genitals be carefully watched, now and then diphtheritic patches will be noticed to form upon them. At first these patches may disappear or yield readily to treatment. When an epidemic has assumed a pestilential form the patches, which may in isolated cases make their appearance at any time in a hospital, are rarely absent in fatal cases. The composition of the patches tells the tale of what it is in the atmosphere which accomplishes the charnel-house work. Favoring conditions have led to the multiplication of disease-germs [p. 1014]in the air, and have fitted them to become the active producers of disease.

In a patient dying in the early stages of an epidemic there may be no diphtheritic manifestations, though the tissues and secretions are filled with bacteria. As, however, the epidemic gains headway, the lesions of the generative apparatus, and especially of the external organs, which are most exposed to air, become covered with patches which swarm with micrococci. Under the conditions named it is certainly more in accord with ordinary scientific reasoning to conclude that the micrococci play an important part in the production of puerperal fever than that the puerperal fever produces the micrococci.

To be sure, bacteria or their spores are always present in the air, and it may be fairly asked how patients are ever spared from their perverse industry. The answer is, that the effect produced by the atmosphere of a hospital is dependent partly upon the quantity, and partly upon the quality, of the suspended germs. Floating spores, when sparsely distributed, rarely possess the power of invading a healthy organism. In the inauguration of an epidemic the first patient severely attacked is usually one whose powers of resistance are broken down by prolonged labor, by hemorrhage, by poverty, or some other condition leading to impaired vitality.

Puerperal-fever epidemics due to contamination of the atmosphere, and not to direct contagion, do not at once reach the maximum of intensity. At first the temperature tables indicate the prevalence of milk fever; next follow cases closely resembling those of mild paludal poisoning; and, finally, if these warnings are unheeded and reliance is placed upon antiperiodic remedies rather than upon prompt closure of the threatened ward, the pestilence develops. In the conduct of lying-in hospitals it should never be forgotten that with the multiplication of the septic germs the danger increases.

At the same time, the quality of the agents which pervade the air where hospital patients are confined is an important element in the genesis of febrile outbreaks. The bacterium termo, which causes putrefaction, is not in itself, as we have already mentioned, a source of danger. A stinking odor is not necessarily incompatible with a low mortality-rate. The importance of the common forms of bacteria, according to Pasteur, results from the fact that by their power to consume oxygen they pave the way for the active development of the pernicious germs, nearly all of which thrive only in media in which that element has been materially diminished. Again, there is reason to believe that the same germs are not[50]always equally active for evil. Gravitz claims that the ordinary varieties of aspergillus and penicillium found everywhere on the surface of the ground, on moistened walls, on food of every variety, on decaying leaves and fruit, and whose spores are universally present in the purest air, can by a succession of cultures be gradually brought to flourish in a warm alkaline fluid, and that they then acquire the capacity to penetrate living tissues, to proliferate in them, to excite local necroses, and to cause death in the course of three days. The resistance of micrococci to carbolic and salicylic acids is found experimentally to depend in a measure upon the[p. 1015]nature of the vehicle in which they are cultivated (Buchholz). The action of septic fluids varies too with the age of the infusions, with the materials employed, and with the conditions under which the poison-germs are generated.

[50] Gravitz, "Ueber Schimmel vegetationen im thierischen organismus,"*Virch. Arch.*, vol. lxxxi, p. 355.

Micrococci multiply in hospitals when organic materials favorable to their growth are present in sufficient quantities. Perrin, Quenquand and others have shown that the hospital wards in Paris, especially those upon the surgical and maternity divisions, contain an infinite number of vibrios, bacteria, and all the coccus forms (Charpentier). Robin[51] has demonstrated the existence of albuminoid matters in water condensed upon vessels containing freezing mixtures and placed in overcrowded wards of hospitals. When the results of crowding become manifest, these albuminoid matters not only impart a fetid odor and putrefy with great rapidity, but rapidly impart putrefaction to healthy muscle and normal blood with which they are brought into contact. Pasteur was able by the microscopic examination of the lochia from patients in the services of Hervieux and Lucas-Champonnière to predict, from the character of the contained organisms, an impending attack of fever in advance of the slightest symptom betokening danger.

[51] *Leçons sur les Humeurs*, Paris, 1867, p. 195.

It is unquestionably the lochial discharge which makes it such a difficult task to keep a maternity ward in a healthful condition. Putrid blood has been found to be the most favorable material for septic experiments. It was noticeable in Bellevue Hospital that febrile outbreaks always arose in, and were usually confined to, the ward in the hospital which, by a bad arrangement, was assigned to patients for the first four or five days following confinement—*i.e.* during the period of the lochia cruenta. As puerperal fever is rare after the fifth day, this at first sight would seem natural. But if a patient was transferred directly after confinement, during one of these unhealthy periods, to the ward containing the patients who had passed the first five days, but had not completed the ten days, she would escape the fever. It was always the same ward that required to be disinfected. In a communicating apartment all the confinements took place, and at all times, therefore, the conditions were present for loading the atmosphere with the products of decomposing blood. In the summer months, so long as the windows were open and the air was diluted by the continuous passage of fresh currents, the patients enjoyed immunity from nosocomial malaria. In the autumn, so soon as it became necessary to close the windows partially on account of the cool nights, it was not uncommon for the more trivial disturbances, such as so-called milk fever, the hospital pulse, and catarrhal affections of the genitalia, to manifest themselves. Through the months of February, March, and April the mortality was usually greatest. During the winter months there was, as a rule, crowding of patients, insufficient ventilation, stagnation of the air, and the rapid accumulation of disease-germs. That the later winter months should prove the most perilous is in accordance not only with the theory of continuous accumulation, but with the experimental fact that weeks sometimes elapse before a decomposing substance acquires the highest degree of virulence.

Apart from the nosocomial malaria of hospitals, there is reason to believe in the influence at times of certain general widespread atmospheric [p. 1016]states which affect the entire community. In the year 1871 the mortality from childbed in New York was 399; in 1872, 503; in 1873, 431; in 1874, 439; and in 1875, 420. Now, the excess in the deaths for 1872 was due wholly to an increase in the cases of metria, those from ordinary accidents remaining nearly the same as in the preceding years. The disease certainly did not extend into the city from the hospitals serving as foci, for the mortality at Bellevue Hospital was hardly more than half the usual average. There was no especial mortality that year from either diphtheria, erysipelas, or scarlatina, but the aggregate mortality was the largest known in the history of the city. There are no positive data connecting the civil deaths from puerperal fever in 1872 with parasiticism, but the prevalence of epizoötics, of epidemic catarrhal affections, of peculiarly fatal forms of pneumonia and other diseases which are now attributed to the presence of minute organisms in the atmosphere, renders such a source highly probable.

It is proper to say here that, though the argument is very strong in favor of regarding the genitalia of puerperal women as the exclusive point of entry of infectious materials into the system, it seems impossible at the present time to make all the facts coincide with such a theory. I have the records of a number of cases occurring during an epidemic of puerperal fever in which patients were either attacked with fever previous to parturition, or in whose cases the unusual length of labor, the frequency of post-partum hemorrhage, and the imperfect contraction of the uterus immediately after confinement were signs of some abnormal influence exercised upon the economy at an early period of labor previous to the existence of traumatism. That deleterious materials may find other channels for entering the system than a wounded surface is evidenced by the cachectic condition not unfrequently produced in physicians by too assiduous attendance in dissecting-rooms and places in which *post-mortem*examinations are conducted. One severe and rapidly fatal case of puerperal fever which occurred in Bellevue Hospital I find it impossible to attribute to any other cause than that the woman for five months previous to her confinement served as a helper in a lying-in ward. The post-mortem examination disclosed no special local lesions, but her symptoms were those of intense septicæmia. French writers report instances of toxæmic conditions developing in young midwives during puerperal-fever epidemics. While we are not prepared to go as far as Tarnier, who says, "It is probable that the lungs, by their extent and activity, offer conditions most favorable to absorption, and that often, if not always, it is by them that poisoning occurs," it does not yet seem time to give up the idea that under exceptional circumstances the respiratory and the digestive tracts may allow the passage of materials of a septic character.

Another and frequent source of puerperal fever is by direct inoculation. Any material of a septic character, introduced into the genital passages of a woman during or after confinement, may produce a general infection of the system. But the point upon which I wish especially to dwell is that it is possible to trace epidemics of puerperal fever directly to the carrying of puerperal poison from patient to patient through the medium of attendants. In such cases changes in wards and the most rigid sanitary precautions avail but little, so long as the affected personnel is continued[p. 1017]in charge. Unless this fact is fully recognized, all the cleverest devices in hospital construction will fail to prevent the occurrence of disasters. In theory, the doctrine of the contagiousness of puerperal fever has ceased to be the subject of dispute; and yet no longer than thirty years ago it was combated as a pernicious heresy by both Meigs and Hodge of Philadelphia, at that time regarded as the best authorities upon obstetrical questions in this country. Hodge, addressing his students, said: "The result of the whole discussion will, I trust, serve not only to exalt your views of the value and dignity of our profession, but to divest your minds of the overpowering dread that you can ever become, especially in women under the extremely interesting circumstances of gestation and parturition, the ministers of evil—that you can ever convey, in any possible manner, a horrible virus so destructive in its effects and so mysterious in its operations as that attributed to puerperal fever;" and Meigs, in his letters to students, writes: "I prefer to attribute them to accident or to Providence, of which I can form a conception, rather than to a contagion of which I cannot form any clear idea, at least as to this particular malady."

Contrasted with these rhetorical utterances, in an essay published in 1843 by Prof. Oliver Wendell Holmes, entitled *Puerperal Fever as a Private Pestilence*, the opposing testimony in favor of contagion was presented with equal literary and scientific skill. The evidence was complete and conclusive, and has exercised a most beneficial influence upon the practice of midwifery in America. With his many claims to our admiration and esteem there is probably no title which Prof. Holmes wears with greater pride than that of pioneer in a movement that has done so much to prevent the slaughter of innocent women and the wrecking of happy homes.

Thanks to changed theoretical views, physicians seem now rarely to be the carriers of contagion. At least, in studying the records of New York City for nine years, I find that the occurrence of two deaths from puerperal disease, following one another so closely as to lead to the suspicion of inoculation, occurred to thirty physicians; a sequence of three cases occurred in the practice of three physicians: one physician lost three cases, and afterward two, in succession; one physician had once two deaths, once three deaths, and twice four deaths, following one another; finally, a physician reported once a loss of two cases near together, then of six patients in six months and then of six patients in six weeks. Thus in the practice of more than twelve hundred physicians in nine years I find, excluding cases occurring in hospitals, that the experience of thirty-six only lends color to the idea that puerperal fever is due to criminal neglect on the part of the medical profession. Undoubtedly in many of these cases, too, the responsibility is only apparent, as when a practitioner has, for example, had the misfortune to lose in one week a woman from puerperal convulsions, and another in the following week from placental hemorrhage. Singularly enough, not one of the sequences mentioned occurred in the practice of a physician connected with a lying-in hospital. In face of the charge that the physicians holding obstetrical appointments in public institutions are active disseminators of puerperal fever through populous communities, I find that the total loss from all puerperal causes, occurring in the private practice of ten physicians intimately associated with such institutions, numbered during the nine years but twenty-one cases. Of these, thirteen were the result of ordinary [p. 1018]accidents, and only eight cases of metria proper, of which one was developed before the physician was called in attendance; whereas a single physician, holding no hospital appointment, lost during the same time twenty-seven cases, of which twenty-one were cases of metria.

There is, however, a survival of the older ideas, chiefly to be seen among the laity, in propositions to secure absolute immunity from puerperal fever in hospital patients by confining them in wooden structures or by conducting births under carbolic acid spray.

I have been interested in endeavoring to ascertain how far experience corresponds with Semmelweis's original theory that puerperal fever owes its origin to poisonous materials obtained from dissecting-rooms and introduced into the genital canal by the hands of physicians attending cases of labor. With this view I have made personal application to a number of gentlemen who have engaged in midwifery practice while performing the functions of demonstrators of anatomy in our medical schools. H. B. Sands, of the College of Physicians and Surgeons, reports that in the five years during which he held the office of demonstrator he attended about sixty cases of labor. All did well. He lost his first patient, from childbed, a short time after he had resigned his position in the dissecting-room. J. W. Wright, the present professor of surgery in the Medical Department of the New York University, who held for one year the position of demonstrator in the Woman's College, writes me that "during the year I attended one hundred and four cases, including twenty-two forceps cases, two of craniotomy, two of podalic version, and four of breech presentation. Of this number I lost two cases, one from phlegmasia dolens complicating uræmia, from both of which troubles the patient had suffered during her previous labor, and one from double pneumonia, the result of unusual exposure following confinement. Out of these one hundred and four cases I can recall but three or four cases of metritis, and those of a mild character; I have never thought they had any special connection with my duties in the dissecting-room. I may add that for ten years I have attended a pretty large number of confinements each year, and that during the whole of this time I have been in the habit of making autopsies as occasion has offered, and of handling and examining pathological specimens both in and out of the dissecting-room, notwithstanding which my death-record among this class of cases has been unusually low." Samuel B. Ward, formerly demonstrator at the Woman's College, at present professor of surgery in the Medical School at Albany, writes: "While I was daily in the dissecting-room during the winter sessions of the school from 1868 to 1872, I attended thirty-two confinements, of which I have notes. All of the patients recovered, nor did any of them suffer from any complication that could be traced to infection." It is familiarly known that after Semmelweis had introduced the practice, among the physicians attending patients at the large lying-in hospital in Vienna, of washing the hands in a solution of chloride of lime, there was a great diminution in the mortality which prevailed, notwithstanding which G. Braun reports, however, that in 1857, in the month of July, in two hundred and forty-five deliveries there were seventeen deaths. The following month Klein gave orders to suspend the use of disinfectants. By chance, in August there were only six deaths out of two [p. 1019]hundred and fifty confinements, and in September, of two hundred and seventy-five patients, none died. From 1857 to 1860 the mortality was slight, though disinfectants were not used, while during the three following years, in spite of the systematic and persistent employment of these agents, the death-rate once more assumed formidable proportions.[52]

[52] Braun, *Rückblicke auf die Gesundheits Verhältnisse unter den Wöchnerinnen*, u. s. w., S. 32, 33.

Of course I do not wish to underrate the importance of Semmelweis's labors. There is no question but that it is a perilous experiment to pass from the dissecting-room to a patient in labor without employing rigorous measures to disinfect the hands and all parts of the person brought into contact with the dead body. But it is well to call attention to the fact that puerperal fever is not due to any single, simple cause, nor can be effectually guarded against by a single precaution; and, again, that an infectious poison does not of necessity exist in every cadaver examined. Hausmann found that injections into the vagina of gravid rabbits, in the latter half of pregnancy, of serum from the corpse of a person who had not died of septicæmia produced no fatal results, while rapid death resulted from injections, under the same conditions, of pus from the abdomen of a woman who had died from puerperal infectious disease.[53]

[53] "Untersuchungen und Versuche über die Entstehung der übertragbaren Krankheiten des Wochenbettes," *Beitr. zur Geb. und Gynaek.*, Bd. iii, Heft 3, S. 374.

Barnes and other English writers lay considerable stress upon cases of puerperal fever due neither to contagion nor to atmospheric conditions, but to the poisoning of the patient by her own secretions. There is justification for this view in the fact that even normal lochia contain bacteria, and when inoculated into animals produce in them affections of an ichorrhæmic and septicæmic nature. When death takes place the tissues of animals thus treated are found to be filled with round bacteria. Furthermore, the disease artificially produced is in itself infectious, and can be continuously propagated in other animals. But it may be asked, "Does not this admission cut both ways? How is it possible, if even normal lochia possess virulent qualities, that childbed is ever unattended by accessions of fever?" To this we can only answer that the reasons for immunity in ordinary cases are only known in part. Karewski[54] and other experimental investigators have shown that the virulence of the lochia increases proportionately to the number of days that have transpired since the birth of the child, and that during the first three days the lochia are comparatively harmless. Meantime, the retraction of the uterus, the closure of the sinuses, and the formation upon the wounded surfaces of protecting granulations, all act as natural barriers to the penetration of poison-germs. But, aside from these reasons, there is undoubtedly an unknown quantity calling for further investigation, which, in the absence of positive knowledge, we are content to term the predisposition of the individual patient. The vagina after childbirth possesses all the conditions most favorable for the production of putrefaction—viz. the access of air, fostering warmth, and stagnating fluids charged with dead tissue. It is probable that the first of these needful conditions is, in normal labors, happily wanting in the uterine cavity. In these days of intra-uterine medication it is well to [p. 1020]bear in mind the relatively greater frequency of infection through vaginal and cervical wounds, as compared with that which takes place through the denuded intra-uterine surface. The term auto-infection may, with propriety, be employed as a distinctive appellation to designate those attacks of fever which, in the absence of any demonstrable cause, occur in the early days of childbed, and which there, quoad vitam, pursue a favorable course, and to cases of so-called late infection— *i.e.* where, after the fifth day, the accidental opening of a healing wound permits the tardy absorption of poisonous secretions; but with the reserve that the primary cause is, in point of fact, atmospheric, and the predisposing condition the susceptibility of the individual. Cases of auto-infection are in this country extremely rare, if not unknown altogether, in salubrious or rural districts.

[54] "Experimentelle Untersuchungen ueber die Einwirkungen puerperaler secrete auf den thierischen organismus," *Zeitschr. f. Geb. und Gynaek.*, Bd. vii, 2te Th., S. 331.

On another occasion I have shown that in New York City the death-rate from puerperal fever is nearly twice as great during the six months from December to May, inclusive, as from June to November. The greatest mortality occurred in February and March, comprising rather more than one-fourth the entire amount. The smallest number of deaths occurred in September and October, in which months but one-thirteenth of the entire number took place.

That puerperal fever, in its harvest of death, does not spare the wealthy and well-to-do classes is too familiar a truth to be worthy of discussion. That, however, the wealthy do enjoy special immunities as compared with the less-favored members of society, I have shown by comparisons made between sections of the city which, though lying side by side, exhibit in a marked degree the two extremes of wealth and poverty. Thus, the mortality among the representatives of the lower social strata, in proportion to population, was from three to six times as great as that among the more fortunate classes.

RELATIONS TO ZYMOTIC DISEASES.—In investigating, some years ago, the nature, causes, and prevention of puerperal fever,[55] I prepared, from the statistics of the Health Board of New York City, tables extending over a period of nine years to answer the inquiry as to whether there was any relation between the frequency of deaths from scarlatina, diphtheria, and erysipelas and those from metria. Previous to their publication I was anticipated in my deductions by a paper upon the same subject by Matthews Duncan.[56] Neither Duncan nor myself found any such relation existing between the statistical frequency of puerperal fever and the zymotic diseases mentioned. There was, however, nothing in our investigations to invalidate any direct testimony which tends to show that, in individual cases, a real connection between puerperal fever and the zymotic diseases may exist. Indeed, it seems to me to be fairly established that a poison may be conveyed from patients suffering from either of the foregoing morbid processes which may be absorbed by the puerperal woman, and may in her give rise to an infectious fever possessing an intense degree of virulence. My friend Prof. Barker has recently drawn attention to the important relations of intermittent fever to the puerperal state. I have not, however, thought it advisable to complicate [p. 1021]the present discussion with any extended notice of his very valuable observations. So far as malarial fever occurs unequivocally as such in puerperal women, there is no more reason for establishing a special category for puerperal malaria than for puerperal typhoid or puerperal small-pox. In the class of cases characterized by sharp chills, intense fever, irregular remissions, and profuse perspiration, which pursue a pernicious course unaffected by antiperiodic remedies, the nature is extremely dubious. The same symptoms are likewise characteristic of certain forms of pyæmia, and I cannot learn that such cases are familiar in the practice of those of our physicians who practise outside of cities in districts where malarial affections are most prevalent.

[55] *Trans. of the International Med. Congress*, Philadelphia, 1876.

[56] "On the Alleged Occasional Epidemic Prevalence of Puerperal Pyæmia, or Puerperal Fever and Erysipelas," *Edinburgh Med. Journal*, March, 1876, p. 774.

PREVENTION.—Of the 3342 deaths from puerperal causes in New York City from 1868 to 1875, inclusive, 420 occurred in hospital, or one-eighth of the entire number. Of the 1947 cases of metria, about 300, or not quite one-sixth, were contributed by the hospitals. After such a showing the first impulse would be to cry out loudly for the suppression of the maternities. But a wiser policy suggests an inquiry as to whether the large mortality mentioned is an evil necessity. The following reports will show how much may be done in the present state of our scientific knowledge to so control the conditions which favor the generation of puerperal diseases in large hospitals as to make them safe asylums for the needy.

Goodell[57] has stated that at the Preston Retreat in 756 cases of labor there have been but 2 deaths from septic disease. Winckel[58] of the Lying-in Institution in Dresden reported, in 1873, 18 deaths from metria, or 1.8 per cent., but from the 10th of January to the 7th of July in 570 births there was but 1 case of septic disease; in the year 1872 the death-rate exceeded 5 per cent. The reduction in mortality was no fortuitous circumstance, but was due to rigid measures for the prevention of disease. Stadfeldt[59] reduced the mortality from puerperal fever in the Maternity Hospital of Copenhagen from 1 to 37, the proportion between the years 1865 and 1869, to 1 in 87 between the years 1870-74. Johnston[60] reports, in the Rotunda Hospital of Dublin, during the seven years of his mastership, 7860 births with 169 deaths, of which 85, or 1 in 91, were from metria. Braun von Fernwald[61] in sixteen years reports 61,949 confinements in the vast Maternity Hospital of Vienna, with 825 deaths from puerperal fever, or 1.3 per cent. In a visit made by me to the Vienna Maternity in 1883, I was informed that the recent mortality, including difficult operations, had been reduced to one-half of 1 per cent. Spiegelberg[62] lost, in 901 confinements at Breslau, only 5 cases of puerperal fever. Beurmann[63] reports that in the Hôpital Lariboisière, under the administration of M. Siredey, the death-rate in 1877 was 1 in 145, and in 1878, 1 in 199, confinements; in the Hôpital Cochin, under the charge of M. Polaillon, the total mortality from 1873 to 1877 was 1 to 108.7. In 1877 there was but 1 death from puerperal causes in 807 confinements. Upon Prof. Streng's division of the magnificent [p. 1022]maternity in Prague, I was told that, in 1882-83, in over 1100 confinements there had been no death from septic causes.

[57] *On the Means employed at the Preston Retreat for the Prevention and Treatment of Puerperal Diseases*, p. 13.

[58] *Berichte und Studien*, Leipsic, 1874, S. 183.

[59] *Les maternités, leur organsation et administration*, Copenhagen, 1876.

[60] *Clinical Reports*, from 1870 to 1876, inclusive.

[61] *Lehrbuch der gesammten Gynaekologie*, S. 885.

[62] *Ibid.*, S. 748.

[63] *Recherches sur la mortalité des femmes en couches dans les hôpitaux*, Paris, 1879.

When the maternity service was transferred in 1872 from Bellevue Hospital to Blackwell's Island, it became necessary to make some provision for so-called street-cases—*i.e.* women taken suddenly in labor without homes, and representing the extremes of penury and want. At first they were received, in part, by the various private institutions of charity in New York City, but these in 1877 decided to exclude them thenceforth, on the ground that their condition at the time of their reception was such as to endanger the lives of the inmates for whom the charities were specially provided. An old engine-house was then put in readiness by the city, and under the name of the Emergency Hospital was placed under the charge of Henry F. Walker[64] and myself. The number of confinements in the Emergency has averaged 220 annually. The death-rate from all causes has been 2 per cent., which, though large, is not an unfavorable showing when we remember that the patients all belong to the homeless class, that all were taken in labor before their entrance, and that many of them were in a deplorable condition at the time of their admission. The hospital, too, receives a considerable number of patients annually who are sent there only after protracted, and often severe, operative measures have been fruitlessly attempted outside its walls.[65] The building possesses, for maternity purposes, two fairly ventilated rooms. Excellent nurses are furnished by the New York Training School for Nurses. Mr. Osborn, a liberal private citizen, has had constructed in the rear, but detached from the main house, a small pavilion, modelled after that of Tarnier, for the reception of infectious cases. The Commissioners of Charities have promptly responded to every call made upon them to extend the facilities for the care of patients.

[64] Dr. Walker has since resigned, and my present colleague is Prof. Wm. M. Polk.

[65] From Oct., 1883, to Aug., 1884, there have been confined 168 women in the hospital. Twenty were brought in from the street just after the birth of the child. Of these 188, not one suffered from any puerperal affection. There were 2 deaths—1 from intestinal

ulcerations, possibly the result of the corrosive sublimate irrigations, and 1 from exhaustion. This latter patient had been thirty-six hours in labor before she was brought to the hospital, and died four hours after admission. Under the admirable management of Miss Hart, the matron, in addition to the slight mortality, there has likewise been almost complete absence of even trivial temperature elevations.

Surely these results do not support the idea that it is better for a woman to be confined in a street-gutter than to enter the portals of a lying-in asylum. Goodell's experience shows that a hospital for respectable married women may be so conducted that its inmates may enjoy absolutely a greater degree of safety than do women in their homes surrounded by all the aids that wealth can command. Equally good results are not to be obtained in hospitals which are open to unfortunates of every class. But there is much misapprehension and confusion of ideas respecting the fate of these women when no charitable provision is made for them. In Copenhagen the Maternity Hospital is closed for from six to eight weeks in the summer-time. During this period unmarried parturient women receive pecuniary assistance from the hospital to enable them to obtain a place in which to be confined. Now, Stadfeldt reports a larger mortality among this class than among those delivered in the hospital. Yet they are confined at a favorable season of the year, without any communication with the furniture, the sage-femmes, or the [p. 1023]physicians of the hospital. As they fortunately receive nothing but money, that can hardly be suspected of communicating contagion. What their fate would be in New York City perhaps may be judged from the following facts: Excluding cases confined in hospitals, nearly one-thirtieth of all the deaths and one-twenty-fourth of the cases of metria between 1867 and 1875 are reported by four practitioners. Ten practitioners out of twelve hundred signed the death-certificates of one-fifteenth of the women dying from puerperal causes, and one-tenth of the cases of metria. But it is not to be supposed that these deaths were all the result of malpractice and incompetence. The true history of most of them probably was that the doctor was engaged to attend the case of confinement for a small fee, with the understanding that he should make no calls subsequently, unless specially summoned by the friends of the patient. The latter, left to ignorant care or perhaps without any assistance whatever, and exposed to all the pernicious influences bred by poverty, when illness supervened probably did not call the physician to her aid until the time for help had passed, so that in the end his professional functions were confined to procuring the requisite permit for burial.

Humanity demands that charity should furnish places of refuge in which poor outcasts can receive assistance during the perils of child-bearing. If we must, then, have maternities, we should make them safe, and this can be in great measure accomplished by remembering the twofold source of danger arising from a poisoned atmosphere and direct inoculation. A hospital must be clean, spacious, and well-ventilated, or its atmosphere will become charged with the spores of septic fungi and produce nosocomial malaria. The most rigid sanitary precautions observed by the attendants will not prevent a badly-ventilated ward from becoming unwholesome, unless unoccupied wards are kept to which patients can be transferred upon the first admonition of danger. Goodell states that at the Preston Retreat the wards are used invariably in rotation. In connection with the Maternity at Copenhagen there are a number of small supplementary hospitals scattered through the city, which serve as safety-valves for the central institution. Artificial methods of ventilation render the task of keeping the wards wholesome comparatively easy. They do not need, however, to be complicated and expensive. The good repute of the Rotunda Hospital, it seems to me, is in large measure due to the natural ventilation afforded by open fireplaces.

In the Vienna Clinic, according to C. Braun, the mortality between 1834 and 1862 averaged 6 per cent., and in 1842 the enormous total of 521 deaths to 3067 confinements was reached. With the introduction in 1862 of what is known as Böhm's heating and ventilation system an immediate improvement was experienced. In the sixteen years from 1863 to 1878, inclusive, the total mortality has been 1.6 per cent., though in that time 5464 practitioners have received an obstetrical training in its wards. In commenting upon this change, Braun says: "I have now from practical experience arrived at the knowledge of the fact that the rapid and thorough prevention of putridity by adequate ventilation is to be regarded as a good preventive measure against puerperal fever; that it is not the number of patients in a lying-in hospital, nor yet the number of patients in a single room, but the deficient circulation of air—a fault [p. 1024]which may inhere to separate compartments in the smallest maternities—which is the important feature in the spread of puerperal fever; that puerperal women are to be protected from childbed diseases not by isolated buildings and gardens, nor by walls, but by the permanent introduction of great quantities of pure, warm air." He then adds, what is in thorough accord with my own experience, "Before new institutions are built greater attention than heretofore should be paid to the ventilation of the old structures, and, where this is found defective, a system should be substituted corresponding to the scientific requirements."

In the year 1872 puerperal fever destroyed 28 women of 156 who were confined in the Bellevue Hospital. The service was then broken up, and a great outcry arose against "tainted hospitals." Wooden pavilions were accordingly erected on Blackwell's Island for the reception of lying-in women. These buildings were constructed upon what is known as the cottage plan. They were favorably situated in an airy location remote from the general hospital. They were, however, heated by large iron stoves, and no means of ventilating the wards was provided, except by lowering the windows. In less than three months from their occupancy an epidemic of puerperal fever made it necessary to remove the service for a time to the Charity Hospital. The same result followed every subsequent attempt to utilize them for maternity purposes, until, after three years' trial, it was found necessary to abandon them altogether.

In private practice it is likewise important that the lying-in room should be provided with plenty of light and air. The physician should insist upon the value of ventilation as a means of contributing to the speedy recovery of childbed women. By hermetically sealing the windows, through false fears of his patient's taking cold, he exposes her to the risk of becoming poisoned with her own exhalations.

But the early experiences of the Hôpital Cochin and the Hôpital Lariboisière, costly, palace-like structures, with every appliance of art, prove that fresh air alone does not protect patients from the consequences of inoculation.

The great improvement in the condition of maternity patients in recent years has been due to the application of Lister's principles to obstetric practice. Complete antisepsis in the surgical sense is, of course, impracticable. Adequate antisepsis has, however, been proved to result from the observance of a variety of precautions which have been the slow outcome of experience. These, in brief, in hospitals, consist in protecting the patient from every known form of contamination, and in the prompt removal and isolation of every puerperal woman who manifests febrile symptoms.

In citing the examples of the Hôpital Cochin and the Hôpital Lariboisière, I was led to the selection because these hospitals most strikingly illustrate the extent of the triumph of the new doctrines. Whereas at the Lariboisière the mortality in 1854, the year of its opening, exceeded 10 per cent., as a result of the prophylactic measures adopted by M. Siredey the mortality was 1 to 145 in 1877, and 1 to 199 in 1878. And at the Hôpital Cochin, in 1878, Lucas-Champonnière, with 770 confinements, was able to report but 2 deaths from puerperal causes.

[p. 1025]As regards details, the bedsteads should be of iron and should be frequently scrubbed with a carbolic solution; after each confinement the palliasse upon which the woman lay should be washed in boiling water and the straw should be burned; in place of the usual rubber covering to the bed, Tarnier recommends tarred paper, which is antiseptic, and costs so little that it need be used in but a single case; all soiled linen should be instantly removed from the ward, either to be burned or disinfected by prolonged boiling; sponges should be banished, as, when they have once been soaked with blood, not even carbolic acid can make them safe; nurses employed in the puerperal wards ought not to have access to cases of labor, as D'Espine and Karewski[66] have shown that the lochia of even a healthy person on the third day will poison a rabbit; a patient attacked with fever should be immediately removed, and the nurse in attendance should go with her. At the Emergency Hospital, with the first appearance of catarrhal affection of the genital organs or of so-called milk fever, the wards are immediately emptied and fumigated with sulphurous acid. In spite of recent scepticism regarding the value of the fumes of sulphurous acid as a germicide and disinfectant, I do not hesitate to express, after long experience, my firm conviction as to their efficacy.

[66] D'Espine, *"Contributions à l'étude de la septicémie puerpérale,"* p. 18; Karewski, *loc. cit.*

Doléris[67] formulates the indications for effective prophylaxis as follows: 1, prevent the introduction of germs (antisepsis before confinement); 2, paralyze their action (antisepsis after confinement); 3, shut up the doors—veins, lymphatics, and Fallopian tubes (employment of means which promote uterine contraction).

[67] *La fièvre puerpérale*, 1880, p. 303.

The first duty of the physician is to refrain from attending a case of labor when fresh from the presence of contagious diseases or from contact with septic materials, whether derived from the dissecting-room or the clinic. Scepticism regarding these sources of danger is sure in the long run to be severely punished. In a doubtful case the least concession should consist in a full bath and a complete change of clothing. A special coat for confinement purposes, stained with blood and amniotic fluid, is liable to convey infection. In every case of labor, whether in hospital or private practice, the hands and forearms should be freely bathed in a carbolic solution before making a vaginal examination. A nail-brush should form a part of the ordinary obstetric equipment. Frequent examinations during labor should be avoided. All instruments employed during or subsequent to confinement should be carefully disinfected. In prolonged labors, after operation, in cases of dystocia, or where the membranes have ruptured prematurely and the foetus is dead, it is a useful precaution after delivery to wash both uterus and vagina with warm carbolized water or solution of corrosive sublimate (1:2000). In Vienna both Spaeth and Braun after difficult labors introduce a suppository of iodoform, 2 to 2½ inches in length, into the uterine cavity. The formula recommended consists of—

x. | Iodoformi, | 20 grammes;
Gummi Arabici, |
Glycerinæ, |
Amyli puri, | *aa.* 2 grammes;
Ft. Bacilli, | No. iij.

[p. 1026]In their introduction the half-hand (left) should be passed to the cervix; the iodoform bacillus should be seized by a pair of polypus forceps and pushed into the cervical canal. The hand in the vagina should then be used to shove the suppository upward past the internal os. No symptoms of poisoning from the iodoform have been observed. The disinfection is complete and prolonged. In hospitals the woman should be bathed before entering the lying-in ward, and the vagina should in all cases be disinfected with carbolic acid or corrosive sublimate both before and immediately after labor. The conduct of labor under carbolic acid spray is commended by Fancourt Barnes. Doléris advises the application of a compress soaked in carbolic fluid to the external genitals during the progress of labor. Tarnier advises dressing the vulva, so soon as the head begins to emerge, with a pledget soaked in carbolized oil (1:10). With the recession of the head during the interval between pains a portion of the oil is carried upward into the vagina.

In the puerperal period the warm carbolized douche stimulates uterine retraction and promotes the rapid healing of wounds in the vaginal canal; in hospital practice it possesses the additional advantage of preventing the accumulation of putrid albuminoid matters in the air. In private practice the patient should employ a new syringe; in hospitals every woman should be supplied with a glass tube to be attached to the irrigator. When not in use these tubes should be immersed in carbolic acid. The stream injected into the vagina should be continuous, like that furnished by the fountain syringe. With my hospital patients, in place of cloths to the vulva I have been in the habit of using oakum. By soaking the latter in a solution of carbolic acid the vulva is surrounded by an antiseptic atmosphere.[68]

[68] I know that of late there has been a strong reaction against the use of vaginal injections in normal childbed, but personally I have experienced none of the disagreeable effects ascribed to them. Indeed, both my hospital and private patients alike speak of them as soothing and grateful. I therefore have had no ground to discontinue them. That they are indispensable I do not claim. They are no longer used in Vienna, in Prague, nor in the New York Maternity, and yet, none the less, their results have since been in the highest degree satisfactory. At these institutions, however, vaginal disinfection is vigorously resorted to during and immediately subsequent to labor, and during childbed some form of antiseptic pad over the vulva is employed.

Pedantic as these directions may seem, they are justified by experience, and the carrying out of the details given easily becomes a matter of habit. That by such precautions puerperal fever is destined to be erased from the list of dangerous diseases attacking the woman in childbed is saying more than is warranted. Nevertheless, it is true that a physician ought never to lose the sense of personal responsibility for its occurrence. Indeed, puerperal fever ought to be regarded as a preventable disease, and an attack as the evidence that some source of danger has been overlooked, though, owing to the imperfection of our knowledge, it may easily happen that even with the keenest scrutiny the precise cause in an individual case may escape detection.[69]

[69] Since the above was written Dr. Garrigues has furnished a most extraordinary example of the efficacy of the antiseptic treatment at the New York Maternity Hospital. From the years 1875 to 1882, inclusive, the number of confinements was 2827; the deaths 116, or a little over 4 per cent. The highest percentage was reached in 1877—viz. 6.67; the lowest in 1881, when it fell to 2.36. In 1883, of 345 women confined, 30 died. In September of that year there were 9 deaths, and of 5 puerperæ who were seriously ill, 1 died later. At this time he introduced a series of reforms of which the following, omitting details, gives the essentials: Wards fumigated with sulphurous acid fumes, and the floors and furniture washed with a solution of corrosive sublimate (1:1000). Every patient, on entering the lying-in ward after the bath, had her abdomen, buttocks, genitals, and thighs washed with sublimate solution (1:2000). During labor vagina irrigated with latter solution. In prolonged labors irrigation repeated every three hours. Great care of hands on part of doctor and nurses. Glycerine and corrosive sublimate (1:1000) used for lubricating fingers before making internal examinations. Antiseptic pad applied to the head during its egress, and to the vulva until the secondines had been expelled. Absorbent cotton covered with netting soaked in corrosive sublimate solution applied to external genitals during childbed period. This latter applied and removed with the same care as in dressing a wound after a capital operation. Irrigation, first of the vagina and afterward of the uterus, immediately after labor in cases where the hand or instruments had been passed into the uterine cavity.

When the details of this treatment were first published by Garrigues, many took a humorous view of it, but mark the result: In the following 162 confinements there were no deaths, and from October to July, inclusive, of the present year, of 409 patients confined, though many operations were performed, 5 died; but of these, 3 only were from septic causes, and they, Garrigues believes, were the result of the neglect of certain of the prescribed details.

[p. 1027]Before terminating this section upon the prophylaxis of puerperal fever, I take great satisfaction in furnishing from Tarnier's recent treatise the following description, by Pinard, of the ingenious pavilion designed by Tarnier to make it possible to secure for hospital patients, at the minimum expense, the benefits of isolation, and to provide for each room in the pavilion all the conditions favorable to rapid and complete disinfection.

The pavilions are two-storied and of a rectangular shape, twenty-four feet in width by forty-six feet in length. The front and rear face to the north and south, the ends to the east and west. Two main partitions divide the interior into three divisions. Each end division is subdivided by a central partition into two chambers, so that each story has five compartments—a central one for the attendants, and four at the four corners destined for the reception of patients. On the ground floor the central compartment consists of a vestibule facing to the north, and an office facing to the south. On the former are placed the staircase, the water-closet, and a reception-closet. In addition to the main entrance there are three interior doors—one leading to the water-closet, one to the closet, and one to the office. The latter, for the occupation of the person on duty, contains a heater, a portable bath, a table, chairs, and wardrobe. Two windows face the south. The office has two doors, one opening into the vestibule, and the other, in the opposite side, opens directly outward. The four corner rooms for patients have each a door and a window, the latter looking from the end of the partition and reaching to the floor, and the former opening out from the façade. These four rooms are therefore not only independent of one another, but have no communication with the vestibule or the central office. On the second floor the arrangement is similar, except that the rooms open upon a balcony, by means of which communication from the outside is rendered possible. Upon each façade a glazed screen furnishes shelter in rainy weather. The screen extends to the roof, but is not in direct contact with the walls, a space being left for a current of air. The eight rooms for patients, four on each story, are severally fourteen feet long, eleven and a half feet wide, and ten feet high. Below, the floors are of asphaltum; above, of flags or slates. The walls and ceilings are stuccoed and covered with oil paint. The corners are rounded to prevent the accumulation of dust. To facilitate [p. 1028]washing, the floors slant toward a gutter communicating by means of a pipe with the sewer. In each room panes of glass enable patients and the office attendant to see one another, so that surveillance is secured without sacrificing the principle of isolation. The furniture of the rooms consists of an iron bedstead with metallic springs. The pillow, bolster, and palliasse are stuffed with straw. In addition, each room is provided with a night table, a round table, a chair, a stool, and a crib—all of iron. A bell-rope at the bedside, the wire of which passes to the office by the outside of the building, enables the patient to summon assistance. Each room likewise contains a washstand, with faucets for hot and cold water, the latter supplied from a cistern on the roof, the former from the office heater. The patients remain in the rooms where they are confined until they are discharged. When this takes place the chamber is aired, the furniture is removed and washed with care, the straw is burned, and the walls are washed with an abundant supply of water. If a patient is taken ill, she is carefully isolated, and has assigned to her her own especial attendant and physician, who do not come into contact with other puerperal patients.

That the plans of construction in the Tarnier pavilions would require some modification to adapt them to the rigor of our winters seems probable, but the principles which they illustrate are sufficiently vindicated by the results so far reported—viz. 6 deaths in 1062 confinements, whereas in the old Maternity the death-rate, formerly amounting to 5 per cent., still aggregates 2 to the 100.

TREATMENT.—When the septic germs characteristic of putrid infection have once entered the blood, they are beyond the reach of the physician. Except, however, in cases of acute septicæmia, where the quantity of poison introduced at the outset is excessive, the patient rallies from the immediate shock, and, provided no fresh pyrogenic material finds its way into the system, recovery is to be anticipated. The indications for treatment are, therefore, to neutralize the puerperal poison at the point of production, in order to prevent its causing further mischief, and to adopt measures calculated to enable the patient to tolerate its presence, when once absorbed, until it is either eliminated or loses its harmful properties.

Toward the fulfilment of the first indication it is to be recommended that in every case of fever of puerperal origin the vagina be cleansed with a 2 to 3 per cent. solution of carbolic acid or corrosive sublimate (1:3000) every four to six hours. The douche in itself is absolutely harmless. In most cases the infection starts from the wounds of the vagina and of the cervix. Then, too, the tendency of the secretions to stagnate in the vaginal cul-de-sac, bathing as they do the cervical portion, is a prolific source of septic trouble. In all but the mildest cases the vaginal orifice should be examined with reference to the existence of puerperal ulcers. All necrotic patches should be touched with hydrochloric acid, with a 10 per cent. solution of carbolic acid, with iodoform, or, what I personally prefer, a mixture composed of equal parts of the solution of the persulphate of iron and the compound tincture of iodine. The latter acts as a powerful antiseptic, while the former, by corrugating the tissues, closes the lymphatics and shuts up the portals through which the septic germs penetrate into the system.

[p. 1029]Intra-uterine injections should be resorted to with extreme circumspection. They are not indicated by a simple rise of temperature. A very large proportion of the febrile attacks which occur in childbed run an absolutely favorable course. Unless the infection—and this is not the rule, but the exception—proceeds from the uterine cavity, they are unnecessary. In circumscribed inflammations, where the morbific poison loses its virulence at a short distance from the puerperal lesion, they are often injurious. It is difficult, if not impossible, to so conduct them as to avoid opening up afresh recent granulating wounds. Yet the practice of local disinfection is warmly advocated by Fritsch, Schüller, Langenbuch, and Schroeder as a prophylactic against puerperal affections. On the other hand, Braun von Fernwald, with his vast opportunities for judging obstetrical questions, writes with reference to this: "We must protest against injections made by physicians into the uterine cavity. Such meddlesomeness is more likely to do harm than good." This corresponds with my own experience. In theory, the proposition to treat the uterus as one would any other pus-secreting cavity seems rational, but I have found that every attempt to carry the theory to its logical conclusion in hospital practice has been followed by a rise in the puerperal death-rate. Runge reports an epidemic of puerperal fever in Gusserrow's clinic brought about by the employment of intra-uterine irrigations, during which the mortality rose to 3.8 per cent. With the abolition of the irrigations the mortality sank to .39 per cent. In 1880, Fischel[70] introduced the so-called permanent irrigations into the Prague maternity. Of 880 patients, 9 died of sepsis. The irrigations were then prohibited. The following year, of 933 patients, only 2 died from the same cause, and in 1882, of 521 patients, there were no deaths from sepsis. Fehling, who limited the use of intra-uterine injections to special momentary indications, reported, in 1880, 415 confinements without a single death.

[70] "Zur Therapie der Puerperalen Sepsis," *Arch. f. Gynaek.*, vol. xx. p. 41.

Among the accidents which have been referred to the use of injections are convulsions, shock, and carbolic-acid or corrosive-sublimate poisoning; but the chief danger lies in the possibility of conveying the infectious materials from the vagina to the previously normal uterus. There seems to be no question as to the superior effectiveness of corrosive sublimate as a germicide. It not only acts more rapidly than carbolic acid, but its action is more permanent. In the usual proportion of 1:2000 it is apt, when repeated frequently as a vaginal douche, to corrugate the vagina and cervix. When used for intra-uterine irrigation great pains should be taken that no portion of the fluid remain behind in the uterine cavity. Since its introduction into the Emergency Hospital there has been one death from ulceration in the colon, which possibly was attributable to its use. It is to be hoped the claim that corrosive sublimate is an efficient antiseptic in the proportion of 1:10,000 may prove well founded.

In pressing the necessity of caution and discrimination, I have not, however, intended to discourage the employment of intra-uterine antisepsis in cases where it is strictly indicated. Thus, it would be folly, in a fever due to the decomposition of placental débris, of shreds of decidua, of strips of membrane, or of retained coagula, or in diphtheritis of the mucous membrane, to treat the general symptoms and neglect [p. 1030]the local cause of difficulty. In a specific case it may prove difficult to decide as to the correct course to pursue. In general it may be stated that it is proper to wash out the entire length of the genital canal when fever follows prolonged operations conducted within the uterine cavity or the birth of a dead foetus, and in cases of fever associated with a fetid discharge which persists in spite of the vaginal douche, with the presence of recognizable portions of the ovum or its dependencies in the lochia, with the repeated discharge of decomposed coagula, or with a large, flabby uterus. It will, however, be seen that with proper disinfection during and immediately after labor, the occasions for late intra-uterine injections are extremely rare.

The operation of cleansing the uterus should be conducted with the most scrupulous care. The syringe employed should produce a continuous and not an interrupted stream, and all air should be expelled from the pipe. The tube to be passed through the cervix should be of glass, of the size of the little finger, and bent somewhat to conform to the pelvic curve. The vagina should first be subjected to a thorough disinfection, by way of precaution against conveying septic materials into the uterus. The introduction of the tube should be made with the guidance of two fingers passed through the external os. But slight force is requisite to reach the internal os. It is neither necessary nor desirable to push the tube to the fundus. The fluid injected should be tepid, and, if carbolic acid is used, of the strength of two or three drachms to the pint; if corrosive sublimate is employed, the strength should not exceed 1:3000. It should be introduced very slowly, and pains should be taken to ensure its unimpeded escape, which can usually be accomplished by pressing the anterior wall of the cervix forward by means of the glass tube. Langenbuch recommends securing permanent drainage by leaving a bit of rubber tubing in the cervical canal—a plan concerning the merits of which I am not able to speak from experience. The tube is said to be well tolerated, and to possess the advantage of enabling subsequent injections to be performed without disturbing the patient.

In many cases the results of intra-uterine treatment are very striking. Often the temperature falls notably within an hour or two of the operation. This result is, however, rarely permanent. Usually the fever recurs, and the operation has to be repeated. The patient should be carefully watched, and with the first sign of returning danger the injection should be repeated. Two or three injections may thus be called for in twenty-four hours, and they may require to be continued for a week. Still, by the means indicated a certain pretty large proportion of women seemingly destined to destruction in the end make favorable recoveries.[71]

[71] The admirable monograph of Dr. T. G. Thomas, entitled *The Prevention and Treatment of Puerperal Fever*, has already done much good in calling the attention of the profession at large to the practice of local disinfection. His experience, however, based upon a very large consulting practice, has perhaps been of a kind to furnish him with an undue proportion of puerperal cases calling for intra-uterine treatment. With increasing care in the management of labor and of the birth of the child there seems reason to hope that the necessity for the treatment he so eloquently advocates may, in the near future, disappear entirely.

Ehrendorfer[72] relates a case of septic endometritis and erysipelas [p. 1031]starting from the genital organs, in Spaeth's Clinic, where, after seven days of ineffective uterine irrigations, two bacilli, containing together ten grains of iodoform, were introduced into the uterus. The washings with carbolic acid were then stopped. On the next day the discharge was diminished and the odor was less marked. On the fourth day two new iodoform bacilli were introduced. The patient, in spite of the fact that the erysipelas spread over nearly the entire body, eventually recovered.

[72] "Ueber die Verwendung der Jodoform staebchen bei der intrauterinen nach behandlung im Wochenbette," *Arch. f. Gynaek.*, vol. xxii. S. 88.

Of the symptoms, the first in order which calls for treatment is usually the peritoneal pain. It is, as we have seen, commonly of a lancinating character, and is associated with hurried breathing and extreme frequency of the pulse. So soon as the pain is once fairly under control the violence of the onset begins to abate. It should be met, therefore, by the hypodermic injection of from one-sixth to one-third grain of morphia in solution. The anodyne action should be maintained by doses administered by the mouth in quantities and at intervals suited to the severity of the case. The most important object to be secured is freedom from spontaneous pain. It is, moreover, good practice to push the opiate until pain elicited by pressure is likewise controlled, provided it can be accomplished without producing narcosis. In susceptible patients and in localized inflammations the quantity required may not be very great, while in acute general peritonitis the tolerance of the drug exhibited by puerperal women is sometimes extraordinary. Thus, a patient of Alonzo Clark took the equivalent of 934 grains of opium in four days; a patient of Fordyce Barker 13,969 drops of Magendie's solution in eleven days; and one of my own, at the Maternity, the equivalent of over 1700 grains of opium in seven days.[73] In this latter instance the patient was to all appearance moribund when the treatment was begun. Thus, the features were pinched, the face was drawn, the pupils were dilated, the finger-tips were blue and cold, the respirations were rapid, and the pulse was scarcely perceptible. In this condition the large doses of opium did not produce narcosis, but were followed by restoration of the circulation, by normal breathing, and by the disappearance of the symptoms of shock. Any attempt to relax the treatment was at once succeeded by a recurrence of the alarming symptoms. At the expiration of the disease the opium was discontinued abruptly without detriment to the patient.

[73] The details of this case have been reported in the *Am. Jour. of Obst.*, Oct., 1880, p. 864, by Dr. F. M. Welles, who conducted the administration of the opium.

In contrast to cases of acute peritonitis an extreme susceptibility to opium is often observed in the pyæmic variety. Here opiates seem to me rarely to do good. They do not hinder the migrations of the round bacteria, there is rarely pain to relieve, and I have sometimes thought that their administration was simply the addition of a second poison to the one which already was overwhelming the nervous system.

In pelvic peritonitis, in the course of forty-eight hours plastic exudation is thrown out and the pain to a great extent subsides. From this time very moderate doses of opium, as a rule, are needed to make the patient comfortable.

In France leeches applied to the abdomen are much used as a means of relieving peritoneal sensitiveness. That they do this is beyond question.[p. 1032]Their disuse in this country is due probably more to popular prejudice than to their inefficacy.

In the beginning of an attack a turpentine stupe to the abdomen is a source of comfort to many women, while the sharp counter-irritation exercises possibly a favorable influence upon the course of the disease. At a later period I commonly employ flannels wrung out in water and covered with oil-silk to prevent speedy evaporation. It is an old experience that in the beginning of a puerperal fever the provocation of loose stools by purgatives is frequently followed by a fall in the temperature and a great improvement in the patient's condition. The result, however, is far from uniform, as in other cases these artificial diarrhoeas have a tendency to aggravate the peritoneal symptoms. Owing to this uncertainty in their action, purgative remedies should be administered with caution, not from any theory as to their eliminative powers, but because of the ascertained existence of fecal accumulation. In pelvic inflammations castor oil in two- or three-tablespoonful doses, or five to ten grains of calomel rubbed up with twenty grains of bicarbonate of sodium, as recommended by Barker, may be given when thus indicated. After the bowels have once been freed, however, the purgative should not be repeated. In cases of intense local inflammation and in general peritonitis enemata should alone be employed for the removal of constipation.

Every increase of body-heat is associated with rapid tissue-waste, with enfeebled heart-action and with exhaustion of the nerve-centres. Since the modern recognition of the deleterious effects of high temperatures per se, antipyretic remedies in place of the old-time cardiac sedatives have come to play the leading rôle in the treatment of fevers.

Of internal antipyretic agents quinia enjoys a deservedly high repute. In the remitting forms of fever it may be administered in five-grain doses at intervals of four to six hours. Given thus in medium doses, it moderates the fever, diminishes the sweating, and in most patients lessens gastric and intestinal disturbances. In continued fevers it should, on the contrary, be given in a single dose large enough to procure a distinct remission. By making a break in the febrile symptoms, if only of a few hours' duration, a retardation of the destructive processes is accomplished. At the first administration twenty to thirty grains may be given. In favorable cases the temperature falls in the course of a few hours below 101°. When the high temperature is only temporarily held in check, at the end of twenty-four hours, if all symptoms of cinchonism have disappeared, the same dose should be repeated. If the doses mentioned, given in the manner prescribed, produce no perceptible effect upon the fever, their continuance may be regarded as unnecessary.

C. Braun and Richter speak favorably of the action of salicylate of sodium.[74] It possesses antipyretic properties, though in a less degree than quinia. It is, however, rapidly absorbed, circulates through all the parenchymatous organs, and finally is discharged unchanged in the urine. It is said by Binz, in small doses, to hinder the action of the disease-producing ferments, while it leaves untouched the normal ferments of the organism. It is of special service where quinia is not well tolerated, or when given fifteen to twenty grains at a time every four to six hours as [p. 1033]an adjuvant to large single doses of quinia. The remedy should be continued until all traces of febrile disturbance have disappeared.

[74] Richter, "Ueber intrauterine Injectionen," etc., *Zeitschr. für Geburtsk. und Gynaek.*, Bd. ii. Heft 1, p. 146.

A more powerful remedy than salicylic acid, where quinia has failed, is the Warburg's tincture. Some patients find, however, that it is somewhat difficult to retain upon the stomach.

Not many years ago, owing to the encomiums of Fordyce Barker,[75] the tincture of veratrum viride was in great favor in puerperal fever as a means of reducing the excited pulse of inflammation. The plan recommended was to administer five drops hourly, in conjunction usually with morphia, until the pulse was brought down to 70 or 80 beats to the minute. If the pulse had once been reduced, then three, two, or one drop hourly would be found sufficient to control it. Vomiting and collapse from its use were no cause for alarm, as they were temporary symptoms, and were followed by a fall of the pulse to 30 or 40 a minute, which was rather of favorable prognostic significance. In the rapid pulse of exhaustion, however, veratrum should not be given. Since the introduction of the thermometer into practice the reduction of the pulse by veratrum has been found to be associated with a fall in the temperature of the body. Of late, however, veratrum has gone rather out of vogue, not because it is not a very effective agent, but because its administration is an art to be acquired, and cannot safely be entrusted to an unskilled assistant. Then, too, in the last ten years there has grown up a better acquaintance with less dangerous remedies.

[75] *The Puerperal Diseases*, p. 347.

Braun recommends in severe cases, where quinia alone is without effect, to give in addition from twelve to twenty-four grains of digitalis in infusion per diem until its specific action is produced. Unlike veratrum, digitalis effects a permanent slowing of the heart. By prolonging the cardiac diastole and contracting the arterioles it allows the left ventricle to fill, restores the arterial tension, diminishes correspondingly the intravenous pressure, and promotes absorption. Its tendency to produce gastric disturbances and the distrust felt as to its safety have prevented its becoming popular in practice.

Alcohol as an adjuvant to treatment is indicated in all cases, whether quinia or salicylic acid or veratrum be simultaneously employed. It stimulates and sustains the heart, it retards tissue-waste, and is in itself an antipyretic of no mean value. Usually I give it in conjunction with quinia, one or two teaspoonfuls hourly of either whiskey, rum, or brandy, in accordance with the recommendation of Breisky.[76] But many years before I had learned from my friend Prof. Barker that the specific influence of veratrum was in many cases not obtained until the use of alcohol was combined with it.

[76] *Ueber Alcohol und Chinin-behandlung*, Bern, 1875.

The antipyretic action of drugs is probably due for the most part to some direct influence they exert upon the oxygenation of the tissues. Of course the less the fire the less the heat. It is well, however, to support their internal administration by the external employment of cold. Cold owes its effect in fevers partly to the abstraction of heat from the body-surface, and in a still more important degree to the impression which it produces upon the nervous system. In healthy persons the action of cold is to increase the consumption of oxygen and the production of carbonic [p. 1034]acid. The additional heat thus generated renders it possible to sustain the vicissitudes of climate. In fevers the primary effect of cold is similar in character. Its main therapeutical action is derived from its secondary influence upon the nerve-centre which regulates the body-heat. If the cold employed be sufficiently intense or sufficiently prolonged, there follows, not always immediately, but in the course of an hour or two, a marked lowering of the temperature, which can only be accounted for by assuming an indirect influence exerted through the sympathetic nerve and the medulla oblongata. This peculiarity renders the external application of cold a most valuable addition to the therapeutical resources available in fevers.

In cases of moderate severity frequently sponging the patient with cold water will be found to be a grateful practice. An ice-cap to the head, where the blood lies near the surface, will often affect the entire temperature of the body. From immemorial times it has been employed to control delirium and promote sleep. An ice-bag placed over the inguinal region is locally beneficial to deep-seated pelvic inflammations, and, according to Braun, is capable of effecting a rapid fall of temperature. Ice-cold drinks should be freely allowed.

Schroeder recommends a permanent stream of cold water in the uterine cavity by means of a large irrigator and a drainage-tube; others advise cold rectal injections maintained for long periods by the aid of a tube with a double current.

In fevers of great violence the systematic application of cold by means of baths or the wet pack is capable in some cases of rendering important service. The temperature of the bath should range from 70° to 80°. Its duration should not exceed ten minutes. The patient should, when removed to the bed, be wrapped in a sheet without drying, and should be comfortably covered. In employing the wet pack two beds should be placed side by side. The body and thighs of the patient should be wrapped in a sheet wrung out in cold water, and be allowed to remain in the pack from ten to twenty minutes. As the sheet becomes heated the patient should be placed in a fresh one upon the second bed, and the transfers should be continued until the desired fall of temperature is effected. Braun claims that four packs are equivalent in action to one full bath.

Both these methods are, however, open to the objection that they cannot be carried out without considerable disturbance of the patient—a point of no small importance in cases of peritonitis. G. B. Kibbie has invented a fever-cot which obviates the ordinary difficulties of this mode of treatment. The cot is covered with "a strong, elastic cotton netting, manufactured for the purpose, through which water readily passes to the bottom below, which is of rubber cloth so adjusted as to convey it to a vessel at the foot." T. G. Thomas,[77] who has employed this apparatus extensively to reduce high temperatures after ovariotomies, explains as follows the modus operandi: "Upon this cot a folded blanket is laid, so as to protect the patient's body from cutting by the cords of the netting, and at one end is placed a pillow covered with india-rubber cloth, and a folded sheet is laid across the middle of the cot about two-thirds of its extent. Upon this the patient is now laid; her [p. 1035]clothing is lifted up to the armpits, and the body enveloped by the folded sheet, which extends from the axillæ to a little below the trochanters. The legs are covered by flannel drawers and the feet by warm woollen stockings, and against the soles of the latter bottles of warm water are placed. Two blankets are then placed over her, and the application of water is made. Turning the blankets down below the pelvis, the physician now takes a large pitcher of water, at from 75° to 80°, and pours it gently over the sheet. This it saturates, and then, percolating the network, it is caught by the india-rubber apron beneath, and, running down the gutter formed by this, is received in a tub placed at its extremity for that purpose. Water at higher or lower degrees of heat than this may be used. As a rule, it is better to begin with a high temperature, 85°, or even 90°, and gradually diminish it. The patient now lies in a thoroughly soaked sheet, with warm bottles to her feet, and is covered up carefully with dry blankets. Neither the portion of the thorax above the shoulders nor the inferior extremities are wet at all. The water is applied only to the trunk. The first effect of the affusion is often to elevate the temperature—a fact noticed by Currie himself—but the next affusion, practised at the end of an hour, pretty surely brings it down. It is better to pour water at a moderate degree of coldness over the surface for ten or fifteen minutes than to pour a colder fluid for a shorter time. The water slowly poured robs the body of heat more surely than when used in the other way. The water collected in the tub at the foot of the bed, having passed over the body, is usually 8° or 10° warmer than it was when poured from the pitcher. On one occasion Dr. Van Vorst, my assistant, tells me that it had gained 12°. At the end of every hour the result of the affusion is tested by the thermometer, and if the temperature has not fallen another affusion is practised, and this is kept up until the temperature comes down to 100°, or even less. It must be appreciated that the patient lies constantly in a cold wet sheet, but this never becomes a fomentation, for the reason that as soon as it abstracts from the body sufficient heat to do so it is again wet with cold water and goes on still with its work of heat-abstraction. I have kept patients upon this cot enveloped in the wet sheet for two and three weeks, without discomfort to them and with the most marked control over the degree of animal heat. Ordinarily, after the temperature has come down to 99° or 100°, four or five hours will pass before affusion again becomes necessary."

[77] "The Most Effectual Method of Controlling the High Temperature occurring after Ovariotomy," *N.Y. Med. Jour.*, August, 1878.

Since reading this account, I have made a good many trials of the method upon puerperal women, and have not found that it agrees with all in an equal degree. In some instances the affusions have been followed, in spite of hot bottles to the feet and the administration of stimulants, by such a degree of depression and impairment of cardiac force, as shown by the persistent coldness of the extremities, that it has been necessary to discontinue them. On the other hand, I can look back upon cases, apparently so desperate that the condition of the patients was looked upon as hopeless, where they proved the means of saving life as by a miracle. Of course, the difference depends upon whether the high temperature is the sole cause of the alarming symptoms, or whether the latter are in part due to blood-dissolution and secondary changes in the parenchymatous organs.

[p. 1036]The use of the coil in fever, whether of rubber or of metal tubing, I can highly recommend. Either the night-dress or a towel should be placed between the coil and the skin. A current of cold water passing through the tube rapidly abstracts the surface heat, and is usually grateful to the patient. The lowering of the temperature by this means is much slower than by cold affusions. Disturbance of the patient is, however, avoided, and the method, so far as I have tried it, has been free from the objections incident to the direct application of water to the skin.

It is hardly necessary to state that in puerperal, as in other fevers, the patient's strength requires to be sustained and the waste of tissue to be repaired, as far as possible, by the regulated administration of liquid food, as milk and beef-tea, in such quantities as can be borne by the stomach, and at one to two hours' intervals.

In the treatment of encysted peritoneal effusions, and in inflammatory exudations into the pelvic and adjacent cellular tissue, after the acute symptoms have subsided the attention should be directed to the afternoon fever and to promoting the assimilation of food. So soon as the sweating and fever are checked the absorption of the plastic materials begins. The most important agents for accomplishing this object are quinia, in moderate doses, combined with some form of alcohol and with tepid sponging. Deep-seated pain in the iliac region is best relieved by a large blister upon the side over the point where the tenderness is felt. Prolonged rest in bed should be enjoined. Even after convalescence is well advanced, so long as the exudation remains unabsorbed the resumption of household duties is pretty certain to be followed by a relapse or by the development of a chronic condition of a most intractable description. The sooner the patient's stomach can be got to digest and absorb beefsteak and iron the more speedy will be her recovery.

In pelvic exudations the hot vaginal douche, warm baths, and the application of flannels wrung out in water to the abdomen aid in diminishing the local pain, and, perhaps, in causing a disappearance of the tumor. The action of mercurials or of iodide of potassium in melting away plastic inflammatory materials is sometimes very striking, but more frequently they either do no good or else do harm by disturbing the digestion.

If fever, chills, and sweating announce the presence of pus, the most careful exploration should be made to determine, if possible, the seat of suppuration. It is of great advantage to treat pelvic abscesses as abscesses are treated elsewhere in the body. If the redness of the skin above Poupart's ligament indicates a tendency to point in that direction, an aspirator-needle should be introduced to make sure of the diagnosis. If the sac is near the surface, a free incision should be made and the pus should be allowed to escape. In many cases I make these incisions three to four inches in length. The redness of the external skin makes it certain that the abscess has become adherent to the abdominal wall, and that the incision consequently will not communicate with the peritoneum. After the abscess has been opened it should be cleansed twice daily, and the cavity should be filled with oakum. If, after a time, the granulations become flabby, Peruvian balsam or iodoform should be introduced into the sac at each change of the dressing. I can recommend this plan as essentially a mild procedure. With a large opening for the discharge of [p. 1037]pus the fever and sweating disappear, the appetite returns, and the abscess fills rapidly by granulation. With a small incision hectic is apt to persist, and the abscess to end in the formation of interminable fistulæ.

If softening and bagginess or distinct fluctuation indicate that the pus can be reached through the vaginal cul-de-sac, the aspirator-needle should be inserted deeply at the suspected point, and if a large amount of pus is detected, an incision should be made with a long-handled bistoury, using the needle as a director, and making the opening large enough to permit the introduction of a drainage-tube. I prefer for this purpose a self-retaining Nélaton catheter, which is easily passed by means of a uterine sound inserted into the eye at the extremity. Through the tube—without disturbing the patient—the pus-cavity can be washed as frequently as required, and with drainage and cleanliness cases of the longest standing may be expected to recover.

P. F. Mundé[78] has reported a number of cases of chronic character where the aspiration of pus has been followed by rapid absorption of the intra-pelvic exudation. The presence of pus was suspected because of a boggy, doughy feeling in the exudation tumor.

[78] "Diagnosis and Treatment of Obscure Pelvic Abscess," etc., *Arch. of Med.*, December, 1880.

[p. 1038]

BERIBERI.
BY DUANE B. SIMMONS, M.D.

DEFINITION.—Beriberi is a disease of inanition, most common in tropical countries, though found in high latitudes (41° N.), especially in low-lying seaboard towns, during the summer months, and is both endemic and epidemic. It is usually chronic in form, but is subject to exacerbations of varying degrees, and has for its characteristic symptoms anæsthesia of the skin, hyperæsthesia and paralysis of the muscles, anasarca, palpitation, cardiac and arterial murmurs (in the wet form), præcordial oppression, and abdominal pulsation.

HISTORY AND GEOGRAPHICAL DISTRIBUTION.—It was for a long time confounded with a great variety of other diseases. The Anglo-Indian physicians of Ceylon and the Malabar coast were no doubt the first to recognize the specific nature of the disease, though it is claimed that Chinese medical works of the thirteenth century contain a fairly accurate description of it.

The literature of beriberi, at the first glance, appears to be very meagre, as some of the most popular medical works make no mention of the disease at all, while others only give it a passing notice. Its bibliography, however, is very considerable, as may be seen in the exhaustive list in Billings' *Index Catalogue*, but for want of space we refer only to the most recent contributions to the subject. These are—an article by A. LeRoy de Mericourt;[1] an essay by Tarissan, entitled *Beriberi in Brazil;* an article by Anderson,[2] and an essay by myself.[3]

[1] *Dictionnaire Encyclopédique des Sciences Médicales*, Paris, 1876.
[2] *Guy's Hospital Reports*.
[3] *Chinese Maritime Customs Medical Report* (1880).

For a long time beriberi was supposed to have a peculiar territorial limitation. It is now known to be more or less prevalent on all the islands and shores of Eastern Asia and Africa from Japan to the Cape of Good Hope, and in Brazil.

ETIOLOGY.—I know of no disease in regard to which a greater diversity of opinion exists as to its cause. Indeed, as one has observed, "autant d'auteurs, autant d'opinions diverses." Ten years' study and observation of the malady under a great variety of circumstances and conditions have led me to the definite conclusion that its exciting cause is a specific poison or germ, having many striking resemblances in its mode of production to paludal or marsh miasm, though entirely distinct and separate from it. A great variety of predisposing causes, however, exert a powerful influence in rendering individuals or classes susceptible to the [p. 1039]disease, such as age, sex,[4] occupation, race, mode of life, diet, and climate.

[4] Women suffer from the disease much less frequently than men.

CLINICAL HISTORY AND SYMPTOMS.—There are three forms of the disease: 1st. Beriberi hydrops (wet beriberi), in which there is a hydræmic condition of the blood, distension of the general areolar tissue, with serum, and effusion into the serous cavities. 2d. Beriberi atrophia (dry or atrophic beriberi), in which there is a notable deficiency of fluids in the vessels and areolar tissue, and atrophy of the muscles. 3d. Mixed beriberi, in which the above forms lose the sharp lines of distinction and merge into each other. Cases complicated with dysentery, diarrhoea, and especially with continued fevers of the typhoid type, are not uncommon.[5] These last, besides being of grave prognosis, are frequently very embarrassing and difficult of diagnosis.

[5] Some authors have designated fatty or convulsive forms of the disease, which I think unnecessary.

In general terms, wet beriberi may be divided into two stages—the prodromic stage and the stage of attack; and into several types—the acute or pernicious, and the chronic. From the very insidious nature of the approach of the disease, sometimes extending over a period of several weeks, it is often very difficult, or even impossible, to determine the exact time of its invasion. It is generally admitted that a residence of some weeks in an infected locality is necessary before any decided symptoms make their appearance. As in many other diseases of slow development, the symptoms of the prodromic stage are certain not easily defined feelings of indisposition, such as an occasional sense of chilliness, inaptitude for mental exertion, and especially a tired feeling in the lower extremities. A period of uncertain length now intervenes, during which the characteristic symptoms appear and constitute the stage of attack. The first of these symptoms is, generally, anæsthesia of the skin over the anterior tibial muscles, in the tips of the fingers, and around the mouth, in the order given. Paralysis in varying degrees next declares itself in certain groups of muscles, usually those immediately underlying the regions of anæsthesia. One of the consequences of this is a drooping of the toes, causing the patient while walking to lift the feet high so as to clear the ground, thus occasioning the peculiar gait noticed by many observers as characteristic of the disease. A sense of constriction in the muscles of the calves is experienced at the same time, arising from a veritable contraction, which causes their apparent enlargement and hardening, with tension of the tendo achillis. A feeling of tightness in the chest usually accompanies this condition, due, no doubt, to partial paralysis of the muscles of respiration. If firm pressure be now made upon the muscles in various parts of the body, a greater or less degree of tenderness will be found to exist in many of them, and especially those occupying the posterior part of the leg, back of the forearm, inside of the arm, and upper part of the chest. Tenderness of the periosteum of the long bones and a peculiar roughness of their surfaces often exist also. Palpitation of the heart, especially on making any considerable exertion, is a frequent and often troublesome symptom, even at this stage of the disease.

Up to this point the above symptoms are common to both the wet and [p. 1040]dry forms of the malady, and to them the characteristic features either of beriberi hydrops or atrophia are now added. The first manifestation of anasarca, the pathognomonic symptom of wet beriberi, is in an oedematous condition of the areolar tissue of the anterior part of the legs. This, in reality, is more or less general even at an early stage of the disease, as is evident from the plump appearance of the patient and a certain sallow-white color of the skin, especially of that of the face. In uncomplicated cases the temperature is normal, or it may be at times a little below the normal point. There is also little or no increase in the frequency of the pulse. Its quality, however, is changed, and somewhat characteristic for both forms of the disease. Thus in the wet form it is full, large, and easily compressible, indicating a great diminution of arterial tone, while in the dry form there is nearly an opposite condition. If the heart be now examined, a decided systolic murmur will be heard, most distinctly over the pulmonary valves; and in most cases of wet beriberi it exists in all the large arterial trunks. The heart furnishes the usual signs of dilatation and want of tone. In the dry form the cardiac murmurs are either slight or wanting altogether, and the area of cardiac dulness is variable, and frequently diminishes as the disease advances.

In both wet and dry beriberi the appetite is little impaired in the earlier stages, but if in the former the stomach is over-distended, there is increased præcordial oppression, and sometimes sudden death. The bowels in the wet form are sluggish, and urine scanty; in the other there is but little deviation from the normal in these respects.

The cases of the subacute type are by far the most numerous. From this it is evident that the acute or pernicious type of the malady is, in most cases, only an exaggeration of the subacute, as observed in some other diseases, notably rheumatism and those of marsh malarial origin. The term pernicious is, strictly speaking, applicable to the wet form of the disease only, as the dry form is rarely, if ever, rapidly fatal. A marked case of wet beriberi is always to be regarded as dangerous, from the suddenness with which pernicious symptoms often declare themselves. In these the anasarca (which, as has been stated, constitutes the leading clinical difference between the two forms of the malady) plays an important rôle. It often happens that in the course of a few hours the local oedema in the extremities and the slight puffiness of the face become general and extreme, and the neck is enormously swollen by the distension of the veins, both deep and superficial. The pleural and pericardial sacs are more or less distended with serum, thus mechanically embarrassing the action of the organs they contain. The action of the heart now becomes laborious, the lungs oedematous and filled with coarse râles, and a terrible sense of suffocation comes over the patient, causing him to seek relief by constant change of position. The stomach is irritable, a greenish-yellow fluid is vomited, and death closes the scene. The acute stage of dry beriberi, on the contrary, is characterized by a rapid diminution of the fluids of the body and muscular atrophy.

The annual appearance in the same individual of either wet or dry beriberi, and its long continuance, constitute the chronic type of the disease.

MORBID ANATOMY.—The morbid anatomical changes in beriberi vary considerably with its form. Few, if any, observers claim seriously to [p. 1041]have found in either the wet or dry form of the disease evidences of acute inflammatory action in any of the tissues or organs. The blood undoubtedly undergoes important morbid changes, whereby its nutritive and oxygenating power is impaired, indicating that this is a disease of inanition. This shows itself most markedly in necrobiotic and degenerative changes, especially in the muscular tissues, which are the seat of the leading morbid phenomena in all stages of both forms of this disease. The respiratory, digestive, and glandular systems rarely undergo morbid changes other than those of a secondary or passive kind, such as engorgement with serum and venous blood.

The condition of the organs contained in the cranial and spinal cavities is variable and inconstant. According to some observers, the substance of the brain and spinal cord is hardened. The greater number by far, however, have found it more or less softened.[6] The heart in wet beriberi is habitually large and flabby, its muscular tissue softened and of a pale-yellow and macerated appearance. Its cavities are engorged with dark blood, sometimes fluid, but more often clotted. These clots are often voluminous in the right heart, semi-fibrinous, and extend into the pulmonary artery and great venous trunks, which are enormously enlarged. The cardiac muscular tissue I always found to have undergone metamorphic changes, varying from granular clouding to advanced fatty degeneration.[7] The tissue of the paralyzed voluntary muscles undergoes degenerative changes in both forms of the disease. In the extreme atrophy of dry beriberi I have not unfrequently found many of the sarcolemma sheaths completely emptied of their contents. The power of regeneration in these cases is often wonderfully displayed by an almost complete restoration of the lost elements, and, in a corresponding degree, of the function of the part.

[6] The former condition was undoubtedly observed in autopsies made of the dry or atrophic form of the disease, though this fact is not mentioned. The latter, or softened, condition of the cerebro-spinal contents belongs to the wet form of the disease (my own cases being of this kind). I regard this softening as not ante-mortem, but as consecutive to serous imbibition (as observed by Eismann and Sanders in chlorosis), and as taking place during the last moments of life or after death, when the vital forces no longer oppose themselves to the mechanical disintegrating power of the fluid with which the nervous as well as all the other tissues of the body are engorged.

[7] I believe this to be the condition of the heart-muscle in all cases of death from the wet form of beriberi. In this opinion I am supported by Oudenhoven and many of the Dutch observers.

It would appear that in wet beriberi the heart is first weakened by paresis of the cardiac ganglia, with consequent incomplete emptying of its cavities. This, in connection with rapid degenerative changes in its muscular tissue, causes the walls to yield to the blood-pressure, producing dilatation and tricuspid insufficiency, with regurgitation and consequent capillary stasis and dropsy. Vaso-motor nerve-paralysis, acting at the same time on the pulmonary artery and arterioles, and on other large arterial trunks, probably gives rise to the murmurs heard in them. In the dry form of the disease the vaso-motor nerve-paralysis is less pronounced, and the degenerative changes in the muscular tissue of the heart slower, while the marked decrease in the fluids of the system and the great failure of nutrition tend toward atrophic changes. From this it follows that we usually have, instead of a large dilated heart, a small weak one, with a narrow tricuspid orifice instead of a dilated one; little or no [p. 1042]intercostal pulsation, and hence less cardiac dulness; no venous distension or capillary stasis, and hence no dropsy.

PROGNOSIS.—In temperate climates the prognosis of uncomplicated beriberi is favorable in a majority of cases. In seasons of its epidemic prevalence, however, all cases of the wet form of the disease must be carefully watched, as it not unfrequently happens that grave symptoms suddenly appear at a time when no danger has been anticipated. An unfavorable prognosis may be ventured when, in a case of wet beriberi, relief is not obtained by free purging or when vomiting sets in. In dry beriberi the termination in death is exceedingly rare as a direct result of the action of the poison producing the disease, so that when death does occur it is chiefly from exhaustion. The time of recovery depends on the amount of muscular degeneration, and also upon the season of the year when the attack occurred, as all cases of both forms of beriberi usually get well without treatment during the winter months.

TREATMENT.—The well-established fact of the influence of certain localities in the production of beriberi makes the removal of the patient from them a hygienic measure of great importance, and this is frequently the only treatment necessary if it can be done early. The effect of the change is often almost magical, especially if it be made to an elevated locality and among the mountains.

Diet is an important element in the treatment of beriberi. At the head of the list of foods to be avoided is rice. Coarsely prepared grains, such as wheat, barley, certain kinds of beans,[8] apparently because of more or less laxative properties, are preferable as articles of food.

[8] A small red bean called adzuke, possessing both laxative and diuretic properties, is a favorite remedy with the Japanese for beriberi. It is used alone or mixed with rice, and is not unfrequently the only means resorted to for the successful cure of mild cases.

No drug has been discovered possessing specific properties in this disease. In the wet form, medication consists in the administration of drugs calculated to draw off the excess of serum in the areolar tissues and in the serous sacs. First in point of efficacy for this purpose are the hydragogue cathartics. In my own practice the sulphate of magnesia, in large and repeated doses, has given the best results; elaterium, a powder of jalap, squill, and digitalis, and, in fact, any medicine which will give frequent and copious stools, are sure to afford marked relief to the more urgent symptoms, and in many cases will alone effect a cure. Care must be taken, however, not to exhaust the patient, though I have never seen the judicious use of this method of treatment do harm.

Copious bleeding is recommended by Anderson, especially in the stage of greatest danger, but I have never been able to convince myself of its safety.

The almost specific virtue claimed by the old Indian physicians for treeak farook is no doubt due to its cathartic properties.

Diuretics are indicated for the same reason as cathartics, and any of the more active are productive of good results. They are too slow in their action, however, to be relied on otherwise than as adjuvants to cathartics. I have found juniper gin to answer an excellent purpose, both as a stimulant and diuretic, where there was danger of exhaustion from the free use of cathartics.

The medical treatment of dry beriberi differs materially from that of [p. 1043]the wet disease. Cathartics and diuretics are alike useless, and the former injurious. The ordinary means, such as electricity, strychnia, frictions, etc., employed in cases of muscular atrophy and paralysis from other causes, are indicated when the active stage has passed, but they are useless, and even injurious, before this time. The muscular hyperæsthesia common to both forms of the disease may be generally greatly relieved by anodyne liniments containing aconite. The internal use of the latter is highly recommended by some. Hypodermic injections of morphia afford relief to the painful sense of constriction in the calves of the legs so often complained of.

www.ingramcontent.com/pod-product-compliance
Lightning Source LLC
Chambersburg PA
CBHW072046190526
45165CB00019B/1954